Wheater's FUNCTIONAL HISTOLOGY

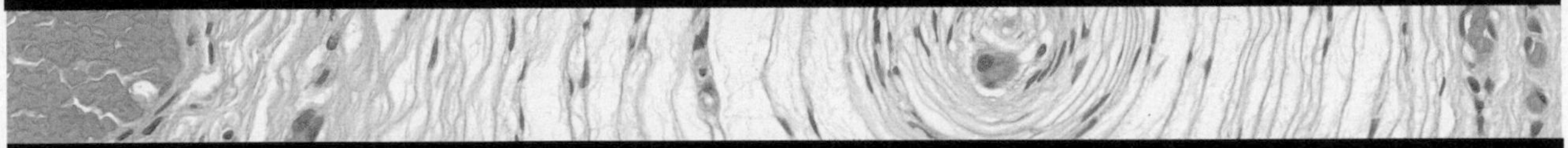

A TEXT AND COLOUR ATLAS

Seventh EDITION

Wheater's FUNCTIONAL HISTOLOGY

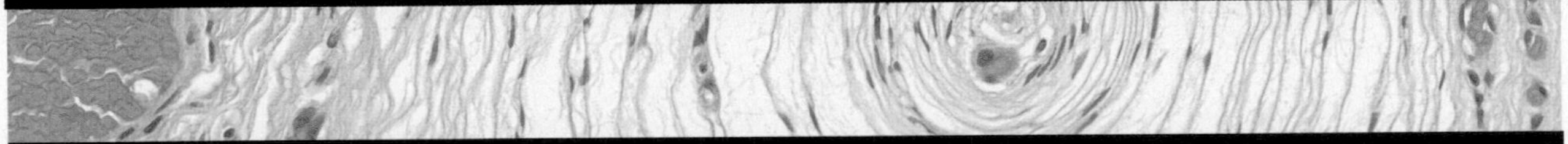

A TEXT AND COLOUR ATLAS

Dr Geraldine O'Dowd
BSc (Hons), MBChB (Hons), FRCPath
Consultant Diagnostic Pathologist
Lanarkshire NHS Board
Honorary Clinical Senior Lecturer
University of Glasgow
Glasgow, UK

Dr Sarah Bell
BSc Med Sci (Hons), MBChB (Hons), DipFMS, FRCPath, MSc (Mol Path)
Consultant Pathologist
Department of Pathology
Queen Elizabeth University Hospital
Glasgow, UK

Dr Sylvia Wright
BSc (Hons), MBChB (Hons), DipFMS, FRCPath, MSc (Mol Path)
Consultant Pathologist
Department of Pathology
Queen Elizabeth University Hospital
Glasgow, UK

ELSEVIER London New York Oxford Philadelphia St Louis Sydney 2024

ISBN: 978-0-7020-8334-1

Previous editions copyrighted 2014, 2006, 2000, 1993, 1987 and 1979.

Notice

Practitioners and researchers must always rely on their own experience and knowledge in evaluating and using any information, methods, compounds or experiments described herein. Because of rapid advances in the medical sciences, in particular, independent verification of diagnoses and drug dosages should be made. To the fullest extent of the law, no responsibility is assumed by Elsevier, authors, editors or contributors for any injury and/or damage to persons or property as a matter of products liability, negligence or otherwise, or from any use or operation of any methods, products, instructions, or ideas contained in the material herein.

IE ISBN: 978-0-7020-8335-8
eISBN: 978-0-7020-8336-5

Senior Content Strategist: Alexandra Mortimer
Senior Content Development Specialist: Joanie Milnes
Senior Project Manager: Joanna Souch
Designer: Patrick Ferguson
Marketing Manager: Deborah Watkins

Printed in Scotland

Last digit is the print number: 9 8 7 6 5 4 3 2 1

For John Paul, Francis and Patrick, with all my love.
GO'D

For Mum/Nana, who is greatly missed.
SB

In loving memory of Dad, Gran and Pablo. Missed every day.
SW

PREFACE *to the seventh edition*

In preparing this latest edition of *Wheater's Functional Histology*, we have in large part retained the layout that has proven so popular with generations of histology students. *Wheater's* remains primarily an atlas of histology, with only short sections of introductory text in each section, followed by numerous high-quality annotated light micrographs, electron micrographs and line drawings. The text has been updated to improve clarity and to reflect newer advances and we have once more aimed to enhance the quality of the illustrations with the addition of many new and improved micrographs, as well as some updated line drawings.

The availability of new, electronic platforms has allowed us to provide significant additional content for students, without producing a large and unwieldy tome. We recognise that many of our readers will be involved in medicine and have therefore built upon the clinical correlation sections from the previous edition by adding further detail and relevant electronic links to the companion textbook, *Wheater's Basic Pathology*. We hope that these links will prove useful in aiding retention of seemingly abstract histological features, by building understanding of the links between structure and function and, in turn, dysfunction and disease. We have revised and updated the end of chapter reviews and have added an expanded bank of self-assessment questions, which we hope will be helpful study aids.

In order to ensure that the text remains accessible to the absolute beginner, we have greatly improved and expanded the appendices at the back of the book, outlining the basics of tissue preparation, microscopy and various histological staining techniques, as well as a basic glossary. For those who are entirely new to microscopy, these appendices should prove helpful in understanding the various types of image which are used throughout the text.

Two new authors have joined us for the production of this edition. Our colleague of many years, Dr Barbara Young, has recently retired following her career-long involvement in the *Wheater's* series and Dr Phillip Woodford has also left the team as he retires from his diagnostic practice. We wish them both well for the future. Our new authors, Dr Sarah Bell and Dr Sylvia Wright, have previously been involved in updating the companion text, *Wheater's Basic Pathology*, and have brought their great energy and drive to this new production, as well as their considerable expertise in teaching and in molecular pathology.

We hope that we have succeeded in producing a concise but up-to-date introduction which will help to make histology relevant and memorable for students of medicine and the life sciences.

Geraldine O'Dowd
Sarah Bell
Sylvia Wright

Glasgow, 2022

PREFACE *to the first edition*

Histology has bored generations of students. This is almost certainly because it has been regarded as the study of structure in isolation from function; yet few would dispute that structure and function are intimately related. Thus, the aim of this book is to present histology in relation to the principles of physiology, biochemistry and molecular biology.

Within the limits imposed by any book format, we have attempted to create the environment of the lecture room and microscope laboratory by basing the discussion of histology upon appropriate micrographs and diagrams. Consequently, colour photography has been used since it reproduces the actual images seen in light microscopy and allows a variety of common staining methods to be employed in highlighting different aspects of tissue structure. In addition, some less common techniques such as immunohistochemistry have been introduced where such methods best illustrate a particular point.

Since electron microscopy is a relatively new technique, a myth has arisen amongst many students that light and electron microscopy are poles apart. We have tried to show that electron microscopy is merely an extension of light microscopy. In order to demonstrate this continuity, we have included resin-embedded thin sections photographed around the limit of resolution of the light microscope; this technique is being applied increasingly in routine histological and histopathological practice. Where such less conventional techniques have been adopted, their rationale has been outlined at the appropriate place rather than in a formal chapter devoted to techniques.

The content and pictorial design of the book have been chosen to make it easy to use both as a textbook and as a laboratory guide. Wherever possible, the subject matter has been condensed into units of illustration plus relevant text; each unit is designed to have a degree of autonomy whilst at the same time remaining integrated into the subject as a whole. Short sections of non-illustrated text have been used by way of introduction, to outline general principles and to consider the subject matter in broader perspective.

Human tissues were mainly selected in order to maintain consistency, but when suitable human specimens were not available, primate tissues were generally substituted. Since this book stresses the understanding of principles rather than extensive detail, some tissues have been omitted deliberately, for example the regional variations of the central nervous system and the vestibulo-auditory apparatus.

This book should adequately encompass the requirements of undergraduate courses in medicine, dentistry, veterinary science, pharmacy, mammalian biology and allied fields. Further, it offers a pictorial reference for use in histology and histopathology laboratories. Finally, we envisage that the book will also find application as a teaching manual in schools and colleges of further education.

Paul R. Wheater
H. George Burkitt
Victor G. Daniels

Nottingham 1979

ACKNOWLEDGEMENTS

This new edition of *Wheater's Functional Histology* could not have been completed without the input of the many individuals who have helped and supported us. Colleagues in our local laboratories have very kindly allowed us access to their cases for slide photography and, in some instances, have recommended suitable material for us to illustrate specific features. We are immensely grateful also to the biomedical scientists and technical staff, far too many to name individually, in our laboratories (the Departments of Pathology at Queen Elizabeth University Hospital [QEUH], Glasgow, and at University Hospital Monklands, NHS Lanarkshire). Without your high-quality sections, production of this illustrated work would have been impossible.

Particular thanks are due to the following for their contributions to specific figures used in the text and as online resources: Dr Lorna Cooper of the Department of Pathology, QEUH, Glasgow, for e-Fig. 17.7 and Dr Fraser Duthie of the Department of Pathology, QEUH, Glasgow, for Figs 15.17a and b. We also extend our thanks to the many contributors who provided material for earlier editions, as mentioned previously.

It is appropriate to reiterate our appreciation for the efforts of our colleague, Dr Barbara Young, who has retired from writing the text with this edition. Her commitment and personal contribution to the *Wheater's* books throughout her career in pathology should not be understated and we are immensely grateful for her support, as well as privileged that she has entrusted to us the continuance of these works. Over many years, her skill as a teacher and her excellent photomicrography skills have helped shape *Wheater's* into a highly respected resource for those beginning their studies of microscopy. We have aimed to retain these key features in this new edition and hope that we have produced a text worthy of the *Wheater's* title.

Finally, we are grateful to the staff of Elsevier for their help and support in the writing of this edition during the difficult period of the COVID-19 pandemic. The team at Elsevier deserves our heartfelt appreciation, both for giving us the opportunity to write this new edition and for all the hard work they have put in to making this happen in very challenging times.

Finally, we thank our families and friends for their immense patience and support throughout this project which has consumed so much of our time and energy. Without you, we could not have completed this work.

CONTENTS

PART

I

THE CELL

1 Cell structure and function

INTRODUCTION TO THE CELL

Histology is the study of normal cells and tissues, mainly using microscopes. This book describes the histology of normal human tissues, although much of the material applies to other mammals and, indeed, non-mammals. Structure and function are interdependent. Histological structure determines and is determined by the functions of different organs and tissues; the study of one has enriched the understanding and study of the other. When diseases such as cancer or inflammation affect a tissue, there are often specific changes in the microscopic structure of the tissue. The microscopic study of these changes is known as ***histopathology, anatomical pathology*** or sometimes just ***pathology***. Obviously a sound knowledge of normal structure is essential for an understanding of pathology.

The ***cell*** is the functional unit of all living organisms. The simplest organisms, such as bacteria and algae, consist of a single cell. More complex organisms consist of many cells as well as extracellular matrix (e.g. the matrix of bone). The term ***eukaryote*** refers to organisms whose cells consist of ***cytoplasm*** and a defined ***nucleus*** bounded by a ***nuclear membrane***; this includes plants, fungi and animals, both unicellular and multicellular. The ***cytoplasm*** contains variable numbers of several different recognisable structures called organelles, each with a defined function. The nucleus may be considered to be the largest organelle.

Prokaryote refers to bacteria and archaea, whose cells do not have a membrane-bound nucleus; they also have other major structural differences and will not be discussed further here.

The cells of multicellular organisms, such as humans, show a great variety of functional and morphological specialisation, with amplification of one or another of the basic functions common to all living cells. The process by which cells adopt a specialised structure and function is known as ***differentiation***. Despite an extraordinary range of morphological forms, all eukaryotic cells conform to a basic structural model, which is the subject of this chapter.

The major tool in the study of histology is the microscope. The basic techniques used in histology, including tissue preparation, slide production, light microscopy and electron microscopy, are outlined in Appendix 1. Various staining techniques are used to prepare tissues to make them visible through the microscope and these are described in Appendix 2. The student is strongly urged to read these appendices first; it really will make all that follows more comprehensible. Appendix 3 is a glossary of common histological terms and, like the other appendices, can be dipped into at any time.

FIG. 1.1 The cell *(illustrations opposite)*
(a) EM ×16 500 (b) Schematic diagram

The basic structural features common to all eukaryotic cells are illustrated in this electron micrograph (Fig. 1.1a) of a fibroblast and diagram (Fig. 1.1b). All cells are bounded by an external lipid membrane, called the ***plasma membrane*** or ***plasmalemma*** **PM**, which serves as a dynamic interface with the external environment. Most cells interact with two types of external environment: adjacent cells **C** and ***extracellular matrix*** as represented by collagen fibrils **F**. The space between cells is designated the ***intercellular space*** **IS**. The functions of the plasma membrane include transfer of nutrients and metabolites, attachment of the cell to adjacent cells and extracellular matrix, and communication with the external environment.

The ***nucleus*** **N** is the largest organelle and its substance is bounded by a membrane system called the ***nuclear envelope*** or ***membrane*** **NE**. The nucleus contains the genetic material of the cell in the form of ***deoxyribonucleic acid*** (***DNA***). The cytoplasm contains a variety of other organelles, many of which are also bounded by membranes. An extensive system of flattened membrane-bound tubules, saccules and flattened cisterns, collectively known as the ***endoplasmic reticulum*** **ER**, is widely distributed throughout the cytoplasm. A second discrete system of membrane-bound saccules, the ***Golgi apparatus*** **G**, is typically located close to the nucleus (best seen in the adjacent cell). Scattered free in the cytoplasm are a number of relatively large, elongated organelles called ***mitochondria*** **M**, which have a smooth outer membrane and a convoluted inner membrane system. In addition to these major organelles, the cell contains a variety of other membrane-bound structures, including ***intracellular transport vesicles*** **V** and ***lysosomes*** **L**. The cytoplasmic organelles are suspended in a gel-like medium called the ***cytosol***, in which many metabolic reactions take place. Within the cytosol, there is a network of minute tubules and filaments, collectively known as the ***cytoskeleton***, which provides structural support for the cell and its organelles, as well as providing a mechanism for transfer of materials within the cell and movement of the cell itself.

Thus the cell is divided into a number of membrane-bound compartments, each of which has its own particular biochemical environment. Membranes therefore serve to separate incompatible biochemical and physiological processes. In addition, enzyme systems are found anchored in membranes so that membranes are themselves the site of many specific biochemical reactions. Membrane-enclosed compartments occupy approximately half the volume of the cell.

C adjacent cell **ER** endoplasmic reticulum **F** collagen fibrils **G** Golgi apparatus **IS** intercellular space **L** lysosome **M** mitochondrion **N** nucleus **NE** nuclear envelope **PM** plasma membrane **V** transport vesicles

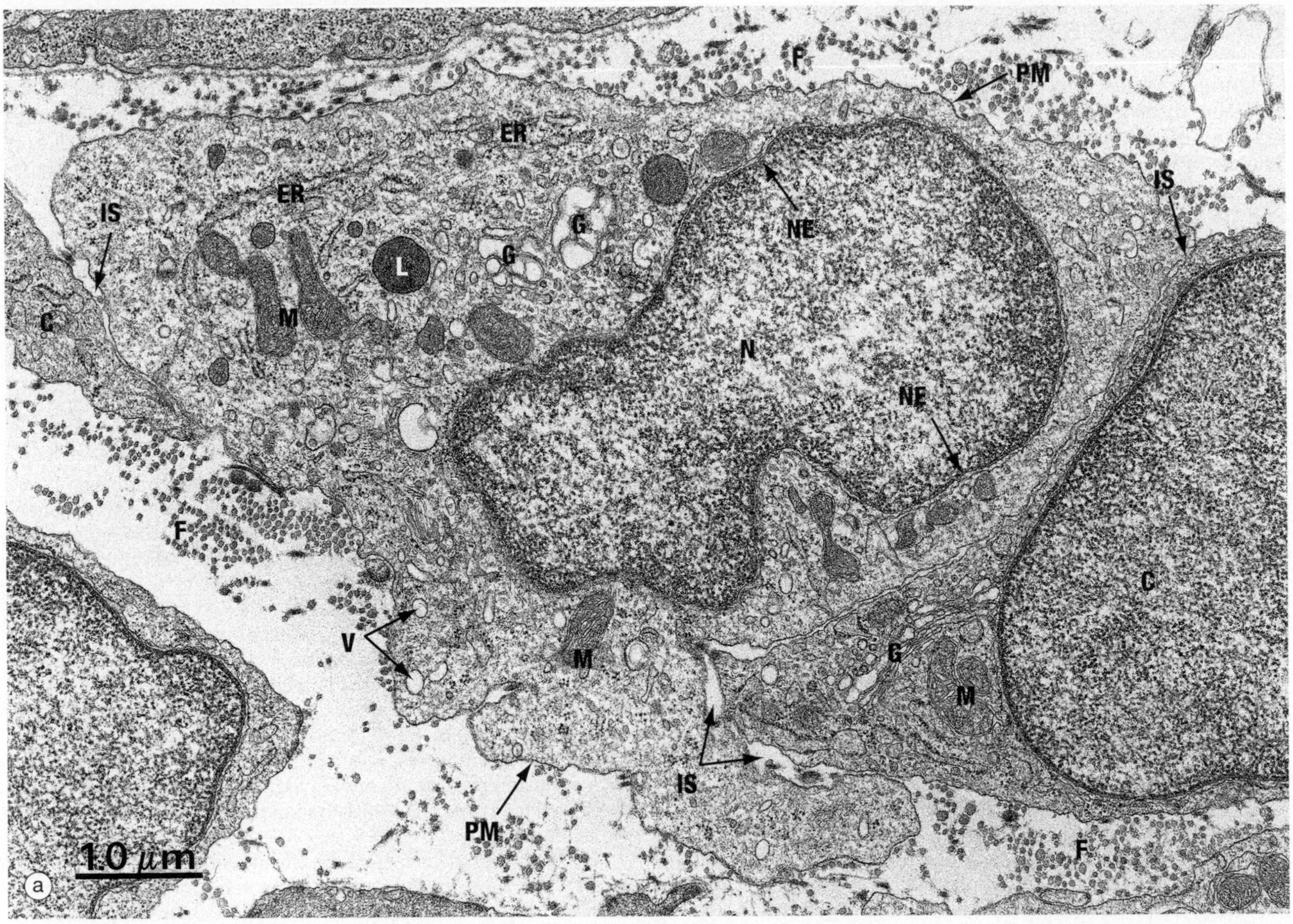

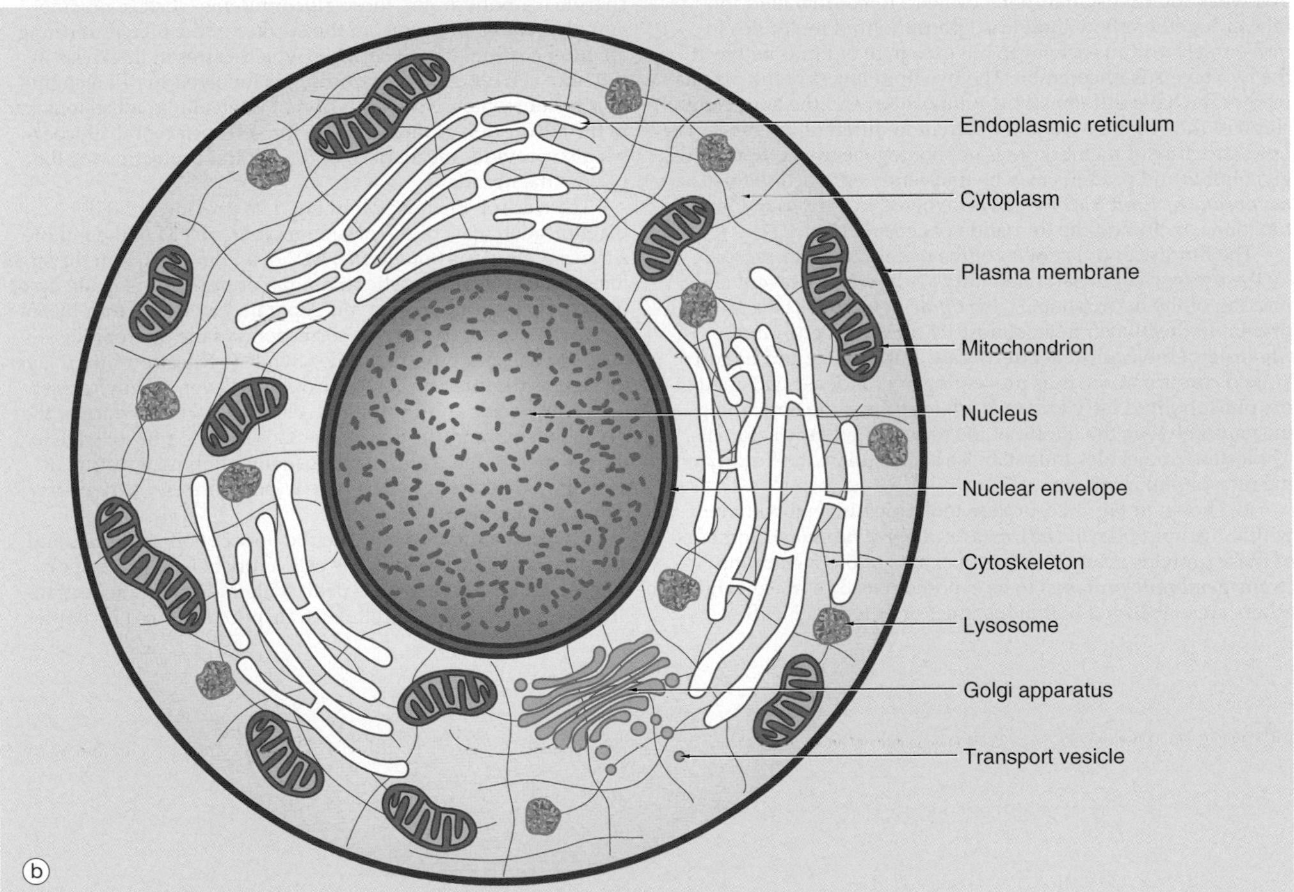

FIG. 1.1 The cell ***(caption opposite)***
(a) EM ×16 500 (b) Schematic diagram

MEMBRANE STRUCTURE

Cell membranes, including the outer plasma membrane and the internal membranes, are composed of approximately equal amounts (by weight) of lipids and proteins. The unique properties of cell membranes allow them to separate the interior of the cell from the external milieu and the internal compartments of the cell from each other. Most of the chemical reactions of cells take place in aqueous polarised solution. The immiscibility of lipids with water leads them to form ***lipid bilayers***, which effectively prevent passage of polarised ions and molecules; thus the contents of different compartments are kept separate and ion gradients between different compartments are maintained. Proteins embedded within the lipid bilayer act as channels to allow selective passage of particular ions and molecules. Some types of cell signalling are also mediated by membrane proteins.

FIG. 1.2 Membrane structure *(illustrations opposite)*
(a) EM ×210 000 (b) Phospholipid structure (c) Membrane structure

The ***phospholipid*** molecules that make up the lipid bilayers are ***amphiphilic***, i.e. they consist of a polar, ***hydrophilic*** (water-loving) head and a non-polar, ***hydrophobic*** (water-hating) tail. Most often, the polar heads consist of glycerol conjugated to a nitrogenous compound such as choline, ethanolamine or serine via a phosphate bridge as shown in Fig. 1.2b. The phosphate group is negatively charged, whereas the nitrogenous group is positively charged. The non-polar tail of the phospholipid molecule consists of two long-chain fatty acids, each covalently linked to the glycerol component of the polar head. In most mammalian cell membranes, one of the fatty acids is a straight-chain saturated fatty acid, while the other is an unsaturated fatty acid which is 'kinked' at the position of the unsaturated bond.

Sphingomyelin is another important and plentiful phospholipid in cell membranes.

Phospholipids in aqueous solution will spontaneously form a bilayer with the hydrophilic (polar) heads directed outwards and the hydrophobic (non-polar) tails forced together inwards. The weak intermolecular (non-covalent) forces that hold the bilayer together allow individual phospholipid molecules to move freely within each layer, but exchange of lipids between the two layers is uncommon. The two lipid layers of the plasma membrane have different lipid composition and the lipid composition of the cell membrane is different in different cell types. The lipid structure of membranes is not homogeneous; certain lipids, glycolipids and proteins may be transiently enriched to form a ***membrane*** or ***lipid 'raft'*** which is involved in various membrane functions, including the formation of ***caveola*** (Fig. 1.12).

The fluidity and flexibility of the membrane is increased by the presence of unsaturated fatty acids, which prevent close packing of the hydrophobic tails. ***Cholesterol*** molecules are also present in the bilayer in an almost 1:1 ratio with phospholipids. Cholesterol molecules themselves are amphiphilic and have a kinked conformation, thus preventing overly dense packing of the phospholipid fatty acid tails while at the same time filling the gaps between the 'kinks' of the unsaturated fatty acid tails. Cholesterol molecules thus stabilise and regulate the fluidity of the phospholipid bilayer.

As shown in Fig. 1.2c, protein molecules are embedded within the lipid bilayer (***intrinsic*** or ***integral proteins***). Some of these proteins span the entire thickness of the membrane (***transmembrane proteins***) to be exposed to each surface, while others are embedded within the inner or outer lipid leaflet.

Membrane proteins are held within the membrane by a hydrophobic zone which allows the protein to move in the plane of the membrane. The parts of these proteins protruding beyond the lipid bilayer are hydrophilic. Some membrane proteins are anchored to cytoplasmic structures by the cytoskeleton. ***Peripheral membrane proteins*** are attached to the inner or outer membrane leaflet by weak non-covalent bonds to other proteins or lipids. Membrane proteins are important in cell–cell adhesion, cell–matrix adhesion, intercellular signalling and for the formation of transmembrane channels for transport of materials into and out of the cell. In many cases, the transmembrane proteins assemble into complexes of two or more protein molecules to form a transmembrane channel or signalling complex; one example is the ***aquaporins*** which transport water molecules across the cell membrane.

On the external surface of the plasma membranes of animal cells, most of the membrane proteins and some of the membrane lipids are conjugated with short chains of polysaccharide (carbohydrate); these ***glycoproteins*** (surface mucins) and ***glycolipids*** project from the surface of the bilayer forming an outer coating, the ***glycocalyx***, which varies in thickness in different cell types. The glycocalyx is involved in cell recognition phenomena, in the formation of intercellular adhesions and in the adsorption of molecules to the cell surface; the glycocalyx also provides mechanical and chemical protection for the plasma membrane.

The electron micrograph in Fig. 1.2a provides a high-magnification view of the plasma membrane **PM** of the minute surface projections (***microvilli***) **MV** of a lining cell from the small intestine. The characteristic trilaminar appearance is made up of two outer electron-dense layers separated by an electron-lucent layer. The outer dense layers correspond to the hydrophilic heads of phospholipid molecules, while the electron-lucent layer represents the intermediate hydrophobic layer, mainly consisting of fatty acids and cholesterol. On the external surface of the plasma membrane, the glycocalyx **G** is seen as a fuzzy edge to the cell membrane. This is an unusually prominent feature of small intestinal lining cells where it incorporates a variety of digestive enzymes.

Plasma membranes mediate the flow of both materials and information into and out of the cell, a function of vital importance to the cell. This topic is dealt with in detail in the section 'Import, export and intracellular transport' later in this chapter.

G glycocalyx **MV** microvilli **PM** plasma membrane

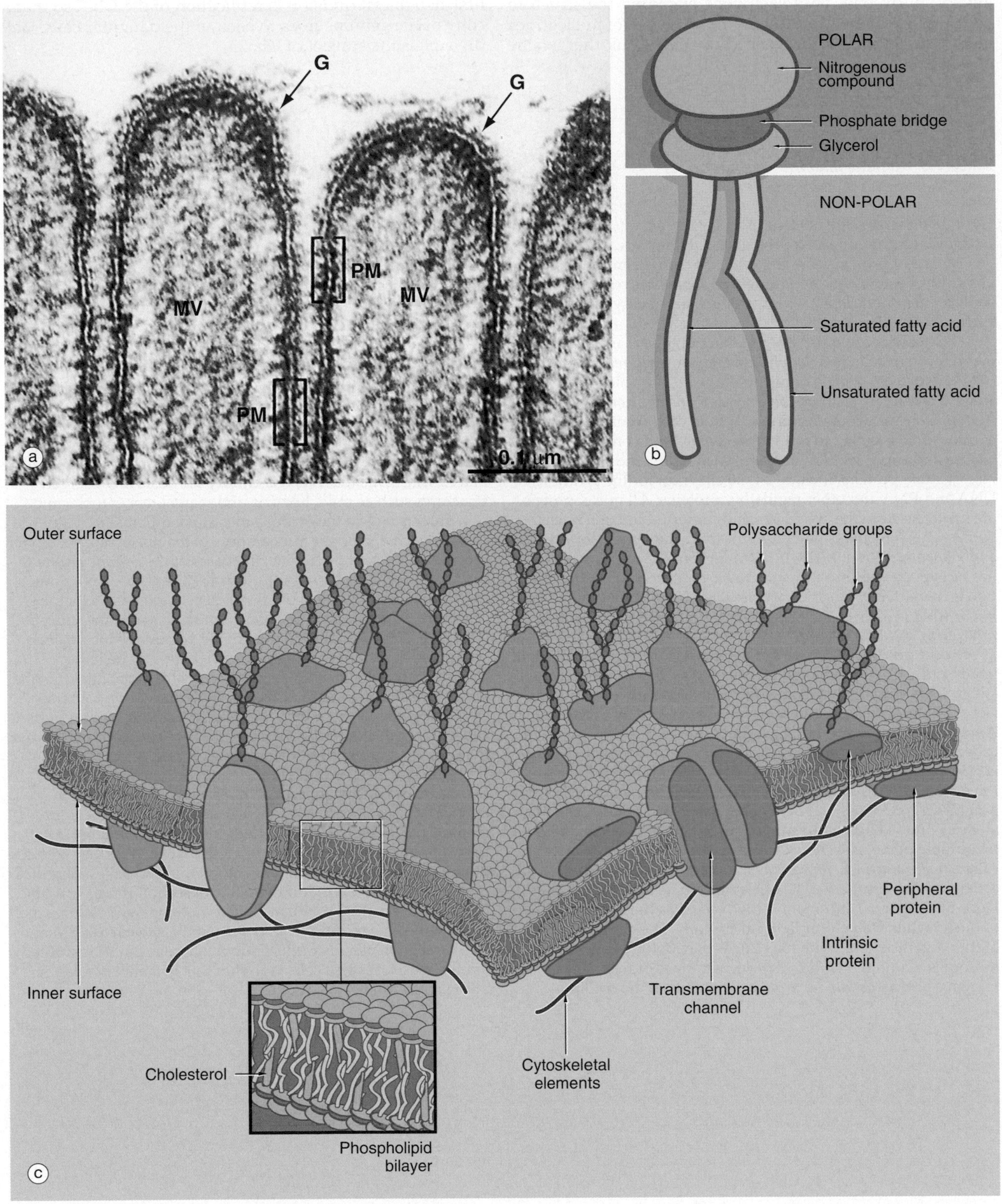

FIG. 1.2 Membrane structure *(caption opposite)*
(a) EM ×210 000 (b) Phospholipid structure (c) Membrane structure

THE NUCLEUS

The *nucleus* is the largest organelle in the cell and is usually the most obvious feature of the cell seen by light microscopy. The nucleus contains the genetic material of the cell, *deoxyribonucleic acid (DNA)*, arranged in the form of chromosomes. Each chromosome contains a number of genes joined end to end, with each gene encoding the structure of a single protein according to the sequence of nucleotides along the length of the gene (Fig. 1.6). Thus the genetic blueprint for all proteins, whether structural or enzymes, is contained within the nucleus of every cell in the body except for red blood cells, which have no nucleus (see Ch. 3). The substance of the nucleus is known as the *nucleoplasm* and it is surrounded by the nuclear membrane. The first step in cell division is replication of the DNA so that a copy of the genome goes to each of the daughter cells. Cell division is the subject of Ch. 2.

FIG. 1.3 Nucleus *(illustrations opposite)*
(a) EM × 15000 (b) H&E (HP)

Fig. 1.3a illustrates the nucleus of a plasma cell, a type of cell that secretes large amounts of a protein called antibody.

Typical of protein-secreting cells, the cytoplasm contains plentiful ribosome-studded ***(rough) endoplasmic reticulum*** **ER** as well as ***mitochondria*** **M**, which produce the energy required for such a metabolically active cell.

The nucleus contains DNA (making up less than 20% of its mass), protein called ***nucleoprotein*** and some ***ribonucleic acid (RNA)***. Nucleoprotein is of two major types: low molecular weight, positively charged ***histone proteins*** and ***non-histone proteins***. Histone proteins form a protein core around which the chromosome is coiled to form ***nucleosomes*** and control the uncoiling and expression of the genes encoded by the DNA strand. Non-histone proteins include all the enzymes for the synthesis of DNA and RNA and other regulatory proteins. All nucleoproteins are synthesised in the cytoplasm and imported into the nucleus. Nuclear RNA includes newly synthesised ***messenger, transfer*** and ***ribosomal RNA*** (***mRNA, tRNA*** and ***rRNA***, respectively) that has not yet passed into the cytoplasm. Control of DNA transcription is mediated by a variety of small RNA molecules including ***micro RNA (miRNA), small nuclear RNA (snRNA)*** and ***small interfering RNA (siRNA)***.

Except during cell division, the chromosomes, each a discrete length of DNA with bound histone proteins, exist as coiled and supercoiled strands that cannot be visualised individually. Nuclei are heterogeneous structures with electron-dense (dark, see Appendix 1) and electron-lucent (light) areas. The dense areas, called ***heterochromatin*** **H**, consist of tightly coiled inactive ***chromatin*** found in irregular clumps, often around the periphery of the nucleus. In females, the inactivated X-chromosome may form a small discrete mass, the ***Barr body***. Barr bodies are occasionally seen at the edge of the nucleus in female cells when cut in a favourable plane of section. The electron-lucent nuclear material, called ***euchromatin*** **E**, represents that part of the DNA that is active in RNA synthesis. The nucleolus **Nu** is also evident (see Fig. 1.5). The name chromatin is derived from the strong colour of nuclei when stained for light microscopy. The chromatin is a highly organised but dynamic structure, with individual chromosomes tending to clump in particular areas of the nucleus, known as ***chromosome territories***. Segments of the chromosome are coiled and uncoiled as different genes are brought into contact with the enzymes that make the RNA copy of the DNA, i.e. ***transcription***. Histone proteins also exist as variant forms or can be chemically modified in ways that promote or suppress expression of a particular gene. Permanent switching on or off of a particular set of genes leads to differentiation of the cell.

The shape, appearance and position of cell nuclei can be very helpful in identifying particular cell types. Fig. 1.3b shows part of the wall of the colon (see also Fig. 14.29), which has been stained with haematoxylin and eosin (H&E, see Appendix 2), the 'standard' histological staining method. Haematoxylin is blue in colour and eosin is pink. Haematoxylin, a basic dye which binds to negatively charged DNA and RNA, stains nuclei dark blue. Eosin, an acidic dye, has affinity for positively charged structures such as mitochondria and many other cytoplasmic constituents and so the cytoplasm is stained pink. Fig. 1.3b shows the characteristic appearances of the nuclei of various cell types. At the top of the image, the bases of the ***colonic crypts*** **C** can be seen. The epithelial cells forming the crypts have round to ovoid nuclei **N**, typical of epithelial cells. Note also that the nuclei are positioned at the bases of the cells while the superficial cytoplasm is filled with mucin; the position of the nucleus within a cell, the ***polarity***, may also be highly characteristic. Deep to the crypts, running across the centre of the image, is the ***muscularis mucosae*** **MM**, which is composed of smooth muscle cells. Smooth muscle cell nuclei **SN** are elongated with rounded ends, often called ***spindle shaped***. This is of course only apparent if they are cut in the right plane of section; if cut perpendicular to the long axis of the cell, they appear rounded (see also Fig. 6.15). The nuclei are typically placed in the centre of the cell, although this is not always easy to see as the cell borders are indistinct. Eosinophils scattered within the ***lamina propria*** **LP** have a unique bilobed nuclear form **BN** which, together with the prominent coral red granules in the cytoplasm, makes identification easy. Note again that if the plane of section is unfavourable, the bilobed structure of the nucleus is not apparent. A very small blood vessel, a ***capillary*** **Cap**, is seen in the ***submucosa*** **SM** and the flattened nuclei **FN** of the endothelial cells can be identified; the cytoplasm of these cells is so thin that it cannot be seen at this magnification.

BN bilobed eosinophil nucleus **C** colonic crypt **Cap** capillary **E** euchromatin **ER** endoplasmic reticulum
FN flattened endothelial cell nucleus **H** heterochromatin **LP** lamina propria **M** mitochondrion **MM** muscularis mucosae
N crypt epithelial cell nucleus **Nu** nucleolus **SM** submucosa **SN** smooth muscle cell nucleus

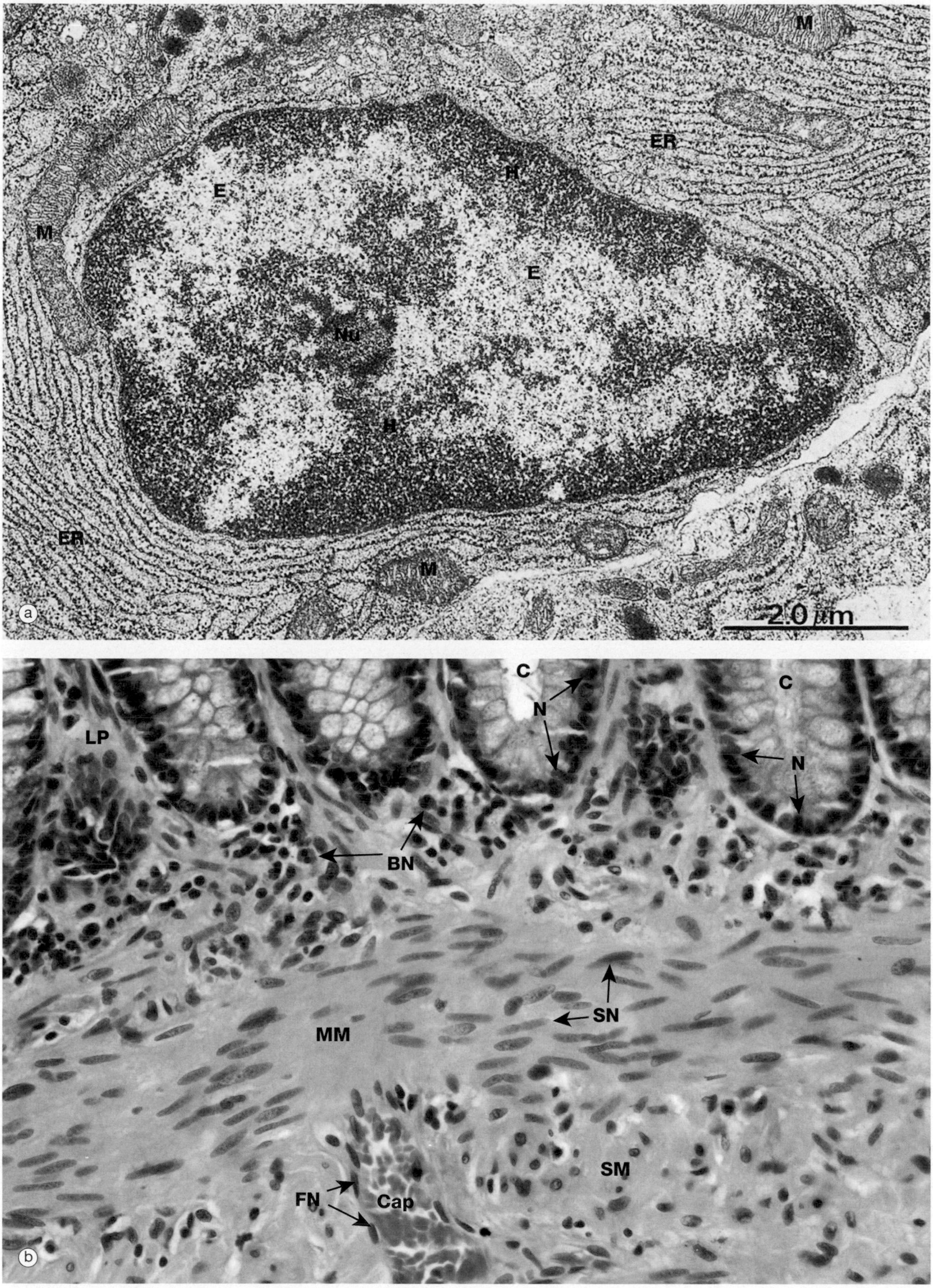

FIG. 1.3 Nucleus ***(caption opposite)***
(a) EM ×15 000 (b) H&E (HP)

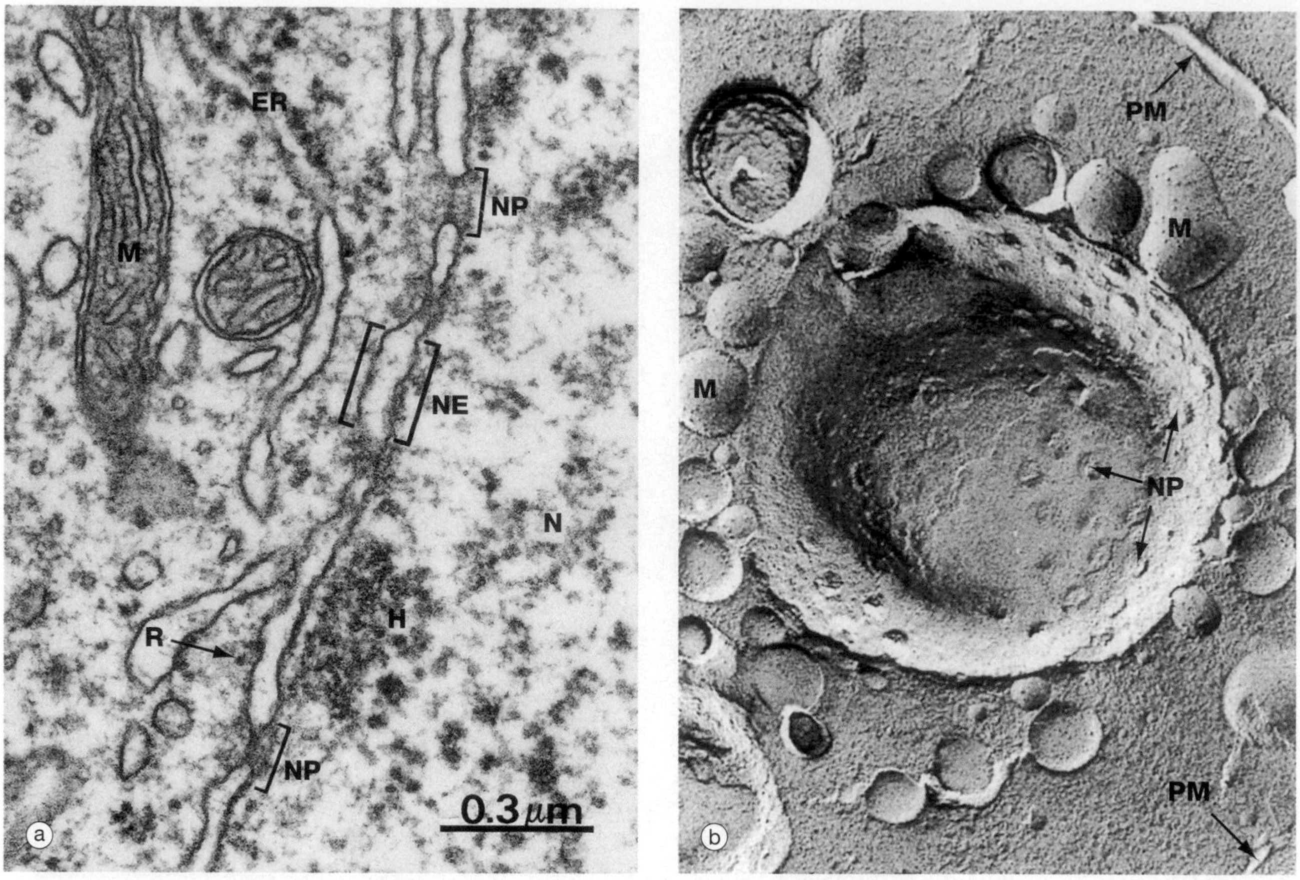

FIG. 1.4 Nuclear envelope
(a) EM ×59 000 (b) Freeze-etched preparation, SEM ×34 000

The ***nuclear envelope*** **NE**, which encloses the nucleus **N**, consists of two lipid bilayers with the ***intermembranous*** or ***perinuclear space*** between. The inner and outer nuclear membranes have the typical phospholipid bilayer structure but contain different integral proteins. The outer lipid bilayer is continuous with the endoplasmic reticulum **ER** and has ribosomes **R** on its cytoplasmic face. The intermembranous space is continuous with the lumen of the endoplasmic reticulum. On the inner aspect of the inner nuclear membrane, there is an electron-dense layer of intermediate filaments, the ***nuclear lamina***, consisting of intermediate filaments called ***lamins*** that link inner membrane proteins and ***heterochromatin*** **H**.

The nuclear envelope contains numerous ***nuclear pores*** **NP**, at the margins of which the inner and outer membranes become continuous. Each pore contains a ***nuclear pore complex***, an elaborate cylindrical structure consisting of approximately 30 proteins known as ***nucleoporins***, forming a central pore approximately 125 nm in diameter. Nuclear pores permit and regulate the exchange of metabolites, macromolecules and ribosomal subunits between nucleus and cytoplasm. Ions and small molecules diffuse freely through the nuclear pore. Larger molecules, such as mRNA moving from nucleus to cytoplasm and histones from cytoplasm to nucleus, dock to the nuclear pore complex by means of a targeting sequence and are moved through the pore by an energy-dependent process. The nuclear pore complex may also hold together the two lipid bilayers of the nuclear envelope. Note that ***mitochondria*** **M** are also identifiable in the cytoplasm.

Fig. 1.4b shows an example of a technique called ***freeze-etching***. Briefly, this method involves the rapid freezing of cells which are then fractured. Internal surfaces of the cell are exposed at random, the fracture lines tending to follow natural planes of weakness. Surface detail is obtained by 'etching' or sublimating excess water molecules from the specimen at low temperature. A thin carbon impression is then made of the surface and this mirror image is viewed by scanning electron microscopy. Freeze-etching provides a valuable tool for studying internal cell surfaces at high resolution. In this preparation, the plane of cleavage has included part of the nuclear envelope in which nuclear pores **NP** are clearly demonstrated. Note also the outline of the plasma membrane **PM** and mitochondria **M**.

DFC dense fibrillar component **E** euchromatin **ECS** extracellular space **ER** endoplasmic reticulum **FC** fibrillar centre **GC** ganglion cell **G** granular component **H** heterochromatin **M** mitochondrion **N** nucleus **NE** nuclear envelope **NP** nuclear pore **PM** plasma membrane **R** ribosome **ST** sustentacular cell nucleus

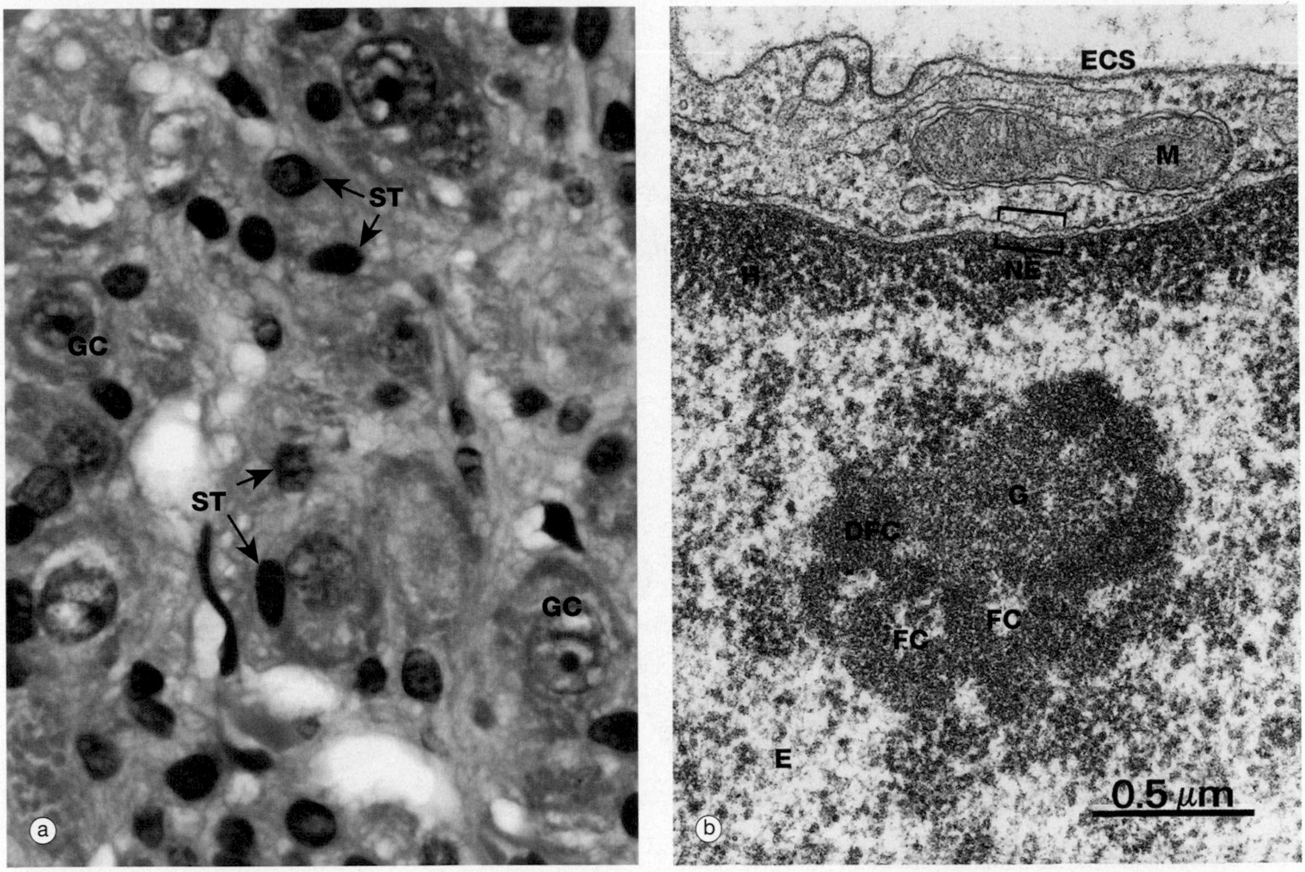

FIG. 1.5 The nucleolus
(a) H&E (HP) (b) EM ×37 000

Most nuclei contain a dense structure called the ***nucleolus***, which is the site of ribosomal RNA (rRNA) synthesis and ribosome assembly. Transfer RNA (tRNA) is also processed in the nucleolus. More recently discovered roles include control of the cell cycle and stress responses. The nucleolus may be very prominent in some cell types and quite inconspicuous in others, as shown in Fig. 1.5a which is a high power photomicrograph of an autonomic ganglion (see also Figs 7.21 and 7.22). In this micrograph, the nuclei of the ***ganglion cells*** **GC** contain large purple nucleoli, while the smaller ***sustentacular cell nuclei*** **ST** have small nucleoli that are only just visible at this magnification.

Furthermore, the nucleolus may change appearance depending on the state of the cell, so that an inactive fibroblast usually has a very small nucleolus while an activated fibroblast, for instance in a healing wound, has a prominent nucleolus.

Remember that this is a thin slice of the tissue and that the plane of section does not go through the nucleolus of every cell, so that some nuclei appear to lack nucleoli.

The nucleolus is not membrane bound but consists of an aggregate of ribosomal genes, newly synthesised rRNA, ribosomal proteins and ribonucleoproteins. The ribosomal genes are found on five chromosomes and are called the ***nucleolar organiser regions*** (***NORs***). The rRNA is transcribed from the DNA template and then modified in the nucleolus and combined with ribosomal proteins. The subunits then pass back to the cytoplasm through the nuclear pore complex (NPC) to aggregate into complete ribosomes when bound to an mRNA molecule. Fig. 1.5b is a high-power electron micrograph of a typical nucleolus. Nucleoli can be variable in appearance, but most contain ***dense fibrillar components*** **DFC** and paler ***fibrillar centres*** **FC** surrounded by the ***granular component*** **G**. The fibrillar components are the sites of ribosomal RNA synthesis, while ribosome assembly takes place in the granular components. Note also euchromatin **E** and heterochromatin **H** within the nucleus, which is bounded by the nuclear envelope **NE**. A thin rim of cytoplasm containing a mitochondrion **M** separates the nucleus from the extracellular space **ECS**.

PROTEIN SYNTHESIS

Proteins are not only a major structural component of cells, but, as enzymes, transport and regulatory proteins, they mediate many metabolic processes. The nature and quantity of proteins within a cell determine its activity and thus the study of ***proteomics*** can be very informative about the functions of a particular cell. All cellular proteins are replaced continuously. Many cells also synthesise proteins for export, including glandular secretions and extracellular structural proteins like collagen. Protein synthesis is therefore an essential and continuous activity of all cells and the major function of some cells. The ***ribosome*** is the protein factory of the cell. Every cell contains within its DNA the code for every protein that individual could produce. Production or ***expression*** of selected proteins only is characteristic of differentiated cells.

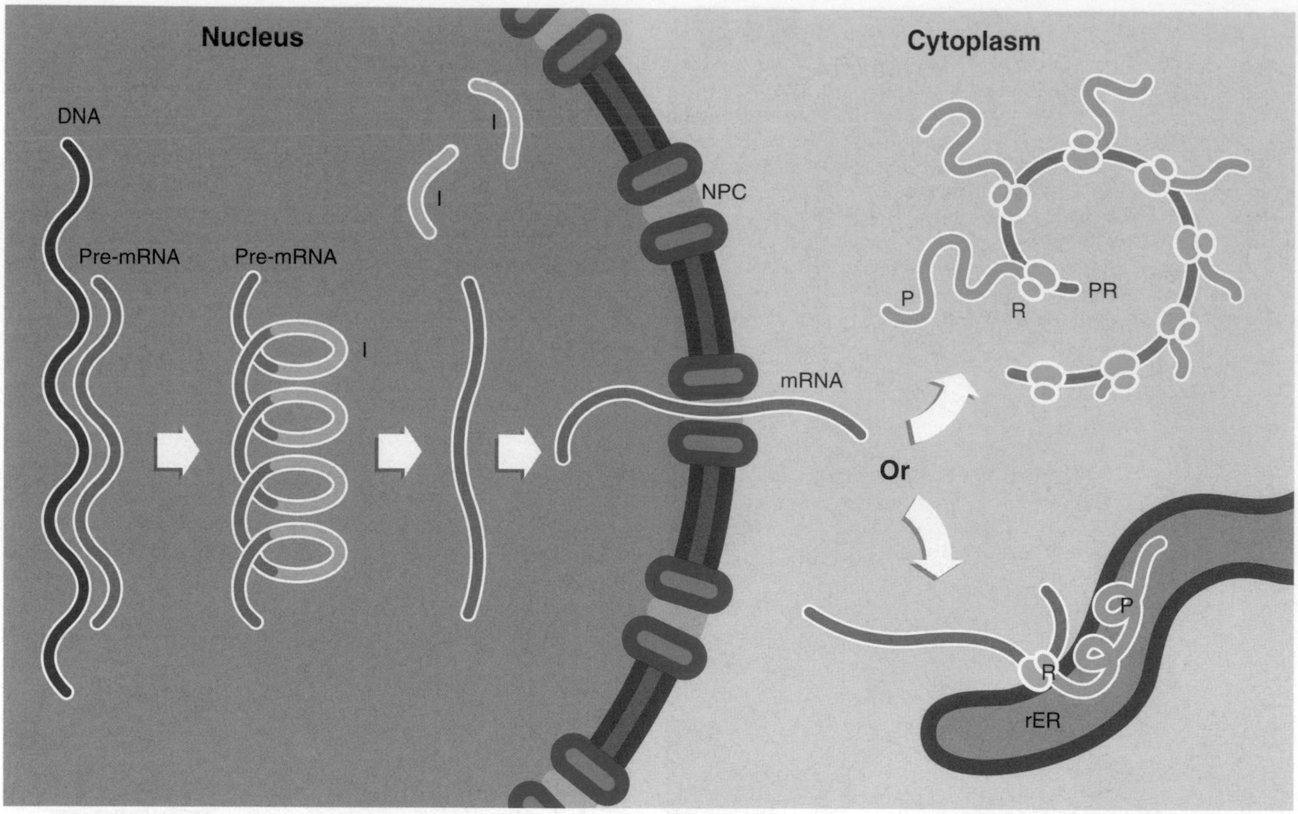

FIG. 1.6 Protein synthesis and degradation

Protein synthesis occurs in several steps. First, the **DNA** template (the ***gene***) of a particular protein is copied to form a complementary ***pre–messenger RNA*** (**pre-mRNA**) copy, a process known as ***transcription***. Post-transcriptional processing of the mRNA results in excision of ***introns*** **I** (non-coding regions of the mRNA strand). This step is controlled by ***small nuclear RNAs*** (***snRNA***) which in combination with various proteins form the ***spliceosome***. The ***messenger RNA*** (**mRNA**) then passes through the nuclear pore complex **NPC** into the cytoplasm. Here the mRNA binds to ***ribosomes*** **R**, organelles that synthesise proteins using the mRNA strand as a template to determine the specific amino acid sequence of the protein; this is known as ***translation***. Ribosomes, which are synthesised in the nucleolus, comprise two subunits of unequal size. Each subunit consists of a strand of RNA, ***ribosomal RNA*** (***rRNA***) molecules, with associated ribosomal proteins forming a globular structure.

Ribosomes align mRNA strands so that ***transfer RNA*** (***tRNA***) molecules may be brought into position and their amino acids added sequentially to the growing polypeptide chain **P**. Some of the RNA molecules in ribosomes catalyse peptide bond formation between amino acids and are sometimes called ***ribozymes*** to indicate this enzymatic function. Most enzymes are proteins. Thus the DNA code is converted first into RNA and then into a specific protein. Ribosomes are often found attached to mRNA molecules in small circular aggregations called ***polyribosomes*** or ***polysomes*** **PR**, formed by a single strand of mRNA with ribosomes attached along its length. Each ribosome in a polyribosome is making a separate molecule of the protein.

Ribosomes and polyribosomes may also be attached to the surface of ***endoplasmic reticulum***. The ER consists of an interconnecting network of membranous tubules, vesicles and flattened sacs (***cisternae***) which ramifies throughout the cytoplasm. Much of its surface is studded with ribosomes, giving a 'rough' appearance, leading to the name ***rough endoplasmic reticulum*** **rER**. Proteins destined for export, as well as lysosomal proteins, are synthesised by ribosomes attached to the surface of the rER and pass through the membrane into its lumen. Integral membrane proteins are also synthesised on rER and inserted into the membrane at this point, the extracellular part of the protein protruding into the lumen of the rER and the intramembranous part held firmly in place by hydrophobic attraction. It is within the rER that many proteins are folded to form their ***tertiary structure***, intrachain disulphide bonds are formed and the first steps of glycosylation take place. In contrast, proteins destined for the cytoplasm, nucleus and mitochondria are synthesised on free ribosomes and folding and other post-translational modifications take place there.

Proteins that are damaged or no longer required by the cell are degraded to short peptides. The first step in this process is binding of the protein ***ubiquitin*** to the damaged protein. This acts as a signal that allows the protein to be taken up by a ***proteasome***. Proteasomes are non–membrane bound arrays of proteolytic enzymes that are plentiful in all cells. Other proteins are degraded by proteolytic enzymes within lysosomes.

DNA deoxyribonucleic acid **I** intron **M** mitochondrion **mRNA** messenger ribonucleic acid **N** nucleus **NE** nuclear envelope **NPC** nuclear pore complex **Nu** nucleolus **P** polypeptide chain **PR** polyribosome **pre-mRNA** pre–messenger RNA **R** ribosome **rER** rough endoplasmic reticulum

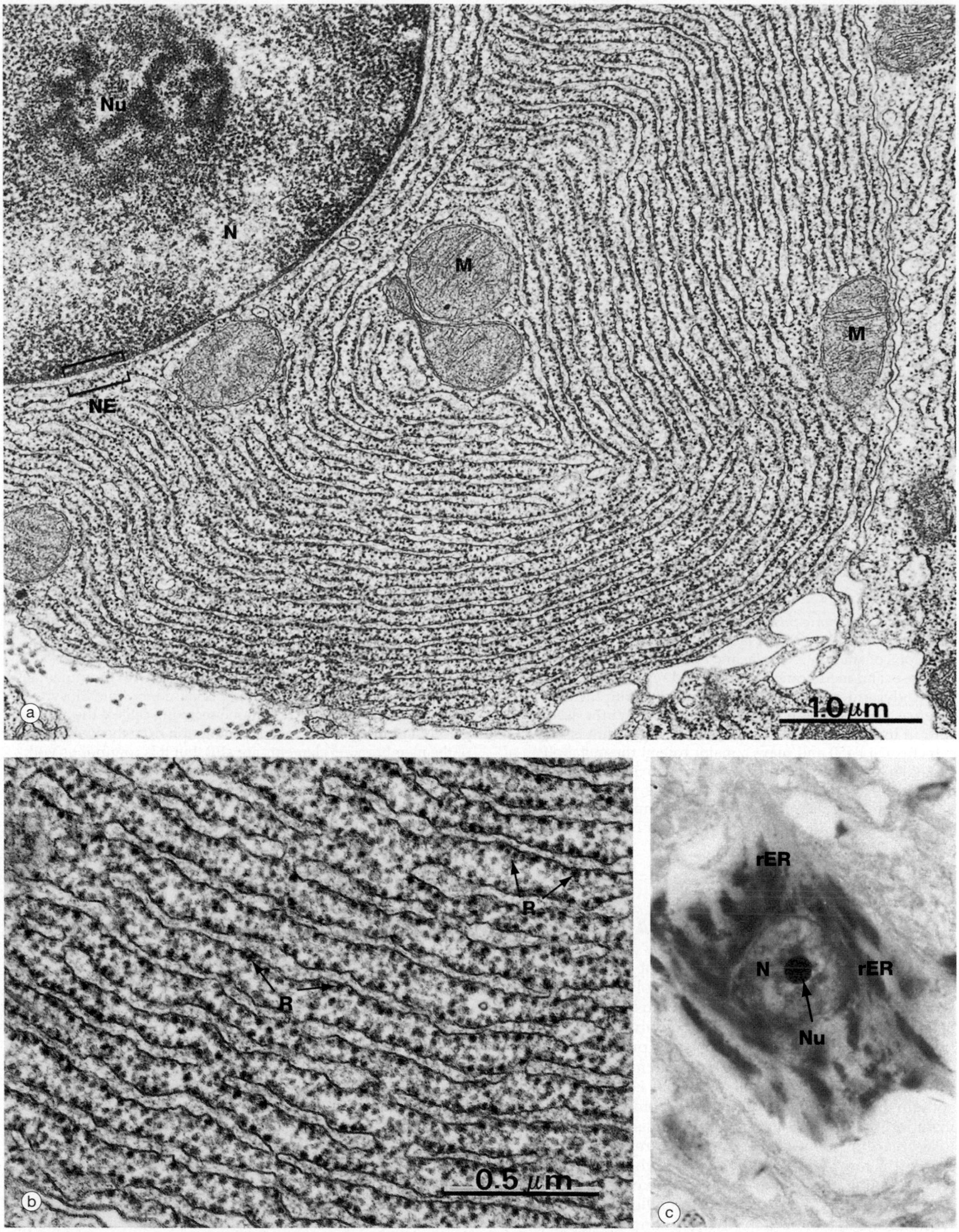

FIG. 1.7 Rough endoplasmic reticulum

These micrographs illustrate ***rough endoplasmic reticulum*** **rER** in a cell specialised for the synthesis and secretion of protein; in such cells, rER tends to be profuse and to form closely packed parallel laminae of flattened cisternae. In Fig. 1.7a, the dimensions of the rER can be compared with that of mitochondria **M** and the nucleus **N**. The nucleus typically contains a prominent nucleolus **Nu**. Note the close association between the rER and the outer lipid bilayer of the nuclear envelope **NE** with which it is in continuity. The chromatin in the nucleus is mainly dispersed (euchromatin), consistent with prolific protein synthesis.

Fig. 1.7b shows part of the rER at high magnification. Numerous ribosomes **R** stud the surface of the membrane system and there are plentiful ribosomes lying free in the intervening cytosol. Fig. 1.7c shows a nerve cell at high magnification stained by the basophilic dye cresyl violet. The basophilic clumps in the cytoplasm represent areas of plentiful **rER**. The nuclear envelope can be distinguished due to the basophilia of the numerous ribosomes that stud its outer surface. The nucleus **N** contains a prominent nucleolus **Nu** and dispersed chromatin.

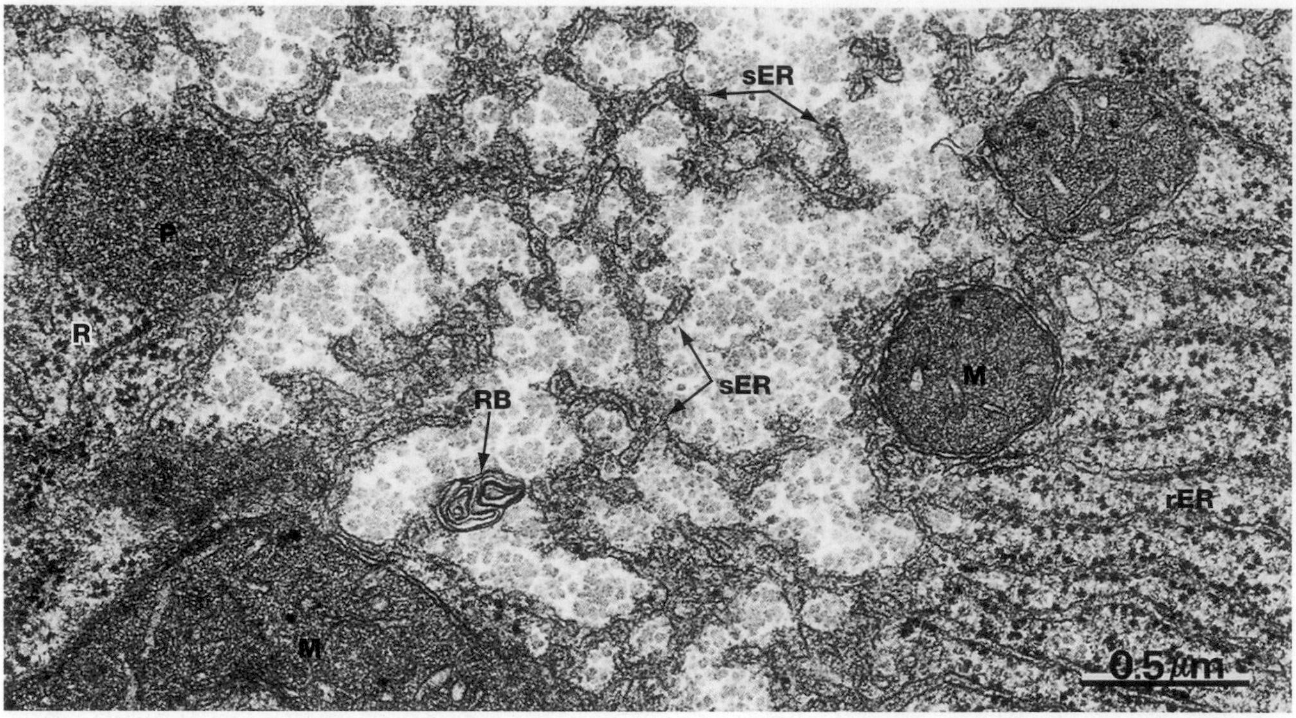

FIG. 1.8 Smooth endoplasmic reticulum
EM ×40 000

Smooth endoplasmic reticulum **sER** is continuous with and similar to rER except that it lacks ribosomes. The principal functions of smooth endoplasmic reticulum are lipid biosynthesis and membrane synthesis and repair. Fatty acids and triglycerides are mostly synthesised within the cytosol, whereas cholesterol and phospholipids are synthesised in sER. In liver cells, smooth endoplasmic reticulum is rich in cytochrome P450 and plays a major role in the metabolism of glycogen and detoxification of various noxious metabolic by-products, drugs and alcohol. In most cells, sER is involved in the storage and release of Ca^{2+} ions, an important mechanism of cell signalling. In muscle cells, where it is called ***sarcoplasmic reticulum***, release and reuptake of Ca^{2+} ions activates the contractile mechanism (see Ch. 6).

Most cells contain only scattered elements of sER interspersed with the other organelles. Cell types with prominent sER include liver cells and those cells specialised for lipid biosynthesis, such as the steroid hormone secreting cells of the adrenal glands and the gonads. In this micrograph from the liver, most of the membranous elements are **sER**, but it is continuous with rough endoplasmic reticulum **rER** in the lower right of the field. This field also includes several mitochondria **M**, a peroxisome **P** (Fig. 1.25), free ribosomes and polyribosomes **R** and a whorl of membrane in a residual body **RB** (Fig. 1.12).

IMPORT, EXPORT AND INTRACELLULAR TRANSPORTATION

Movement of materials into and out of cells and between separate compartments of a cell involves crossing lipid membranes. The plasma membrane thus controls the interaction of the cell with the external environment, mediating the exchange of nutrients and waste products, secretions and signalling mechanisms. Lipid membranes also separate different compartments within the cell, many of which contain mutually incompatible biochemical reactions. For instance, the process of protein synthesis and export which takes place in the rough endoplasmic reticulum and Golgi apparatus must be kept separate from the garbage disposal and recycling plant, the ***lysosome***. Likewise, microorganisms phagocytosed by cells must be killed and disposed of without damage to normal structures and mechanisms.

Information must also cross membranes, telling the cell when to divide, release secretions, contract or perform many other functions. Many of the mechanisms used for transport of cargo also serve to transmit messages to the interior of the cell. There are also dedicated mechanisms for the transfer of information, such as the transient ***depolarisation*** of the plasma membrane along the length of a nerve axon in the conduction of a nerve impulse. Histologically, these transport processes can only be observed indirectly: for example, cells suspended in hypotonic solutions swell due to passive uptake of water, whereas cells placed in hypertonic solutions tend to shrink due to outflow of water. Radioisotope labelling techniques can be used to follow active transport processes. Bulk transport, however, is readily observable by microscopy (Fig. 1.13). Both active and passive transport processes are enhanced if the area of the plasma membrane is increased by folds or projections of the cell surface, as exemplified by the absorptive cells lining the small intestine (Fig. 1.2).

M mitochondrion **P** peroxisome **R** ribosomes **RB** residual body **rER** rough endoplasmic reticulum
sER smooth endoplasmic reticulum

The main mechanisms by which materials and information are transported across cell membranes are:

- **Passive diffusion**. This type of transport is dependent on the presence of a concentration gradient across the membrane and also on the size and polarity of the molecule. Lipids and lipid-soluble molecules such as the hormones oestrogen and testosterone pass freely through lipid membranes, as do gases such as oxygen, nitrogen and carbon dioxide. Uncharged but polar small molecules such as water and urea diffuse through lipid membranes slowly, but charged molecules such as sodium (Na^+) and potassium (K^+) ions diffuse through very slowly indeed.
- **Facilitated diffusion**. This type of transport involves the movement of hydrophilic molecules such as water, ions, glucose and amino acids. This process is strictly passive, moving polar or charged substances along an electrochemical gradient, but requires the presence of protein carrier molecules. There are two types of protein carrier molecule: the first type (known as ***pores*** or ***channels***) form a water-filled channel across the membrane through which selected molecules or ions can pass depending on concentration, size and electrical charge, while the second type binds a particular molecule or ion and then undergoes a change in conformation, moving the substrate to the other side of the membrane (a ***transporter*** or ***carrier***). Aquaporins, which allow water to cross membranes at a much faster rate than by diffusion alone, are an important and common example of a transmembrane channel. There are many different aquaporin molecules, some of which are highly specific for water molecules, while others allow the passage of other small molecules such as urea or glycerol. Some facilitated diffusion pores are ***gated***, which means that the pore is open or closed depending on different physiological conditions (e.g. open only at a particular pH).
- **Active transport**. This mode of transport is not only independent of electrochemical gradients, but also often operates against extreme electrochemical gradients. The classic example of active transport is the continuous movement of Na^+ out of the cell and K^+ into the cell by the Na^+-K^+ pump, which moves Na^+ ions out of the cell and K^+ ions into the cell across the plasma membrane. Adenosine triphosphate (ATP) is converted to adenosine diphosphate (ADP) in the process to generate the energy required, hence the name ***Na^+-K^+ ATPase***.
- **Bulk transport**. Transport of large molecules or small particles into, out of or between compartments within the cell is mediated by subcellular, transient membrane-bound vesicles. These vesicles transport proteins embedded in the membrane of the vesicle (e.g. proteins destined for the plasma membrane) and soluble cargo within the lumen. ***Transport vesicles*** are formed by the assembly of a protein 'coat,' leading to budding of a section of membrane which is pinched off to form a vesicle. At their destination, the reverse process takes place when the transport vesicle fuses with the target membrane, incorporating into it and releasing its contents. These mechanisms are dependent on the fluidity and deformability of lipid membranes and the mobility of intrinsic membrane proteins within the plane of the membrane. Specific examples such as endocytosis, exocytosis and intracellular transport vesicles are given in Figs 1.10–1.13.
- **Transmembrane signalling**. There are various ways in which signals may cross a plasma membrane to deliver information to a cell. One example is lipid-soluble molecules, such as the hormone oestrogen, which diffuse through the plasma membrane to bind to an intracellular receptor. Non–lipid soluble molecules, such as the hormone insulin, bind to a protein receptor embedded in the plasma membrane, which is thus activated, and pass the signal on to an intracellular signalling pathway. Other signalling molecules, such as neurotransmitters at nerve synapses (see Ch. 7), bind to an ion channel in the postsynaptic membrane, allowing ions to enter the cell and initiating depolarisation of the membrane.

Abnormal receptors can cause disease

Drugs that modify membrane receptors can be used in the treatment of disease. One example of this is the use of drugs such as trastuzumab in the treatment of some breast cancers. Normal breast epithelium expresses a signalling molecule called ***human epidermal growth factor type 2*** (***Her2***, also known as ***Her2/neu*** or ***ErbB-2***) on the plasma membrane. Her2 (along with Her1, Her3 and Her4) regulate growth and survival of normal breast epithelium cells. Her2 is a transmembrane protein with three functional domains: an extracellular receptor component, a hydrophobic transmembrane component and an intracellular enzyme, a tyrosine kinase, that passes on the received signal within the cell. When a ligand binds to Her2 it passes a signal to the cell to divide and also promotes longer survival of the cell.

In approximately 20% to 30% of breast cancers there is ***gene amplification*** of the *HER2* gene, i.e. there are more than the normal number of copies of the gene in the nucleus. This results in more than the normal number of molecules of Her2 at the cell surface, i.e. ***overexpression***, which seems to be one of the mechanisms whereby the cells undergo uncontrolled growth and survival to form a cancer. The excess Her2 expression can be detected by various techniques (Fig. 1.9 and e-Fig. 1.1). Patients with cancers that overexpress Her2 are treated with drugs such as trastuzumab, a monoclonal antibody that binds to the extracellular domain of Her2 and blocks its activation. Thus the effects of Her2 overexpression by the tumour cells are blocked and the patient survives for longer.

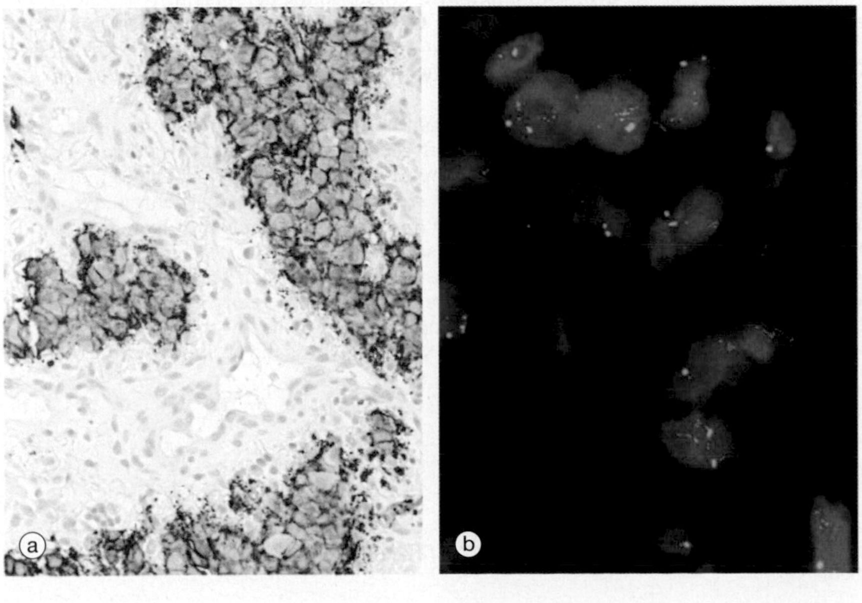

FIG. 1.9 Testing for *HER2* amplification (a) Immunohistochemistry for Her2 (HP) (b) Fluorescence in situ hybridisation for *HER2* (HP)

Fig. 1.9a illustrates a breast cancer showing a positive ***immunohistochemical*** test for Her2. The principles of this technique are outlined in Appendix 2. The over-expressed protein is found on the cell surface and so strong brown membrane staining is required for a positive result, as seen here. Note that the cell nucleus is not stained. The test is typically validated or, in borderline cases, confirmed by ***in situ hybridisation*** to demonstrate gene amplification by highlighting multiple copies of the *HER2* gene in the nucleus (Fig. 1.9b). The cancer cell nuclei are stained blue. The gene target normally shows a single orange and green signal but multiple signals are seen in each nucleus here, indicating *HER2* gene amplification.

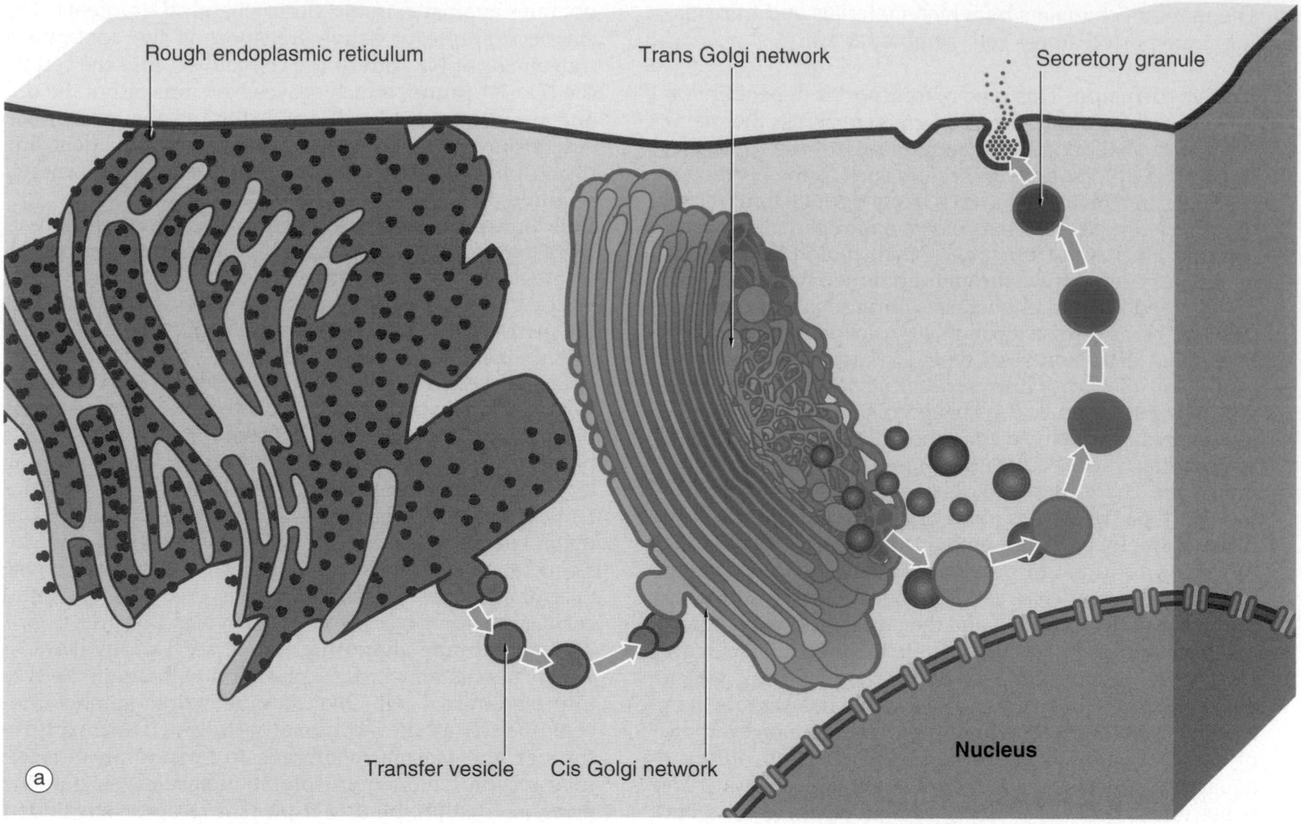

FIG. 1.10 Golgi apparatus *(illustrations (b) to (e) opposite)*
(a) Schematic diagram (b) EM ×30 000 (c) H&E (HP) (d) Iron haematoxylin (HP) (e) H&E (HP)

The ***Golgi apparatus, complex*** or ***stack*** is an important site of protein and lipid glycosylation, as well as the site of synthesis of many glycosaminoglycans that form the extracellular matrix. Fig. 1.10a illustrates the main structural features of the Golgi apparatus and summarises the mechanism by which secretory products are packaged within membrane-bound vesicles. A cell may contain one or more Golgi stacks, and these may break up and reform during different phases of the cell cycle or in different physiological states. The Golgi apparatus consists of 4 to 6 saucer-shaped membrane-bound ***cisternae***. The outermost cisternae take the form of a network of tubules known as the ***cis*** and ***trans Golgi network*** (***CGN*** and ***TGN***, respectively).

Proteins synthesised in the rER are transported to the Golgi apparatus in ***coated vesicles*** (Fig. 1.11); the coat protein in this case is known as ***coat protein complex II (COP II)***. Soon after the coated vesicles bud off from the rER, the coat proteins disengage and are recycled. On arrival at the convex forming face or CGN, the vesicles fuse with the CGN. In the Golgi apparatus the glycosylation of proteins, begun in the rER, is completed by sequential addition of sugar residues and the proteins are packaged for transport to their final destination.

Each cisterna is enriched for the specific enzyme to add a specific sugar.

There appear to be two mechanisms by which proteins pass through the Golgi apparatus. In the first, proteins are passed from cisterna to cisterna in coated vesicles (***COP I*** in this instance). However, for very large proteins such as collagen rods, the medial cisternae mature, with specific enzymes being moved backwards to less mature cisternae by coated vesicles. On arrival at the concave maturing face or TGN, the proteins are accurately sorted into secretory vesicles destined for the extracellular space (e.g. hormones, neurotransmitters, collagen) or the plasma membrane (e.g. cell surface receptors, adhesion molecules) or intracellular organelles such as lysosomes. The sorting of cargo into secretory vesicles is dependent on binding of specific adapter molecules to the cargo, which then bind to specific coat proteins. Secretory vesicles become increasingly condensed as they migrate through the cytoplasm to form mature ***secretory granules***, which are then liberated at the cell surface by ***exocytosis***. A group of membrane proteins called SNAREs regulate docking and fusion of coated vesicles to their target membrane.

Fig. 1.10b illustrates a particularly well-developed Golgi apparatus. Transfer vesicles **T** and elements of the rough endoplasmic reticulum **rER** are seen adjacent to the forming face. A variety of larger vesicles **V** can be seen in the concavity of the maturing face, some of which appear to be budding from the Golgi cisternae **C**; such vesicles could be either secretory granules or lysosomes. Note the proximity of the Golgi apparatus to the nucleus **N**. The nuclear membrane **NM** is particularly well demonstrated in this micrograph.

Fig. 1.10c illustrates a group of plasma cells from inflamed tissue; these cells are responsible for antibody production as part of the body's immune defences (see Ch. 11). The plentiful rER is strongly basophilic and the protein is acidophilic so that there is staining with both eosin and haematoxylin, giving a purple or ***amphiphilic*** colour to the cytoplasm. The well-developed Golgi complex **G** consists of lipid (membranes), which is dissolved out during preparation. Thus the Golgi is unstained and appears as a pale area (negative image) adjacent to the nucleus **N**.

Fig. 1.10d demonstrates secretory granules in the acinar cells of the pancreas, which secretes digestive enzymes. The secretory cells are grouped around a minute central duct **D** and the secretory granules, which are stained black, are concentrated towards the luminal aspect of the cell. The nuclei **N** are arranged around the periphery of the secretory unit.

Fig. 1.10e demonstrates a very similar secretory acinus in a salivary gland. The purple-stained secretory granules **SG** are seen in the superficial cytoplasm of the cells towards the central duct **D**. The nuclei **N** are pushed towards the periphery of the cells.

C Golgi cisternae **D** central duct **G** Golgi apparatus **N** nucleus **NM** nuclear membrane **rER** rough endoplasmic reticulum **SG** secretory granules **T** transfer vesicles **V** vesicles

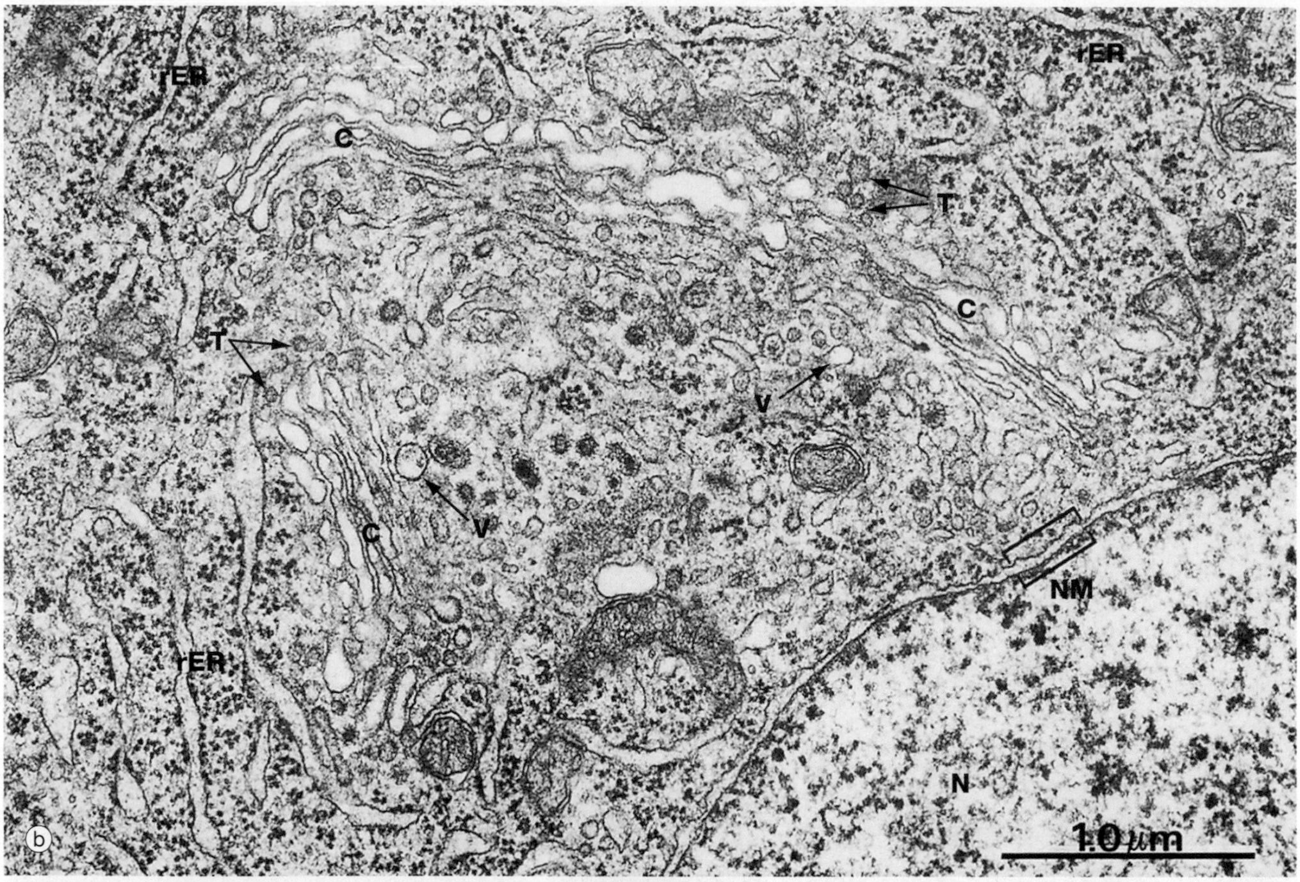

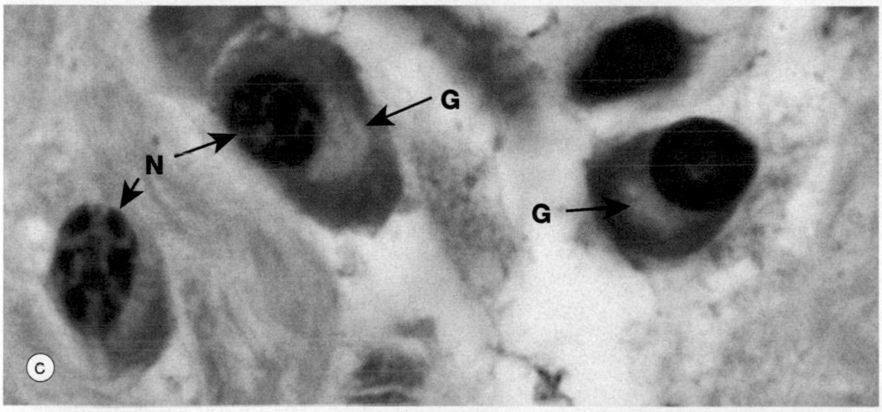

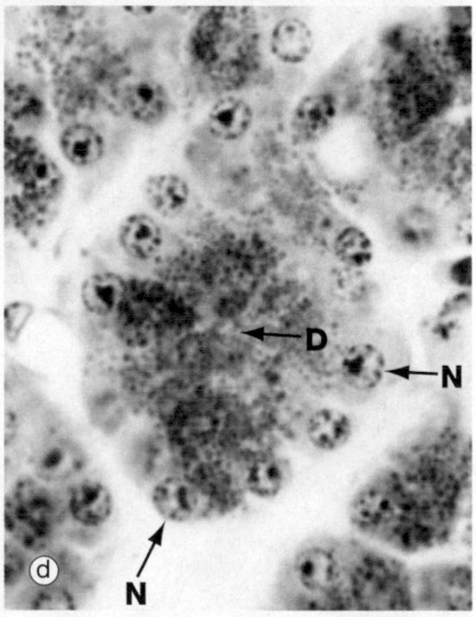

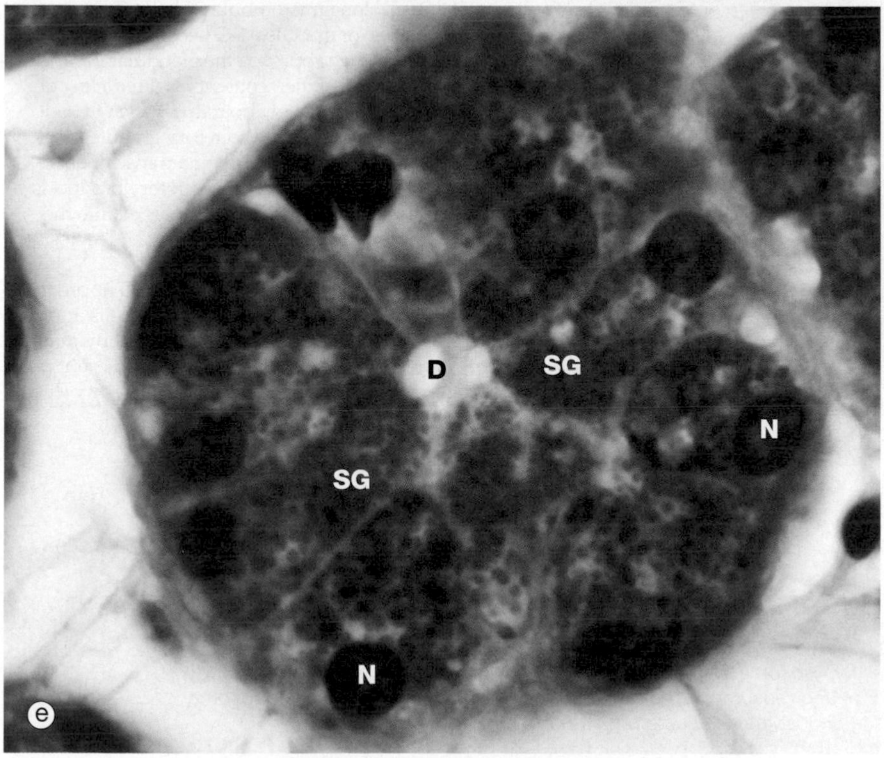

FIG. 1.10 Golgi apparatus *(caption and illustration (a) opposite)*
(a) Schematic diagram
(b) EM ×30 000 (c) H&E (HP) (d) Iron haematoxylin (HP) (e) H&E (HP)

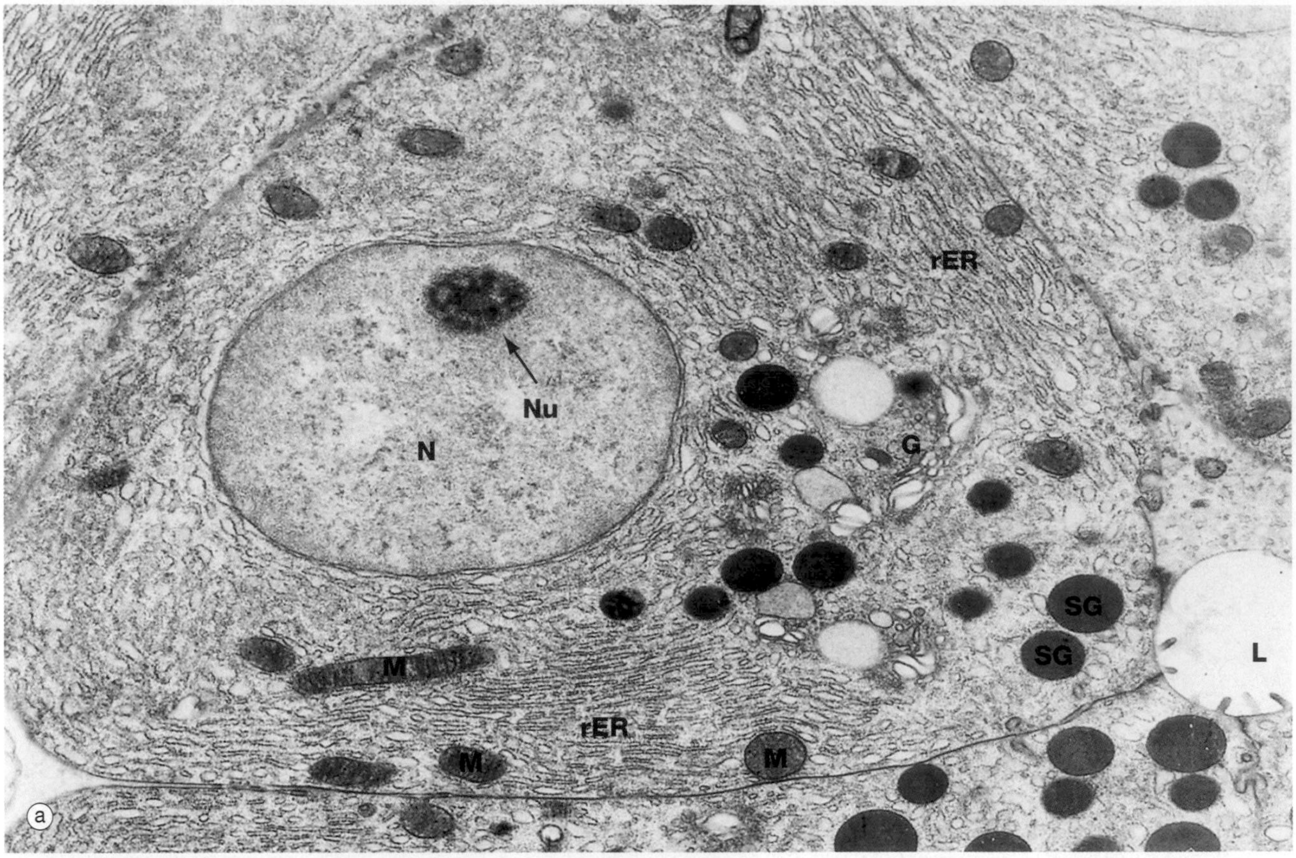

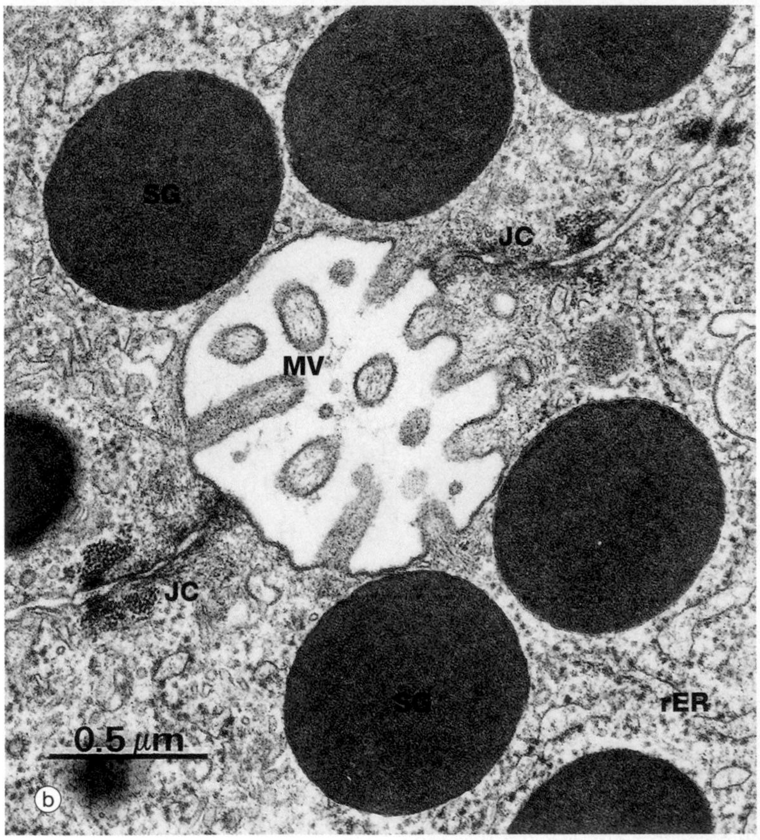

FIG. 1.11 Exocytosis
(a) EM ×14 000 (b) EM ×41 500

Fig. 1.11a and b illustrate typical protein-secreting cells from the pancreas, which produces digestive enzymes. All cells undergo continuous exocytosis (***constitutive secretion***) but, in specialised secretory cells, there is also signal-dependent exocytosis (***regulated secretion***), as in this case where digestive enzymes are secreted in response to food in the duodenum. In Fig. 1.11a the nucleus **N** has dispersed chromatin and a prominent nucleolus **Nu**. The rough endoplasmic reticulum **rER** and Golgi apparatus **G** are prominent. Mitochondria **M** supply energy. Small secretory vesicles leave the Golgi apparatus as coated vesicles (***clathrin-coated*** in this case) but soon uncoat and may fuse together to form larger vesicles. Vesicles are moved towards the plasma membrane of the cell along microtubules (Fig. 1.17). Immature secretory vesicles (or granules) **SG** become increasingly electron dense as they approach the glandular lumen **L**, due to concentration of their contents and recycling of membrane back to the Golgi apparatus. When the cell receives a signal to secrete, the secretory granules dock with the plasma membrane, forming a transient opening (***porosome***) through which the secretory product is discharged. The vesicle membrane is merged into the plasma membrane but is later recycled by endocytosis to maintain the normal cell size.

Fig. 1.11b shows secretory granules **SG** approaching the apices of two pancreatic secretory cells and converging on a tiny excretory duct formed by ***junctional complexes*** **JC** (see Fig. 5.9) joining adjacent cells. Short microvilli **MV** protrude into the excretory duct.

B bacterium **CL** clathrin **CP** coated pit **CV** coated vesicle **EL** endolysosome **G** Golgi apparatus **JC** junctional complex **L** gland lumen **LE** late endosome **Li** ligand **Ly** lysosome **M** mitochondrion **MV** microvilli **MVB** multivesicular body **N** nucleus **Nu** nucleolus **P** phagosome **PL** phagolysosome **R** receptor **RB** residual body **RE** recycling endosome **rER** rough endoplasmic reticulum **SE** sorting endosome **SG** secretory granules

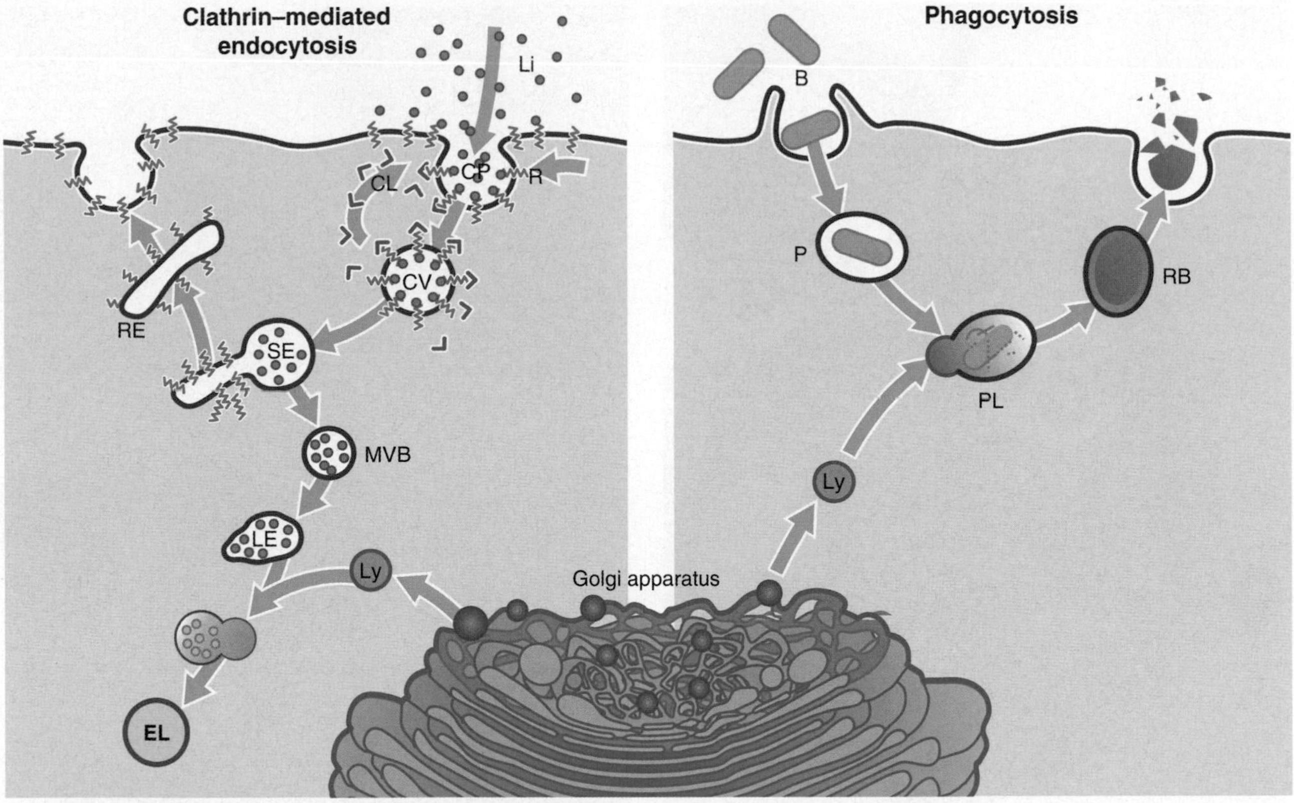

FIG. 1.12 Endocytosis

Cells take up particulate matter and large macromolecules by a variety of processes collectively known as ***endocytosis***. The best known of these mechanisms is ***phagocytosis***, which is used by specialised phagocytic cells to ingest particulate matter, usually larger than 0.5 µm, such as bacteria, fungi and apoptotic cells. ***Pinocytosis*** is used by all cells to take up fluid and solutes.

Several mechanisms of pinocytosis are known, including ***clathrin-mediated pinocytosis***, ***caveolae-mediated pinocytosis*** (see Fig. 6.19) and ***macropinocytosis***. This diagram summarises the main steps of clathrin-mediated pinocytosis and phagocytosis.

Clathrin-mediated endocytosis

Clathrin-mediated endocytosis takes place continuously, with ***clathrin-coated pits*** **CP** constantly forming and pinching off to form coated vesicles. ***Clathrin*** **CL** binds to specialised areas of the plasma membrane and shapes them into vesicles. Thus the cell takes up extracellular fluid and molecules. In addition, specific molecules (***ligands*** **Li**) that bind to cell surface receptors **R** are taken into the cell by this mechanism. A well-known example is the low-density lipoprotein (LDL) receptor, an intrinsic membrane protein with extracellular and cytoplasmic domains. Receptors with bound ligand concentrate into the coated pit by diffusion in the plane of the membrane. The coated pit then buds off to form a ***coated vesicle*** **CV**. Many different types of receptors may be found in a single clathrin-coated pit, although only one type is shown here for simplicity. The vesicles very quickly lose their coat and fuse with ***sorting endosomes*** **SE**, which are dynamic tubulovesicular structures, usually found close to the plasma membrane. The acid pH in the lumen of sorting endosomes encourages dissociation of receptor and ligand; these are then quickly separated so that most of the membrane and its intrinsic receptors are shuttled to ***recycling endosomes*** **RE** and from there back to the cell surface. Some membrane receptors may go through this cycle up to 300 times and the expression of receptors on the cell surface can be regulated by this mechanism. The remaining part of the sorting endosome, which contains the unbound LDL, converts into a ***multivesicular body*** **MVB**. Multivesicular bodies are moved towards the Golgi apparatus where they become ***late endosomes*** **LE** and fuse with ***lysosomes*** **Ly**. Degradative enzymes within the lysosomes, now called ***endolysosomes*** **EL**, digest the protein component of the LDL, freeing cholesterol for incorporation into membranes.

Vesicles leaving the sorting endosome may also migrate to another part of the cell membrane, such as the basal membrane of an epithelial cell. There, the vesicle fuses with the plasma membrane, releasing its contents to the extracellular space; this process is called ***transcytosis*** and is important, for instance, in the gastrointestinal tract for absorption of nutrients from food.

Phagocytosis

Bacteria **B** are taken up by specialised phagocytic cells, such as ***neutrophils*** and ***macrophages***, by phagocytosis. The bacterium binds to cell surface receptors, triggering the formation of ***pseudopodia*** that extend around the organism until they fuse, leaving the engulfed bacterium in a membrane-bound ***phagosome*** **P** within the cytoplasm. At this stage, recycling of membrane and receptors back to the plasma membrane takes place. The phagosome then fuses with a lysosome **Ly** to become a ***phagolysosome*** **PL** (or secondary lysosome) and the bacterium is subjected to the toxic activities of the lysosomal enzymes.

These enzymes also break down the components of the dead bacteria, which may be released into the cytoplasm, expelled from the cell by exocytosis or remain in the cytoplasm as a ***residual body*** **RB**. Lysosomes are also involved in the degradation of cellular organelles, many of which have only a finite lifespan and are therefore replaced continuously; this lysosomal function is termed ***autophagy***. Most autophagocytic degradation products accumulate and become indistinguishable from the residual bodies of phagocytosis. With advancing age, residual bodies accumulate in the cells of some tissues and appear as brown ***lipofuscin*** granules (Fig. 1.26).

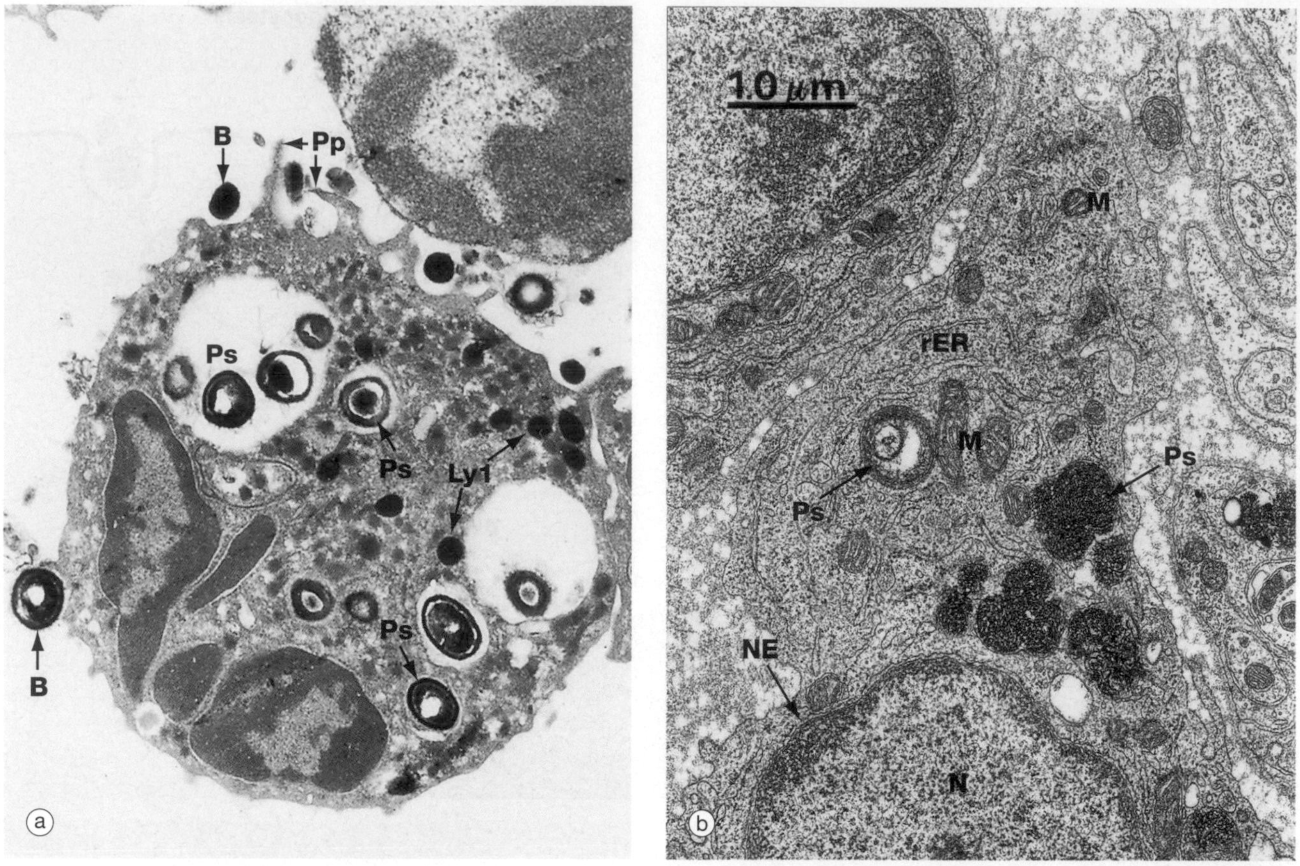

FIG. 1.13 Phagocytosis
(a) EM ×11 750 (b) EM ×14 000 (c) H&E (HP)

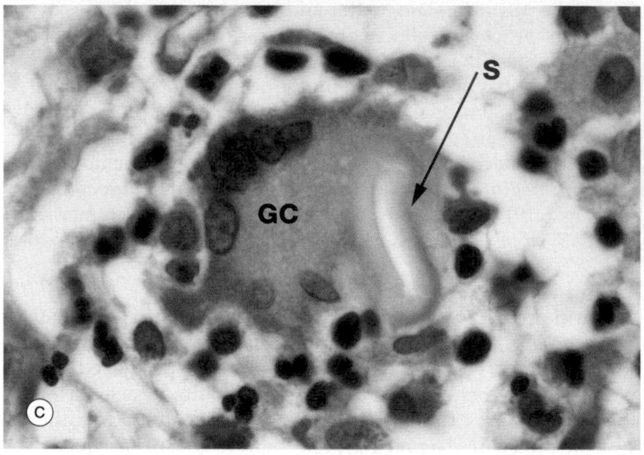

Fig. 1.13a illustrates a professional phagocytic white blood cell, a ***neutrophil polymorph*** (see Ch. 3), in the process of engulfing and destroying bacteria **B**. Note the manner in which ***pseudopodia*** **Pp** embrace the bacteria before engulfment. Note also phagosomes **Ps** containing bacteria in various stages of degradation. Several lysosomes **Ly1** are also visible.

Fig. 1.13b is a high-power view of phagosomes **Ps** in the cytoplasm of a ***macrophage***, another professional phagocyte found in almost all tissues. The large, irregularly shaped membrane-bound phagosomes contain coiled fragments of plasma membrane and other cellular constituents derived from damaged cells. This macrophage is performing its function as a scavenger cell by phagocytosing dead and damaged cells and recycling their components. Note also the cell nucleus **N** with its easily identified nuclear envelope **NE**, as well as mitochondria **M** and rough endoplasmic reticulum **rER**.

Fig. 1.13c shows a light micrograph of a similar process at a site of inflammation (a healing scar in this case). The large cell in the centre is a ***multinucleate giant cell*** **GC** (a modified macrophage) that has phagocytosed a fragment of suture material used to suture the wound. The fragment of suture material **S** is easily seen as a pale, elongated shape within the giant cell. Collections of such multinucleate giant cells are often seen at sites where foreign material has entered the tissues.

Microbial tricks in intracellular infections

Phagocytosis is a vital component of the ***innate immune system*** (see Ch. 11). Phagocytosis of bacteria in most cases results in bacterial cell death with lysis of the dead organisms within a phagolysosome. However, some pathogenic organisms have learned to use the phagocytic mechanism to their own advantage to gain entry to the cell and grow there in a protected environment, safe from other elements of the immune system. For instance, *Mycobacterium tuberculosis*, the agent responsible for the important worldwide infection tuberculosis, is able to grow and divide within macrophages.

M. tuberculosis does this by preventing the phagosome from fusing with a lysosome and thus lives and divides safely within the phagosome. *Listeria monocytogenes*, a rare cause of food poisoning, is able to disrupt the phagosomal membrane and escape into the cell cytoplasm. *Legionella pneumophila* modifies the membrane of the phagosome so that it resembles ER and thus remains untouched. Some viruses, on the other hand, gain entry to the cell by receptor-mediated endocytosis. Both Poliovirus and Adenovirus use this mechanism, casting their protein coats inside the endosome and allowing their genome to escape into the cytoplasm.

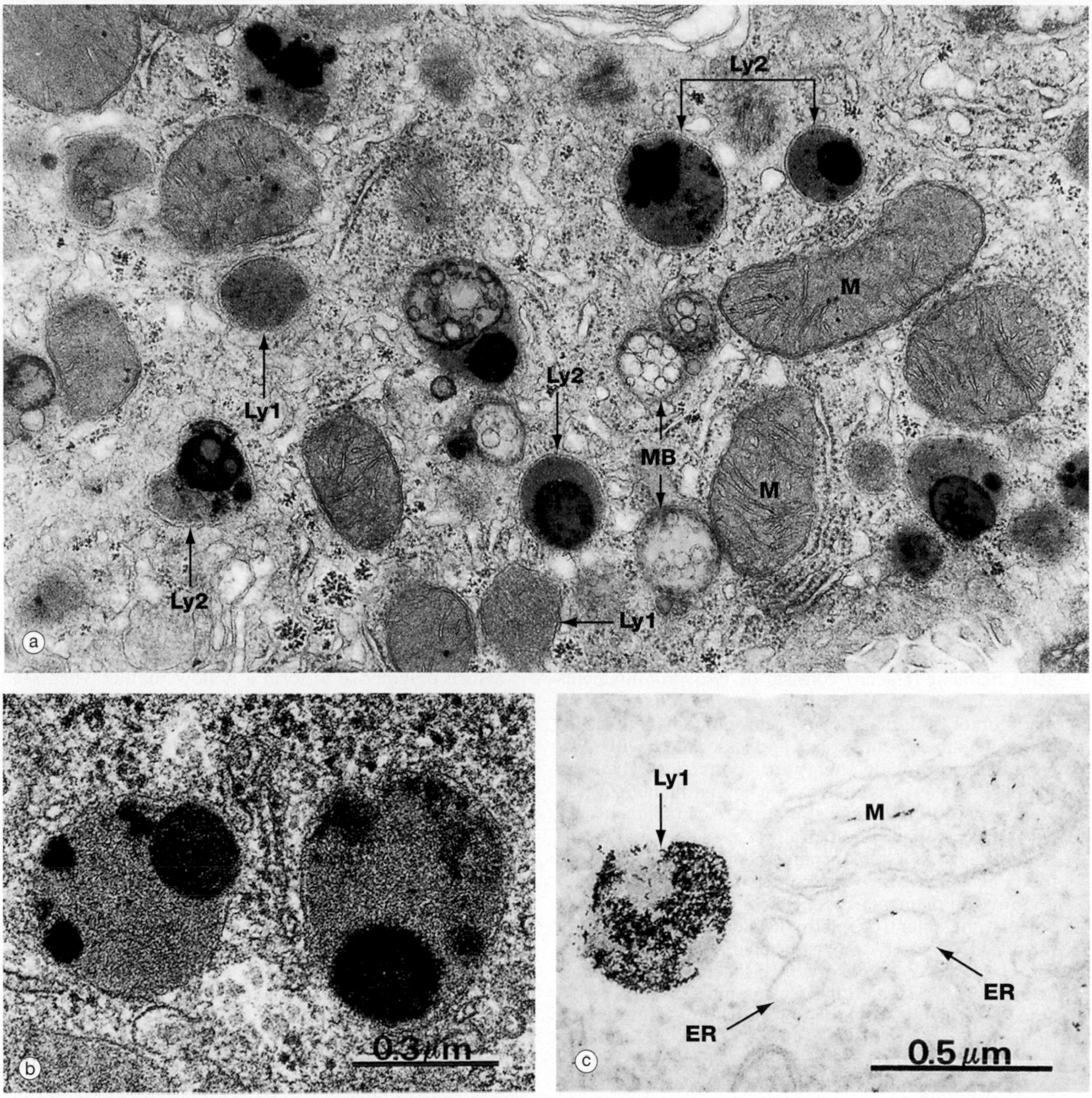

FIG. 1.14 Lysosomes
(a) EM ×27 000 (b) EM ×60 000 (c) Histochemical method for acid phosphatase, EM × 50 000

Lysosomes are the site of degradation of material taken up into the cells by phagocytosis or endocytosis and of old or unnecessary cellular constituents (***autophagy***). These micrographs show the typical features of ***lysosomes*** and ***residual bodies***. Fig. 1.14a shows part of the cytoplasm of a liver cell. Lysosomes **Ly1** vary greatly in size and appearance but are recognised as membrane-bound organelles containing an amorphous granular material. ***Phagolysosomes*** or ***secondary lysosomes*** **Ly2** are even more variable in appearance but are recognisable by their diverse particulate content, some of which is extremely electron-dense. The distinction between residual bodies and secondary lysosomes is often difficult. ***Late endosomes*** or ***multivesicular bodies*** **MB** are also seen in this micrograph. Note the size of lysosomes relative to mitochondria **M**.

Fig. 1.14b shows two phagolysosomes at higher magnification, allowing the limiting membrane to be visualised. Both contain electron-dense particulate material and amorphous granular material.

The lysosomal enzymes comprise more than 40 different degradative enzymes including proteases, lipases and nucleases. These are collectively known as ***acid hydrolases*** because they are optimally active at a pH of about 5.0. This protects the cell should lysosomal enzymes escape into the cytosol where they would be inactive at the higher pH. Histochemical methods can be used to demonstrate sites of enzyme activity within cells and thus act as markers for organelles that contain these enzymes. Such a method has been used in Fig. 1.14c to demonstrate the presence of acid phosphatase, a typical lysosomal enzyme; enzyme activity is represented by the electron-dense area within a lysosome **Ly1**. Other organelles remain unstained, but the outline of a mitochondrion **M** and profiles of endoplasmic reticulum **ER** can nevertheless be identified.

B bacterium **ER** endoplasmic reticulum **GC** multinucleate giant cell **Ly1** lysosomes **Ly2** secondary or phagolysosome **M** mitochondrion **MB** multivesicular body **N** nucleus **NE** nuclear envelope **Pp** pseudopodia **Ps** phagosome **rER** rough endoplasmic reticulum **S** suture material

THE CYTOSKELETON AND CELL MOVEMENT

Every cell has a supporting framework of minute filaments and tubules, the ***cytoskeleton***, which maintains the shape and polarity of the cell. Nevertheless, the cell membrane and intracellular organelles are not rigid or static structures but are in a constant state of movement to accommodate processes such as endocytosis, phagocytosis and secretion. Some cells (e.g. white blood cells) propel themselves about by ***amoeboid movement***; other cells have actively motile membrane specialisations such as ***cilia*** and ***flagella*** (see Ch. 5); while other cells (e.g. muscle cells) are highly specialised for contractility. In addition, cell division is a process that involves extensive reorganisation of cellular constituents. The cytoskeleton incorporates features that accommodate all these dynamic functions.

The cytoskeleton of each cell contains structural elements of three main types: ***microfilaments***, ***microtubules*** and ***intermediate filaments***. The cytoskeleton structures are made up of protein subunits (***monomers***) that are non-covalently bound together into filaments (***polymers***). Many accessory proteins link these structures to one another, to the plasma membrane and to the membranes of intracellular organelles. Other associated proteins are the ***motor proteins*** responsible for movement, the best known of which are the ***myosin***, ***dynein*** and ***kinesin*** protein families.

- **Microfilaments**. Microfilaments are extremely fine strands (5 to 9 nm in diameter) of the protein ***actin***. Each actin filament (F-actin) consists of two protofilaments twisted together to form a helix. The ***protofilaments*** are made up of multiple globular actin monomers (G-actin) joined together head to tail and associated with ATP molecules to provide energy for contraction. The actin filament is then assembled into larger filaments, networks and 3-dimensional structures. Actin filaments are best demonstrated histologically in skeletal muscle cells where they form a stable arrangement of bundles with the motor protein myosin. Contraction occurs when the actin and myosin filaments slide relative to each other due to the rearrangement of intermolecular bonds, fuelled by the release of energy from associated ATP molecules (see Ch. 6). However, all eukaryotic cells contain a dynamic actin network. Beneath the plasma membrane, actin, in association with various transmembrane and linking proteins, forms a robust supporting meshwork called the ***cell cortex***, which protects against deformation and yet can be rearranged to accommodate changes in cell morphology. Membrane specialisations such as ***microvilli*** (see Fig. 5.14) also contain a skeleton of actin filaments. Actin plays a central role in cell movement, pinocytosis and phagocytosis. Actin may also bind to intrinsic plasma membrane proteins to anchor them in position.
- **Intermediate filaments**. Intermediate filaments (approximately 10 nm in diameter) are, as their name implies, intermediate in size between microfilaments and microtubules. These proteins have a purely structural function and consist of filaments that self-assemble into larger filaments and bind intracellular structures to each other and to plasma membrane proteins. In humans, there are more than 50 different types of intermediate filament, but these can be divided into different classes, with some classes characteristic of particular cell types. This feature is used in diagnostic pathology to identify different varieties of tumour. For example, the ***keratin*** (or ***cytokeratin***) intermediate filament family is characteristic of epithelial cells, where they form a supporting network within the cytoplasm and are anchored to the plasma membrane at intercellular junctions. Specific keratin types form hair and nails. Likewise, ***vimentin*** is found in cells of mesodermal origin, ***desmin*** in muscle cells, ***neurofilament proteins*** in nerve cells and ***glial fibrillary acidic protein*** in glial cells. ***Lamin*** intermediate filaments form a structural layer on the inner side of the nuclear membrane.
- **Microtubules**. Microtubules (25 nm in diameter) are much larger than microfilaments but, like them, are made up of globular protein subunits which can readily be assembled and disassembled to provide for alterations in cell shape and position of organelles. The microtubule subunits are of two types, α- and β-tubulin, which polymerise to form a hollow tubule; when seen in cross-section, thirteen tubulin molecules make up a circle. Microtubules originate from a specialised ***microtubule organising centre***, the ***centriole***, found in the ***centrosome*** (see below), and movement may be effected by the addition or subtraction of tubulin subunits from the microtubules, making them longer or shorter. ***Microtubule-associated proteins (MAPs)*** stabilise the tubular structure and include ***capping proteins***, which stabilise the growing ends of the tubules. The motor proteins dynein and kinesin move along the tubules towards and away from the cell centre, respectively. These motors attach to membranous organelles (e.g. mitochondria, secretory vesicles) and move them about within the cytoplasm, rather like an engine pulling cargo along a railway track. The function of the spindle during cell division is a classic example of this process on a large scale (Fig. 2.3). The centrosome, consisting of a pair of centrioles, each of nine triplets of microtubules, organises the microtubules of the ***cell spindle*** during cell division (Figs 1.17 and 1.18). In cilia, nine pairs of microtubules form a cylindrical structure and movement occurs by rearrangement of chemical bonds between adjacent microtubule pairs (see Fig. 5.13).

Abnormalities of the cytoskeleton can produce life-threatening diseases

A number of blistering diseases of the skin are caused by abnormalities of the cytoskeleton. In the rare congenital disorder epidermolysis bullosa simplex, mutations have been found in the genes coding for cytokeratins 5 and 15. These intermediate filaments normally provide basal epidermal cells of the skin with resistance to friction and, in this condition, clumps of abnormal intermediate filaments can be seen within the cells. The result is a loss of cohesion between the basal epithelial cells and the underlying basement membrane, causing blister formation and fluid loss. Mutations in the gene for plectin, a cross-linking protein for intermediate filaments, give rise to various syndromes of epidermolysis bullosa and muscular dystrophy (see e-Fig. 1.2) or epidermolysis bullosa and pyloric atresia.

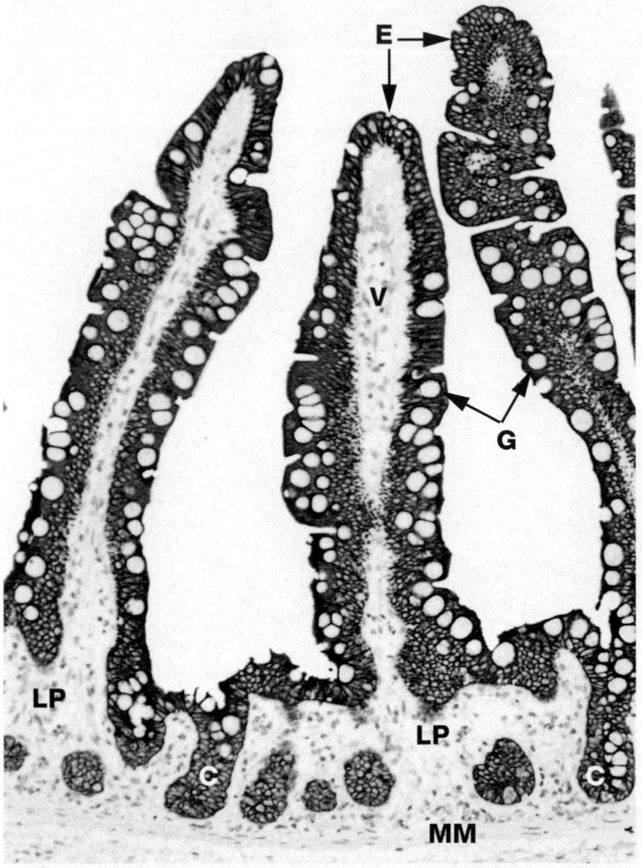

FIG. 1.15 Cytoskeleton
Immunohistochemical method for keratin (MP)

Individual elements of the cytoskeleton are not easily visualised by routine light microscopy, but immunostaining techniques can indirectly identify cellular constituents and are commonly used to do so in research and in diagnostic histopathology. The principles of the method are explained in Appendix 2. In brief, this section of small bowel mucosa (see also Fig. 14.19) has been treated with an antibody that is specific for keratin. The antibody binds to the keratin and is then further treated with a chromogen (a colour-producing chemical) which turns areas with bound antibody a different colour. In this case, the intermediate filament keratin is present in the epithelial cells **E** that form the surface of the villi **V** and line the crypts **C** of the small bowel mucosa. The cytoplasm of these cells is stained a strong brown colour. Notice that the mucous vacuoles of the goblet cells **G** are unstained as they do not contain keratin and the nuclei can be seen as a blue area in each cell (stained by the haematoxylin counterstain), as again they do not contain keratin intermediate filaments. The stromal cells of the lamina propria **LP** and the smooth muscle cells of the muscularis mucosae **MM** are also demonstrated only by the haematoxylin counterstain that highlights their nuclei.

Immunohistochemistry for cytoskeletal proteins is useful in the pathological diagnosis of disease

Cytokeratins are the main intermediate filaments present in epithelial tissues. There are many different keratin molecules, often identified by numbers, e.g. CK7, CK20, and these are typically expressed in specific tissues and organs. In diagnostic pathology, a broad stain covering many different cytokeratin molecules can be used to confirm that a poorly differentiated tumour is of epithelial origin and is a ***carcinoma***. More specific cytokeratin stains can help in identifying the likely site of origin of a carcinoma. For example, cytokeratin 20 (CK20) is mainly found in glandular epithelium of the intestine whilst CK5 is associated with squamous epithelial cells.

Different intermediate filaments are typical of other tissue types and immunohistochemical staining for these molecules can be used to confirm tissue type. For example, ***desmin*** is found in muscle cells as part of the sarcomere (see Ch. 6) whilst ***neurofilaments*** are associated with neurones (see Ch. 7). Staining for these structural proteins is often helpful in diagnosing tumours, and in other inherited diseases such as muscular dystrophy, as described above (see textbox 'Abnormalities of the cytoskeleton can produce life-threatening diseases').

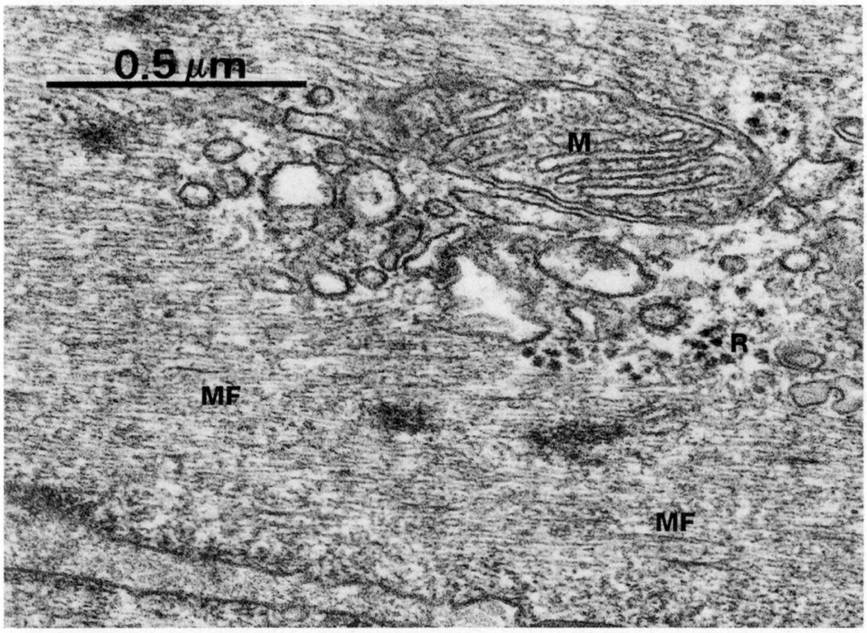

FIG. 1.16 Microfilaments
EM × 76 500

In general, individual microfilaments are difficult to demonstrate due to their small diameter (approximately 7 nm) and their diffuse arrangement among other cytoplasmic components. In this example from a smooth muscle cell, a cell type in which cytoplasmic microfilaments are a predominant feature, parallel arrays of microfilaments **MF** are readily seen. The diameter of microfilaments may be compared with the diameter of a mitochondrion **M** and ribosomes **R**.

C crypt **E** epithelial cells **G** goblet cells **LP** lamina propria **M** mitochondrion **MF** microfilaments **MM** muscularis mucosae **R** ribosomes **V** villus

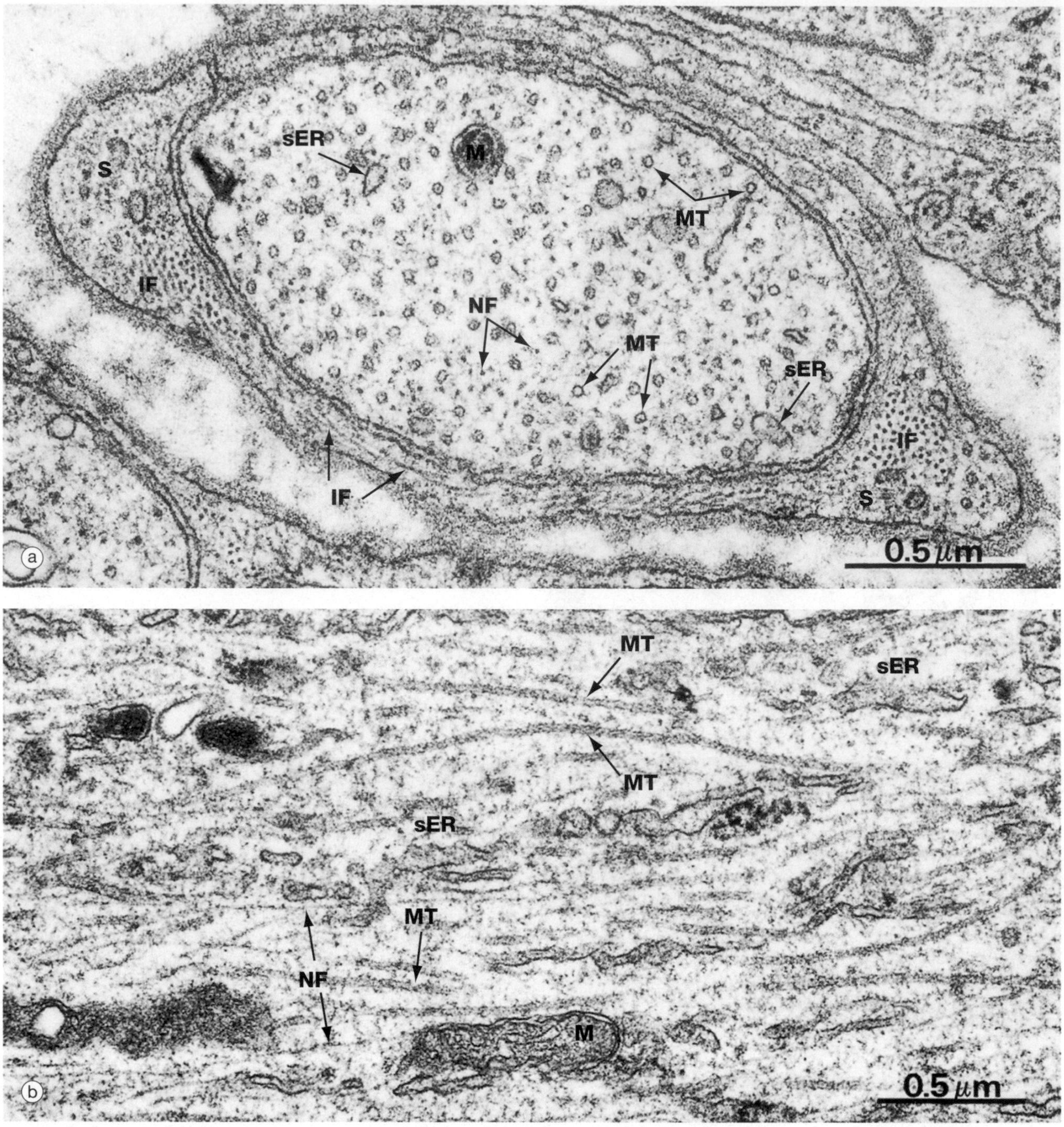

FIG. 1.17 Intermediate filaments and microtubules
(a) EM, TS ×53 000 (b) EM, LS ×40 000

These micrographs are taken from nerve tissue; nerve cells contain both intermediate filaments and microtubules, allowing comparison of size and morphology. Each nerve cell has an elongated cytoplasmic extension called an ***axon*** (see Ch. 7) which, in the peripheral nervous system, is ensheathed by a supporting Schwann cell. Fig. 1.17a shows an axon in transverse section wrapped in the cytoplasm of a Schwann cell **S**. Fig. 1.17b shows part of an axon in longitudinal section. The axonal microtubules provide structural support and transport along the axon.

In longitudinal section, microtubules **MT** appear as straight, unbranched structures and, in transverse section, they appear hollow. Their diameter can be compared with small mitochondria **M** and smooth endoplasmic reticulum **sER**.

Intermediate filaments (known as ***neurofilaments*** in this case) are a prominent feature of nerve cells, providing internal support for the cell by cross-linkage with microtubules and other organelles. The neurofilaments **NF** are dispersed among and in parallel with the microtubules, but are much smaller in diameter and are not hollow in cross-section. Intermediate filaments **IF** are also seen in the Schwann cell cytoplasm in Fig. 1.17a, both in transverse and longitudinal view.

C centriole **F** filament **G** Golgi apparatus **IF** intermediate filament **M** mitochondrion **MT** microtubule **N** nucleus **NF** neurofilament **S** Schwann cell **sER** smooth endoplasmic reticulum **T** triplet

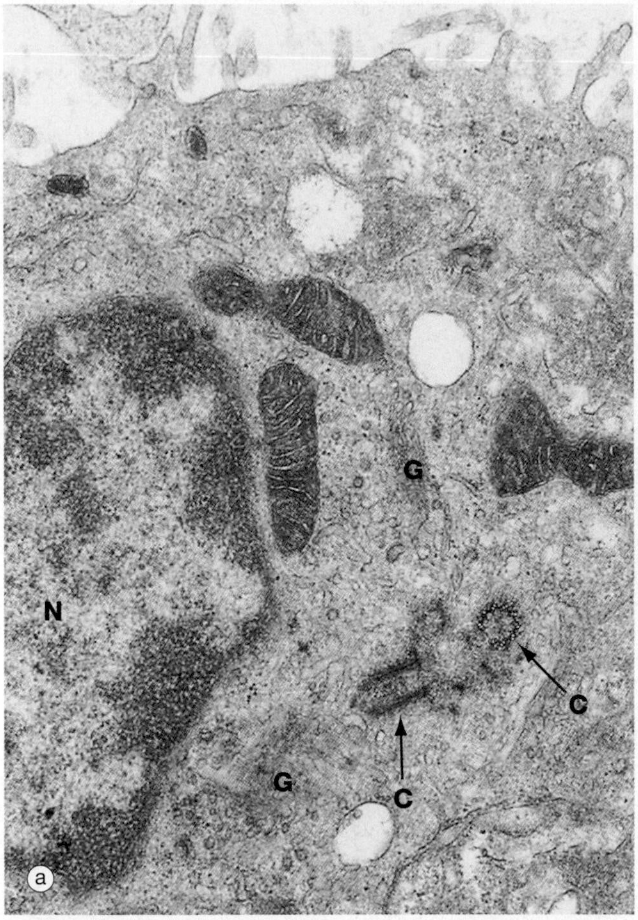

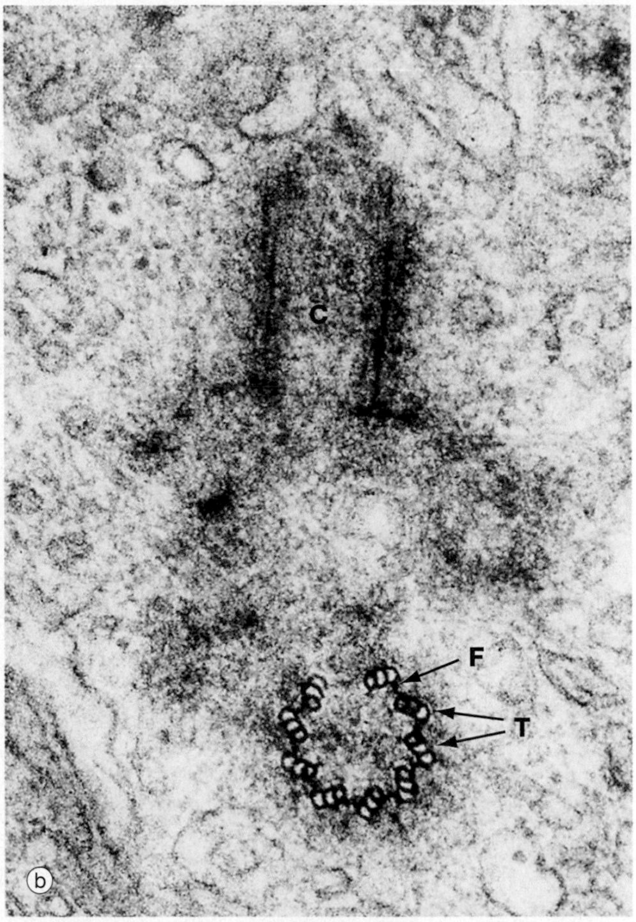

FIG. 1.18 Centrosome
(a) EM ×9200 (b) EM ×48 000 (c) Schematic diagram

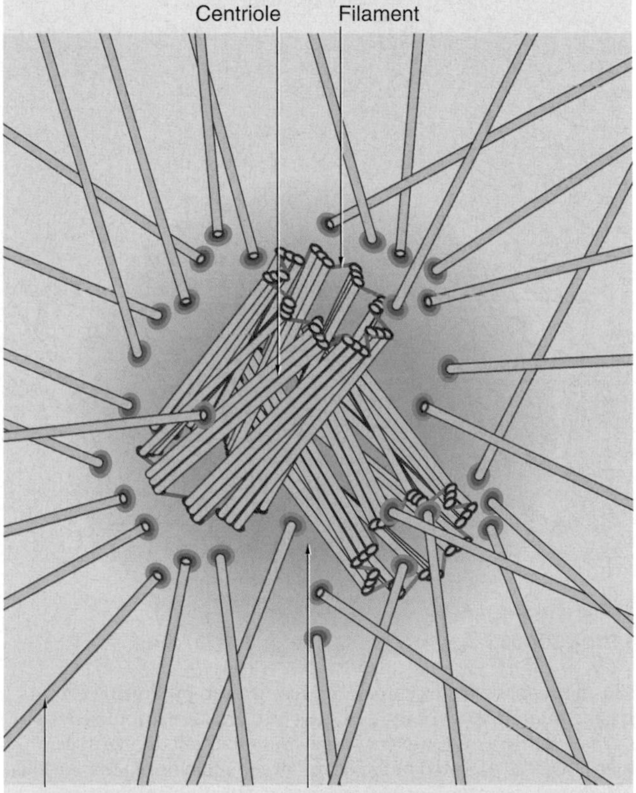

The centrosome includes a pair of ***centrioles*** **C** and the ***centrosome matrix*** or ***pericentriolar material***. The centrosome matrix is a zone of cytoplasm distinguishable by its different texture. It is usually centrally located in the cell, adjacent to the nucleus **N** and often surrounded by the Golgi apparatus **G**. The pair of centrioles are also known as a ***diplosome***. There are also 50 or more δ-tubulin ring complexes, which form a nucleus for the polymerisation of microtubules. Thus the centrioles, themselves composed of microtubules, act as a ***microtubule organising centre***. Microtubules radiate outwards from the centrioles in a star-like arrangement, often called an ***aster***.

Each centriole is cylindrical in form, consisting of nine triplets of parallel microtubules. In transverse section, as in the lower half of Fig. 1.18b and in Fig. 1.18c, each triplet **T** is seen to consist of an inner microtubule, which is circular in cross-section, and two further microtubules, which are C-shaped in cross-section. Each of the inner microtubules is connected to the outermost microtubule of the adjacent triplet by fine filaments **F**, thus forming a cylinder. The two centrioles of each diplosome are arranged with their long axes at right angles to each other, as can be seen in these micrographs.

Structures apparently identical to centrioles form the ***basal bodies*** of ***cilia*** and ***flagella*** (see Figs 5.13, 18.6 and 18.7), both of which are moved by microtubules. Cilia are a cell surface specialisation, each cilium comprising a minute hair-like cytoplasmic extension containing microtubules. Cilia move in a wave-like fashion for the purpose of moving secretions across a tissue surface. Flagella are the long tails responsible for the motility of sperm.

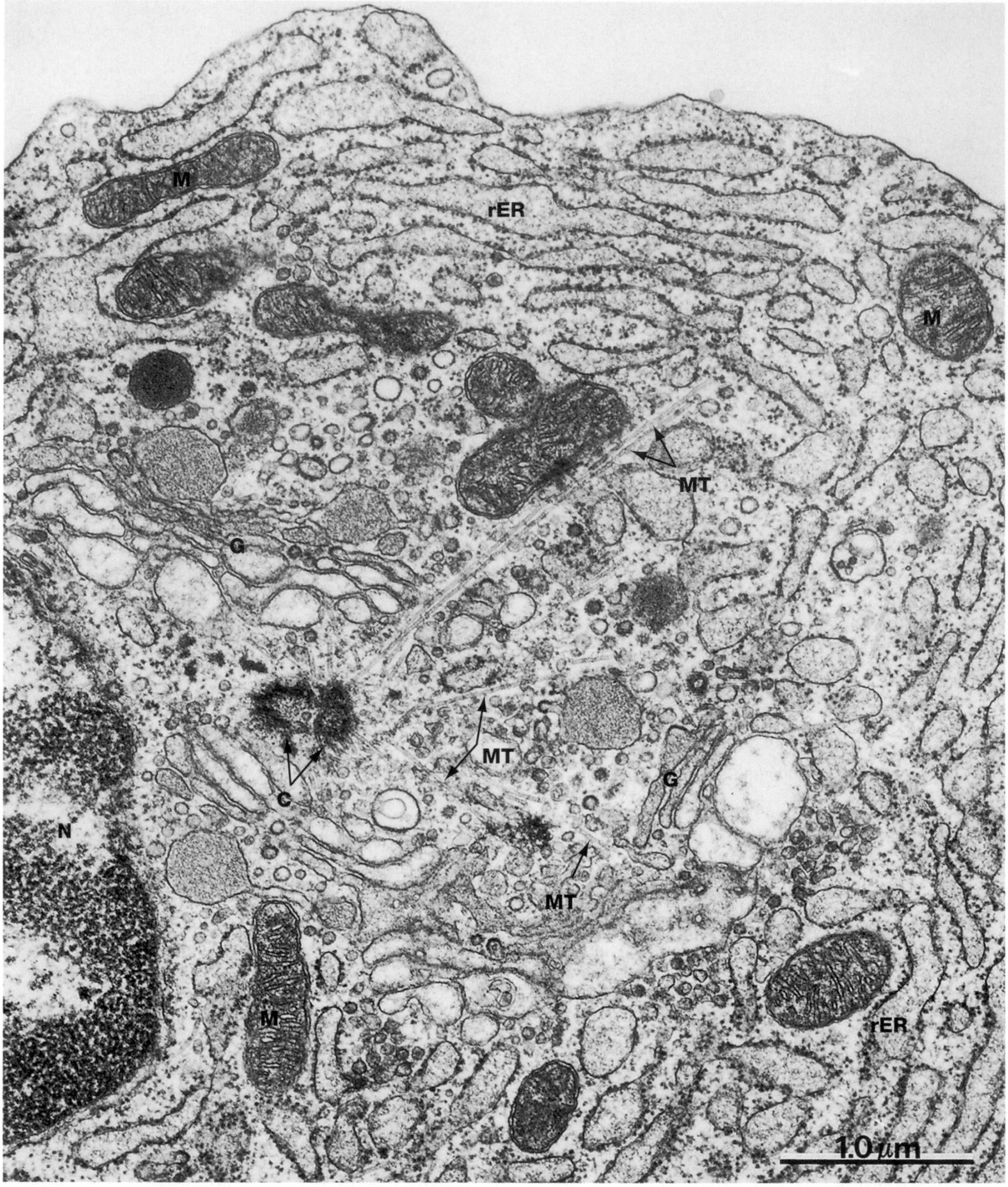

FIG. 1.19 Centrosome and microtubules
EM ×30 000

This figure shows the centrosome acting as an organising centre for the microtubules of the cytoskeleton. The centrosome consists of two centrioles **C** (both cut somewhat obliquely in this specimen), typically located at the centre of the cell close to the nucleus **N**. Several microtubules **MT** are seen radiating from the centrosome towards the cell periphery. Centrioles appear to be necessary for microtubule function. For example, prior to cell division the pair of centrioles is duplicated, the pairs migrating towards opposite ends of the cell. Here they act as organising centres for the microtubules of the spindle that controls distribution of chromosomes to the daughter cells (see Ch. 2). Likewise, a centriole known as a ***basal body*** is found attached to the microtubules at the base of cilia.

Other features of this micrograph, which is from an antibody-secreting plasma cell, include profuse rough endoplasmic reticulum **rER** distended with secretory product, several saccular profiles of an extensive Golgi complex **G** and scattered mitochondria **M**.

C centriole **G** Golgi complex **M** mitochondrion **MT** microtubules **N** nucleus **rER** rough endoplasmic reticulum

ENERGY PRODUCTION AND STORAGE

All cellular functions are dependent on a continuous supply of energy, which is derived from the sequential breakdown of organic molecules during the process of ***cellular respiration***. The energy released during this process is ultimately stored in the form of ATP molecules. In all cells, ATP forms a pool of readily available energy for all the metabolic functions of the cell. The main substrates for cellular respiration are simple sugars and lipids, particularly glucose and fatty acids. Cellular respiration of glucose (***glycolysis***) begins in the cytosol, where it is partially degraded to form pyruvic acid, yielding a small amount of ATP. Pyruvic acid then diffuses into specialised membranous organelles called ***mitochondria*** where, in the presence of oxygen, it is degraded to carbon dioxide and water; this process yields a large quantity of ATP. In contrast, fatty acids pass directly into mitochondria where they are also degraded to carbon dioxide and water; this also generates a large amount of ATP. Glycolysis may occur in the absence of oxygen and is then termed ***anaerobic respiration***, whereas mitochondrial respiration is dependent on a continuous supply of oxygen and is therefore termed ***aerobic respiration***. Mitochondria are the principal organelles involved in cellular respiration in mammals and are found in large numbers in metabolically active cells, such as those of liver and skeletal muscle.

When there is excess fuel available, most cells convert glucose and fatty acids into glycogen and triglycerides, respectively, for storage. The amounts of each vary in different cell types. For example, nerve cells contain very little of either; most of the body's limited store of glycogen is found in muscle and liver cells and triglycerides can be stored in almost unlimited amounts in fat (***adipose***) cells.

FIG. 1.20 Mitochondria

Mitochondria vary considerably in size and shape and change shape over time but are most often elongated, sausage-shaped organelles. Mitochondria are very mobile, moving around the cell by means of microtubules. They tend to localise at intracellular sites of maximum energy requirement. The number of mitochondria in cells is highly variable; liver cells contain as many as 2000 mitochondria whereas inactive cells contain very few. The number of mitochondria in a cell are modified by mitochondrial division and fusion and by autophagy. In some cells, fused mitochondria may form an interconnected network throughout the cytoplasm.

Each mitochondrion consists of four compartments:

- The ***outer membrane*** is relatively permeable as it contains a pore-forming protein known as ***porin***, which allows free passage of small molecules. The outer membrane contains enzymes that convert certain lipid substrates into forms that can be metabolised within the mitochondrion.
- The ***inner membrane***, which is thinner than the outer, is thrown into complex folds and tubules called cristae that project into the inner cavity. In some cell types, mitochondria typically have tubular cristae (see Fig. 17.16).
- The ***inner cavity*** filled by the ***mitochondrial matrix***. The matrix is the site of the mitochondrial DNA and ribosomes. The matrix also contains a number of ***dense matrix granules***, the function of which is unknown.
- The ***intermembranous space*** between the two membranes also contains a variety of enzymes.

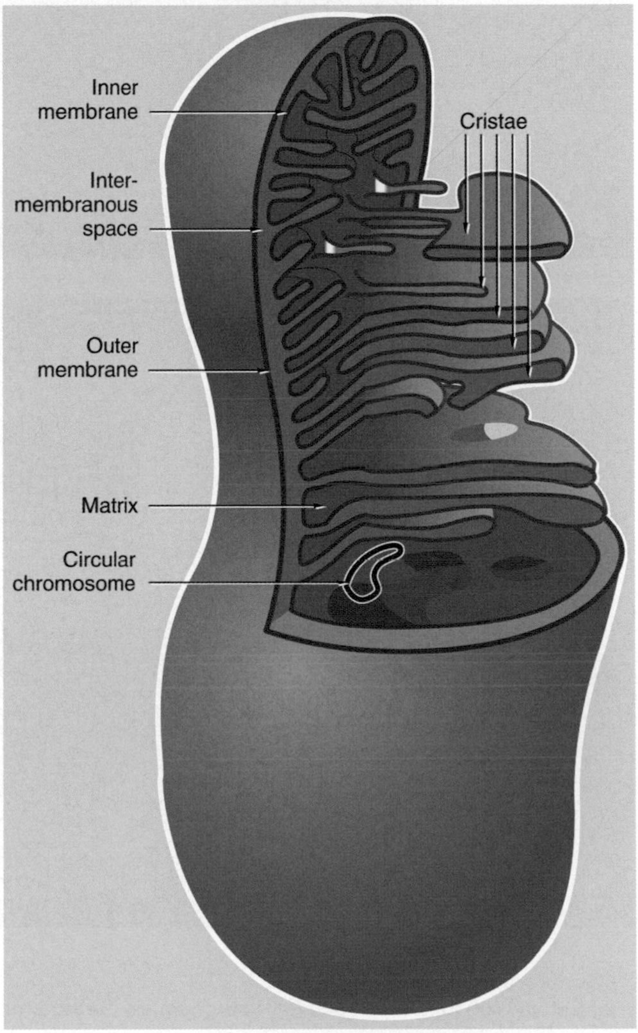

Aerobic respiration takes place within the matrix and on the inner membrane, a process enhanced by the large surface area provided by the cristae. The matrix contains most of the enzymes involved in oxidation of fatty acids and the Krebs cycle. The inner membrane contains the cytochromes, the carrier molecules of the electron transport chain, and the enzymes involved in ATP production.

As organelles, mitochondria have several unusual features. The mitochondrial matrix contains one or more circular strands of DNA resembling the chromosomes of bacteria. The matrix also contains ribosomes with a similar structure to bacterial ribosomes. Mitochondria synthesise 13 of their own constituent proteins, others being synthesised by the usual protein synthetic mechanisms of the cell and imported into the mitochondrion. Mitochondrial DNA also encodes another protein called humanin which does not remain in the mitochondria and has a role in cytoprotection. In addition, mitochondria undergo self-replication in a manner similar to bacterial cell division. Mitochondria are thought to be derived from bacteria which formed a symbiotic relationship with eukaryotic cells during the process of evolution.

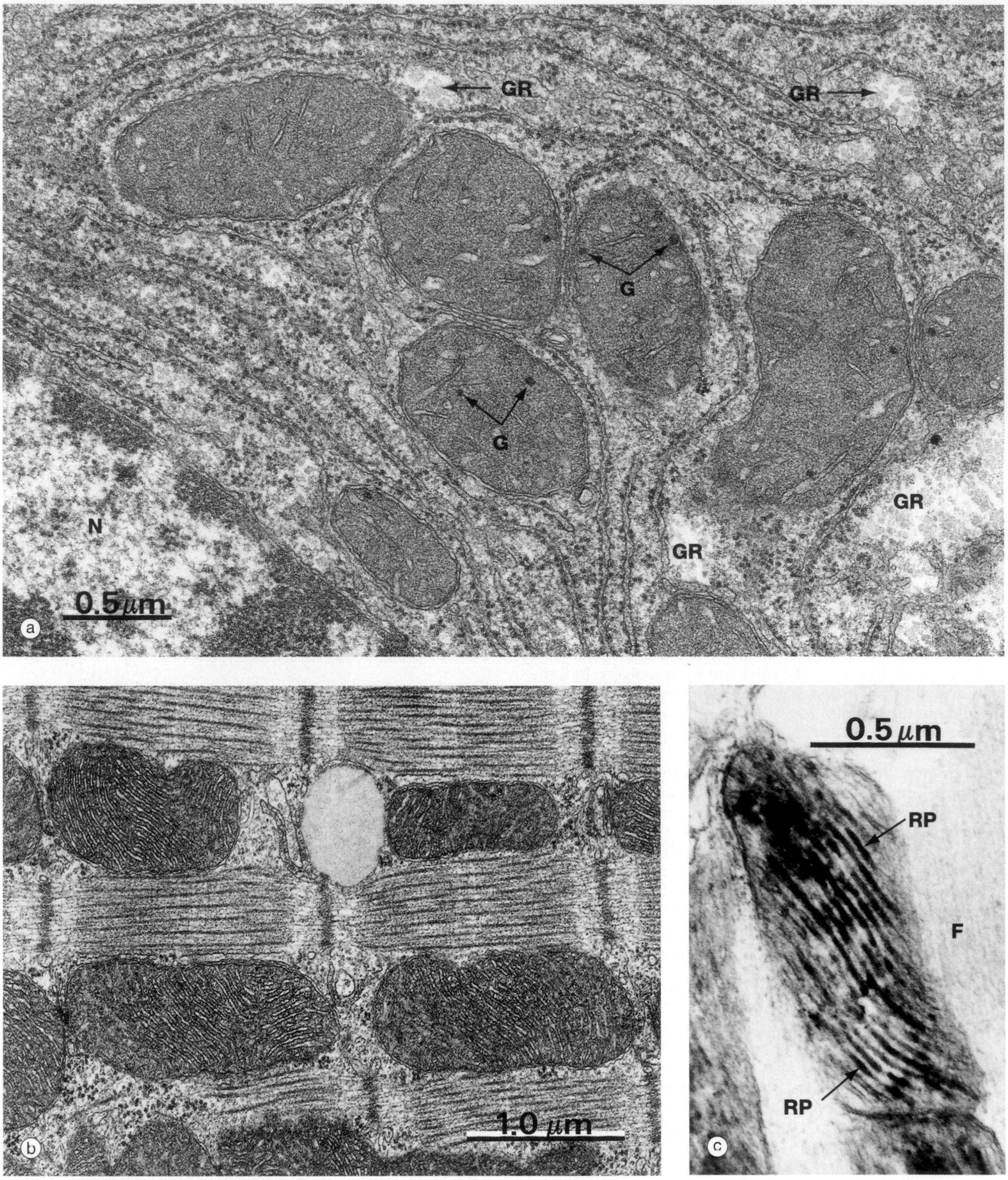

FIG. 1.21 Mitochondria
(a) EM ×34 000 (b) EM ×25 000 (c) Histochemical method for cytochrome oxidase, EM ×50 000

All mitochondria conform to the same general structure but vary greatly in size, shape and arrangement of cristae; these variations are often characteristic of the cell type. Mitochondria move freely within the cytosol and tend to aggregate in intracellular sites with high energy demands, where their shape often conforms to the available space.

Fig. 1.21a of liver cell cytoplasm shows the typical appearance of mitochondria when cut in different planes of section; note their relatively dense matrix containing a few matrix granules **G**. ***Glycogen rosettes*** **GR** are also seen in this micrograph (see also Fig. 1.23). Part of the nucleus **N** is seen in the bottom left corner.

Mitochondria from heart muscle cells can be seen in Fig. 1.21b and Fig. 1.21c. The cristae are densely packed, reflecting the metabolic activity of the cell. In some cells the cristae have a characteristic shape, those of heart muscle being laminar. Fig. 1.21c uses a histochemical technique to localise a mitochondrial enzyme, cytochrome oxidase. The electron-dense reaction product **RP** is located in the intermembranous space. The actin and myosin filaments **F** are essentially unstained in this preparation.

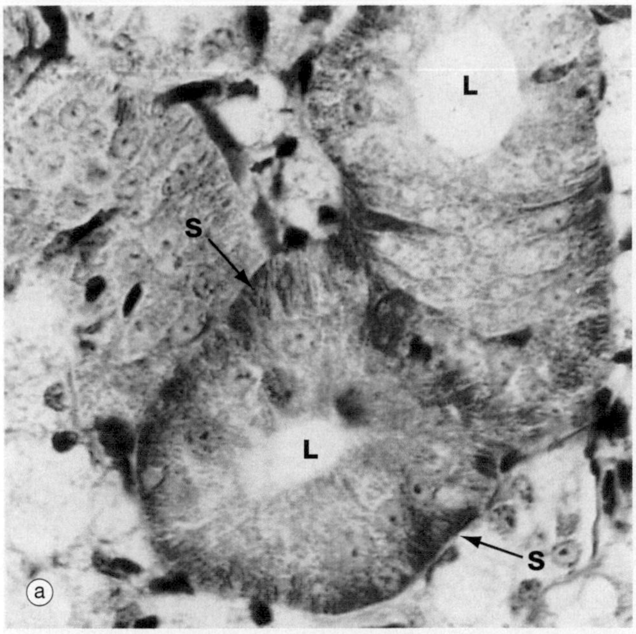

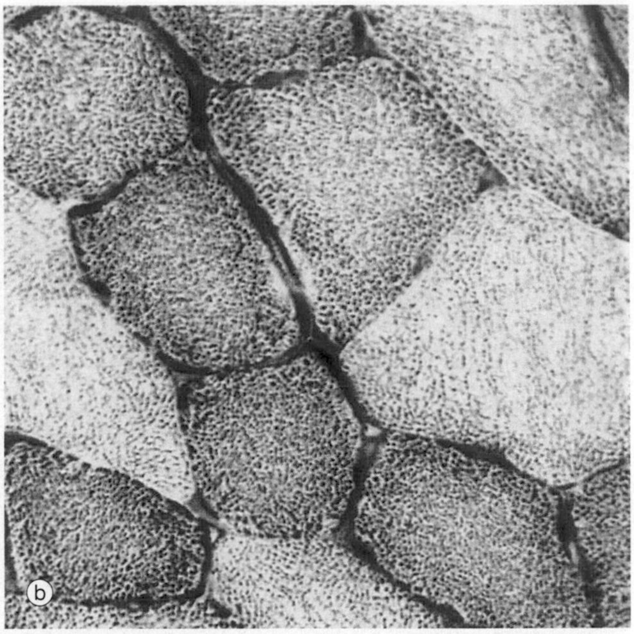

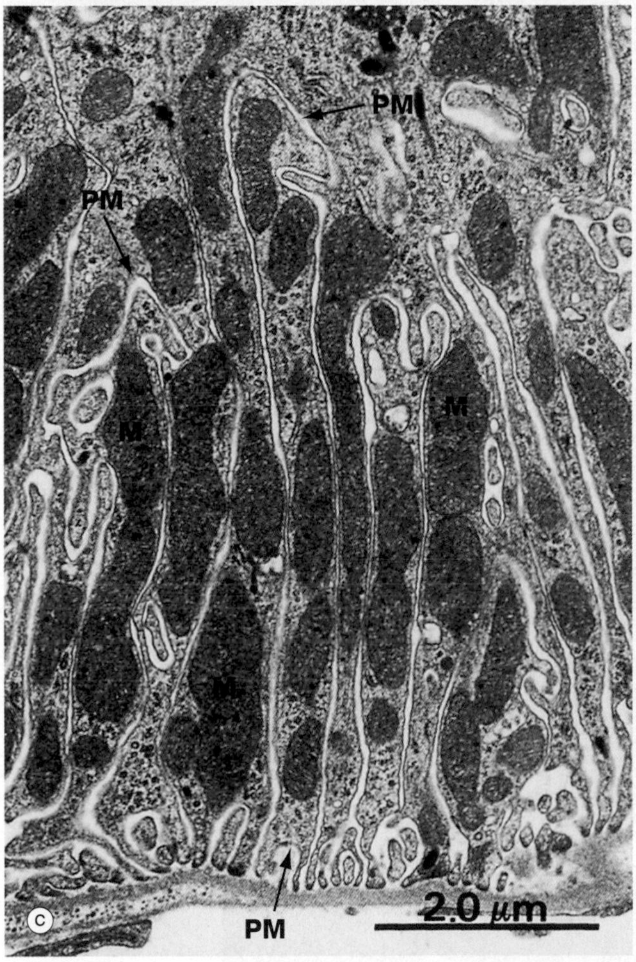

FIG. 1.22 Mitochondria
(a) Iron haematoxylin (HP) (b) Succinate dehydrogenase (HP) (c) EM ×13 000

Mitochondria are, in general, not seen individually by light microscopy. However, they are acidophilic and, with the standard H&E stain, are responsible for much of the eosinophilia (pink staining) of cytoplasm. In some cells, the mitochondria are profuse and may be concentrated in one region of the cell where they can be demonstrated directly and indirectly by various staining methods.

Fig. 1.22a shows a salivary gland duct made up of cells that are extremely active in secretion and reabsorption of a variety of inorganic ions. This takes place at the base of the cells (i.e. the surface away from the lumen **L**) and is powered by ATP produced by elongated mitochondria associated with numerous basal plasma membrane interdigitations between adjacent cells. This strategy greatly increases the plasma membrane surface area. The cells have been stained by a modified haematoxylin method which stains not only basophilic structures (i.e. DNA and RNA) but also acidophilic structures such as mitochondria that can be seen as striations **S** in the basal aspect of the cells.

Fig. 1.22b shows skeletal muscle cells in transverse section. An enzyme histochemical method for succinate dehydrogenase has been employed. Succinate dehydrogenase is an enzyme of the citric acid cycle that is exclusive to mitochondria and therefore provides a marker for them. In skeletal muscle there are three muscle cell types, which differ from each other in mitochondrial concentration. Such a staining method can be used to demonstrate their relative proportions (see also Fig. 6.14), as shown here by the different intensity of staining for mitochondria in different cells.

Fig. 1.22c shows the base of an absorptive cell from a kidney tubule where there is intense active transport of ions. The basal plasma membranes **PM** of adjacent cells form interdigitations that greatly increase their surface area, and elongated mitochondria **M** are packed into the intervening spaces. Fig. 1.22a and Fig. 1.22c demonstrate an example of the same structure, interdigitation of a membrane, being used for the same purpose in two different situations to maximise ion transportation.

F actin and myosin filaments **G** matrix granules **GR** glycogen rosettes **L** lumen **M** mitochondrion **N** nucleus
PM plasma membrane **RP** reaction product **S** striations

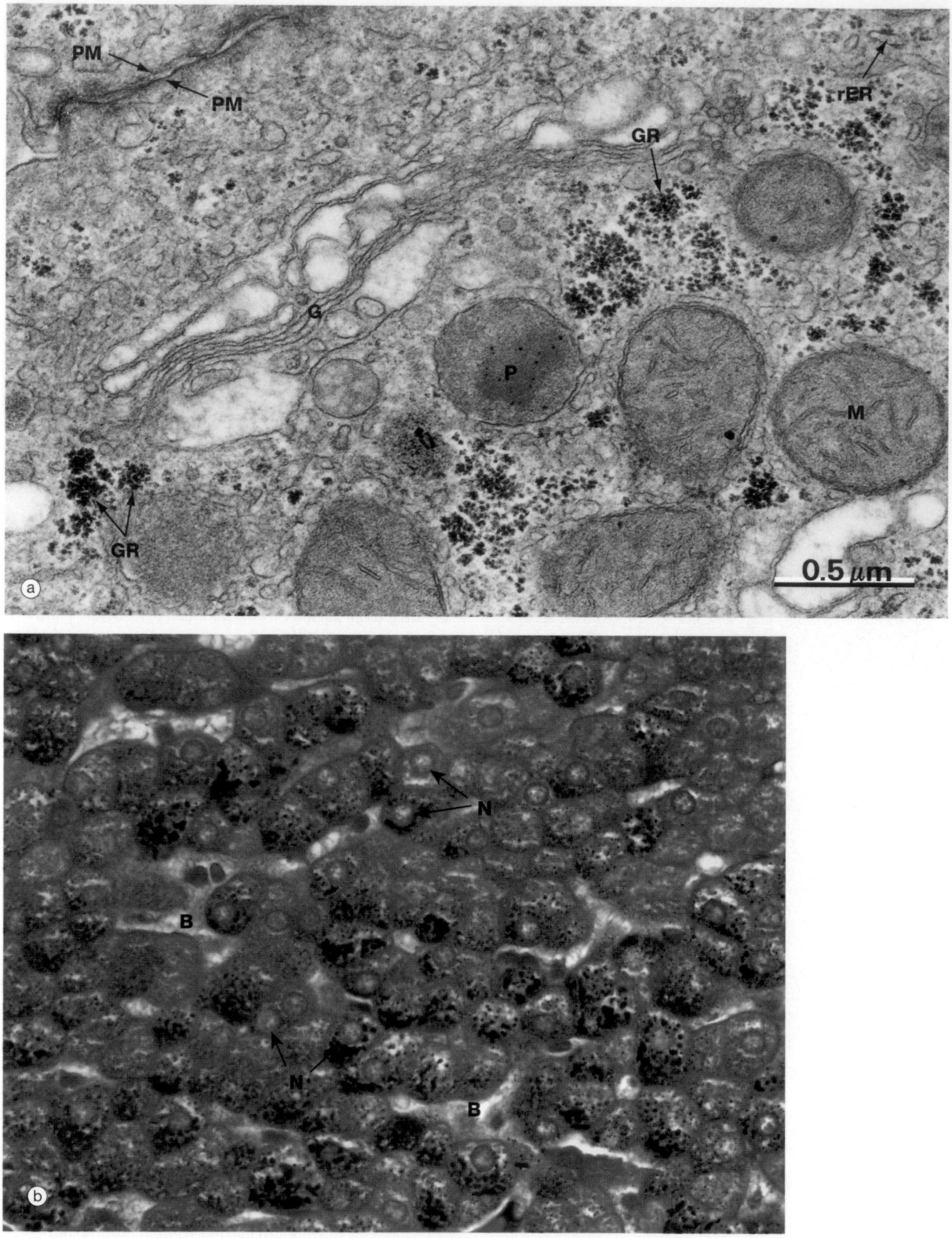

FIG. 1.23 Glycogen
(a) EM ×47 000 (b) PAS/haematoxylin (MP)

Glycogen is found in the cytoplasm of many cell types but is most prominent in muscle cells and liver cells (***hepatocytes***). In Fig. 1.23a, plentiful glycogen granules are present, appearing either as irregular single granules (called ***β particles***) or as aggregations termed ***glycogen rosettes*** **GR** (also called ***α particles***). Compare the size of the ribosomes on the rough endoplasmic reticulum **rER** with glycogen granules, which are slightly larger on average. A prominent Golgi apparatus **G** can be seen near the plasma membrane **PM**. Note that although the Golgi apparatus is classically found near the nucleus, it is not at all unusual to find it in other areas of the cytoplasm, especially in cells like hepatocytes which contain multiple Golgi stacks. Several mitochondria **M** and a peroxisome **P** can also be seen in this field.

Fig. 1.23b has been stained by a histochemical method to demonstrate the presence of glycogen, which is stained magenta (see Appendix 2). The specimen is of liver, the cytoplasm of each liver cell being packed with glycogen which is easily identified as granules. The section has been counterstained (i.e. stained with a second dye) to demonstrate the liver cell nuclei **N** (blue). It also stains the nuclei of the cells lining the blood channels **B** (***sinusoids***) between the rows of liver cells; these nuclei are smaller and more condensed and hence stain more intensely.

LIPID BIOSYNTHESIS

Lipids are synthesised by all cells in order to maintain the constant turnover of cell membranes. Cells may also synthesise lipid as a means of storing excess energy as cytoplasmic droplets, for lipid transport, e.g. chylomicron production by cells of the small intestine, and in the form of steroid hormones, for sending information to other cells. The precursor molecules (***fatty acids, triglycerides*** and ***cholesterol***) are available to the cell from dietary sources, from mobilisation of lipid stored in other cells or can be synthesised by most cells using simple sources of carbon such as acetyl CoA and other intermediates of glucose catabolism. Fatty acids and triglycerides are mostly synthesised within the cytosol, whereas cholesterol and phospholipids are synthesised in areas of smooth endoplasmic reticulum (Fig. 1.8).

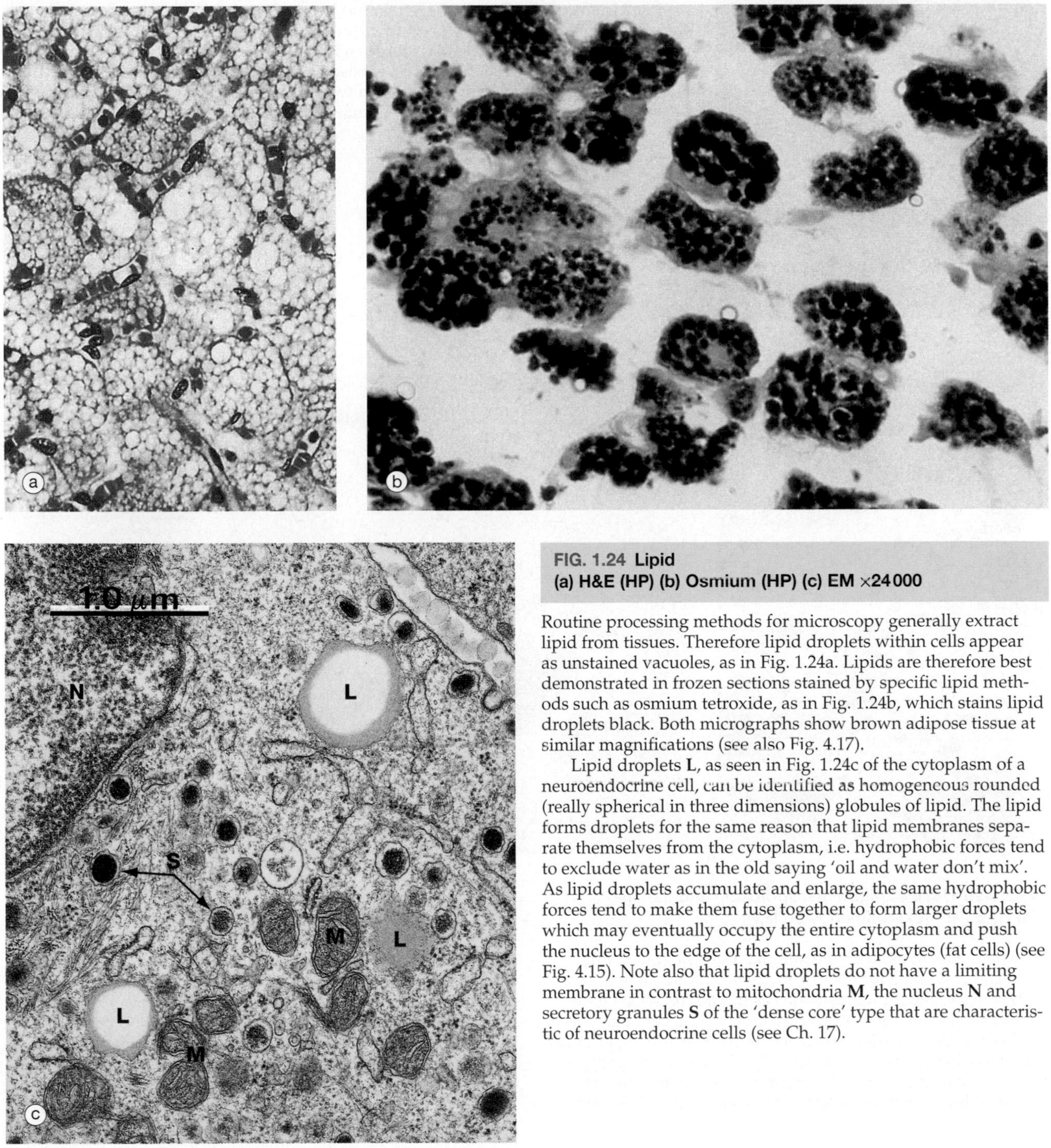

FIG. 1.24 Lipid
(a) H&E (HP) (b) Osmium (HP) (c) EM ×24 000

Routine processing methods for microscopy generally extract lipid from tissues. Therefore lipid droplets within cells appear as unstained vacuoles, as in Fig. 1.24a. Lipids are therefore best demonstrated in frozen sections stained by specific lipid methods such as osmium tetroxide, as in Fig. 1.24b, which stains lipid droplets black. Both micrographs show brown adipose tissue at similar magnifications (see also Fig. 4.17).

Lipid droplets **L**, as seen in Fig. 1.24c of the cytoplasm of a neuroendocrine cell, can be identified as homogeneous rounded (really spherical in three dimensions) globules of lipid. The lipid forms droplets for the same reason that lipid membranes separate themselves from the cytoplasm, i.e. hydrophobic forces tend to exclude water as in the old saying 'oil and water don't mix'. As lipid droplets accumulate and enlarge, the same hydrophobic forces tend to make them fuse together to form larger droplets which may eventually occupy the entire cytoplasm and push the nucleus to the edge of the cell, as in adipocytes (fat cells) (see Fig. 4.15). Note also that lipid droplets do not have a limiting membrane in contrast to mitochondria **M**, the nucleus **N** and secretory granules **S** of the 'dense core' type that are characteristic of neuroendocrine cells (see Ch. 17).

B blood channels **G** Golgi apparatus **GR** glycogen rosette **L** lipid droplets **M** mitochondrion **N** nucleus **P** peroxisome **PM** plasma membrane **rER** rough endoplasmic reticulum **S** secretory granule

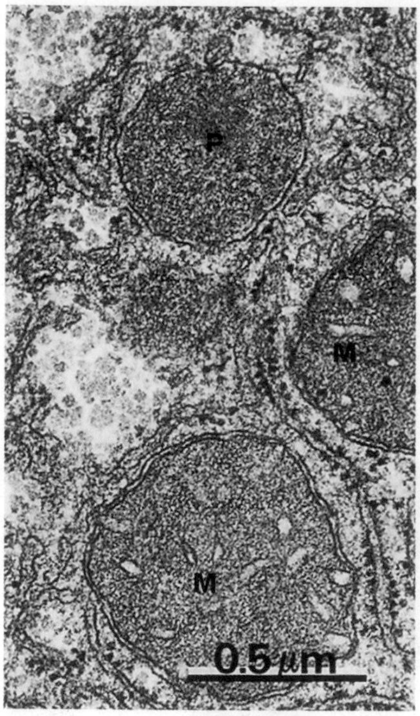

FIG. 1.25 Peroxisomes
EM ×40 000

Peroxisomes (sometimes called ***microbodies***) are unusual organelles: they are present in all cells but have different functions in different cell types and in the same cell type in different species. Broadly speaking, peroxisomes perform enzymatic oxidation and contain a range of oxidative enzymes. Functions include β-oxidation of certain long chain fatty acids, some steps in the synthesis of plasmalogens (lipids found in the myelin sheath of nerve axons) and some steps in the synthesis of bile acids (in the liver). Hydrogen peroxide is a by-product in some of these reactions and peroxisomes commonly contain catalase which utilises the hydrogen peroxide to detoxify other substances such as phenols and alcohol by peroxidation.

Peroxisomes appear somewhat similar to lysosomes by electron microscopy but vary greatly in size, ranging from 0.1 to 0.9 μm in different tissues. The peroxisomes in the liver and kidney are particularly large and abundant. In this figure, note the fine, granular, electron-dense contents of a peroxisome **P**, the size of which can be compared to that of adjacent mitochondria **M**. Like mitochondria, peroxisomes self-replicate, and the numbers of peroxisomes within a cell may change over the lifetime of the cell.

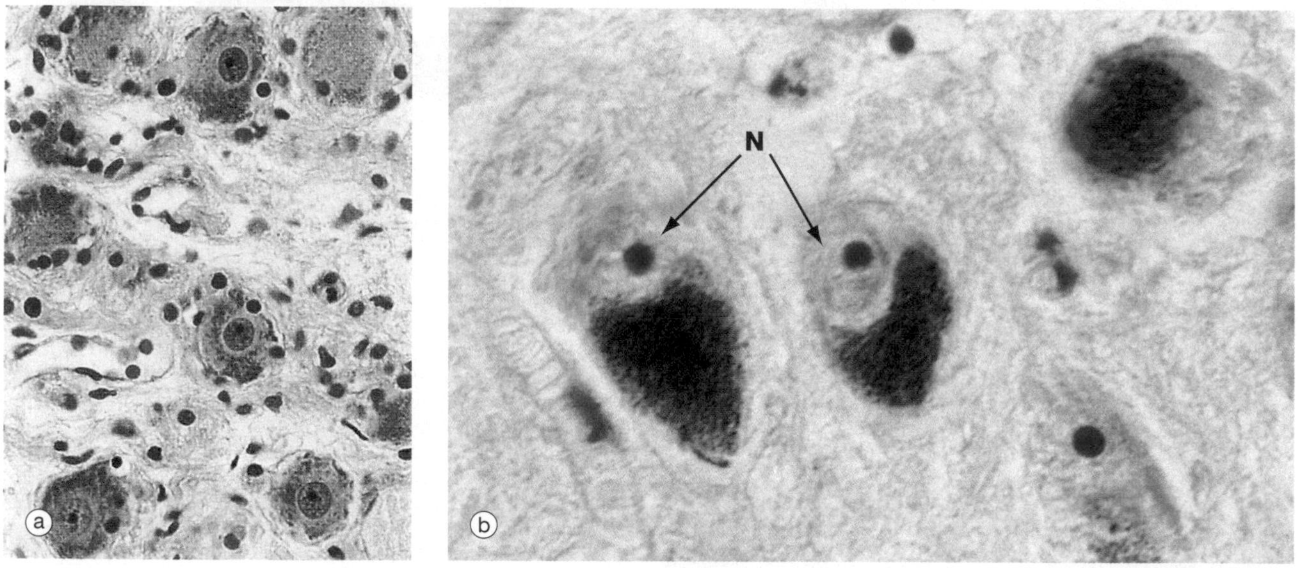

FIG. 1.26 Cellular pigments: lipofuscin and melanin
(a) H&E (HP) (b) Modified Azan (HP)

Most mammalian tissues have minimal intrinsic colour, thus the need for staining for microscopy. A few tissues, however, contain intracellular pigments such as ***lipofuscin***, which probably represents an insoluble degradation product of organelle turnover. With increasing age, it accumulates as brown, granular material in the cytoplasm, particularly of sympathetic ganglion cells as seen in Fig. 1.26a, other neurones and cardiac muscle cells; it is thus sometimes referred to as 'age pigment'. Another natural pigment is ***melanin***, which is mainly responsible for skin colour (see Ch. 9). This brown pigment is also present in nerve cells in certain brain regions such as the ***substantia nigra***, shown in Fig. 1.26b, where the cell cytoplasm is largely obscured by its content of brown melanin pigment. This specimen has been stained by the Azan method to pick out the nuclei **N** which are stained pale blue with prominent magenta nucleoli.

M mitochondrion **N** nucleus **P** peroxisome

Mutation in a single gene may have widespread effects

Lysosomal storage diseases are rare congenital disorders mainly caused by a mutation in the gene coding for one or other lysosomal enzyme. This may lead to either production of a defective enzyme or no enzyme at all. Predictably, the enzyme substrate collects in cells and in some cases can be identified in tissues submitted for a diagnostic biopsy (e.g. Tay–Sachs disease, Gaucher's disease). Some of these conditions are associated with a typical ***phenotype*** or appearance of the affected person (e.g. Hurler syndrome).

THE INTEGRATED FUNCTION OF CELLS IN TISSUES, ORGANS AND ORGAN SYSTEMS

As mentioned at the outset, cells are the functional units of all living organisms; indeed the most primitive organisms merely consist of single cells. In multicellular organisms, however, individual cells become specialised (*differentiated*) and grouped together to perform specific functions. Multicellular organisms would obviously disintegrate if the cells were not organised into specific structures and held together by ***intercellular junctions*** (see Ch. 5) and ***extracellular matrix*** (see Ch. 4). Cells of similar morphology and function along with extracellular matrix form ***tissues***, which are relatively homogeneous in overall structure; examples include cartilage, bone and muscle. Extracellular matrix, such as the calcified matrix of bone and the fibrous matrix of the deep layer of the skin (the dermis), can impart great strength to tissues. Other cell types, such as blood cells and tissue macrophages, migrate throughout the body either in the blood or other body fluids or through the extracellular matrix. ***Organs*** are anatomically discrete collections of tissues that together perform certain specific functions (e.g. liver, kidney, eye and ovary). Tissues and organs may constitute integrated functional ***systems*** forming major anatomical entities (e.g. central nervous system, female reproductive tract, gastrointestinal tract, urinary system) or be more diffusely arranged (e.g. immune defence system, diffuse neuroendocrine system). Despite the foregoing, the terms *tissue*, *organ* and *system* are not necessarily mutually exclusive and may in some cases be used interchangeably, depending on the functional implications. Section 2 of this book describes five basic tissues: ***blood, supporting/connective tissue, epithelia, muscle*** and ***nervous tissues***. These are constituents of all organs and organ systems. In tissues and organs, the functionally specialised cells are often called the ***parenchyma*** and the less specialised supporting tissue, the ***stroma***.

Within tissues and organs, cells interact with one another in numerous ways during embryological development and growth, maintenance of structural integrity, response to injury (inflammation and repair), integration and control of tissue and organ functions and the maintenance of overall biochemical and metabolic integrity (***homeostasis***). Various types of intercellular junctions also serve as conduits for information exchange in the form of electrical excitation or chemical messengers. Within tissues, cellular functions are integrated by a great variety of local chemical mediators (***paracrine signalling***) or by direct contact between cells and interaction between messaging molecules bound to the cell surface. At the level of systems and of the whole body, functions are coordinated via circulating chemical messengers (***hormones***) and/or via the nervous system (***synaptic signalling***). The great pleasure to be derived from the study of histology is that all structures, from the subcellular to organ systems, reflect these functional requirements and interrelationships; it really is all very cleverly arranged.

REVIEW

TABLE 1.1 Review of cell structure and function

Organelle	Brief description	Functions	Figure
Nucleus	Double membrane-bound large structure containing chromatin	Chromosomes (DNA) contain the genetic blueprint for every protein in the body	1.3
Nuclear envelope/ membrane	Double lipid bilayer with nuclear pore complexes	Separates and mediates transport between nucleus and cytoplasm	1.4
Nucleolus	Dense non-membrane-bound structure in nucleus	Ribosomal RNA synthesis and ribosome assembly	1.5
Ribosomes	Small structures free in cytoplasm or bound to endoplasmic reticulum. Consist of two subunits of ribosomal RNA.	Protein synthesis – formation of peptide bonds between amino acids to make polypeptide chains using messenger RNA as template	1.7
Endoplasmic reticulum	Extensive membrane system within the cell; may be rough (rER) with associated ribosomes, or smooth (sER)	Modification and folding of proteins synthesised on ribosomes (rER), synthesis of some lipids (sER)	1.8
Golgi apparatus/stack	Stacks of flattened membrane-bound cisternae	Final assembly and glycosylation of proteins and dispatch to their ultimate destination	1.10
Mitochondria	Double membrane-bound organelles with folded inner membrane	Energy production, mainly in the form of ATP	1.20–1.22
Plasma membrane	Lipid bilayer containing intrinsic proteins and with an external coat of carbohydrate	Divides cell from external environment and mediates interactions with external environment	1.2
Cytoskeleton	Microfilaments, intermediate filaments and microtubules	Maintain cell shape and orientation, cell movement, movement of organelles around the cell, movement of chromosomes during cell division	1.15–1.17
Transport/secretory vesicles	Membrane-bound vesicles often with a protein coat, e.g. COP I, clathrin	Transport materials between different cell compartments and to plasma membrane for export	1.11–1.12
Phagosomes/ endosomes – including sorting and recycling endosomes	Membrane-bound vesicles containing material imported into cell	Phagocytosis/endocytosis and transport of cargo to intracellular destination, e.g. lysosome	1.12–1.13
Lysosomes	Membrane-bound vesicles containing hydrolytic enzymes	Killing of pathogenic organisms (in phagocytic cells) and degradation of waste products	1.14
Peroxisomes	Membrane-bound vesicles containing oxidases and catalase	Production of hydrogen peroxide for killing pathogens, detoxification of certain toxic materials, β-oxidation of long chain fatty acids, synthesis of bile acids (in liver)	1.25
Lipid droplets	Non-membrane-bound spherical aggregates of lipid of variable size	Energy storage	1.24
Glycogen granules	Non-membrane-bound granules and aggregates of granules (rosettes)	Energy storage	1.23
Lipofuscin	Brown pigment in cytoplasm	Waste product	1.26
Melanin	Brown pigment in cytoplasm	Skin pigmentation	1.26

2 Cell cycle and replication

INTRODUCTION

The development of a single fertilised egg cell to form a complex multicellular organism involves cellular replication, growth and progressive specialisation (***differentiation***) for a variety of functions. The fertilised egg (***zygote***) divides by a process known as ***mitosis*** to produce two genetically identical daughter cells, each of which divides to produce two more daughter cells and so on. Some of these daughter cells progressively specialise and eventually produce the ***terminally differentiated cells*** of mature tissues, such as muscle or skin cells. Most tissues, however, retain a population of relatively undifferentiated cells (***stem cells***) that are able to divide and replace the differentiated cell population as required. The interval between mitotic divisions is known as the ***cell cycle***. All body cells divide by mitosis except for male and female germ cells, which divide by ***meiosis*** to produce ***gametes*** (Fig. 2.6).

In the fully developed organism, the terminally differentiated cells of some tissues, such as the neurones of the nervous system, lose the ability to undergo mitosis. In contrast, the cells of certain other tissues, such as the stem cells of gut and skin, undergo continuous cycles of mitotic division throughout the lifespan of the organism, replacing cells lost during normal wear and tear. Between these extremes are cells such as liver cells that do not normally divide but retain the capacity to undergo mitosis should the need arise (***facultative dividers***). Cell division is tightly controlled to meet the needs of the organism; uncontrolled cell division is one of the features of cancer.

Cell division and differentiation are balanced by cell death, both during the development and growth of the immature organism and in the mature adult. In these circumstances, cell death occurs by a mechanism known as ***apoptosis*** (Fig. 2.7).

FIG. 2.1 The cell cycle

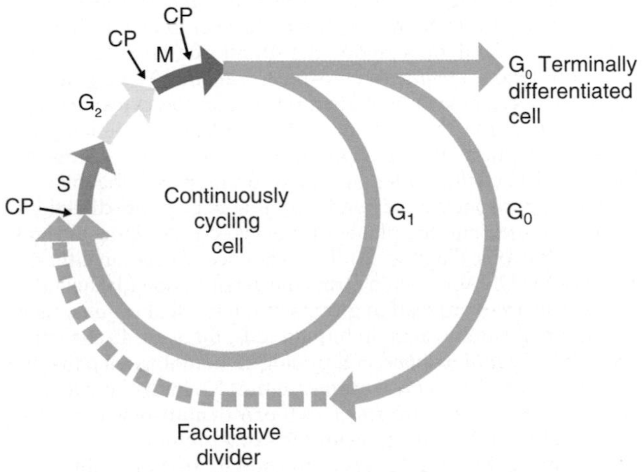

Historically, only two phases of the cell cycle were recognised: a relatively short ***mitotic phase (M phase)*** and a non-dividing phase (***interphase***), which usually occupies most of the life cycle of the cell. However, there is a discrete period during interphase when nuclear DNA is replicated; this phase, described as the ***synthesis*** or ***S phase***, is completed some time before the onset of mitosis. Thus interphase may be divided into three separate phases. Between the end of the M phase and the beginning of the S phase is the ***first gap*** or ***G_1 phase***; this is usually much longer than the other phases of the cell cycle. During the G_1 phase, cells differentiate and perform their specialised functions as part of the whole tissue. The interval between the end of the S phase and the beginning of the M phase, the ***second gap*** or ***G_2 phase***, is relatively short and is the period in which cells prepare for mitotic division.

Stem cells in some tissues progress continually through the cell cycle to accommodate tissue growth or cell turnover, whereas terminally differentiated cells leave the cell cycle after the M phase and enter a state of continuous differentiated function designated as ***G_0 phase***. Facultative dividers enter the G_0 phase but retain the capacity to re-enter the cell cycle when suitably stimulated. Liver cells are a prominent example of facultative dividers with differentiated hepatocytes acting as stem cells in cases of massive liver injury. Some liver cells appear to enter a protracted G_2 phase in which they perform their normal differentiated functions despite the presence of a duplicated complement of DNA. These cells may be seen histologically as ***binucleate cells***.

In general, the S, G and M phases of the cell cycle are relatively constant in duration, each taking up to several hours to complete, whereas the G_1 phase is highly variable, in some cases lasting for several days or weeks. M phase typically lasts about 1 hour, while S phase takes 10 to 12 hours to complete. The G_0 phase may last for the entire lifespan of the organism.

During mitosis, various ***checkpoints*** **CP** prevent progression to the next phase before the previous one is completed (see textbox). For example, the ***metaphase checkpoint*** prevents progression to anaphase before all the chromosomes are properly connected to the mitotic spindle and lined up at the cell equator; this prevents unequal distribution of the chromosomes to the two daughter cells.

CP checkpoint **G_0** continuous differentiated function **G_1** gap phase 1 **G_2** gap phase 2 **M** mitotic phase **S** synthesis phase

Cell cycle checkpoints and disease

Cell cycle checkpoints are critical in regulating the process of cell division and involve a series of processes which aim to avoid incomplete or damaged DNA being passed on to daughter cells. This involves various regulatory proteins, mainly cyclin-dependent kinases, which control progression through the cell cycle. There are 3 main checkpoints, occurring at ***G_1/S***, ***G_2/M*** and in ***metaphase***. The G_1/S checkpoint is known as the ***restriction point*** and indicates the point at which cells are committed to entering cell cycle, after ensuring the raw materials are available to allow DNA replication. Disruption of this signalling pathway may cause cells to enter cycle inappropriately and this dysregulation can give rise to uncontrolled cell division and ***cancer***. The G_2/M checkpoint involves checking for DNA damage and effecting repair if necessary. If DNA damage is not repaired before entering M phase, ***apoptosis*** can be triggered. The metaphase checkpoint is known as the ***spindle checkpoint*** and aims to ensure equal distribution of chromosomes between the two daughter cells. Failures in these checkpoints can lead to accumulation of damaged DNA and uncontrolled cellular proliferation, as occurs in cancer. Some evolving cancer therapies aim to target cyclin-dependent kinase pathways in order to disrupt cell division and inhibit tumour growth.

MITOSIS

Division of ***somatic cells*** (all body cells except for the ***germ cells***) occurs in two phases. Firstly, the chromosomes duplicated in S phase are distributed equally between the two potential daughter cells; this process is known as ***mitosis***. Secondly, the dividing cell is cleaved into genetically identical daughter cells by cytoplasmic division or ***cytokinesis***.

Although mitosis is always equal and symmetrical, cytokinesis may, in some situations, result in the formation of two daughter cells with grossly unequal amounts of cytoplasm or cytoplasmic organelles. In other circumstances, mitosis may occur in the absence of cytokinesis, as in the formation of binucleate and multinucleate cells.

FIG. 2.2 Chromosomes during mitosis *(illustrations opposite)*

The nuclei of all somatic cells of an individual contain the same fixed complement of ***deoxyribonucleic acid (DNA)***, a quantity called the ***genome***. The DNA is arranged into ***chromosomes***, with each species having a set number. DNA is a very large molecular weight polymer consisting of many ***deoxyribonucleotides*** with a double-stranded structure. Each strand consists of a backbone of alternating ***deoxyribose* S** and ***phosphate* P** moieties. Each deoxyribose unit is covalently bound to a ***purine*** or ***pyrimidine*** base, which is in turn non-covalently linked to a complementary base on the other strand, thus linking the strands together. The bases are of four types, ***adenine* A**, ***cytosine* C**, ***thymine* T** and ***guanine* G**, with adenine only linking to thymine and cytosine only linking to guanine, thus making each strand complementary to the other, diagram (a). Linked in this way, the strands assume a double helical conformation around a common axis, the internucleotide phosphodiester bonds running in opposite directions (i.e. antiparallel) and the planes of the linked bases lying at right angles to the axis, diagram (b). The sequence of bases in either strand of the DNA molecule forms the genetic code for the individual. The bases are read in groups of three called ***codons***, each coding for one amino acid. In human cells, there are 46 chromosomes (the ***diploid number***) comprising 22 homologous pairs, the ***autosomes***, and 2 ***sex chromosomes***, either XX in the female or XY in the male. The members of each pair of autosomes have the same length of DNA and code for the same proteins.

Histologically, individual chromosomes are not visible within the cell nucleus during interphase. During S phase, each chromosome is duplicated, as shown in diagram (c). The resulting identical chromosomes, now known as ***sister chromatids***, remain attached to one another at a point called the ***centromere*** and become even more tightly coiled and condensed when they may be visualised with the light microscope (Figs 2.3 and 2.4). Accurate reproduction of the DNA strand is vital and multiple complex mechanisms exist to prevent mistakes (***mutations***) from occurring.

The extremely long DNA molecule making up each chromosome binds to a range of ***histone proteins*** that hold the chromosome in a supercoiled and folded conformation, compact enough to be accommodated within the nucleus (not illustrated). Thus the 2 nm diameter double helix is coiled and packed through several orders of three-dimensional complexity to form an elongated structure some 300 nm in diameter and very much shorter in length than the otherwise uncoiled molecule would be. This is the form in which the chromosome is structured during the G_1 and G_0 phases of the cell cycle, during which ***gene transcription*** (the prerequisite for protein synthesis) occurs. Histone proteins are also reduplicated during S phase so that the sister chromatids will have their own complement of histones.

Diagram (d) shows further detail of the structure of mitotic chromosomes and their supercoiled three-dimensional structure. Note the position of the ***kinetochore*** (Fig. 2.3) that provides attachment for the microtubules of the ***cell spindle*** during cell division and seems also to control the progression of mitosis. Examination of the chromosomes of dividing cells, ***karyotyping***, can give diagnostic information about the chromosomal complement of an individual or of a malignant tumour (Fig. 2.5).

Stem cells

In tissues with a regular turnover of cells, the dividing cells are relatively undifferentiated cells and are known as ***stem cells***. Some of the progeny of these cells undergo further cell division and finally differentiate to become the various types of mature cells, while others remain undifferentiated to maintain the pool of stem cells.

Stem cell research is currently a very controversial area. Embryonic stem cells are theoretically ***totipotent***, i.e. able to differentiate into any other cell type, while many stem cells found in adults are either ***multipotent***, able to produce cells of several lineages, or ***unipotent***, producing only a single cell type. Thus multipotent haematopoietic stem cells can produce all the formed elements of the blood, whereas unipotent epidermal stem cells of the skin can produce only epithelial cells. Recent research has hinted that, under certain circumstances, haematopoietic stem cells can produce other cell types. The advantages of such cells in the treatment of degenerative diseases are obvious – imagine being able to grow a new kidney or even a new limb to order. However, the ethical minefield created by the possible applications of such technology, especially the use of embryonic cells, is equally apparent.

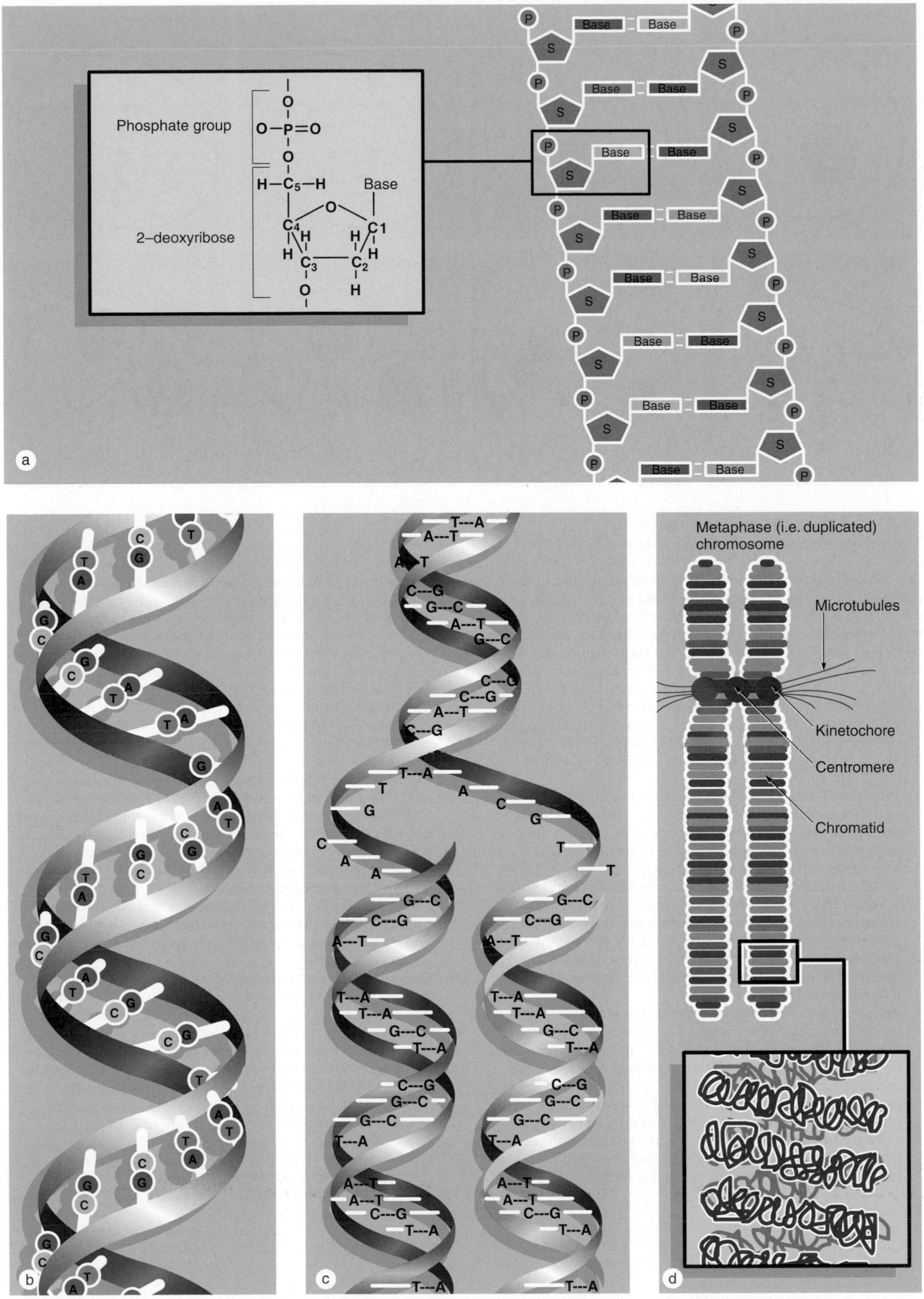

FIG. 2.2 Chromosomes during mitosis *(caption opposite)*

A adenine **C** cytosine **G** guanine **P** phosphate **S** deoxyribose **T** thymine

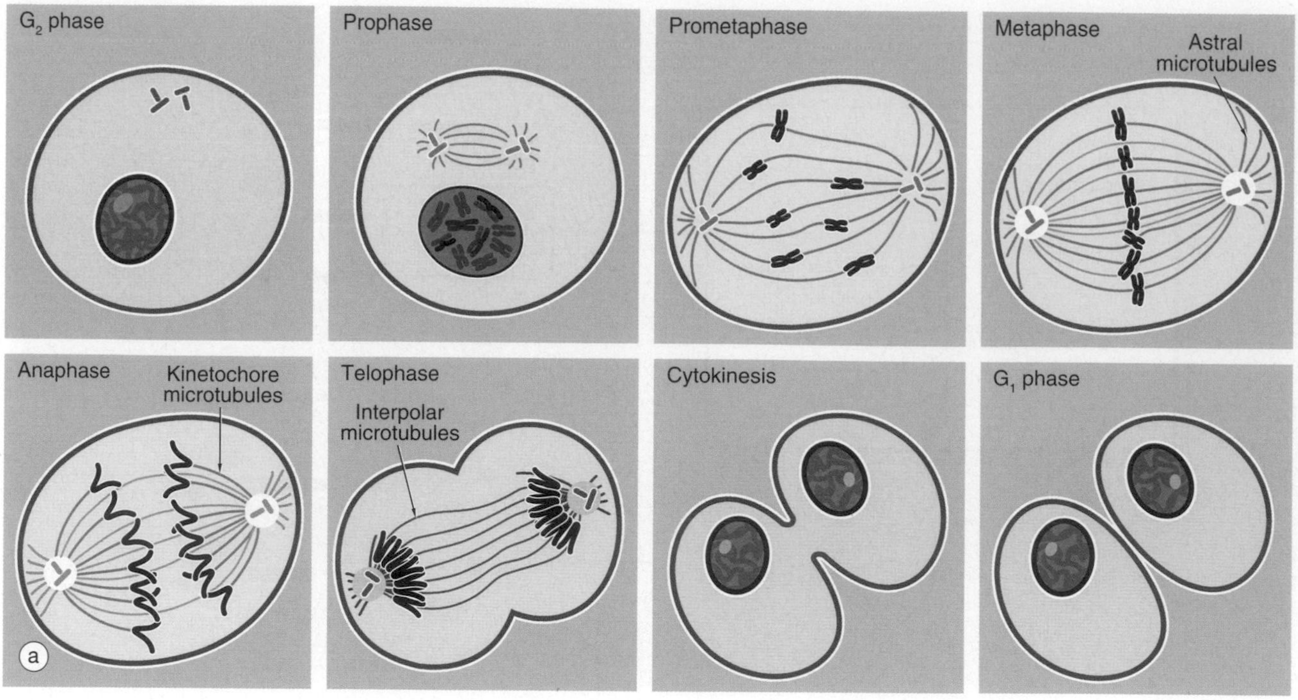

FIG. 2.3 Mitosis *(illustration (b) opposite)*
(a) Schematic diagram (b) Mitotic series Giemsa (HP)

The series of micrographs shown opposite illustrates the mitotic process in actively dividing immature blood cells from a smear preparation of human bone marrow. Mitosis is a continuous process that is traditionally divided into five phases, ***prophase***, ***prometaphase***, ***metaphase***, ***anaphase*** and ***telophase***, each stage being readily recognisable with the light microscope. Cell division requires the presence of a structure called the ***mitotic apparatus***, which comprises a spindle of longitudinally arranged microtubules extending between a pair of centrioles (see Figs 1.18 and 1.19) at each pole of the dividing cell. The mitotic apparatus is visible within the cytoplasm only during M phase as it disaggregates shortly after completion of mitosis.

- **Prophase**. The beginning of this stage of mitosis is defined as the moment when the chromosomes (already duplicated during the preceding S phase) first become visible within the nucleus. As prophase continues, the chromosomes become increasingly condensed and shortened and the nucleolus disappears. During prophase, the microfilaments and microtubules of the cytoskeleton disaggregate into their protein subunits. The centrosome has already divided during the preceding interphase and, in prophase, the two pairs of centrioles migrate towards opposite poles of the cell while simultaneously a spindle of microtubules is formed between them (***interpolar microtubules***).
- **Prometaphase**. Dissolution of the nuclear envelope marks the beginning of prometaphase. The mitotic spindle then moves into the nuclear area and each duplicated chromosome becomes attached at a site called the ***kinetochore*** to another group of microtubules of the mitotic spindle (***kinetochore*** or ***chromosome microtubules***). The kinetochore is a DNA and protein structure on each duplicated chromosome, located at the ***centromere***, the structure which binds the duplicated chromosomes (***chromatids***) together (see also Fig. 2.2d). Other microtubules attach the chromosome arms to the spindle.
- **Metaphase**. The chromosomes are then dragged to the plane of the spindle equator, known as the ***equatorial*** or ***metaphase plate***. The kinetochore also controls entry of the cell into anaphase so that the process of mitosis does not progress until all chromatid pairs are aligned at the cell equator. This is called the ***metaphase checkpoint*** and prevents the formation of daughter cells with unequal numbers of chromosomes.
- **Anaphase**. The splitting of the centromere marks this stage of mitosis. The mitotic spindle becomes lengthened by the action of the motor protein kinesin 5 on the interpolar microtubules; meanwhile ***astral microtubules***, joining the centrosome to the cell cortex (the area underlying the plasma membrane), shorten. The centrioles are thus pulled apart and the chromatids of each duplicated chromosome drawn to opposite ends of the cell, thus achieving an exact division of the duplicated genetic material. By the end of anaphase, two groups of identical chromosomes are clustered at opposite poles of the cell.
- **Telophase**. During the final phase of mitosis, the chromosomes begin to uncoil and to regain their interphase conformation. The nuclear envelope reassembles and nucleoli again become apparent.
- **Cytokinesis**. The plane of cytoplasmic division is usually defined by the position of the spindle equator, thus producing two cells of equal size. The plasma membrane around the spindle equator becomes indented to form a circumferential furrow around the cell, the ***cleavage furrow***, which progressively constricts the cell until it is cleaved into two daughter cells. A ring of microfilaments is present just beneath the surface of the cleavage furrow and cytokinesis occurs as a result of contraction of this filamentous ring. In early G_1 phase, the mitotic spindle disaggregates and, in many cell types, the single pair of centrioles begins to duplicate in preparation for the next mitotic division.

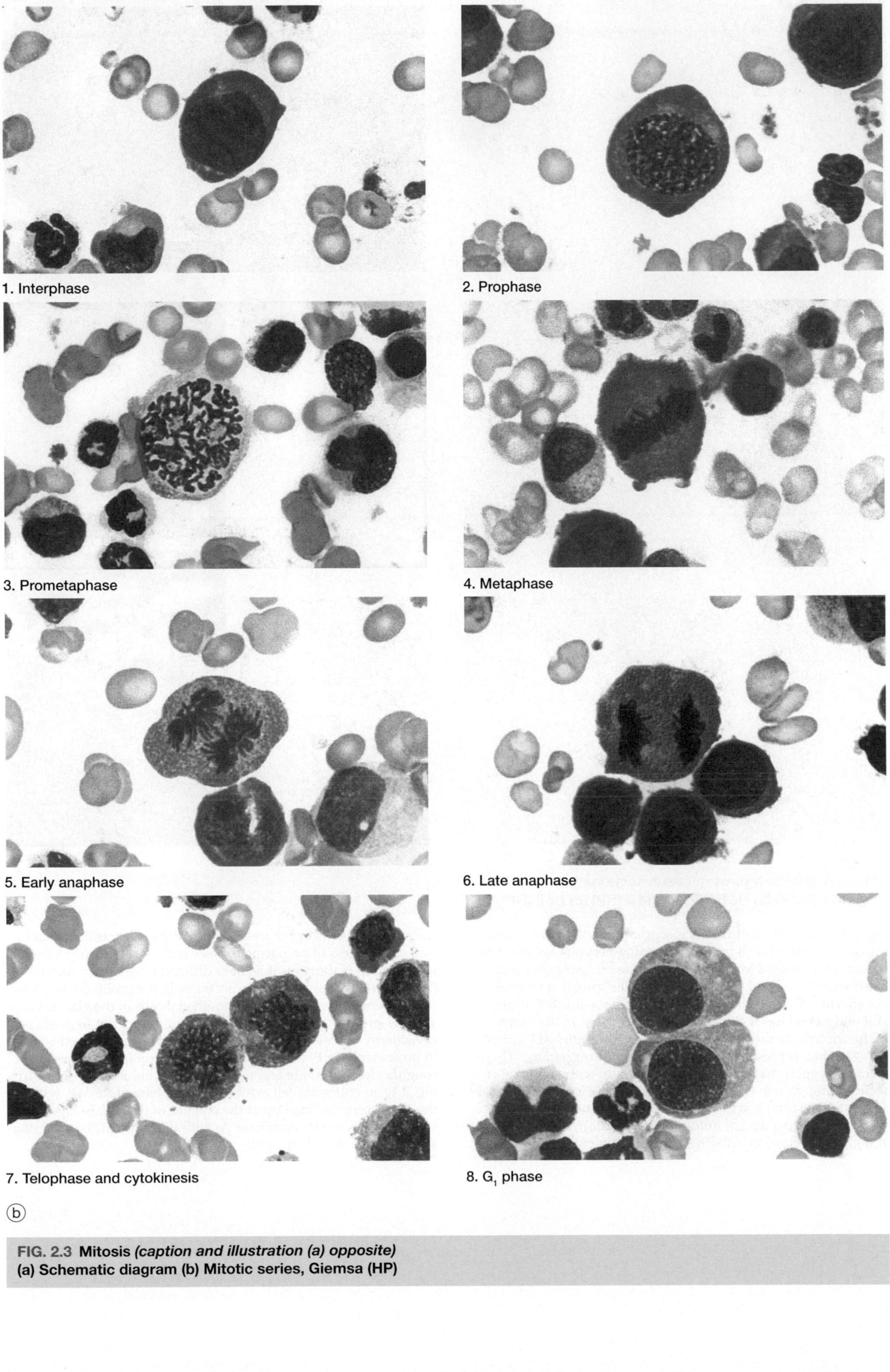

FIG. 2.3 Mitosis *(caption and illustration (a) opposite)*
(a) Schematic diagram (b) Mitotic series, Giemsa (HP)

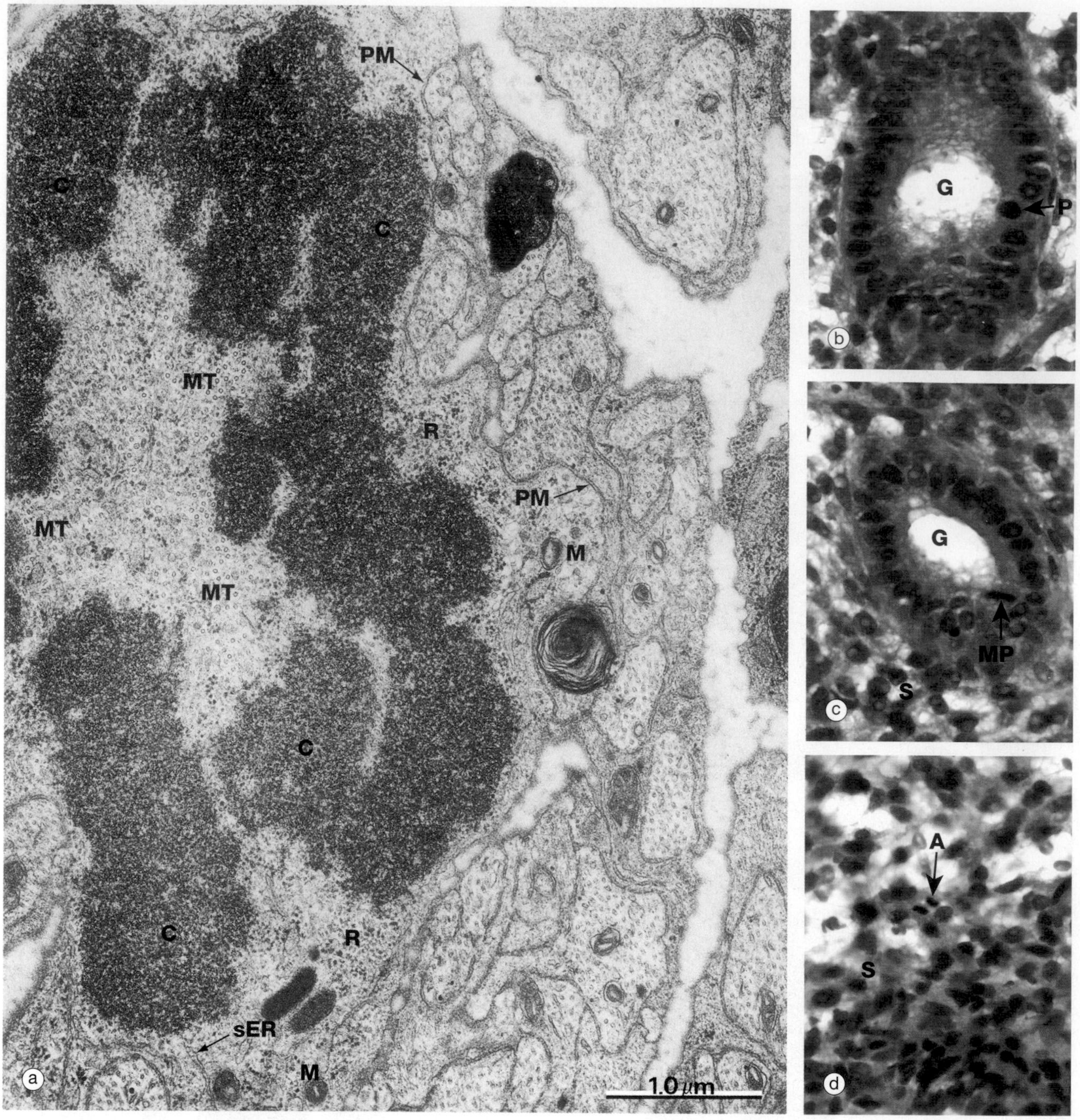

FIG. 2.4 Mitotic figures in tissue sections
(a) EM ×30 000 (b) H&E (HP) (c) H&E (HP) (d) H&E (HP)

Fig. 2.4a shows an electron microscopic view of part of a dividing cell, a Schwann cell in the developing nervous system. The plasma membrane **PM** is evident, but the nuclear membrane has disintegrated and the chromatin **C** has spread out into the cytoplasm. Mitochondria **M**, smooth endoplasmic reticulum **sER** and ribosomes **R** are seen at the periphery. In the centre of the chromatin, there are numerous microtubules **MT** cut in cross-section, representing part of the spindle apparatus. These features suggest that this cell is in anaphase, with the plane of section through one end of the dividing nuclear material at right angles to the spindle axis. Fig. 2.4b, Fig. 2.4c and Fig. 2.4d show the typical appearance of mitotic figures in normal tissue sections at high magnification. All three are of endometrium (see Ch. 19).

In contrast to smear preparations where the entire cell is visualised, the process of preparing a tissue section cuts through the cell in a random plane; thus it is more difficult to recognise mitotic figures with certainty in tissue sections. In the proliferative phase of the menstrual cycle, both the epithelial cells of the glands **G** and the stromal cells **S** of the endometrium undergo frequent cell division by mitosis. In Fig. 2.4b, a glandular epithelial cell is seen in prometaphase **P**, with the duplicated chromosomes forming a roughly circular tangle and the nuclear membrane dispersed. In Fig. 2.4c an epithelial cell exhibits a ***metaphase plate*** **MP**, with the chromosomes lined up at the equator of the cell. In Fig. 2.4d a stromal cell is in ***late anaphase*** **A**, with the chromatids separated and moving towards the poles of the spindle.

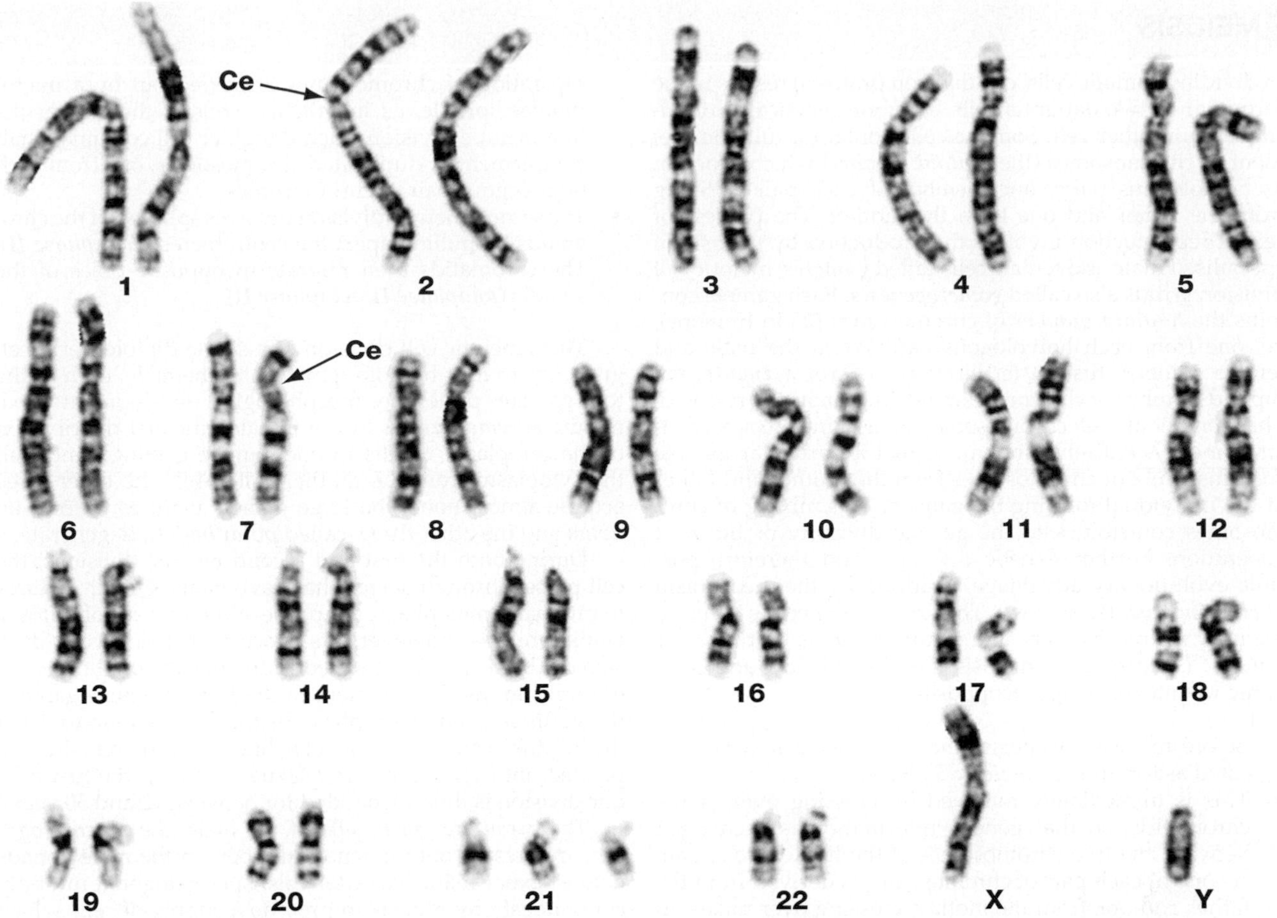

FIG. 2.5 Human karyotype
Leishman (HP)

Fig. 2.5 illustrates the chromosomes of a human cell grown in vitro and harvested at the onset of mitosis. The cell has been disrupted and the chromosomes stained to reveal their characteristic cross-banding pattern. This approach allows the investigator to identify chromosomes 1, 2 etc. At this stage the chromosomes are duplicated and the two chromatids (not visible at this magnification) are joined at the centromere **Ce**. Each member of a homologous pair of mitotic chromosomes is identical in length, centromere location and banding pattern. Study of the chromosomes in this fashion, ***karyotyping***, can reveal structural and numerical chromosomal abnormalities, known as ***cytogenetic abnormalities***. In this particular case there are three copies of chromosome 21, i.e. this is a trisomy 21 karyotype. All the other chromosomes are normal. There is one X and one Y chromosome demonstrating that the fetus is male.

Common cytogenetic abnormalities

The complex processes of meiotic cell division sometimes malfunction. It is unknown how many fetuses are conceived each year with genetic abnormalities so serious that the condition is lethal in utero and results in an early, perhaps even unrecognised, miscarriage. Most cytogenetic defects are thought to be lethal in this way and only a very few such as trisomy 21 (i.e. three copies of chromosome 21, also known as Down syndrome), trisomy 18 (Edward syndrome) and trisomy 13 (Patau syndrome) give rise to live births. In the two latter conditions, the infant usually dies within the first year, but individuals with Down syndrome may live to middle age or longer.

Trisomies arise usually due to failure of the homologous chromosome pairs to separate during the first meiotic division (***nondisjunction***) or failure of the two sister chromatids to separate during the second meiotic division (***anaphase lag***). Thus the resulting gamete has two copies of the relevant chromosome and, when fertilisation occurs, a third copy is added. In most cases, the extra chromosome is from the mother and there is a greatly increased incidence of Down syndrome with increasing maternal age, although the exact mechanism is as yet unclear.

Other types of chromosomal abnormalities that may be detected by karyotyping include ***translocation***, both balanced and unbalanced, abnormal chromosome structures, such as ***ring chromosomes***, and ***amplification*** or ***deletion*** of parts of a chromosome.

Karyotyping of fetal cells is widely available to detect cytogenetic abnormalities by the techniques of ***amniocentesis*** or ***chorionic villous sampling***. These are invasive diagnostic tests which present some fetal and maternal risks.

More recently, novel techniques have been developed to allow ***non invasive prenatal testing*** for certain genetic conditions, including fetal trisomies. ***Cell free fetal DNA*** is detectable in maternal plasma during pregnancy and these DNA fragments, obtained from a simple blood test in the mother, can be amplified, sequenced and then mapped to the human genome to detect fetal genetic abnormalities. In Down syndrome, genetic material from chromosome 21 is over-represented.

A late anaphase **C** chromatin **Ce** centromere **G** gland **M** mitochondrion **MP** metaphase plate **MT** microtubules
P prometaphase **PM** plasma membrane **R** ribosomes **S** stroma **sER** smooth endoplasmic reticulum

MEIOSIS

In dividing somatic cells, cell division (mitosis) results in the formation of two daughter cells, each one genetically identical to the mother cell. Somatic cells contain a full complement of chromosomes (the ***diploid number***) which function as homologous pairs, one member of each pair deriving from the father and one from the mother. The process of sexual reproduction involves the production by ***meiosis*** of specialised male and female cells called ***gametes***; meiotic cell division is thus also called ***gametogenesis***. Each gamete contains the ***haploid number*** of chromosomes (23 in humans), i.e. one from each homologous pair. When the male and female gametes fuse at fertilisation to form a ***zygote***, the diploid number of chromosomes (46 in humans) is restored. The member of each chromosome pair assigned to a particular gamete is entirely random, so that a particular gamete contains a mix of chromosomes from the mother and father of the individual forming the gamete. This mixing of chromosomes contributes to the genetic diversity of the next generation. Further genetic diversity, and therefore possible evolutionary advantage, is added by the mechanism of ***crossing over*** (see below). The process of meiosis involves many of the mechanisms and control systems that regulate mitosis. The process of meiosis is outlined below and compared to mitosis in Fig. 2.6 opposite.

- Before meiosis can begin, the chromosomes are duplicated as for mitosis (***meiotic S phase***).
- This is immediately followed by crossing over of the chromatids, so that genetic information is exchanged between the two chromosomes of the homologous pair. As one of each pair of chromosomes is derived from the father and one from the mother, crossing over mixes up these paternally and maternally derived ***alleles*** (alternative forms of the same gene) so that the haploid gamete ends up with only one of each chromosome pair, but each individual chromosome includes alleles from each parent (Fig. 2.5). The mechanism of crossing over is called ***chiasma formation***. This phase is known as ***prophase I***. As well as generating great genetic diversity, this mixing up of genes explains the conviction of many teenagers that they must be adopted!
- The first meiotic division then proceeds, involving separation of the homologous pairs of chromosomes, each one consisting of a pair of chromatids still joined together at the centromere (***metaphase I*** and ***anaphase I***). This separation of chromosomes is carried out by a microtubules spindle, as in mitosis. Thus at the end of the first meiotic division, each daughter cell contains a half complement of duplicated chromosomes, one from each homologous pair of chromosomes.
- The second meiotic division involves splitting of the chromatids by pulling apart the centromeres (***metaphase II***). The chromatids then migrate to opposite poles of the spindle (***anaphase II, telophase II***).

Thus, meiotic cell division of a single diploid germ cell gives rise to four haploid gametes. In the male, each of the four gametes undergoes morphological development into a mature ***spermatozoon***. In the female, unequal distribution of the cytoplasm results in one gamete gaining almost all the cytoplasm from the mother cell, while the other three acquire almost none; the large gamete matures to form an ***ovum*** and the other three, called ***polar bodies***, degenerate.

During both the first and second meiotic divisions, the cell passes through stages that have many similar features to prophase, metaphase, anaphase and telophase of mitosis. Unlike mitosis, however, the process of meiotic cell division can be suspended for a considerable length of time. For example, in the development of the human female gamete, the germ cells enter prophase of the first meiotic division during the fifth month of fetal life and then remain suspended until some time after sexual maturity; the first meiotic division is thus suspended for between 12 and 50 years!

The primitive germ cells of the male, the ***spermatogonia***, are present only in small numbers in the male gonads before sexual maturity. After this, spermatogonia multiply continuously by mitosis to provide a supply of cells which then undergo meiosis to form male gametes. In contrast, the germ cells of the female, called ***oogonia***, multiply by mitosis only during early fetal development, thereby producing a fixed complement of cells with the potential to undergo gametogenesis.

Chromosomes are not the only source of genes in the germ cells. Mitochondria also contain DNA that codes for some intrinsic mitochondrial proteins required for energy production. Because the spermatozoa shed their mitochondria at the time of fertilisation, only maternal mitochondrial genes are passed on to the offspring. A number of inherited diseases are known to be transmitted through mitochondrial DNA (see textbox).

Mitochondrial diseases

Mitochondria include circular stands of DNA which encode some of the mitochondrial proteins involved in cellular energy production. Mutations in these genes can cause serious illnesses. Mitochondrial DNA is maternally inherited because all of the cytoplasm of the fertilised cell is derived from the oocyte. As a result, these diseases do not follow typical Mendelian inheritance patterns and their clinical features vary widely depending upon the proportion of abnormal mitochondria in particular tissues, as well as the energy requirements of those tissues.

Most commonly, mitochondrial diseases present with features such as muscle weakness, loss of co-ordination, poor growth or a range of neurological symptoms, including autonomic dysfunction, visual and hearing problems. Examples of some mitochondrial diseases include ***mitochondrial myopathies***, ***Leber's hereditary optic neuropathy*** and ***MERRF syndrome (myoclonic epilepsy with ragged red fibres)***. The age of onset of symptoms varies greatly and these conditions may be difficult to diagnose.

Muscle biopsy is often used in diagnosis and typically reveals the presence of so-called 'ragged red fibres', muscle cells with clumps of diseased mitochondria beneath the sarcolemma (see e-Fig. 2.1). It is worth noting that some forms of mitochondrial myopathy occur due to mutations in mitochondrial proteins which are encoded by nuclear DNA and these disorders show more conventional patterns of inheritance.

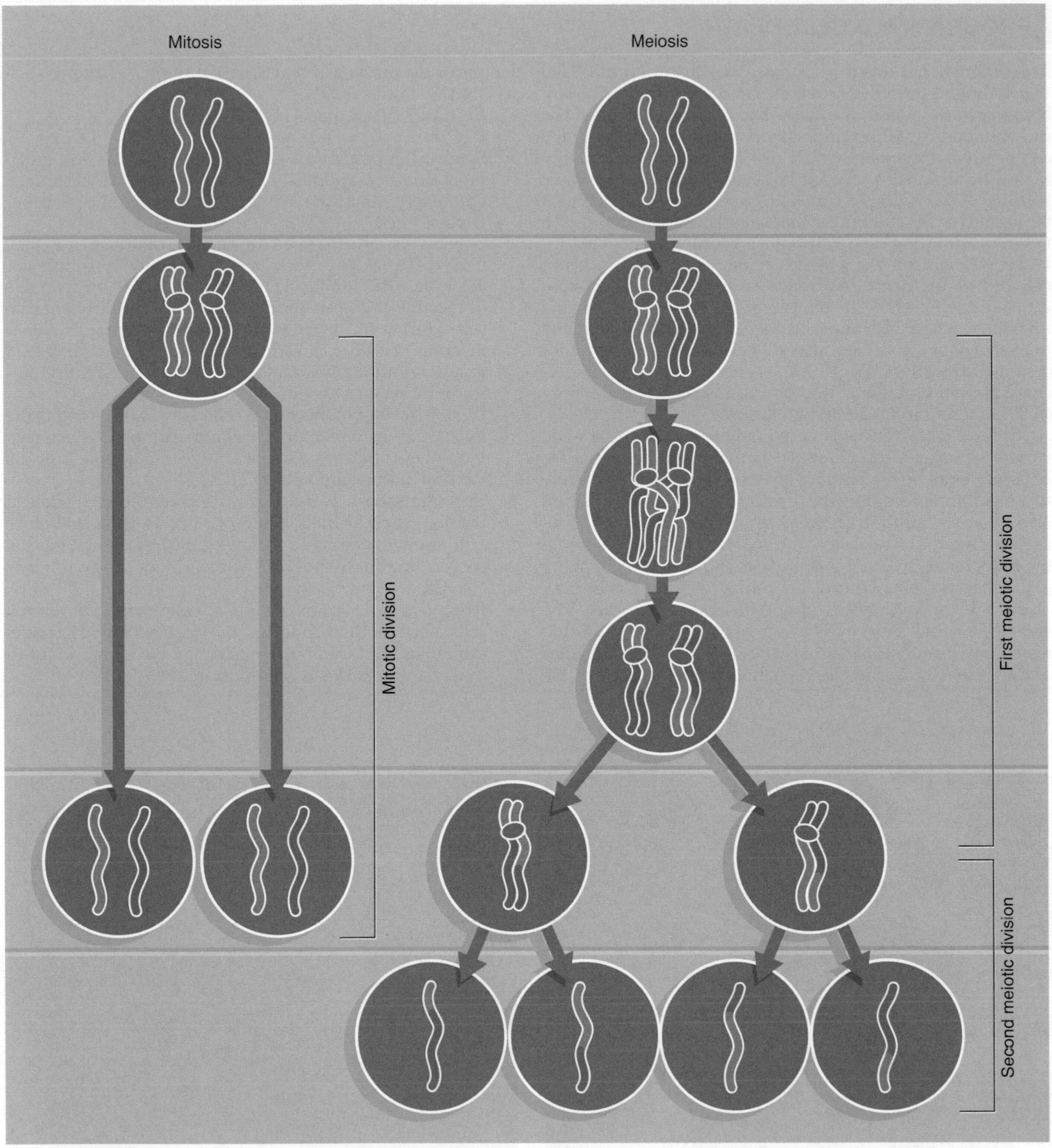

FIG. 2.6 Comparison of mitosis and meiosis

This diagram compares the behaviour of each homologous pair of chromosomes during mitosis and meiosis. For simplicity, the progress of only one homologous pair is represented here. The key differences between the two forms of cell division are as follows:

- Meiosis involves one reduplication of the chromosomes followed by two sequential cell divisions. Thus a diploid cell produces four haploid germ cells (gametes).
- Crossing over occurs only in meiosis, to rearrange alleles such that every gamete is genetically different. In contrast, the products of mitosis are genetically identical.

PROGRAMMED CELL DEATH

Programmed cell death is an essential part of normal fetal development, growth of juveniles and control of cell numbers in adults, where it exactly balances cell division. The most common and best understood method of programmed cell death is ***apoptosis***, which also occurs in certain pathological conditions. Apoptosis has characteristic microscopic features and is a highly controlled and ordered mechanism that removes cells in a way that causes minimal disruption to the surrounding tissue. Apoptosis is brought about by different mechanisms than those causing ***necrosis***, a mode of cell and tissue death that occurs only in pathological conditions. A well-known example of necrosis is myocardial infarction, where heart muscle dies from lack of oxygen due to blockage of a coronary artery. Apoptosis is an active process requiring the expenditure of energy, while necrosis is characterised by the inability of cells to produce the energy (ATP) required to maintain homeostasis.

Control of apoptosis is very finely balanced and a wide variety of triggers may initiate the process. The signal for apoptosis may be the binding of an external signal molecule to a membrane receptor (the 'death receptor' known as Fas) or may arise from intracellular signals such as DNA damage, leading to the release of the enzyme cytochrome c from the mitochondria into the cytoplasm. Within the cell, many regulatory proteins control apoptosis, including members of the bcl-2 and inhibitors of apoptosis (IAP) families. The end result of all these various signals is a common mechanism known as the ***caspase cascade***. The activated enzymes of the caspase cascade cleave cellular proteins such as the lamins of the nucleus and activate additional enzymes such as DNAase to cleave DNA.

Examples of apoptosis include:

- Some cell types have a preset limited lifetime and inevitably undergo apoptosis as part of their life cycle (e.g. epithelial cells in the skin or the lining of the gastrointestinal tract).
- Other cells are triggered to destroy themselves if they behave in ways which are potentially harmful; for example, developing T lymphocytes that are capable of reacting to normal body components are triggered to self-destruct in the thymus, a process known as ***clonal deletion*** (see Ch. 11). Failure of clonal deletion may lead to autoimmune disorders such as autoimmune thyroiditis or pernicious anaemia.
- During development certain cells are programmed to die by apoptosis; for example, in humans the webs between the fingers and toes disappear and the tadpole loses its tail as it matures into a frog.
- Certain tissues in adults grow and regress in a cyclical fashion, such as the growth of ovarian follicles before ovulation in females, followed by regression of the corpus luteum by apoptosis to form a corpus albicans (see Ch. 19).
- Apoptosis is a common mode of cell death of abnormal cells, such as those infected by viruses or with genetic mutations. Failure of apoptosis may be as important in cancer as unrestricted cell division.

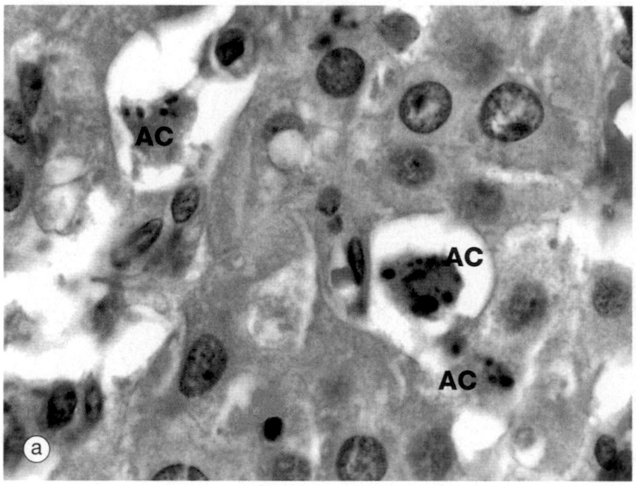

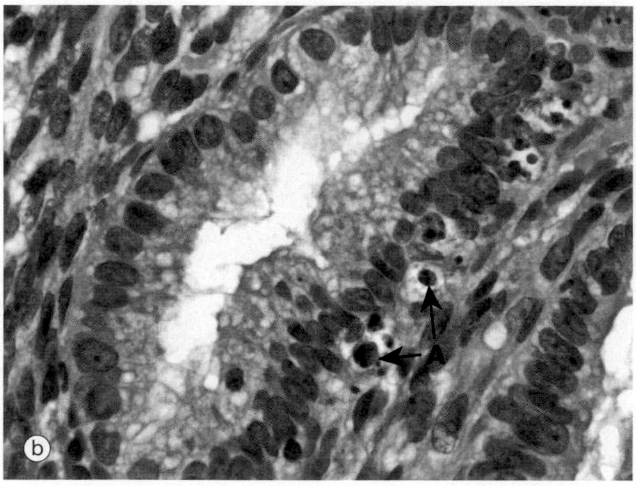

FIG. 2.7 Apoptosis in normal tissues
(a) H&E (HP) (b) H&E (HP)

These two micrographs illustrate the typical features of apoptotic cells in normal tissues. Fig. 2.7a is a corpus luteum, formed from an ovarian follicle after discharge of an ovum (see Ch. 19). If the ovum is not fertilised, the corpus luteum will involute, a process that involves progressive death of its constituent cells, leaving a fibrotic scar known as a ***corpus albicans***. In this micrograph several apoptotic cells **AC** can be identified by their condensed nuclei and eosinophilic cytoplasm.

Fig. 2.7b shows a later stage of apoptosis in epithelial cells of endometrial glands at the beginning of menstruation (see Ch. 19). Several cells have undergone apoptosis and reached the stage of forming easily identified apoptotic bodies **A**. The apoptotic bodies have been phagocytosed by adjacent cells, which are themselves about to undergo the same process as the superficial part of the endometrium is shed.

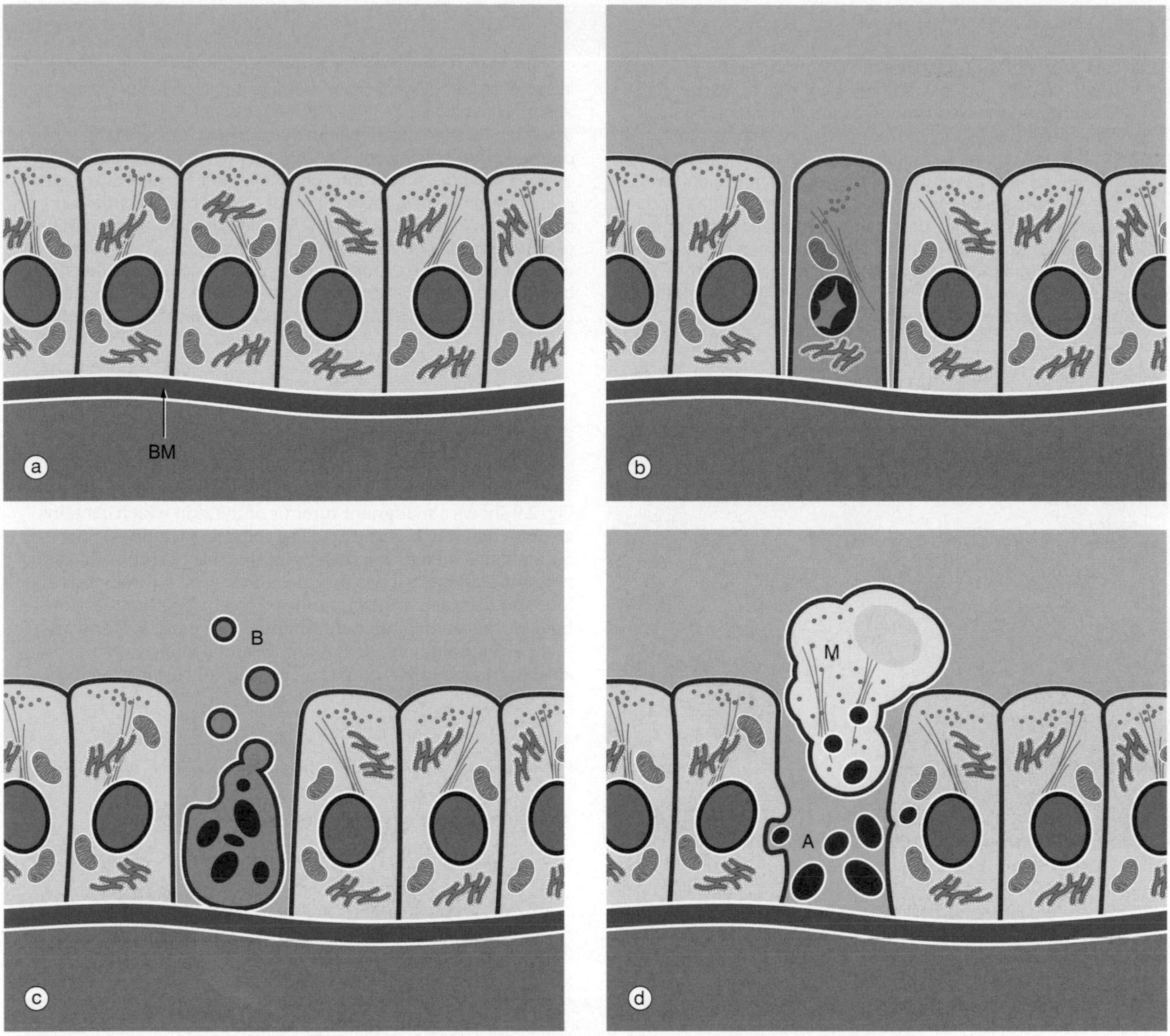

FIG. 2.8 The mechanism of apoptosis

Although a variety of extrinsic and intrinsic triggers may initiate apoptosis, at the molecular level the final common pathway is the activation of the ***caspase cascade***. Caspases are a set of enzymes found in inactive form in all cells. When the first in the series is activated, by cleaving off a short peptide sequence it is then able to activate the next enzyme in the series and so on. Because each enzyme is able to activate many copies of the next enzyme, the reaction is greatly amplified. This ***enzyme cascade*** mechanism is also seen in other situations requiring a rapid but controlled response, such as the blood clotting mechanism (the ***coagulation cascade***) and the ***complement cascade***.

The process of apoptosis is shown in this diagram of simple columnar epithelial cells resting on a ***basement membrane*** **BM**. When a normal cell (Fig. 2.8a) receives a signal to initiate apoptosis, the characteristic change by light microscopy (Fig. 2.8b) is condensation of the nuclear chromatin (***pyknosis***) to form one or more dark-staining masses found against the nuclear membrane. At the same time, the cell shrinks away from its neighbours, with loss of cell–cell contacts and increasing ***eosinophilia*** (pink staining) of the cytoplasm. The cytoplasmic organelles are still preserved at this stage. As the process continues (Fig. 2.8c), the nuclear material breaks into fragments (***karyorrhexis***). This is accompanied by dissolution of the nuclear membrane. ***Cytoplasmic blebs*** **B** break away from the cell surface, and eventually the entire cell breaks up (***karyolysis***) (Fig. 2.8d) to form membrane-bound fragments. Some of the cell fragments contain nuclear material and are known as ***apoptotic bodies*** **A**. These apoptotic bodies may be phagocytosed by adjacent cells or by tissue macrophages **M**, scavenger cells derived from the bone marrow and found in virtually every tissue in the body.

In some circumstances, part of the cell remains as a normal tissue component after apoptosis. For instance, in the skin, epithelial cells undergo apoptosis as part of their normal life cycle, but for some considerable time after the nucleus has disappeared, the cell cytoplasm filled with keratin intermediate filaments remains as an anucleate 'squame' to form a waterproof coating on the surface of the skin (see Ch. 9).

A apoptotic bodies **AC** apoptotic cell **B** cytoplasmic blebs **BM** basement membrane **M** macrophage

Cancer

Cancers or ***malignant tumours*** are common causes of illness and death in most societies and the diagnosis of cancer is an important part of the workload of diagnostic histopathology. Cancers cause disease by growing in an uncontrolled fashion within the body and replacing or destroying normal tissues. Importantly, as well as growing at their site of origin, cancers are able to ***metastasise*** or spread to other areas of the body such as the lungs or liver. Thus a primary cancer of the breast can spread to the lungs, causing death from respiratory failure, or a cancer of the prostate may replace the bone marrow, with consequent failure of production of white blood cells, causing death from overwhelming infection.

The many features of malignant tumours are well described in standard pathological texts, but one common feature is the abnormal mitotic figure (Fig. 2.9), which is not seen in normal tissue but is frequently a feature of malignant tumours (and some ***premalignant*** conditions). Abnormal mitotic figures are a visually obvious example of the many genetic abnormalities that are found in cancer cells, where there is loss of control of cell division and of cell death (see Figs. 2.7 and 2.8). These genetic abnormalities or mutations may be caused by infections (e.g. Epstein–Barr virus), toxins (e.g. cigarette smoke), radiation (e.g. sunlight) or may be inherited. Intensive research in this area continues and more causes and mechanisms of cancer are uncovered almost daily.

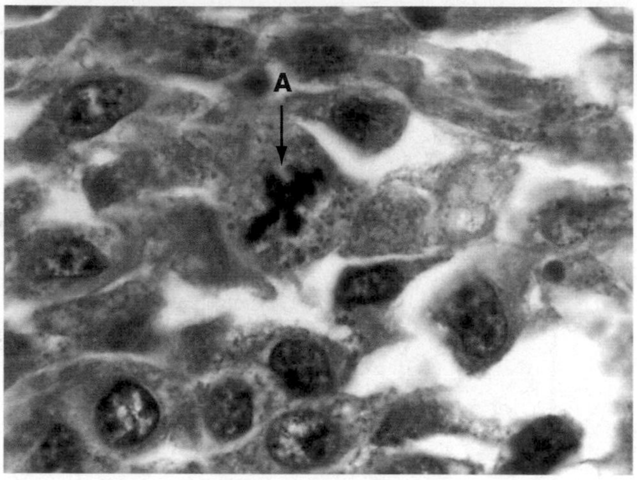

FIG. 2.9 Abnormal mitotic figure
H&E (HP)

Fig. 2.9 shows a malignant tumour of the skin which contains an abnormal mitotic figure **A**. The cell is in metaphase, but rather than a metaphase plate with two sets of chromatids and two spindles, the cell has produced four sets of chromatids and four spindles, a quadripolar mitosis. Such abnormalities are frequently seen in malignant tumours (see e-Fig. 2.2) and are virtually never found in normal tissues and benign tumours; thus an abnormal mitotic figure can be a helpful clue in diagnostic pathology.

REVIEW

TABLE 2.1 Review of cell cycle and replication

Process	Definition	Key features	Figures
The cell cycle	The period of time it takes for a cell to complete one cell division	May last a few hours in certain continuously dividing cells May last years in stable, terminally differentiated cells Consists of gap phase 1 (G_1), synthesis phase (S), gap phase 2 (G_2) and mitosis phase (M) Some cells enter G_0 phase, a prolonged non-dividing phase	2.1
Mitosis	Cell division of somatic cells	Results in two identical diploid daughter cells Phases are prophase, prometaphase, metaphase, anaphase, telophase and cytokinesis	2.2–2.4
Meiosis	Division of germ cells to produce zygotes	Results in four haploid cells – four spermatogonia in males and one oogonium and three polar bodies in females Crossing over during meiosis results in greatly increased genetic diversity in offspring	2.6
Apoptosis	Controlled cell death to remove unnecessary or potentially harmful cells	Various internal or external receptors may trigger apoptosis Cell death occurs by activation of the caspase cascade Histologically, apoptotic bodies may be seen Cell death occurs and the cell is removed without disruption or damage to the adjacent tissue	2.7, 2.8
Abnormal mitosis	Abnormal cell division, a common feature of cancer	Commonly seen in tissue sections from malignant tumours, often with abnormal tripolar and quadripolar forms	2.9

A abnormal mitotic figure

PART

II

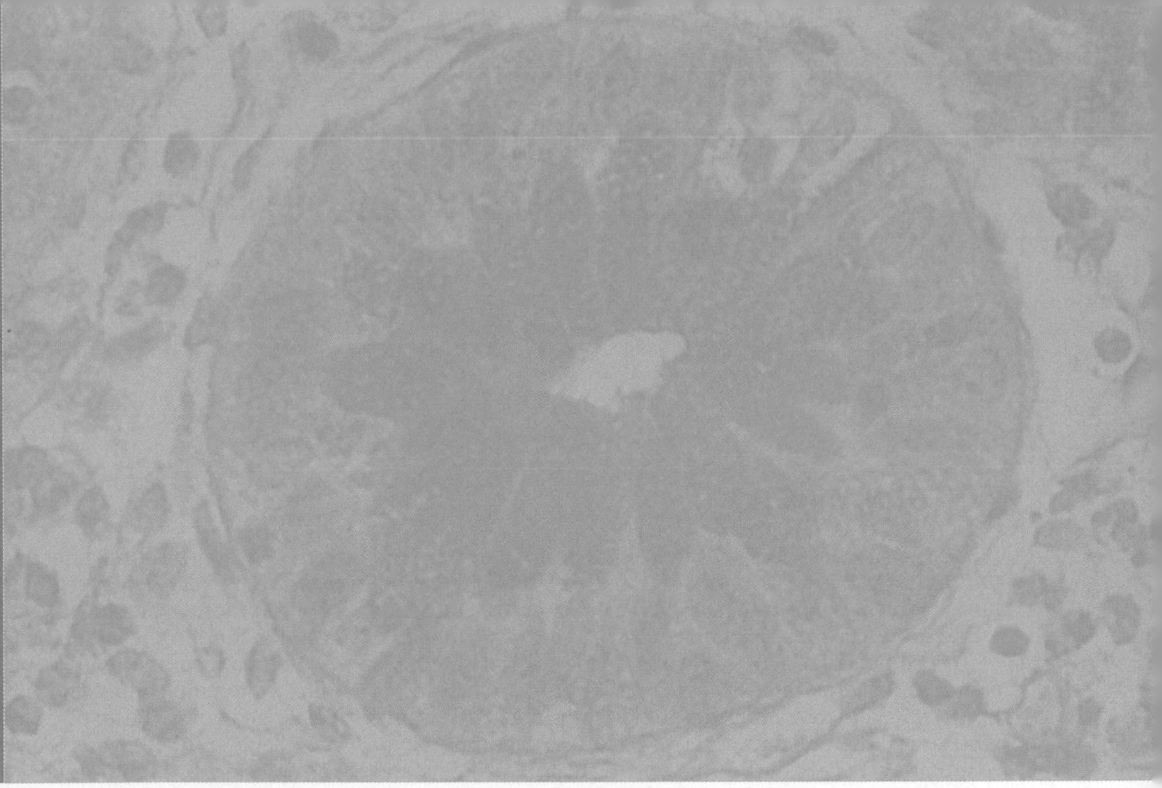

BASIC TISSUE TYPES

3 Blood, haematopoiesis and bone marrow

INTRODUCTION

Blood is a suspension of cells in fluid. It is circulated around the body by the heart and, as a result of this circulation, blood serves as the transport vehicle for gases, nutrients, waste products, cells and hormones.

The fluid is known as ***plasma*** and a typical sample is composed of 90% water, 8% protein, 1% inorganic salts, 0.5% lipids, 0.1% glucose and other minor components. The proteins are numerous and diverse, including albumin, blood coagulation factors, anti-proteases, transport proteins and antibodies (immunoglobulins). Collectively, these proteins exert a water-binding effect known as ***colloidal osmotic pressure*** which helps regulate the distribution of fluid between the plasma and the extracellular space, serving to keep the fluid in the circulation.

Plasma components, including hormones, lipids, salts, water molecules and small proteins, are constantly exchanged with the extracellular fluid of body tissues in accordance with the blood's transport functions. Proteins and plasma are not demonstrated by light microscopy except as a background colour.

BLOOD CELL TYPES

The cellular components of the blood are:

- **Red blood cells** (***erythrocytes***) are specialised cells containing the red pigment ***haemoglobin***. They provide most of the oxygen transport from the lungs and much of the return carbon dioxide carriage. They are immotile and serve their function only as the result of being passively circulated around the vascular system. The fraction of blood (by volume) occupied by erythrocytes is called the ***haematocrit*** and is in the range of 0.35 to 0.50 in adults.
- **White blood cells** (***leukocytes***) constitute an important part of the defence and immune systems of the body but undertake these functions mainly in the tissues; leukocytes in circulating blood are in transit or are simply waiting in reserve. There are five main subtypes of leukocytes.
- **Platelets** (***thrombocytes***) are specialised cells which bind to and coat damaged vessel walls, plug small defects in blood vessel walls and help activate the blood-clotting cascade. They are essential for ***haemostasis***, the system that controls bleeding.

In adults these cells are formed in the bone marrow, a process known as ***haemopoiesis*** or ***haematopoiesis***.

METHODS USED TO STUDY BLOOD AND BONE MARROW CELLS

Blood cell numbers are now usually counted by sophisticated laboratory analysers. Blood cell morphology is examined by microscopy using cytological methods. A standard method is to place a drop of blood on a glass slide and spread (smear) it into a very thin layer one cell thick. This smear is then air dried, which results in the cells spreading like fried eggs, making the cells appear larger and giving a clear view into the thinned cytoplasm. These smears are alcohol fixed and stained with Romanowsky-type stains which use polychromatic dyes containing multiple molecular variants to give subtle complexity in the staining. These are the best stains for morphology of blood and bone marrow; common examples are Giemsa and Wright. Distinctive staining characteristics are easily identified and reflect the affinity of the various cellular organelles for different stain components:

- ***Basophilia*** (deep blue) – affinity for the basic dye methylene blue; DNA in nuclei and RNA in ribosomes.
- ***Azurophilia*** (purple) – affinity for azure dyes; typically lysosomes, one of the granule types in leukocytes.
- ***Eosinophilia*** (pink/red) – affinity for the acidic dye eosin, thus also described as ***acidophilia***.
- ***Neutrophilia*** (salmon pink/lilac) – affinity for a dye once erroneously believed to be of neutral pH; characteristic of the specific cytoplasmic granules of neutrophil leukocytes.

Examination of haematopoietic bone marrow in adults involves sampling from the axial skeleton, usually the iliac crest in the pelvis, with an aspiration sample and often a bone core (also called a trephine). Aspiration samples can also be obtained from the sternum. Aspirated tissue fragments are smeared and stained like blood. Larger tissue pieces and cores of bone are examined as histology preparations, requiring decalcification and often stained with haematoxylin and eosin.

Clinical use of blood tests

Laboratory analysis of many components of blood, including cells, salts, various proteins, hormones, etc., are a convenient way of examining many body functions. 'Blood tests' have a large role in diagnosis and management of disease.

For example, a build-up of ***creatinine***, a breakdown product of wear and tear on muscle, can indicate renal failure. The ***HbA1c*** test gives an average blood glucose level to monitor compliance in patents with diabetes mellitus.

WHITE CELL SERIES

Five types of leukocytes are normally present in human blood and are classified into two groups:

Granulocytes
- Neutrophils
- Eosinophils
- Basophils

Mononuclear leukocytes
- Lymphocytes
- Monocytes

Granulocytes

Granulocyte types are named for the staining characteristics of their prominent type-specific cytoplasmic granules: ***neutrophil*** (lilac), ***eosinophil*** (red) and ***basophil*** (blue). Granulocytes have a single nucleus segmented into multiple lobes, assuming variable shapes that led to the use of the term ***polymorphonuclear leukocytes*** or ***polymorphs***, mainly because early microscopists mistook the multi-lobed nuclei for multiple nuclei. The term polymorph is sometimes used as a synonym for granulocyte. To confound matters further, polymorph is often used specifically for neutrophils as they are the commonest granulocyte. Granulocytes are also referred to as ***myeloid cells*** due to their origin from bone marrow, but they are not the only white blood cells to be formed in bone marrow.

Granulocytes are important components of the innate (non-learned) defences against infection (see Ch. 11); however, this role usually takes place in the tissues, not in blood (see e-Fig. 3.1). All leukocytes carry surface proteins which can bind to receptors on the endothelial cells of blood vessels (see Ch. 8) and, via this binding, granulocytes actively adhere to vessel walls and then migrate into the tissues using ***pseudopodial movement***.

With the exception of eosinophils entering intestinal mucosa, granulocytes do not normally enter tissues in any number; they simply circulate. They enter tissues in response to ***chemotactic signals*** and due to changes in the expression of endothelial cell surface receptors, induced by mediators of ***acute inflammation***.

Neutrophils are highly ***phagocytic***. They engulf and kill micro-organisms and ingest cell debris and particulate matter (see e-Fig. 3.2). These cells release multiple important proinflammatory chemical signals and regulators contributing to the overall inflammatory process. Granulocytes have a short functional life; having left the circulation they ***apoptose*** in the tissues and do not re-enter the blood.

Lymphocytes and monocytes

Lymphocytes and ***monocytes*** have non-lobulated nuclei and were described as mononuclear leukocytes by early microscopists to distinguish them from the polymorphs.

Lymphocytes play a key role in all immune responses, facilitating and regulating inflammation. In contrast to other leukocytes, their activity is directed toward specific foreign agents (antigens), providing a learned and targeted response, both antibody- and cell-mediated. Lymphocytes routinely traffic through tissues, then through lymphatics and lymph nodes and finally re-enter the circulation, providing routine surveillance against foreign antigens. They have an indefinite lifespan and are capable of proliferation.

Monocytes are highly phagocytic cells, ingesting micro-organisms, cell debris and particulate matter (see e-Fig. 3.3). They routinely enter some tissues, can mature into ***macrophages*** (including becoming resident ***tissue macrophages***) and can have extended tissue survival.

Monocytes and lymphoid cells produce, secrete and have receptors for a large number of inflammation-related chemical mediators.

White cell count

The white cells in blood are a cell population in waiting, a reserve pool. When stimulated by chemotaxins and aided by expression of leukocyte receptors on the endothelial cells, the blood leukocytes exit into tissue and become part of the inflammatory process. Numbers in blood might be expected to fall as a result, but a number of mature granulocytes are ready to respond, attached to the lining of small vessels. These form a functional reserve, not included in the blood count, but rapidly mobilised by the chemotaxins and cytokine signals of inflammation.

The same chemical signals stimulate movement of mature and almost mature cells in bone marrow into the circulating blood, forming an additional functional reserve. These signals will also stimulate faster maturation of the existing immature granulocytes in the marrow, which forms yet another reserve, and stimulate increased cell production in marrow from stem cells but this is a slower process.

In most cases of inflammation or infection, the granulocyte blood count will rise. Examples include:

- A raised neutrophil count (***neutrophilia***) indicating acute inflammation, especially seen in bacterial infections.
- Increased eosinophils (***eosinophilia***) – associated with allergy and parasitic infections.
- High lymphocyte counts (***lymphocytosis***) are particularly seen in viral infections.

Transient reduction in neutrophils in the blood (***neutropenia***) can occur due to cytokines produced in early viral infections.

Continued reduction in numbers (***cytopenia***), however, implies that the demand is greater than the supply. This can arise from either increased utilisation or disrupted marrow production.

In very sudden and extremely severe infections, the blood count may fall as the reserve granulocytes are drained faster than increased production can replace them. In these circumstances, immature granulocyte precursors such as ***band forms, metamyelocytes*** and ***myelocytes*** (see Fig. 3.8) may be mobilised to enter the circulation. This is a phenomenon called ***left shift***. A low neutrophil count (***neutropenia***) can be a blood count finding in overwhelming or severe sepsis, especially if there is left shift or in the setting of chemotherapy.

Malignant and pre-malignant diseases of white cell precursors can lead to circulating abnormal white cells (***leukaemias***) (see e-Fig. 3.4), or the disruption of normal white cell production, leading to ***cytopenias***. In both settings, the normal homeostasis is lost and there are clinical features relating to loss of white cell function, such as repeated infections or an enlarged spleen (***splenomegaly***).

HAEMATOPOIESIS

Haematopoiesis is the process of production of mature blood cells from precursors. This is a major task as an adult produces 100×10^9, i.e. a hundred billion, granulocytes each day. This production is ultimately derived from the ***pluripotential stem cells*** and their more differentiated offspring, the ***haematopoietic stem cells***. Stem cells are the cells which provide the lifelong reserve; they actively maintain their own population (self-renewing). They also proliferate and differentiate, contributing to the maintenance of the next level of more mature differentiated populations of stem cells or progenitors. As we move through the process, the emphasis for these cells progressively shifts from self-renewal to proliferation and differentiation.

These cells have been extensively studied in animal transplantation models and in laboratories, in short- and long-term culture systems. Many of the identified precursors have been named ***colony forming units*** (***CFU***) or ***burst forming units*** (***BFU***) and the regulatory molecules have been named ***colony-stimulating factors*** (***CSF***), reflecting this laboratory background. Other regulatory molecules have been called ***interleukins***, ***cytokines*** or ***growth factors***, depending on their laboratory histories.

The stem cells, progenitors and the later differentiated forms all depend on a complex microenvironment for growth, proliferation and differentiation. This microenvironment is physical, with cell–cell attachments, signalling by these attachments and local secretion of growth factors. The analogy of seed (stem cell) and soil (microenvironment) has often been used.

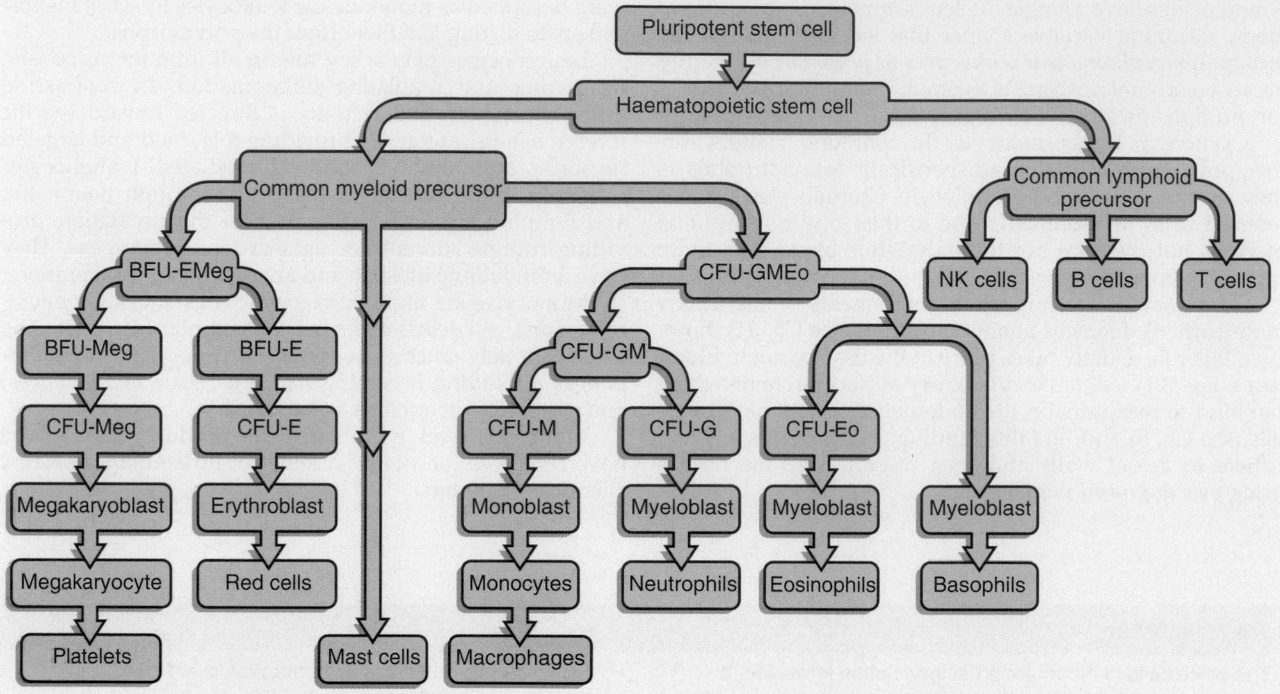

FIG. 3.1 Haematopoietic stem cells and progenitors

This diagram illustrates some of the identified stem cells and precursors in haematopoiesis. The haematopoietic stem cell (HSC) differentiates into a common ***lymphoid precursor*** and a ***common myeloid precursor*** (**CMP**) also known as the CFU-GEMM (CFU–granulocyte, erythroid, monocyte, megakaryocyte).

This common myeloid precursor differentiates into a common erythroid and megakaryocyte progenitor, the **BFU-EMeg** (***BFU–erythroid megakaryocyte***) and into a combined granulocyte and monocyte precursor, the **CFU-GMEo** (***CFU–granulocyte, monocyte, eosinophil***).

These precursors differentiate as shown in the diagram into a committed precursor type for each individual lineage.

BFU- and CFU-GM precursors produce large numbers of progeny (hundreds to thousands), while the individual lineage CFU-precursors may only have 20 to 50 progeny.

Each recognisable blast in a bone marrow smear (other than megakaryocyte lineage) might average 16 offspring when counted as the final differentiated cells.

The mast cell derivation pathway is unclear but is believed to be of early myeloid lineage. Mast cell progenitors are released into the blood and, once activated, they mature in the connective tissues.

BFU burst forming unit **CFU** colony forming unit **E** erythroid **EMeg** erythroid megakaryocyte **Eo** eosinophil **G** granulocyte **GM** granulocyte monocyte **GMEo** granulocyte monocyte eosinophil **M** monocyte **Meg** megakaryocyte

Major haematopoietic growth factors

Haematopoiesis is tightly controlled by growth factors and the microenvironment. Growth factors, with the possible exception of ***erythropoietin***, are multifunctional. A single growth factor will influence several different stages of several lineages and promote proliferation and/or differentiation, maturation, egress from bone marrow and survival in tissue. The differences in effect are due to the developmental stage of the cell on which the growth factor is acting, combined with its differentiation, surface receptors and the multitude of other signals it is receiving (see Table 3.1).

The haematopoietic stem cell (HSC) is particularly influenced by ***stem cell factor (SCF)***, ***Flt-3 ligand*** and ***vascular endothelial growth factor (VEGF)***, while the supporting stromal cells of the microenvironment are responsive to ***interleukin-1 (IL-1)*** and ***tumour necrosis factor (TNF)***. These stem cells are not geographically constrained; they normally circulate in blood in small numbers. ***Granulocyte-CSF (G-CSF)*** will mobilise stem cells into the circulation in large numbers. These circulating stem cells then home to sources of stromal derived factor-1 (SDF-1), a product of the haematopoietic microenvironment.

Major generic drivers for haematopoiesis in general are ***interleukin 3*** (***IL-3***), ***granulocyte-monocyte CSF*** (***GM-CSF***) and ***stem cell factor*** (***SFC***); these promote most lineages at most stages. ***Thrombopoietin***, produced in the kidney and liver, is important for megakaryocyte and platelet production and also promotes the early stages of red cell production. ***Erythropoietin***, a protein hormone produced mostly in the kidneys, drives the later part of red cell production (from CFU-E) but has little effect on the early red cell progenitors. Granulocyte CSF (G-CSF) and ***monocyte CSF (M-CSF)*** promote granulocyte and monocyte lineages while ***interleukin-5 (IL-5)*** helps drive eosinophil production.

These stem cells and progenitor cells are not recognisable by microscopy. Many resemble lymphocytes and are only identifiable by their expression of different combinations of cell surface molecules. The earliest committed cells recognised in marrow smears are the blasts e.g. myeloblasts, proerythroblasts, monoblasts, etc. These are quite late in the process, about to undertake final proliferation and differentiation. A BFU-E takes about 7 days to become very many CFU-E; each CFU-E takes about 7 days to become many recognisable proerythroblasts and each proerythroblast will form about 16 mature red cells, taking 6 to 7 days. Note that the adult requirement is for about 2.5 billion red cells/kg body weight each day. Many of these growth factors are now available and are used therapeutically; for example, erythropoietin can be used to treat anaemia.

TABLE 3.1 Major haematopoietic growth factors

Factor	Abbreviation	Cells affected
Stem cell factor	SCF	All
Granulocyte–monocyte colony-stimulating factor (CSF)	GM-CSF	Most
Interleukin-3	IL-3	All
Interleukin-11	IL-11	Megakaryocyte production
Interleukin-5	IL-5	Eosinophil production
Granulocyte CSF	G-CSF	Granulocyte production
Monocyte CSF	M-CSF	Monocyte production
Thrombopoietin	TBO	Megakaryocyte and red cell production
Erythropoietin	EPO	Red cell production

Bone marrow transplantation

Bone marrow transplantation (BMT) is really haematopoietic stem cell (HSC) transplantation, with the aim of providing a new system of haematopoiesis and, via the lymphocyte pathway, a new immune system. The stem cells are collected either as anticoagulated aspirates of bone marrow from multiple sites or as white cell concentrates collected from peripheral blood after mobilisation of stem cells via injections of G-CSF.

The patient's original haematopoietic system is destroyed by cytotoxic drugs and radiotherapy. The collected stem cell–containing material is then transfused and the stem cells return to the haematopoietic microenvironment where they grow, re-establishing haematopoiesis and an immune system.

The donor source may be other people, called allogenic transplantation, or self, called autologous transplantation. When allogenic cells are used, HLA matching is important to minimise graft versus host disease (GVHD), a condition where mature lymphoid cells in the graft recognise the patient as foreign and attack, causing a number of clinical scenarios.

BMT is used to treat severe genetic immunodeficiencies and haematopoietic disorders. Examples include aplastic anaemia, a condition of acquired failure of haematopoiesis, and leukaemia. Autologous transplantation is used to enable survival following very high doses of marrow-toxic drugs, thereby allowing higher-dose anti-cancer therapy.

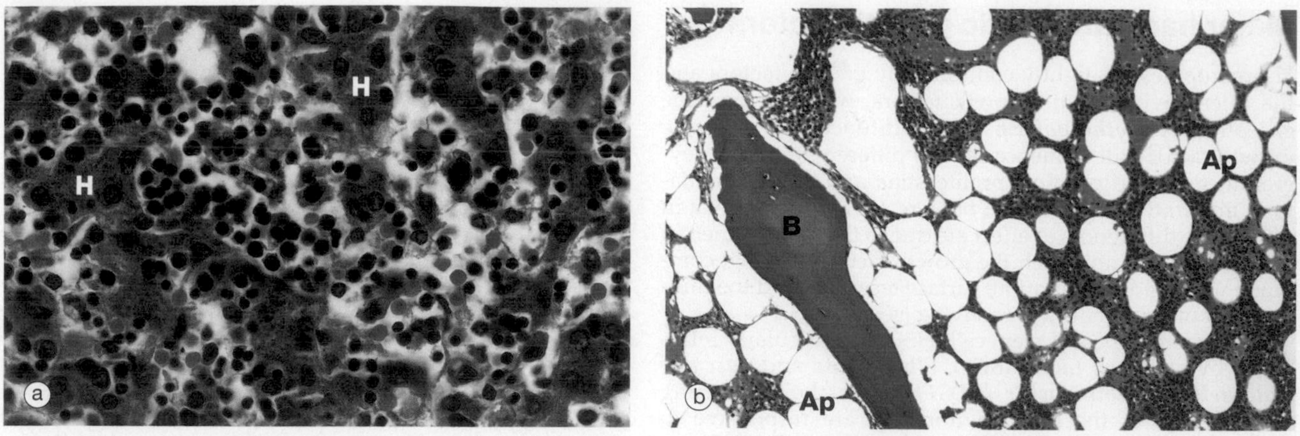

FIG. 3.2 Haematopoiesis in liver and bone marrow
(a) H&E (MP) (b) H&E (LP)

Haematopoiesis begins in early intrauterine life in an embryonic organ, the ***yolk sac***. It soon becomes established in the liver sinusoids. These are the vascular spaces between the hepatocytes **H**, in Fig. 3.2a, where numerous small, darkly staining haematopoietic cells are seen. This is the dominant site of haematopoiesis from 3 to 7 months' gestation. As bones develop, haematopoiesis establishes in the spaces between bone trabeculae **B** in all bones and, by birth, this provides sufficient space for all the haematopoiesis so that ***extramedullary haematopoiesis*** (see e-Fig. 3.5) comes to an end.

With growth through childhood, bone marrow space increases faster than total body growth and, increasingly, the marrow becomes occupied by adipocytes **Ap** (fat cells). Haematopoietic marrow has a macroscopic red colour, while adipocyte-dominated marrow is yellow. By early adulthood, most of the marrow in the limb bones is yellow marrow, while the axial skeleton remains red and haematopoietic, although usually with 30% to 60% of the volume being admixed adipocytes. Fig. 3.2b shows adult vertebral marrow with moderate numbers of adipocytes.

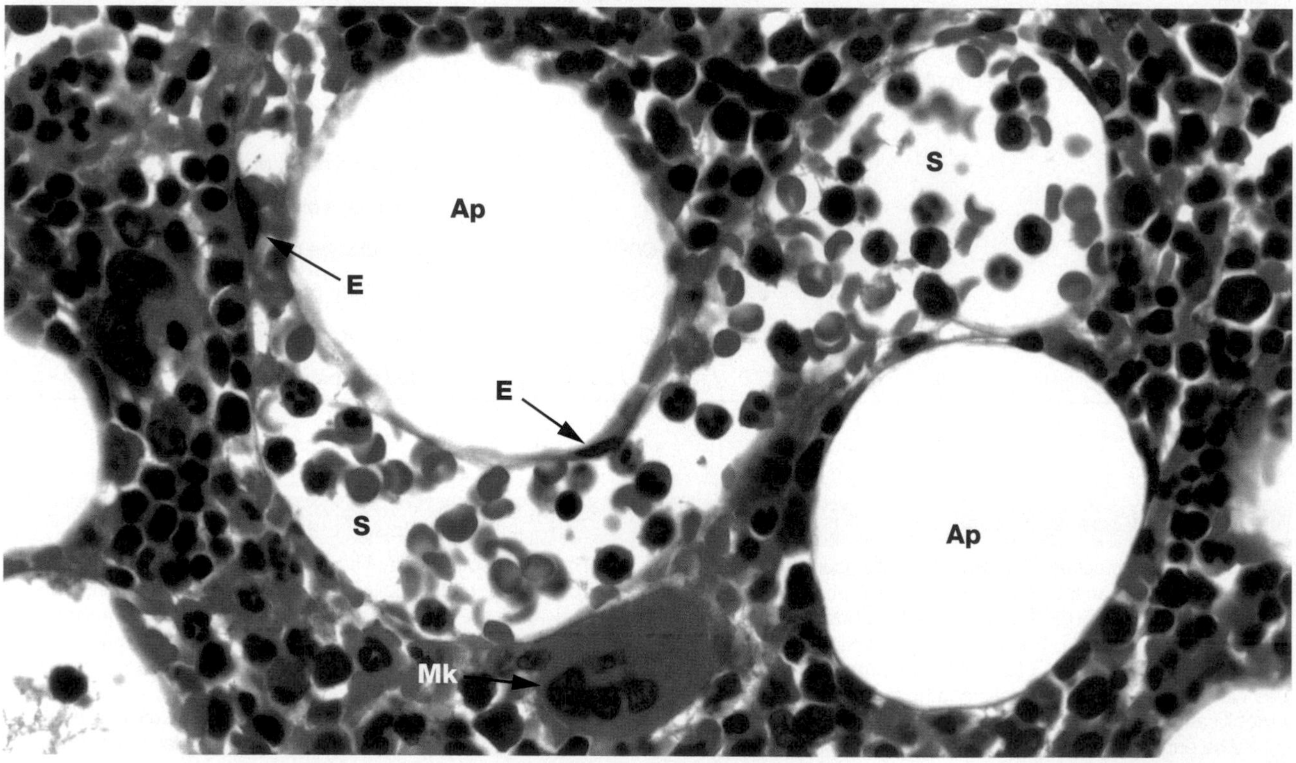

FIG. 3.3 Bone marrow sinusoids
H&E (HP)

Bone marrow has a framework of vascular ***sinusoids*** lined by endothelial cells **E** and intervening spaces called ***marrow cords***, supported by a meshwork of fibroblastic cells with long, branched cytoplasmic processes (***reticular cells***) and reticulin fibres (type III collagen). Macrophages are numerous and may also have long, branched processes. Adipocytes **Ap** and plasma cells are present in significant numbers. The result is a microenvironment which supports haematopoiesis and the marrow cords are correspondingly cellular. Megakaryocytes **Mk** sit next to the sinusoids **S** so their cytoplasmic processes, ***proplatelets***, can be released into the circulation. ***Erythroblastic islands*** also sit next to sinusoids, with red cell precursors adhering to long macrophage processes that direct red cells to, and control egress into, the sinusoids. Granulocyte precursors tend to sit away from the sinusoids, but these are motile cells which can migrate into sinusoids.

Ap adipocyte **B** bone trabeculae **E** endothelial cell nucleus **H** hepatocyte **Mk** megakaryocyte **S** sinusoid

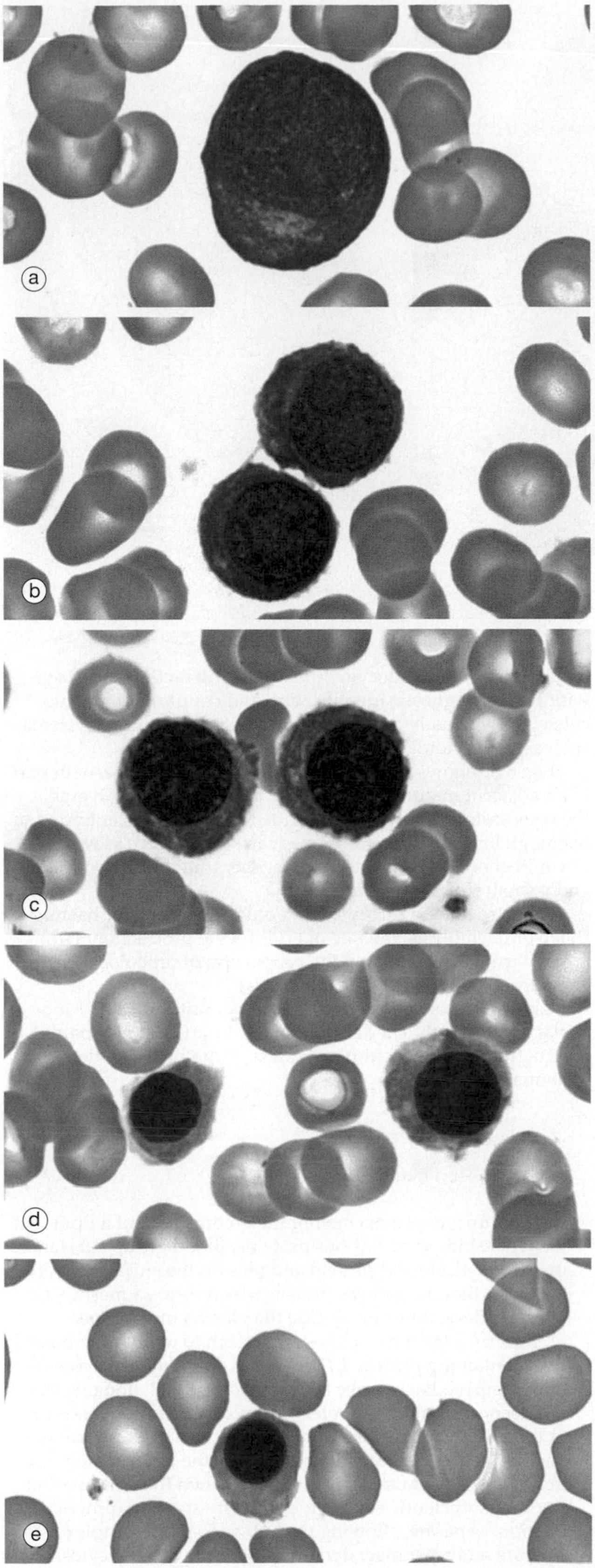

FIG. 3.4 Erythropoiesis
Giemsa (HP)

These micrographs from a bone marrow smear illustrate the stages of erythropoiesis. The process of erythropoiesis involves:

- Progressive reduction in size and cytoplasmic organelles, helped by cell divisions diluting cytoplasmic contents in the early stages.
- Inactivation and ultimately extrusion of the nucleus.
- Progressive haemoglobin synthesis by ribosomes.

The ***proerythroblast***, Fig. 3.4a, is the first recognisable erythrocyte precursor; the cell is large with fine, granular nuclear chromatin containing one or more paler nucleoli. The relatively sparse cytoplasm is strongly basophilic due to its high content of RNA and ribosomes. A narrow, pale zone of cytoplasm close to the nucleus represents the Golgi apparatus. Proerythroblasts divide and differentiate, producing smaller cells called ***basophilic erythroblasts*** or ***early normoblasts***, Fig. 3.4b. These are smaller cells with some condensation and clumping of chromatin.

The next morphological forms are called ***polychromatic erythroblasts*** (***intermediate normoblasts***). In these cells the cytoplasm develops a grey colouration due to increasing cytoplasmic haemoglobin. As this is a mixture of basophilia and eosinophilia, the term ***polychromasia*** is applied. The nuclear chromatin becomes increasingly condensed. These cells are no longer capable of division. Fig. 3.4c shows an early example and parts of several white cell precursors while Fig. 3.4d shows two late examples.

The final nucleated form, Fig. 3.4e, is the ***orthochromatic erythroblast*** (***late normoblast***). The cytoplasm is rich in haemoglobin but still contains ribosomes with continuing haemoglobin synthesis. Cytoplasmic organelles are degenerate. The nuclear chromatin, and nucleus, becomes extremely condensed; the nucleus is then extruded. The result is an anucleate early red cell, the ***reticulocyte*** (Fig. 3.5).

The process of nuclear condensation and extrusion may be incomplete, leaving small, spherical, condensed nuclear remnants in the red cells. These are known as ***Howell–Jolly bodies***; they are normally pinched off from red cells in a small envelope of plasma membrane by splenic macrophages and are not found in blood. However, in persons who have had a splenectomy, it is normal to find small numbers of red cells containing Howell–Jolly bodies in a blood smear.

Red cells share a common progenitor with megakaryocytes.

Proliferation and differentiation to produce red blood cells is stimulated by the growth factor ***erythropoietin***, produced mostly in kidneys, although early stages are also supported by thrombopoietin and some interleukins.

In bone marrow histology, red cell precursors are found in small, scattered clusters called ***erythroblastic islands***. Each of these is centered on a macrophage with long cytoplasmic processes and membrane folds which accommodate the precursors. Precursors move outward along the processes as they mature, reaching the sinusoidal endothelium whence they enter the circulation. These macrophages provide cell–cell contact and signalling and control the release of maturing red cells into sinusoids.

Each proerythroblast will generally become 16 red blood cells over 5 to 7 days. Each of these micrographs shows numerous mature red blood cells in the smears, with absence of nuclei and often central pallor.

Anaemia

Anaemia is a reduction in blood haemoglobin below normal. Reduced marrow production can occur from lack of required nutrients, including iron, vitamin B_{12}, vitamin B_9 (folate); from primary marrow failure, known as aplastic anaemia; or from a genetic abnormality in the red cell production system (e.g. thalassaemia).

The red cells produced can be destroyed (haemolytic anaemia) by various mechanisms, most commonly mediated by autoimmune antibodies, or they may be lost by haemorrhage. Anaemia may present clinically with pallor, fatigue and breathlessness.

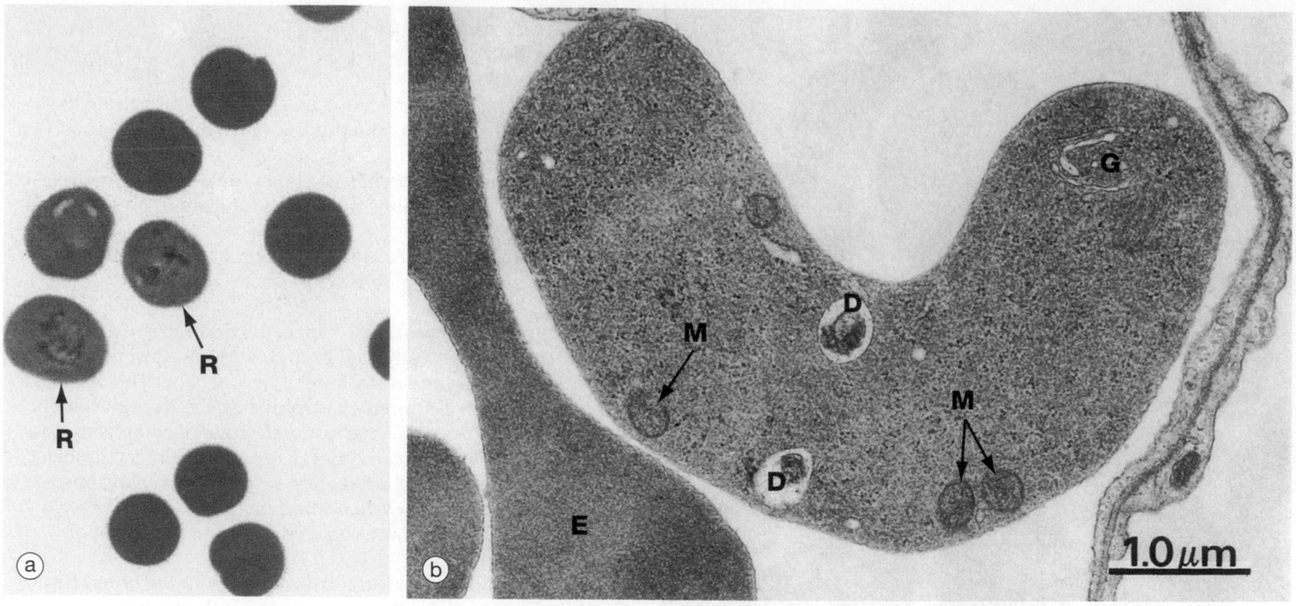

FIG. 3.5 Reticulocytes
(a) Cresyl blue/eosin (HP) (b) EM ×16 000

Reticulocytes are immature red blood cells and are the form in which erythrocytes are released from the bone marrow. They still contain mitochondria, ribosomes and Golgi elements and continue to synthesise haemoglobin. Final maturation into erythrocytes occurs within 48 hours of release. The rate of release of reticulocytes into the circulation generally equals the rate of removal of spent erythrocytes by spleen and liver. Since the lifespan of circulating erythrocytes is about 120 days, reticulocytes constitute slightly less than 1% of circulating red blood cells. Reticulocytes are slightly larger than mature erythrocytes and their staining is slightly basophilic due to the ribosomes and RNA. Increased reticulocytes can be suspected from a blood film by the varying basophilia of the cells on a smear, a finding called polychromasia (many colours).

Reliable reticulocyte identification and counting requires special techniques such as supravital staining, illustrated in Fig. 3.5a. A fresh blood sample is incubated with the basic dye, brilliant cresyl blue, resulting in a blue-stained reticular precipitate **R** in reticulocytes, due to the interaction of the dye with RNA. Diagnostic identification and counting of reticulocytes is now usually done using automated laboratory systems such as flow cytometry.

Fig. 3.5b shows the ultrastructure of a reticulocyte, with part of an adjacent mature erythrocyte **E** for comparison. Overall, the cytoplasmic density is lower due to a lower concentration of haemoglobin. Scattered ribosomes can still be seen, as well as a few mitochondria **M**, occasional degenerating mitochondria **D** and a small Golgi remnant **G**.

When severe erythrocyte loss occurs, such as after haemorrhage or haemolysis, the rate of erythrocyte production in the bone marrow increases and the proportion of reticulocytes in circulating blood rises (***reticulocytosis***).

Clinically, an elevated reticulocyte count indicates functional marrow, while a decreased count may mean impaired production. This is an important test in the investigation of anaemia.

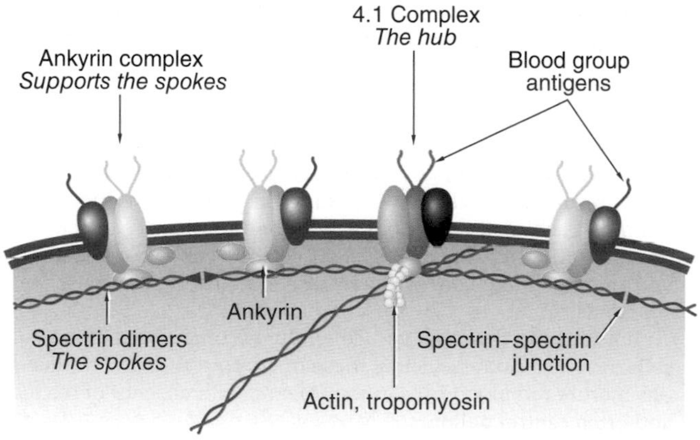

FIG. 3.6 Red cell cytoskeleton

The erythrocyte plasma membrane is composed of a lipid bilayer, stabilised by various proteins. Blood group substances are carbohydrate and protein antigens on the surface. ***Spectrin*** is a long, dimeric, springy protein which forms a meshwork like a geodesic dome just inside the plasma membrane.

Spectrins form the spokes and attach to membrane-bound hubs containing ***protein 4.1, actin*** and ***tropomyosin*** proteins among others. Each spoke is further supported along its length by a second membrane protein complex containing ***ankyrin***. At the end away from the hubs, the spectrin spokes form non-covalent spectrin–spectrin junctions. As the red cell membrane bends, the spectrin molecules stretch. When the deformation becomes sufficiently severe, the spectrin–spectrin dimeric junctions separate, allowing the hub and spoke complexes to separate and rearrange, dynamically reshaping the cytoskeleton. Actin is part of a contractile segment, possibly applying tension to the spectrins.

D degenerating mitochondrion **DB** dumbbell-shaped erythrocyte **E** mature erythrocyte **G** Golgi remnants **M** mitochondrion **P** platelet **R** reticular precipitate in reticulocyte

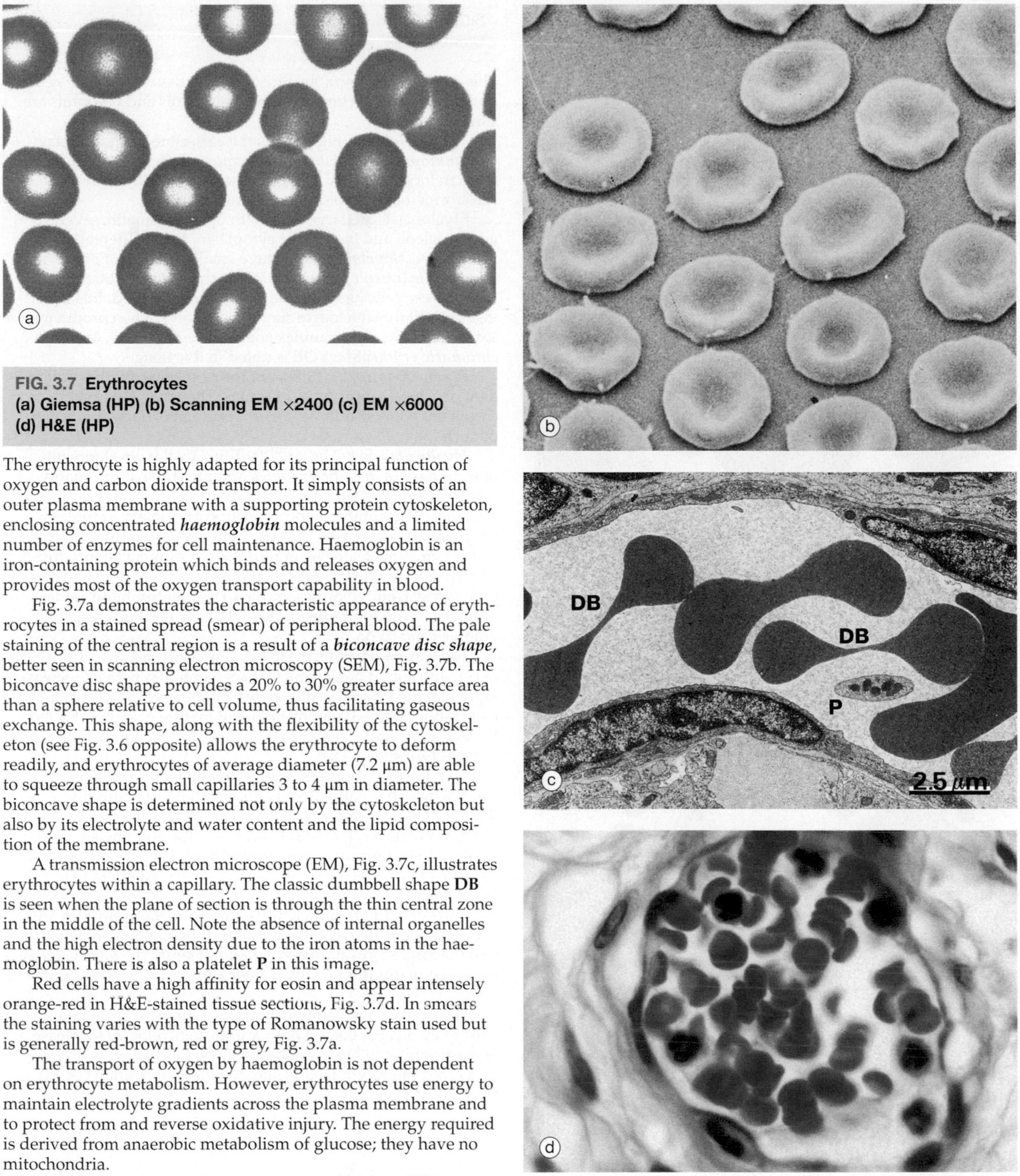

FIG. 3.7 Erythrocytes
(a) Giemsa (HP) (b) Scanning EM ×2400 (c) EM ×6000 (d) H&E (HP)

The erythrocyte is highly adapted for its principal function of oxygen and carbon dioxide transport. It simply consists of an outer plasma membrane with a supporting protein cytoskeleton, enclosing concentrated ***haemoglobin*** molecules and a limited number of enzymes for cell maintenance. Haemoglobin is an iron-containing protein which binds and releases oxygen and provides most of the oxygen transport capability in blood.

Fig. 3.7a demonstrates the characteristic appearance of erythrocytes in a stained spread (smear) of peripheral blood. The pale staining of the central region is a result of a ***biconcave disc shape***, better seen in scanning electron microscopy (SEM), Fig. 3.7b. The biconcave disc shape provides a 20% to 30% greater surface area than a sphere relative to cell volume, thus facilitating gaseous exchange. This shape, along with the flexibility of the cytoskeleton (see Fig. 3.6 opposite) allows the erythrocyte to deform readily, and erythrocytes of average diameter (7.2 μm) are able to squeeze through small capillaries 3 to 4 μm in diameter. The biconcave shape is determined not only by the cytoskeleton but also by its electrolyte and water content and the lipid composition of the membrane.

A transmission electron microscope (EM), Fig. 3.7c, illustrates erythrocytes within a capillary. The classic dumbbell shape **DB** is seen when the plane of section is through the thin central zone in the middle of the cell. Note the absence of internal organelles and the high electron density due to the iron atoms in the haemoglobin. There is also a platelet **P** in this image.

Red cells have a high affinity for eosin and appear intensely orange-red in H&E-stained tissue sections, Fig. 3.7d. In smears the staining varies with the type of Romanowsky stain used but is generally red-brown, red or grey, Fig. 3.7a.

The transport of oxygen by haemoglobin is not dependent on erythrocyte metabolism. However, erythrocytes use energy to maintain electrolyte gradients across the plasma membrane and to protect from and reverse oxidative injury. The energy required is derived from anaerobic metabolism of glucose; they have no mitochondria.

The lifespan of an erythrocyte averages 120 days. Without the appropriate organelles, erythrocytes are unable to replace deteriorating enzymes and membrane proteins and repair damage. Misshapen red cells and cells with inflexible cytoskeletons are removed from the circulation by spleen and liver macrophages.

Examination of blood can help determine the cause of anaemia

In iron deficiency, production of haemoglobin is impaired and the red cells produced are small. Their appearance is described as ***hypochromic*** and ***microcytic***, meaning of pale colour and small cell size.

Vitamins B_{12} and B_9 (folic acid) are necessary for the nuclear divisions and nuclear maturation. When these are deficient, nuclear maturation and cell divisions lag behind the cytoplasm development, giving large red cell precursors with inappropriately large nuclei and open chromatin for the cytoplasmic maturation. These have been called megaloblasts and the process megaloblastic anaemia. The final red cells are large and are named macrocytes.

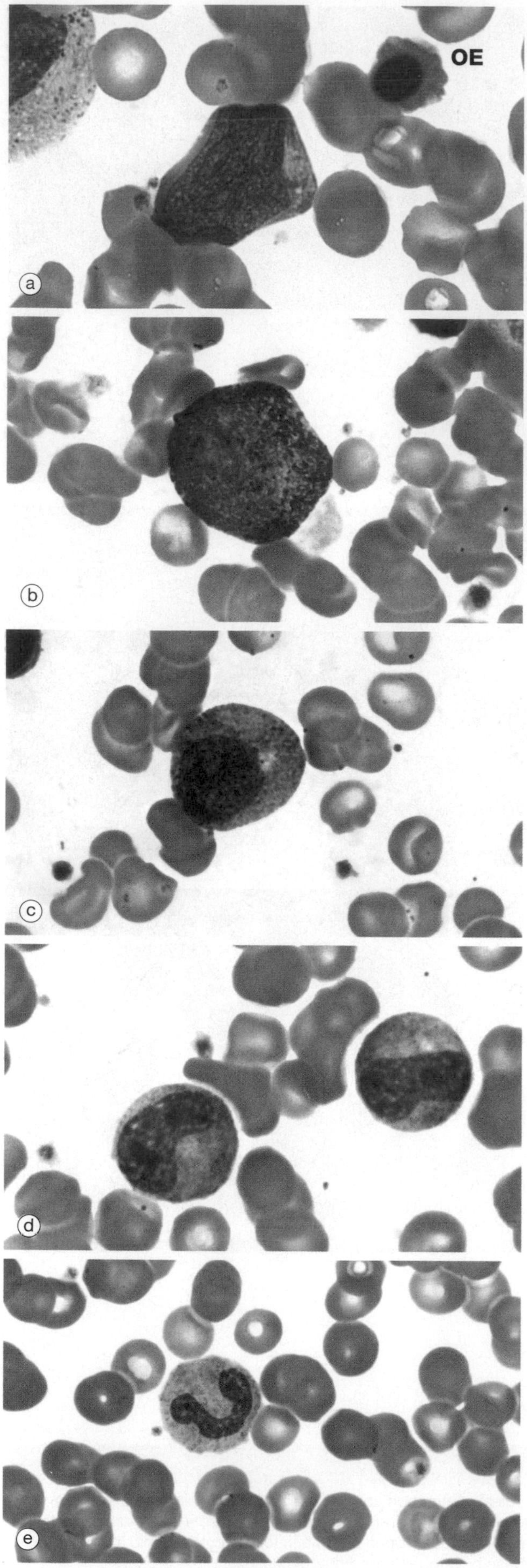

FIG. 3.8 Granulopoiesis
Giemsa (HP)

This series of photographs illustrates the development of neutrophil granulocytes. The stages for eosinophils and basophils are similar.

The ***myeloblast***, Fig. 3.8a, is the earliest recognisable stage in ***granulopoiesis***. This name is inappropriate and was derived from an incorrect view that granulocytes were the only white cells formed in myeloid tissue (bone marrow).

Myeloblasts are large cells with open chromatin, several large nucleoli and basophilic cytoplasm. More differentiated myeloblasts (***myeloblasts II***) have small numbers of ***primary azurophilic*** (purple) ***granules***. While the ultimate differentiation of these cells has been biologically determined, this is not visible until the myelocyte stage (see below), when production of secondary (specific) granules enables identification. An ***orthochromatic erythroblast*** **OE** is noted in this image.

Promyelocytes, Fig. 3.8b, are the next stage and have abundant primary (azurophilic) granules. They may show slight chromatin condensation in an otherwise fine, open chromatin pattern.

Myelocytes, Fig. 3.8c, are identified by the development of ***secondary*** or ***specific granules*** and progressive chromatin condensation; this process continues through several further cell divisions. The number and proportion of primary granules is progressively decreased, diluted by the repeated divisions of the cytoplasm, whilst specific granules are progressively produced. The myelocyte illustrated is a neutrophilic myelocyte and shows pink cytoplasmic colouration due to the neutrophil secondary granules. Eosinophil myelocytes will have eosinophil-specific granules and so on.

The ***metamyelocyte***, Fig. 3.8d, is now an end cell, incapable of cell division. It begins nuclear segmentation with an increasingly indented nucleus and shows progressive cytoplasmic maturation. Immediate precursors of mature granulocytes tend to have an irregular horseshoe nucleus and are termed ***stab cells*** or ***band forms***, Fig. 3.8e.

Immature neutrophils enter a functional ***reserve pool*** in the marrow which is equivalent to about 5 days of neutrophil production. Then, on entry to the circulation, about half these band forms circulate whilst the rest adhere to the endothelial walls of small vessels, forming a ***marginated pool***. These pools provide sizeable reserve resources and are mobilised on demand (e.g. by chemotaxins).

If the demand is sufficiently extreme, metamyelocytes and myelocytes are also mobilised into the circulation and hence into the tissues; this has been called ***left shift***. The alternative of increased maturation is called ***right shift*** but is not commonly seen.

The normal development process in marrow from myeloblast to myelocyte takes 6 days and from myelocyte to release of neutrophil into blood another 7 days. Production is driven by a range of growth factors and cytokines, including G-CSF, GM-CSF, IL-3, and IL-5.

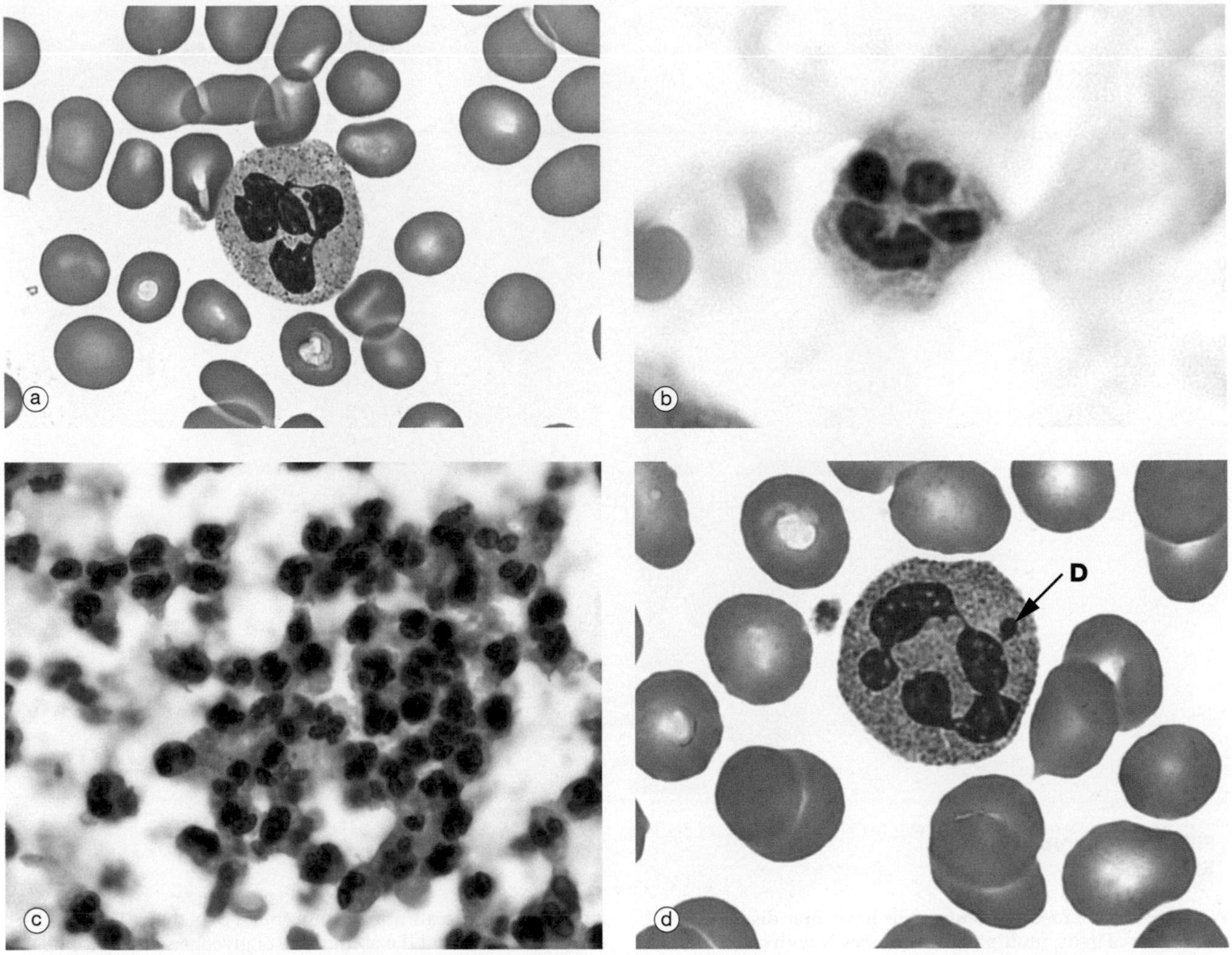

FIG. 3.9 Neutrophils
(a) Giemsa (HP) (b) H&E (HP) (c) H&E (MP) (d) Giemsa (HP)

Neutrophils account for 40% to 60% of the leukocytes in the circulating blood, with 1.0 to 5.0×10^9/L. They are 12 to 14 µm in diameter. The lifespan of a neutrophil is a few days and they are rarely found in normal tissue.

Neutrophils exhibit progressive segmentation of their nucleus, with a young cell having 2 lobes, the average cell 3 to 4 lobes and older cells 5 lobes. They have a lightly stippled granular pink cytoplasmic appearance due to numerous small membrane-bound granules (0.2 to 0.8 µm in diameter) (Fig. 3.9a). These granules include the azurophilic ***primary granules*** (purple) and the specific ***secondary granules*** (pink/lilac), ***tertiary granules*** and ***secretory granules***. In H&E stains, they have pink or pale red cytoplasm, Fig. 3.9b.

Neutrophils leave the vascular space in response to chemotactic signals generated by inflammation. They are highly motile, phagocytose bacteria and kill them by fusing the phagosome with neutrophil primary granules and producing activated oxygen derivatives. Under certain conditions, they degranulate, releasing granule contents including inflammatory mediators, antibacterial enzymes and tissue matrix breakdown enzymes. Massed neutrophils and their debris in tissue are visually recognised as pus, Fig. 3.9c (see e-Fig. 3.2). Neutrophils do not re-enter the blood stream from tissue but undergo lysis or apoptosis in tissues.

As an incidental finding the inactivated X chromosome in females is seen as a small drumstick-shaped appendage **D** in a few (3%) percent of neutrophils (Fig. 3.9d).

TABLE 3.2 Functional products of neutrophil granules

Granule type	Main active components	Actions
Primary granules	Myeloperoxidase Neutrophil defensins	Killing and degradation of engulfed micro-organisms
Specific secondary granules	Lysozyme, gelatinase, collagenase, lactoferrin, cathelicidins, transcobalamin I	Anti-microbial substances and tissue (matrix) breakdown
Tertiary granules	Gelatinase Adhesion molecules	Matrix (tissue) breakdown Fused into cell membrane
Secretory granules	Membrane proteins Enzymes, alkaline phosphatase, etc.	Fused into cell membrane; receptors for endothelial binding Tissue breakdown

D drumstick appendage **OE** orthochromatic erythroblast

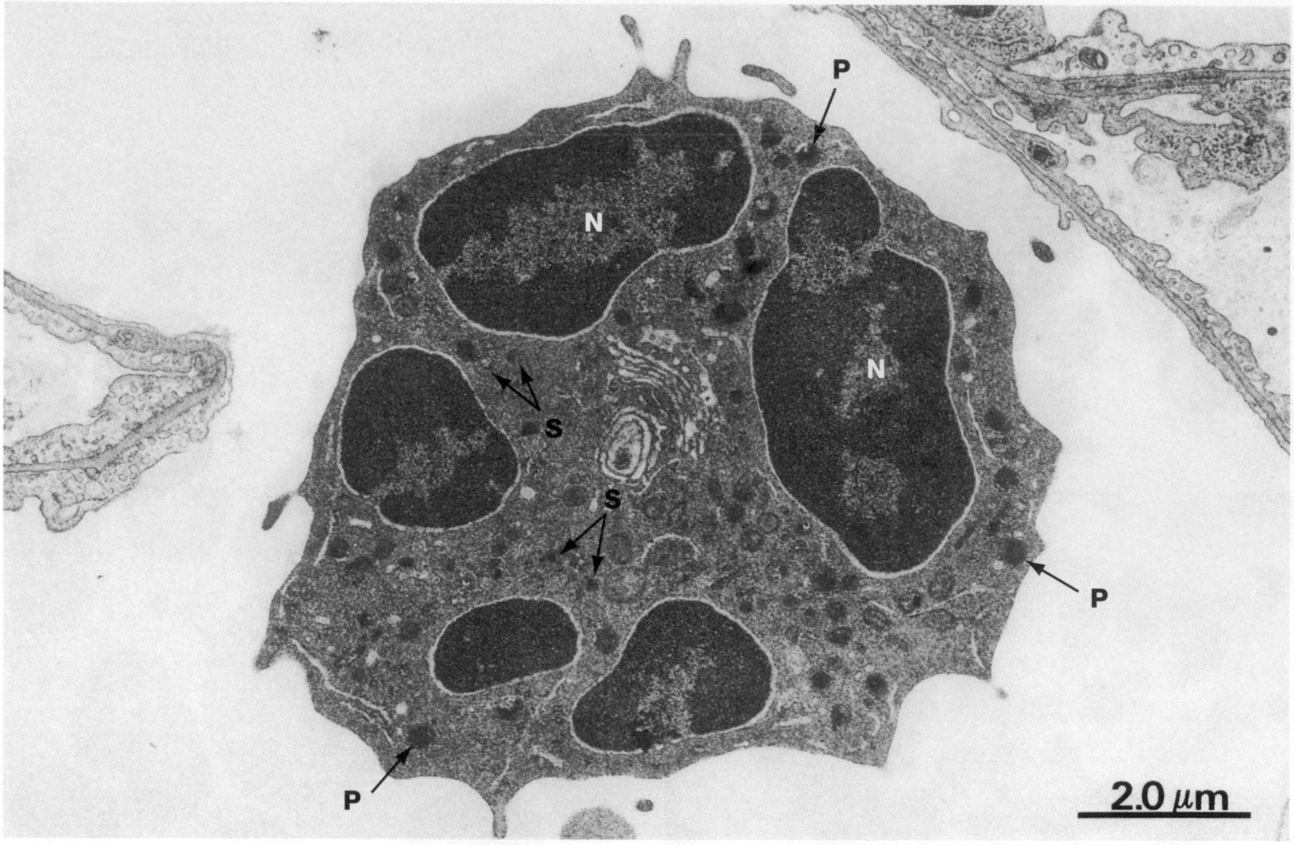

FIG. 3.10 Neutrophil
EM ×10 000

With electron microscopy, neutrophils have three distinguishing features. Firstly, multiple nuclear lobes **N** with condensed chromatin; these lobes are seen as separate in the thin EM sections. Secondly, the cytoplasm contains many membrane-bound granules. The ***primary granules*** **P** are large, spheroidal and electron-dense. The ***secondary*** or ***specific granules*** **S** are more numerous, small and often rod-like and are of variable density and shape. ***Tertiary*** and ***secretory granules*** cannot be readily distinguished from other membrane-bound vesicles on ultrastructure. The third feature is that other cytoplasmic organelles are scarce. Additionally, the cytoplasm is particularly rich in dispersed glycogen.

The mature neutrophil has few organelles for protein synthesis and has a limited capacity to regenerate secreted proteins; it tends to degenerate after a single burst of activity. The paucity of mitochondria and the abundance of glycogen in neutrophils reflect the importance of the anaerobic mode of metabolism. Energy production via glycolysis permits neutrophils to function in the poorly oxygenated environment of damaged tissues. Neutrophils are highly motile cells, moving through the extracellular spaces in a crawling fashion with an undulating ***pseudopodium*** typically thrust out in the line of advance. Motility and endocytotic (phagocytic) activity are reflected in a large content of the contractile proteins, actin and myosin, as well as tubulin and microtubule-associated proteins.

Neutrophil function

Neutrophils in the circulation are attracted by chemotactic factors (***chemotaxins***) released from damaged tissue or generated by the interaction of antibodies with antigens on the surface of the micro-organisms (see Ch. 11). Chemotaxins stimulate neutrophils and signal them to fuse secretory granules with the cell surface, thereby expressing stored cell adhesion proteins that allow the neutrophil to adhere to vascular endothelial cells and start to move into the tissues.

As the first step in ***phagocytosis***, an organism is surrounded by pseudopodia which then fuse to completely enclose it in an endocytotic vesicle called a ***phagosome***. This then fuses with cytoplasmic granules, in particular the primary granules, which discharge their contents, exposing the organism to a potent mixture of antimicrobial proteins. Killing is greatly enhanced by the generation of hydrogen peroxide and superoxide by enzymatic reduction of oxygen (respiratory burst oxidase).

Coating of organisms with antibodies and complement components (***opsonins***) enhances neutrophil (and monocyte) phagocytic activity. Neutrophils have surface receptors for the Fc (constant) portion of immunoglobulin molecules and for various complement proteins. These receptors bind to opsonins and stimulate internalisation by phagocytosis. This enhancement of phagocytosis is called ***opsonisation***.

If there is sufficient stimulation of neutrophil receptors, they will secrete their granule contents by degranulation, fusing the granule membranes with the plasma membrane, thereby externalising the contents (***exocytosis***). Tertiary granules are most readily released, followed by specific (secondary) granules and rarely primary granules.

N nuclear lobe **P** primary granule **S** secondary granule

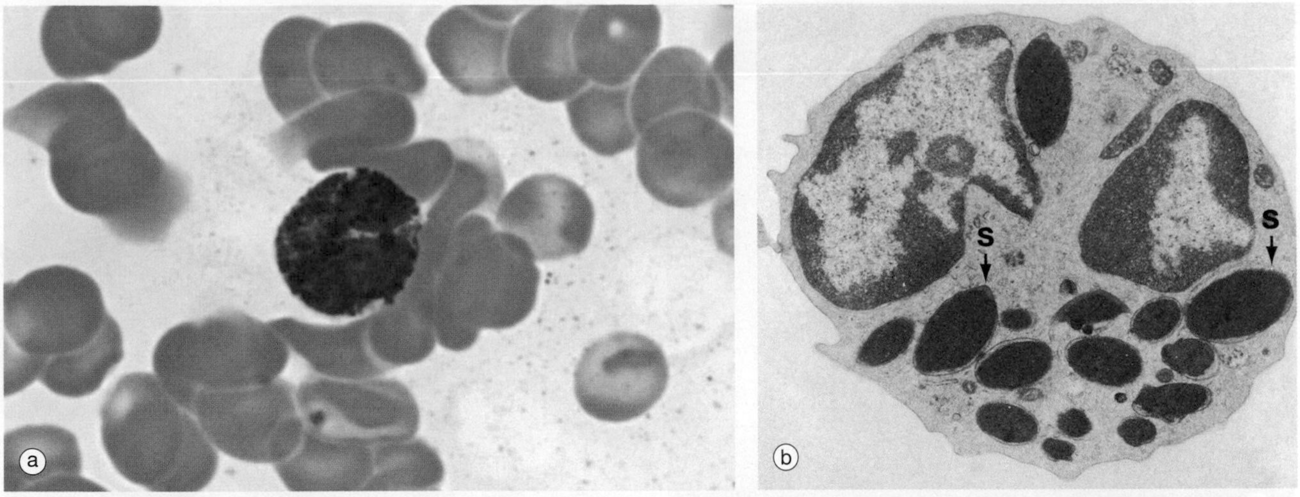

FIG. 3.11 Basophils
(a) Giemsa (HP) (b) EM ×10 500

Basophils, Fig. 3.11a, are the least common leukocyte, constituting <0.5% of leukocytes in blood; they are intermediate in size (14–16 μm in diameter) between neutrophils and eosinophils. A mature basophil has a bilobed nucleus, but this is usually obscured by numerous large, densely basophilic (deep blue) specific granules which are larger, but fewer in number, than those of eosinophils. The granule contents are highly soluble in water and may be dissolved away during preparation. Basophils are formed in the bone marrow, sharing a common precursor with eosinophils and develop through stages analogous to neutrophils and eosinophils. Basophils enter tissue in response to inflammation and chemotaxins. They are not believed to re-enter the blood. Their tissue half-life is uncertain.

When stained with the basic dye toluidine blue, the granules of basophils bind the blue dye but stain a purple colour. The phenomenon of staining a different colour to that of the dye is called ***metachromasia*** (see Fig. 4.20).

With electron microscopy, Fig. 3.11b, the basophils show their large, slightly variable, oval specific **S** (secondary) granules filled with electron-dense material. Crystalloids, lipid whorls and dense inclusions can be found in the granules (not illustrated).

The granules have a core of sulfated glycosaminoglycans, specifically chondroitin sulfate and some heparan sulfate; this is responsible for their staining characteristics. Functionally, the granules contain histamine, other vasoactive chemicals and enzymes (see Table 3.3).

Mast cells are tissue cells with many similarities to basophils, also derived from bone marrow, while remaining a different and distinct cell type (see Fig. 4.20).

TABLE 3.3 Functional products of basophils

Products	Actions
Major basic protein	Same protein as eosinophils; toxic to parasites
Charcot–Leyden protein	As per eosinophils, but in small amounts
Histamine and other vasoactive amines	Vasoactive; congestion and oedema
Tryptase	Enzyme, useful blood marker for basophils and mast cell activity
Carboxypeptidase	Enzyme
Leukotrienes and prostaglandins	Lipid mediators
Interleukin (IL)-4, IL-13, exotaxins	Cytokine release
Vascular endothelial growth factor (VEGF)	Growth factor release

Functions of basophils and mast cells

Basophils and mast cells have high-affinity IgE Fc receptors and thus bind IgE, a class of immunoglobulins involved in allergy. Cross-linking of these receptors and their attached IgE by antigen causes degranulation of the cells with an ***immediate hypersensitivity reaction***. This includes allergic rhinitis (hay fever), extrinsic asthma, skin urticaria and anaphylactic shock (common antigens include peanuts, bee sting and penicillin).

These cells are also part of the innate immune response to infection (see Ch. 11) and help recruitment of neutrophils prior to the development of the adaptive immune responses. They also have a role in reaction to parasites, such as a response to larvae of some worm species migrating through skin (cutaneous lava migrans).

An increase in blood basophils is a common finding in patients with pre-malignant bone marrow genetic mutations, known as myelodysplasia, myelofibrosis (see e-Fig. 3.5) and in chronic myeloid leukaemia (CML) (see e-Fig. 3.6).

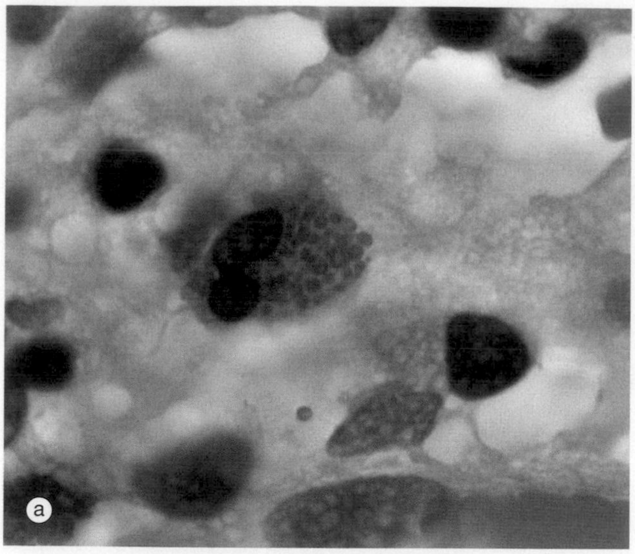

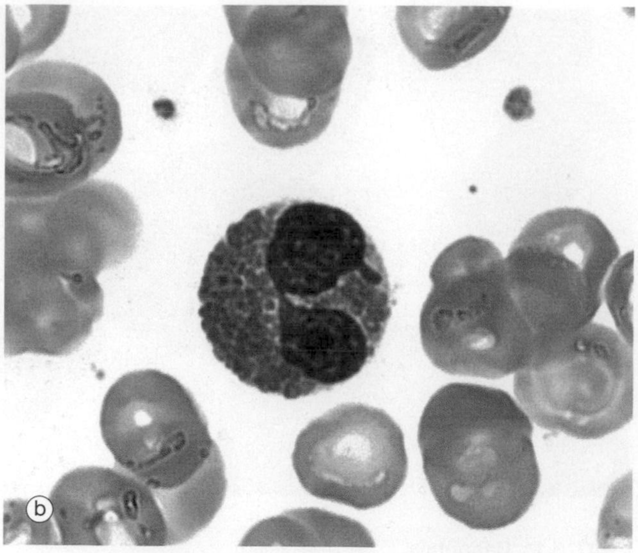

FIG. 3.12 Eosinophils
(a) H&E tissue (HP) (b) Giemsa blood (HP)

Eosinophils account for 1% to 6% of leukocytes in circulating blood; their numbers exhibit diurnal variation, being greatest in the morning and least in the afternoon. The production of eosinophils by the bone marrow is controlled by the cytokine interleukin 5 (IL-5) and to a lesser extent, interleukin 3 (IL-3) and granulocyte–monocyte colony-stimulating factor (GM-CSF). Eosinophils circulate in the blood for approximately 18 hours and exit from capillaries to enter the tissues, where the majority (>95%) of eosinophils reside.

Under normal conditions, tissue-based eosinophils are found in the mucosa of the gastrointestinal tract, mainly the intestine. Small numbers, probably in transit, are found in the spleen and lymph nodes.

Eosinophils enter other tissues in response to chemotactic signals generated by mucosal inflammatory or allergic responses; these signals include chemokines eotaxin-1 and eotaxin-2, IL-5 and some leukotrienes. The process of egress from vessels partially activates the eosinophils and they are further activated by mediators released as part of T helper cell type 2 immune responses (T_H2), including IL-5, IL-3 and GM-CSF. Appropriate stimuli cause granule and mediator release. Unlike neutrophils, they are not phagocytic cells.

Eosinophils are believed to survive in tissues for extended periods (8–12 days and longer), but experimental data are limited. Eosinophils do not generally recirculate; from the intestine they exit into the bowel lumen or otherwise undergo lysis.

The eosinophil (12–17 µm in diameter) is larger than the neutrophil and is easily recognised by its numerous large ***specific granules***, which stain bright red with eosin, Fig. 3.12a, and a more brick-red with Romanowsky methods, Fig. 3.12b. Most cells have a bilobed nucleus, but as cells mature in tissue, the nucleus can further segment. The densely packed cytoplasmic granules may partially obscure the nucleus.

The specific granules are membrane bound, of uniform size, with a matrix and a crystalloid cubic lattice structure (see Fig. 3.13 opposite). They contain extremely alkaline (i.e. basic) proteins, especially the ***major basic protein***. Other proteins include ***eosinophil cationic protein*** (***ECP***), ***eosinophil-derived neurotoxin*** (***EDN***) and an ***eosinophil peroxidase*** (***EPO***). These proteins are toxic to parasites, some RNA viruses and, in certain circumstances, tissues.

TABLE 3.4 Functional products of eosinophils

Product	Function
Major basic protein	Toxic to parasites; degranulates mast cells and basophils
Eosinophil-derived neurotoxin (EDN)	Ribonuclease with antiviral activity
Eosinophil cationic protein (ECP)	Cell membrane injury; mast cell degranulation
Eosinophil peroxidase (EPO)	Generation of reactive oxygen species, including superoxide, and hypobromic acid (from bromide ions)
Histaminase, phospholipase, acid phosphatase, arylsulphatase, cathepsin	Enzyme
Leukotrienes and prostaglandins	Lipid mediators
Interleukin (IL)-1, IL-2, IL-4, IL-5, IL-8, IL-13, tumour necrosis factor (TNF)-α	Cytokines
Transforming growth factor beta (TGF-β), TGF-α, vascular endothelial growth factor (VEGF) and platelet-derived growth factor (PDGF)	Growth factors
Charcot–Leyden crystal protein (galectin-10)	Unknown, but can form crystals in tissue

M mitochondrion **N** nucleus **R** ribosomes **rER** rough endoplasmic reticulum **S** specific granules
sER smooth endoplasmic reticulum

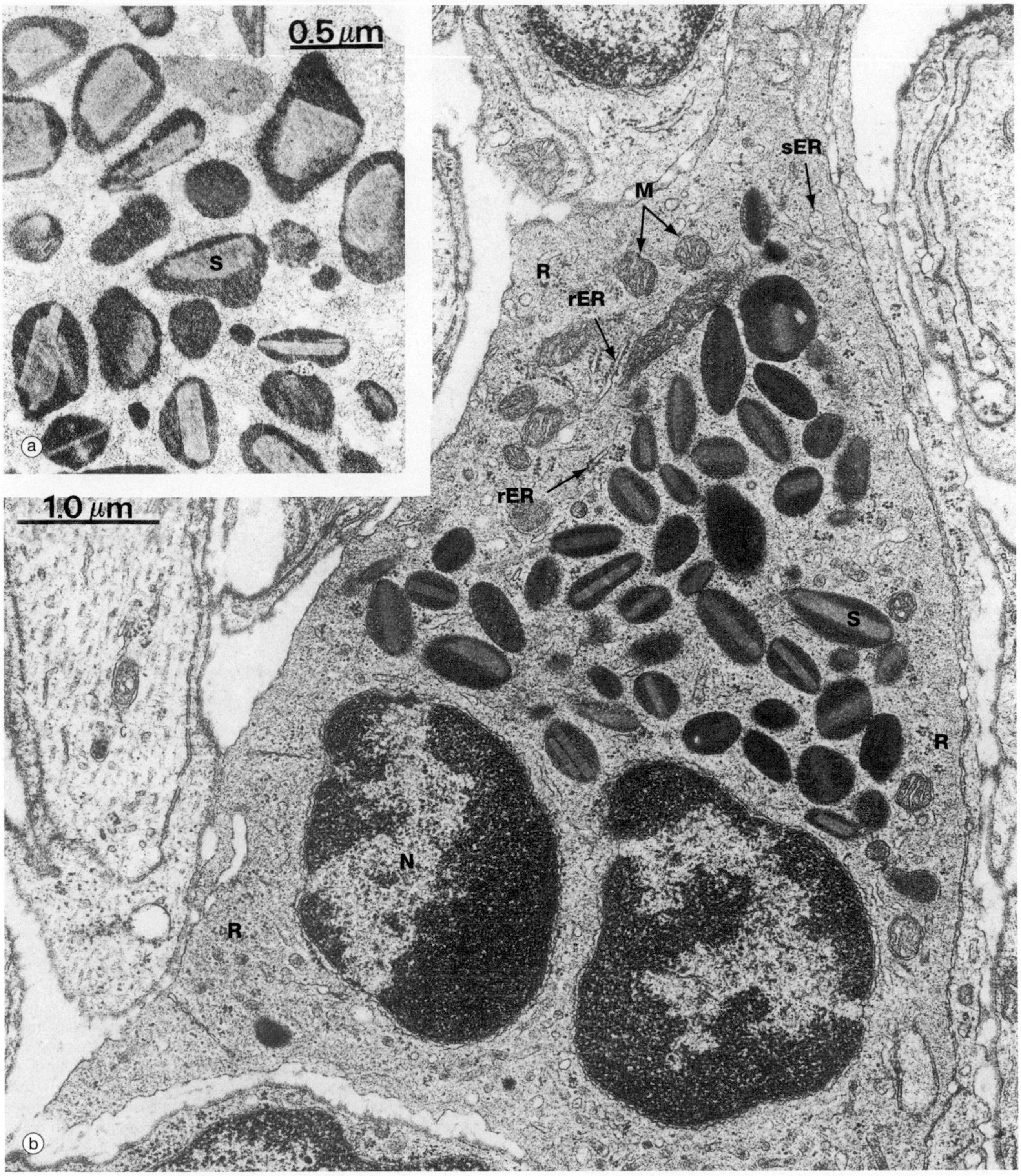

FIG. 3.13 Eosinophil
(a) EM ×25 000, human (b) EM ×20 000, mouse

On electron microscopy, these cells are dominated by the large, ovoid, specific granules **S**, each containing an elongated crystalloid. In humans, as illustrated in Fig. 3.13a, the crystalloids are relatively electron-lucent and irregular in form, but in many other mammals they have a more regular discoid shape.

Fig. 3.13b shows an eosinophil within the tissues of a mouse; in this species the crystalloids are also relatively electron-lucent. Eosinophils have only small numbers of mitochondria **M** and extensive smooth and some rough endoplasmic reticulum **sER** and **rER**. Note the free ribosomes **R** and the bilobed nucleus **N**.

Eosinophils in disease

Eosinophils are multifunctional inflammatory cells. They have a central role in response to parasites, especially worms (helminths), and a central role in the induction and maintenance of inflammatory responses due to allergy; examples include allergic rhinitis (hay fever) and asthma. They also have a role in viral infections and a lesser role in many inflammatory processes (see e-Fig. 3.7). Eosinophils have a minor role as antigen presenting cells.

Inflammatory processes involving eosinophils can often result in an increase in eosinophils in the blood (>0.5 × 10^9/L) known as ***eosinophilia***, and this may be a clinical clue to parasitic and allergic conditions.

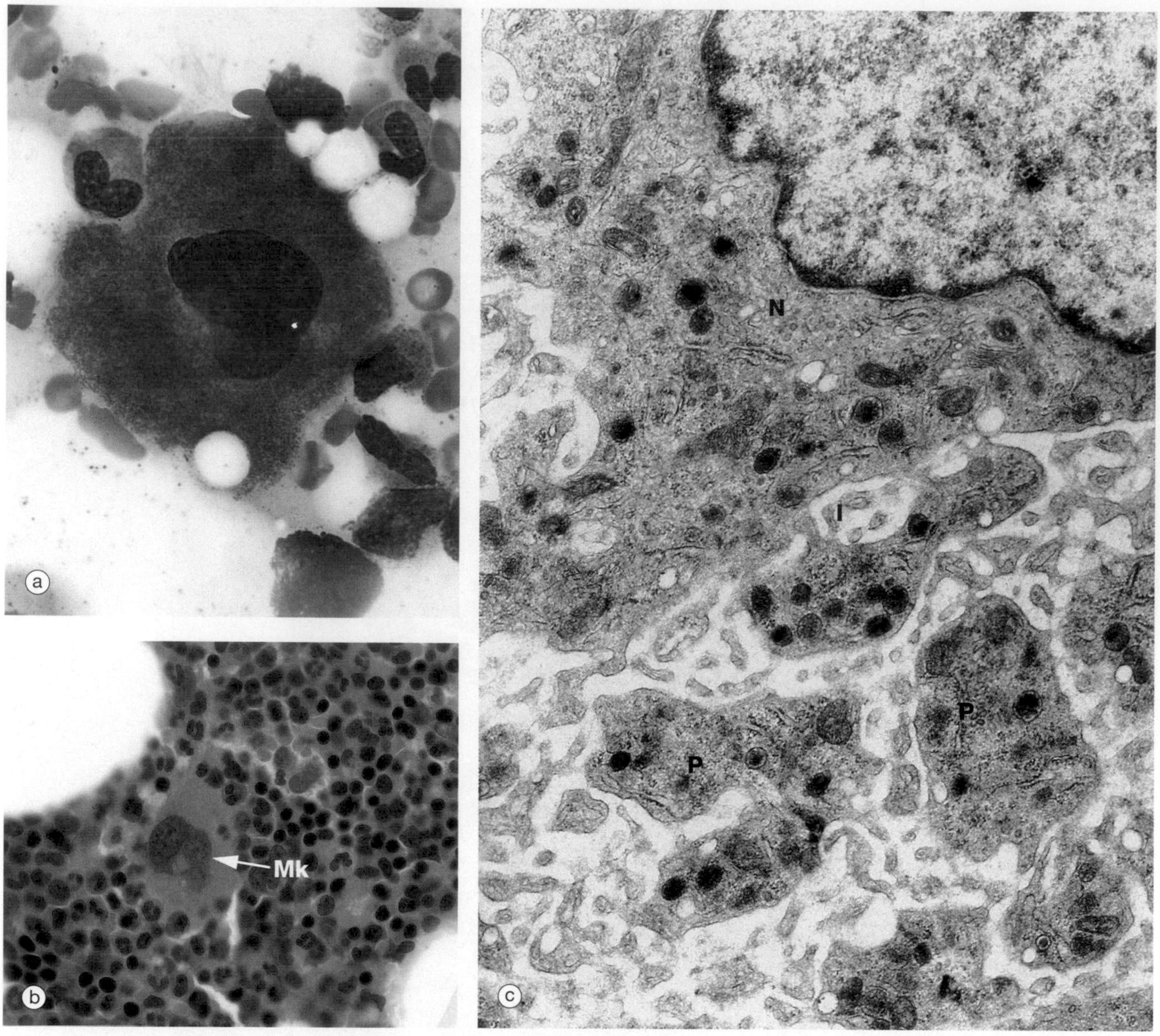

FIG. 3.14 **Platelets and megakaryocytes**
(a) Giemsa (HP) (b) H&E (MP) (c) EM ×6000

Megakaryocytes are responsible for platelet production and are the largest cells found in the bone marrow (30–100 μm). In smears, Fig. 3.14a, they have large polylobated nuclei containing clumped dispersed chromatin, inconspicuous nucleoli and abundant cytoplasm filled with fine basophilic granules. In H&E-stained histology preparations, Fig. 3.14b, megakaryocytes **Mk** are easily recognised by their size, lobulated nuclei and abundant pale eosinophilic cytoplasm.

The development and maturation of megakaryocytes is complex and the early precursors are not reliably recognisable on light microscopy. The precursor of the megakaryocyte in the bone marrow is called a ***megakaryoblast***.

The mature cells are ***polyploid***, having undergone repeated nuclear replication without cell division (***endomitosis***). A mature cell may have undergone as many as seven reduplications of nuclear and cytoplasmic constituents without cell division; hence the huge cell size and multilobed nucleus.

As they mature, the extensive cytoplasm becomes filled with fine basophilic granules, reflecting a profusion of cytoplasmic organelles, granules, vesicles and tubules. There is also an extensive system of ***demarcation membranes***, complex invaginations of the plasma membrane, which forms the basis for ultimate fragmentation into individual platelets.

Megakaryocytes sit adjacent to bone marrow sinusoids and, when mature, extrude pseudopodia known as ***proplatelets*** into the sinusoid lumens. These pseudopodia fragment, releasing platelets. Whole megakaryocytes are known to enter the sinusoid lumens, as they are occasionally found in pulmonary capillaries, where some platelets are presumably also released. The proportions released from these two sites are not known although marrow is believed to be dominant.

Each megakaryocyte will release 2000 to 4000 platelets. Each day about 100 million megakaryocytes (10^8) are needed to supply 2×10^{11} platelets for the average adult.

On electron microscopy of mature cells, Fig. 3.14c, there is a ***perinuclear zone* N** with usual organelles (Golgi apparatus, rough and smooth endoplasmic reticulum, developing granules, centrioles), an ***intermediate zone* I** with an extensive system of interconnected demarcation membranes and an ***outer zone* P** of yet more extensive membranes and cytoskeletal filaments.

Megakaryocytes and red cells have a common precursor. Megakaryocyte production, differentiation and maturation is partially driven by thrombopoietin, a growth factor produced mainly in the liver, together with interleukins (IL-3 and IL-11) and other growth factors.

I intermediate zone **Mk** megakaryocyte **N** perinuclear zone **P** incipient and mature platelets (outer zone) **Plt** platelet

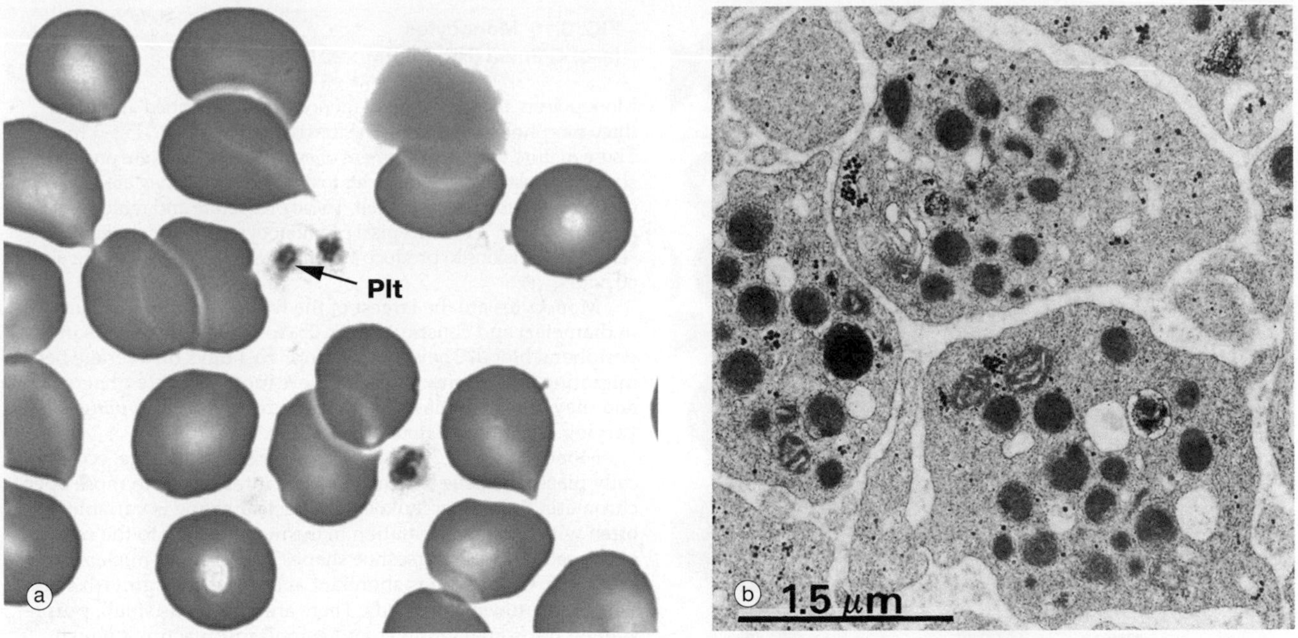

FIG. 3.15 Platelets
(a) Giemsa (HP) (b) EM ×18 000

Fig. 3.15a shows several platelets **Plt**. Platelets (***thrombocytes***) are small, non-nucleated fragments of cytoplasm released from megakaryocytes. Platelets are small, round or oval, biconvex cytoplasmic discs, varying in size from 1.5 to 3.5 μm diameter. In blood smears, they have a central purple-stained granular appearance, due to their numerous organelles and a poorly seen pale-staining periphery. Platelet numbers in circulating blood range from 150 to 500 × 10^9/L, and they survive there for 5 to 10 days.

Platelets have most of the organelles of other cells except nuclei. The conspicuous granules/organelles when seen on EM (b) can be classified into several types:

- ***Alpha granules*** are variable in size and shape. These contain many proteins related to adhesion, blood clotting and growth factors for repair.
- ***Dense granules*** are very electron-dense. They contain serotonin, ADP, ATP, Ca^{2+} and Mg^{2+}.
- ***Lysosomes*** are membrane-bound vesicles as found elsewhere, containing the usual enzymes (see Ch. 1).

Platelets are surprisingly complex. They have a marginal band of microtubules in their peripheral cytoplasm, associated with abundant contractile proteins, actin and myosin; this is a contractile system.

Located deep to the marginal band of microtubules and scattered throughout the cytoplasm is the ***dense tubular system*** (***DTS***), consisting of narrow membranous tubules with homogeneous electron-dense contents; these contain Ca^{2+} and enzymes related to the synthesis of lipid mediators of platelet activation, specifically cyclooxygenase and thromboxane synthetase.

Platelets also contain a system of interconnected membrane channels, the ***surface-connected canalicular system*** (***SCCS***), which is in continuity with the external environment via external pits; granules fuse with this system to release their contents to the exterior.

Platelets are functionally complex. They have over 50 different types of surface receptors. They respond to vessel injury to prevent bleeding and are active in blood clotting and tissue repair. On exposure to damaged tissue, platelets adhere to exposed collagen and other basement membrane proteins via their surface membrane receptors. Activation leads to contraction of the microtubule system and degranulation with release of granule contents, serotonin and ADP. Activated platelets also produce the lipid mediator thromboxane. These signals recruit adherence of additional platelets, with formation of a ***platelet plug***.

Degranulation leads to transfer of membrane proteins from storage in the granule membranes, via the membrane fusion, onto the platelet surface. This includes the glycoprotein (GP) Ib-IX-V complex and platelet integrin αIIbβ3 (GPIIb-IIIa), both important receptors. Release of coagulation factors and Ca^{2+}, and the exposure of negatively charged platelet lipids, provides a surface for assembly of coagulation factor enzyme complexes. This facilitates the coagulation cascade with production of fibrin fibrils which bind the platelets together, strengthening the platelet plug. On a larger scale, this fibrin entraps red cells and results in a blood clot.

Activated platelets take on a stellate shape, with long pseudopodia. Subsequent contraction of the cytofilaments pulls the plug or clot tighter, a process known as ***clot retraction***.

Platelets also release an array of growth factors to simulate repair; ***platelet-derived growth factor*** (***PDGF***) and ***transforming growth factor beta*** (TGF-β) amongst others. Many of the platelet functional products are inherited from the parent megakaryocyte, but some are obtained from plasma via membrane receptors, subsequent endocytosis and then storage in granules e.g. 5-HT (serotonin).

Disorders of platelets

Reduced platelet numbers is called ***thrombocytopenia***. Low levels, especially <20 × 10^9/L, are associated with spontaneous small vessel bleeding (petechiae) usually in skin and in the bowel wall; this is a life-threatening situation.

There are many genetic disorders with mutations in various proteins affecting platelet function. The commonest is von Willebrand disease, which is due to defects in von Willebrand factor (FVIII-VWF), a complex adhesion molecule produced in endothelium and megakaryocytes.

Drugs can affect platelet function. Aspirin (acetylsalicylic acid) blocks the enzyme cyclooxygenase, inhibiting thromboxane production, and thereby impairing platelet function.

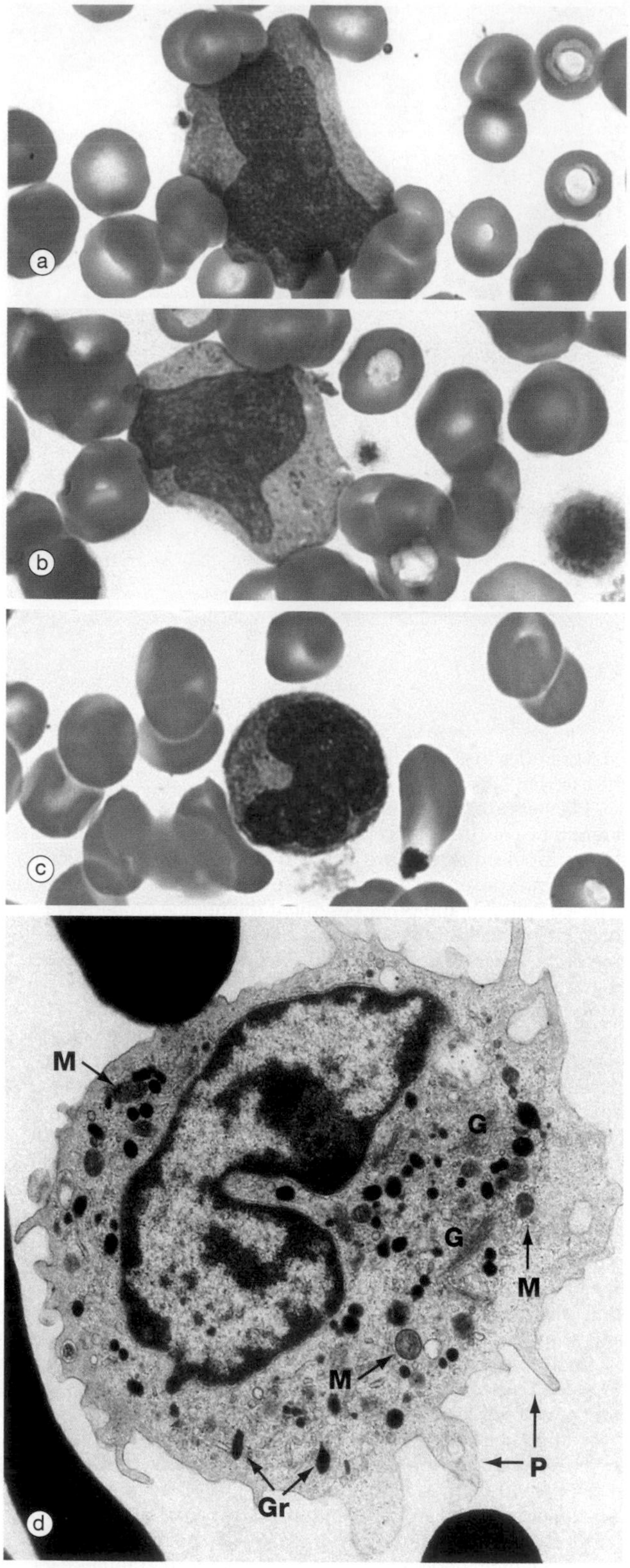

FIG. 3.16 Monocytes
(a–c) Giemsa (HP) (d) EM ×20 000

Monopoiesis, the formation of monocytes, is described as having three morphological stages. The first is the ***monoblast***, Fig. 3.16a. These mature with development of cytoplasmic granules and the start of a 'frosted glass' character to the cytoplasm; they are then called ***promonocytes***, Fig. 3.16b. These proliferate and mature into ***monocytes***, Fig. 3.16c. A typical promonocyte will undertake two serial cell divisions to produce 4 monocytes in a process taking about 60 hours.

Monocytes are the largest of the white cells (up to 20 μm in diameter) and constitute from 2% to 10% of leukocytes in peripheral blood. They circulate for 3 to 4 days on average before migrating into tissues. These cells are motile, highly phagocytic and may mature in tissues into tissue resident ***macrophages*** of varying kinds with extended lifespans.

Monocytes, Fig. 3.16c, are characterised by a large, eccentrically placed nucleus which stains less intensely with more open chromatin than other leukocytes. Nuclear shape is variable but often with a deep indentation in the nucleus near to the centre of the cell, giving a horseshoe shape. Two or more nucleoli may be visible. Cytoplasm is abundant and stains pale greyish-blue with Romanowsky methods. There are numerous small, purple-stained lysosomal granules and cytoplasmic vacuoles which confer a 'frosted-glass' appearance.

With the electron microscope, Fig. 3.16d, the cytoplasm is seen to contain a variable number of ribosomes, polyribosomes and little rough endoplasmic reticulum. The Golgi apparatus **G** is well developed and is located with the centrosome in the vicinity of the nuclear indentation. Small elongated mitochondria **M** are prolific. Small pseudopodia **P** extend from the cell, reflecting phagocytic ability and amoeboid movement.

The cytoplasmic granules **Gr** of monocytes are electron-dense and homogeneous. Half resemble primary (azurophilic) granules of neutrophils and these contain myeloperoxidase, acid phosphatase, elastase and cathepsin G. The other half are secretory granules containing plasma proteins, membrane adhesion proteins and tumour necrosis factor alpha (TNF-α).

Monocytes are capable of continuous lysosomal activity and regeneration and utilise aerobic and anaerobic metabolic pathways, depending on the availability of oxygen in the tissues.

Monocyte function

Monocytes circulate in the blood. They respond to chemotactic signals from damaged tissue, micro-organisms and inflammation by migration into the tissues and differentiation into ***macrophages***. With their capacity for phagocytosis and their content of hydrolytic enzymes, they engulf and destroy tissue debris and foreign material.

Monocytes survive and proliferate in tissue as macrophages if they are stimulated by growth factors, such as macrophage colony-stimulating factor (M-CSF), granulocyte-macrophage colony-stimulating factor (GM-CSF) or IL-3, but do not re-enter the circulation.

Macrophages have receptors for numerous chemokines and cytokines, including interferon gamma (IFN-γ), a cytokine produced by T lymphocytes (Ch. 11). They can process antigens and present antigen to T cells to promote an adaptive immune response. They can secrete numerous chemokines, cytokines and growth factors involved in inflammation, immunity, tissue healing and repair.

Lb lymphoblast **Lc** lymphocyte **G** Golgi apparatus **Gr** granules **M** mitochondrion **P** pseudopodia

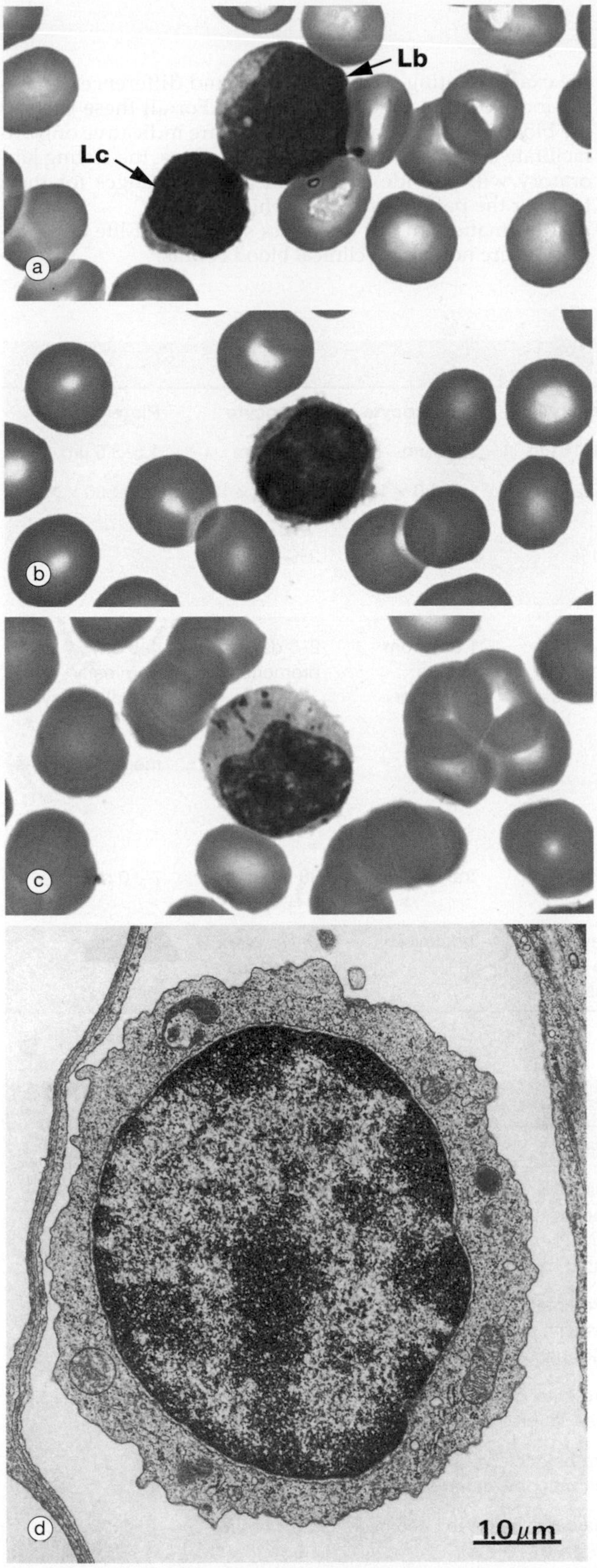

FIG. 3.17 Lymphocytes
(a–c) Giemsa (HP) (d) EM ×15 000

Lymphocytes have a central role in immunological defence mechanisms and are described in detail in Ch. 11. Lymphocyte production from haematopoietic stem cells occurs in marrow. An early recognisable form is the ***lymphoblast*** **Lb**, illustrated in Fig. 3.17a, with an adjacent lymphocyte **Lc**. The lymphoblast is larger than a lymphocyte, with fine, open nuclear chromatin, a few pale inconspicuous nucleoli and scant cytoplasm. Some lymphoblasts mature in bone marrow into B cells, others mature via the thymus into T cells, while yet others differentiate into natural killer cells (NK cells) in bone marrow.

The lymphocytes circulate between various lymphoid tissues and other tissues of the body via the blood and lymphatic vessels. They continuously transit through tissues and back into the circulation as part of immune surveillance. Lymphoid cells have a variable lifespan ranging from weeks to an indefinite lifespan and, unlike granulocytes, are not end cells; they can proliferate, with most proliferation occurring in tissues. Lymphopoiesis is a constant but relatively inconspicuous activity in bone marrow.

Lymphocytes constitute 20% to 40% of the circulating leukocytes, with 1.0 to 4.5×10^9/L. Lymphocytes are the smallest of the white cells, being only slightly larger than erythrocytes. They generally have a round or oval, densely stained nucleus with clumped chromatin and a relatively small amount of pale, basophilic, non-granular cytoplasm **Lc**, Fig. 3.17a. These small lymphocytes are 'inactive' forms.

A proportion of the normal lymphoid cells are larger with bigger nuclei, more cytoplasm and small numbers of cytoplasmic granules. These are known as ***large granular lymphocytes*** (***LGL***) and represent natural killer cells or cytotoxic T lymphocytes, Fig. 3.17b.

The state of the nucleus and the amount of cytoplasm depends upon the activity of the cell. When activated or proliferating, the lymphocytes increase in size with larger nuclei, open chromatin, visible large nucleoli and more cytoplasm (Fig. 3.17c). Some of these reactive cells circulate in the blood, particularly during inflammatory processes; activated B cells may settle in tissue, maturing into long-lived antibody-secreting ***plasma cells***.

Fig. 3.17d is an electron micrograph of a small circulating lymphocyte in a pulmonary capillary. The nucleus is rounded but slightly indented and the chromatin moderately condensed and clumped; nucleoli are not present. The sparse cytoplasm contains a few mitochondria, a rudimentary Golgi apparatus, minimal endoplasmic reticulum and a comparatively large number of free ribosomes. The plasma membrane exhibits small cytoplasmic projections which appear as short microvilli.

Disorders of lymphocytes

Infectious mononucleosis is a viral infection due to Epstein–Barr virus. Among many effects it manifests lymphadenopathy (enlarged lymph nodes) and often prominently increased blood lymphocyte counts (lymphocytosis). Marked activation/reactive changes are seen in the blood lymphocytes, hence the name for the disease. Increased uniform-appearing small lymphocytes are found in blood in chronic lymphocytic leukaemia (CLL), a common disease in the elderly (see e-Fig. 3.4).

REVIEW

Clinical blood cell tests (the ***full blood count***) usually include counts of cells in blood and size information about red cells and platelets. These vary. Neonatal normal values vary with the time since birth, differing from one day of life to the next. Normal values in children differ from normal values in adults, and male and female values differ after adolescence until at least menopause. There are also population-based differences, subtle differences with the exact counting technology used and differences due to the individual machine's calibration. For all these reasons the blood count numbers in Table 3.5 are indicative only. To facilitate interpretation of full blood counts, the testing laboratory will provide appropriate normal ranges for their tests for the patient's demographic.

Information on cell dynamics such as half-life and production are not part of clinical blood counts.

TABLE 3.5 Review of mature blood cell types

	Erythrocyte	Neutrophil	Eosinophil	Basophil	Lymphocyte	Monocyte	Platelet
Size	6.7–7.7 μm	12–14 μm	12–17 μm	14–16 μm	5–20 μm	16–20 μm	1.5–3.5 μm
Numbers in blood	$3.9–6.0 \times 10^{12}$/L	$1.5–7.5 \times 10^9$/L	$0.04–0.5 \times 10^9$/L	$<0.2 \times 10^9$/L	$1.5–4.0 \times 10^9$/L	$0.2–0.8 \times 10^9$/L	$150–500 \times 10^9$/L
Proportion of total white cells		40%–75%	1%–6%	<1%	20%–50%	2%–10%	
Development time (normal)	5–7 days from proerythroblast	7 days from myelocyte	6–9 days from myelocyte	6–9 days from myelocyte	1 day from mature precursor	2–3 days from promonocyte	4–5 days from early megakaryocyte
Marrow production per day per Kg body weight	3×10^9	1.5×10^9	0.22×10^9			0.17×10^9	2.5×10^9~10^6 megakaryocytes
Blood transit time	120 days	8–12 hours	18 hours	3 days	Transit only	30 hours	7–10 days
Normal lifespan ex-marrow	120 days	3–4 days	3–12 days	Days; may be greater in tissue?	Indefinite	Days; years as a tissue macrophage	7–10 days

TABLE 3.6 Review of blood cell functions

Cell type	Key features	Functional attributes	Figure
Red blood cell (erythyrocyte)	Oxygen and carbon dioxide carriage	End anucleate cells Specialised for mechanical flexibility 120 day lifespan Contain concentrated haemoglobin	3.1–3.7
Neutrophils	Acute inflammation and defence against bacteria	End cells; cannot re-enter blood Numerous granules with proinflammatory and antibacterial products Phagocytose and kill bacteria	3.8–3.10
Eosinophils	Inflammation, allergy and defence against parasites	End cells; cannot re-enter blood Numerous granules with proinflammatory and anti-parasite products	3.12, 3.13
Basophils	Inflammation, allergy and defence against parasites	End cells; cannot re-enter blood Numerous granules with proinflammatory products	3.11
Monocytes	Inflammation and defence against infections	Can mature into macrophages (can become long-term tissue macrophages) Ingest organisms and debris Major cytokine producers	3.16
Lymphocytes	Adaptive immune system	After formation can proliferate in tissue and lymph nodes and recirculate through blood	3.17
Platelets (thrombocytes)	Blood clotting (haemostasis)	Cell fragments produced by fragmentation of megakaryocyte cytoplasm Major source of growth factors at sites of injury	3.14, 3.15

4 Supporting/connective tissues

INTRODUCTION

Supporting/connective tissue is the term applied to tissues which provide general structure, mechanical strength, space filling (sculpting body shape), and physical and metabolic support for more specialised tissues.

Connective tissues usually have three structural properties with corresponding construction materials:

- ***Tensile strength*** to resist pulling, stretching and tearing. This is provided by strong fibres of structural proteins from the ***collagen*** family.
- ***Elasticity*** to facilitate return to original shape after mechanical distortion. This is provided mostly by specialised ***elastin*** fibrils which function like rubber.
- ***Volume*** (i.e. bulk/substance). This is provided by ***glycoproteins*** and ***complex carbohydrates*** with profound water-binding ability, forming a wet gel known as ***ground substance***.

The combined mix of fibres and ground substance is called ***extracellular matrix*** and this determines the physical properties of the tissue. Matrix is produced and assembled under the control of ***support cells***, most commonly ***fibroblasts***. The cells of supporting tissue are derived from precursor cells in primitive (fetal) supporting tissue called ***mesenchyme***.

Supporting tissues occur with diverse physical properties. In most organs, loose connective tissue (also known as ***areolar tissue***) acts as a biological packing and wrapping material. Tissue with a greater density of fibres provides a structural framework. Dense forms of supporting tissue provide tough physical support in the dermis of the skin, comprise the robust capsules of organs such as the liver and spleen, and the specialised high–tensile strength ligaments and tendons. ***Cartilage*** and ***bone***, both major skeletal components, are specialised forms of connective tissue that are considered separately in Ch. 10.

Specialised fat storage is a further function, with ***adipose tissues*** having important metabolic roles. ***White adipose tissue*** also provides a structural fill and forms part of shock-absorbing padding. Highly metabolically active ***brown adipose tissue*** helps in the regulation of body temperature and body weight.

In addition, supporting tissues usually contain blood vessels, lymphatic vessels and associated nerves. Repair of tissue damage, especially wound closure and scar formation, is also largely a function of supporting tissues, involving both the support cells and blood and lymphatic vessels.

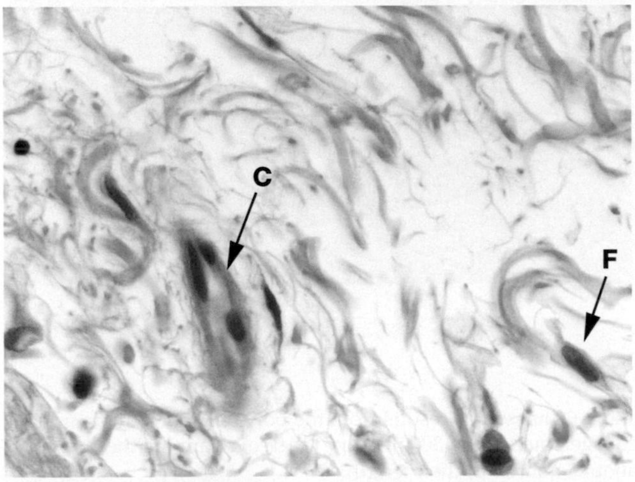

FIG. 4.1 Components of connective tissue
H&E (HP)

The components of connective tissue are seen in Fig. 4.1 which shows tissue from the submucosa of the bowel wall. The main component is extracellular matrix material which is largely composed of organised bundles of fibrous proteins, seen as wavy bundles of pink-stained material. Ground substance is unstained and is seen as the pale spaces between the pink-staining fibrous proteins.

The cell density of support tissues is generally low, reflected by the scattered cell nuclei seen in this type of tissue. The cells seen here are fibroblasts **F** with a few cells of the immune defence system. In the centre of this micrograph is a blood vessel **C**.

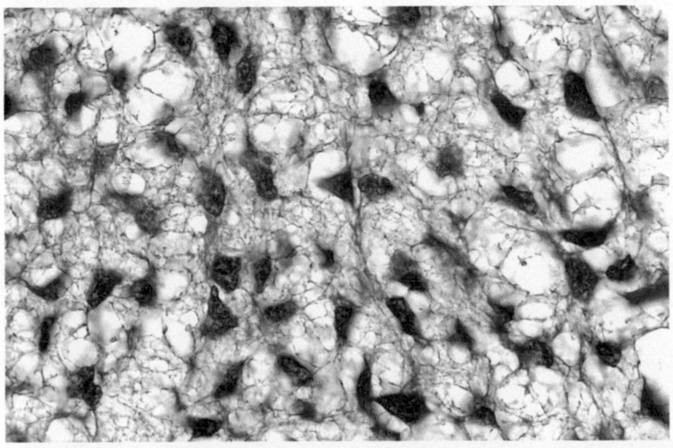

FIG. 4.2 Mesenchyme
H&E (HP)

Mesenchyme is the embryological tissue from which all types of supporting/connective tissue are derived. Mesenchymal cells are relatively unspecialised and are capable of differentiation into all supporting tissue cell types. Some mesenchymal cells remain in mature supporting tissue and act as stem cells (see Ch. 2).

Mesenchymal cells have an irregular, star (***stellate***) or spindle (***fusiform***) shape, with delicate branching cytoplasmic extensions which form an interlacing network throughout the tissue. The nuclei have dispersed chromatin and visible nucleoli. The matrix consists almost exclusively of blue-staining ground substance without mature fibres, facilitating diffusion of metabolites to and from developing tissues.

C capillary blood vessel **F** fibroblast

FIBRES OF CONNECTIVE TISSUE

The fibrous components of connective tissues are of two main types: ***collagen*** (including ***reticulin***, which was formerly considered a separate fibre type) and ***elastin***.

Collagen

Collagen is the main fibre type found in most supporting tissues and is the most abundant protein in the human body. Its notable function is the provision of tensile strength to resist pulling, stretching and tearing.

Collagen is secreted into the extracellular matrix by connective tissue cells (e.g. fibroblasts) in the form of a ***tropocollagen monomer***. This consists of three polypeptide chains (each called an ***alpha chain*** and not necessarily all identical), bound together to form a helical protein structure 300 nm long and 1.5 nm in diameter. In the extracellular matrix, these tropocollagen molecules polymerise longitudinally and also side-to-side, forming ***collagen fibrils*** which are cross-linked by the enzyme lysyl oxidase.

At least 28 different types of collagen (designated by Roman numerals I to XXVIII) have now been delineated in the collagen super-family on the basis of morphology, amino acid composition and physical properties. Collagens can be fibre forming, mesh/network forming or cell membrane–associated proteins.

- **Type I collagen** is the main structural collagen and is found in fibrous supporting tissue, skin (dermis), tendons, ligaments and bone. The tropocollagen molecules polymerise longitudinally and also side-to-side to form fibrils, and these are strengthened by numerous intermolecular bonds. Parallel collagen fibrils are further arranged into strong fibre bundles 2 to 10 μm in diameter, which confer great tensile strength to the tissue. These collagen fibres are visible with the light microscope, staining pink with H&E, with fibres in varying patterns of orientation, size and density according to the mechanical support required in the tissue.
- **Type II collagen** is the main structural collagen of hyaline cartilage and consists of fibrils in the cartilage ground substance.
- **Type III collagen** forms the delicate branched 'reticular' supporting meshwork which is prominent in highly cellular tissues such as the liver, bone marrow and lymphoid organs. This fibre was initially recognised by its affinity for silver salts and was (and often still is) called reticulin.
- **Type IV collagen** is a network/mesh-forming collagen and is an important constituent of ***basement membranes***.
- **Type VII collagen** forms special anchoring fibrils that link extracellular matrix to basement membranes.

The remaining collagen types are present in various specialised situations.

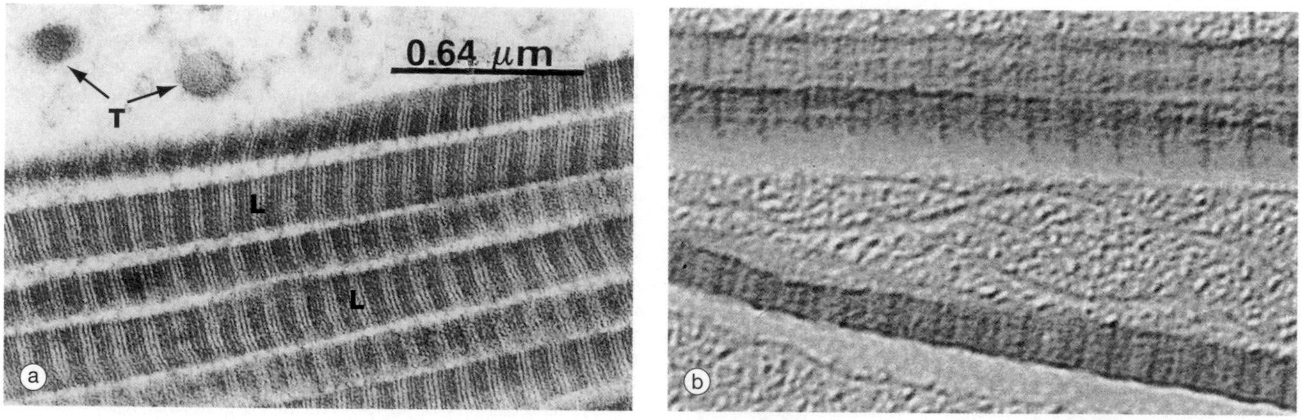

FIG. 4.3 Collagen
(a) EM ×32 000 (b) SEM ×32 000, teased preparation

The typical appearance of type I collagen is shown here. The fibres are seen in transverse **T** and longitudinal **L** sections. A characteristic feature is the cross-banding, with a periodicity of about 64 nm which results from the polymerisation of the tropocollagen molecules (300 nm long) each overlapping the next by about a quarter of their length.

Ap adipocytes **BV** blood vessels **E** elastin fibres **F** fibroblasts **L** longitudinal collagen fibres **SM** smooth muscle **T** transverse collagen fibres

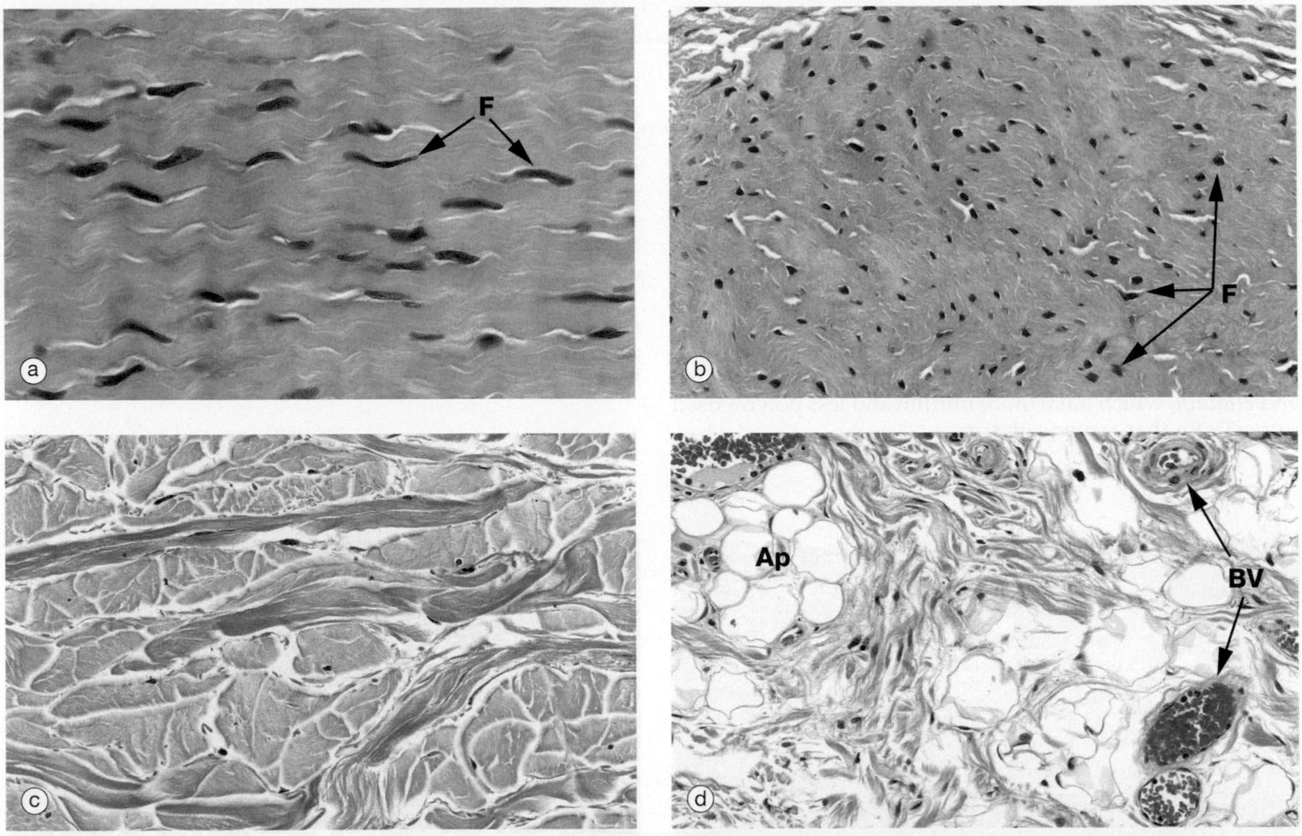

FIG. 4.4 Collagen
(a) H&E (HP) (b–d) H&E (MP) (e) Trichrome (HP)

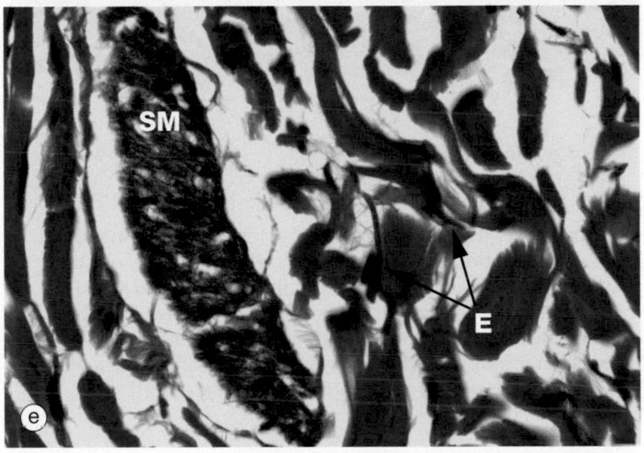

These micrographs show variations in the size and packing of collagen fibres (type I collagen) and demonstrate fibroblasts **F**. Fig. 4.4a and b are from a fascia in the hand, with (a) longitudinal and (b) transverse; in these the collagen fibres are large, tightly packed and oriented in one direction for maximal tensile strength. Fig. 4.4c is from the dermis of the skin, with less tightly packed collagen fibres running perpendicular to each other (longitudinal and transverse) to give strength in both directions. Fig. 4.4d is fibroadipose tissue from a finger, with fine collagen fibres coursing between adipocytes **Ap** and blood vessels **BV**. Fig. 4.4e is a trichrome stain of skin; collagen stains blue, smooth muscle **SM** red, and elastin fibres **E** red.

FIG. 4.5 Reticulin fibres (type III collagen)
Silver impregnation method/neutral red (HP)

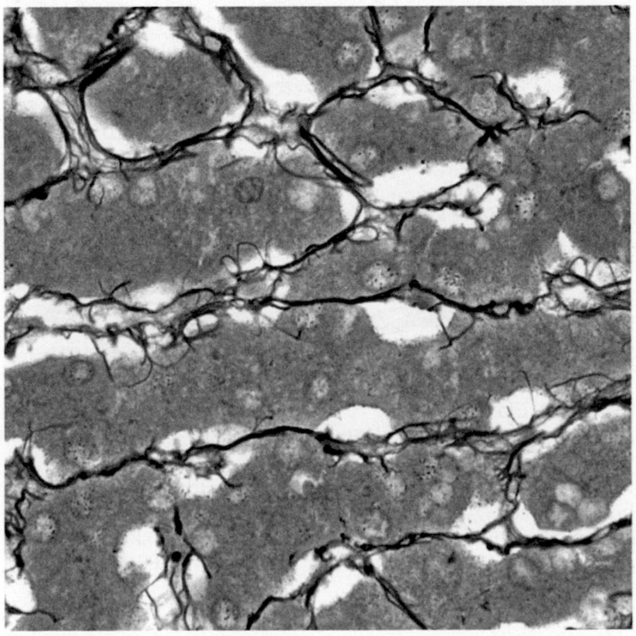

Reticulin fibres form a delicate supporting framework for many cellular organs such as endocrine glands, lymph nodes, bone marrow and liver. A fine network of branching fibres ramifies throughout the parenchyma, often anchored to collagenous septa which traverse the tissue. Reticulin is a non-banded form of collagen, type III collagen.

Reticulin fibres stain poorly in H&E preparations but are able to absorb metallic silver, staining them black. Reticulin is the earliest type of collagen fibre to be produced during the development of all supporting tissues. It is found in varying quantities in most mature supporting tissues.

Fig. 4.5 shows the fine reticulin scaffolding of the liver; the framework supports the hepatocytes (the purple-stained plates of cells) and the sinusoids through which blood flows.

Elastin

Elastin is arranged as fibres and/or discontinuous sheets in the extracellular matrix where it confers the properties of stretching and elastic recoil. Elastin is a protein synthesised by fibroblasts in the form of a precursor monomer known as ***tropoelastin***. The monomers are polymerised in the extracellular matrix by the enzyme lysyl oxidase, with extensive cross-linking of lysine amino acid side chains. Deposition of elastin in the form of fibres requires the presence of a template of microfibrils of the structural glycoprotein ***fibrillin*** and associated glycoproteins. These become incorporated around and within the ultimate elastic fibre.

Elastin is the name of both the fibre and the polymerised protein. There are also two named related fibres, ***oxytalan*** and ***elaunin***, which have more fibrillin and less polymerised tropoelastin than generic elastin.

Elastin is found in varying proportions in most supporting tissues, conferring elasticity to enable recovery of tissue shape following normal physiological deformation. Elastin is present in large amounts in tissues such as lung, skin and urinary bladder. It is an important constituent of the wall of blood vessels; in arteries, elastin provides the stretch and recoil to smooth and transmit the pulse pressure generated by each heartbeat. In the lung, the stretch and recoil of the elastin is basic to that organ's function.

Elastic fibres are eosinophilic and when large they are slightly ***refractile***, meaning they bend light differently to other tissue components. This may enable their recognition; however, special elastin stains are usually needed.

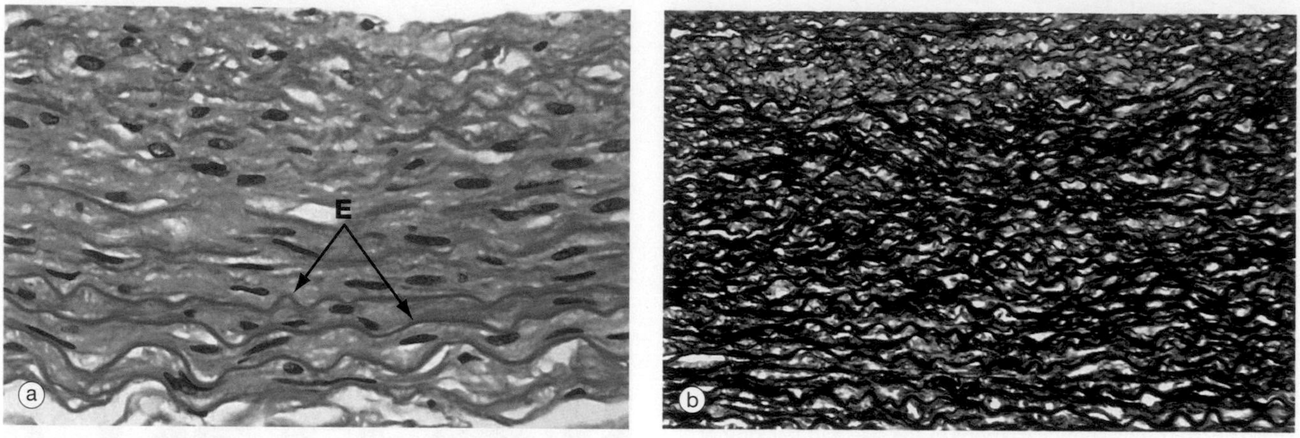

FIG. 4.6 Elastin fibres
(a) H&E (HP) (b) Elastin stain (HP)

Fig. 4.6a shows the wall of an elastic artery, made up mainly of alternating smooth muscle cells and thick sheets of elastin admixed with collagen (see Ch. 8). Like collagen and smooth muscle cytoplasm, elastin **E** is eosinophilic; it is recognisable here because the elastin sheets are thick and slightly refractile, slightly more eosinophilic than the other components and have a wave-like conformation due to relaxation of the vessel wall.

Fig. 4.6b shows a histological section of an elastic artery stained specifically for elastin; with this method, elastin is stained black and collagen red. The functional properties of large arteries are mainly determined by the amount of elastin in their walls, which allows stretching and recoil with the pulse pressure generated by the heart.

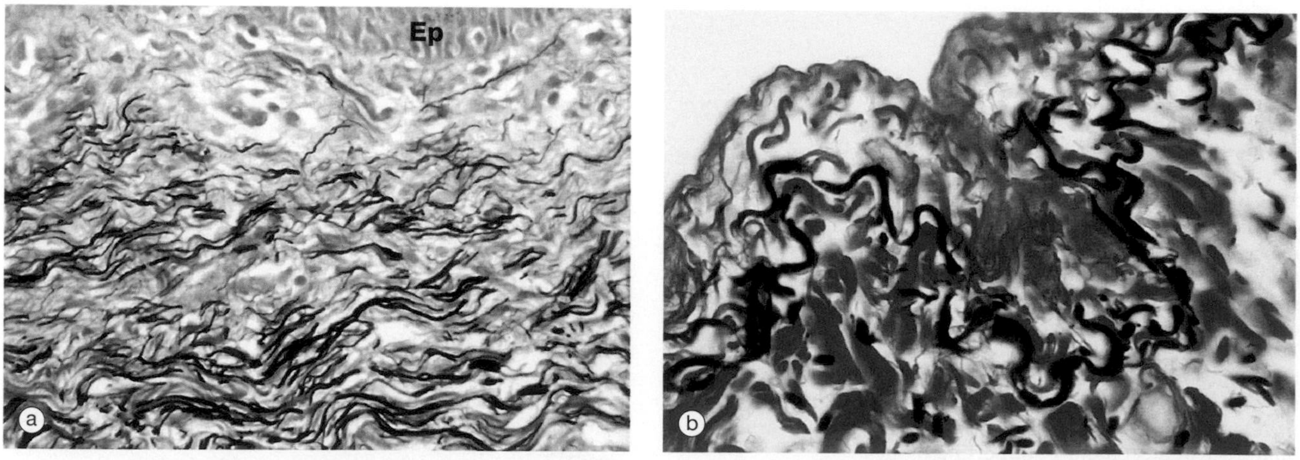

FIG. 4.7 Elastin fibres
(a) Elastin stain (MP) (b) Elastin stain (HP)

In Fig. 4.7a of skin, the pink-stained, coarse, closely packed bundles of collagen in the dermis are interwoven by elastic fibres, stained black. Elastic fibres in the dermis allow the skin to stretch and recoil, keeping it wrinkle-free. The epidermis **Ep** is just visible.

Fig. 4.7b shows pleura (see Ch. 12) where a layer of elastic fibres, stained black, is woven into the collagen supporting tissues (stained red). The lung contains abundant elastic fibres which help to expel air in expiration.

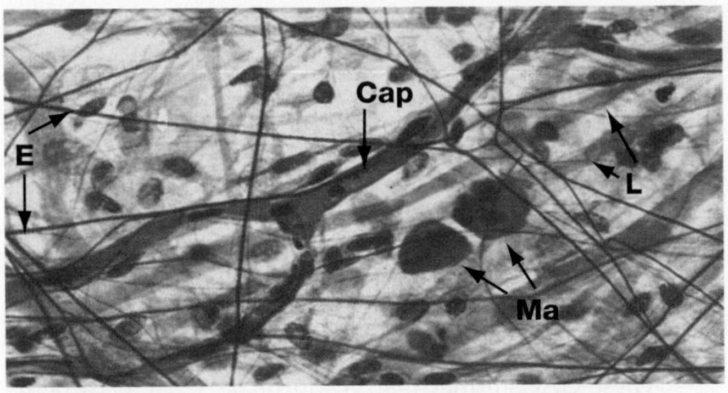

FIG. 4.8 Elastin fibres (spread preparation) Elastin H&E (HP)

In most tissues, elastin occurs as short, branching fibres which form an irregular network throughout the tissue. This is not easily seen in tissue sections. It can be better demonstrated in ***spread preparations*** as in Fig. 4.8 in which elastin fibres **E** are stained dark purple, collagen fibres **L** are stained pink and nuclei are stained blue. A branched capillary **Cap** crosses the field and two densely stained mast cells **Ma** are also seen (see Fig. 4.20).

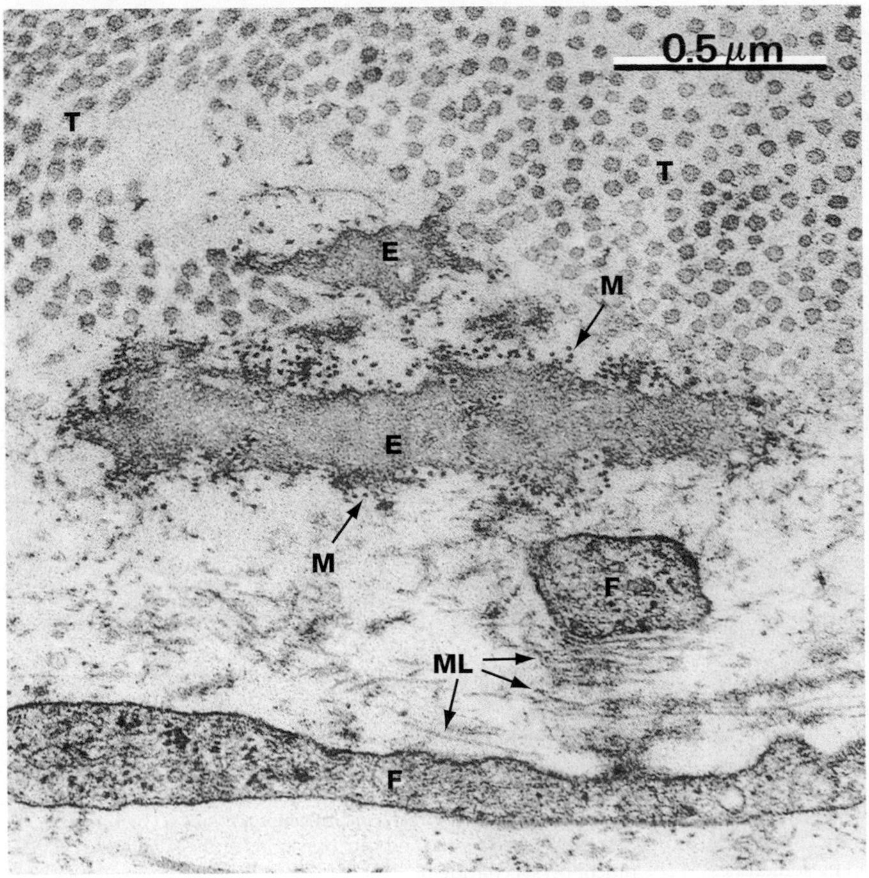

FIG. 4.9 Elastin EM ×50 000

Fig. 4.9 shows elastin **E** in the delicate supporting tissue underlying the epithelium of mouse trachea. The field also contains collagen fibrils **T** (cut in transverse section) and the fine cytoplasmic extensions of fibroblasts **F**, responsible for elaboration of the extracellular constituents.

The elastin is mostly an amorphous mass of polymerised tropoelastin. Microfibrils **M** of the structural glycoprotein fibrillin, which is involved in the process of elastin deposition, can just be discerned at this magnification as dots (in transverse section) lying within and around the elastin.

Microfibrils can also be seen in the lower part of the field cut in longitudinal section **ML** in association with small amounts of elastin protein.

Diseases due to disorders of collagen

Scurvy is a classical disease, historically of sailors, where defective collagen formation from lack of vitamin C results in loose teeth, skin haemorrhages and death. Small haemorrhages around skin hair follicles are an early sign.

There are several inherited diseases caused by mutations in genes coding for types I and III collagen. Their main effects are in reduced tensile strength in supporting tissues, leading to abnormal tissue laxity or susceptibility to injury. Ehlers–Danlos syndromes, for example, are characterised by abnormal skin laxity and hypermobility of joints which can predispose to recurrent joint dislocations. Thirteen forms have been described, which have distinct clinical associations. The vascular subtype of Ehlers–Danlos syndrome can lead to bulges in the walls of arteries (***aneurysms***) (e-Fig. 4.1). These can rupture, causing death.

Cap capillary **E** elastin fibres **Ep** epidermis **F** fibroblasts **L** longitudinal collagen fibres **M** microfibrils (fibrillin) **Ma** mast cells **ML** longitudinal microfibrils **T** transverse collagen fibres

GROUND SUBSTANCE

Ground substance derived its name from being an amorphous transparent material with the physical character of semi-solid gel. It is a mixture of glycoproteins and complex carbohydrates with profound water-binding ability. Extra-cellular fluid, both water and salts (particularly sodium), are bound to these molecules, providing volume and compression resistance to the tissue and its tissue turgor (i.e. the internal pressure). They form the physical milieu and indirectly control the passage of both molecules and cells through the tissue and the exchange of metabolites with the circulatory system.

The carbohydrates are long, unbranched polysaccharide chains of seven different types, each composed of repeating units of two sugar derivatives, usually a uronic acid and an amino sugar such as N-acetyl glucosamine. This gives rise to the term ***glycosaminoglycan*** (***GAG***).

Hyaluronate, also known as ***hyaluronic acid***, consists of repeating d-glucuronate (β1,3)-N-acetyl-d-glucosamine units and is the predominant GAG, forming huge unbranching linear molecules of 100,000 to 10,000,000 molecular weight.

The other GAGs include ***chondroitin-4-sulphate, chondroitin-6-sulphate, dermatan sulphate, keratan sulphate, heparan sulphate*** and ***heparin sulphate***. Each of these molecules contains sulphated N-acetyl groups substituted onto galactosamine sugars in the repeating carbohydrate units, making them highly negatively charged (acidic). These charged groups prevent the carbohydrate chains from folding into globular aggregates, causing them to remain in an expanded linear form, thereby occupying a large volume for a small mass. The charged side groups also render them extremely hydrophilic, attracting a large volume of water and positive ions, particularly sodium.

These GAGs (other than hyaluronate) exist as carbohydrate chains covalently linked to various protein molecules, forming a range of molecular structures containing up to 90% to 95% carbohydrate. These are called ***proteoglycans***. There are numerous specific proteins, including ***perlecan, syndecan, decorin, lumican*** and ***aggrecan***. Proteoglycans have various specific functions. Some bind to hyaluronic acid producing massive quaternary structures, others interact with collagens or bind to various other matrix molecules including remodelling enzymes, enzyme inhibitors, growth factors, cytokines and cell surface receptors.

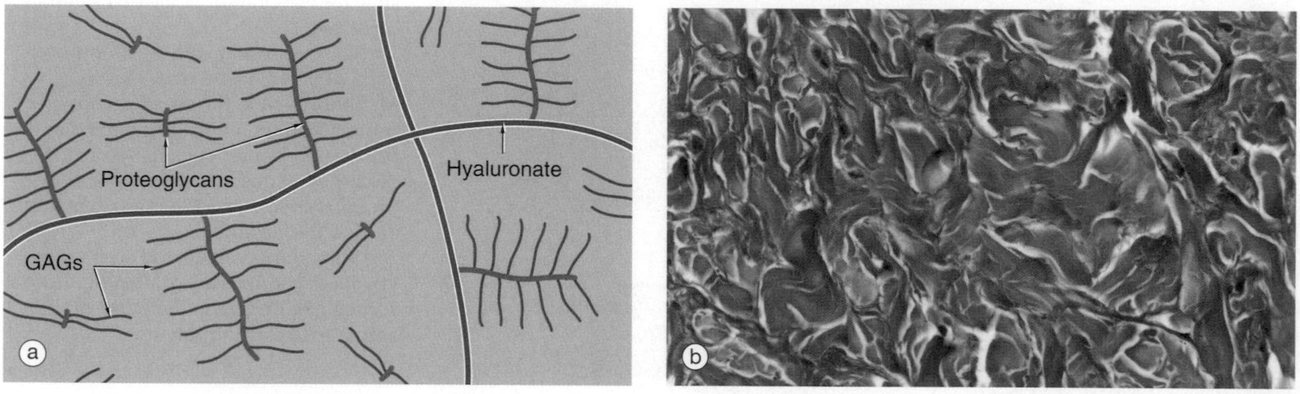

FIG. 4.10 Ground substance
(a) Diagram (b) Alcian blue PAS (HP)

Fig. 4.10a represents long, linear hyaluronate molecules and proteoglycans with their covalently attached glycosaminoglycans (GAGs) in a gel. Fig. 4.10b shows ground substance in the form of the wispy blue-staining material between pink collagen fibres in a micrograph of skin. Ground substance can be sometimes seen in H&E sections of connective tissue as a background pale blue colour between collagen fibres, but it can be seen more clearly with appropriate special stains as shown here. It was, and sometimes still is, referred to as ***tissue mucin*** (historically, proteoglycans were called mucoproteins and GAGs were called mucopolysaccharides).

Structural glycoproteins

In addition to the proteoglycans, there are further glycoprotein molecules important in ground substance. These include two fibril-forming molecules, ***fibrillin*** (discussed in the section on elastin) and ***fibronectin***.

Fibronectin has binding sites for many connective tissue components and plays a part in controlling the deposition and orientation of collagen in extracellular matrix. Fibronectin molecules bind to collagens, to heparan sulphate (a GAG) and to specific membrane receptors on cells.

Cell membranes incorporate a group of transmembrane protein complexes called ***integrins***, which act as cell adhesion molecules. One of these acts as a fibronectin receptor; it binds internally within the cytoplasm to actin filaments of the cytoskeleton and externally binds with the fibronectin. This interaction forms part of a specialised layer of extracellular matrix called ***basement membrane*** where cells meet matrix. Here, other non-filamentous glycoproteins also play a structural role (see opposite).

BASEMENT MEMBRANES

Basement membranes are sheet-like arrangements of extracellular matrix proteins which act as an interface between the support tissues and epithelial or parenchymal cells. Basement membranes are also associated with blood vessels and muscle cells and form a limiting membrane around the central nervous system. The term derives from the initial recognition of membranes lying beneath the basal cells of epithelia. In the context of muscle and nervous tissue, the term ***external lamina*** is often applied.

Basement membranes have several functions:

- Provide physical binding of the epithelium to the underlying tissue and physical support
- Control of epithelial growth and differentiation, they form a barrier to downward epithelial growth; this is only breached if epithelia undergo malignant transformation (cancer).
- Permit the flow of nutrients, metabolites and other molecules to and from an epithelium, as epithelium is devoid of blood vessels
- Where a cell layer acts as a selective barrier to the passage of molecules from one compartment to another (e.g. between the lumen of blood vessels and adjacent tissues), the basement membrane assumes a critical role in regulating permeability. This role of forming a selective barrier reaches an extreme level of sophistication in the kidney, where the glomerular basement membrane is part of the highly selective filter for molecules passing from the bloodstream into the urine.

The main components of basement membranes and external laminae are the glycosaminoglycan ***heparan sulphate***, ***type IV collagen***, and the structural glycoproteins ***fibronectin***, ***laminins*** and ***nidogen-1***. While fibronectin appears to be produced by fibroblasts of the supporting tissue, the rest are at least partly elaborated by the tissues being supported.

The structural framework is a fine meshwork of type IV collagen, a mesh/network-forming collagen found exclusively in basement membranes. The glycoprotein laminin, in concert with nidogen (also called ***entactin***), binds the type IV collagen and links to other basement membrane constituents and to laminin receptors on the basal plasma membranes of the epithelial cells.

Type III collagen (reticulin) is bound via the fibrillar glycoprotein fibronectin to integrins in the epithelial basal plasma membrane. Fibronectin also binds the GAG heparan sulphate. Basement membranes vary in their molecular details between sites and between types of epithelia.

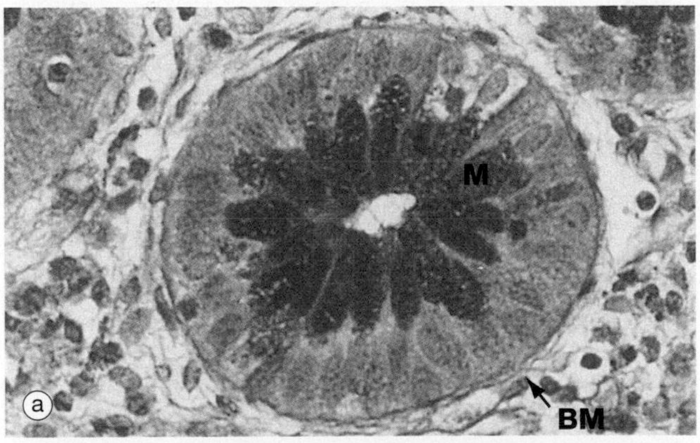

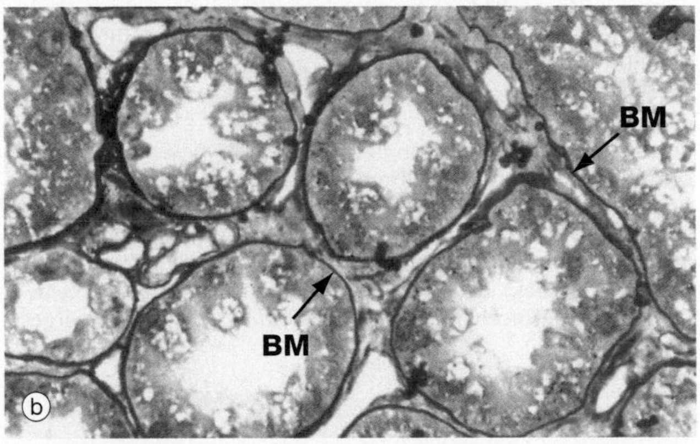

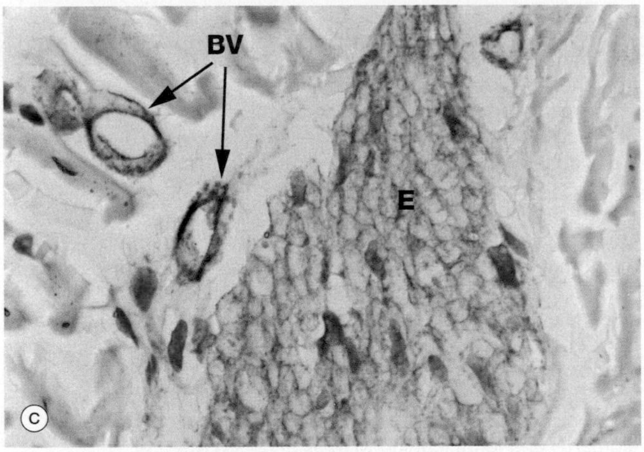

FIG. 4.11 Basement membrane
(a) PAS haematoxylin (HP)
(b) Jones methenamine silver (MP)
(c) Immunohistochemical stain for type IV collagen (MP)

Basement membranes can be seen beneath epithelia when the membrane is relatively thick or when histochemical or other methods for basement membrane components are used.

Fig. 4.11a is of a duodenal crypt lined by mucus-secreting cells stained with PAS. The PAS reacts with the complex carbohydrates in the proteoglycans of the basement membrane **BM** and with the mucin **M** in secretory vacuoles in the apical cytoplasm of the epithelial cells. In Fig. 4.11b, a silver impregnation method with affinity for reticulin highlights the basement membrane **BM** of renal tubules. In Fig. 4.11c, an immunohistochemical stain using an antibody to type IV collagen shows the basement membrane around blood vessels **BV** and external laminae **E** around individual smooth muscle cells in a hair-related muscle in skin; the muscle cell cytoplasm is unstained, although the muscle cell nuclei can be seen.

BM basement membrane **BV** blood vessels **E** external laminae **M** mucin

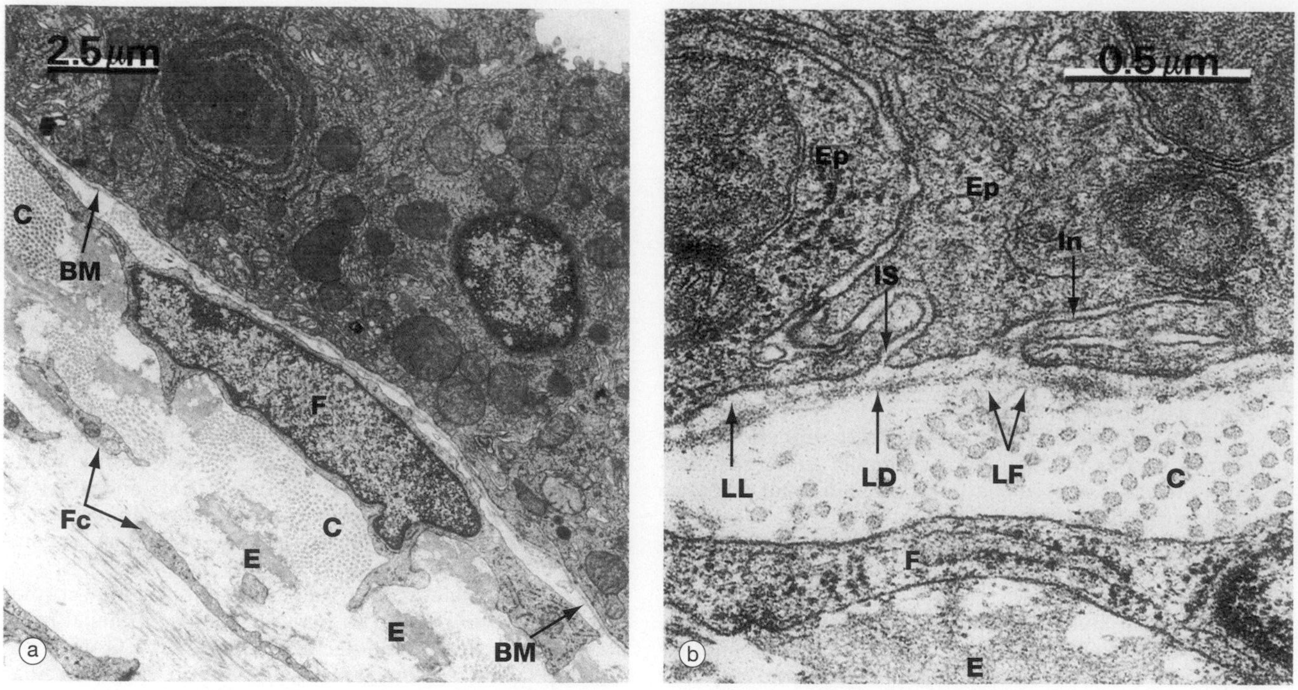

FIG. 4.12 Basement membrane
(a) EM ×5000 (b) EM ×45 000

Fig. 4.12a shows the epithelial lining of mouse trachea. A basement membrane **BM** can be seen separating it from the underlying supporting tissue which contains the cell body and nucleus of a fibroblast **F**, numerous fine fibroblast cytoplasmic processes **Fc**, bundles of collagen fibrils **C** (cut in transverse section) and elastin fibres **E**.

At higher magnification in Fig. 4.12b, the basement membrane can be seen to have three layers. The relatively electron-lucent ***lamina lucida*** **LL** (ranging from 10–50 nm in width) abuts the basal epithelial cell plasma membrane. The intermediate layer is electron-dense and is called the ***lamina densa*** **LD** (20–300 nm thick). Beyond the lamina densa is the broad, relatively electron-lucent ***lamina fibroreticularis*** **LF**, which merges with the fibrous and fibrillary (reticular) components of the underlying supporting tissue. In this field, note collagen fibrils **C**, part of a fibroblast **F**, and elastin **E**. The basement membrane typically passes uninterrupted beneath the intercellular space **IS** between two epithelial cells **Ep** and beneath a basal invagination **In** in of one of these cells. The lamina densa was formerly known as the ***basal lamina***.

The terms ***basal lamina*** and ***basement membrane*** were used interchangeably until it was realised that the single layer seen with the light microscope corresponded to the combination of all three layers seen with the electron microscope. If used, the term basal lamina should be confined to meaning lamina densa.

Disorders of basement membranes

Basement membranes are involved in several disease processes.

Renal function

In the kidney (see Ch. 16) the fused basement membranes of endothelial cells and podocytes form the filtration barrier for the ultrafiltrate in the glomerulus. If the glomerular basement membrane becomes abnormal then renal function is impaired. In patients with diabetes mellitus, there is thickening of the glomerular basement membrane, which becomes abnormally permeable to proteins.

Cancer

Epithelial tissues grow and regenerate and are anchored to, but separated from, support tissues by a basement membrane.

Mutations in epithelial cells lead to abnormal growth (***neoplasia***), forming cancers. A malignant tumour can grow from the site of origin and spread into local tissues (invasion). This is achieved by cancer cells secreting factors that facilitate destruction of basement membrane, allowing cells to grow into the extracellular matrix.

Genetic diseases

Mutations in genes coding for components of basement membrane have been shown in renal disease (Alport disease), muscle disease (congenital muscular dystrophy) and skin disease (junctional epidermolysis bullosa).

Autoimmune disease

In Goodpasture syndrome, autoantibodies are produced which target a component of the basement membrane common to glomeruli and lung, leading to renal and lung disease.

BM basement membrane **C** collagen **E** elastin **Eo** eosinophil **Ep** epithelial cell **F** fibroblast **Fc** fibroblast cytoplasmic process **In** basal invagination **IS** intercellular space **LD** lamina densa **LF** lamina fibroreticularis **LL** lamina lucida **L** lymphocyte **M** myofibroblast

THE CELLS OF SUPPORTING/CONNECTIVE TISSUE

The cells of supporting tissue are derived from precursor cells in primitive (fetal) supporting tissue called ***mesenchyme***. Their dominant common function is synthesis, maintenance and recycling of extracellular matrix material.

- ***Fibroblasts*** secrete, maintain and recycle the matrix in most tissues.
- ***Myofibroblasts*** are an activated form of fibroblast associated with repair. They have a contractile function as well as a role in secretion of matrix.
- ***Adipocytes*** are modified support cells specialised in the storage and metabolism of fat; collectively they form ***adipose tissue***.
- ***Chondrocytes, osteoblasts*** and ***osteocytes*** are responsible for secreting and maintaining the matrix in cartilage and bone, respectively (see Ch. 10).

With the important exception of cartilage, supporting tissues are vascularised, containing arteries, capillaries, veins and lymphatics with associated cells of the innate immune system, such as mast cells and tissue macrophages. Cells of the adaptive immune system access the tissues via the blood vessels.

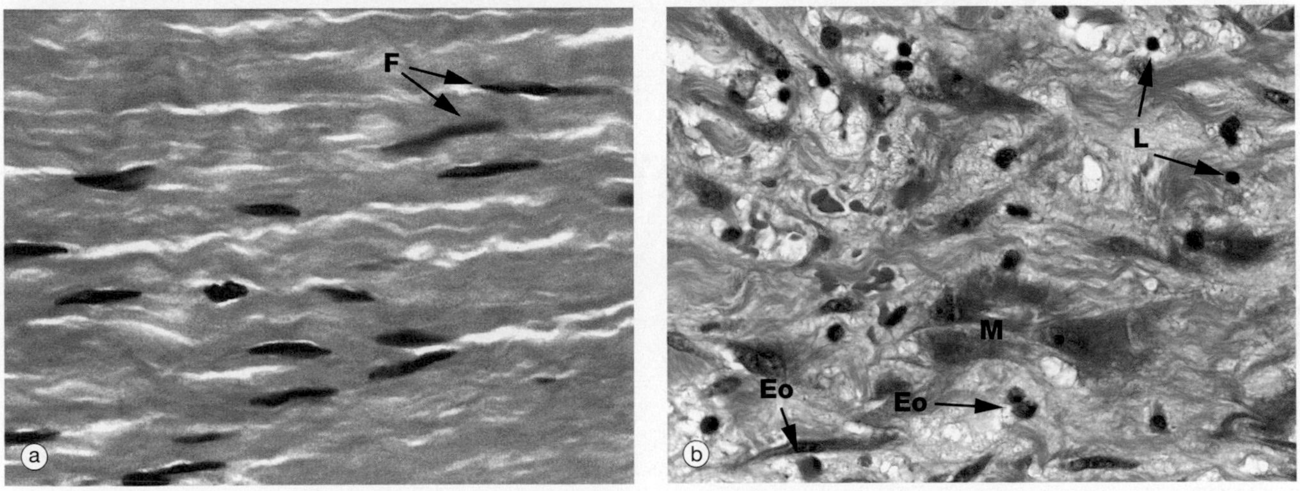

FIG. 4.13 Fibroblasts (a) H&E (MP) Myofibroblasts (b) H&E (MP)

Fig. 4.13a demonstrates the typical histological appearance of mature fibroblasts in collagenous tissue; collagen fibres are stained pink. The fibroblast nuclei **F** are condensed and elongated in the direction of the collagen fibres. The cytoplasm is relatively scanty and barely visible. The cell is long and thin with fine cytoplasmic processes extending into the matrix. The function of fibroblasts is to maintain the integrity of supporting tissue, including continuous turnover of its constituents.

Fig. 4.13b demonstrates active fibroblasts called myofibroblasts **M** in repair of damaged tissue with early fibrosis/scarring. The nuclei are large with prominent nucleoli and the cytoplasm is extensive and basophilic. The basophilic extracellular matrix is prominent. A few eosinophils **Eo** and lymphocytes **L** are present. These myofibroblasts have a contractile function and play an important role in the contraction and shrinkage of the resultant scar tissue.

Repair with fibrosis

Following damage to cells and tissues, there is an inflammatory reaction which is responsible for eliminating the damaging agent and clearing away dead tissue.

Further repair to damaged tissues is mainly delivered by support cells from connective tissues. Briefly, there is a local proliferation of mesenchymal cells from the margins of residual normal tissue to form fibroblasts and myofibroblasts. These grow to replace the area of tissue damage. This proliferation is also associated with florid growth of new capillary blood vessels. This combination is known as ***granulation tissue***. The fibroblasts and myofibroblasts secrete extracellular matrix and replace the damaged area with fibro-collagenous material. This is the basis of a ***collagenous scar***. Over time there is progressive remodelling to maximise the strength of the collagen and to reduce capillary vessel numbers.

This has been called ***healing by repair*** as it often allows good function, but it may be better described as scarring as it does not restore tissue to normal.

Epithelial–mesenchymal transition is a process by which epithelial cells in organs such as liver, kidney and lung can transform into a mesenchymal phenotype and contribute to fibrosis in repair. This process is also important in tumour invasion and metastasis.

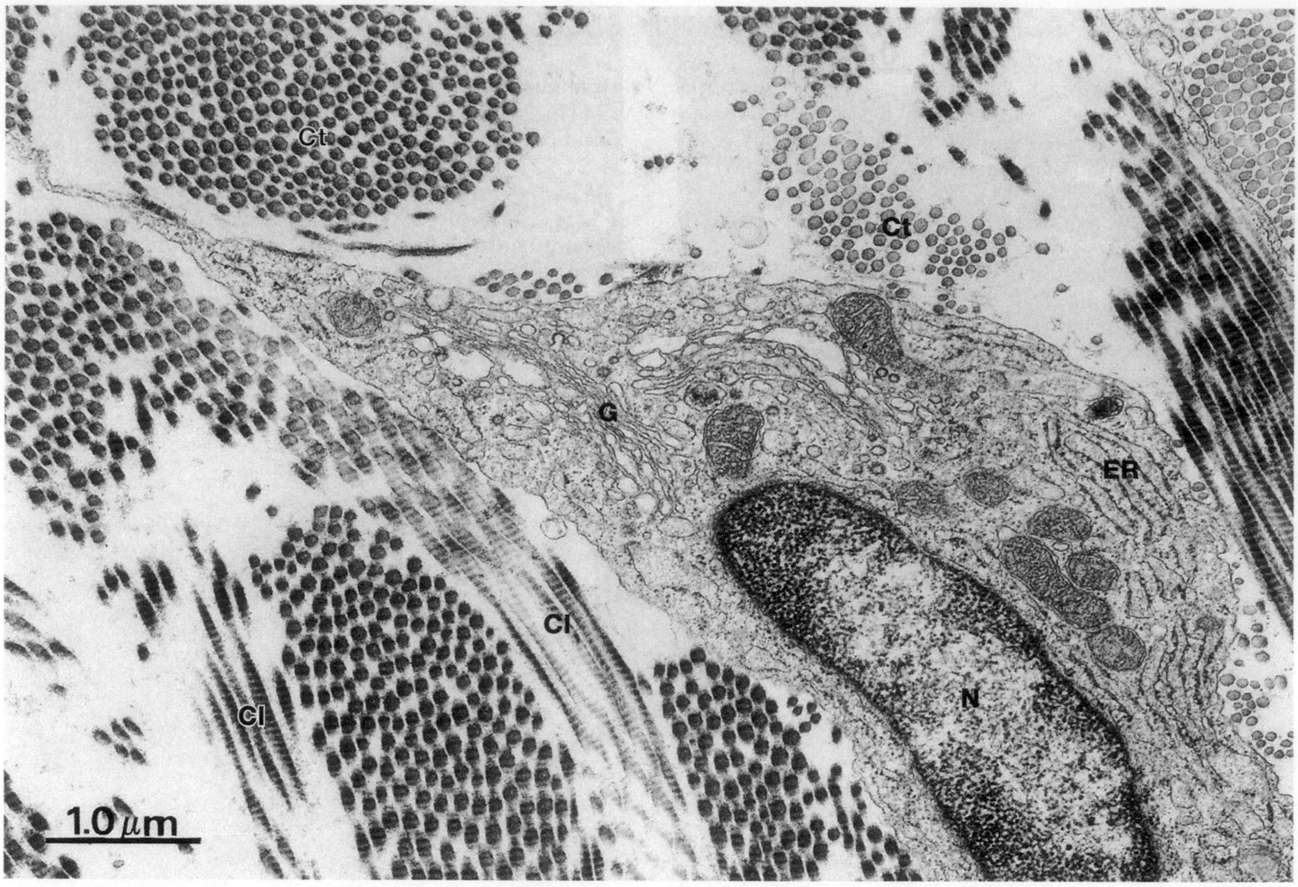

FIG. 4.14 Fibroblasts
EM ×18 500

Fig. 4.14 illustrates the body of a mature fibroblast within supporting tissue. The nucleus **N** is moderately condensed and nucleoli are not seen here. The small quantity of cytoplasm is mostly occupied by rough endoplasmic reticulum **ER**, reflecting the dominant protein-secreting function of this type of cell. The Golgi apparatus **G** is visible and a few mitochondria are present. Bundles of collagen fibrils are seen in transverse **Ct** and longitudinal section **Cl** in the extracellular matrix.

During active synthesis of extracellular fibres, fibroblast cytoplasm becomes markedly expanded, with the rough ER and Golgi apparatus becoming prominent features. Fibroblasts synthesise and secrete the glycosaminoglycans, collagen, elastin and all other extracellular constituents; however, in mature fibroblasts, few secretory vesicles are found.

ADIPOSE TISSUE

Many supporting tissues contain cells specialised for the storage of fat; these cells are called ***adipocytes***. They are ultimately derived from mesenchyme. The recognisable precursors to adipocytes are called ***lipoblasts***. Adipocytes are found in isolation or in small clusters throughout loose supporting tissues and are found as the main cell type in adipose tissues.

The fat in adipocytes is stored as triglycerides and is derived from three main sources: dietary fats circulating in the bloodstream as ***chylomicrons***, triglycerides synthesised in the liver and transported in blood in ***lipoproteins***, and triglycerides synthesised from glucose within adipocytes. Adipose tissue was regarded as an inactive energy store, but it is an extremely important participant in general metabolic processes, acting as a store of substrate for the energy-generating processes of almost all tissues.

Reflecting this metabolic importance, adipose tissue generally has a rich blood supply, although the capillaries can be collapsed and inconspicuous in tissue sections. The rate of fat deposition and utilisation within adipose tissue is largely determined by dietary intake and energy expenditure, but a number of hormones profoundly influence metabolism. Adipocytes have receptors for ***insulin, glucocorticoids, growth hormone*** and ***noradrenaline (norepinephrine***) that modulate uptake and release of fat.

In addition, adipocytes have an endocrine role. Adipocytes modulate energy metabolism and influence general metabolism through secretion of several protein messengers and, in coordination with hormones such as insulin, contribute to regulation of body mass. The protein messengers from adipose tissue have been collectively called ***adipokines*** and include ***leptin, resistin, adiponectin, tumour necrosis factor (TNF)-α***, and ***plasminogen activator inhibitor type 1***. Note that this includes proteins from both adipocytes and tissue macrophages. The protein hormone leptin is involved in the regulation of appetite.

There are two main types of adipose tissue, which have been called white and brown. ***White adipose tissue*** is often macroscopically a pale yellow, while ***brown adipose tissue*** is so named as it has a darker brown tint. Triglycerides are liquid at body temperature and the mobility and feel of adipose tissue to palpation is determined by the amount of fibrous supporting tissue components at the individual sites.

White adipose tissue

This type of adipose tissue comprises up to 20% of total body weight in normal (target weight) well-nourished male adults and up to 25% in females but can reach more than 50% in obesity. It is distributed throughout the body, particularly in the deep layers of the skin. Its roles include:

- Triglyceride storage and mobilisation
- Structural fill; fills in spaces such as in pelvic and perirectal areas and axilla. Contributes to sculpting body shape and outline.
- Acts as a thermal insulator under the skin
- Forms part of shock-absorbing padding e.g. around kidneys. Fat divided into lobules, each surrounded by fibrous tissue, forms a flexible and deformable cushion against compression, essentially a biological bubble wrap. The skin generally uses this architecture, but it is particularly prominent in finger pulps and the soles of feet.

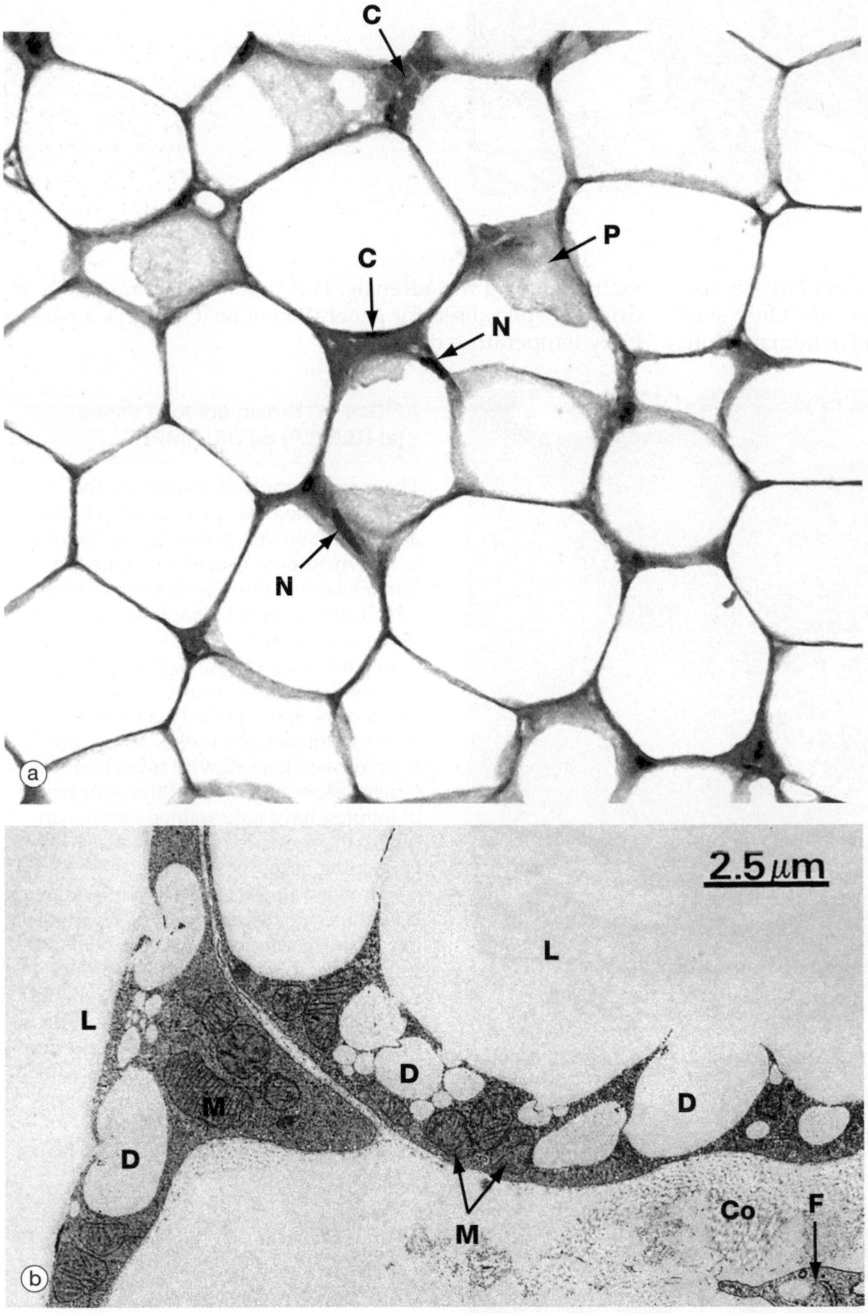

FIG. 4.15 White adipose tissue (a) H&E (HP) (b) EM ×6000

The typical appearance of white adipose tissue is illustrated in Fig. 4.15a. Adipose tissue is pale staining because virtually all the cell is occupied by lipid, which is dissolved out in paraffin-embedded tissue preparations. The cell membrane, a thin rim of peripheral cytoplasm and the external lamina collectively give a 'chicken-wire' appearance.

Fat stored in adipocytes accumulates as lipid droplets that fuse to form a single large droplet which distends and occupies most of the cytoplasm. The adipocyte nucleus **N** is compressed and displaced to one side of the stored lipid droplet and the cytoplasm is reduced to a small rim around the periphery. In some cells, tangential slicing of the top or bottom of a cell is seen as a sheet of pink-stained cytoplasm **P**. Note the minute-appearing blood capillaries **C** compared with the size of the surrounding adipocytes.

Fig. 4.15b shows the periphery of two adjacent adipocytes. Contrary to the impression given by light microscopy, the main lipid droplet **L** in each cell has an irregular outline with numerous tiny droplets **D** at the periphery in the process of fusion with the main droplet. The lipid is not bounded by a membrane. The thin rim of cytoplasm contains the usual organelles, most notably mitochondria **M**. Each adipocyte is surrounded by an external lamina. In the adjacent extracellular tissue, a fibroblast cytoplasmic process **F** and collagen fibrils **Co** can be seen.

C capillary **Cl** collagen fibrils, longitudinal **Co** collagen fibrils **Ct** collagen fibrils, transverse **D** small lipid droplet **ER** endoplasmic reticulum **F** fibroblast cytoplasmic process **G** Golgi apparatus **L** large lipid droplet **M** mitochondrion **N** nucleus **P** cytoplasm of adipocyte

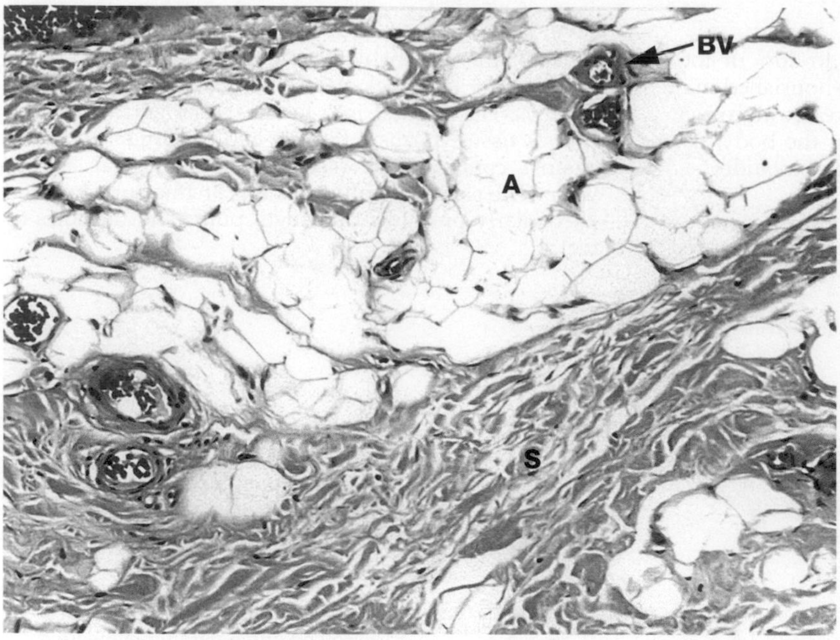

FIG. 4.16 Fibroadipose tissue H&E (MP)

Fig. 4.16 demonstrates the typical appearance of adipocytes **A** scattered within collagenous supporting tissue. Adipocytes occur here either singly or in small groups. There are several small blood vessels **BV** with thin walls, and abundant collagen fibres both as fine fibres dividing the adipocytes into small groups and in broad arrays called ***septa*** **S** which provide structural strength.

Brown adipose tissue

This variant of adipose tissue is found particularly in newborn mammals and some hibernating animals. Only small amounts of brown adipose tissue are found in human adults, mainly around the adrenals. This tissue is rich in mitochondria and specialised for generation of heat; it plays a part in body temperature regulation.

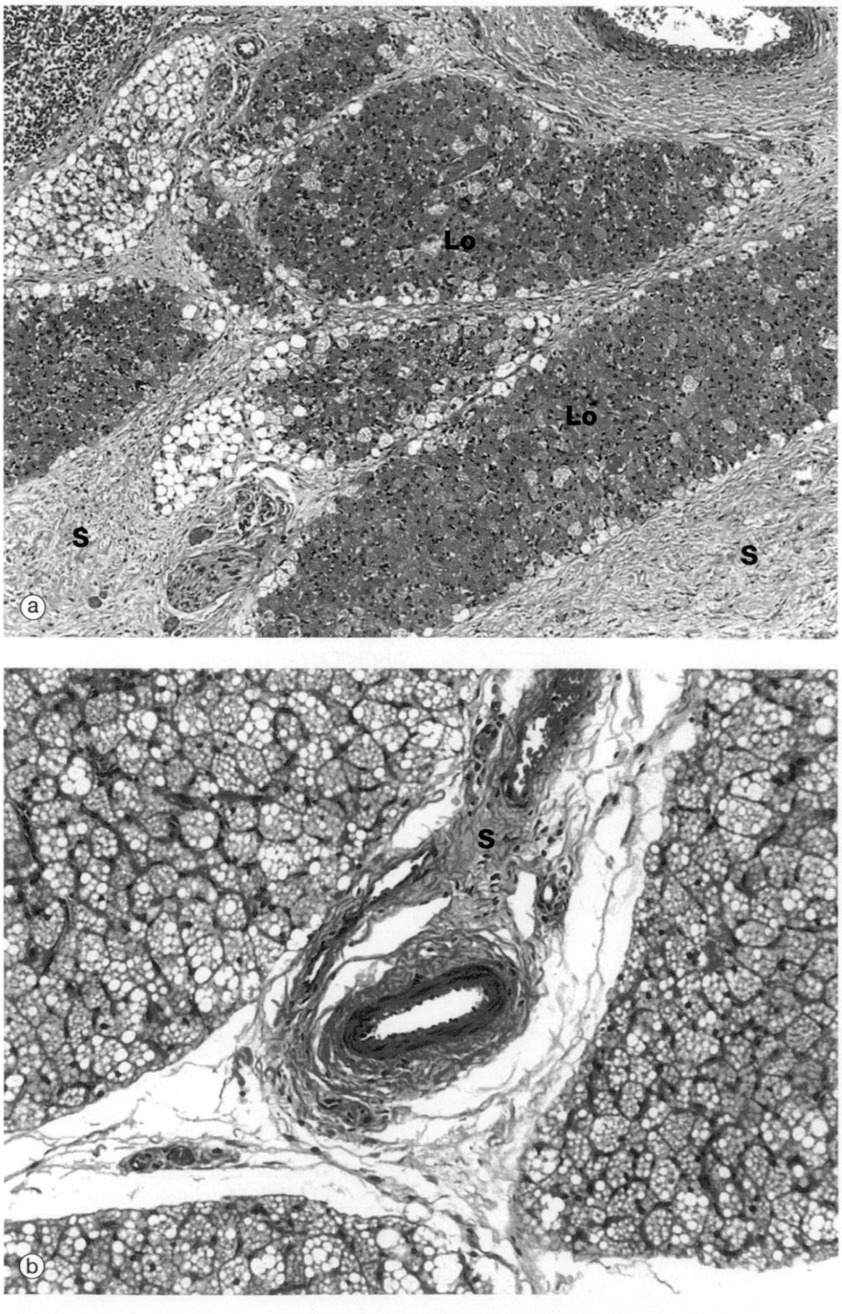

FIG. 4.17 Brown adipose tissue (a) H&E (LP) (b) H&E (MP)

These micrographs demonstrate the typical histological appearance of brown adipose tissue. As seen in Fig. 4.17a and b, brown adipose tissue is arranged in ***lobules*** **Lo** separated by fibrous septa **S** which convey blood vessels and sympathetic nerve fibres.

At low magnification, two cell morphologies (appearances) can be seen. Many cells, and especially cells at the centre of lobules, are pink-stained due to cytoplasm packed with mitochondria. Others, especially those at the periphery of lobules, have pale-stained cytoplasm due to the presence of multiple vesicles containing lipid.

Brown adipose tissue is involved in ***non-shivering thermogenesis***, an increase in metabolic activity producing heat and induced by cold stress. Brown adipose tissue is characterised by expression of a unique uncoupling protein, UCP1 (uncoupling protein 1, previously called thermogenin). This protein, in association with several other modulating factors, serves to uncouple mitochondrial metabolism from production of ATP to produce heat.

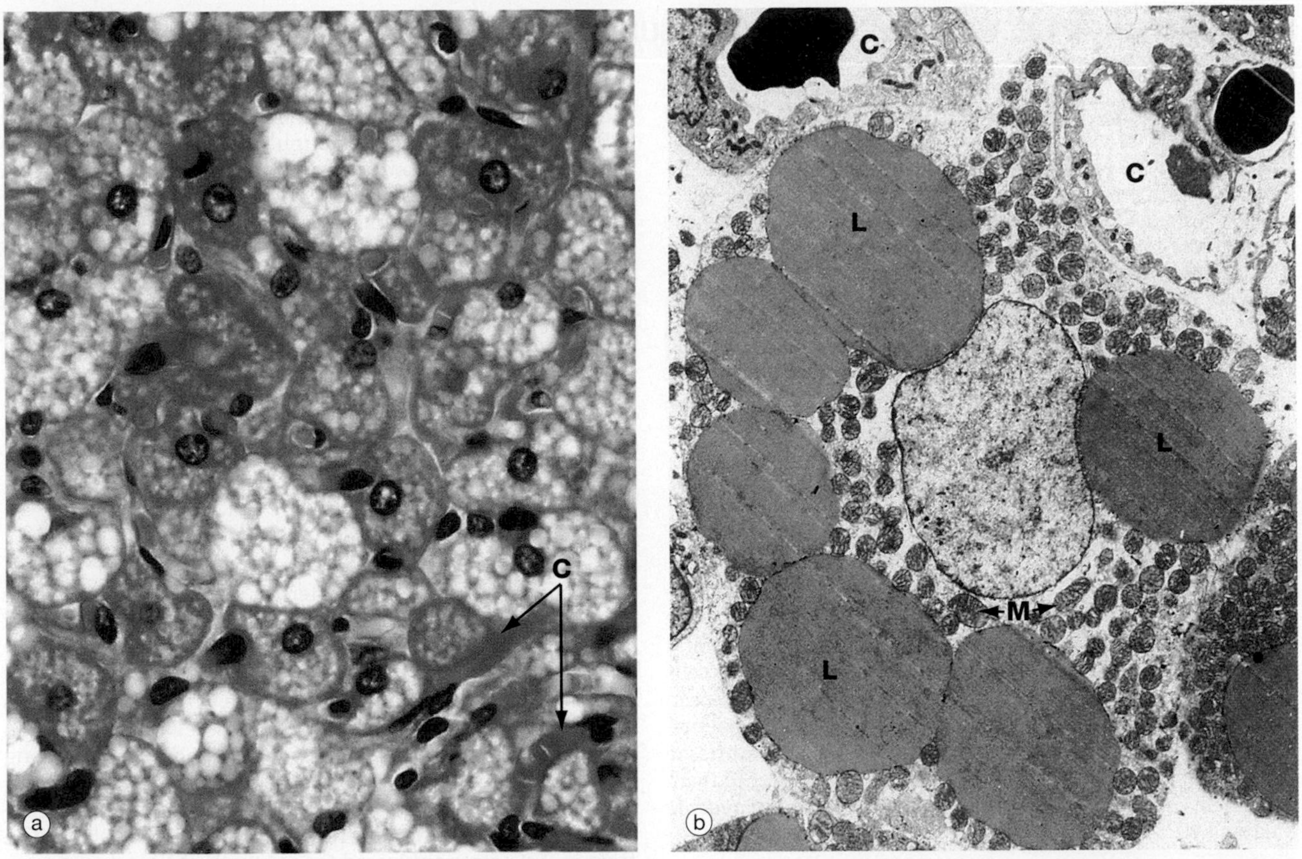

FIG. 4.18 Brown adipose tissue
(a) H&E (HP) (b) EM ×4070, rabbit

At high magnification in Fig. 4.18a, the nuclei of brown adipocytes are seen to be eccentrically located within the cell but, unlike those of white adipocytes, the nuclei are large and surrounded by a significant quantity of strongly eosinophilic cytoplasm. The stored lipid is contained within multiple droplets, all of which have been dissolved away during tissue processing. Note the rich network of capillaries **C** between the brown adipocytes.

Fig. 4.18b shows brown adipose tissue taken from a newborn rabbit and readily demonstrates the multilocular nature of stored lipid **L**. The cytoplasm of brown adipocytes is crammed with mitochondria **M** which have numerous closely packed cristae. These mitochondria are extremely rich in cytochromes, part of the electron transport chain involved in oxidative energy production; this accounts for the brown colour of brown adipose tissue when examined macroscopically.

Unlike the metabolism of other tissues, in brown adipose cells the process of electron transport is readily uncoupled from the phosphorylation of ADP to form ATP. The energy derived from oxidation of lipids, and energy released by electron transport in the uncoupled state, is dissipated as heat which is conducted to the rest of the body by the rich vascular network. Note the intimate association of capillaries **C** with the brown adipocyte in this electron micrograph.

Human neonates and other baby mammals utilise brown adipose tissue to generate body heat during the vulnerable period after birth. Brown adipose tissue undergoes involution in early infancy and in adult humans is found only in restricted sites such as around the adrenal gland and great vessels in retroperitoneal fat. The production of heat by brown adipose tissue is controlled directly by the sympathetic nervous system.

Obesity

Obesity is one of the greatest challenges to public health in the modern age. Complications of obesity include type 2 diabetes mellitus, coronary artery atheroma, stroke and some types of cancer.

Adipose tissues are not merely fat stores and have complex metabolic roles, including secretion of a variety of wide-acting cytokines. Tissue macrophages, present in numbers proportionate to the total mass of adipose tissue, produce proinflammatory cytokines and adipocytes produce a range of hormones.

Obesity has been mainly linked to environmental factors such as increased intake of energy dense foods that are high in fat and sugars and physical inactivity due to the increasingly sedentary nature of many forms of work, changing modes of transportation and increasing urbanisation.

A adipocyte **BV** blood vessels **C** capillary **L** lipid droplet **Lo** lobule of adipose tissue **M** mitochondrion **S** septum

THE DEFENCE CELLS IN SUPPORTING TISSUE

The supporting tissues not only contain cells responsible for their synthesis, maintenance and metabolic activity, but also a variety of cells with defence and immune functions. Traditionally, these cells have been divided into two categories: fixed (intrinsic) cells and wandering (extrinsic) cells.

The intrinsic defence cells of supporting tissue are the ***tissue-fixed macrophages*** (***histiocytes***) and ***mast cells***. Tissue-fixed macrophages are now generally believed to be derived from circulating monocytes (see Fig. 3.16) which have become at least temporarily resident in supporting tissues. Mast cells are similar to basophils in structure and function (see Figs 3.11 and 4.20), but there are structural differences which show that mast cells are not merely basophils resident in the tissues.

The wandering category of defence and immune cells includes all the remaining members of the white blood cell series (see Ch. 3). Although leukocytes (white blood cells) are usually considered as a constituent of blood, their principal site of activity is outside the blood circulation, within tissues. Leukocytes are normally found only in relatively small numbers but, in response to tissue injury and other disease processes, their numbers increase greatly. The supporting tissues of those regions of the body which are subject to the constant threat of pathogenic invasion, such as the gastrointestinal and respiratory tracts, contain a larger population of leukocytes, maintaining constant surveillance.

Macrophage phagocyte system

Particulate matter injected into circulation and normal constituents such as old red blood cells are cleared from the circulation by cells of the bone marrow, liver, spleen and lymph nodes. The common function of the responsible cells is their ability to phagocytose particulate matter; they can be called ***phagocytes***. These cells are derived from haematopoietic stem cells in the marrow and are also called ***tissue macrophages*** (see Fig. 4.19). It is convenient to refer to them and their functions as a group, the ***macrophage phagocyte system*** (***MPS***).

Historically, these were referred to as the ***reticuloendothelial system*** (***RES***). Phagocytic cells are found associated with vascular and lymphatic spaces in liver, bone marrow and spleen and were incorrectly thought to have features in common with the endothelial cells (see Ch. 8). These organs also tend to be rich in a supporting framework of reticulin fibres (see Fig. 4.5) upon which are draped cells with long cytoplasmic processes described as ***reticulum*** or ***reticular cells***. Given these associations they were thought to represent a single functional 'reticuloendothelial' system. The term is still commonly used to refer to the MPS.

Dendritic cells and histiocytes

Amongst the cell types found in tissues, particularly those in contact with the external environment (e.g. skin, nose, lung, stomach, intestines) are cells which may have long, branched cytoplasmic processes called ***dendrites***, hence ***dendritic cells***, but with a specific function as ***antigen-presenting cells*** (***APCs***). These cells phagocytose, partially digest and present antigen to T cells with co-expressed membrane T cell–activating molecules, thereby inducing immune responses to antigens (see Ch. 11). They migrate to lymph nodes when stimulated.

Dendritic cells of skin are named ***Langerhans cells***. The APCs have an origin from haematopoietic stem cells in the bone marrow, many with a monocyte lineage (***myeloid dendritic cells***), while some have a plasma cell–like appearance (***plasmacytoid dendritic cell***). Dendritic cells express ***Toll-like receptors*** (***TLRs***), a type of receptor that recognises molecules common to several bacterial species.

Other cells such as reticular cells may have long dendritic processes but are mesenchymal supporting cells, not APCs. There is thus a potential difficulty with terminology due to overlap between morphology (dendritic shape) and function (APC). Because APCs are phagocytic, they have historically been called histiocytes, a term also used for macrophages.

Tumours of supporting cells

Tumours are caused by changes in the cells that lead them to undergo poorly regulated growth. Local overgrowth produces a mass of cells termed a ***neoplasm*** or ***tumour***.

Tumours may be confined to the body part in which they arise or may develop further loss of growth control that allows cells to invade local tissues or spread widely in the body. Tumours of support cells are commonly seen. They are often collectively referred to as soft tissue tumours.

An overgrowth of adipocytes is responsible for the commonly encountered benign tumour termed a lipoma (e-Fig. 4.2). Although these can arise in almost any site in the body, the commonest presentation is as a subcutaneous soft mass.

Histologically, lipomas are composed of mature white adipose tissue, indistinguishable from normal adipose tissue. Malignant tumours of adipocytes are rare and are called liposarcomas (e-Fig. 4.3). These malignant tumours often arise deep within the retroperitoneal tissues.

Benign tumours of fibroblasts are sometimes seen, termed fibromas, while malignant tumours of fibroblasts are termed fibrosarcomas and may arise at any site.

Soft tissue tumours may have a prominent myxoid background in tissue sections due to ground substance and be associated with an inflammatory cell population throughout the tumour; a myxoid inflammatory myofibroblastic tumour is an example (e-Fig. 4.4).

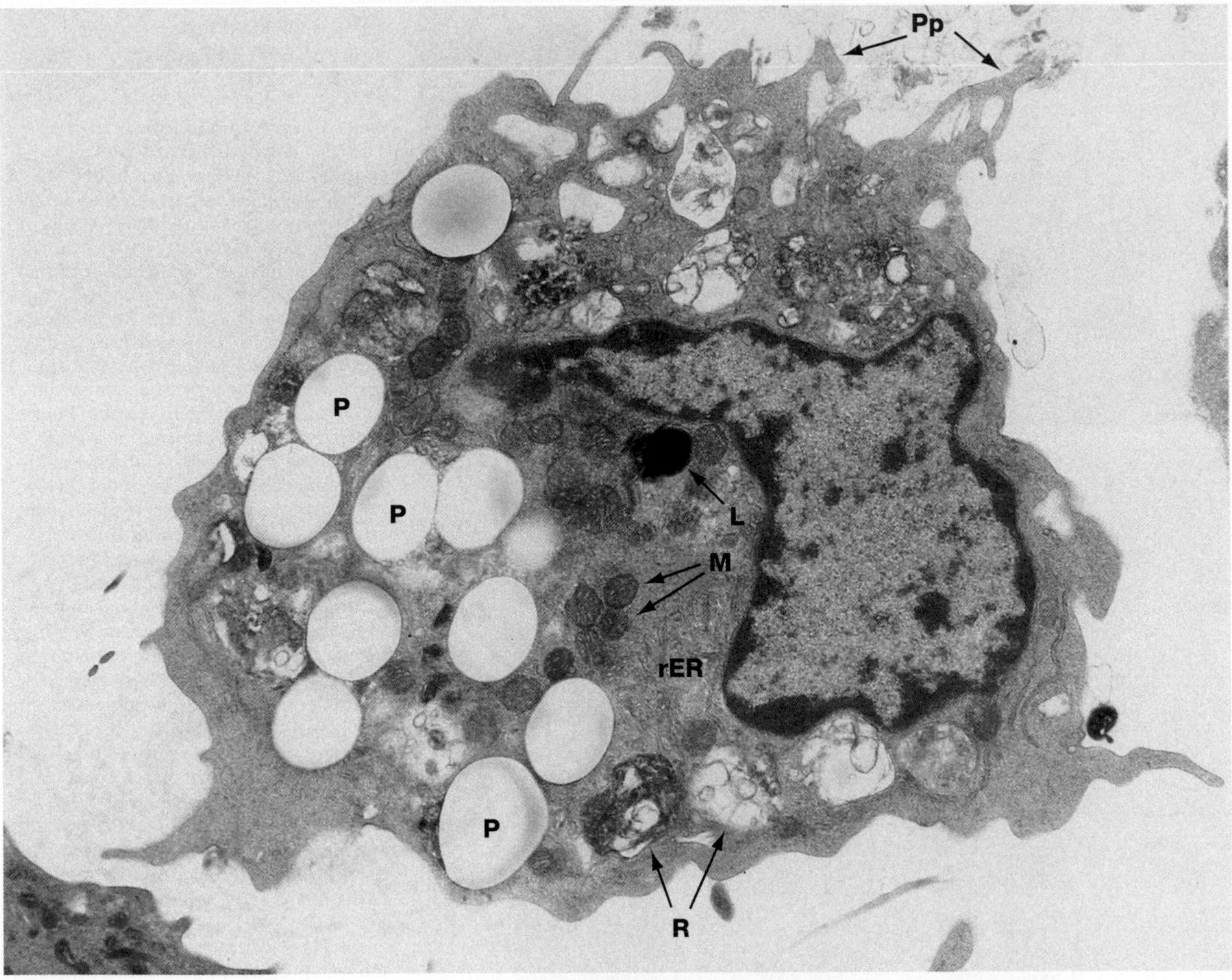

FIG. 4.19 Macrophage
EM ×11 600

The ultrastructural features of macrophages vary widely according to their state of activity and tissue location. Fig. 4.19 shows an active macrophage obtained from the peritoneum of a rat which had previously been injected intraperitoneally with latex particles; a number of particles **P** have been engulfed by the macrophage.

The macrophage nucleus is irregular, with heterochromatin typically clumped around the nuclear envelope. The cytoplasm contains a few mitochondria **M** and a variable amount of free ribosomes and rough endoplasmic reticulum **rER**. In quiescent macrophages, lysosomes **L** are abundant, but their number is much reduced in actively phagocytic cells; additional lysosomes are later produced via the Golgi apparatus. The macrophage cytoplasm contains an assortment of phagosomes and residual bodies **R**. Residual material may be released from the macrophage by exocytosis or may remain sequestered in the tissues, as occurs with the dyes used in tattooing of the skin. Actively phagocytic cells exhibit irregular cytoplasmic projections or pseudopodia **Pp** which are involved in amoeboid movement and phagocytosis.

In addition to their role as tissue scavengers, macrophages play an important role in the adaptive immune system (see Ch. 11). Macrophages process antigenic material before presenting it to memory lymphocytes, thus acting as APCs; lymphocytes are then stimulated to undergo specific immune responses. As a result of various immune mechanisms, antigenic material may become combined or coated with substances such as ***antibodies*** and ***complement***, which are then collectively known as ***opsonins***, a process known as ***opsonisation***. Opsonins are recognised by surface receptors on the macrophage surface and this greatly enhances the phagocytic ability of macrophages and other phagocytes such as neutrophils (see Chs 3 and 11). Cytokines released during the immune response, especially cytokines from activated T cells, act directly on macrophages to increase greatly their metabolic and phagocytic activity. Macrophages also secrete a variety of cytokines that act to enhance local and systemic immune responses.

In some disease states, under cytokine stimulation macrophages may develop an enhanced phenotype for killing microorganisms, the ***epithelioid macrophage***, particularly seen in diseases such as tuberculosis and leprosy. Macrophages can also fuse to form ***multinucleated histiocytes/giant cells***.

L lysosome **M** mitochondrion **P** latex particle **Pp** pseudopodia **R** residual bodies **rER** rough endoplasmic reticulum

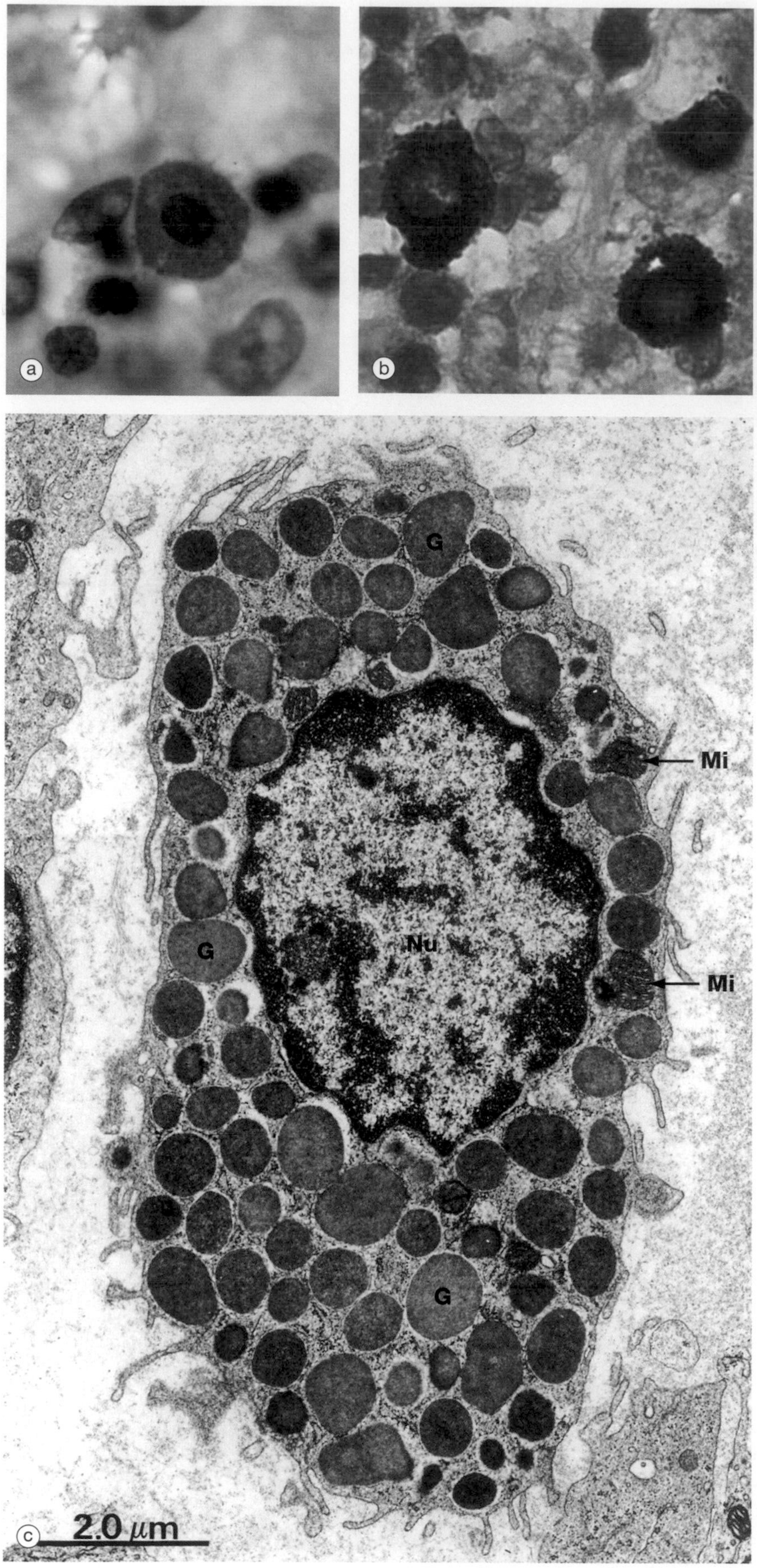

FIG. 4.20 Mast cells
(a) H&E (HP) (b) Toluidine blue (HP)
(c) EM ×12 000

Mast cells are found in all supporting tissues but are particularly prevalent in the skin, gastrointestinal lining, the serosal lining of the peritoneal and pleural cavities and around blood vessels. Their major constituents and functions are very similar to those of basophils, to which they are related (see Fig. 3.11). Mast cells are long-lived with the ability to proliferate in the tissues. Mast cell degranulation results in the release of ***histamine*** and other vasoactive mediators which induce the ***immediate hypersensitivity*** (***anaphylactoid***) ***response*** characteristic of urticaria, allergic rhinitis, asthma and anaphylactic shock.

Mast cells may be inconspicuous in routine histological sections due to the water solubility of their densely basophilic granules, which tend to be lost during preparation. Special techniques of fixation, embedding and staining may be employed. With suitable preparation, Fig. 4.20a, however, the characteristic feature of mast cells is an extensive cytoplasm packed with large granules; these are smaller in size, though more numerous, than those of basophils. When stained with certain blue basic dyes such as ***toluidine blue***, the granules bind to the dye, changing its colour. This property of staining a different colour to the dye is known as ***metachromasia***, Fig. 4.20b.

In Fig. 4.20c, mast cell granules **G** are seen to be membrane bound and to contain a dense amorphous material. The granules are liberated from the cell by exocytosis when stimulated during an inflammatory or allergic response. The cytoplasm contains a few rounded mitochondria **Mi** and a little rough endoplasmic reticulum. The non-segmented nucleus **Nu** has less condensed chromatin than that of basophils. Other differences from basophils include a more uniform distribution of their thin surface processes, a greater number of cytoplasmic filaments and a lack of glycogen granules.

Eo eosinophil **F** fibroblast **G** mast cell granule **L** lymphocyte **Ma** mast cell **Mc** macrophage **Mi** mitochondrion **N** neutrophil **Nu** nucleus **PC** plasma cell

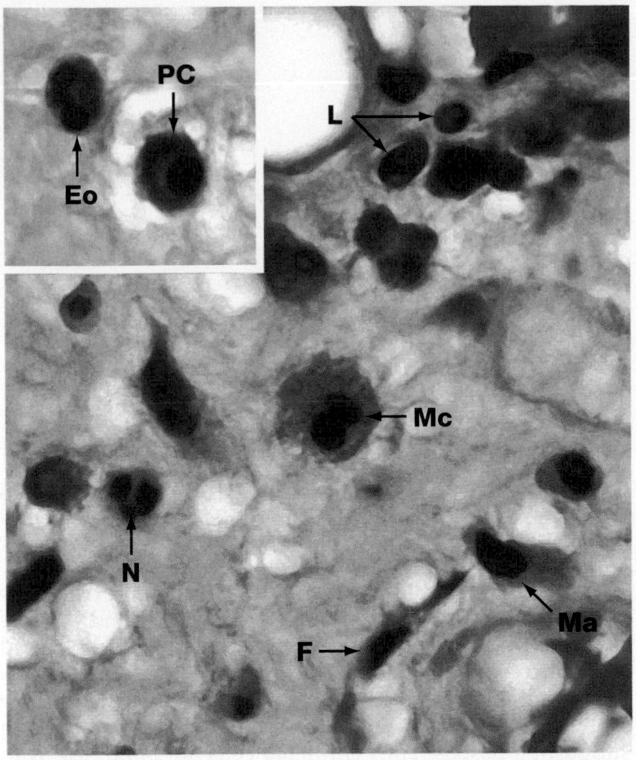

FIG. 4.21 Leukocytes in loose connective tissue H&E (HP)

The appearance of leukocytes in tissue sections differs from their appearance in blood smears (see Ch. 3). In Fig. 4.21, a variety of leukocytes are seen in the loose supporting tissue beneath the nasal epithelium. Fibroblasts **F** are identified by their elongated nuclei. Neutrophils **N** have multilobed nuclei and pale-staining cytoplasm. Eosinophils **Eo** are recognised by their bilobed nuclei and strongly eosinophilic cytoplasmic granules. Mast cells **Ma** show finely granular cytoplasm and often an eccentric rounded nucleus.

Lymphocytes **L** have small, densely stained nuclei and a thin halo of poorly stained cytoplasm. Lymphocyte nuclei are approximately 7 to 8 µm in diameter and provide a useful reference for the size of other cells in tissue sections. Plasma cells **PC** have eccentric round nuclei, abundant amphophilic cytoplasm and a pale-stained perinuclear area (***perinuclear hof***) which represents a well-developed Golgi apparatus.

When they have been actively phagocytic, macrophages may be recognised by their large size and cytoplasmic content of engulfed material. Note, however, that active macrophages have an extremely variable appearance depending on the nature of their phagocytic activity. The macrophage shown in this tissue **Mc** has a granular pale purple cytoplasm, possibly representing mucous material phagocytosed from the local environment.

REVIEW

TABLE 4.1 Review of supporting/connective tissue

Specialised tissue type	Tissue type subcategory	Key features	Functional attributes	Figure
Matrix fibres	Collagen fibres	Type I collagen, type II collagen, etc	Strength and structure	4.3, 4.4
	Elastin	Elastin and fibrillin	Stretch and elasticity; elastin is formed on fibrillin microfibres	4.6–4.9
Ground substances	Glycosaminoglycans (GAGs)	Hyaluronate, proteoglycans	Water-binding gel, provides volume, structure and interacts with supporting cells, epithelial cells, blood vessels and immune cells	4.10
	Structural glycoproteins	Fibronectin	Structural glycoproteins; binds and interacts with many connective tissue molecular components	
Basement membrane	Interface of cells with connective tissue	Type IV collagen, nidogen, heparan sulphate, etc	Specialised structures formed where epithelia and other cells meet connective tissue matrix Binds epithelial cells to connective tissue Connective tissue and epithelial cells contribute to formation and maintenance	4.11, 4.12
Cells	Mesenchyme	Mesenchymal cells	Embryological and fetal cells which form connective tissue	4.2
	Fibroblasts	Fibroblast	Creates and maintains connective tissue, fibres and matrix	4.1, 4.13, 4.14
		Myofibroblast	Activated fibroblast specialised for tissue repair with contractile ability; generates repair/healing with scar	4.13
	Adipocytes	White adipose	Specialised tissue for storage of triglycerides (fat) as an energy reserve; also has metabolic and structural roles	4.15, 4.16
		Brown adipose	Specialised form of adipose tissue most prominent in babies; metabolises triglycerides for heat under the control of the nervous system	4.17, 4.18
	Haematopoietic stem cell-derived	Mast cells	Tissue resident immune cells involved in immediate hypersensitivity and allergy	4.20
		Tissue macrophages	Tissue resident immune cells with prominent phagocytic abilities and major roles in the immune system	4.19
		Lymphocytes, eosinophils, neutrophils, plasma cells	Other immune cells (usually in transit or in response to inflammation)	4.21 Ch. 3

5 Epithelial tissues

INTRODUCTION

The ***epithelia*** (singular: ***epithelium***) are a diverse group of tissues that include both ***surface epithelia*** and ***solid organs***. Surface epithelia cover or line all body surfaces, cavities and tubes and form the interface between different biological compartments. For instance, the epidermis of the skin is exposed to the external environment and the epithelial lining of the gastrointestinal tract is exposed to partially digested food and bacteria in the lumen of the gut. Functions of epithelia include: forming a protective barrier, regulation of the exchange of molecules between compartments (selective diffusion and absorption) and synthesis and secretion of glandular products. Many of these major functions may be exhibited at a single epithelial surface. For example, the epithelial lining of the small intestine is primarily involved in absorption of the products of digestion, but the epithelium also protects itself from noxious intestinal contents by secreting a surface coating of mucus. Epithelial cells are characterised by the production of ***keratin intermediate filaments*** (see Ch. 1), and this can be used to recognise epithelial cells using immunohistochemistry, a technique often used in diagnostic histopathology to classify difficult malignant tumours (see Appendix 2).

Surface epithelia form continuous sheets comprising one or more layers of cells. Epithelial cells are bound to adjacent cells by a variety of ***cell junctions*** that provide physical strength and mediate exchange of information and metabolites. All epithelia are supported by a ***basement membrane*** (see Ch. 4) which separates the epithelium from underlying supporting tissues. Thus epithelial cells are ***polarised***, with one side facing the basement membrane and underlying supporting tissues (the basal surface) and the other facing outwards (the apical surface).

Blood vessels never cross epithelial basement membranes, so epithelia depend on the diffusion of oxygen and metabolites from adjacent supporting tissues.

CLASSIFICATION OF SURFACE EPITHELIA

Surface epithelia are traditionally classified according to three morphological characteristics: number of cell layers, type of cell (profile perpendicular to basement membrane) and special features. Special features include adaptations such as ***cilia*** or ***goblet cells*** that may be characteristic of particular sites (e.g. the epithelium of the upper respiratory tract is a ciliated pseudostratified columnar epithelium).

TABLE 5.1 Classification of epithelia

Number of cell layers	Type of cell	Special features	Example
Simple (one layer)	Squamous (flattened)		Peritoneum, vascular endothelium
	Cuboidal		Collecting tubule of kidney
		Microvilli	Proximal convoluted tubule of kidney
	Columnar		Gallbladder
		Microvilli	Small intestine
		Surface cilia	Fallopian tube
		Pseudostratification	Respiratory tract
		Goblet cells	Small and large bowel
		Stereocilia	Vas deferens
Stratified (multiple layers)	Squamous		Oral cavity
		Keratinisation	Epidermis of skin
	Cuboidal		Exocrine gland ducts
	Transitional		Bladder

GLANDULAR EPITHELIA

Epithelium that is primarily involved in secretion is often arranged into structures called ***glands***. Glands are merely invaginations of epithelial surfaces which are formed during embryonic development by proliferation of epithelium into the underlying tissues. For example, glandular epithelium is characteristic of the lining of much of the gastrointestinal tract.

However, some solid organs are composed largely of epithelial cells with a supporting tissue framework. Some of these organs are connected to the surface epithelium of the gastrointestinal tract by a branching system of ducts and belong to the category of ***exocrine glands*** (e.g. salivary glands). ***Endocrine glands*** on the other hand have lost their connection to the epithelial surface from which they developed and release their secretions directly into the blood (e.g. thyroid gland). Most of the solid epithelial organs such as liver, pancreas and thyroid are described in detail in the relevant organ system chapter and only a few examples are described here.

SIMPLE EPITHELIA

Simple epithelia are defined as surface epithelia consisting of a single layer of cells. Simple epithelia are almost always found at interfaces involved in selective diffusion, absorption and/or secretion. They provide little protection against mechanical abrasion and thus are not found on surfaces subject to such stresses. The cells comprising simple epithelia range in shape from flattened to tall columnar, depending on their function. For example, flattened simple epithelia are ideally suited to diffusion and are therefore found in the air sacs of the lung (***alveoli***), the lining of blood vessels (***endothelium***) and lining body cavities (***mesothelium***). In contrast, highly active epithelial cells, such as the cells lining the small intestine, are generally tall since they must accommodate the appropriate organelles. Simple epithelia may exhibit a variety of surface specialisations, such as ***microvilli*** and ***cilia***, which facilitate their specific surface functions.

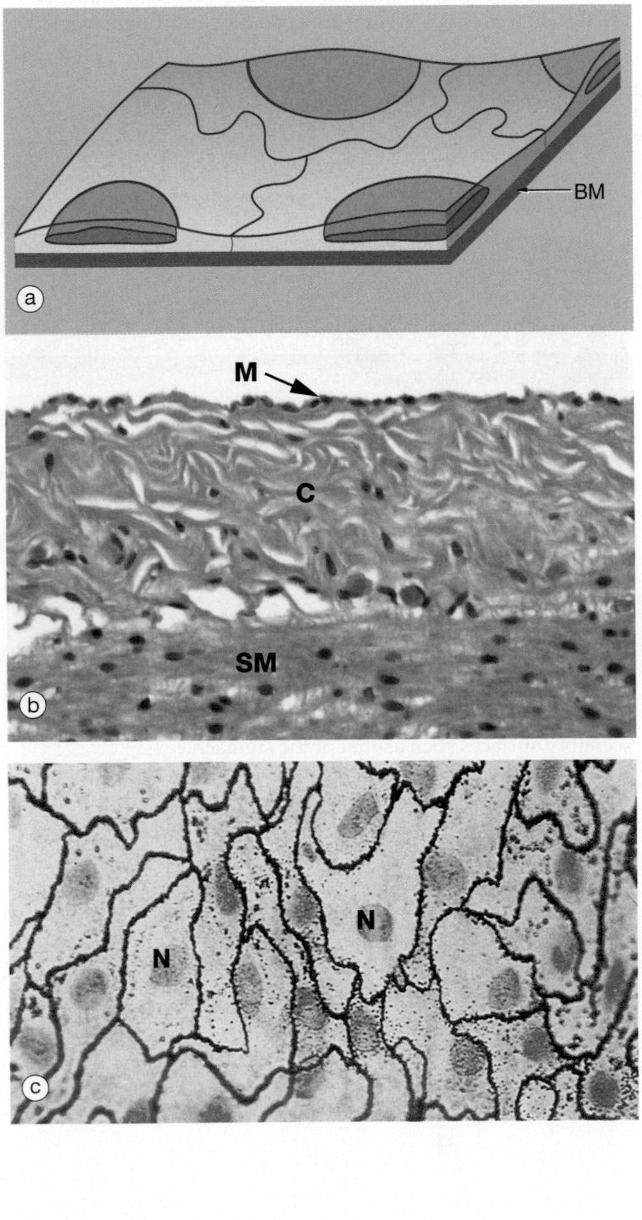

FIG. 5.1 Simple squamous epithelium
(a) Diagram (b) H&E (HP) (c) Spread preparation, silver method/neutral red (HP)

Simple squamous epithelium is composed of flattened, irregularly shaped cells forming a continuous surface that is sometimes called ***pavemented epithelium***; the term ***squamous*** derives from the comparison of the cells to the scales of a fish. Like all epithelia, this delicate lining is supported by an underlying basement membrane **BM** as shown diagrammatically in Fig. 5.1a.

Simple squamous epithelium is found lining surfaces involved in passive transport (diffusion) of either gases (as in the lungs) or fluids (as in the walls of blood capillaries). Simple squamous epithelium also forms the delicate lining of the pleural, pericardial and peritoneal cavities where it allows passage of tissue fluid into and out of these cavities. Although these cells appear simple in form they have a wide variety of important roles.

Fig. 5.1b shows a ***mesothelium*** (peritoneum) covering the surface of the appendix and illustrates the typical appearance of simple squamous epithelium in section. The mesothelial lining cells **M** are so flattened that they can only be recognised by their nuclei, which bulge on the surface. The supporting basement membrane is thin and, in H&E stained preparations, has similar staining properties to the underlying collagenous supporting tissue **C**; hence it cannot be seen in this micrograph. Deeper in the wall of the appendix, the smooth muscle **SM** of the muscularis propria can be identified.

In the preparation used in Fig. 5.1c, the mesothelial lining of the peritoneal cavity has been stripped from the underlying tissues and spread onto a slide, thus permitting a surface view of simple squamous epithelium. The intercellular substance has been stained with silver thereby outlining the closely interdigitating and highly irregular cell boundaries. The nuclei **N** are stained a slightly darker pink.

BM basement membrane **C** collagenous supporting tissue **M** mesothelial lining cells **N** nucleus **SM** smooth muscle

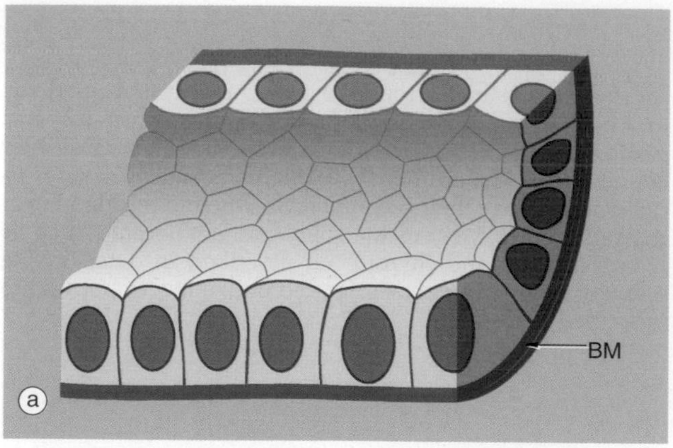

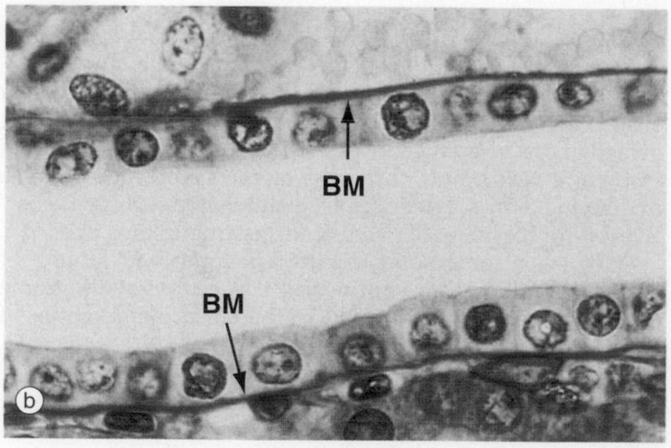

FIG. 5.2 Simple cuboidal epithelium
(a) Diagram (b) Azan (HP)

Simple cuboidal epithelium represents an intermediate form between simple squamous and simple columnar epithelium; the distinction between tall cuboidal and low columnar is often arbitrary and is of descriptive value only. In the section perpendicular to the basement membrane **BM**, the epithelial cells appear square, leading to its traditional description as cuboidal epithelium; on surface view, however, the cells are actually polygonal in shape, as shown in Fig. 5.2a. The nucleus is usually round and located in the centre of the cell.

Simple cuboidal epithelium usually lines small ducts and tubules that may have excretory, secretory or absorptive functions; examples are the collecting tubules of the kidney and the small excretory ducts of the salivary glands and pancreas.

Fig. 5.2b shows the cells lining a collecting tubule in the kidney. Although the boundaries between individual cells are indistinct, the nuclear shape provides an approximate indication of the cell size and shape. The underlying basement membrane **BM** appears as a prominent blue line with the Azan staining method, in contrast to basement membranes stained with the standard H&E stain (see Fig. 5.3b) that are generally indistinguishable.

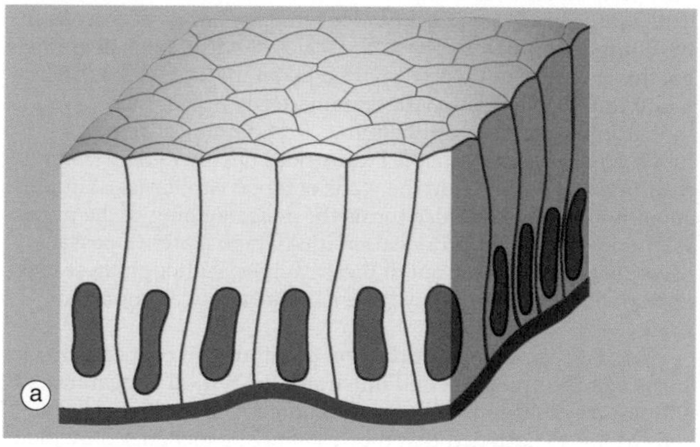

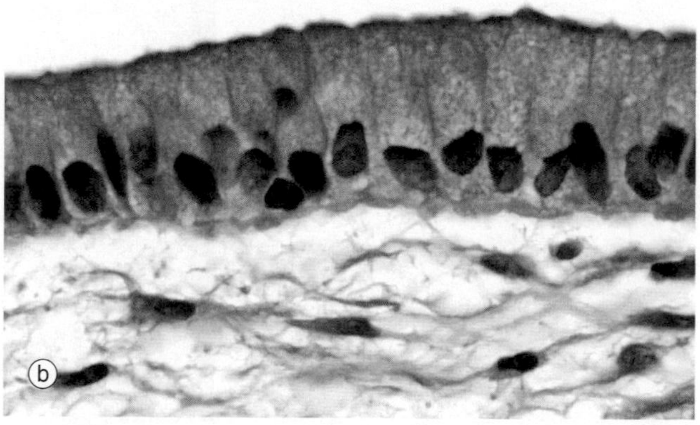

FIG. 5.3 Simple columnar epithelium
(a) Diagram (b) H&E (HP)

Simple columnar epithelium is similar to simple cuboidal epithelium except that the cells are taller and appear columnar in sections perpendicular to the basement membrane (Fig. 5.3a). The height of the cells may vary from low to tall columnar, depending on the site and/or degree of functional activity. The nuclei are elongated and may be located towards the base, the centre or occasionally the apex of the cytoplasm; this is known as the ***polarity*** of the nucleus. Simple columnar epithelium is found on absorptive surfaces such as in the small intestine, as well as at secretory surfaces such as that of the stomach.

Fig. 5.3b shows simple columnar epithelium taken from the endocervix where it has the function of secreting mucus. Note the typically basally located nuclei.

BM basement membrane **C** cilia

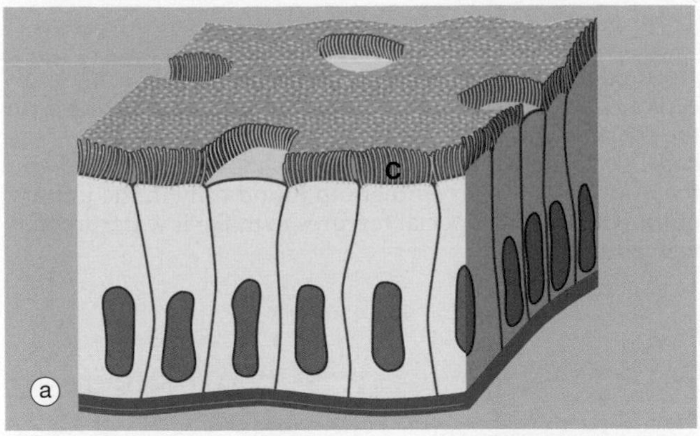

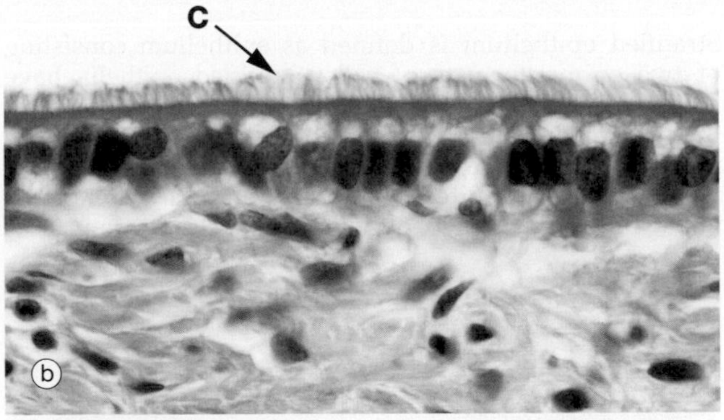

FIG. 5.4 Simple columnar ciliated epithelium
(a) Diagram (b) H&E (HP)

Some simple columnar epithelia (Fig. 5.4a) have surface cilia **C** on the majority of the cells (see also Fig. 5.13). Among the ciliated cells are scattered non-ciliated cells that usually have a secretory function.

Cilia are much larger than microvilli (see Fig. 5.14) and are readily visible with the light microscope. Each cilium consists of a finger-like projection of the plasma membrane, its cytoplasm containing modified microtubules. Each cell may have up to 300 cilia that beat in a wave-like manner, synchronised with the adjacent cells. The waving motion of the cilia propels fluid or minute particles over the epithelial surface. Simple columnar ciliated epithelium is found mainly in the female reproductive tract. Fig. 5.4b, taken from the Fallopian tube (oviduct), shows one of its numerous folds covered by simple columnar ciliated epithelium. The predominant cell type in this epithelium is tall columnar and ciliated, the nuclei being located towards the midzone of the cells. The less numerous blue-stained cells with basally located nuclei are not ciliated and have a secretory function. Ciliary action facilitates transport of the ovum from the ovary towards the uterus.

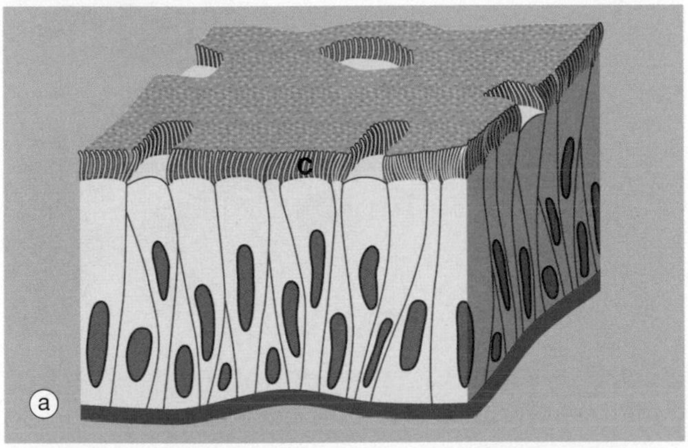

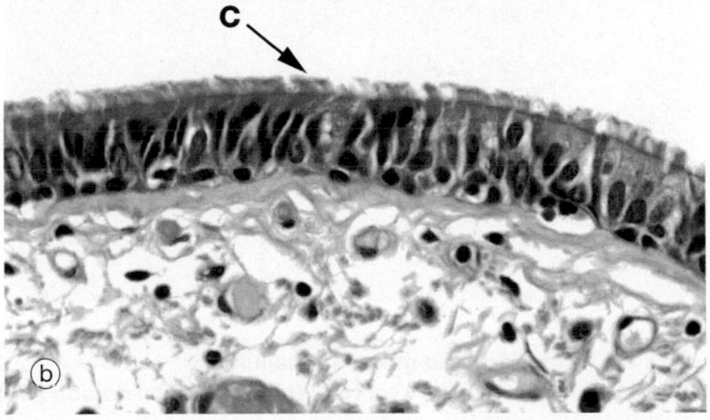

FIG. 5.5 Pseudostratified columnar ciliated epithelium
(a) Diagram (b) H&E (MP)

Another variant of simple columnar epithelium is described in which the majority of cells are also usually ciliated **C**. The term ***pseudostratified*** is derived from the appearance of this epithelium in section, which conveys the erroneous impression that there is more than one layer of cells. In fact, this is a true simple epithelium, since all the cells rest on the basement membrane. The nuclei of these cells, however, are disposed at different levels, thus creating the illusion of cellular stratification (Fig. 5.5a). Scattered stem cells (see Ch. 2) are found throughout the epithelium; these generally are devoid of cilia (i.e. less differentiated) and do not extend to the luminal surface.

Pseudostratified columnar ciliated epithelium may be distinguished from true stratified epithelia by two characteristics. Firstly, the individual cells of the pseudostratified epithelium exhibit polarity, with nuclei being mainly confined to the basal two-thirds of the epithelium. Secondly, cilia are never present on true stratified epithelia.

Pseudostratified epithelium is almost exclusively confined to the airways of the respiratory system in mammals and is therefore often referred to as ***respiratory epithelium***. Fig. 5.5b illustrates the lining of a bronchus. In the respiratory tract, the cilia propel a surface layer of mucus containing entrapped particles towards the pharynx in what is often described as the ***mucociliary escalator***. The mucus is secreted by non-ciliated goblet cells found amongst the ciliated cells (not seen in this micrograph, see Figs 5.16 and 5.17).

STRATIFIED EPITHELIA

Stratified epithelium is defined as epithelium consisting of two or more layers of cells. Stratified epithelia have mainly a protective function and the degree and nature of the stratification are related to the kinds of physical stresses to which the surface is exposed. In general, stratified epithelia are poorly suited for absorption and secretion by virtue of their thickness, although some stratified surfaces are moderately permeable to water and other small molecules. The classification of stratified epithelia is based on the shape and structure of the surface cells, since cells of the basal layer are usually cuboidal in shape. Transitional epithelium is a stratified epithelium found only in the urinary outflow tract, with special features to make it waterproof as well as expansile.

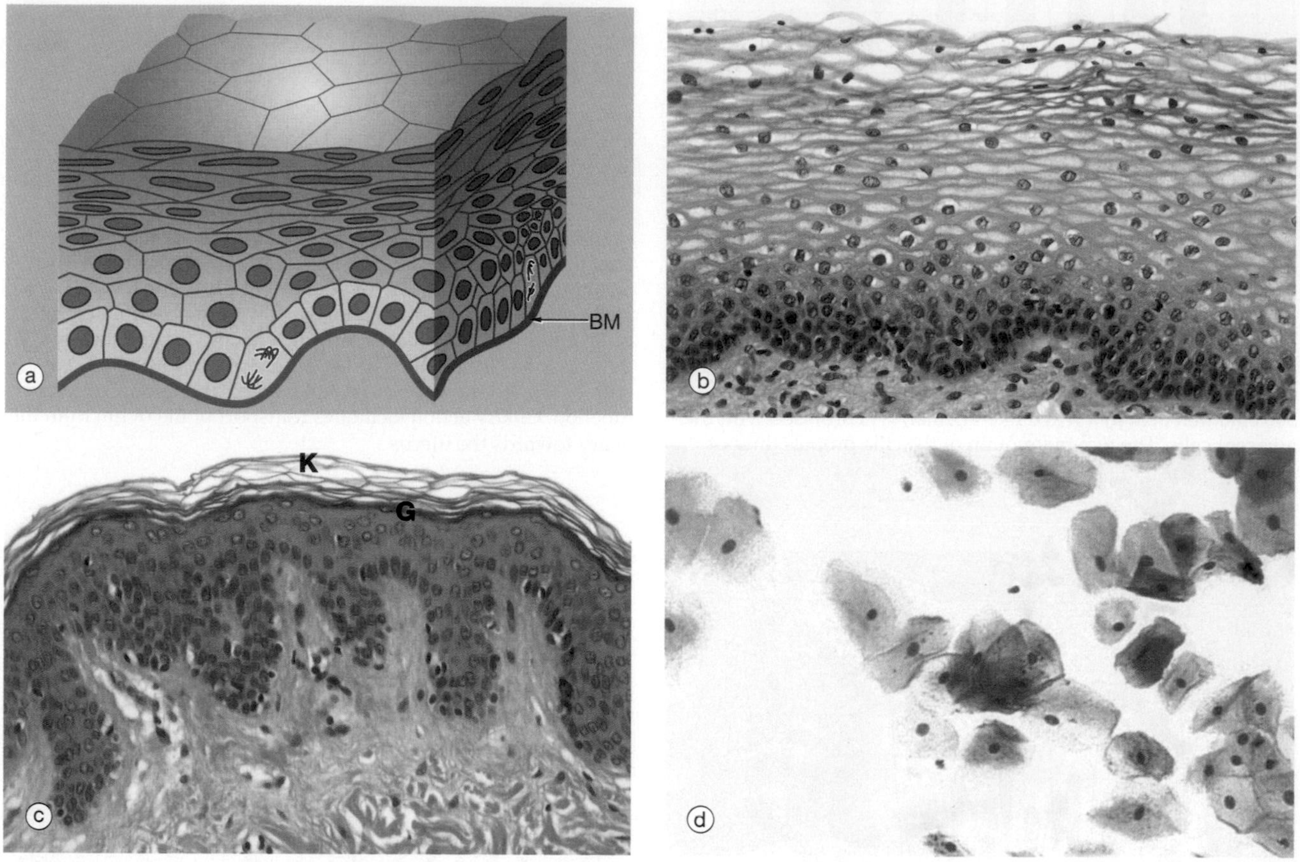

FIG. 5.6 Stratified squamous epithelium
(a) Diagram (b) H&E (HP) (c) H&E (MP) (d) Papanicolaou (HP)

Stratified squamous epithelium (Fig. 5.6a) consists of a variable number of cell layers that exhibit maturation from a cuboidal basal layer to a flattened surface layer. The basal cells which are adherent to the underlying basement membrane **BM** include continuously dividing stem cells, their offspring migrating towards the surface where they are ultimately shed as anucleate ***squames***.

Stratified squamous epithelium is adapted to withstand abrasion, with plentiful cell junctions and a prominent intermediate filament (***keratin***) cytoskeleton. This type of epithelium lines the oral cavity, pharynx, oesophagus, anal canal, uterine cervix and vagina, sites which are subject to mechanical abrasion but which are kept moist by glandular secretions, such as the salivary glands of the mouth.

The epithelium in Fig. 5.6b is from the uterine cervix. Note the cuboidal basal layer and the maturation through the large polygonal cells of the intermediate layers to the flattened superficial squamous cells. The cytoplasm in these cells often appears clear due to the glycogen content.

Keratinising stratified squamous epithelium (Fig. 5.6c) constitutes the epithelial surface of the skin (the ***epidermis***) and is adapted to withstand the constant abrasion and desiccation to which the body surface is exposed. During maturation, the epithelial cells accumulate keratin intermediate filaments which are cross-linked with proteins such as involucrin and loricrin in a process called ***keratinisation*** (or ***cornification***). This results in the formation of a tough, non-living surface layer (***stratum corneum***) consisting of a compacted cross-linked keratin matrix **K** interspersed with specialised lipids (see Ch. 9). The underlying granular cell layer **G** consists of epithelial cells with extensive tight junctions, forming a waterproof barrier.

The nuclei of the maturing epithelial cells become progressively condensed (***pyknotic***) and eventually disappear along with the other cellular organelles. Keratinisation may be induced in normally non-keratinising stratified squamous epithelium such as that of the oral cavity when exposed to excessive abrasion (e.g. poorly fitting false teeth).

Fig. 5.6d shows a smear made from normal cells scraped from the uterine cervix as it projects into the vagina. The degenerate, scaly superficial cells stain pink with this staining method, while the living cells from deeper layers stain blue. This is the basis of the well-known 'Pap smear' which examines cytological preparations of cervical cells for pre-cancerous changes (see e-Fig. 5.1).

BM basement membrane **G** granular layer **K** keratin layer **U** umbrella cell

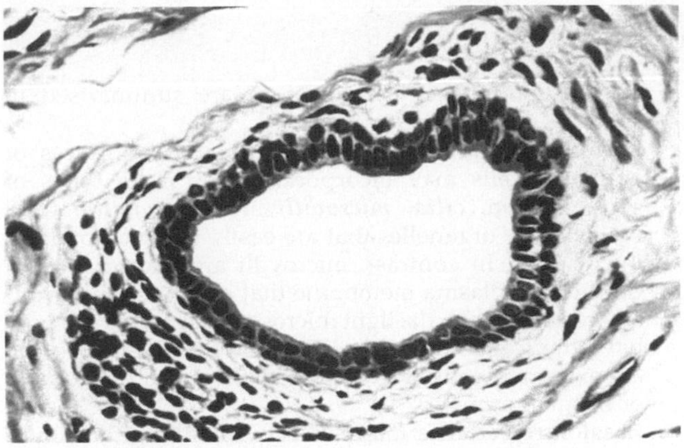

FIG. 5.7 **Stratified cuboidal epithelium H&E (HP)**

Stratified cuboidal epithelium is a thin, stratified epithelium that usually consists of only two or three layers of cuboidal cells. This type of epithelium is usually confined to the lining of the larger excretory ducts of exocrine glands such as the salivary glands. Stratified cuboidal epithelium is probably not involved in significant absorptive or secretory activity but merely provides a more robust lining than would be afforded by a simple epithelium.

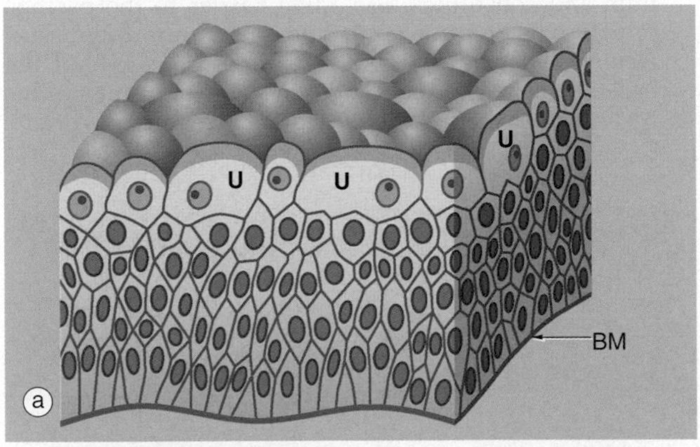

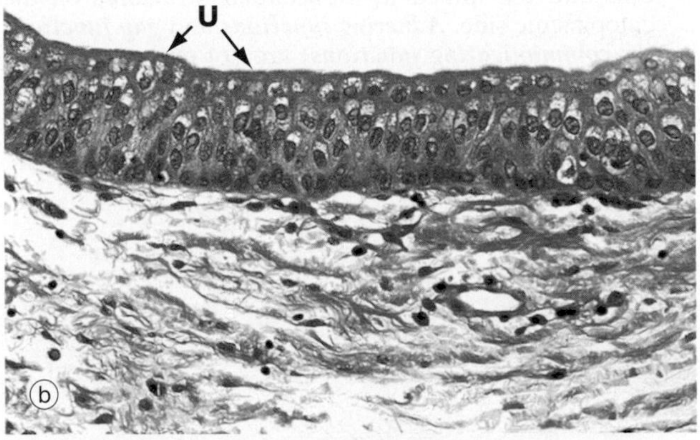

FIG. 5.8 **Transitional epithelium (a) Diagram (b) H&E (HP)**

Transitional epithelium (or ***urothelium***) is a form of stratified epithelium found only in the urinary tract in mammals, where it is highly specialised to accommodate a great degree of stretch and to withstand the toxicity of urine. This epithelial type is so named because it has some features intermediate (transitional) between stratified cuboidal and stratified squamous epithelia. In the non-distended state, transitional epithelium appears to be about four to five cell layers thick. The basal cells are roughly cuboidal, the intermediate cells are polygonal and the surface cells (***umbrella*** or ***dome cells*** **U**) are large and rounded and may contain two nuclei. In the stretched state, transitional epithelium often appears only two or three cells thick (although the actual number of layers remains constant) and the intermediate and surface layers are extremely flattened.

Fig. 5.8b shows the appearance of transitional epithelium from the lining of a non-distended bladder. The shape and apparent size of the basal and intermediate cells vary considerably depending on the degree of distension, but the cells of the surface layer usually retain characteristic features. Firstly, the surface umbrella cells are large and pale stained with a scalloped surface outline often overlapping two or more of the underlying cells. Secondly, the luminal surface of the cells appears thickened and more densely stained.

Keratins

Keratin intermediate filaments (also called ***cytokeratins, CK***) are the characteristic intermediate filaments of epithelial cells. Keratins may be subclassified into α- and β-keratins. α-Keratins are the only types found in mammals and may be further subdivided into acidic and basic subtypes (type I and type II, respectively). β-Keratins are typical of feathers, scales, beaks and claws of birds and reptiles and do not occur in mammals. Humans have 54 genes for keratins found on chromosomes 17 and 12. Keratins are vital for the maintenance of cell shape and polarity, and different keratin types are found in different epithelia and indeed in different layers of stratified epithelia. For instance, the basal cells of epidermis produce keratins K5 and K14 (commonly referred to as CK5 and CK14 in clinical practice), while the suprabasal layers exhibit K1 and K10, and hair is characterised by K31–40 and K81–86.

Keratins confer mechanical strength on epithelia, so it is not surprising that those epithelia subjected to the greatest mechanical stresses contain large amounts of keratins which are connected to the intercellular junctions (***desmosomes***), thus linking the cytoskeletons of adjacent cells and cell–basement membrane junctions (***hemidesmosomes***).

Simple epithelia also contain characteristic keratins, usually K8 and K18 as well as others that are sometimes restricted to particular sites. For instance, colonic mucosa characteristically contains K20 while gastric epithelium expresses K7. In diagnostic histopathology, this differential expression of cytokeratins can be used to classify poorly differentiated metastatic tumours where there is no known primary site (see e-Table 5.1). This may be very important to enable decisions about treatment to be made, as different tumours may respond better to different types of chemotherapy and/or radiotherapy.

MEMBRANE SPECIALISATIONS OF EPITHELIA

The plasma membranes of epithelial cells exhibit a variety of specialised structures that allow them to perform their function as a barrier with selective permeability. In some cases, the epithelial barrier is very impermeable, such as the transitional epithelium of the bladder, while other epithelia, such as the lining of the small intestine or the convoluted tubules of the kidney, promote movement of selected ions and molecules across the epithelium.

- **Intercellular surfaces**. The adjacent or lateral surfaces of epithelial cells are linked by ***cell junctions*** so that the epithelium forms a continuous, cohesive layer. Cell junctions also operate as communication channels governing such functions as growth and cell division. The various types of cell junction are composed of transmembrane proteins that interact with similar proteins on adjacent cells and are linked to intracellular structures on the cytoplasmic side. ***Adhering junctions*** and ***gap junctions*** (or ***communicating junctions***) are not exclusive to epithelia and are also present in cardiac and visceral muscle where they appear to serve similar functions. The main features of intercellular junctions are summarised in Table 5.2.
- **Luminal surfaces**. The luminal or apical surfaces of epithelial cells may incorporate three main types of specialisation: ***cilia, microvilli*** and ***stereocilia***. Cilia are hair-like organelles that are easily resolved by light microscopy. In contrast, microvilli are shorter projections of the plasma membrane that cannot be individually resolved with the light microscope. A single cell may have thousands of microvilli or only a few. Stereocilia are extremely long microvilli usually found only singly or in small numbers.
- **Basal surfaces**. The interface between all epithelia and underlying supporting tissues is marked by a non- cellular structure known as the ***basement membrane*** (see Ch. 4) that provides structural support for the epithelium and constitutes a selective barrier to the passage of materials between epithelium and supporting tissue. ***Hemidesmosomes***, a variant of ***desmosomes***, bind the base of the cell to the underlying basement membrane by linking to the cell's intermediate filament network.

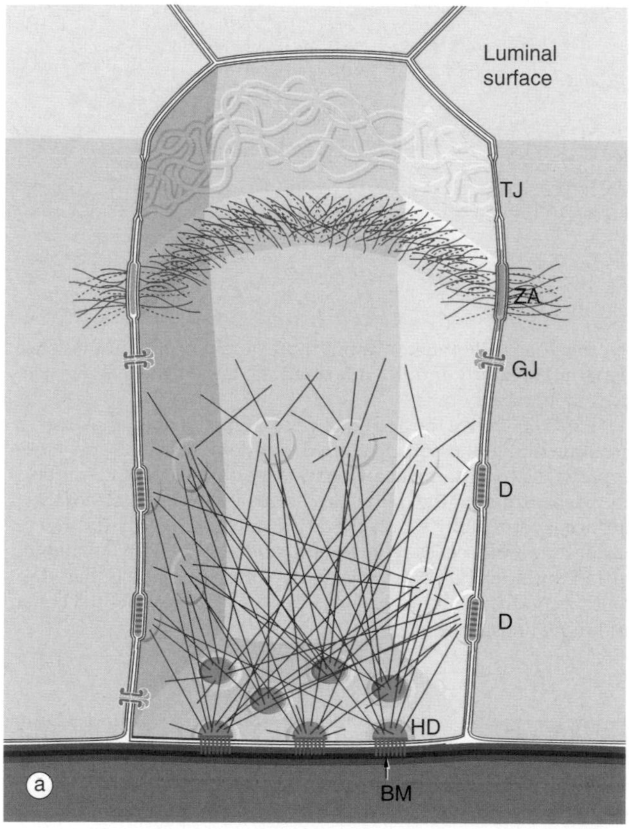

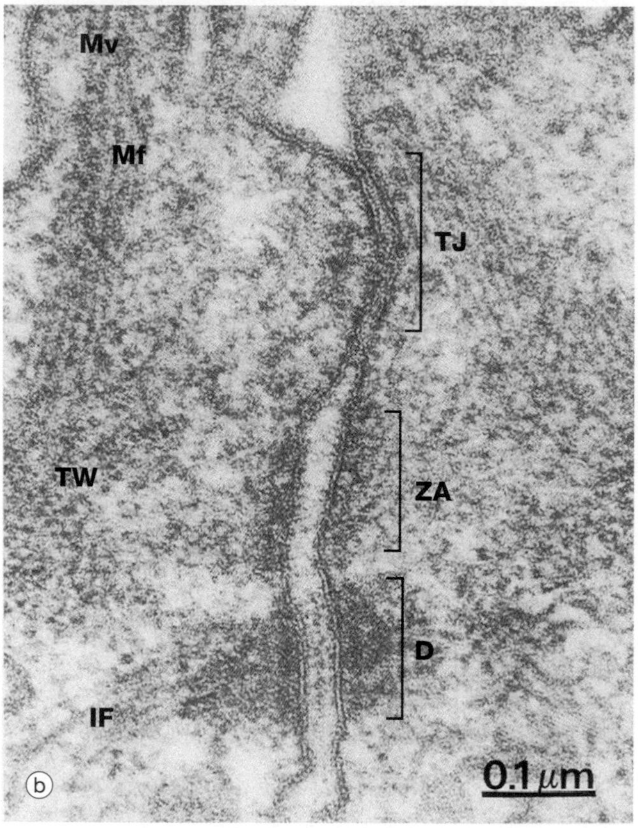

FIG. 5.9 Intercellular junctions
(a) Schematic diagram (b) Junctional complex, EM ×125 000

Fig. 5.9a outlines the three-dimensional organisation of the various intercellular junctions and their interaction with the cytoskeleton. In simple cuboidal and simple columnar epithelia, a ***junctional complex*** encircles each cell, sealing the intercellular spaces and holding the cells tightly together. Also illustrated are the basement membrane **BM** with associated hemidesmosomes **HD**. Gap junctions **GJ** are also present (see Fig. 5.12).

As seen in Fig. 5.9b of intestinal columnar epithelium, the junctional complex at the luminal end of the lateral plasma membrane is made up of three components: a ***tight junction*** **TJ** (***zonula occludens***), an ***adhering belt*** (***zonula adherens***) **ZA** and a row of ***desmosomes*** **D**. The bases of microvilli **Mv** covering the surface of the small intestinal lining cells can be identified. Each microvillus contains a core of actin microfilaments **Mf** which insert into the ***terminal web*** **TW** (see Fig. 5.14). Actin microfilaments are anchored to the zonula adherens, and keratin intermediate filaments **IF** bind to desmosomes.

BM basement membrane **D** desmosome **GJ** gap junction **HD** hemidesmosome **IF** intermediate filaments **Mf** actin microfilaments **Mv** microvillus **TJ** tight junction **TW** terminal web **ZA** zonula adherens

TABLE 5.2 Intercellular junctions

Intercellular junction type	Main protein components	Cytoskeleton connections	Site	Main functions
Tight junction (occluding junction, zonula occludens)	Claudins, occludins, tricellulin	Actin microfilaments	Found at luminal end of lateral cell membrane	Control of paracellular diffusion Prevents exchange of intrinsic proteins and lipids between apical and basolateral plasma membrane
Adhering belt (zonula adherens)	Classic cadherins, catenins	Actin microfilaments Microtubules	Lateral plasma membrane, immediately deep to tight junction	Link cytoskeletons of adjacent cells to form strong cohesive epithelium
Desmosome (macula adherens)	Cadherins	Intermediate filaments (keratins in epithelia)	Lateral plasma membrane	Link cytoskeletons of adjacent cells to form strong cohesive epithelium
Hemidesmosomes	Integrins Laminins of basement membrane	Intermediate filaments (keratins in epithelia)	Basal plasma membrane	Link cells to underlying basement membrane
Gap junctions	Connexins	None	Lateral plasma membrane	Passage of ions and small molecules between cells Intercellular signalling

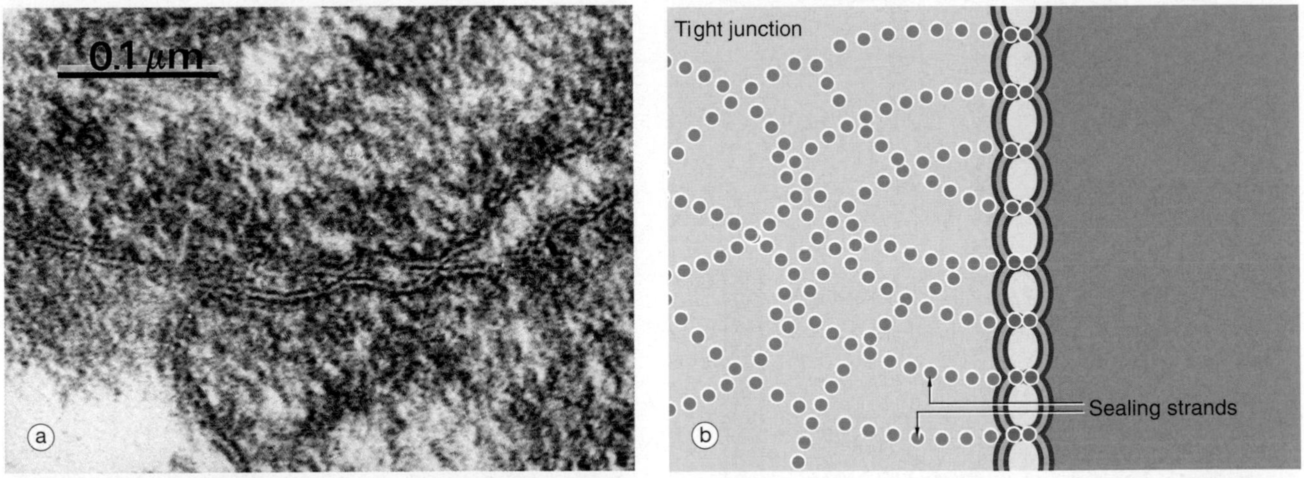

FIG. 5.10 Tight junctions
(a) EM ×190 000 (b) Schematic diagram

The tight junction (occluding junction or zonula occludens) forms a collar around each cell immediately beneath the apical surface, blocking passage of luminal contents between cells and also lateral movement of plasma membrane proteins and lipids in the plane of the membrane between the apical and the basolateral plasma membrane. As seen in Fig. 5.10a, the outer electron-dense layers of opposing cell membranes come extremely close together and, in places, appear to fuse completely. At the molecular level, members of the transmembrane protein families, the ***claudins*** and ***occludins***, form tight links between adjacent cells. Claudins allow passage of selected cations between cells, acting as ion channels (the ***paracellular pathway***). The presence of different claudin molecules in different epithelia explains the variability in permeability between epithelia. ***Tricellulin*** is also present at junctions where three cells meet. Multiple aggregates of tight junction proteins form a branching network known as ***sealing strands*** (Fig. 5.10b). On the cytoplasmic side of the plasma membrane, the tight junctions are linked to the actin cytoskeleton.

Structurally similar but discontinuous strips of tight junction, called ***fascia occludens***, are found between the endothelial cells lining blood vessels, except in the vessels of the brain where they are of the continuous (zonula occludens) type.

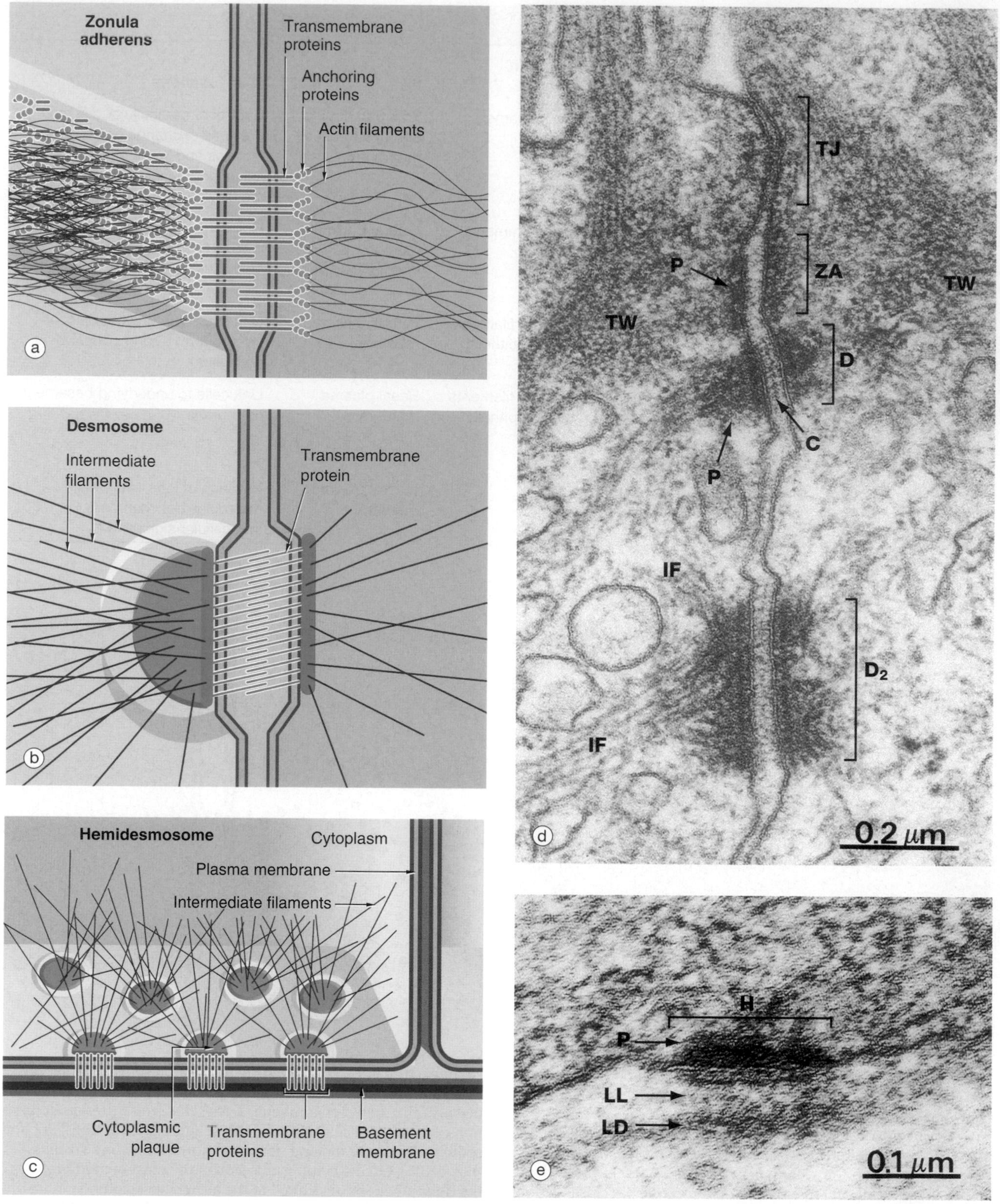

FIG. 5.11 Adhering junctions *(caption continues opposite)*
(a–c) Diagrams (d) EM ×95 000 (e) EM ×150 000

Adhering junctions provide anchorage points for cytoskeletal elements, linking the cytoskeletons of individual cells into a strong transcellular network. These junctions are of three types; the ***adhesion belt (zonula adherens)*** and the ***desmosome*** (***macula adherens***) link adjacent cells, and the ***hemidesmosome*** links the cell to the underlying basement membrane. The zonula adherens forms a single continuous band lying deep to the tight junction at the luminal end of the lateral plasma membranes of columnar epithelium. Deep to the zonula adherens there is ring of desmosomes, the third component of the junctional complex. Larger desmosomes are also scattered over the intercellular surfaces of all epithelial cells. Adhering junctions consist of three components: transmembrane proteins bind to similar proteins on adjacent cells (zonula adherens and desmosomes) or to extracellular matrix (hemidesmosomes), and anchoring proteins on the cytoplasmic side of the junction that link the transmembrane proteins to the third component, the cytoskeleton.

Zonula adherens (Fig. 5.11a) consist of cadherin transmembrane proteins linked to intracellular catenins and actin microfilaments. The cadherins (mainly E-cadherin) span the plasma membranes of the cells and bind to identical cadherins on adjacent cells. The cytoplasmic tails of the cadherins bind to anchor proteins (catenins, vinculin and α-actinin) which in turn bind to actin microfilaments. The intracellular component of the zonula adherens can be seen in Fig. 5.11d as a small electron-dense plaque **P** on the cytoplasmic side of the plasma membrane.

Desmosomes (Fig. 5.11b) employ different members of the cadherin superfamily as transmembrane proteins. The overlapping segments of the cadherin molecules in the intercellular space form an electron-dense line **C**. On the cytoplasmic side,

FIG. 5.11 Adhering junctions ***(illustrations and start of caption opposite)***
(a–c) Diagrams (d) EM ×95 000 (e) EM ×150 000

anchoring proteins (desmoplakin and plakoglobin) bind to intermediate filaments **IF** forming a prominent electron-dense plaque **P**. Desmosome numbers are greatest in stratified squamous epithelia that have to withstand the greatest friction.

Hemidesmosomes (Fig. 5.11c) are modified desmosomes that are found at the basal surface of the cell. In this case, the transmembrane proteins are integrins, the extracellular components of which bind to extracellular laminins in the basement membrane (see Ch. 4). The intracellular component of the integrins binds to the anchor protein plectin and thus to the intermediate filament keratin. Again the intracellular component can be seen as an electron-dense plaque **P**.

Fig. 5.11d from the intestinal lining illustrates a junctional complex comprising tight junction **TJ**, zonula adherens **ZA** and desmosome **D**. At a deeper level, a larger desmosome $\mathbf{D_2}$ is seen. Note the small electron-dense plaque **P** of the zonula adherens and the larger plaques **P** of the desmosomes. The electron-dense line created by overlapping cadherin molecules **C** is also visible in the desmosomes. The terminal web **TW** of the surface microvilli is also evident.

Fig. 5.11e illustrates a hemidesmosome **H** along the basal plasma membrane of an epithelial cell. On the cytoplasmic aspect of the plasma membrane is the protein plaque **P**. The underlying lamina densa **LD** is thickened and more electron-dense than usual, as is the lamina lucida **LL** which contains an electron-dense line. This appearance is the result of binding of the extracellular component of the integrins to the laminins of the basement membrane.

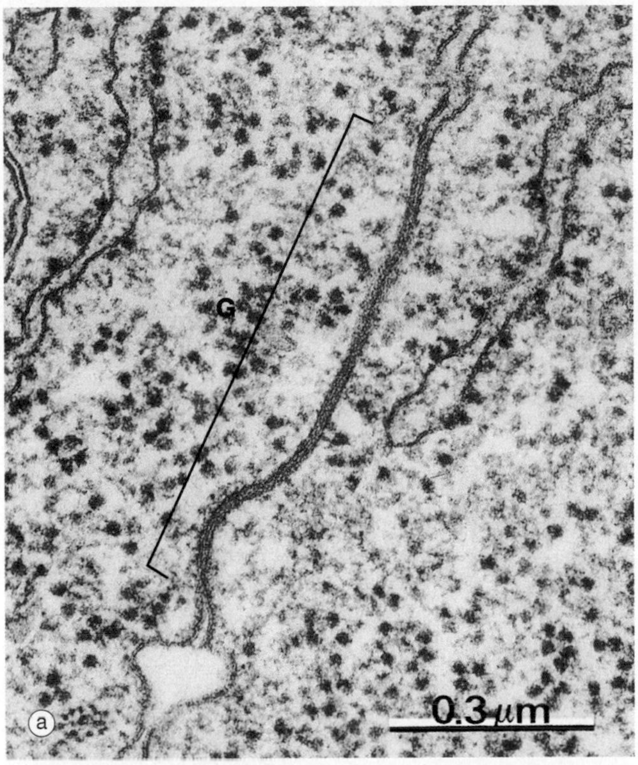

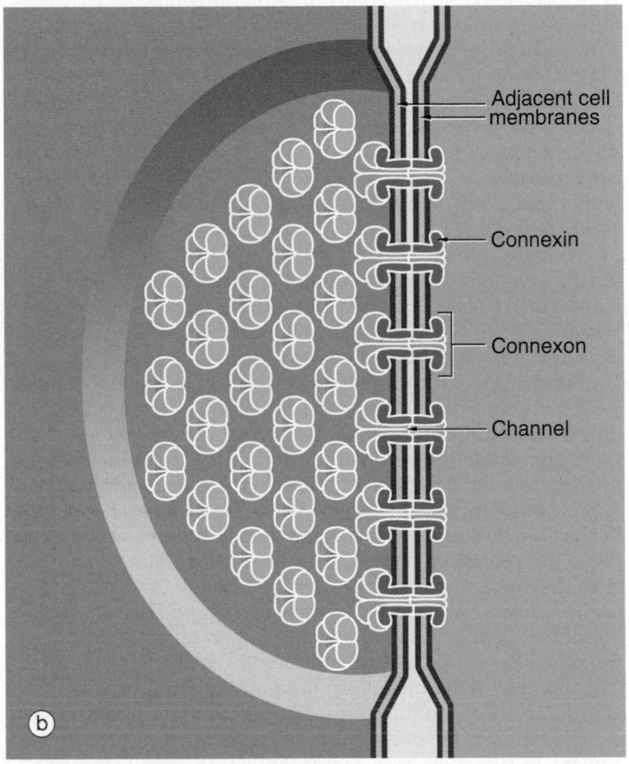

FIG. 5.12 Gap junctions
(a) EM ×80 000 (b) Diagram

Communicating or gap junctions are broad patches where adjacent plasma membranes are closely opposed, leaving a narrow intervening gap 2 to 4 nm in diameter. A gap junction **G** is demonstrated in Fig. 5.12a, taken from intestinal epithelium.

As seen in Fig. 5.12b, each gap junction contains numerous transmembrane channels (***connexons***) that permit the passage of inorganic ions and other small molecules (approximately 1.5 nm in diameter) from the cytoplasm of one cell to another. Large molecules and negatively charged ions are denied access. Gap junctions are thought to be important in the control of growth, development, cell recognition and differentiation. Gap junctions also provide the means of electrical coupling of visceral and cardiac muscle cells, permitting synchronous contraction.

Each connexon is made up of six transmembrane proteins known as ***connexins***. Each connexon aligns with a connexon of a neighbouring cell to form a direct channel between the two cells. There are more than 20 different connexin proteins in humans and these form specific connexons in different tissues with specificity for different molecules and ions. Connexons may be opened or closed depending on the intracellular concentration of calcium ions, the pH or on extracellular signals. For instance, the neurotransmitter dopamine closes gap junctions between certain nerve cells in the retina. A rise in intracellular calcium concentration, a feature of cell death, also closes connexons and this mechanism appears to provide a means of sealing off apoptotic cells and their potentially noxious contents from adjacent viable cells.

Communicating junctions are more numerous in embryonic epithelia, where they appear to be involved in exchange of chemical messengers, as well as in cell recognition, differentiation and control of cell position. They are also probably involved in the passage of nutrients from cells deep in the epithelium (adjacent to supporting tissues and blood vessels) to cells more remote from the nutritional supply.

C overlapping cadherins **D** spot desmosome $\mathbf{D_2}$ individual desmosome **G** gap junction **H** hemidesmosome
IF intermediate filaments **LD** lamina densa **LL** lamina lucida **P** cytoplasmic plaque **TJ** tight junction **TW** terminal web
ZA zonula adherens

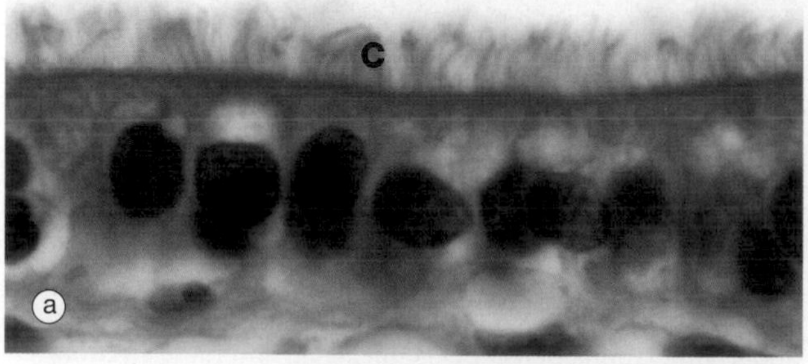

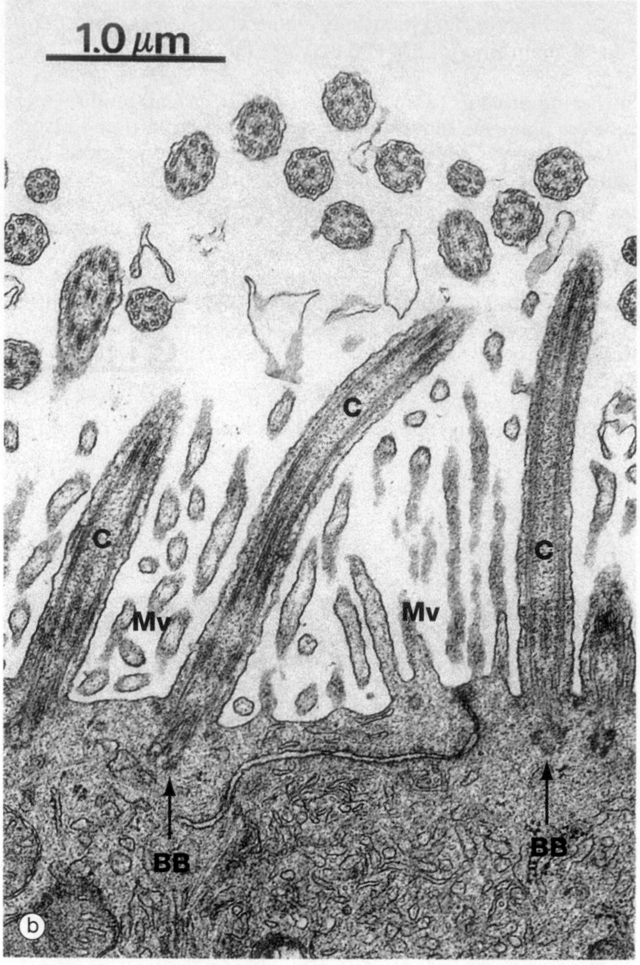

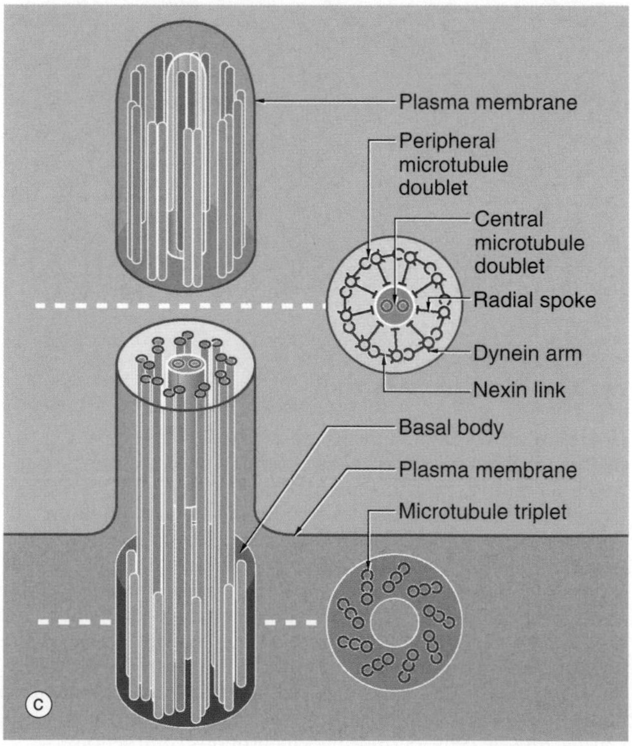

FIG. 5.13 Cilia
(a) H&E (HP) (b) EM ×20 000 (c) Schematic diagram

There are two types of ***cilia***: motile and non-motile. Motile cilia project from the apical surfaces of certain epithelial cells, notably in the respiratory and female reproductive tracts. These cilia beat with a wave-like synchronous rhythm, propelling surface films of mucus or fluid in a consistent direction over the epithelial surface. In the airways, mucus traps debris from inspired air and the cilia move the mucus towards the throat where it is swallowed, thus keeping the airways clear. In the Fallopian tubes, ciliary action propels the ovum from the ovary to the uterus. In the ventricles of the brain, the cilia of ependymal cells move the cerebrospinal fluid. Cilia are up to 10 μm long (up to half the height of the cell). The ***flagellum*** of spermatozoa is a modified cilium (see Ch. 18).

A single epithelial cell may have up to 300 cilia, usually of similar length. A single non-motile cilium is found on most mammalian cells and is often called the ***primary cilium*** or ***sensory cilium***; as suggested by the name, these cilia function as sensors for mechanical and chemical signals.

Fig. 5.13a and b show ciliated cells from the Fallopian tube. Cilia **C** are readily visible at the apical surface of the cell by light microscopy. In Fig. 5.13b, the proximal parts of three cilia **C** are seen in longitudinal section and, more superficially, the tips of a number of others otherwise lying outside the plane of section. Small surface microvilli **Mv** are seen between the cilia. Each cilium is bounded by plasma membrane and, as shown in Fig. 5.13c, contains a central core called the ***axoneme***. In motile cilia, the axoneme consists of 20 microtubules arranged as a ***central doublet*** surrounded by nine ***peripheral doublets***. The peripheral doublets are linked by a protein called ***nexin*** and ***radial spokes*** extend towards the central doublet. In non-motile cilia, the central doublet, nexin links and radial spokes are absent. At the base of the cilium, the microtubule doublets are continuous with the ***basal body***, consisting of nine microtubule triplets. Basal bodies have a very similar structure to the centriole. Each peripheral doublet of the cilium axoneme is continuous with the two inner microtubules of the corresponding triplet of the basal body. The basal bodies **BB** are easily seen in Fig. 5.14b.

Each doublet consists of one complete microtubule closely applied to a second incomplete C-shaped tubule. From each complete tubule, pairs of 'arms' consisting of the protein ***dynein***, a motor protein, extend towards the incomplete tubule of the adjacent doublet. Ciliary action results from bending of the doublets first in one direction and then in the other and is fuelled by dynein-catalysed conversion of ATP to ADP.

Ciliary dysfunction

A wide range of genetic disorders causing ciliary dysfunction have been described. Perhaps the best known of these is Kartagener syndrome (or primary ciliary dyskinesia) which leads to bronchiectasis, sinusitis and situs inversus along with infertility in affected males. These abnormalities arise due to inherited abnormalities in cilia, including lack of the dynein arms, missing central microtubule pairs or absence of one of the many other proteins critical for ciliary function. The lung and sinus problems arise due to infections caused by ineffective clearance of mucus. The infertility in males is due to malfunction of the flagella of spermatozoa. The situs inversus is due to an inability to determine the right–left axis, a function also mediated by ciliary motion during embryonic development.

Other ciliary disorders include hydrocephalus due to lack of flow of cerebrospinal fluid, Bardet–Biedl syndrome and cystic disease of the kidneys, among many others.

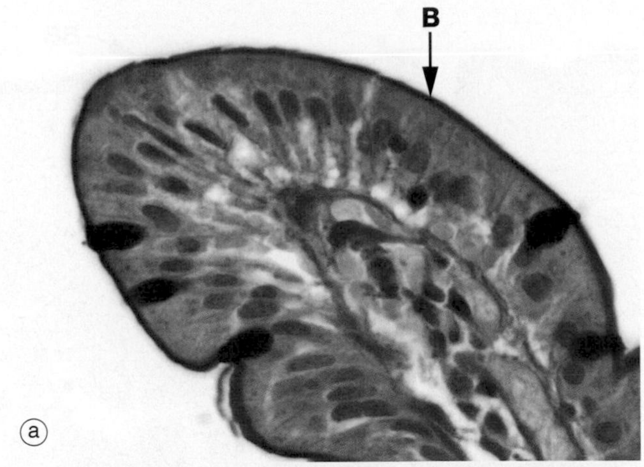

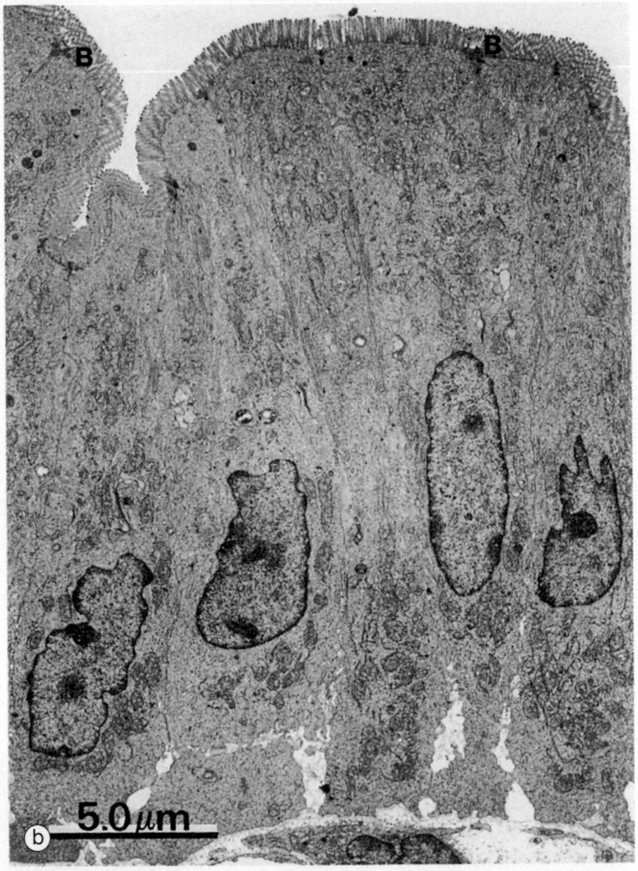

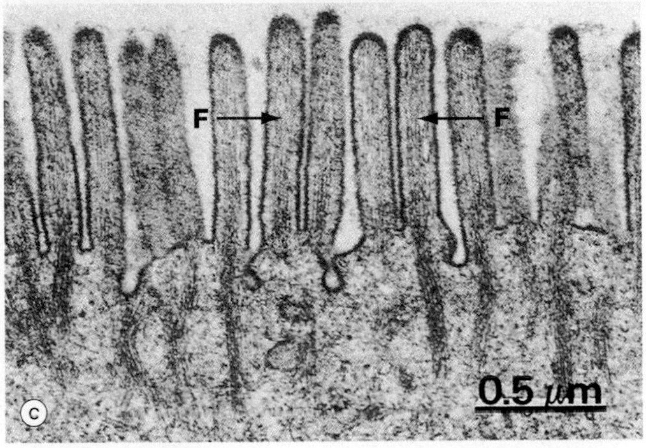

FIG. 5.14 Microvilli
(a) PAS (HP) (b) EM ×4000 (c) EM ×30 000

Microvilli are minute finger-like projections of the plasma membrane found in many epithelia, particularly those specialised for absorption, where their presence may increase the surface area as much as 30-fold. Most epithelia have only a small number of irregular microvilli. However, in the small intestine and proximal renal tubules, the epithelial cells have up to 3000 regular microvilli at the apical surface of each cell, and these can be seen with the light microscope as ***striated*** or ***brush borders*** (see also Figs 14.25 and 16.17). Fig. 5.14a and b illustrate the typical features of microvilli constituting the brush border **B** of cells lining the small intestine. Microvilli are only 0.5 to 1 μm in length and are thus very short in relation to the size of the cell, in contrast with cilia. Individual microvilli are too small to be resolved by light microscopy, as can be seen in Fig. 5.14a which shows the tip of an intestinal villus. The microvilli can only be seen as a magenta-stained band on the surface of the epithelium. Note also the scattered goblet cells containing magenta-stained mucus which fills the apical part of the cell (Fig. 5.16).

As seen at higher magnification in Fig. 5.14c, the cytoplasmic core of each microvillus contains parallel bundles of actin microfilaments **F** which insert into the ***terminal web***, a specialisation of the actin cytoskeleton lying immediately beneath the cell surface. The actin filaments are tightly packed in a hexagonal array and held together by ***actin binding proteins*** such as villin. At the periphery of the cell, the terminal web is anchored to the zonula adherens (Fig. 5.11). At the tip of the microvillus, the filaments attach to an electron-dense part of the plasma membrane. The microfilaments maintain stability of microvilli and may also mediate some contraction and elongation of the microvilli.

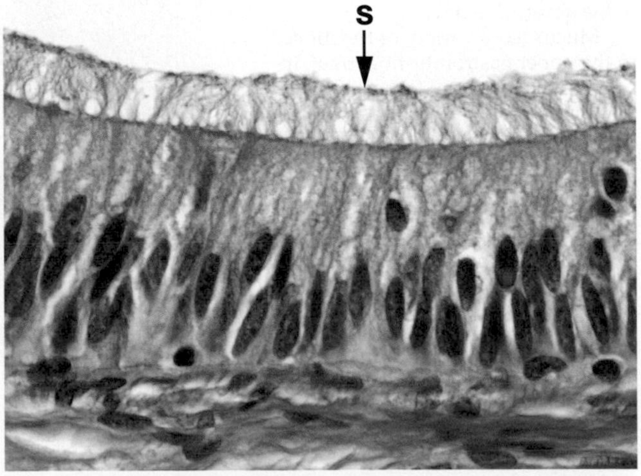

FIG. 5.15 Stereocilia
H&E (HP)

Stereocilia are long microvilli (1.5 to 5.5 μm), readily visible with light microscopy; they are found in the epididymis (shown in this micrograph, see also Ch. 18) and also in the inner ear (see Ch. 21). Originally these structures were thought to be an unusual form of cilia and were termed 'stereocilia'; however, electron microscopy has shown that they have an actin microfilament skeleton similar to that of microvilli. Stereocilia **S** are thought to facilitate absorptive processes in the epididymis, but the reason for their unusual form is not known. In the inner ear, they have an important role in hearing and balance, responding to bending movements by causing cellular depolarisation or hyperpolarisation (see Ch. 21).

B brush border **BB** basal body **C** cilia **F** actin microfilaments **Mv** microvilli **S** stereocilia

FIG. 5.16 Goblet cell
PAS (HP)

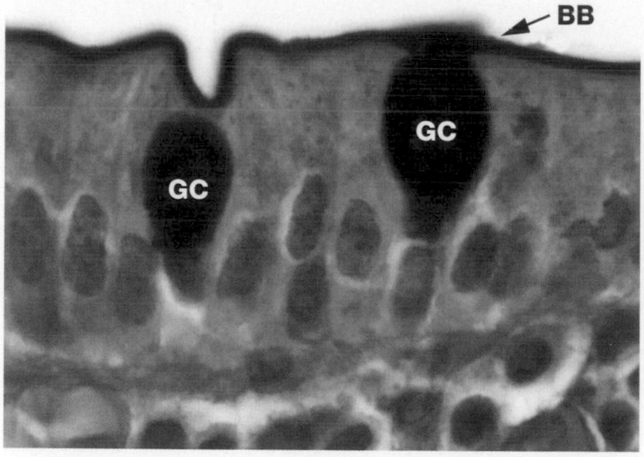

Goblet cells are modified columnar epithelial cells that synthesise and secrete mucus. They are scattered amongst the cells of many simple epithelial linings, particularly those of the respiratory and gastrointestinal tracts and are named for their resemblance to drinking goblets. Goblet cells are terminally differentiated and do not divide.

The distended apical cytoplasm contains a dense aggregation of ***mucigen granules*** which, when released by exocytosis, combine with water to form the viscid secretion called ***mucus***. Mucigen is composed of a mixture of neutral and acidic glycoproteins (mucopolysaccharides) and therefore can be readily demonstrated by the PAS method, which stains carbohydrates magenta. The 'stem' of the goblet cell is occupied by a condensed basal nucleus and is crammed with other organelles involved in mucin synthesis.

In this example from the lining of the small intestine showing two goblet cells **GC**, note the tall columnar nature of the surrounding absorptive cells. The PAS-positive brush border **BB** is composed partly of membrane-bound mucins on the numerous microvilli, which characterise small intestine absorptive cells, and a surface layer of free mucin (see Figs 1.2 and 5.14).

FIG. 5.17 Goblet cell
EM ×5000

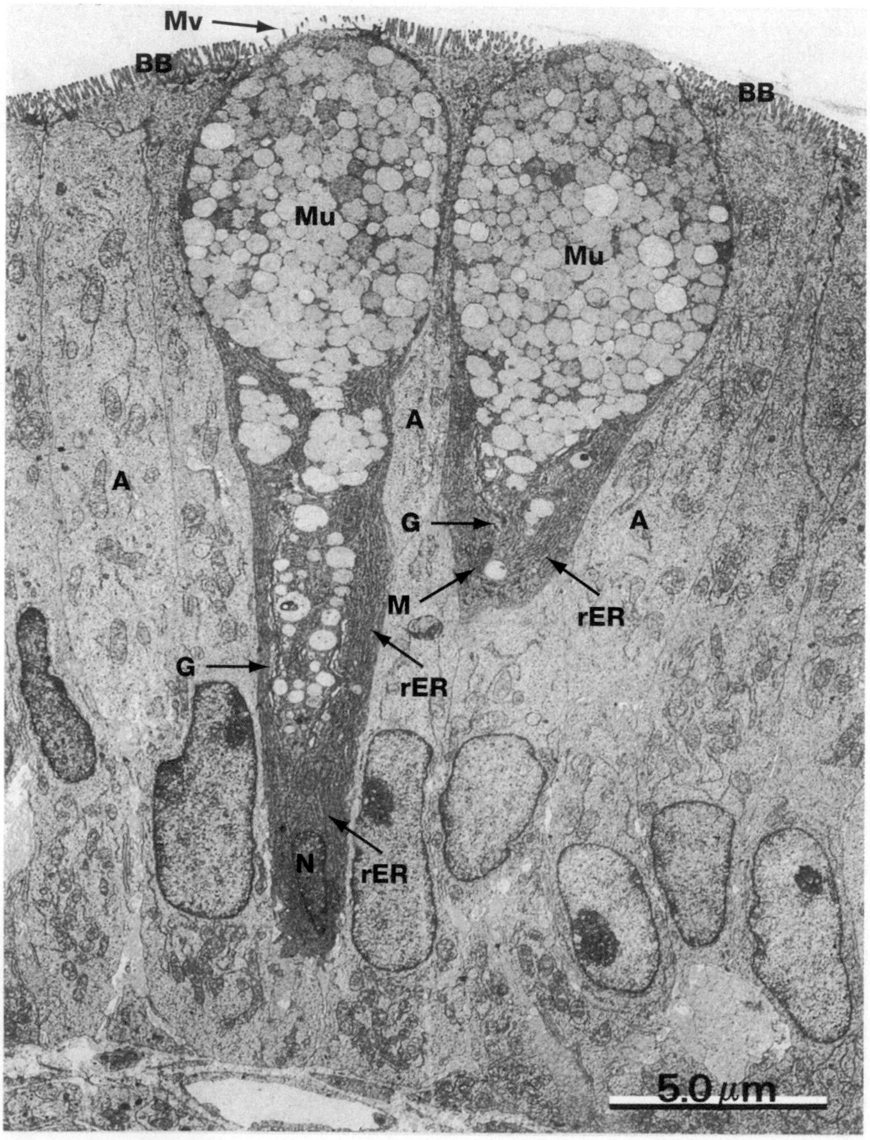

This micrograph shows two goblet cells among columnar absorptive cells **A** (or ***enterocytes***) of the small intestine. The nucleus of the goblet cell on the right is outside the plane of section, the nucleus **N** of the other being typically highly condensed (see also Fig. 14.23 showing a goblet cell in horizontal section). The cytoplasm is packed with rough endoplasmic reticulum **rER** and a few mitochondria **M**. A prominent Golgi apparatus **G** is found in the supranuclear region, although it is barely visible at this magnification.

The protein component of mucigen is synthesised by the rough endoplasmic reticulum and passed to the Golgi apparatus where it is combined with carbohydrate and packaged into membrane-bound secretory granules containing mucigen **Mu**. Goblet cells secrete at a steady basal rate and may be stimulated by local irritation to release their entire mucigen contents. Sparse microvilli **Mv** are seen at the surface of the goblet cell. Note the microvilli forming the brush border **BB** of the absorptive cells.

Mucus has a variety of functions. In the upper gastrointestinal tract, it protects the intestinal lining cells from autodigestion, whilst in the lower tract, it lubricates the passage of faeces. In the respiratory tract it protects the lining from drying, contributes to the humidification of inspired air and acts as a sticky surface trap for fine dust particles and microorganisms. Goblet cells also secrete various anti-microbial factors.

A absorptive cell **BB** brush border **G** Golgi apparatus **GC** goblet cell **M** mitochondrion **Mu** mucigen granules **Mv** microvilli **N** nucleus **rER** rough endoplasmic reticulum

EXOCRINE GLANDS

As discussed earlier in this chapter, epithelial cells are the major component of all the glands of the body. The simplest glands can be easily recognised as an invagination of a surface epithelium. However, increasingly complex glandular structures have evolved over time, and some of the most elaborate have lost contact with the epithelial surface completely. Thus there are two major subdivisions in the classification of glands: ***exocrine glands***, which release their contents onto an epithelial surface either directly or via a duct, and ***endocrine glands***, which have no duct system but by releasing their secretions into the bloodstream can act on distant tissues. Endocrine glands are dealt with briefly at the end of this chapter and in much more detail in Ch. 17.

This section deals with exocrine glands, which vary from microscopic, such as sweat glands of the skin, to large solid organs such as the liver, weighing approximately 1.2 kg. The duct system of the liver ramifies throughout the solid gland and empties its secretions (***bile***) into the duodenum. In contrast, the simple tubular glands (***crypts***) of the large bowel (see also Ch. 14) consist entirely of the secretory component and empty directly onto the surface of the bowel. Indeed, the simplest exocrine glands of all are single mucus-secreting cells such as goblet cells.

Exocrine glands may be subclassified according to the morphology and the means of secretion of the gland.

1. The morphology of the gland
Exocrine glands can be divided into the secretory component and the duct:

- The duct system may be unbranched (***simple gland***) or branched (***compound gland***).
- The secretory component may be ***tubular*** or ***acinar*** (roughly spherical).
- Both types of secretory component may also be coiled or branched.
- Almost any combination of duct and secretory component may occur (Figs. 5.18 to 5.25).

2. The means of secretion
Secretion from exocrine glands may occur in one of three ways:

- ***Merocrine (eccrine)*** secretion involves the process of ***exocytosis*** and is the most common form of secretion; proteins are usually the major secretory product.
- ***Apocrine secretion*** involves the discharge of free, unbroken, membrane-bound vesicles containing secretory product; this is an unusual mode of secretion and applies to lipid secretory products in the breasts and some sweat glands.
- ***Holocrine*** secretion involves the discharge of whole secretory cells, with subsequent disintegration of the cells to release the secretory product. Holocrine secretion occurs principally in sebaceous glands.

In general, all glands have a continuous basal rate of secretion which is modulated by nervous and hormonal influences. The secretory portions of some exocrine glands are surrounded by contractile cells that lie between the secretory cells and the basement membrane. The contractile mechanism of these cells is similar to that of muscle cells and has given rise to the term ***myoepithelial cells***, as these cells share characteristics of both epithelial and muscle cells.

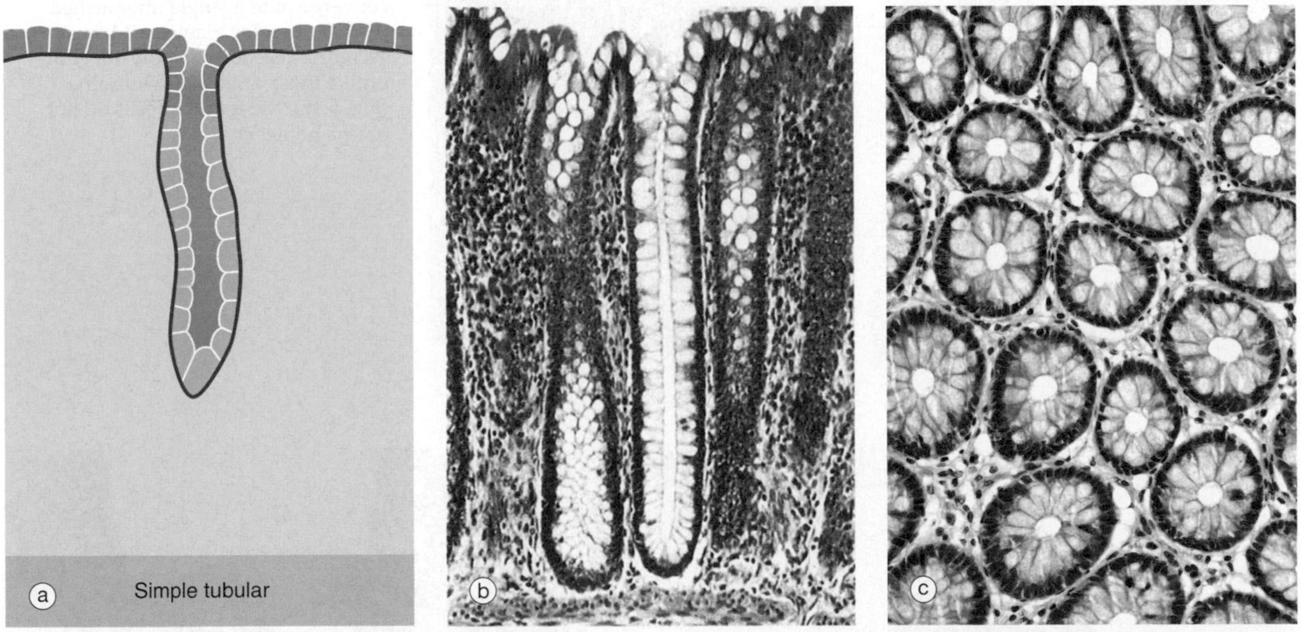

FIG. 5.18 Simple tubular glands
(a) Diagram (b) H&E (LP) (c) H&E (MP)

This example of simple tubular glands is taken from the large intestine. This type of gland has a single, straight tubular lumen into which the secretory products are discharged. In this example, secretory cells line the entire duct; the secretory cells are goblet cells. The glands are shown in longitudinal section in Fig. 5.18b and in transverse section in Fig. 5.18c, which emphasises the regular arrangement of the glands and the large number of mucus-secreting goblet cells in the epithelium. At other sites, mucus is secreted by columnar cells that do not have the classic goblet shape but nonetheless function in a similar manner.

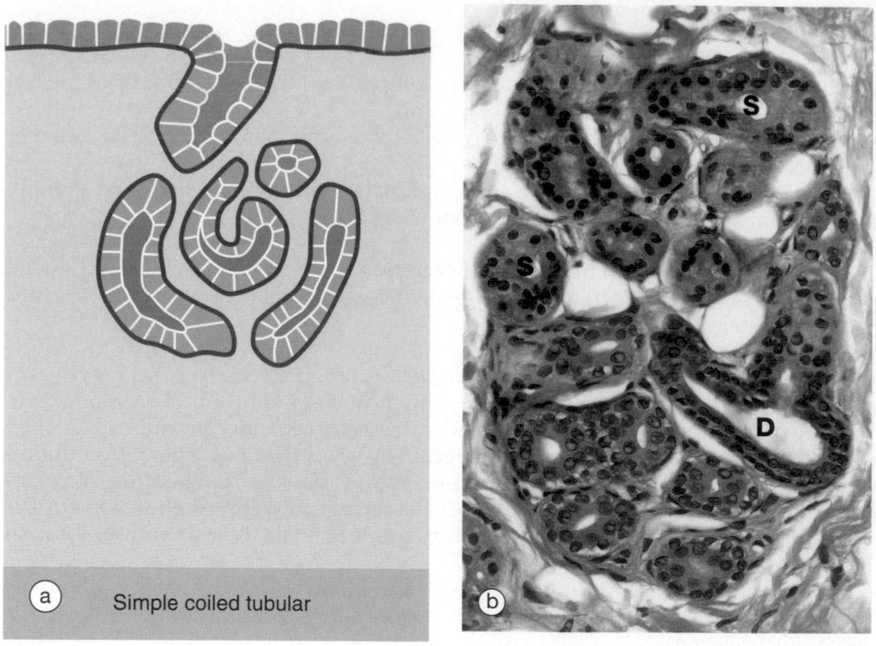

FIG. 5.19 Simple coiled tubular glands
(a) Diagram (b) H&E (LP)

Sweat glands are almost the only example of simple coiled tubular glands. Each consists of a single tube that is tightly coiled in three dimensions; portions of the gland are thus seen in various planes of section. Sweat glands have a terminal secretory portion **S** lined by simple cuboidal epithelium, which gives way to a non-secretory (***excretory***) duct **D** lined by stratified cuboidal epithelium.

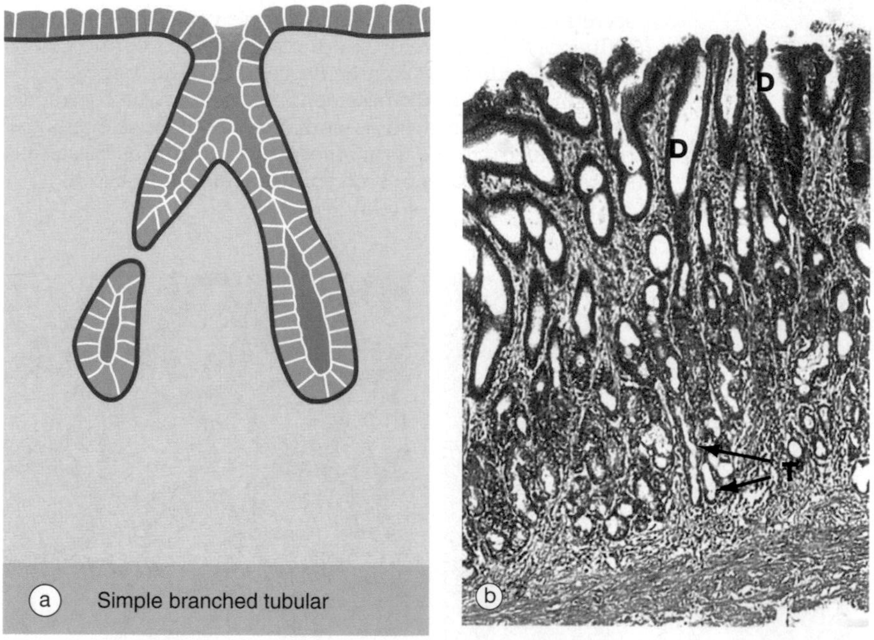

FIG. 5.20 Simple branched tubular glands
(a) Diagram (b) H&E (LP)

Simple branched tubular glands are found mainly in the stomach. The mucus-secreting glands of the pyloric part of the stomach are shown in this example. Each gland consists of several tubular secretory portions **T**, which converge onto a single unbranched duct **D** of wider diameter. Mucus-secreting cells also line the duct but, unlike those of the large intestine (Fig. 5.18), these mucus cells do not have a goblet shape.

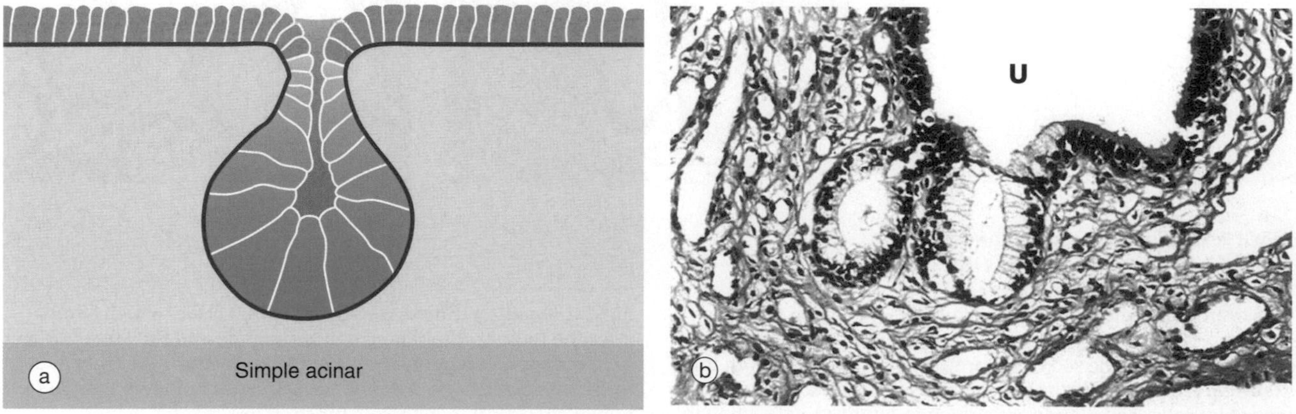

FIG. 5.21 Simple acinar glands
(a) Diagram (b) H&E (LP)

Simple acinar glands occur in the form of pockets in epithelial surfaces and are lined by secretory cells. In this example of the mucus-secreting glands of the penile urethra, the secretory cells are pale stained compared to the non-secretory cells lining the urethra **U**. Note that the term ***acinus*** can be used to describe any rounded exocrine secretory unit.

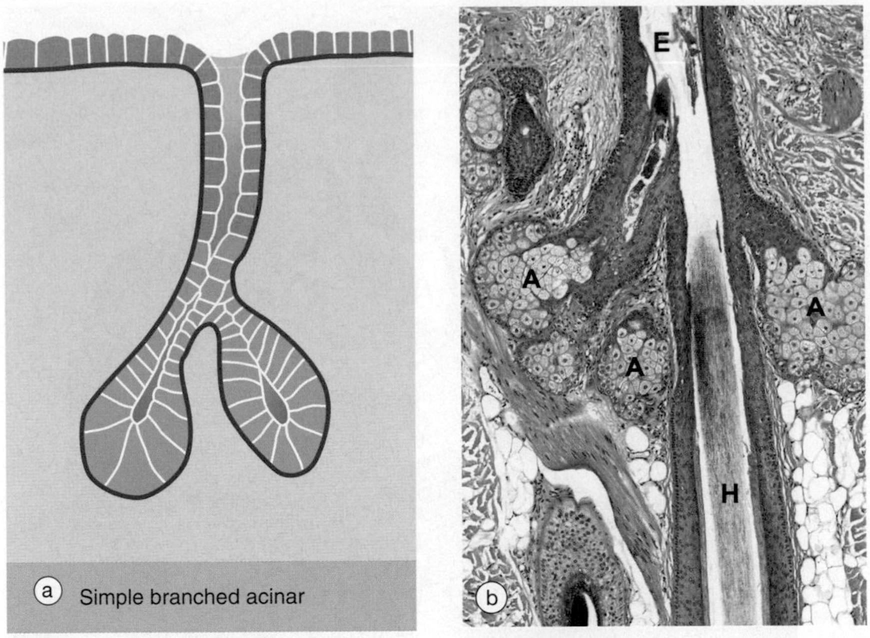

FIG. 5.22 Simple branched acinar gland
(a) Diagram (b) H&E (LP)

Sebaceous glands provide a good example of simple branched acinar glands. Each gland consists of several secretory acini **A** that empty into a single excretory duct; the excretory duct **E** is formed by the stratified epithelium surrounding the hair shaft **H**. The mode of secretion of sebaceous glands is holocrine, i.e. the secretory product, sebum, accumulates within the secretory cells and is discharged by degeneration of the cells.

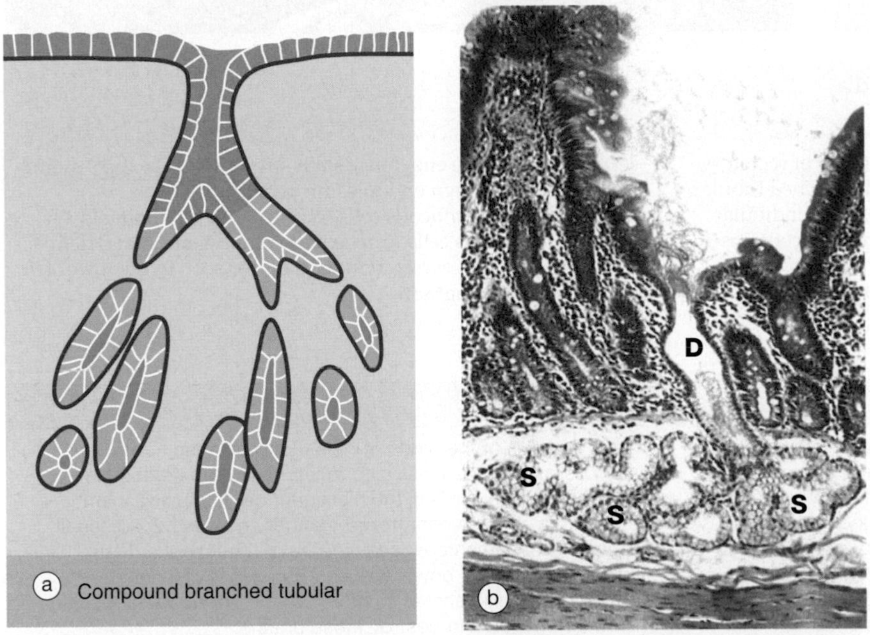

FIG. 5.23 Compound branched tubular gland
(a) Diagram (b) H&E (LP)

Brunner's glands of the duodenum, as shown in this example, are described as compound branched tubular glands. Although difficult to visualise here, the duct system **D** is branched, thus defining the glands as compound glands, and the secretory portions **S** have a tubular form which is branched and coiled.

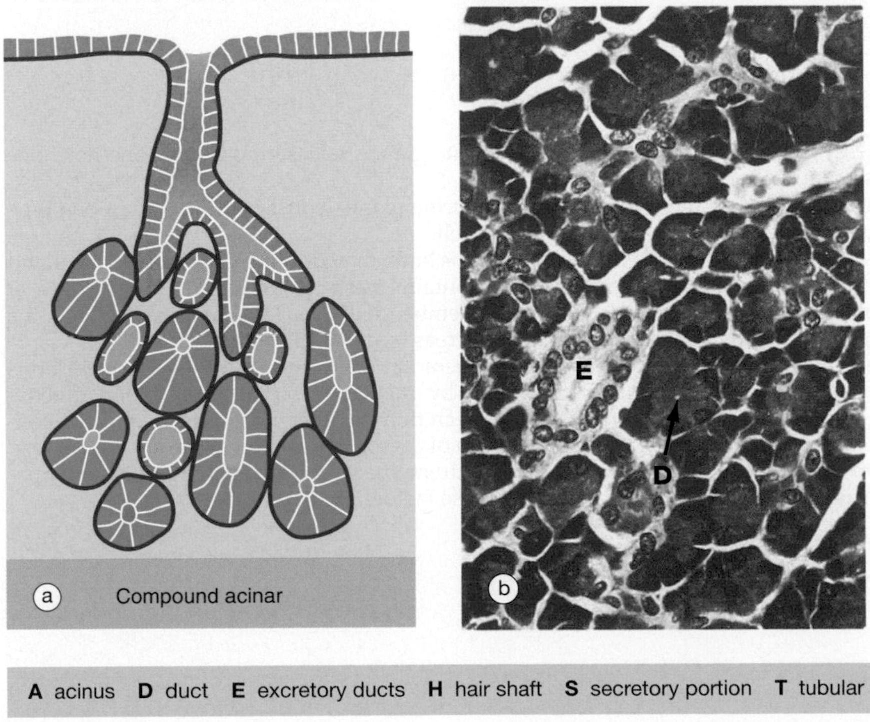

FIG. 5.24 Compound acinar gland
(a) Diagram (b) Chrome alum haematoxylin/phloxine (MP)

Compound acinar glands are those in which the secretory units are acinar in form and drain into a branched duct system. The pancreas shown in this micrograph consists of numerous acini, each of which drains into a minute duct. These minute ducts **D**, which are just discernible in the centre of some acini, drain into a system of branched excretory ducts **E** of increasing diameter which are lined by simple cuboidal epithelium.

A acinus **D** duct **E** excretory ducts **H** hair shaft **S** secretory portion **T** tubular secretory portion of gland **U** urethra

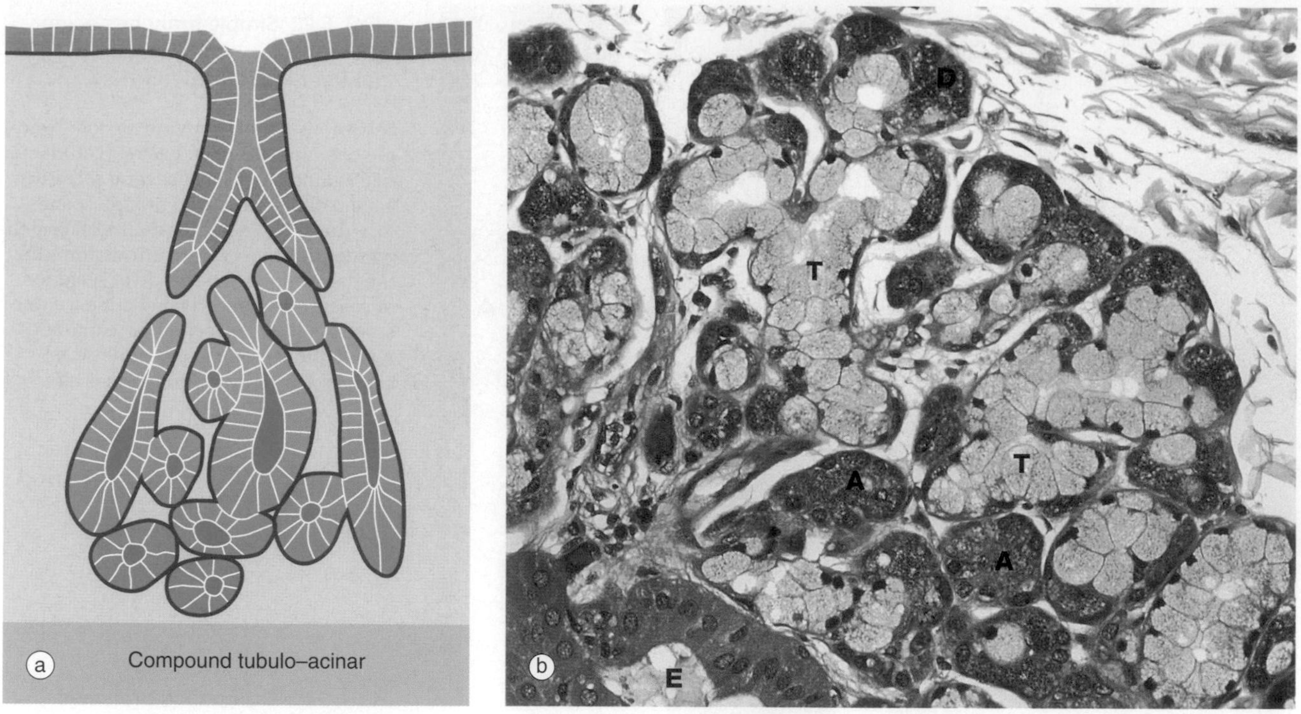

FIG. 5.25 Compound tubulo-acinar gland
(a) Diagram (b) H&E (MP)

Compound tubulo-acinar glands have three types of secretory units: branched tubular, branched acinar and branched tubular with acinar end-pieces called ***demilunes***. The submandibular salivary gland shown here is the classic example. It contains two types of secretory cells, mucus-secreting cells and serous cells; the former are pale but the latter, which have a protein-rich secretion (digestive enzymes), stain strongly due to their prominent content of rough endoplasmic reticulum.

Generally, the mucous cells form tubular components **T**, whereas the serous cells form acinar components **A** and demilunes **D**. Part of an excretory duct **E** is also seen in the lower left corner of the micrograph.

Carcinoma

Malignant tumours (colloquially called 'cancers') may arise from any type of tissue. Malignant tumours arising from epithelial tissues are called ***carcinomas*** and are subclassified according to the tissue from which they are thought to arise or resemble (see e-Table 5.2). Thus carcinomas resembling stratified squamous epithelium are called ***squamous cell carcinomas***, while carcinomas resembling glands are known as ***adenocarcinomas***. In reality, carcinomas arise from the accumulation of mutations in undifferentiated stem cells and show features of the types of cells that may arise from these stem cells. The mutations lead to increased proliferation and inhibition of apoptosis in the malignant cells, causing them to proliferate in an uncontrolled manner and destroy adjacent tissues (as when an adenocarcinoma of the bowel erodes through the normal bowel wall and perforates). Malignant tumours may also spread to other organs (***metastasise***) and likewise overrun and destroy those organs.

ENDOCRINE GLANDS

As described earlier, endocrine (or ductless) glands release their secretions directly into the bloodstream rather than via a duct. Endocrine glands are the source of many of the body's chemical messengers, ***hormones***, that act at a distance from their source. For example, insulin secreted by the pancreas (see Ch. 17) acts on muscle and adipose tissue throughout the body to control the metabolism of glucose. Other hormones may act only on a single tissue; thus thyroid-stimulating hormone (TSH) secreted by the pituitary gland is widely disseminated in the blood, but only the thyroid gland has the necessary receptors to respond.

Endocrine glands are very varied in their size, location and appearance and are described in more detail in Ch. 17.

- Many are solid organs, but some consist of widely distributed single cells.
- Most endocrine glands release more than one hormone product.
- Several endocrine glands consist of more than one type of secretory cell.
- The pancreas is both an endocrine and an exocrine gland because it contains nests of endocrine cells (***islets of Langerhans***) embedded in a large exocrine gland, the exocrine pancreas (see Ch. 15).
- In general, secretion of hormones by endocrine glands is controlled by metabolic factors (e.g. blood glucose levels), the secretion of other hormones (e.g. TSH controls secretion of thyroxine) and the nervous system (e.g. secretion of adrenaline by the adrenal medulla) or a mixture of all these factors.

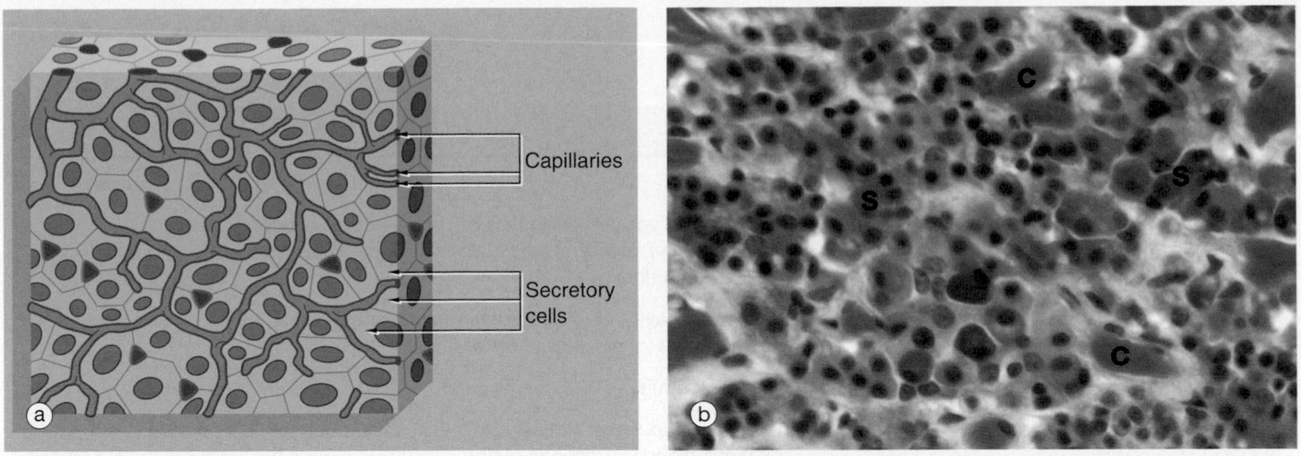

FIG. 5.26 Endocrine gland
(a) Diagram (b) H&E (MP)

Most endocrine glands consist of clusters or cords of secretory cells surrounded by a rich network of small blood vessels. Each cluster of endocrine cells is surrounded by a basement membrane, reflecting its epithelial origin. Endocrine cells release hormones into the intercellular spaces, from which they diffuse rapidly into surrounding blood vessels and from there throughout the body.

Fig. 5.26b of the anterior pituitary gland shows the typical features of endocrine glands. The secretory cells **S** are arranged in cords and clusters and are surrounded by delicate supporting tissue containing a rich network of broad capillaries **C**. The basement membrane surrounding each group of endocrine cells is not visible at this magnification. Like many other endocrine glands, the secretory cells of the pituitary are of several different types; in this case, the majority are acidophilic (red stained), while some stain blue (basophilic) and some stain very little (chromophobes).

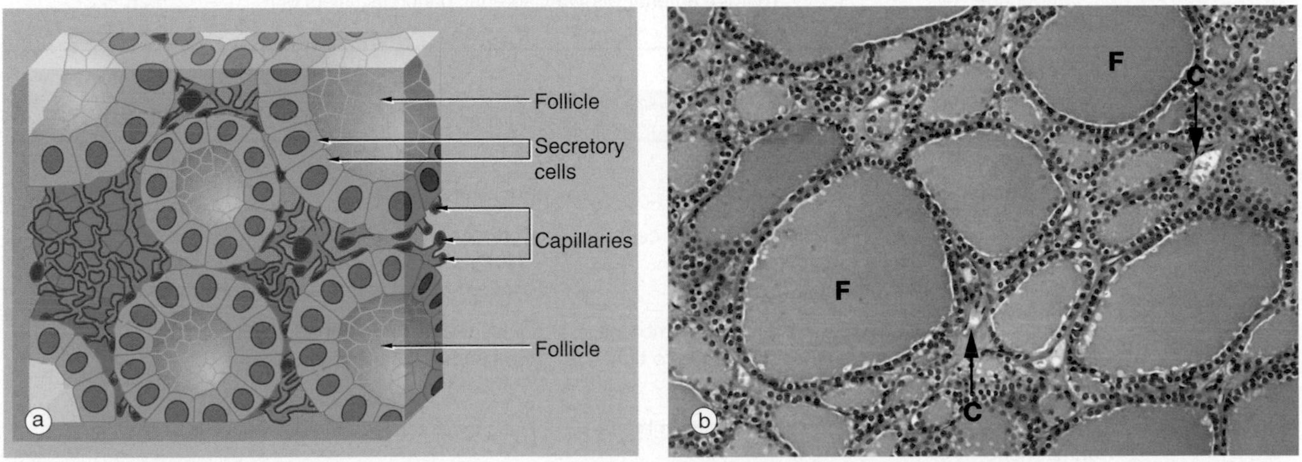

FIG. 5.27 Follicular endocrine gland
(a) Diagram (b) H&E (LP)

The thyroid gland is an unusual endocrine gland in that it stores hormone (***thyroxine***) within roughly spherical cavities enclosed by the secretory cells; these units are called ***follicles***. Secretion of stored hormone involves reabsorption of hormone from the follicular lumen, release into the surrounding interstitial spaces, and then diffusion into the rich capillary network that embraces each follicle.

Fig. 5.27b shows typical thyroid follicles **F**. The secretory cells lining the follicles are of flattened cuboidal shape, although they may vary from low cuboidal to tall columnar depending on the state of activity of the gland. Stored thyroxine is bound to a glycoprotein (***thyroglobulin***), which is strongly eosinophilic and fills the centre of the follicle. The relatively sparse interfollicular supporting tissue is mainly occupied by capillaries **C** (see also Fig. 17.6).

A acinus **C** capillary **D** demilune **E** excretory duct **F** follicle **S** secretory cells **T** tubular secretory component

REVIEW

TABLE 5.3 Review of epithelium: major types and locations

Type of epithelium	Subclassification	Sites	Figures
Squamous	Simple	Lining blood vessels (endothelium), lining body cavities (mesothelium), alveoli of lungs, Bowman's capsule and loop of Henle of kidney	5.1
	Stratified	Lining oral cavity, epiglottis, oesophagus, anus, cervix, vagina, vulva, glans penis, cornea	5.6
	Stratified, keratinising	Skin (epidermis)	5.6
Cuboidal	Simple	Collecting tubules of kidney, rete testis, small ducts of exocrine glands, surface of ovary	5.2
	Stratified	Larger ducts of exocrine glands	5.7
Columnar	Simple	Gallbladder, collecting ducts of kidney, endocervix	5.3
	Simple ciliated	Fallopian tubes	5.4
	Pseudostratified, ciliated	Respiratory tract including nose and sinuses	5.5
Transitional		Lower urinary tract (renal pelvis, ureters, bladder and urethra)	5.8
Glandular	Simple	Colon, stomach, eccrine sweat glands	5.18–5.22
	Compound	Sebaceous glands, Brunner's glands of duodenum, small salivary glands, breast, prostate	5.23–5.25
Glandular – solid organs	Exocrine	Major salivary glands, liver, pancreas (acinar tissue)	13.16–13.18, Ch. 15
	Endocrine	Thyroid, anterior pituitary, adrenal, pancreas (islets of Langerhans)	5.26, 5.27, Ch. 17

TABLE 5.4 Review of membrane specialisations of epithelia

Type of specialisation	Subclassification	Sites/description	Functions	Figures
Intercellular junctions	Tight junction (zonula occludens)	Luminal and lateral cell membranes	Control of paracellular diffusion Prevents exchange of proteins and lipids between apical and basolateral membrane	5.10
	Adhering belt (zonula adherens)	Lateral plasma membrane, immediately deep to tight junction	Links cytoskeletons of adjacent cells to form strong, cohesive epithelium	5.11
	Desmosome (macula adherens)	Lateral plasma membrane	Links cytoskeletons of adjacent cells	5.11
	Hemidesmosome	Basal plasma membrane	Links cells to underlying basement membrane	5.11
	Gap junction	Lateral plasma membrane	Passage of ions and small molecules between cells Intercellular signalling	5.12
Surface specialisations	Cilia	Hair-like surface projections Seen on light microscopy Motile or non-motile	Beat to propel surface films of fluid or mucus in specific direction, e.g. respiratory tract, Fallopian tube	5.13
	Microvilli	Short projections of plasma membrane Not individually seen with light microscope	Increase membrane surface area, especially for absorption, e.g. small intestine	5.14
	Stereocilia	Very long microvilli Usually single or in small numbers	In inner ear, mechanosensing role Facilitate absorptive processes in epididymis	5.15

6 Muscle

INTRODUCTION

Although all cells are capable of some sort of movement, the dominant function of several cell types is to generate force through ***contraction***. In these specialised contractile cells, movement is generated by interaction of the proteins ***actin*** and ***myosin*** (contractile proteins). Certain forms of contractile cell function as single-cell contractile units:

- **Myoepithelial cells** are an important component of certain secretory glands (see Ch. 5), where they function to expel secretions from glandular acini.
- **Pericytes** are smooth muscle-like cells that surround blood vessels (see Ch. 8).
- **Myofibroblasts** are cells that have a contractile role in addition to being able to secrete collagen. This type of cell is generally inconspicuous in normal tissues but becomes important following tissue damage during the process of healing and repair, leading to formation of a scar.

Other forms of contractile cells function by forming multicellular contractile units termed ***muscles***. Such muscle cells can be divided into three types:

- **Skeletal muscle** is responsible for the movement of the skeleton as well as organs such as the globe of the eye and the tongue. Skeletal muscle is often referred to as ***voluntary muscle*** since it is capable of voluntary (conscious) control. The arrangement of the contractile proteins gives rise to the appearance of prominent cross-striations in some histological preparations and so the name ***striated muscle*** is often applied to skeletal muscle. The highly developed functions of the cytoplasmic organelles of muscle cells has led to the use of a special terminology for some muscle cell components: plasma membrane or plasmalemma = ***sarcolemma***; cytoplasm = ***sarcoplasm***; endoplasmic reticulum = ***sarcoplasmic reticulum***.
- **Smooth muscle** is so named because, unlike other forms of muscle, the arrangement of contractile proteins does not give the histological appearance of cross-striations. This type of muscle forms the muscular component of visceral structures such as blood vessels, the gastrointestinal tract, the uterus and the urinary bladder, giving rise to the alternative name of ***visceral muscle***. Since smooth muscle is under inherent autonomic and hormonal control, it is also described as ***involuntary muscle***.
- **Cardiac muscle** has many structural and functional characteristics intermediate between those of skeletal and smooth muscle and provides for the continuous rhythmic contractility of the heart (see Ch. 8). Although striated in appearance, cardiac muscle is readily distinguishable from skeletal muscle and should not be referred to by the term 'striated muscle'.

Muscle cells of all three types are surrounded by an ***external lamina*** (see Ch. 4). In all muscle cell types, contractile forces developed from the internal contractile proteins are transmitted to the external lamina via link proteins which span the muscle cell membrane. The external lamina binds individual muscle cells into a single functional mass.

SKELETAL MUSCLE

Skeletal muscles have a wide variety of morphological forms and modes of action; nevertheless all have the same basic structure. Skeletal muscle is composed of extremely elongated, multinucleate contractile cells, often described as ***muscle fibres***, bound together by collagenous supporting tissue. Individual muscle fibres vary considerably in diameter from 10 to 100 μm and may extend throughout the whole length of a muscle and, in some sites, may be many centimeters in length.

Skeletal muscle contraction is controlled by large motor nerves, individual nerve fibres branching within the muscle to supply a group of muscle fibres, collectively described as a ***motor unit***. Excitation of any one motor nerve results in simultaneous contraction of all the muscle fibres of the corresponding motor unit. The structure of ***neuromuscular junctions*** is described in Fig. 7.12. The vitality of skeletal muscle fibres is dependent on maintenance of their nerve supply which, if damaged, results in ***atrophy*** of the fibres (see below). Skeletal muscle contains highly specialised stretch receptors known as ***neuromuscular spindles*** which are shown in Fig. 7.23.

Muscle changes in health and disease

Atrophy is a decrease in the size of an organ or tissue, usually due to disease or changes in functional requirements (see e-Fig. 6.1). When the nerve supply of skeletal muscle is damaged, the individual muscle fibres innervated by that nerve become smaller and thinner, giving the impression of 'wasting away' of the affected muscle.

A more common example of this process of atrophy is seen when muscles are not used for a period of time (e.g. when a limb is immobilised in plaster to allow healing of a broken bone). The muscles in that area become visibly smaller and, when the plaster is removed, muscle strength is reduced. So long as the nerves supplying the muscle remain intact, exercise can reverse this process and function of the broken limb can be regained.

The opposite process occurs when muscles are exercised over long periods. Muscle bulk in athletes is typically increased. This reflects an increase in the size of individual muscle fibres due to synthesis of more contractile proteins within each cell. The process is known as ***hypertrophy*** (see e-Fig. 6.2). There is no increase in the number of muscle fibres, as these cells do not normally divide. In contrast, increased bulk of smooth muscle can occur due to a combination of hypertrophy (increase in cell size) and ***hyperplasia*** (see e-Fig. 6.3; an increase in the number of cells), since smooth muscle cells retain the ability to divide.

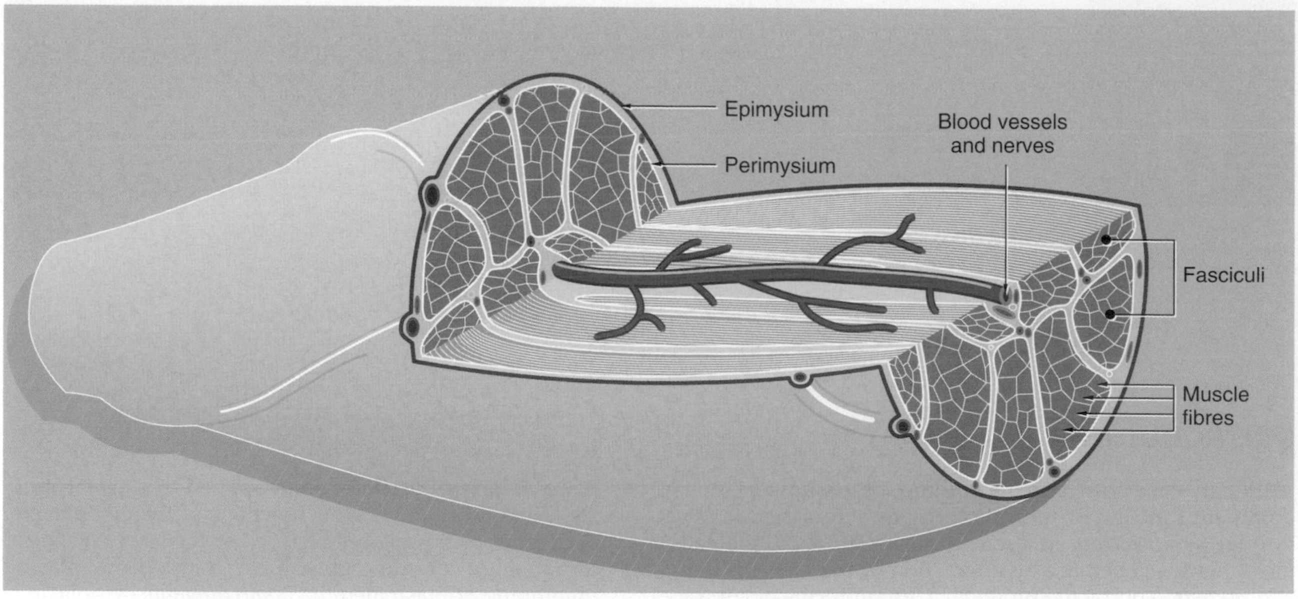

FIG. 6.1 Skeletal muscle

Fig. 6.1 illustrates the arrangement of the basic components which make up a typical skeletal muscle. The individual muscle cells (muscle fibres) are grouped together into elongated bundles called ***fasciculi*** or ***fascicles*** with delicate supporting tissue called ***endomysium*** occupying the spaces between individual muscle fibres.

Each fascicle is surrounded by loose collagenous tissue called ***perimysium***. Most muscles are made up of many fasciculi, and the whole muscle mass is invested in a dense collagenous sheath called the ***epimysium***. Large blood vessels and nerves enter the epimysium and divide to ramify throughout the muscle in the perimysium and endomysium.

The size of the fasciculi reflects the function of the muscle concerned. Muscles responsible for fine, highly controlled movements (e.g. external muscles of the eye) have small fasciculi and a relatively greater proportion of perimysial supporting tissue. In contrast, muscles responsible for gross movements only (e.g. muscles of the buttocks) have large fasciculi and relatively little perimysial tissue. Muscle fibres are anchored to the supporting tissue so that contractile force can be transmitted. The connective tissue framework contains both collagen and elastic fibres. This connective tissue becomes continuous with that of the tendons and muscle attachments (see Ch. 10), which distribute and direct the motive forces of the muscle to bone, skin, etc., as appropriate.

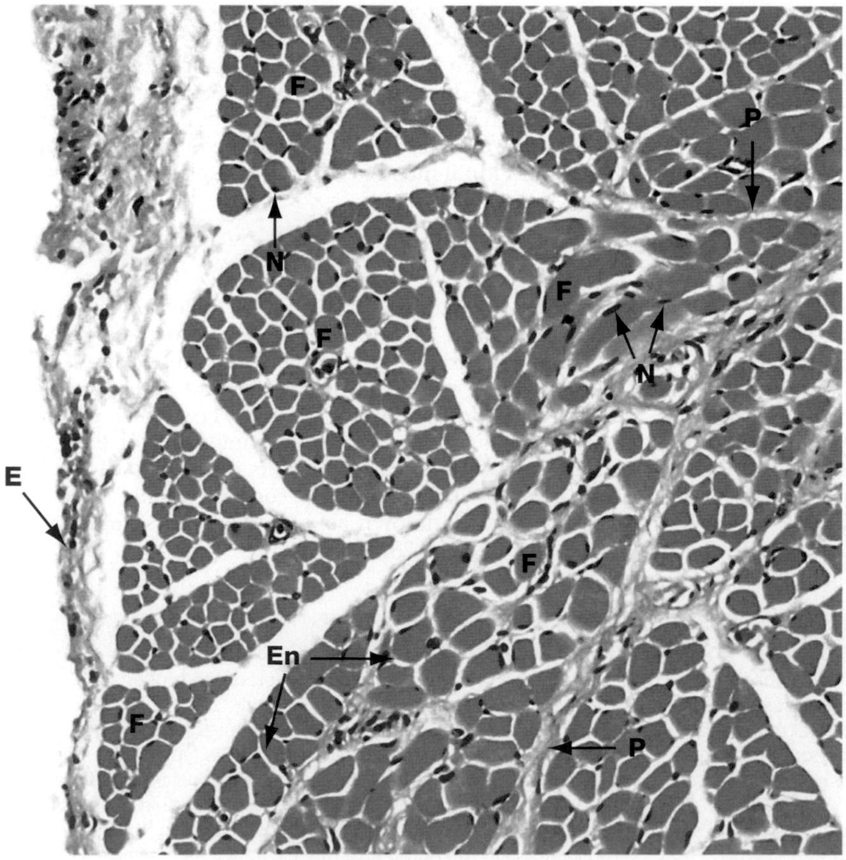

FIG. 6.2 Skeletal muscle H&E (MP)

Fig. 6.2 shows the general arrangement of muscle fibres in skeletal muscle. Here, there are several distinct fasciculi.

The individual pink stained muscle cells (fibres) are cut in transverse section and appear polygonal in shape, with nuclei **N** lying at the peripheries of the cells. The spaces between the cells are occupied by small amounts of barely visible endomysial supporting tissue. The endomysium, which consists mainly of reticulin fibres and a small amount of collagen, conveys numerous small blood vessels, lymphatics and nerves throughout the muscle.

Surrounding the individual fasciculi **F** is the ***perimysium*** **P**, composed of collagen and through which larger vessels and nerves run. The ***epimysium*** **E** is a collagenous sheath that binds the fascicles into a single muscle. The ***endomysium*** **En** is barely visible as the delicate support tissue surrounding each muscle fibre.

B blood vessel **C** capillary **E** epimysium **En** endomysium **F** fascicle **FE** fetal erythrocytes **N** nucleus **P** perimysium

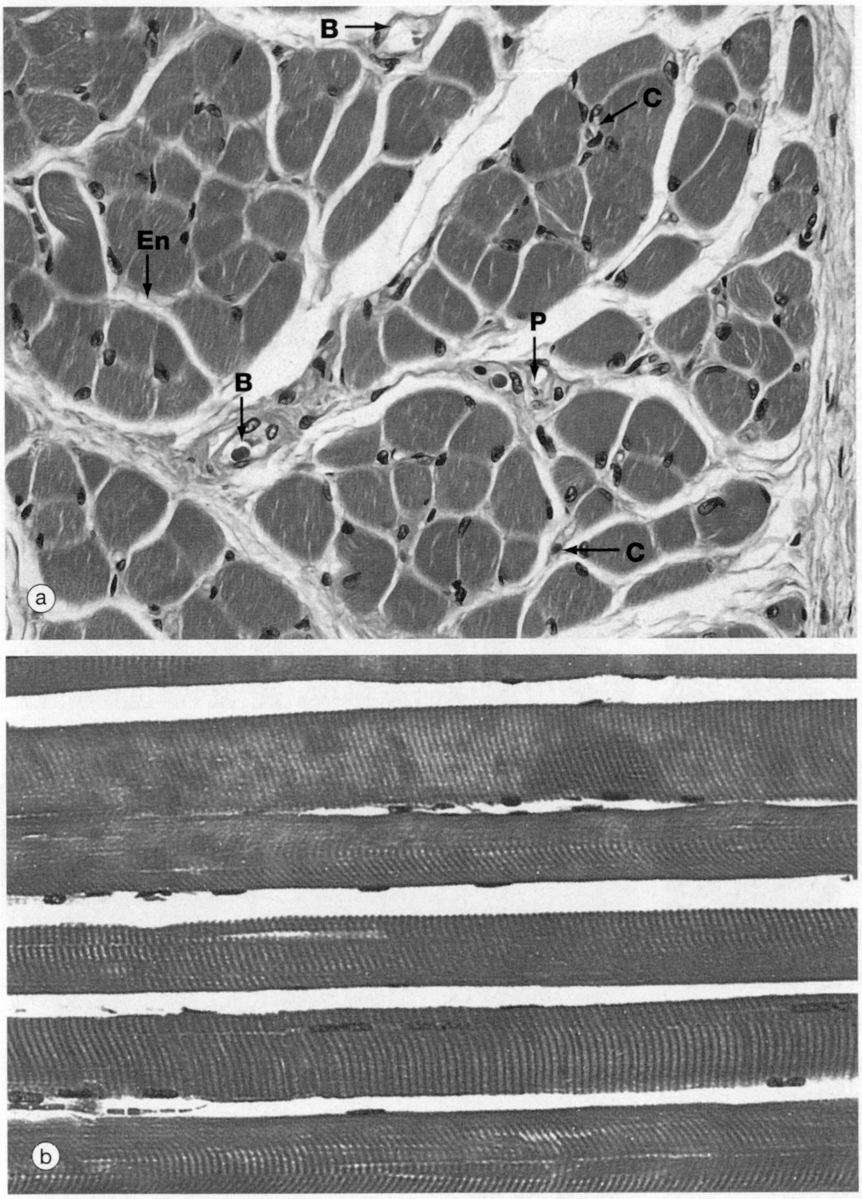

FIG. 6.3 Skeletal muscle (a) H&E, TS (HP) (b) H&E, LS (HP)

These micrographs show skeletal muscle from human limb muscles. Fig. 6.3a in transverse section shows the muscle to be made up of numerous small fasciculi. The spaces between the fasciculi are filled with loose collagenous tissue, the ***perimysium*** **P**, which is continuous with the delicate ***endomysium*** **En**, separating individual muscle fibres in each fasciculus. The supporting tissue of skeletal muscle also contains elastin fibres (not distinguishable in this preparation) which are most numerous in muscles attached to soft tissues as in the tongue and face. Note the rich network of capillaries **C** in the endomysium. Small blood vessels **B** and nerves run in the perimysium.

Fig. 6.3b demonstrates the characteristic histological features of skeletal muscle fibres in longitudinal section. Skeletal muscle fibres are extremely elongated, unbranched cylindrical cells with numerous flattened nuclei located at fairly regular intervals just beneath the ***sarcolemma*** (plasma membrane).

Each muscle fibre has multiple nuclei arranged at the cell periphery. In transverse section, as in Fig. 6.3a, most muscle fibre profiles appear to contain only a single nucleus, while some do not include any because the plane of section has cut between the zones containing a nucleus.

In routine histological preparations stained with H&E, it is often possible to see the striations in skeletal muscle when cut in longitudinal section. Special stains are required for better resolution of these structures (see Fig. 6.6a).

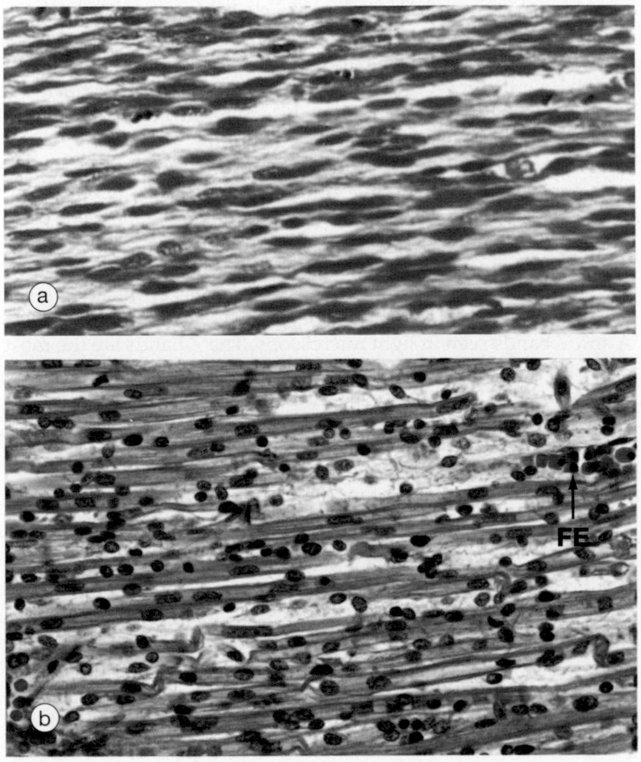

FIG. 6.4 Skeletal muscle embryogenesis (a) H&E (MP) (b) H&E (HP)

During embryological development, mesenchymal cells in each myotome differentiate into long, mononuclear skeletal muscle precursors called ***myoblasts***, which then proliferate by mitosis. Subsequently, the myoblasts fuse end to end forming elongated multinucleate cells called ***myotubes*** which may eventually contain up to 100 nuclei. These myotubes then synthesise contractile proteins to form ***myofilaments*** and so cross-striations gradually become visible. Proliferating myoblasts and early developing myotubes are illustrated in Fig. 6.4a. Fig. 6.4b illustrates a slightly later stage in development and, here, there is a suggestion of very early cross-striation in some of the myotubes. Note the nucleated fetal erythrocytes **FE** within a small vessel on one edge of the image.

Mature muscle cells can regenerate if damaged by proliferation of ***stem cells*** which remain in adult muscles. These muscle stem cells resemble myoblasts and are called ***satellite cells***. They enter mitosis after muscle damage and several fuse to form differentiated muscle fibres. Muscle fibres which have formed as a result of regeneration after damage have nuclei in the centre of the fibre rather than at the periphery.

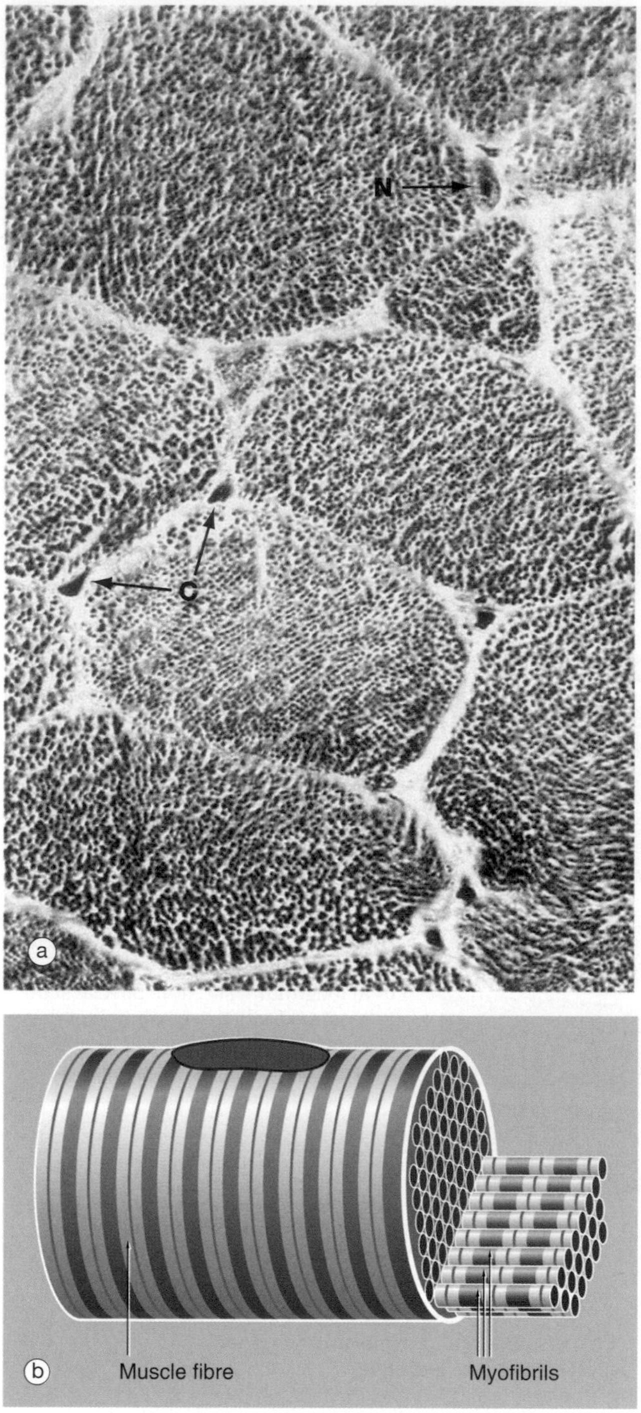

FIG. 6.5 Skeletal muscle
(a) Iron haematoxylin, TS (HP) (b) Schematic diagram

Fig. 6.5a shows a transverse section through several skeletal muscle fibres at very high magnification. The plane of section includes only one skeletal muscle cell nucleus **N**. Note the presence of erythrocytes in endomysial capillaries **C**.

In preparations such as this, the transversely sectioned muscle fibres appear packed with numerous dark dots. These represent the cut ends of myofibrils, elongated cylindrical structures which lie parallel to one another in the sarcoplasm.

Fig. 6.5b shows part of a single muscle fibre. The diagram illustrates that each myofibril exhibits a repeating pattern of cross-striations which is a product of the highly ordered arrangement of the contractile proteins within it; detail of this arrangement can only be seen using electron microscopy (see Fig. 6.6). Furthermore, the parallel myofibrils are each arranged with their cross-striations in register, giving rise to the regular striations which may be seen with light microscopy in longitudinal sections of skeletal muscle as in Fig. 6.3.

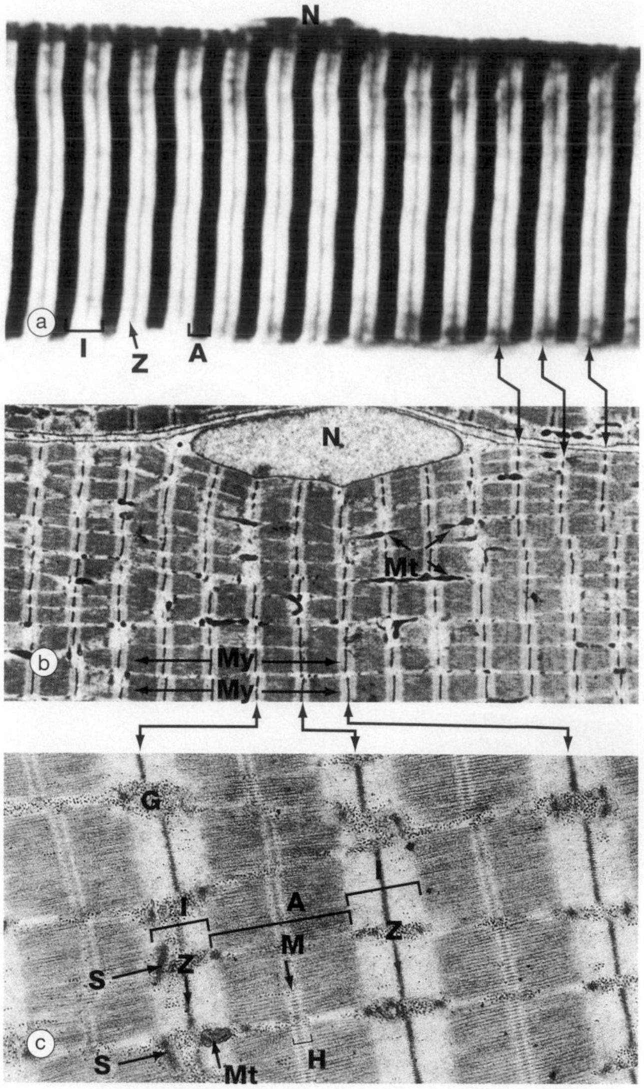

FIG. 6.6 Skeletal muscle
(a) Heidenhain's haematoxylin (HP) (b) EM ×2860
(c) EM ×18 700

This series of micrographs shows the arrangement of the contractile proteins within skeletal muscle and explains the striations seen with light microscopy.

Fig. 6.6a shows the striations of a skeletal muscle fibre at a magnification close to the limit of resolution. They are composed of alternating broad light **I** bands (isotropic in polarised light) and dark (anisotropic) **A** bands. Fine dark lines called ***Z lines*** (Zwischenscheiben) **Z** can be seen bisecting the I bands. Note the nucleus **N** at the periphery of the cell.

Fig. 6.6b shows the electron microscopic appearance of muscle with a nucleus **N** situated in a similar position. The sarcoplasm is filled with myofibrils **My** oriented parallel to the long axis of the cell. These are separated by a small amount of sarcoplasm containing rows of mitochondria **Mt** in a similar orientation. Each myofibril has prominent regular cross-striations arranged in register with those of the other myofibrils and corresponding to the I, A and Z bands seen in light microscopy. The Z bands are the most electron-dense and divide each myofibril into numerous contractile units called sarcomeres, arranged end to end.

With further magnification in Fig. 6.6c, the arrangement of the contractile proteins (myofilaments) may be seen in each sarcomere. The dark **A** band is bisected by the lighter **H** (Heller) band, which is further bisected by a more dense **M** (Mittelscheibe) line. Irrespective of the degree of contraction of the muscle fibre, the A band remains constant in width. In contrast, the **I** and H bands narrow during contraction, and the **Z** lines are drawn closer together. These findings are explained by the sliding filament theory (Fig. 6.7). Mitochondria **Mt** and numerous glycogen granules **G** provide a rich energy source in the scanty cytoplasm between the myofibrils. The mature muscle cell contains little rough endoplasmic reticulum; it contains, however, a smooth membranous system **S** which is involved in activation of the contractile mechanism (see Figs 6.8 to 6.10).

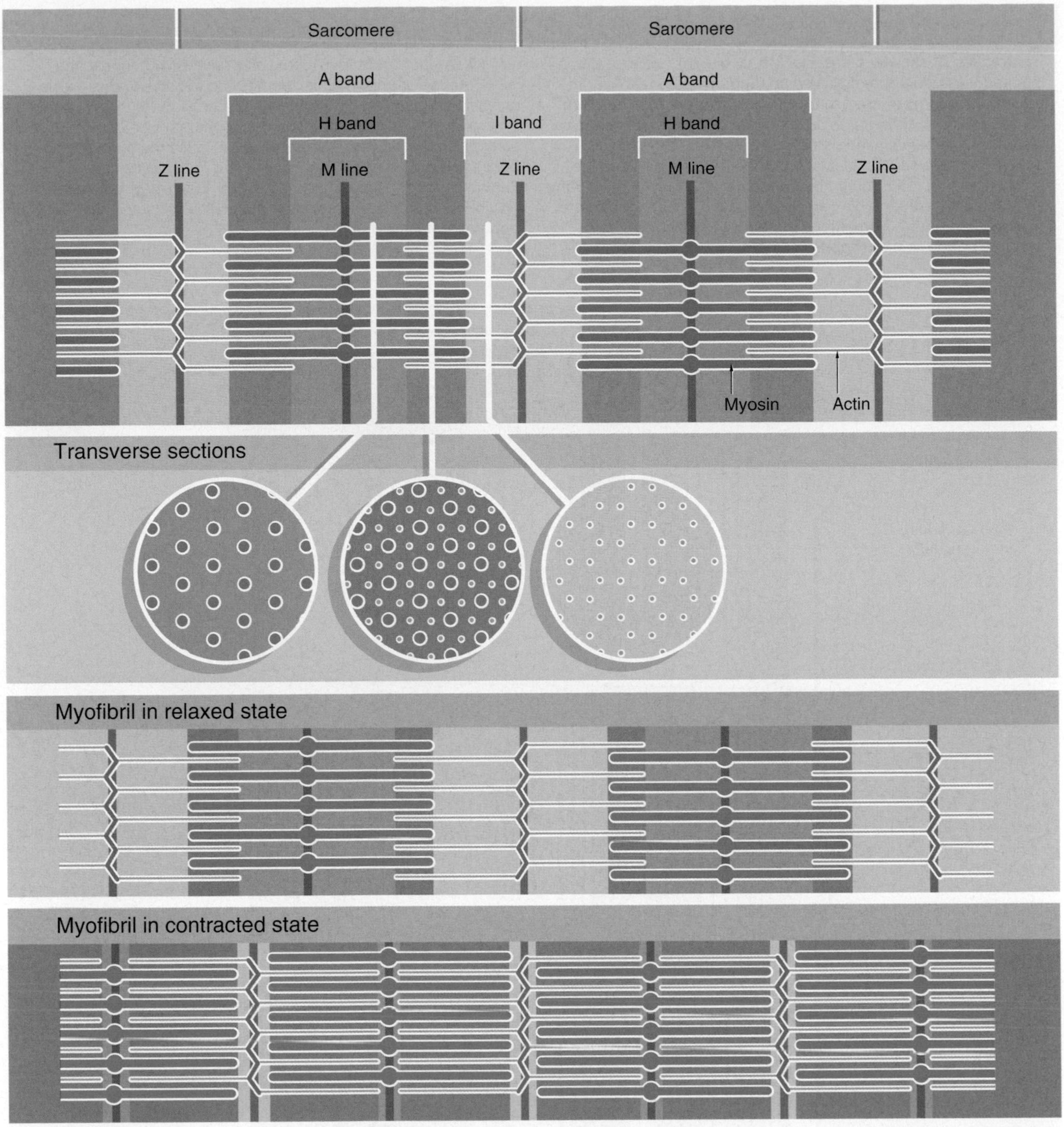

FIG. 6.7 The arrangement of myofilaments in the sarcomere

Muscle function is intimately linked to its microscopic structure. The ***sarcomere*** consists of two types of myofilaments, thick filaments and thin filaments. Each type remains constant in length irrespective of the state of contraction of the muscle. The thick filaments, which are composed mainly of the protein ***myosin***, are maintained in register by their attachment to a disc-like zone represented by the M line. Similarly, the thin filaments, which are composed mainly of the protein ***actin***, are attached to a disc-like zone represented by the Z line. The I and H bands, both areas of low electron density, represent areas where the thick and thin filaments do not overlap one another.

The ***sliding filament mechanism*** of muscle contraction proposes that contraction occurs through a sliding movement of the thick and thin filaments over one another as illustrated above. Myosin molecules possess ATP-activated side projections or head groups which can bind to actin to form ***cross-bridges***, temporary physical linkages between the thick and thin filaments. Once bound to the adjacent actin molecules, these myosin head groups generate movement by a change in protein configuration, triggered by energy from the hydrolysis of ATP, pulling the myosin thick filaments over the thin actin filaments and so shortening the length of the sarcomere. When another ATP molecule binds to the myosin head group, it detaches from actin, breaking the cross-bridge, and the head group then moves back to its original configuration, ready for the next cross-bridge cycle. This process can be likened to multiple small strokes from the oars of a boat steadily producing movement of the craft.

A large number of accessory proteins are also present in the sarcomere where they play roles in filament alignment and in regulation of contraction.

A A band **C** capillary **G** glycogen granules **H** H band **I** I band **M** M line **Mt** mitochondrion **My** myofibril **N** nucleus **S** smooth endoplasmic reticulum **Z** Z line

Muscle function: excitation–contraction coupling

Contraction of skeletal muscle is under voluntary control and is initiated via action potentials in alpha motor neurones. Action potentials are transmitted across the ***neuromuscular junction*** via release of ***acetylcholine*** which binds to ***nicotinic receptors***, resulting in depolarisation of the muscle fibre. Ca^{2+} forms the critical link between the excitation of the muscle fibre and the production of force through the cross-bridge cycle. In the resting state, the cross-bridge binding sites on the actin molecules are masked by another filamentous protein called ***tropomyosin*** which is bound to the ***troponin*** complex.

When Ca^{2+} binds to troponin, this causes a change in the configuration of tropomyosin, unmasking the active sites on the actin filaments and allowing the cross-bridge cycle to commence. When Ca^{2+} levels fall once more due to reuptake of ions into the sarcoplasmic reticulum, the tropomyosin once more blocks the binding sites on the actin molecules and contraction ceases. Extending the boat analogy used earlier, the myosin boat can only row through the sea of actin molecules whilst the layer of tropomyosin ice remains thawed.

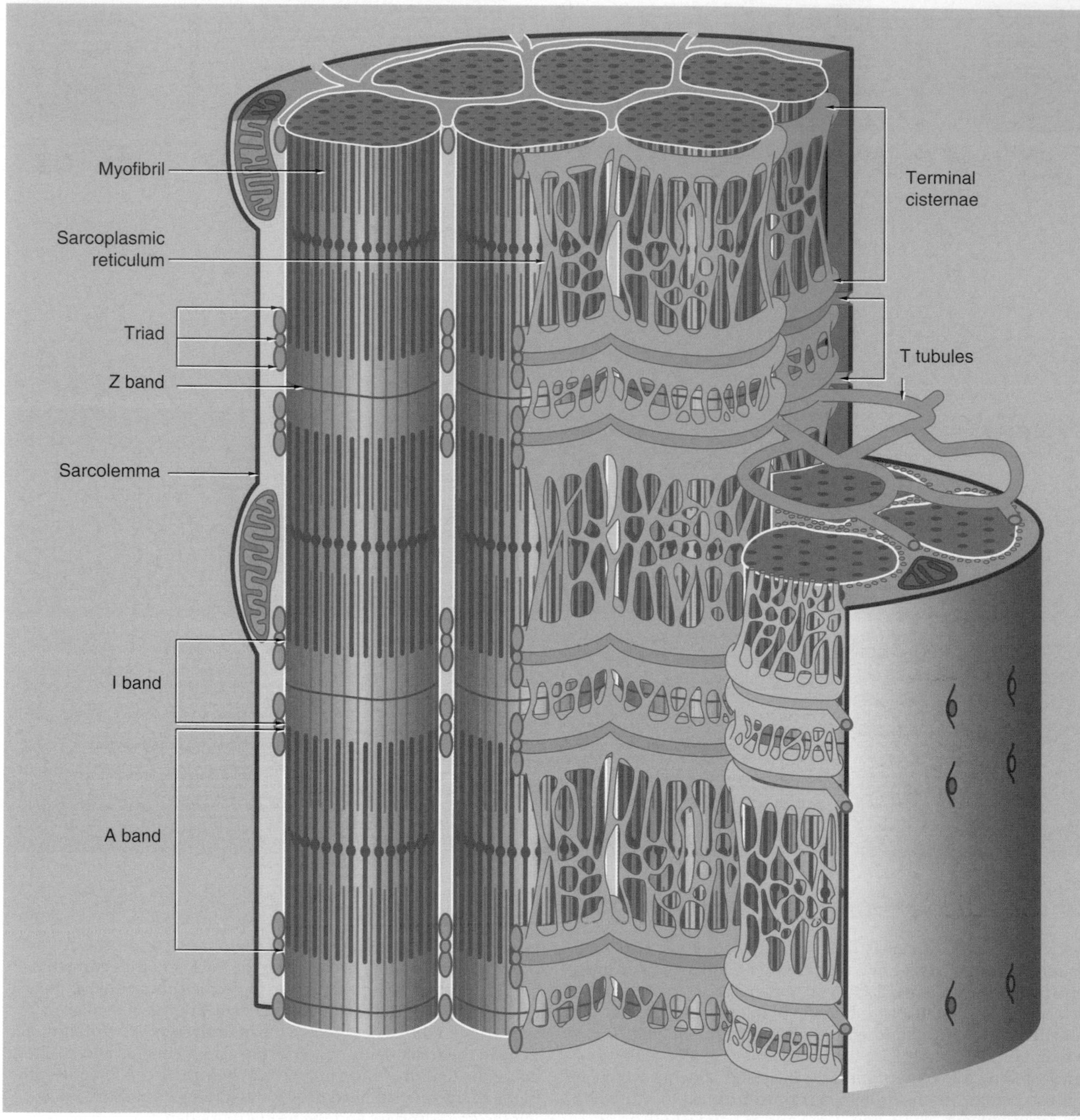

FIG. 6.8 The conducting system for contractile stimuli in skeletal muscle

To permit the synchronous contraction of all sarcomeres in the muscle fibre, a system of tubular extensions of the muscle cell plasma membrane *(sarcolemma)* extends transversely into the muscle cell to surround each myofibril at the region of the junction of the A and I bands. Known as the ***T tubule system***, its lumen is continuous with the extracellular space. (In amphibian skeletal muscle, which was the first to be studied, the T tubules are disposed at the Z bands and the same applies in cardiac muscle.)

Between the T tubules, a second membrane system derived from smooth endoplasmic reticulum, the sarcoplasmic reticulum, forms a membranous network which embraces each myofibril. On either side of each T tubule, the sarcoplasmic reticulum exhibits a flattened cisternal arrangement, each pair of ***terminal cisternae*** and a T tubule forming a ***triad*** near the junction of the I and A bands of each sarcomere.

Calcium ions are concentrated within the lumen of the sarcoplasmic reticulum. Depolarisation of the sarcolemma of the muscle fibre is rapidly disseminated throughout the sarcoplasm by the T tubule system. This promotes the release of Ca^{2+} ions from the sarcoplasmic reticulum into the sarcoplasm surrounding the myofilaments; Ca^{2+} ions then activate the ***sliding filament mechanism*** as described above, resulting in muscle contraction.

Disorders of the neuromuscular junction: myasthenia gravis

Myasthenia gravis occurs due to failure of neuromuscular transmission. Skeletal muscle contraction is entirely dependent upon transmission of the action potential across the neuromuscular junction (see Ch. 7). The action potential in the alpha motor neurone triggers release of acetylcholine into the synaptic cleft at the muscle end plate. Normally, acetylcholine then binds to post-synaptic nicotinic receptors to initiate depolarisation of the muscle fibre. In myasthenia gravis, these post-synaptic receptors are damaged by an ***autoantibody***, an immunoglobulin erroneously produced by the patient's immune system that targets the patient's own tissue. As a result, nerve impulses are not transmitted effectively to the muscle, and the patient experiences weakness and rapid muscle fatigue upon voluntary movement.

FIG. 6.9 Skeletal muscle (LS)
EM ×33 000

Fig. 6.9 is an electron micrograph of mammalian skeletal muscle cut in longitudinal section and demonstrates the main elements of the conducting system. In the vicinity of the junction of the **A** and **I** bands (and depending on the state of contraction) are tubular triads **Td**, each comprising a central flattened tubule of the T tubule system **T** and a pair of terminal cisternae **TC** of the sarcoplasmic reticulum. Within the A bands there are tubular elements of the sarcoplasmic reticulum **SR** connecting the terminal cisternae. Likewise within the I bands, similar though less regular longitudinal tubular profiles of sarcoplasmic reticulum are seen. The conducting system of 'slow-twitch' (red) fibres as shown here (also see Fig. 6.14) is more regular than that of 'fast-twitch' (white) fibres where this pattern is more difficult to discern. Note the distribution of mitochondria **M**, regularly arranged between the sarcomeres within the I bands in immediate association with those parts of the actin and myosin filaments which interact during the process of contraction. The reason for this appearance is evident in Fig. 6.10.

A A band **I** I band **M** mitochondrion **SR** sarcoplasmic reticulum **T** T tubule system **TC** terminal cisternae **Td** tubular triad

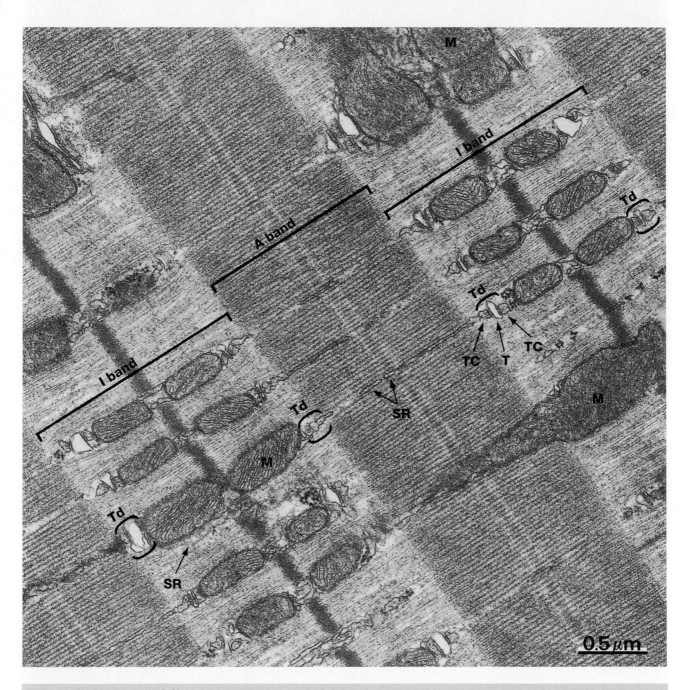

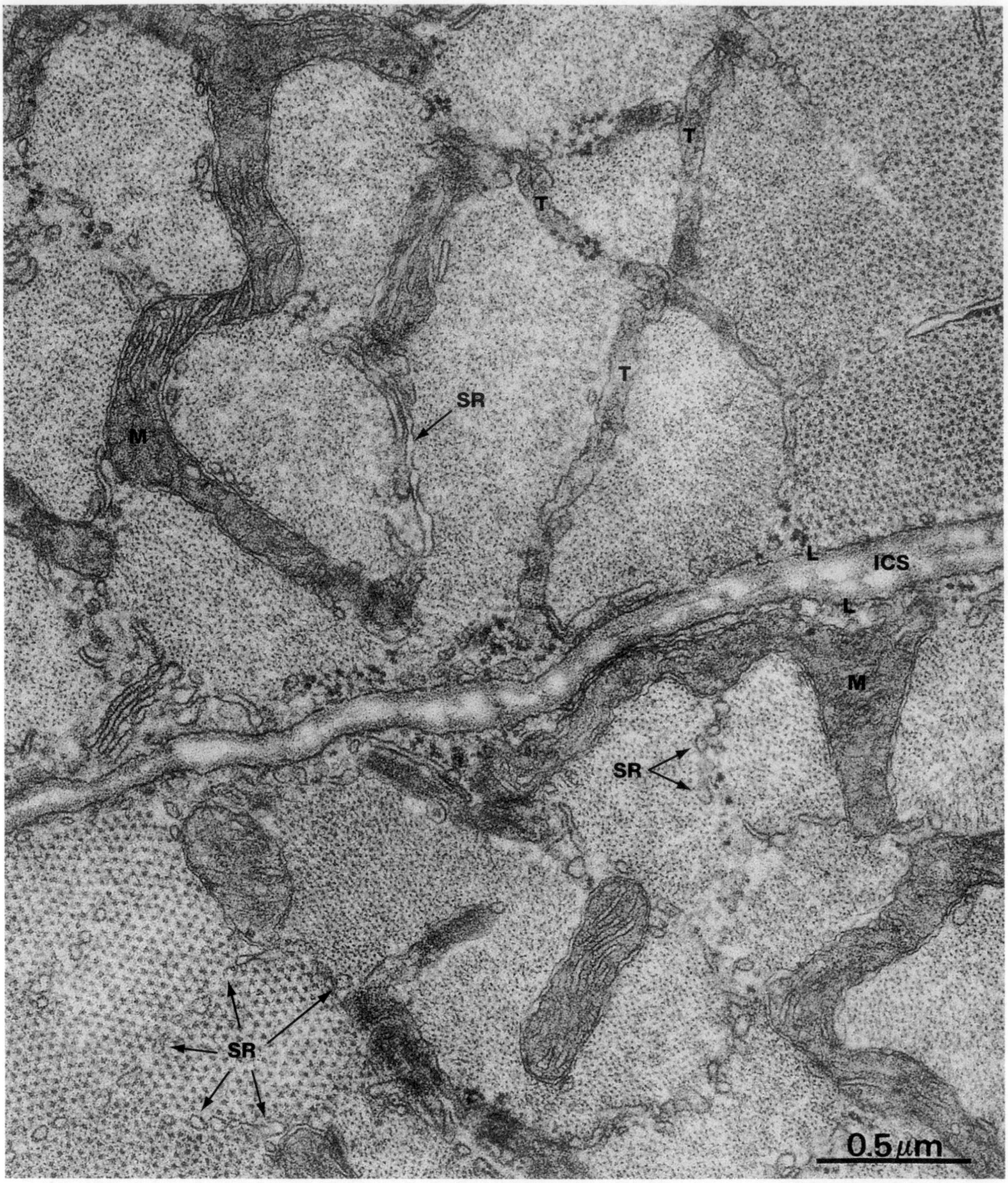

FIG. 6.10 Skeletal muscle
EM ×44 000

Fig. 6.10 shows parts of two skeletal muscle cells cut in transverse section in the vicinity of the junction of A and I bands; the intercellular space **ICS** bisects the field. Note the ***external lamina*** **L** adjacent to the sarcolemma. Sarcomeres at the upper right and lower left of this field have been sectioned through the end part of the A band and thus show both actin and myosin filaments. The remaining sarcomeres are cut through the I band and contain only actin filaments. This results from the fact that the bands of all sarcomeres within any one muscle cell are not exactly in register with one another.

Each sarcomere is ensheathed by a network of tubules of the sarcoplasmic reticulum **SR**. The plane of section has also included a part of a broader diameter T tubule system **T** which branches to encompass several different sarcomeres. Direct communication of T tubules with the intercellular space is difficult to see here, as the tubules appear to ramify into a complex tubular system just beneath the plasmalemma, but continuity of the T tubule lumen and the intercellular space has been convincingly demonstrated by experimental techniques. Note the extraordinary serpentine branched mitochondria **M** which lie between the sarcomeres within the I bands, giving rise to the mitochondrial appearance seen in longitudinal section in Fig. 6.9.

Ar artery **C** capillary **ICS** intercellular space **L** external lamina **M** mitochondrion **SR** sarcoplasmic reticulum **T** T tubule system

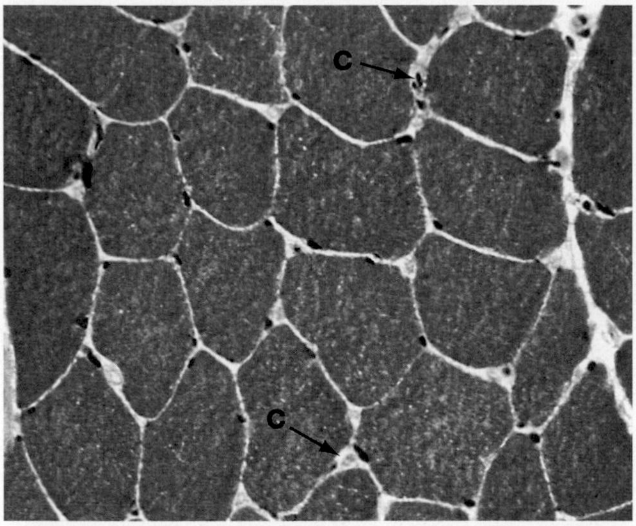

FIG. 6.11 Skeletal muscle
Frozen section, H&E (HP)

In research and clinical diagnosis of muscle disease, formalin-fixed paraffin-embedded tissues are not always used, as they cause artefact to develop and can limit investigation of muscle structure. Fresh frozen section is often the preferred method for preparation of muscle for investigation by light microscopy.

Fig. 6.11 shows a frozen section of skeletal muscle from human vastus lateralis muscle. Tissue shrinkage is minimised. In this transverse section, the extreme peripheral location of the nuclei of the skeletal muscle fibres is well seen. In cross-section, muscle fibres appear polyhedral with flattening of adjacent cells. In normal muscle, the cross-sectional areas of individual fibres are approximately the same. In the endomysial space, numerous minute capillaries **C** are just recognisable.

Compare the huge diameter of the muscle fibres, which may be as great as 0.1 mm in diameter, with that of the capillaries, the latter being approximately 7 μm across.

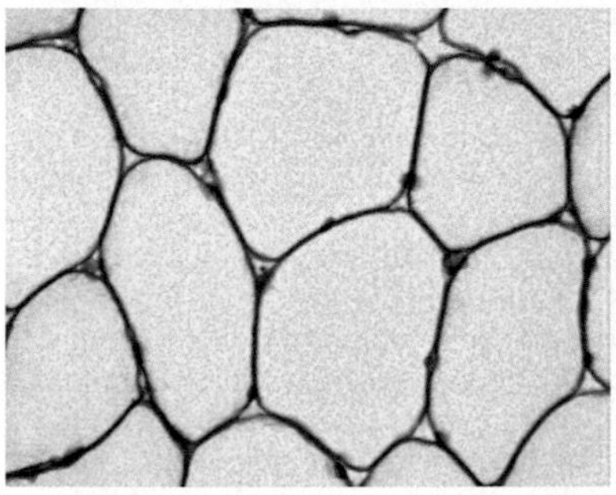

FIG. 6.12 Skeletal muscle
Immunohistochemical stain for dystrophin (HP)

The proteins of the myofilaments actin and desmin are critical for normal muscle function. Another group of proteins which have a key role in muscle function are those associated with the cell membrane of skeletal muscle. A complex of large proteins act to link the contractile proteins within the cell through the cell membrane with structural proteins in the external lamina. Thus, contractile forces within each muscle fibre are transmitted to the collagenous support tissues to bring about movement.

One of the most important and well understood of these linkage proteins is called ***dystrophin***. Immunohistochemical staining for this protein, seen here as a brown stain, shows it to be closely associated with the muscle cell membrane (see textbox 'Muscular dystrophy').

Muscular dystrophy

In muscular dystrophy, there is weakness and wasting of muscles due to a defect in one of the proteins involved in muscle function. Gene mutations affecting proteins of the membrane linkage complex are an important cause of the group of muscular dystrophies. Other genes coding for contractile and other structural proteins may also cause muscular dystrophy.

Some people have a mutation in the gene for dystrophin that results in inefficient linking of contractile forces to the support tissues in muscle (see e-Fig. 6.4). The muscle does not function correctly and fibres undergo progressive damage with repeated contraction, ultimately leading to death of muscle cells.

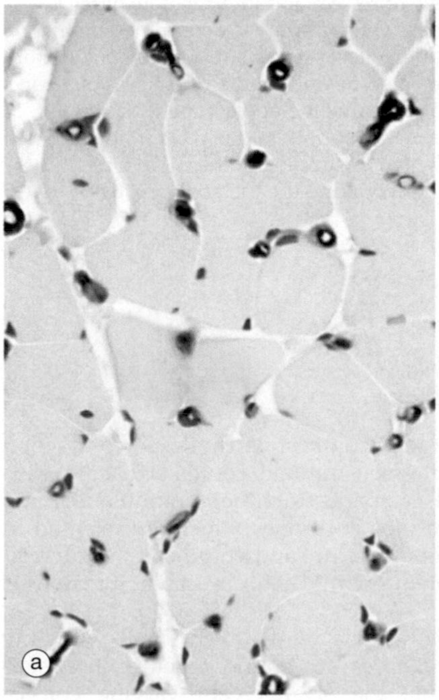

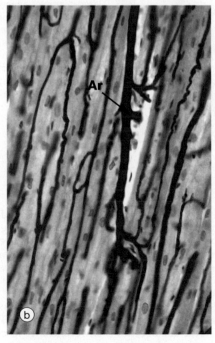

FIG. 6.13 Skeletal muscle blood supply
(a) Immunohistochemical stain for CD 34, TS (HP) (b) Perfusion preparation/haematoxylin, LS (HP)

Fig. 6.13a shows skeletal muscle cut in transverse section and stained to show endothelial cells using an immunohistochemical technique. This highlights capillaries. Each muscle fibre is in close contact with 1 to 3 capillaries, seen as small circular brown profiles.

The capillaries run along the muscle fibres, a feature best illustrated in Fig. 6.13b which is a perfusion preparation of muscle in which the vessels have been injected with red gel.

Muscle nuclei can be seen stained blue with haematoxylin. A small artery **Ar** running in the perimysium can be seen, giving off capillaries which branch out and run along the length of the muscle fibres. The high energy requirement of skeletal muscle demands an extensive capillary network.

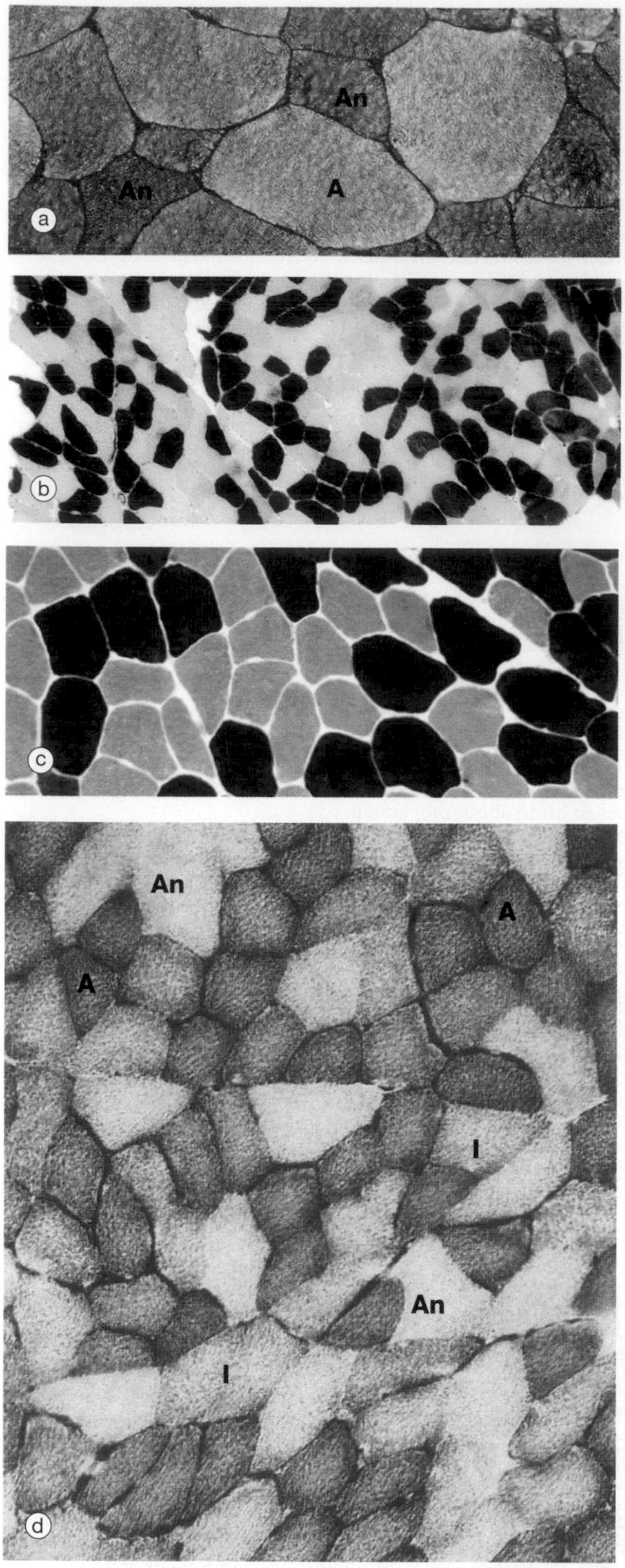

FIG. 6.14 Skeletal muscle
Histochemical techniques, TS
(a) PAS (HP) (b) ATPase pH 4.2 (MP) (c) ATPase pH 9.4 (HP) (d) Succinate dehydrogenase (HP)

The mode of activity of skeletal muscle varies from one part of the body to another. Some muscles, such as those involved in the maintenance of posture, are required to contract almost continuously while others, such as the extra-ocular muscles, make rapid short-lived movements. In humans, distinction between these types cannot be made on gross examination of the muscle. In domestic poultry, however, the extremes are easily identified by a difference in colours; for example, leg muscles are red, and flight (breast) muscles are white.

Correspondingly, 'slow-twitch' and 'fast-twitch' muscle fibre types can be demonstrated by nerve stimulation studies. The metabolic requirements of each fibre type differ markedly, the slow red fibres mainly relying on aerobic metabolism and the fast white fibres using predominantly anaerobic pathways. Most muscles contain a mixture of these extreme fibre types as well as an intermediate type. There are significant interspecies differences.

Aerobic (type I) muscle fibres **A** contain abundant mitochondria. They also have a large content of myoglobin, an oxygen-storage molecule analogous to haemoglobin, which accounts for the red colour of such fibres.

In contrast, ***anaerobic (type II) muscle fibres*** **An** contain few mitochondria and relatively little myoglobin. These muscle fibres are, however, rich in glycogen and glycolytic enzymes.

These characteristics account for the 'white' colour of such fibres. In Fig. 6.14a, the PAS stain demonstrates this difference in glycogen content. The type II fibres stain dark pink due to the presence of abundant glycogen granules, whilst the aerobic type I fibres contain little glycogen and appear paler in colour. Anaerobic fibres predominate in muscles responsible for intense but sporadic contraction such as the biceps and triceps of the arms.

Type I and II fibres can also be identified by the nature of their ***myosin ATPase***, which differs in its protein structure between different fibre types. In the preparation in Fig. 6.14b, type I fibres are dark and type II fibres are light. This low magnification shows the checkerboard pattern of the fibre types within a muscle fascicle. Fig. 6.14c has been stained at a pH that reveals type I fibres as pale and type II fibres as dark (the opposite to Fig. 6.14b). Such histochemical staining is used routinely in diagnosis of muscle disease.

The activity of the specific mitochondrial enzyme ***succinate dehydrogenase***, which catalyses one of the stages of the Krebs cycle, demonstrates the relative proportions of mitochondria within the muscle fibres. In Fig. 6.14d, note the presence of intensely stained small-diameter aerobic fibres **A**, poorly stained large-diameter anaerobic fibres **An** and intermediate fibres **I**.

The type of metabolism of each fibre is determined by the frequency of impulses in its motor nerve supply. Any one motor nerve supplies fibres of one type only, and all the fibres of a particular motor unit are of the same metabolic type.

Indeed, if the motor nerve supply to one type of fibre is experimentally transplanted to supply another fibre type, this fibre type will become converted to the metabolic pattern of the former.

SMOOTH MUSCLE

Skeletal muscle is specialised for relatively forceful contractions of short duration under voluntary control. In contrast, smooth muscle is specialised for continuous contractions of relatively low force, producing diffuse movements through contraction of the whole muscle mass, rather than contraction of individual motor units. Contractility is an inherent property of smooth muscle, occurring independently of innervation, often in a rhythmic or wave-like fashion. Superimposed on this inherent contractility are the influences of the autonomic nervous system, hormones and local metabolites which modulate contractility to accommodate changing functional demands. For example, the smooth muscle of the intestinal wall undergoes continuous rhythmic contraction (***peristalsis***), propelling the luminal contents distally. This activity is enhanced by parasympathetic stimulation and influenced by a variety of hormones which are released in response to changes in the nature and volume of the gut contents. The structure of autonomic neuromuscular junctions is described in Ch. 7.

The cells of smooth muscle are relatively small, with only a single nucleus. The fibres are bound together in irregular branching fasciculi, the arrangement varying considerably from one organ to another according to functional requirements.

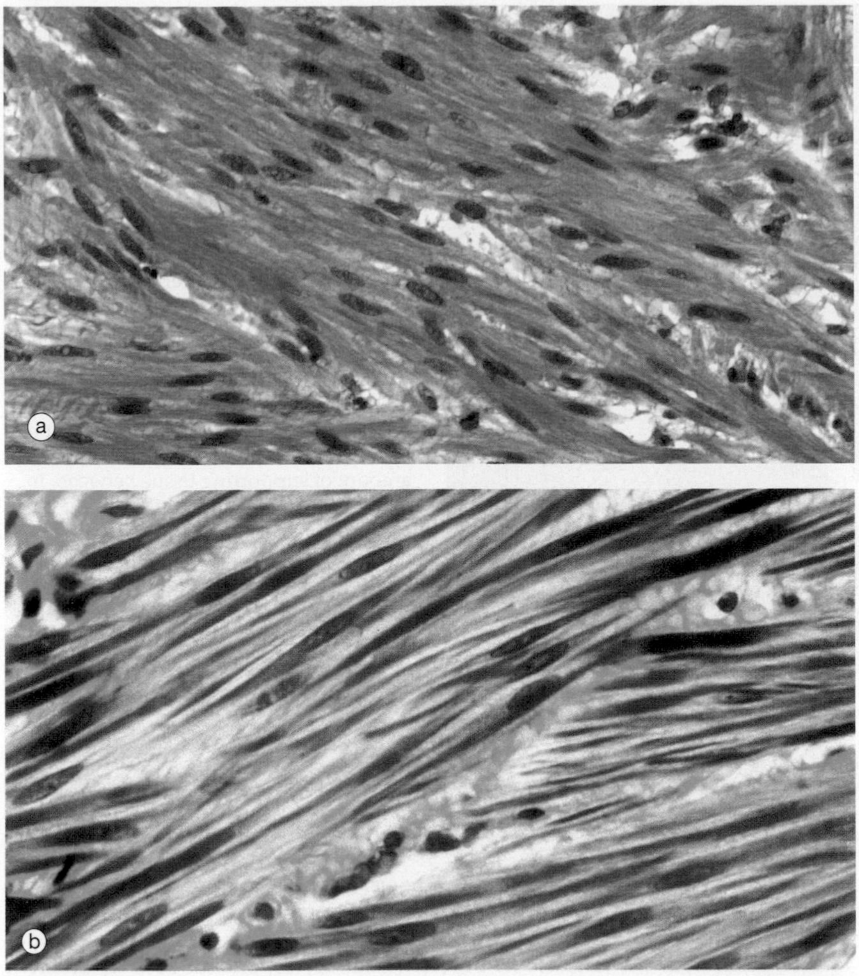

FIG. 6.15 Smooth muscle
(a) H&E, LS (HP)
(b) Masson trichrome, LS (HP)

As seen in Figs 6.15a and b, smooth muscle fibres are elongated, spindle-shaped cells with tapered ends which may occasionally be bifurcated. Smooth muscle fibres are generally much shorter than skeletal muscle fibres and contain only one nucleus which is elongated and centrally located in the cytoplasm at the widest part of the cell; however, depending on the contractile state of the fibres at fixation, the nuclei may sometimes appear to be spiral-shaped.

Smooth muscle fibres are bound together in irregular branching fasciculi and these fasciculi, rather than individual fibres, are the functional contractile units. Within the fasciculi, individual muscle fibres are arranged roughly parallel to one another with the thickest part of one cell lying against the thin parts of adjacent cells.

The contractile proteins of smooth muscle are not arranged in myofibrils, as in skeletal and cardiac muscle, and thus visceral muscle cells are not striated.

Between the individual muscle fibres and between the fasciculi, there is a network of supporting collagenous tissue. This is well demonstrated in Fig. 6.15b in which the collagen is stained blue-green.

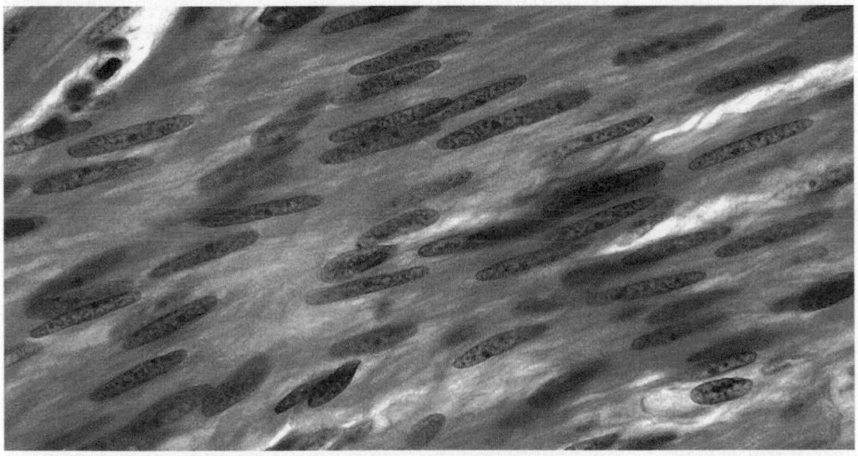

FIG. 6.16 Smooth muscle
H&E, LS (HP)

Fig. 6.16 illustrates smooth muscle from the bowel wall, cut in longitudinal section. In this case, the fibres are arranged in a highly regular manner and packed so closely that it is difficult to identify individual cell outlines, although cell shape can be deduced from that of the nuclei.

Smooth muscle cell nuclei are elongated and are typically described as being 'cigar-shaped' with rather blunt ends.

The cytoplasm is eosinophilic but lacks the cross-striations seen in skeletal and cardiac muscle.

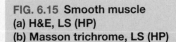

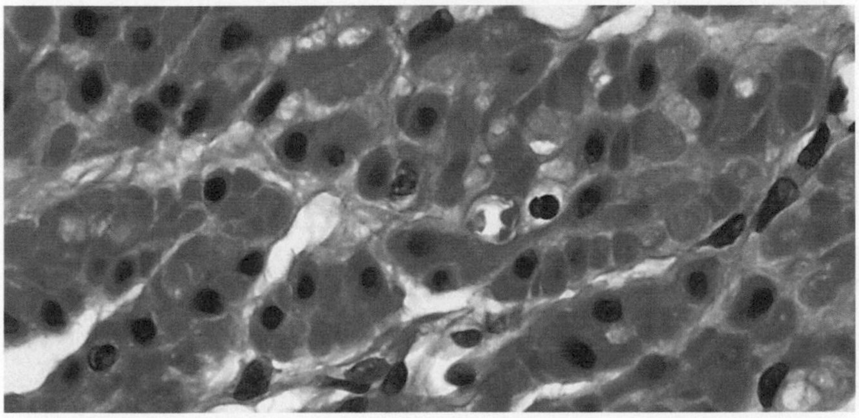

FIG. 6.17 Smooth muscle
H&E, TS (HP)

Fig. 6.17 shows smooth muscle in transverse section at very high magnification. The spindle-shaped cells are sectioned at various different points along their length, which gives the erroneous impression that they are of differing diameters. Nuclei are only included in the plane of section where fibres have been cut through their widest diameter. Note the plump nuclear shape and the central location of the nuclei within the cytoplasm.

A aerobic fibre **An** anaerobic fibre **I** intermediate fibre

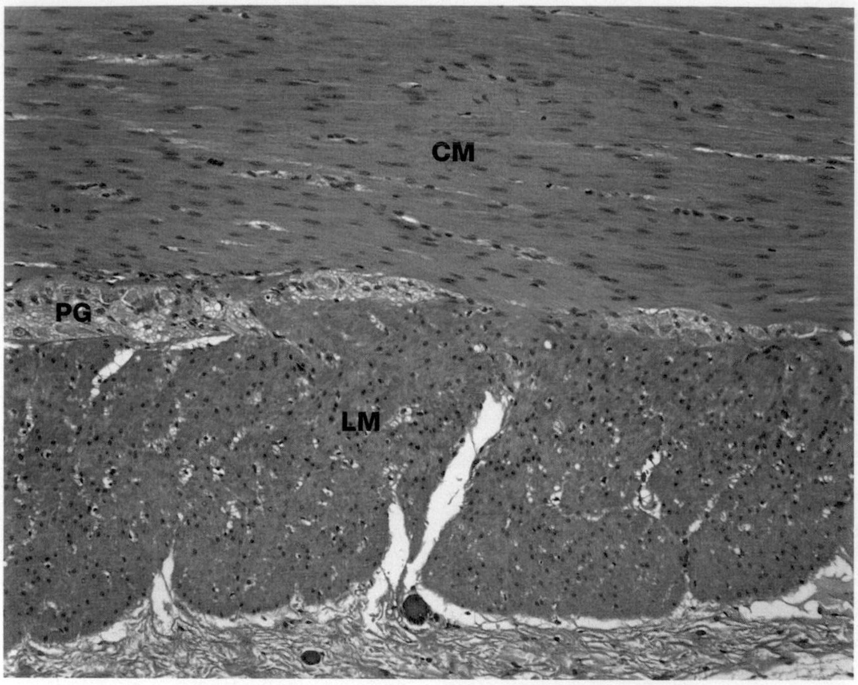

FIG. 6.18 Smooth muscle H&E, TS (MP)

Fig. 6.18 illustrates smooth muscle from the bowel wall, cut in transverse section. In many tubular visceral structures, such as the ileum as shown in this micrograph, smooth muscle is disposed in layers, with the cells of one layer arranged at right angles to those of the adjacent layer.

This arrangement permits a wave of contraction to pass down the tube, propelling the contents forward; this action is called ***peristalsis***.

Typically, the longitudinal outer smooth muscle layer **LM** (cut in transverse section here) is closely applied to the inner circular layer **CM**, with only a minimal amount of supporting tissue between. In this specimen, the collagen is stained blue.

The supporting tissue here contains clumps of large cells with pale nuclei which represent ***parasympathetic ganglia*** **PG** (see Fig. 7.22). The parasympathetic nervous system of the gastrointestinal tract modulates the intensity of peristalsis.

SMOOTH MUSCLE CONTRACTION

Smooth muscle does not show the longitudinally organised system of contractile proteins that is seen in striated muscle, but has an arrangement where bundles of contractile proteins criss-cross the cell, being inserted into anchoring points (***focal densities***) within the cytoplasm, as well as anchoring to the cell membrane as ***focal adhesion densities***. Tension generated by contraction is transmitted through anchoring densities in the cell membrane to the surrounding external lamina, thus allowing a mass of smooth muscle cells to function as one unit. The intermediate filaments of smooth muscle, ***desmin***, are also inserted into the focal densities (Fig. 6.20).

The contraction mechanism of smooth muscle differs from that for striated muscle. Because the contractile proteins are arranged in a criss-cross lattice inserted around the cell membrane, contraction results in shortening of the cell, which assumes a globular shape in contrast to its elongated shape in the relaxed state (see Fig. 6.20).

The mechanism of smooth muscle contraction is as follows:

- Thin filaments of actin are associated with ***tropomyosin***.
- Thick filaments composed of myosin only bind to actin if one chain is phosphorylated.
- Calcium ions in the cytosol of smooth muscle cells cause contraction, as in striated muscle, but the control of Ca^{2+} ion movements is different. In relaxed smooth muscle, free Ca^{2+} ions are normally sequestered in sarcoplasmic reticulum throughout the cell. On membrane excitation, free Ca^{2+} ions are released into the cytoplasm and bind to a protein called ***calmodulin*** (a calcium-binding protein). The calcium–calmodulin complex then activates an enzyme called ***myosin light-chain kinase***, which phosphorylates myosin and permits it to bind to actin. Actin and myosin subsequently interact by filament sliding to produce contraction in a similar way to that for skeletal muscle.
- Contraction of smooth muscle can be modulated by surface receptors activating internal second messenger systems. Expression of different receptors allows smooth muscle in different sites to respond to several different hormones.
- Compared with skeletal muscle, smooth muscle is able to maintain a high force of contraction for very little ATP usage.

Most smooth muscle is present in the walls of hollow viscera (e.g. gut, ureter, Fallopian tube) where it is arranged in sheets with cells aligned circumferentially or longitudinally, with contraction resulting in reduction of the lumen diameter.

In these so-called ***unitary smooth muscles***, cells tend to generate their own low level of rhythmic contraction, which may also be stimulated by stretch and is transmitted from cell to cell via the gap junctions. Such smooth muscle is richly innervated by the autonomic nervous system (see Ch. 7), which increases or decreases levels of spontaneous contraction rather than actually initiating it. Physiologically, this is termed ***tonic smooth muscle*** and is characterised by slow contraction, no action potentials and a low content of fast myosin.

A second arrangement of smooth muscle is typified by that of the iris of the eye. Here, rather than simply modulating spontaneous activity, autonomic innervation precisely controls contraction, resulting in opening and closing of the pupil. Similar neurally controlled or multi-unit smooth muscle is found in the vas deferens and in some large arteries. Physiologically, this is termed ***phasic smooth muscle***, and it is characterised by rapid contraction associated with an action potential.

Tumours of smooth muscle

Benign tumours of smooth muscle are termed ***leiomyomas*** (e-Fig. 6.5). These are typically found in the uterus where they are more commonly known as fibroids but they can be found at other sites such as the skin or gastrointestinal tract. Malignant smooth muscle tumours are known as ***leiomyosarcomas*** (e-Fig. 6.6). These tumours retain the appearance of smooth muscle but also show malignant features such as necrosis, atypia and/or increased mitotic activity.

C caveola **CM** circular smooth muscle layer **D** focal density **ER** endoplasmic reticulum **F** fibroblast **Fi** filaments **G** gap junction **J** attachment junction **LM** longitudinal smooth muscle layer **M** mitochondrion **N** nucleus **PG** parasympathetic ganglion **S** supporting tissue **T** tubular structure

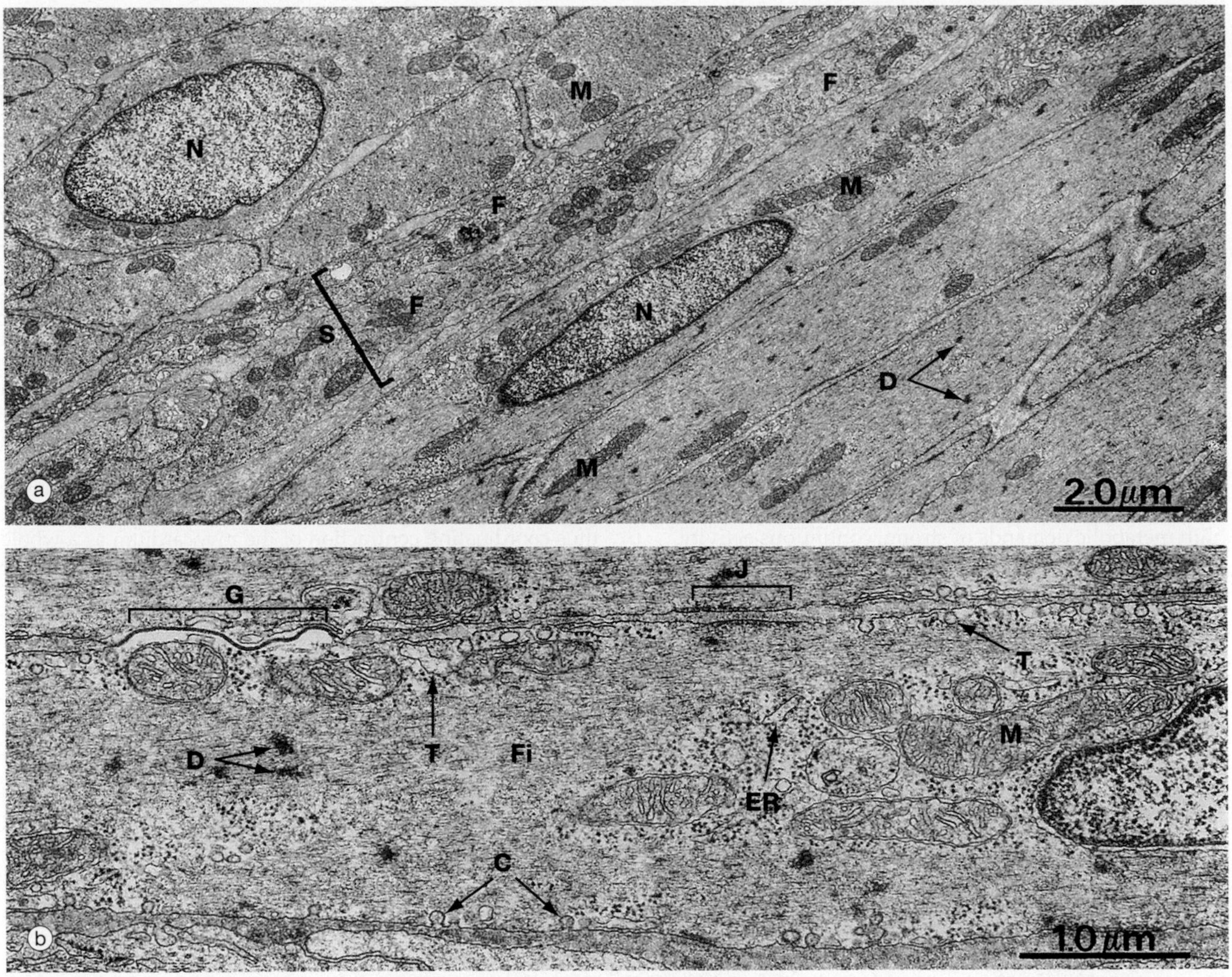

FIG. 6.19 Smooth muscle
(a) EM ×8000 (b) EM ×21 000

At low magnification, Fig. 6.19a demonstrates the spindle-shaped and elongated central nuclei **N** of smooth muscle cells. The cells at the lower right are cut longitudinally, and those at the upper left transversely. Between them is a band of supporting tissue **S** containing the cytoplasmic processes of fibroblasts **F**. Note the relative sparsity of mitochondria **M** and other intracellular organelles.

At high magnification in Fig. 6.19b, details of the plasma membrane and endomembrane system can be seen. The plasma membrane contains numerous flask-shaped invaginations. In some areas, these are irregular in shape and size and may be involved in pinocytosis. In other areas, the invaginations are regular in shape and distribution and are called *caveolae* **C**. The endomembrane system contains some elements which represent a poorly developed Golgi and endoplasmic reticulum **ER**. Other vesicular and tubular structures **T** are seen near the plasma membrane, often in association with caveolae; these probably constitute a system analogous to the sarcoplasmic reticulum of skeletal muscle, with caveolae being analogous to the T tubule system.

Thick and thin filaments **Fi** of myosin and actin criss-cross the cytoplasm of each cell and are anchored to the cell membrane at ***attachment junctions (focal adhesion densities)*** **J**. Filaments are also attached within the cytoplasm to focal densities **D** which are believed to hold filaments in register.

The narrow intercellular spaces are of almost uniform width, but at numerous sites the plasma membranes of adjacent cells form specialised cell junctions. ***Nexus (gap) junctions*** **G** mediate spread of excitation throughout visceral muscle (see Fig. 5.12).

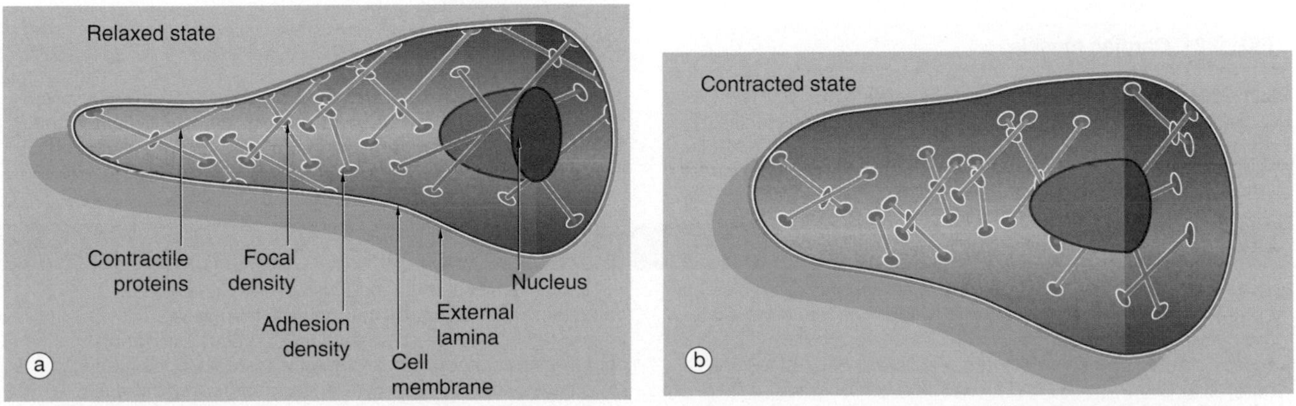

FIG. 6.20 Smooth muscle contraction

Contractile proteins are inserted into focal densities and focal adhesion densities around the cell membrane. In the relaxed state (Fig. 6.20a) the cell is elongated. With contraction (Fig. 6.20b), the smooth muscle cell adopts a globular shape.

CARDIAC MUSCLE

Cardiac muscle or ***myocardium*** exhibits many structural and functional characteristics intermediate between those of skeletal and visceral muscle. Like the former, its contractions are strong and utilise a great deal of energy; like the latter, the contractions are continuous and initiated by inherent mechanisms, although they are modulated by external autonomic and hormonal stimuli.

Cardiac muscle fibres are essentially long, cylindrical cells with one or at most two nuclei which are centrally located within the cell. The ends of the fibres are split longitudinally into a small number of branches, the ends of which abut onto similar branches of adjacent cells, giving the impression of a continuous three-dimensional cytoplasmic network; this was formerly described as a syncytium before the discrete intercellular boundaries were recognised.

Between the muscle fibres, delicate collagenous tissue analogous to the endomysium of skeletal muscle supports the extremely rich capillary network necessary to meet the high metabolic demands of strong, continuous activity.

Cardiac muscle fibres have an arrangement of contractile proteins similar to that of skeletal muscle and are consequently striated in a similar manner. However, this is often difficult to see with light microscopy due to the irregular branching shape of the cells and their myofibrils. Cardiac muscle fibres also have a system of T tubules and sarcoplasmic reticulum analogous to that of skeletal muscle. In the case of cardiac muscle, however, there is a slow leak of Ca^{2+} ions into the cytoplasm from the sarcoplasmic reticulum after recovery from the preceding contraction; this causes a succession of automatic contractions independent of external stimuli. The rate of this inherent rhythm is then modulated by external autonomic and hormonal stimuli.

Between the ends of adjacent cardiac muscle cells are specialised intercellular junctions called ***intercalated discs*** which not only provide points of anchorage for the myofibrils but also permit extremely rapid spread of contractile stimuli from one cell to another. Thus, adjacent fibres are triggered to contract almost simultaneously, thereby acting as a ***functional syncytium***. In addition, a system of highly modified cardiac muscle cells constitutes the pacemaker regions of the heart and ramifies throughout the organ as the ***Purkinje system***, thus coordinating contraction of the myocardium as a whole in each cardiac cycle. This is illustrated and described in more detail in Ch. 8.

Cardiac muscle cells in certain locations in the heart are responsible for secreting hormones into the bloodstream.

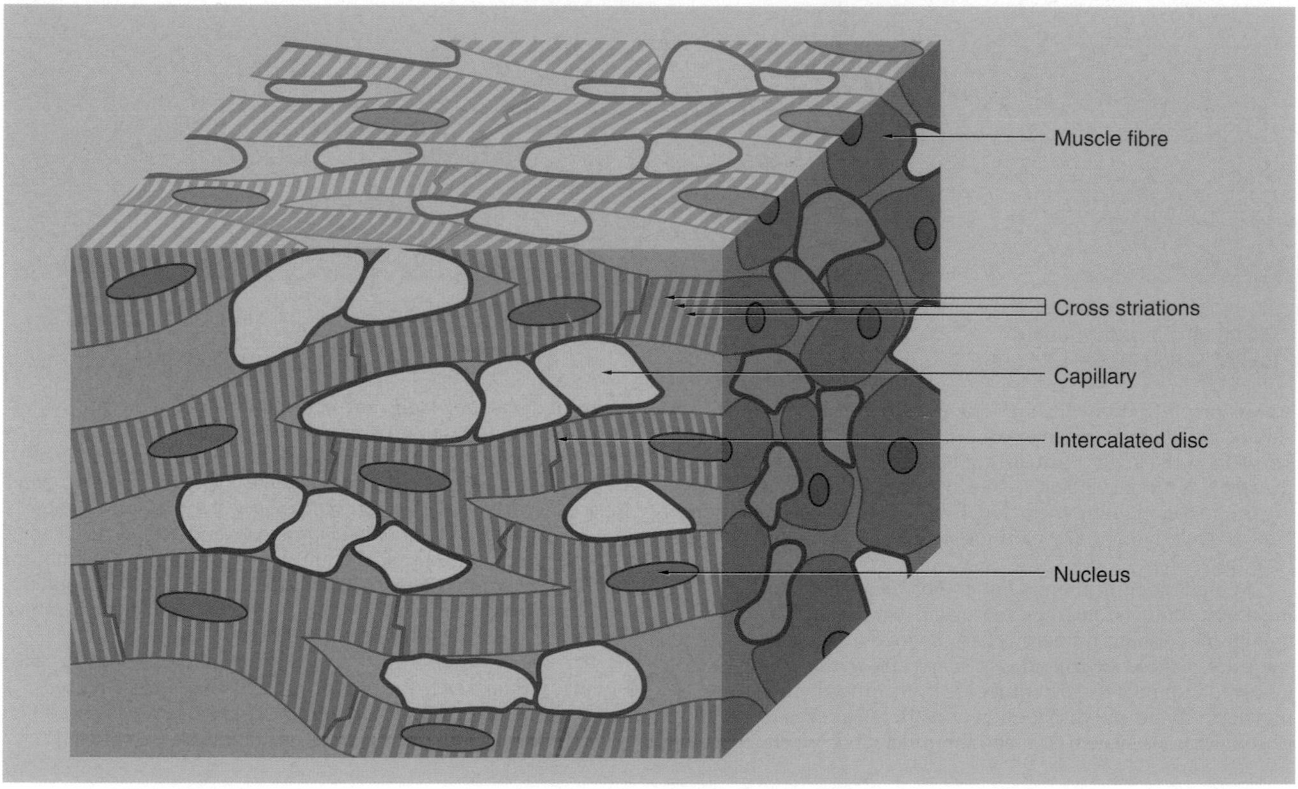

FIG. 6.21 Cardiac muscle

Fig. 6.21 highlights the key features of cardiac muscle. The cardiac myocytes are long, branching cells with central nuclei. The cells are joined together end to end via specialised intercellular junctions termed intercalated discs. These produce both structural and electrical coupling between the myocytes, allowing them to act as a ***functional syncytium***. There are large numbers of capillaries between the cells, reflecting the high metabolic requirements of cardiac muscle.

Cardiac muscle and disease

The heart muscle has high metabolic demands as it is constantly contracting to supply the body with blood. The blood supply to the heart itself is through three main coronary arteries which are prone to ***atheroma*** (see *Wheater's Pathology*, Ch. 8), leading to narrowing of the vessels and a reduction in blood flow. If there is a critical failure of blood flow to the myocardium, the cardiac muscle cells may be deprived of oxygen and other nutrients and may die. Death of cardiac muscle cells causes ***myocardial infarction*** (e-Fig. 6.7).

In the normal heart, conduction of depolarisation for contraction runs along the muscle cells themselves. This is interrupted in the case of an area of infarction. A common complication of a myocardial infarct is the development of disturbances of the heart rhythm, for example ***ventricular fibrillation***. This can lead to sudden cardiac death. If the patient survives myocardial infarction, loss of a significant portion of muscle mass from the heart can cause ***heart failure***, where the heart is unable to pump blood at a sufficient rate to meet the metabolic needs of the tissues.

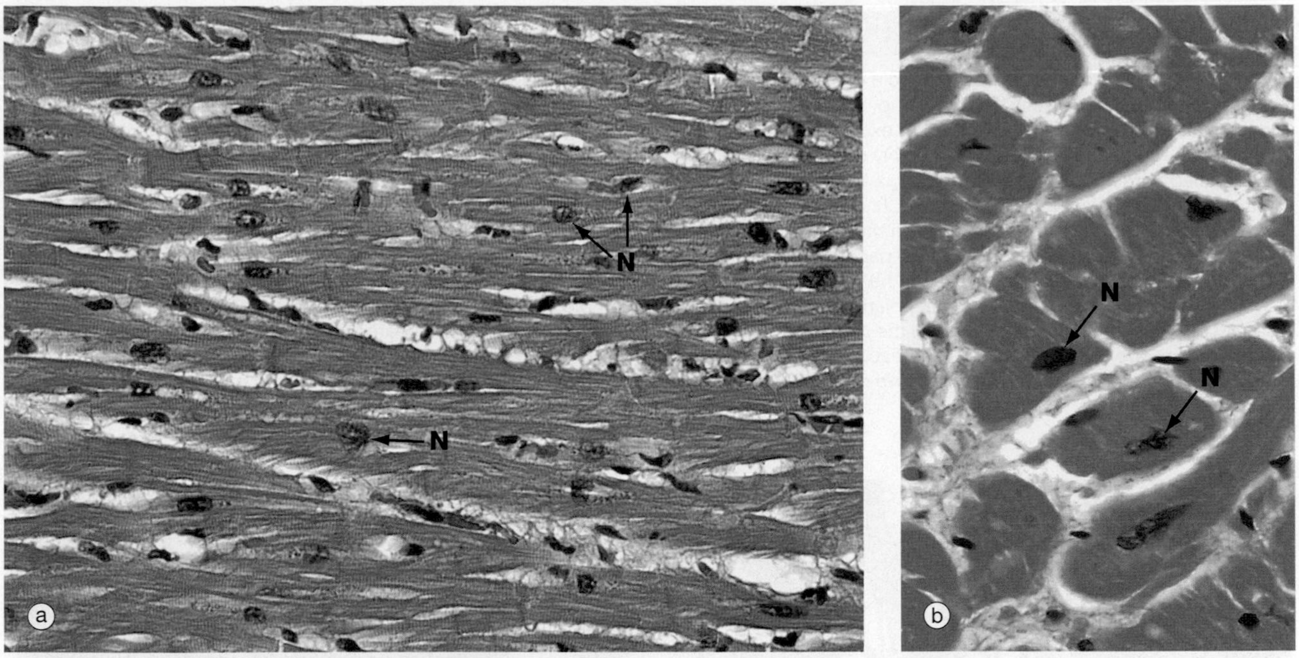

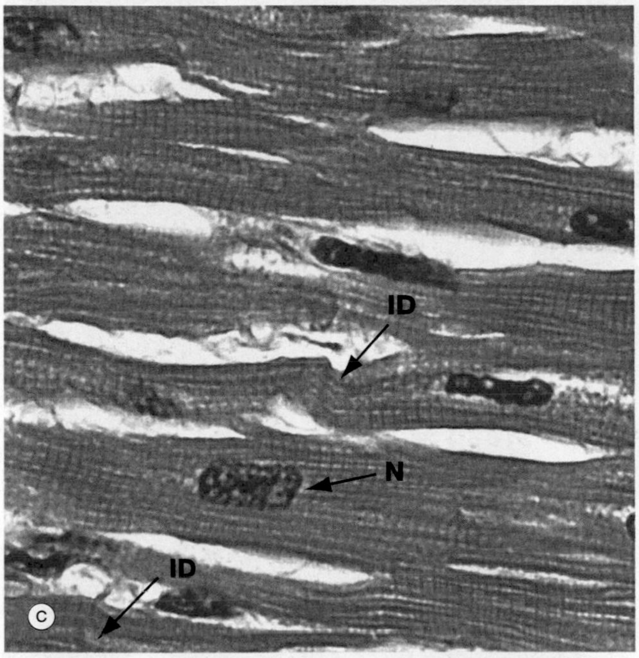

FIG. 6.22 Cardiac muscle
(a) H&E, LS (MP) (b) H&E, TS (HP) (c) H&E, polarised light, LS (HP)

In longitudinal section in Fig. 6.22a, cardiac muscle cells are seen to contain one or two nuclei **N** and an extensive eosinophilic cytoplasm which branches to give the appearance of a continuous three-dimensional network. The elongated nuclei are mainly centrally located, a characteristic well demonstrated in transverse section as shown in Fig. 6.22b.

Fine wisps of collagenous tissue run between fibres, together with an extensive capillary supply which is not seen at this resolution.

Fig. 6.22c has been taken from an H&E-stained section but viewed using polarised light. This creates improved optical contrast so as to reveal the cross-striations. In routine light microscopy, striations in cardiac muscle are generally not as easy to demonstrate as in skeletal muscle. The branching cytoplasmic network is readily seen. Intercalated discs **ID** mark the intercellular boundaries and are just visible in this micrograph. Note the delicate supporting tissue filling the intercellular spaces.

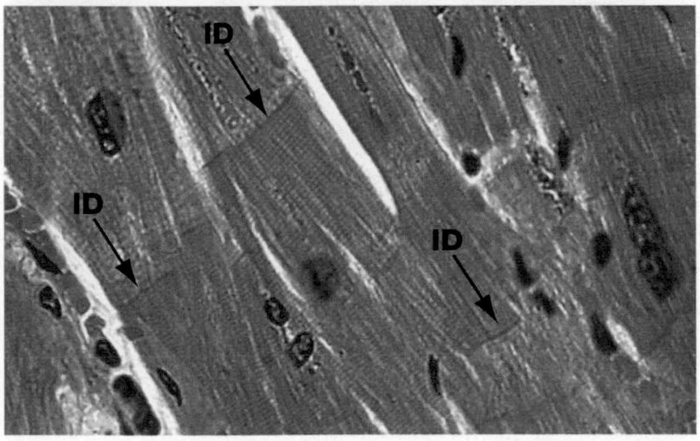

FIG. 6.23 Cardiac muscle
H&E, LS (HP)

The branching pattern of cardiac muscle cells is well demonstrated in this image. Individual cells are attached to each other end to end by specialised cell junctions termed ***intercalated discs*** (see also Figs 6.26 and 6.27). These can just be seen as transverse bands **ID** within the muscle cells. A red- brown pigment seen in these cardiac cells is termed ***lipofuscin*** and is derived from turnover of cell material within lysosomes, so-called wear-and-tear pigment. This pigment gradually accumulates in the human heart with age and can be responsible for the heart muscle appearing brown in colour (see also Ch. 1).

ID intercalated disc **N** nucleus

The conducting system of the heart

Coordinated contraction of cardiac muscle is critical in allowing the heart to function effectively as a pump, supplying blood to the tissues of the body. Rapid spread of excitation through the whole myocardium is achieved via a highly specialised system of modified cardiac muscle cells known as the ***conducting system***. This is discussed more fully in Ch. 8.

In short, electrical excitation begins in the cells of the ***sino-atrial node*** (see Fig. 8.5), also known as 'pacemaker cells', and then spreads through the atria of the heart, initiating atrial contraction before the ventricles are depolarised, so that blood can first be pumped from the atria to fill the ventricles. The ***atrio-ventricular node*** then transmits the cardiac action potential into the ventricles via the ***bundle of His*** or ***atrio-ventricular bundle***.

This electrical pathway runs through the interventricular septum of the heart and allows ventricular depolarisation and contraction to spread from the apex of the heart towards the ventricular outflow tracts, facilitating effective expulsion of blood from the ventricles with each heart beat.

Disorders of heart rhythm may arise due to myocardial ischaemia or infarction, as described previously (see textbox), or may be produced by more specific disorders of the conducting system itself. Abnormal heart rhythm or ***arrhythmia*** is a fairly common medical problem and its clinical features may range from immediately life-threatening medical emergencies requiring a pacemaker, through to other forms which may give rise to only mild or intermittent symptoms.

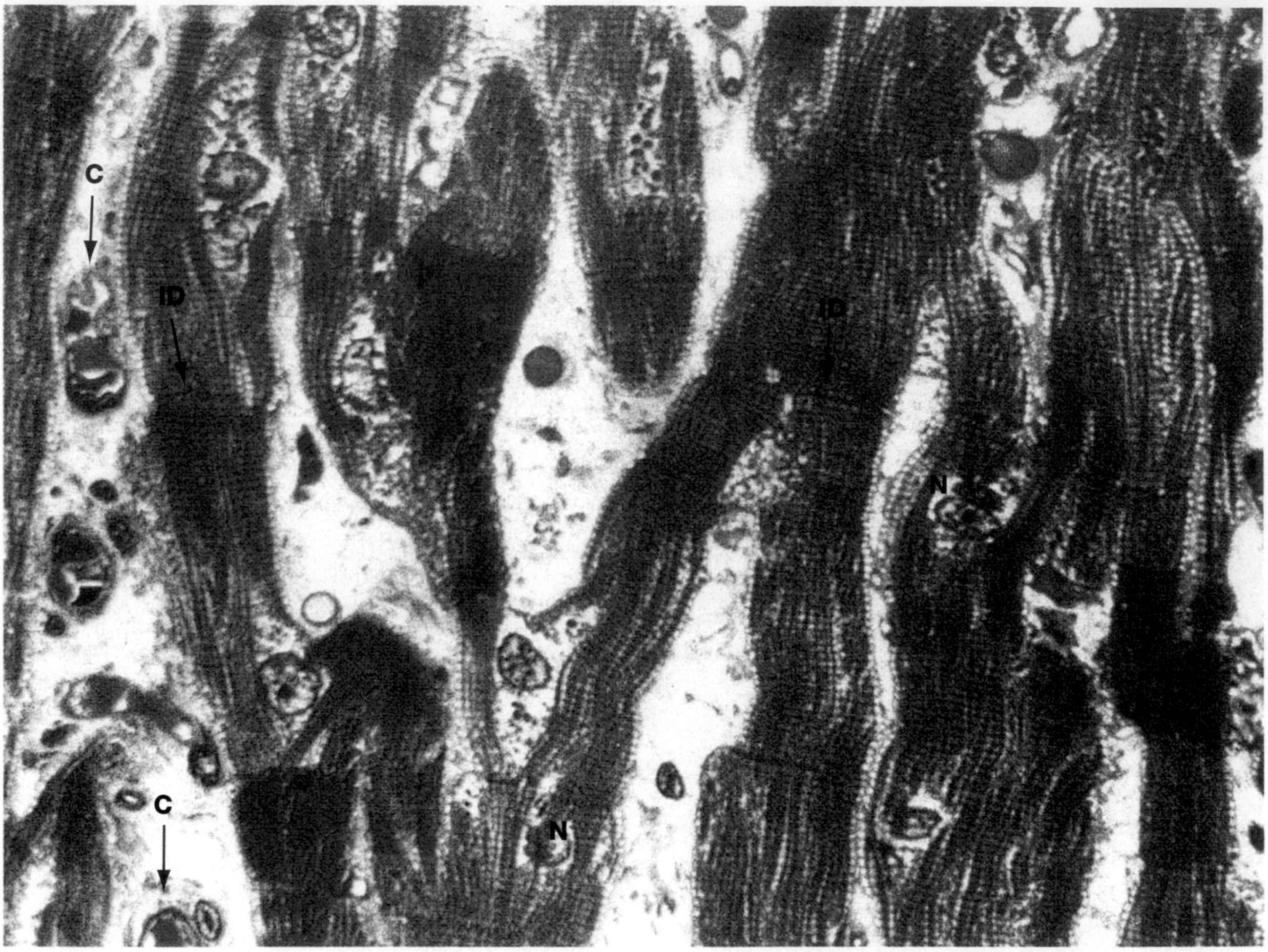

FIG. 6.24 Cardiac muscle
Thin section, toluidine blue, LS (HP)

Fig. 6.24 illustrates an extremely thin, resin-embedded section at very high magnification. The branching cytoplasmic network of cardiac muscle cells is readily seen, with prominent intercalated discs **ID** marking the intercellular boundaries.

With this method of preparation, it is easy to see the typical cross-striations and central nuclei **N**. Also note the delicate supporting tissue filling the intercellular spaces, containing an extensive network of blood capillaries **C**.

C capillary **C1–C6** cardiac muscle cells **F** fibroblast **G** glycogen granules **ID** intercalated disc **L** lipid droplet **M** mitochondrion **N** nucleus **T** T tubule **SR** sarcoplasmic reticulum

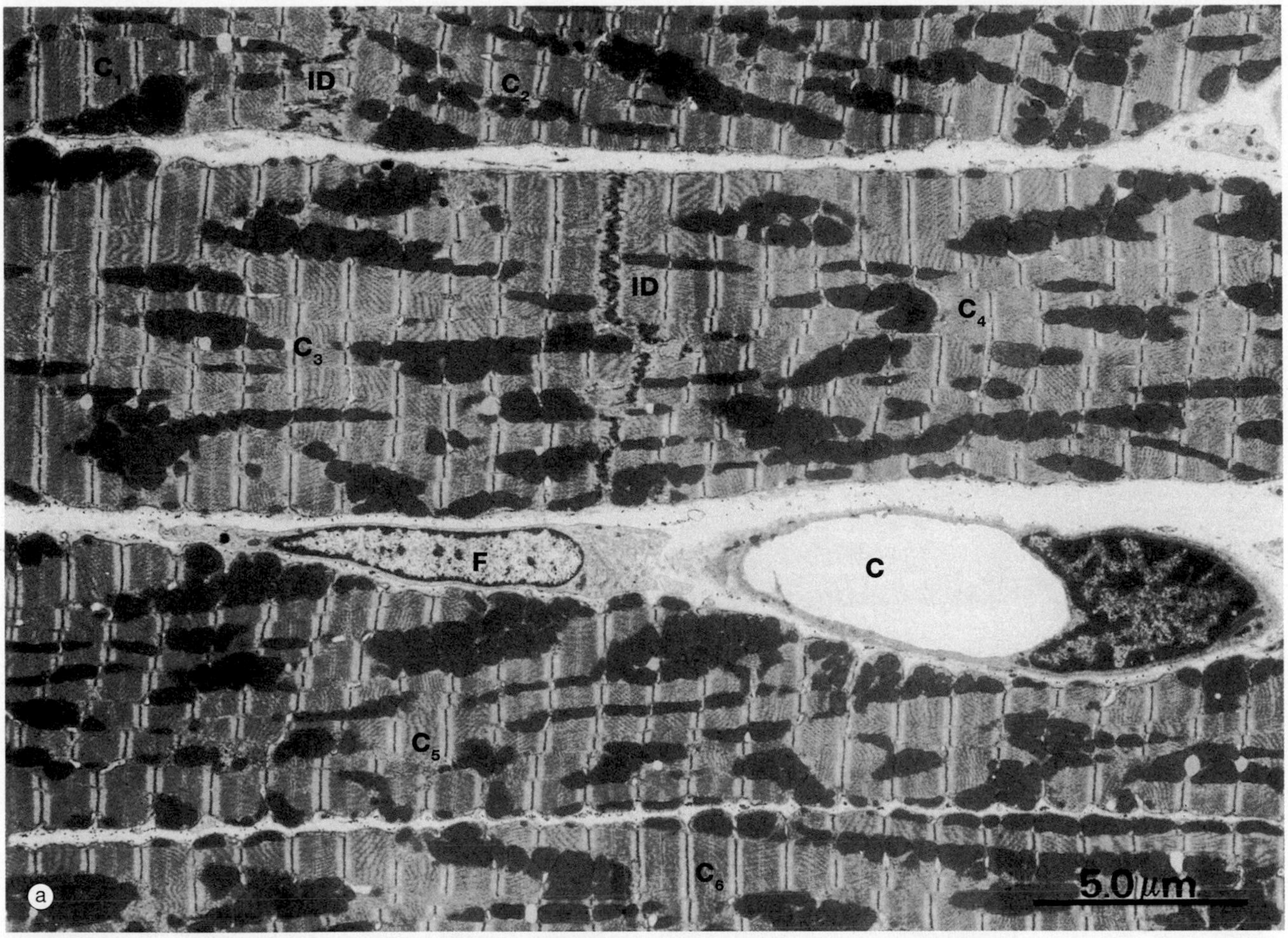

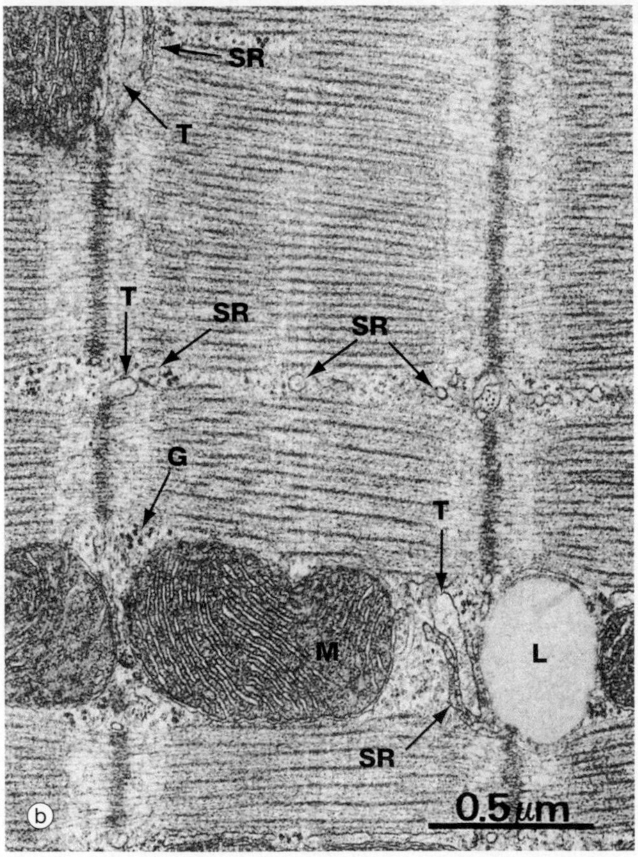

FIG. 6.25 Cardiac muscle
(a) EM ×5000 (b) EM ×38 000

Fig. 6.25a illustrates portions of six cardiac muscle cells labelled **C_1** to **C_6**. None of their nuclei is included in the plane of section. Cells **C_1** and **C_2** abut one another end to end and are demarcated by an intercalated disc **ID**. Cells **C_3** and **C_4** are demarcated similarly. The intercellular space contains a capillary **C** and a fibroblast **F**.

The sarcomeres of cardiac muscle have an identical banding pattern to that of skeletal muscle. The sarcomeres are not, however, arranged into single columns making up cylindrical myofibrils as in skeletal muscle, but form a branching myofibrillar network, continuous in three dimensions throughout the cytoplasm. The branching columns of sarcomeres are separated by sarcoplasm containing rows of mitochondria and sarcoplasmic reticulum. The great abundance of mitochondria in cardiac muscle reflects the enormous metabolic demands of continuous cardiac muscle activity.

Conduction of excitatory stimuli to the sarcomeres of cardiac muscle is mediated by a system of T tubules and sarcoplasmic reticulum, essentially similar in arrangement to that of skeletal muscle. The T tubules, however, ramify throughout the cardiac muscle cytoplasm at the Z lines, and their origins are seen as indentations in the sarcolemma, which thus has a somewhat scalloped outline.

The conducting system of the cardiac myocyte can be seen at high magnification in Fig. 6.25b. T tubules **T** and sarcoplasmic reticulum **SR** form poorly defined triads compared with those of skeletal muscle. Note the typical closely packed cristae of the mitochondria **M**, a lipid droplet **L** and glycogen granules **G**.

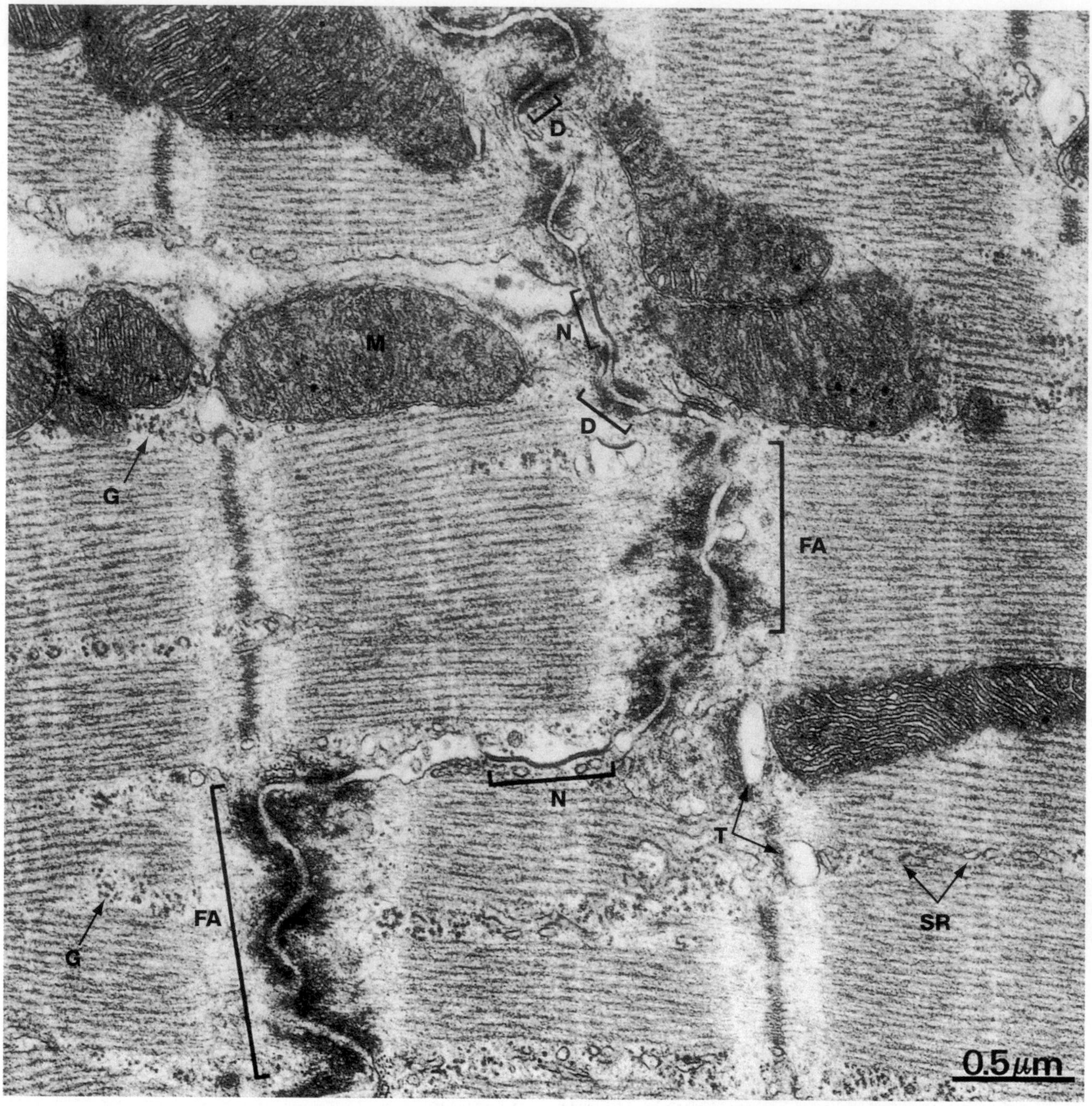

FIG. 6.26 Cardiac muscle, intercalated disc, LS
EM ×31 000

Intercalated discs are specialised transverse junctions between cardiac muscle cells at sites where they meet end to end; they always coincide with the Z lines. Intercalated discs bind the cells, transmit forces of contraction and provide areas of low electrical resistance for the rapid spread of excitation throughout the myocardium.

The intercalated disc is an interdigitating junction and consists of three types of membrane-to-membrane contact. The predominant type of contact, the ***fascia adherens*** **FA**, resembles the ***zonula adherens*** of epithelial junctional complexes (see Fig. 5.11) but is more extensive and less regular. The actin filaments at the ends of terminal sarcomeres insert into the fasciae adherentes and thereby transmit contractile forces from cell to cell. ***Desmosomes*** **D** occur less frequently and provide anchorage for intermediate filaments of the cytoskeleton. ***Gap (nexus) junctions*** **N** (see Fig. 5.12) are present mainly in the longitudinal portions of the interdigitations and are sites of low electrical resistance through which excitation passes from cell to cell.

Note the similarity of the sarcomeres of cardiac and skeletal muscle (see Fig. 6.9). The mitochondria **M** are elongated or spheroidal and have abundant closely packed cristae rich in oxidative enzyme systems. The sarcoplasm within and between the sarcomeres is rich in glycogen granules **G**. Lace-like profiles of sarcoplasmic reticulum **SR** and parts of T tubules **T** can be identified.

D desmosome **E** endothelium of capillary **EL** external lamina **F** fibroblast **FA** fascia adherens **G** glycogen granules **ID** intercalated disc **L** leukocyte **M** mitochondrion **N** nexus junction **S** sarcomere filaments **SR** sarcoplasmic reticulum **T** T tubule

Diseases affecting the heart muscle

Heart disease is an important cause of morbidity and mortality worldwide. Its causes vary dramatically across different geographical areas and, in some parts of the world, conditions such as poor nutrition and infections result in serious cardiac disease. In the developed world, ***coronary artery atheroma*** is the root cause of the vast majority of cardiac pathology, including disorders such as ***angina pectoris*** (crushing chest pain due to ischaemia of the heart muscle), ***arrhythmias*** (see textbox 'The conducting system of the heart') and ***cardiac failure***.

Cardiac failure occurs when the muscle of the heart is unable to pump effectively and cannot deliver enough blood supply to meet the body's metabolic needs. This results in a diverse range of symptoms because of the effects on many other organs of the body, particularly the lungs. Symptoms include fatigue, breathlessness (fluid can build up in the lungs due to back pressure caused by ineffective emptying of blood from the heart) and peripheral oedema (swelling of the tissues occurs because of accumulation of tissue fluid in the interstitial space due to back pressure in the venous system). Treatment options are very diverse but aim to relieve these symptoms, as well as attempting to manage the underlying cause of cardiac failure.

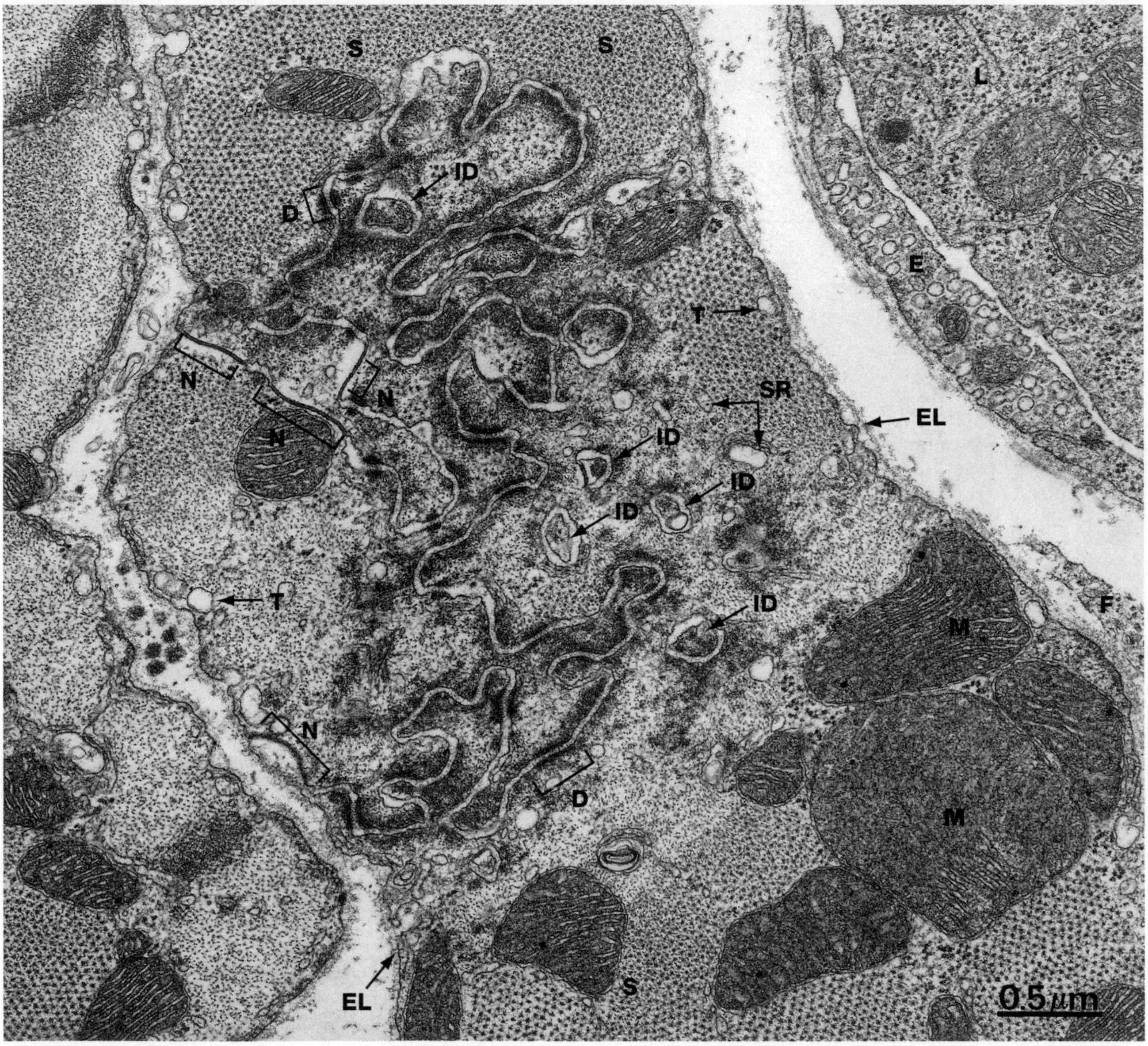

FIG. 6.27 Cardiac muscle, intercalated disc, TS EM ×27 000

The end-to-end junction between cardiac muscle cells is not simply a flat surface. In reality, each junction is a highly convoluted set of finger-like interdigitations, maximising the surface area in contact between each cell.

This rich structure can be appreciated in Fig. 6.27 which shows a transverse section through cardiac muscle in the vicinity of a Z line incorporating an intercalated disc. The tortuous course of the intercellular junction as well as islands of apparently isolated paired cell membranes **ID** reflect the manner in which the ends of the cardiac muscle cells interdigitate with one another. Most of the intercellular junction comprises fasciae adherentes with interspersed desmosomes **D** and some nexus junctions **N**.

The regular dot-like lattice represents the contractile proteins of the sarcomeres **S**, with the thick filaments surrounded by thin filaments cut in transverse section. Mitochondria **M** are prominent.

Beneath the cell membrane are dilated tubules **T** representing part of the T tubule system. Elements of the sarcoplasmic reticulum **SR** can be seen surrounding the sarcomeres. Beyond the plasma membrane lies the external lamina **EL**. A fibroblast cytoplasmic extension **F** is present in the extracellular space at the right of the field. At the upper right is an endomysial capillary, its endothelium **E** containing numerous pinocytotic vesicles. The lumen contains a leukocyte **L**.

REVIEW

TABLE 6.1 Review of muscle

Muscle type	Key features	Functional attributes	Figure
Skeletal muscle	Large cells with multiple peripherally located nuclei Arranged in fascicles Three supporting layers – endomysium, perimysium and epimysium	Myofibrils organised into cross-striations Sliding filament mechanism of contraction Excitation–contraction coupling	6.1–6.14, 6.28a 6.28b 6.28c
Smooth muscle	Small fusiform-shaped cells Single cigar-shaped nucleus	Involuntary, autonomic innervation No striations, myofibril meshwork anchored to dense bodies Cells shorten and broaden on contraction	6.15–6.20 6.28d 6.28e 6.28f
Cardiac muscle	Elongated branching cells joined by intercalated discs Single central nuclei	Involuntary contraction, autonomic innervation and spontaneous contraction Branching, interconnected cells act as a functional syncytium Cross-striations due to organisation of myofibrils Sliding filament mechanism of contraction	6.21–6.27 6.28g 6.28h 6.28i

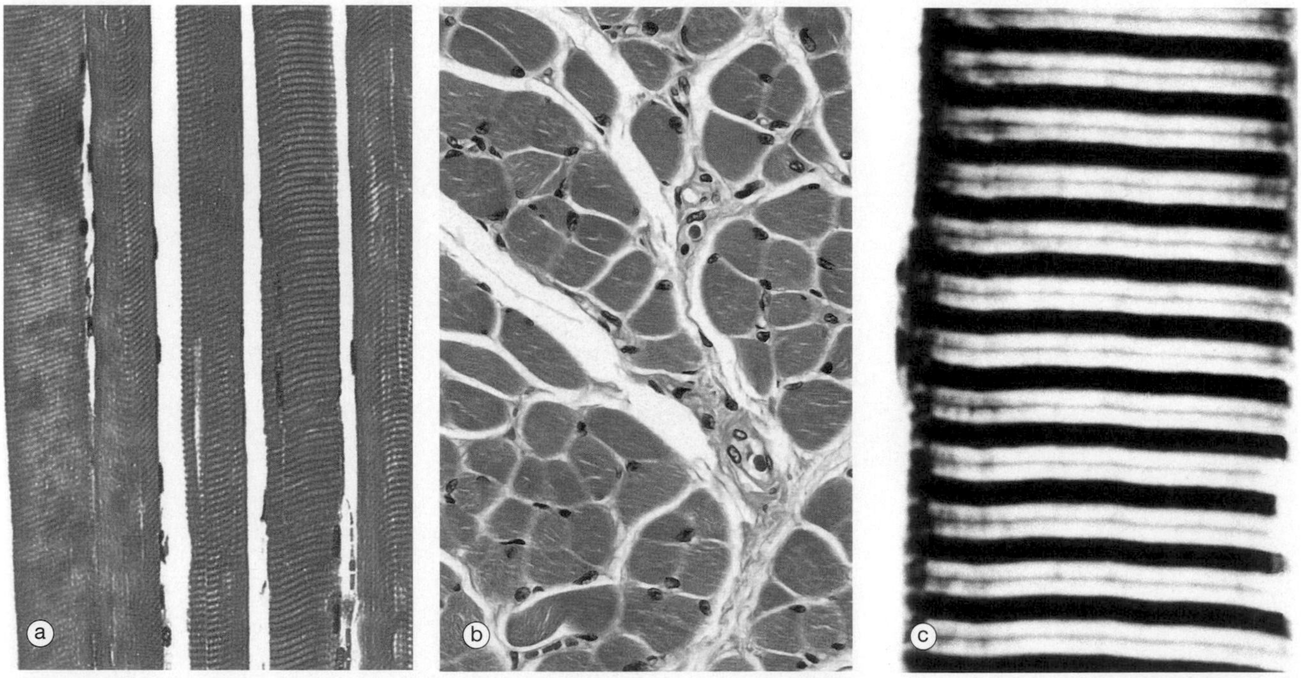

FIG. 6.28 Examples of skeletal, smooth, and cardiac muscle *(illustrations (d) to (i) opposite)*
(a) Skeletal muscle, LS, H&E (HP) (b) Skeletal muscle, TS, H&E (HP) (c) Skeletal muscle, LS, Heidenhain's haematoxylin (HP) (d) Smooth muscle, LS, H&E (HP) (e) Smooth muscle, TS, H&E (HP) (f) Smooth muscle, Masson trichrome (HP) (g) Cardiac muscle, LS, H&E (MP) (h) Cardiac muscle, TS, H&E (HP) (i) Cardiac muscle, EM ×5000

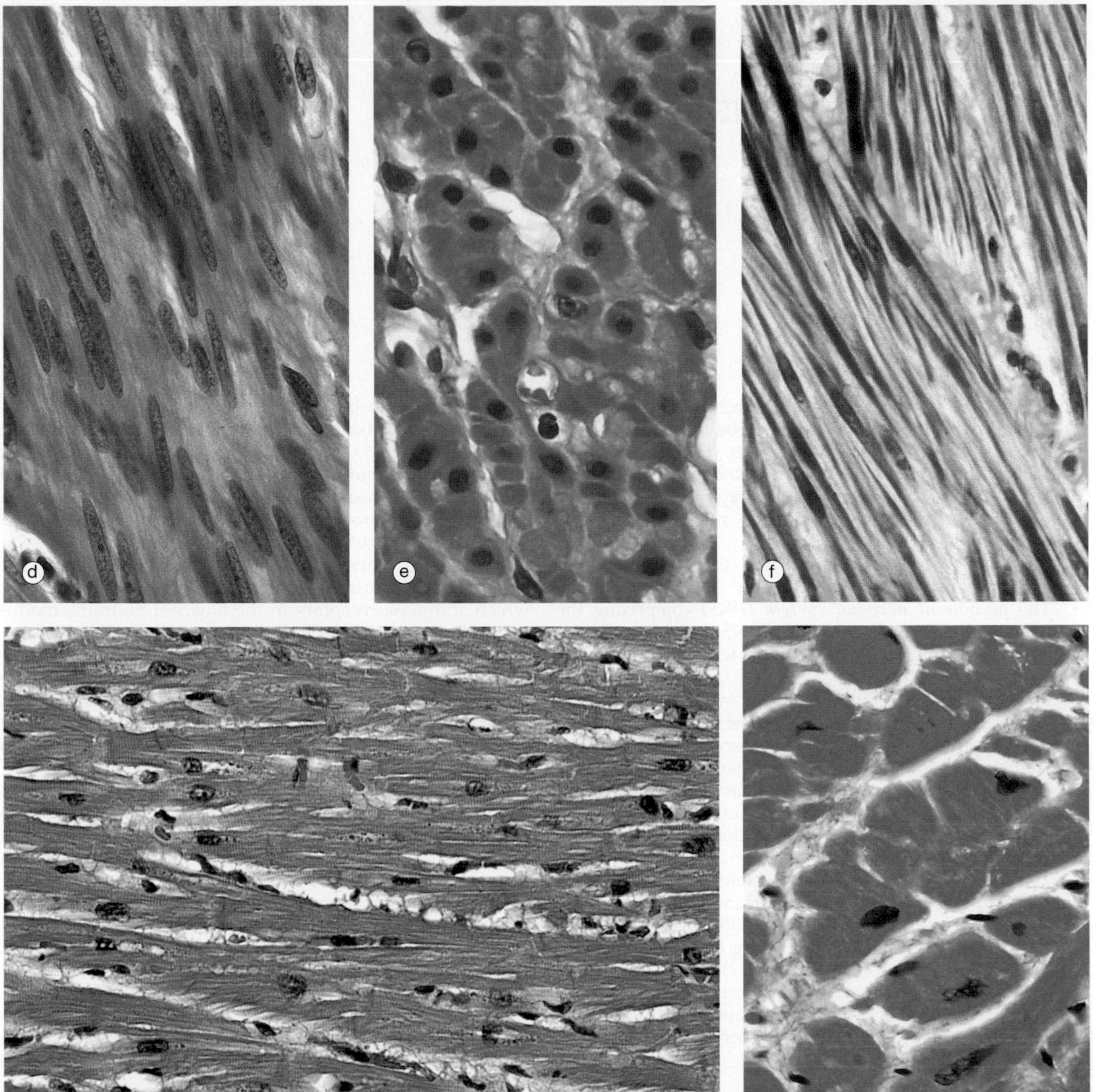

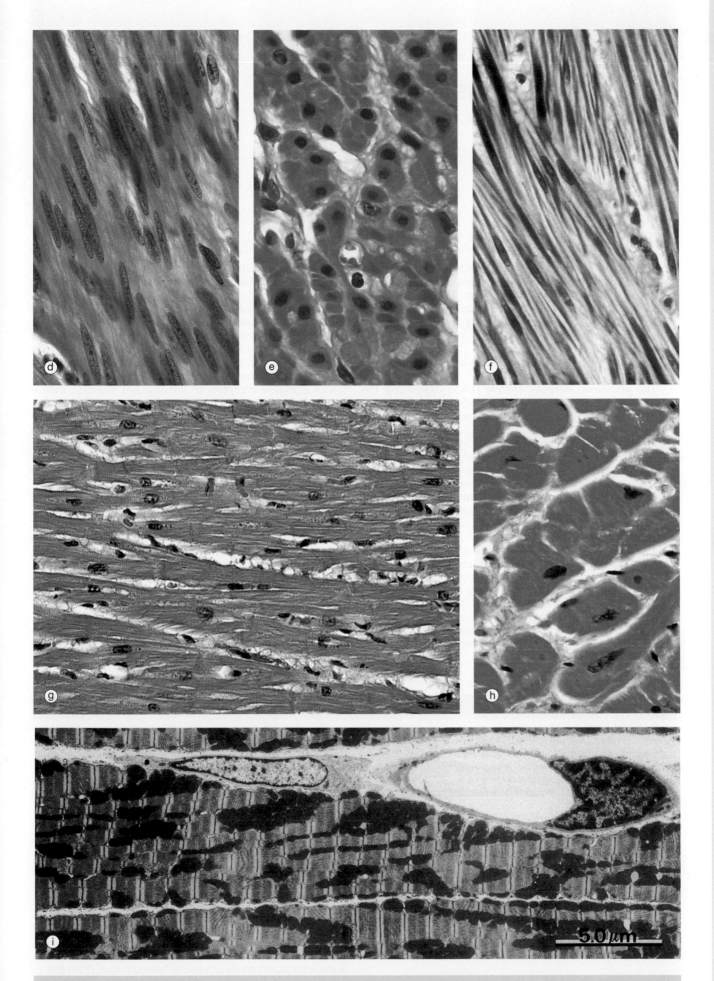

FIG. 6.28 Examples of skeletal, smooth, and cardiac muscle *(illustrations (a) to (c) opposite)*
(a) Skeletal muscle, LS, H&E (HP) (b) Skeletal muscle, TS, H&E (HP) (c) Skeletal muscle, LS, Heidenhain's haematoxylin (HP) (d) Smooth muscle, LS, H&E (HP) (e) Smooth muscle, TS, H&E (HP) (f) Smooth muscle, Masson trichrome (HP) (g) Cardiac muscle, LS, H&E (MP) (h) Cardiac muscle, TS, H&E (HP) (i) Cardiac muscle, EM ×5000

7 Nervous tissues

INTRODUCTION

The nervous system provides rapid and precise communication between different parts of the body via the action of specialised nerve cells called ***neurones***. These highly specialised cells are interconnected and function to gather and process information and then generate appropriate response signals. The nervous system is divided into two main parts:

- The ***central nervous system (CNS)*** comprising the brain and spinal cord
- The ***peripheral nervous system (PNS)*** comprising the nerves which run between the CNS and other tissues, together with nerve 'relay stations' termed ***ganglia***

Histologically, the entire nervous system merely consists of variations in the arrangement of neurones and their supporting tissues. Functionally, the nervous system can be divided into the ***somatic nervous system***, which is involved in voluntary functions, and the ***autonomic nervous system*** which exerts control over many involuntary functions. The autonomic system can be further divided into ***sympathetic*** and ***parasympathetic systems***.

The functions of the nervous system depend on a fundamental property of neurones called ***excitability***. As in all cells, the resting neurone maintains an ionic gradient across its plasma membrane, thereby creating an electrical potential. Excitability involves transiently changing the membrane permeability in response to appropriate stimuli so that the ionic gradient is partially reversed and the plasma membrane loses its electrical potential (i.e. becomes ***depolarised***). Depolarisation itself simulates adjacent plasma membrane to depolarise, causing a wave of depolarisation called an ***action potential*** to spread along the plasma membrane. This is followed by rapid repolarisation in which the membrane re-establishes its resting potential.

At sites of intercommunication between neurones called ***synapses***, transfer of the action potential (the message) is via chemicals. Depolarisation of the neurone causes the release of chemical transmitter substances, ***neurotransmitters***, which stimulate receptors in the adjacent neurone, modulating the potential for or triggering an action potential. Neurones are arranged in pathways, often with many interconnecting neurones, for the conduction of action potentials from receptors to effector (acting) organs. Neurotransmitters serve not only to mediate neurone-to-neurone transmission but also act as chemical signals from neurones to receptors on the effector organs which also exhibit excitability.

The effector organs of the voluntary somatic pathways are generally skeletal muscle causing movement, while those of involuntary pathways are usually smooth muscle, cardiac muscle and muscle-like epithelial cells (myoepithelial cells) within exocrine glands.

This chapter encompasses nerve cells and their supporting cells, focused on the histological structure of the peripheral nervous system and simple types of sensory receptors. Details of the supporting cells and arrangement of nervous tissue in the central nervous system are the subject of Ch. 20, while the structure of the highly specialised organs of sensory reception, eyes and ears, is presented in Ch. 21.

Diseases of the nervous system

Infections
Infections of the CNS are caused by bacterial, viral or fungal organisms and result in inflammation of the brain. Infection can affect the meninges (meningitis), the spinal cord (myelitis) or the brain substance (encephalitis) and can be life threatening. Infection occurs most commonly as a result of haematogenous spread (spread from the blood stream).

Epilepsy
The regulation of neuronal excitability within the brain may become abnormal, leading to an uncontrolled spread of depolarisation, termed an epileptic seizure.

Neurodegenerative diseases
These are a group of diseases mainly seen in old age and characterised by progressive degeneration and death of nerve cells, often limited to specific neuronal systems; Alzheimer's disease (e-Fig. 7.1), motor neurone disease and Parkinson's disease (e-Fig. 7.2) fall in this group.

Demyelinating diseases
The transmission of signals in the nervous system is largely by way of long nerve cell processes which are insulated by cells making a substance called ***myelin***. These specialised myelin-forming cells (Schwann cells) can be the target of specific diseases, leading to loss of function of effective signalling between nerve cells. Multiple sclerosis is the main disease in this group (e-Fig. 7.3).

Cerebral infarction (stroke)
The vascular supply to the brain is vital in maintaining its function. Cerebral infarction (stroke) is one of the major causes of morbidity and death in affluent societies (e-Fig. 7.4). The majority of strokes are due to cerebral artery atheroma, thrombosis or embolism resulting in irreversible ischaemic damage to neurones. Haemorrhagic stroke can also occur as a result of bleeding of small intracerebral vessels or reperfusion following reversal of a blockage (thrombosis).

Intracranial haemorrhage
This can occur as a result of bleeding within the brain itself (intracerebral haemorrhage) or from vessels outside the brain (subarachnoid, extradural or subdural haemorrhage). Often this is due to the effects of trauma or, in subarachnoid haemorrhage, is due to rupture of a cerebral artery aneurysm (a weakness in the vessel wall causing a bulge which may rupture).

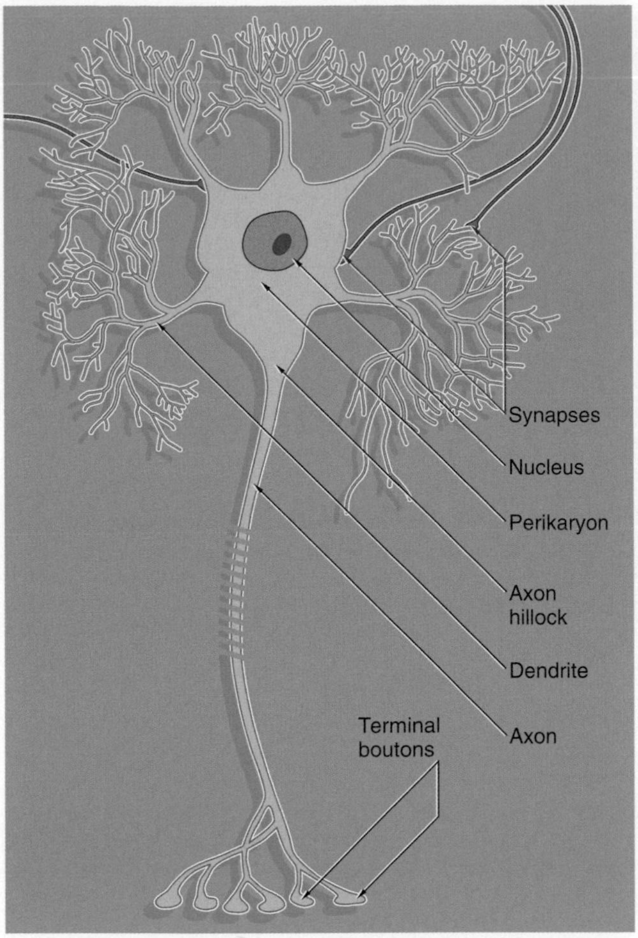

FIG. 7.1 The neurone

Despite great variation in size and shape in different parts of the nervous system, all neurones have the same basic structure as shown in Fig. 7.1. The neurone consists of a large cell body containing the nucleus surrounded by cytoplasm known as the ***perikaryon***. Processes of two types extend from the cell body, namely a single ***axon*** and one or more ***dendrites***. Dendrites are highly branched tapering processes which either end in specialised sensory receptors (as in primary sensory neurones) or form synapses with neighbouring neurones from which they receive stimuli. In general, dendrites function as the major sites of information input into the neurone.

Each neurone has a single axon arising from a cone-shaped portion of the cell body called the ***axon hillock***. The axon is a cylindrical process up to 1 metre in length, terminating on other neurones or effector organs by way of a variable number of small branches which end in small swellings called ***terminal boutons***. Action potentials arise in the cell body as a result of integration of afferent (incoming) stimuli; action potentials are then conducted along the axon to influence other neurones or effector organs by release of ***neurotransmitter*** chemicals. Axons are commonly referred to as ***nerve fibres***.

In general, the cell bodies of all neurones are located in the central nervous system; exceptions are the cell bodies of most primary sensory neurones and the terminal effector neurones of the autonomic nervous system where, in both cases, the cell bodies lie in aggregations called ***ganglia*** in peripheral sites.

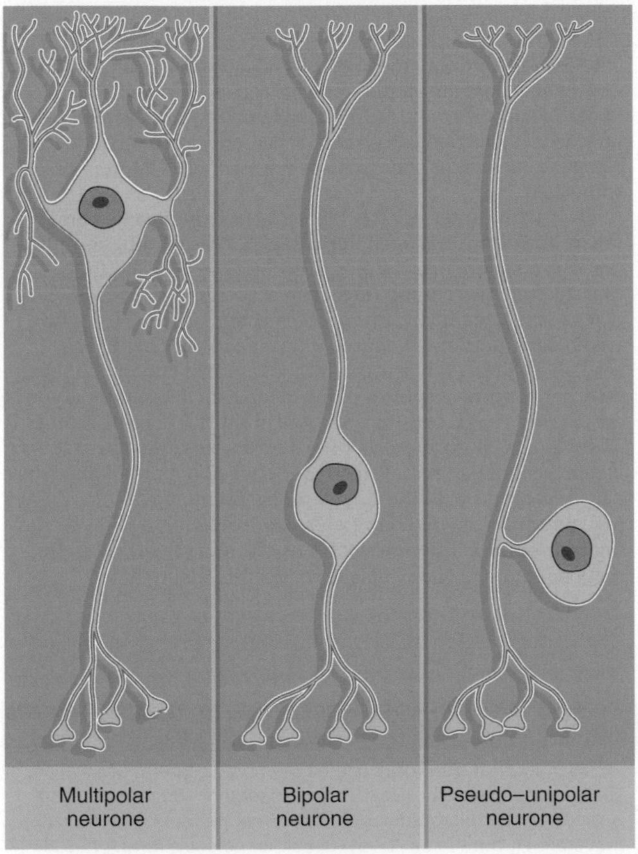

FIG. 7.2 Basic neurone types

Throughout the nervous system, neurones have a wide variety of shapes which fall into three main patterns according to the arrangement of the axon and dendrites with respect to the cell body. These are illustrated in Fig. 7.2.

The most common form is the ***multipolar neurone*** in which numerous dendrites project from the cell body; the dendrites may all arise from one pole of the cell body or may extend from all areas of the cell body surface. In general, intermediate, integratory and motor neurones conform to this pattern.

Bipolar neurones have only a single dendrite which arises from the pole of the cell body opposite to the origin of the axon. These unusual neurones act as receptor neurones for the senses of smell, sight and balance. Most other primary sensory neurones are described as ***pseudo-unipolar*** neurones, since a single dendrite and the axon arise from a common stem of the cell body; this stem is formed by the fusion of the first part of the dendrite and axon of a bipolar type of neurone during embryological development.

As a general rule, neurone impulses are conveyed along dendrites towards the nerve cell body (*afferent*) while axons usually convey impulses away from the nerve cell body (*efferent*).

Origin and regeneration of nerve cells

Neurones are derived in embryogenesis from ***primitive neuroblasts***. Neurones are terminally differentiated cells that, for all practical purposes, do not regenerate in the event of cell death. Studies have shown cell division in neurones in the adult brain, although the biological significance of this remains uncertain. However, regeneration of axons and dendrites can occur in the event of damage, provided the neurone cell body remains viable. This is the basis of nerve grafting used to treat peripheral nerve injuries.

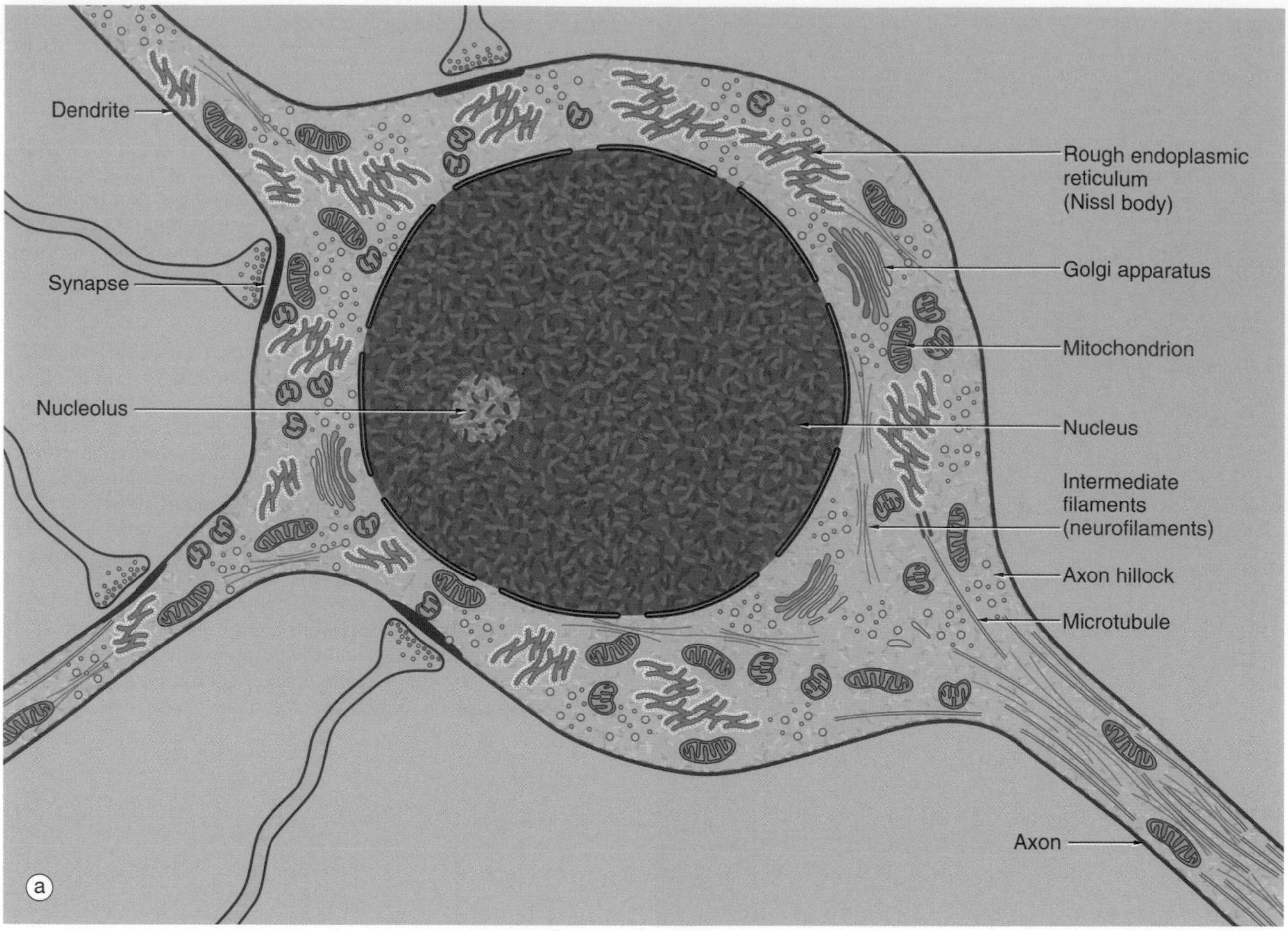

FIG. 7.3 Ultrastructure of the neurone *(illustration (b) opposite)*
(a) Schematic diagram (b) EM ×19 000

Fig. 7.3a illustrates the main ultrastructural features of the neurone, in this case a multipolar neurone with an axon and two dendrites. The nucleus is large, round or ovoid and usually centrally located within the perikaryon. Reflecting the intense metabolic activity of the neurone (and consequent need to replace proteins which are rapidly turned over), the chromatin is completely dispersed and the nucleolus is a conspicuous feature.

The cytoplasm of the cell body contains large aggregations of rough endoplasmic reticulum which correspond to the ***Nissl substance*** of light microscopy (see Fig. 7.4); the rough endoplasmic reticulum extends into the dendrites but not into the axon hillock or axon. Rough endoplasmic reticulum is a much more prominent feature in large neurones, such as somatic motor neurones, than in smaller neurones such as those of the autonomic nervous system. A diffuse Golgi apparatus is found adjacent to the nucleus. Smooth endoplasmic reticulum is not a prominent feature of the perikaryon, but tubules, cisternae and vesicles are prominent in the axon and dendrites. The mitochondria of the perikaryon are numerous and have the usual rod-like appearances; those of the axon are extremely slender and elongated.

Neurones are very metabolically active and expend much energy in maintaining ionic gradients across the plasma membrane. Neurones synthesise neurotransmitter substances or their precursors in the perikaryon from where they are transported along the axon to the synapse to be released when appropriately stimulated.

Numerous intermediate filaments (***neurofilaments***) and microtubules are arranged in parallel bundles throughout the perikaryon and along the length of the axon and dendrites. The electron micrograph (Fig. 7.3b) shows part of the cell body of a neurone and includes a portion of the nucleus **N**. At the lower right, part of the neuronal plasma membrane **PM**, is seen, including a synapse **S** with the terminal bouton **TB** of an adjacent neurone. Features of the cytoplasm of the perikaryon are areas of rough endoplasmic reticulum **rER**, free ribosomes **R** and scattered mitochondria **M**. An extensive Golgi apparatus **G** is represented by several stacks of flattened membranous cisternae. Associated with the Golgi are several multivesicular bodies **MB**, which are involved in transport to other organelles including lysosomes **L**. Microtubules **T** can be identified in oblique section, but neurofilaments are not readily identifiable.

The cytoskeleton of the neurone is vital for axonal transport

The cytoskeleton of neurones is highly organised.

Neurofilaments, the intermediate filaments of nerve cells, act as a scaffold to maintain the shape of the axon and cell body.

There is a highly organised network of microtubules which transport material up and down the axon. ***Slow axonal transport*** carries cytoskeletal elements.

Fast axonal transport carries membrane-bound organelles, such as neurosecretory vesicles, at speeds of 400 mm/day and is mediated by microtubular transport mechanisms. Anterograde movement (from the cell body) uses the molecule ***kinesin*** as a molecular motor, while retrograde movement (to the cell body) uses the molecule ***dynein***.

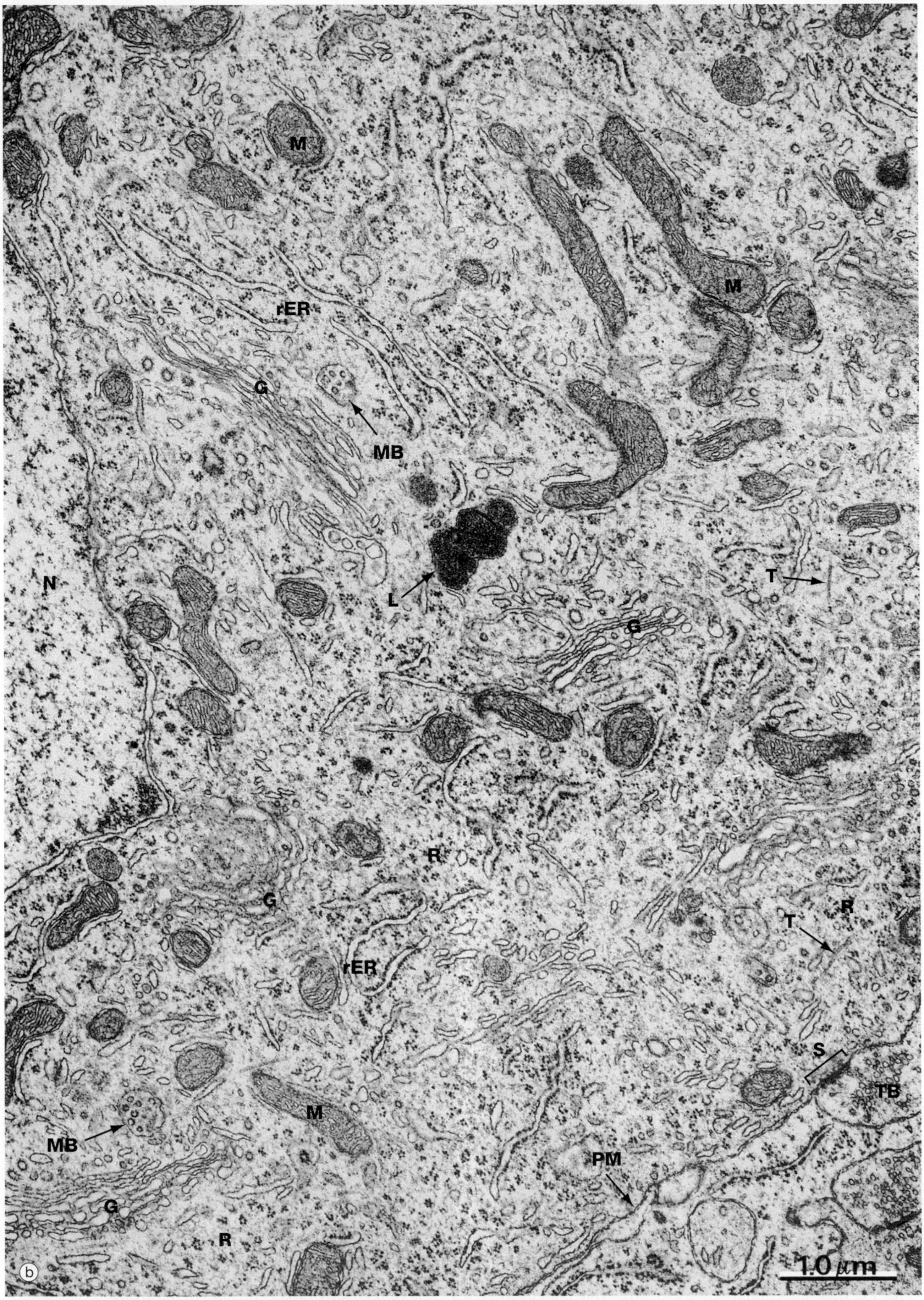

FIG. 7.3 Ultrastructure of the neurone *(caption and illustration (a) opposite)*
(a) Schematic diagram (b) EM ×19 000

G Golgi apparatus **L** lysosome **M** mitochondrion **MB** multivesicular body **N** nucleus **PM** plasma membrane
R free ribosomes **rER** rough endoplasmic reticulum **S** synapse **T** microtubules **TB** terminal bouton

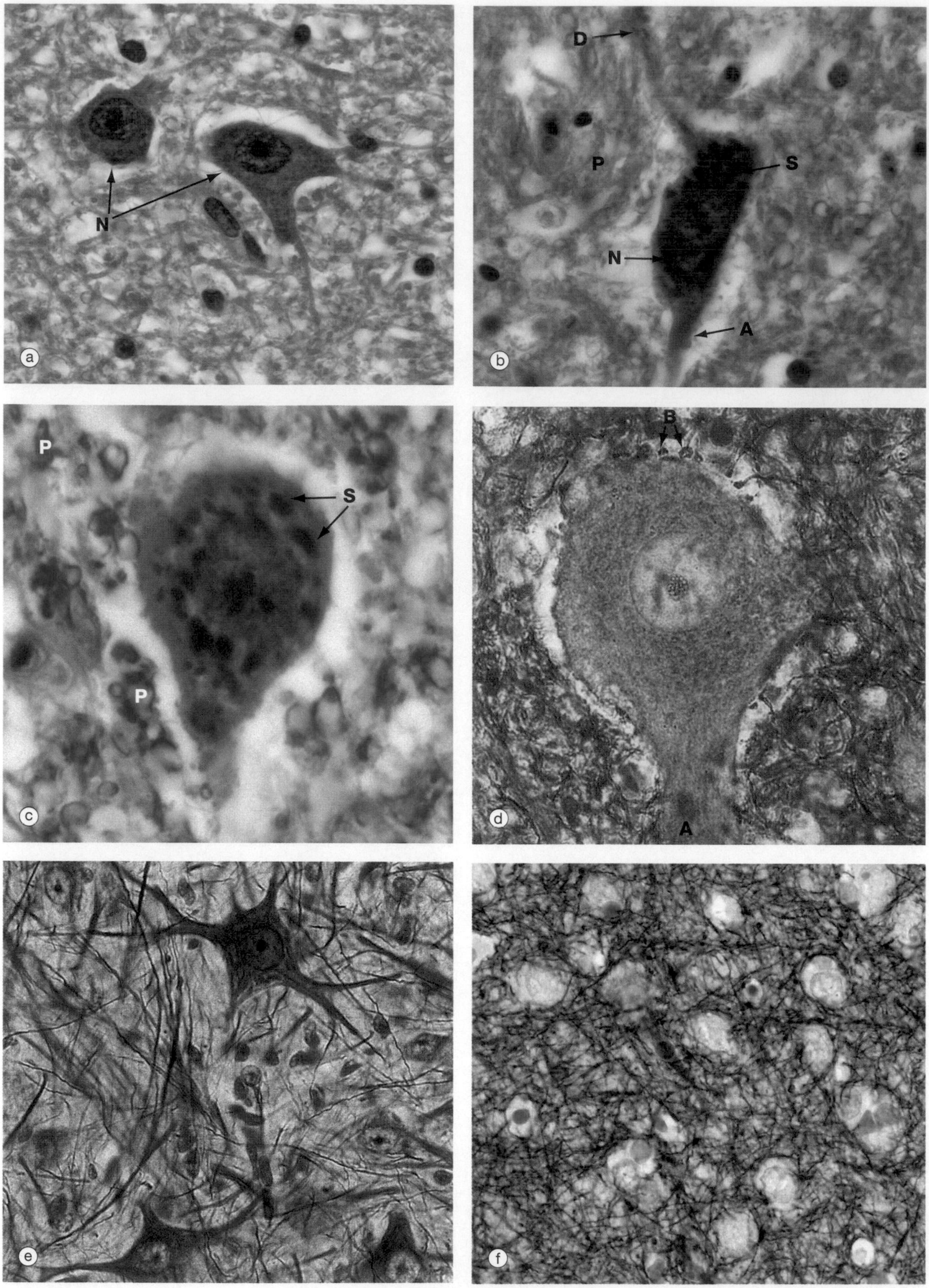

FIG. 7.4 **Neurones and methods of study with light microscopy** ***(caption and illustrations (g) and (h) opposite)***
(a, b) H&E (HP) (c) Luxol fast blue, H&E (HP) (d) Gold method (HP) (e) Gold/toluidine blue (HP) (f) Immunohistochemistry for neurofilament protein (HP) (g) Spread preparation, gold method (MP) (h) Golgi–Cox (HP)

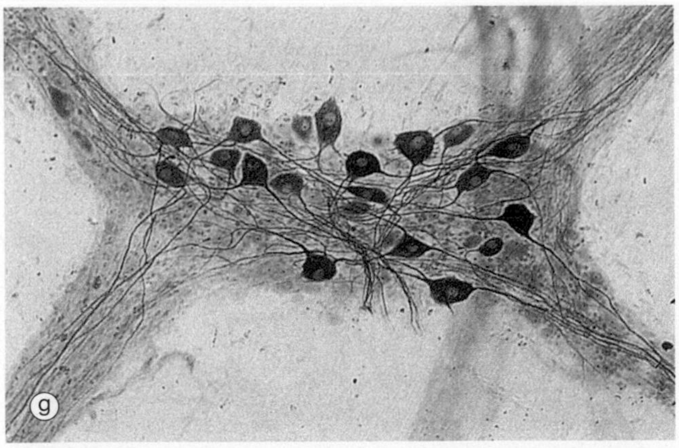

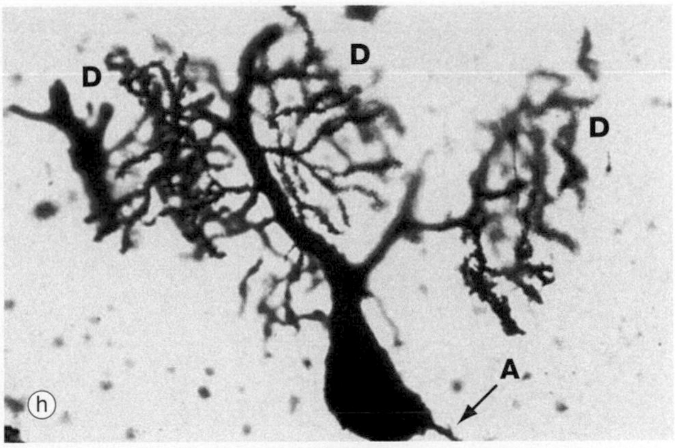

FIG. 7.4 Neurones and methods of study with light microscopy *(illustrations (a) to (f) opposite)*
(a, b) H&E (HP) (c) Luxol fast blue, H&E (HP) (d) Gold method (HP) (e) Gold/toluidine blue (HP) (f) Immunohistochemistry for neurofilament protein (HP) (g) Spread preparation, gold method (MP) (h) Golgi–Cox (HP)

Special staining techniques are required to show the rich structural detail of the nervous system. ***Heavy metal impregnation techniques*** with gold and silver are valuable in the study of neurone morphology and were widely employed by the pioneers of neuroanatomy such as Cajal and Golgi, from whom they take their names. Likewise, ***spread preparations*** often permit the examination of complete neurones and their cytoplasmic processes. ***Immunohistochemistry*** can also be used to identify neurone-specific proteins (e.g. neurofilament protein).

Figs 7.4a and b, stained with H&E, show neurones **N** in the central nervous system; the nuclei are huge in comparison with those of surrounding support cells. Dispersed chromatin and prominent nucleoli reflect a high level of protein synthesis. Neurones have extensive cytoplasm which is basophilic (blue stained) due to extensive ribosomal RNA. Many of the ribosomes are associated with rough endoplasmic reticulum, found gathered in patches called ***Nissl substance*** **S**, which extends into dendrites **D** but not the axon **A**. In H&E preparations, virtually no detail can be seen of cytoplasmic processes, which merge into a fibrillary background termed the ***neuropil*** **P** composed of both nerve cell and support cell processes.

In Fig. 7.4c, the Nissl substance is seen as dark purple material giving the neuronal cytoplasm a mottled appearance. Here the myelin (see below) is stained blue, demonstrating the structure of the neuropil **P**. A very similar neurone is shown in Fig. 7.4d using a heavy metal impregnation technique that highlights small axons. Numerous axons from other neurones with tiny ***terminal boutons*** **B** can be seen forming synapses with the cell body.

Fig. 7.4e employs another gold method providing excellent detail of neuronal shape and showing the cytoskeleton in the dendrites and axons; the blue counter-stain demonstrates the nuclei of surrounding support cells. Note that detail in the neuronal processes is lost as they pass out of the plane of focus.

Fig. 7.4f shows an area of the brain stained with an antibody to neurofilament protein. This highlights the complex network of axons within the neuropil between neurones. Neurones are seen as clear spaces containing a nucleus in this preparation.

Spread preparations, as shown in Fig. 7.4g, also outline the complexity of nerve cell processes, both axons and dendrites. Here, neurones in a small peripheral ganglion and their main cytoplasmic processes are clearly delineated.

Fig. 7.4h illustrates a very thick section stained by a silver impregnation method and shows a Purkinje cell in the cerebellar cortex. These cells have a single small axon **A** at one pole and an extraordinary finely branching dendritic tree **D** at the other pole. Note that the base of the dendritic system is in this case much larger than that of the axon.

Neuronal response to injury

Neurones are less robust than other cells in the CNS such as astrocytes or microglia. As a result, they are vulnerable to environmental changes such as hypoxia. This is known as **selective vulnerability** and leads to neuronal injury and death. Healing in the brain following injury occurs as a result of gliosis as the usual granulation tissue and fibrous scarring that occurs in other tissues in the body is uncommon in the CNS (e-Fig. 7.5).

MYELINATED AND NON-MYELINATED NERVE FIBRES

In the peripheral nervous system, all axons are enveloped by highly specialised cells called ***Schwann cells***, which provide structural and metabolic support. In general, small-diameter axons (e.g. those of the autonomic nervous system and small pain fibres) are simply enveloped by the cytoplasm of Schwann cells; these nerve fibres are said to be ***non-myelinated***. Large-diameter fibres are wrapped by a variable number of concentric layers of the Schwann cell plasma membrane forming a ***myelin sheath***; such nerve fibres are said to be ***myelinated***. Within the central nervous system, myelination is similar to that in the peripheral nervous system except that the myelin sheaths are formed by cells called ***oligodendrocytes*** (see Fig. 20.3). There are distinct chemical differences between central and peripheral myelin. In all nerve fibres, the rate of conduction of action potentials is proportional to the diameter of the axon; however, myelination greatly increases axon conduction velocity compared with that of a non-myelinated fibre of the same diameter.

A axon **B** terminal bouton (synapse) **D** dendrite **N** neurone **P** neuropil **S** Nissl substance

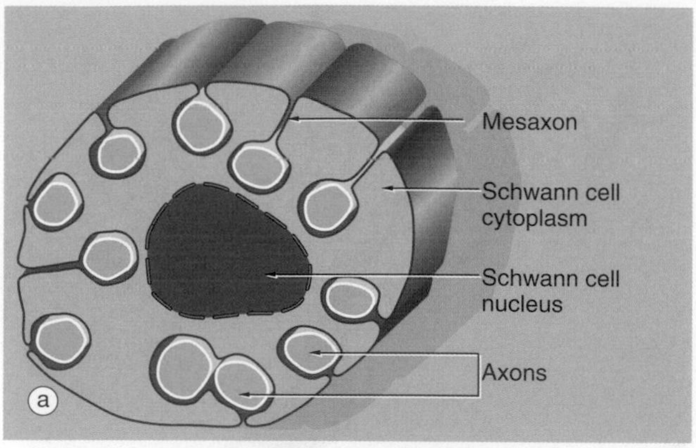

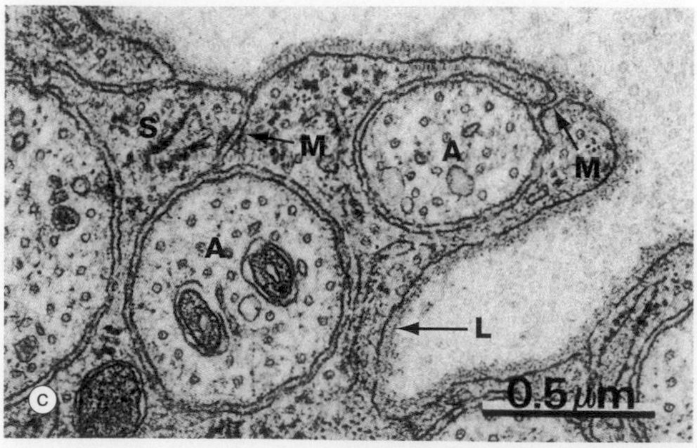

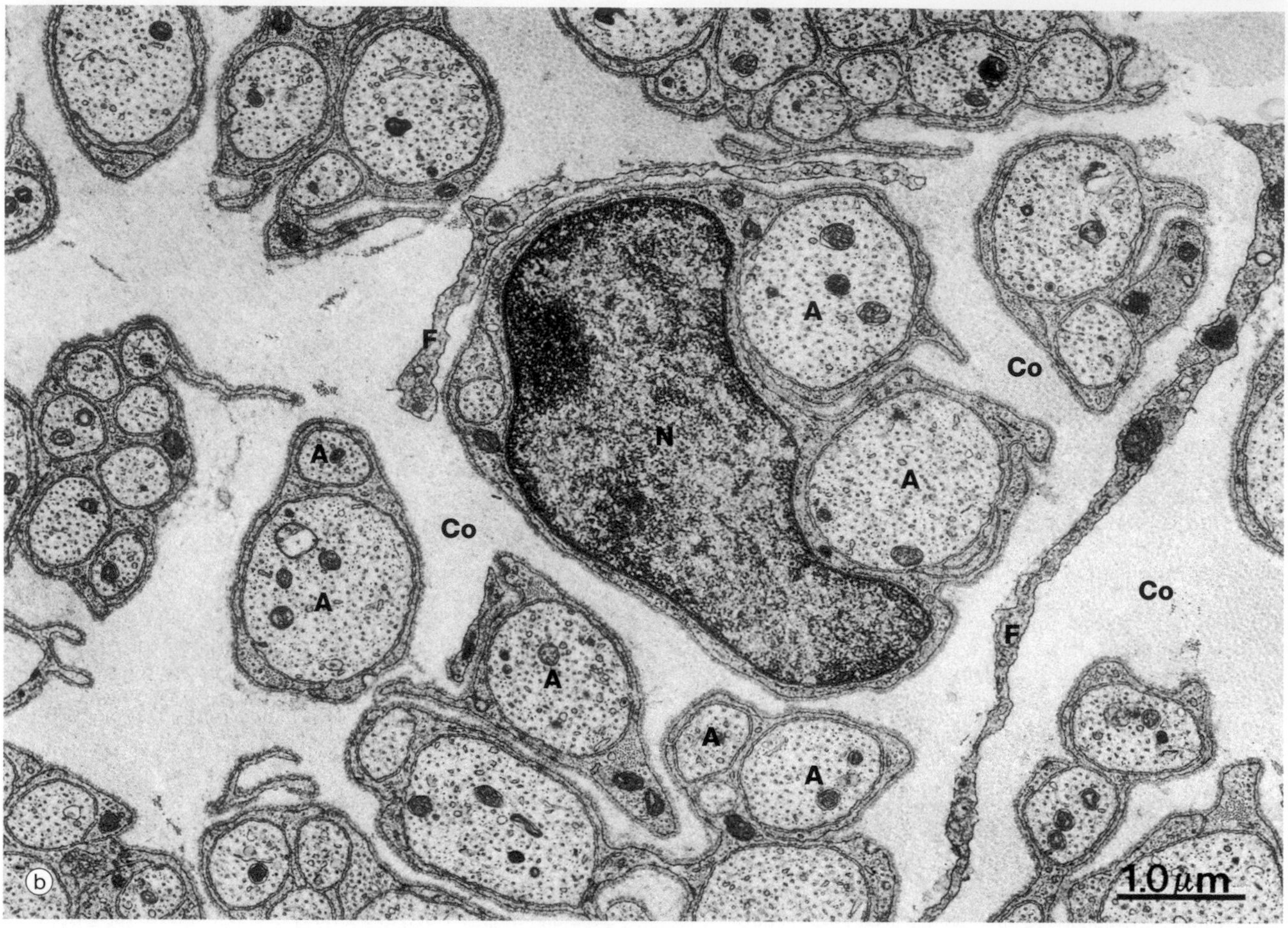

FIG. 7.5 Non-myelinated nerve fibres
(a) Diagram (b) EM ×15 000 (c) EM ×36 000

The relationship of non-myelinated axons with their supporting Schwann cell is illustrated in Fig. 7.5a. One or more axons become longitudinally invaginated into the Schwann cell so that each axon is embedded in a channel, invested by the Schwann cell plasma membrane and cytoplasm. The Schwann cell plasma membrane becomes apposed to itself along the opening of the channel, thus effectively sealing the axon within an extracellular compartment bounded by the Schwann cell.

The zone of apposition of the Schwann cell membrane is called the ***mesaxon***. Note that more than one axon may occupy a single channel within the Schwann cell. Each Schwann cell extends for only a short distance along the nerve tract, and at its termination the ensheathment is continued by another Schwann cell with which it interdigitates closely end to end.

At low magnification in Fig. 7.5b, non-myelinated axons **A** of various sizes are seen ensheathed by Schwann cells **S**; one of the Schwann cells has been sectioned transversely through its nucleus **N**. Note the variable number of axons enclosed by each Schwann cell. Delicate cytoplasmic extensions of fibroblasts **F** and collagen fibrils **Co** cut in cross-section can be seen in the endoneurium.

At high magnification in Fig. 7.5c, part of the cytoplasm of a Schwann cell **S** is shown ensheathing several axons **A**; axons are readily identified by their content of smooth endoplasmic reticulum and microtubules, seen in cross-section. Several mesaxons **M** can be seen. The external surface of the Schwann cell is bounded by an external lamina **L**, equivalent to lamina densa in epithelia.

A axon **C** Schwann cell cytoplasm **Ci** inner Schwann cell cytoplasm **Co** collagen **F** fibroblast cytoplasmic process **L** external lamina **M** mesaxon **My** myelin sheath **N** Schwann cell nucleus **S** Schwann cell

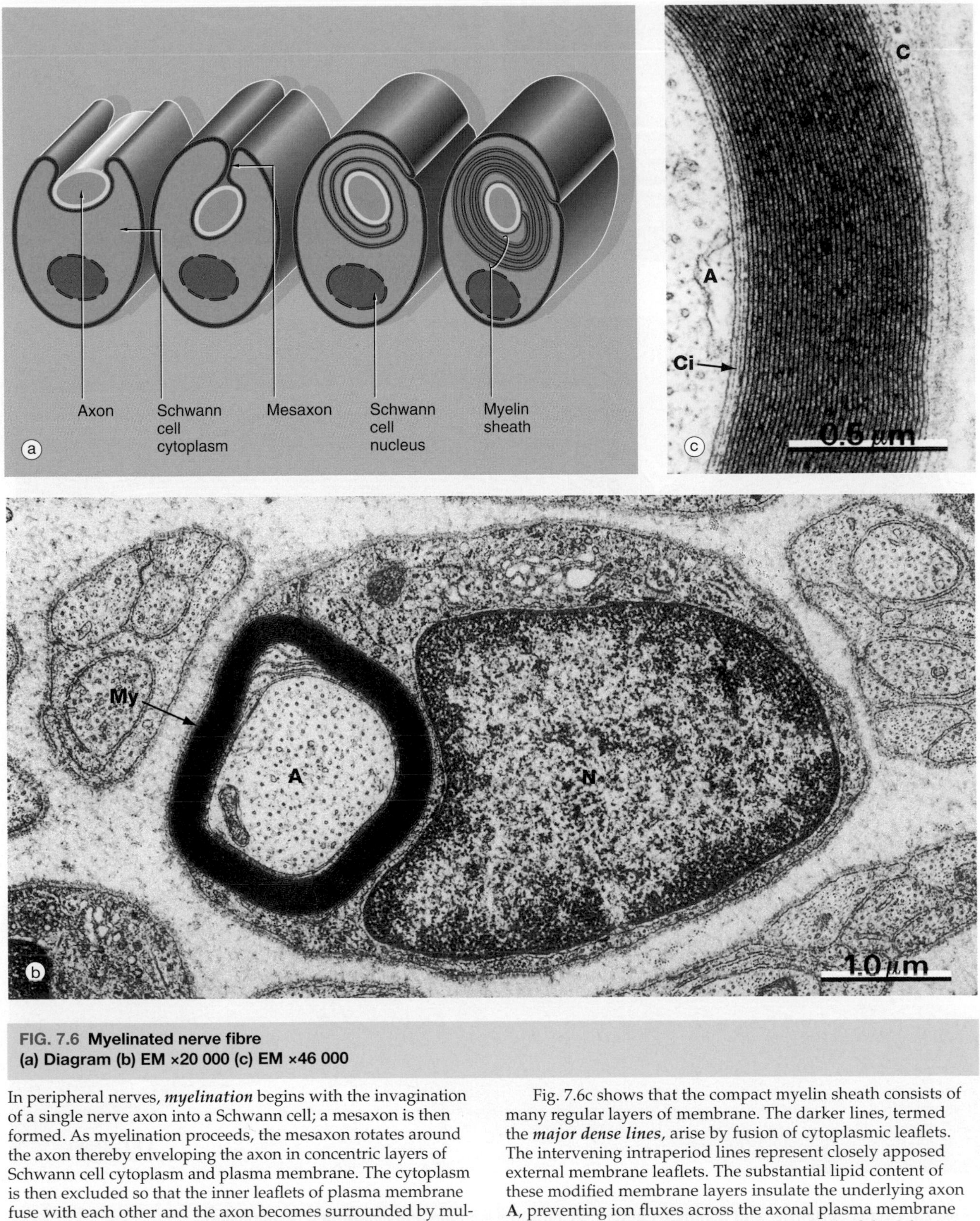

FIG. 7.6 Myelinated nerve fibre
(a) Diagram (b) EM ×20 000 (c) EM ×46 000

In peripheral nerves, ***myelination*** begins with the invagination of a single nerve axon into a Schwann cell; a mesaxon is then formed. As myelination proceeds, the mesaxon rotates around the axon thereby enveloping the axon in concentric layers of Schwann cell cytoplasm and plasma membrane. The cytoplasm is then excluded so that the inner leaflets of plasma membrane fuse with each other and the axon becomes surrounded by multiple layers of membrane which together constitute the ***myelin sheath*** (Fig. 7.6a). The single segment of myelin produced by each Schwann cell is termed an ***internode***; this ensheaths the axon between one ***node of Ranvier*** and the next (see Fig. 7.7).

In Fig. 7.6b, a myelinated nerve fibre from the PNS is sectioned transversely at the level of the nucleus of an ensheathing Schwann cell **N**. The single axon **A** is enveloped by many layers of fused Schwann cell plasma membrane forming the myelin sheath **My**.

Fig. 7.6c shows that the compact myelin sheath consists of many regular layers of membrane. The darker lines, termed the ***major dense lines***, arise by fusion of cytoplasmic leaflets. The intervening intraperiod lines represent closely apposed external membrane leaflets. The substantial lipid content of these modified membrane layers insulate the underlying axon **A**, preventing ion fluxes across the axonal plasma membrane except at the nodes of Ranvier. The main bulk of the Schwann cell cytoplasm **C** encircles the myelin sheath. However, a thin layer of Schwann cell cytoplasm also persists immediately surrounding the axon **Ci**.

In the CNS, oligodendrocytes are responsible for myelination; a single oligodendrocyte, however, forms multiple myelin internodes which contribute to the ensheathment of as many as 50 individual axons (see Fig. 20.3).

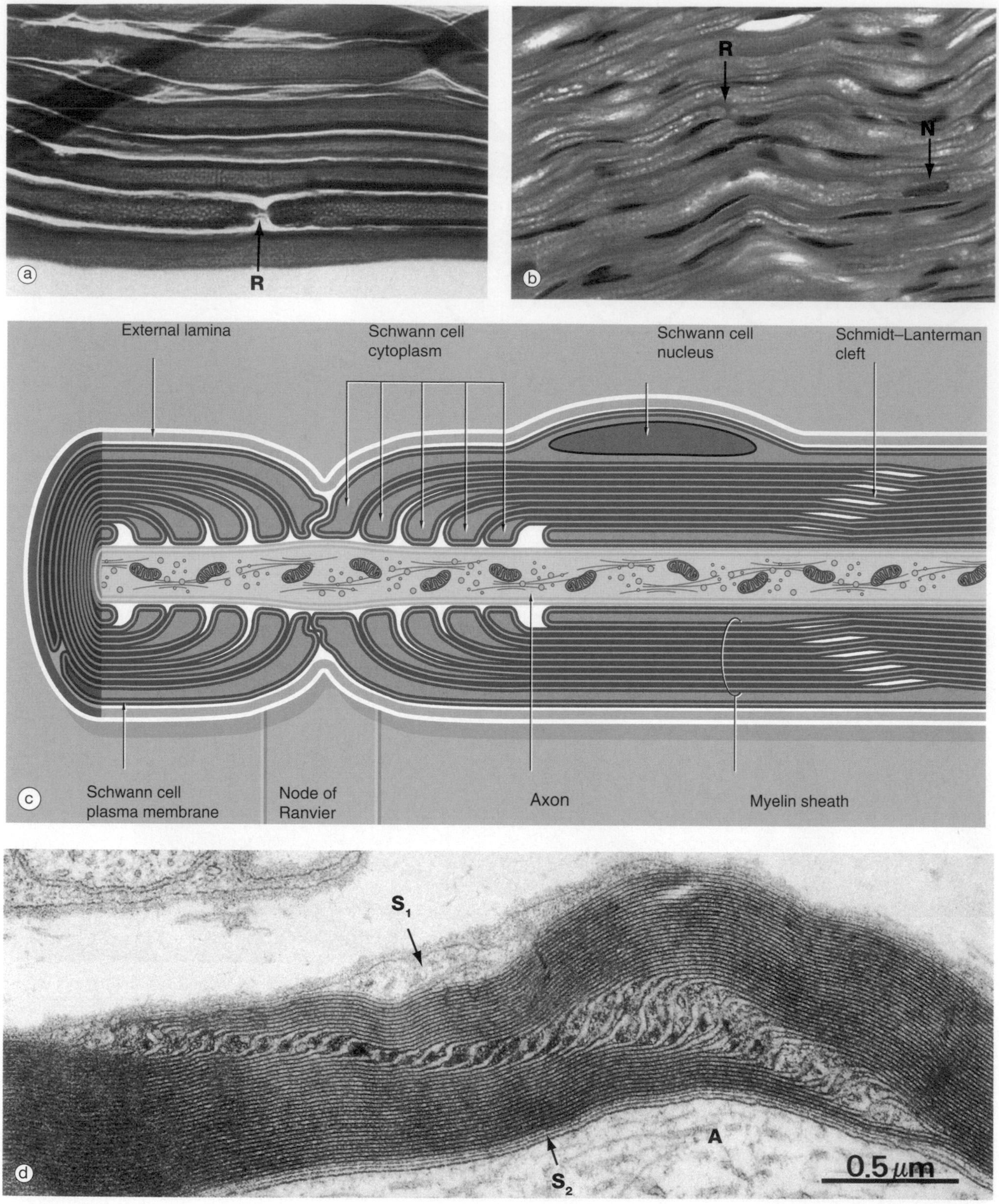

FIG. 7.7 Nodes of Ranvier and Schmidt–Lanterman incisures *(caption and illustration (e) opposite)*
(a) Teased preparation, Sudan black (MP) (b) H&E (MP) (c) Schematic diagram (d) EM ×42 000 (e) EM ×14 000

Disorders of myelin

Diseases can specifically attack myelin in CNS, PNS or both. In **multiple sclerosis**, there is immune-mediated destruction of myelin, confined to the CNS. This leads to slowing of axonal conduction and neurological dysfunction. Signs and symptoms relate to the location of affected white matter. Histological examination of an affected area shows loss of myelin staining in areas called ***plaques of demyelination*** (e-Fig. 7.3).

In Guillain–Barré syndrome, there is immune-mediated destruction of myelin in the PNS. Patients develop rapidly progressive weakness of limbs and weakness of respiratory muscles. Histological examination of affected nerve shows loss of myelin with preservation of axons. Conduction velocity in affected nerves is greatly slowed. Mutation in genes coding for myelin proteins is the basis for several inherited disorders of the nervous system.

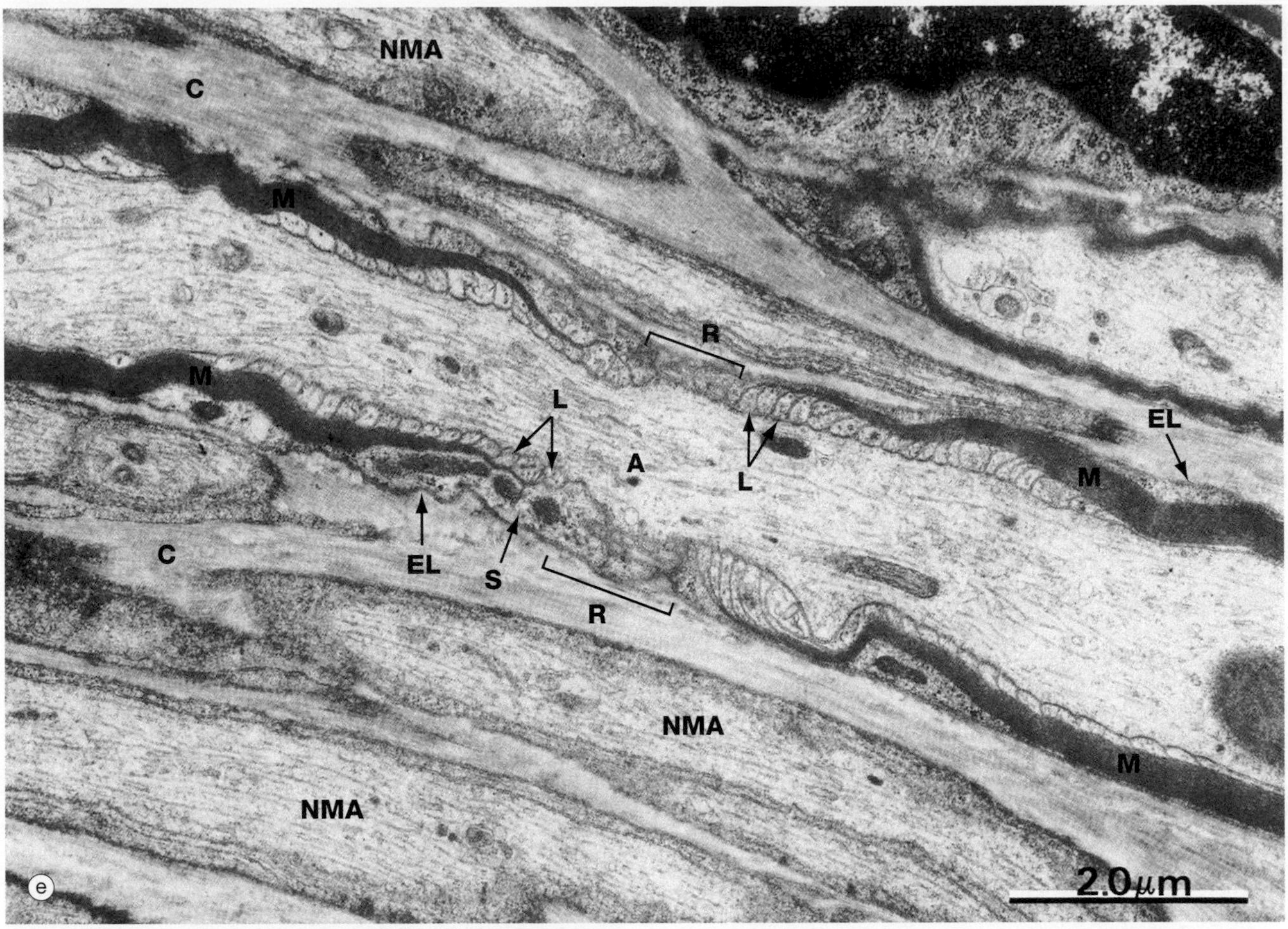

FIG. 7.7 Nodes of Ranvier and Schmidt–Lanterman incisures *(illustrations (a–d) opposite)*
(a) Teased preparation, Sudan black (MP) (b) H&E (MP) (c) Schematic diagram (d) EM ×42 000 (e) EM ×14 000

The myelin sheath of an individual axon is provided by many Schwann cells (oligodendrocytes in the CNS), each Schwann cell covering only a segment of the axon. Between the Schwann cells, there are short intervals where the axon is not covered by a myelin sheath; these points are known as ***nodes of Ranvier***.

Fig. 7.7a shows a node of Ranvier **R** in a teased preparation of myelinated axons. With this method, only the lipid of the myelin has been stained and thus Schwann cell nuclei are not seen.

Fig. 7.7b shows axons in longitudinal section stained with H&E. Due to a fixation artefact, myelin sheaths appear 'bubbly'; the lipid is mostly dissolved out during preparation and is therefore unstained. A node of Ranvier **R** is identifiable in the large axon in midfield. These are very difficult to see in routine preparations. Most of the elongated nuclei **N** are those of Schwann cells.

Fig. 7.7c illustrates the manner in which Schwann cells terminate at the node of Ranvier, so exposing the axon to the surrounding environment. Note the manner in which cytoplasmic processes of adjacent Schwann cells interdigitate at the node; also note the continuation of the Schwann cell basement membrane (external lamina) across the node. The myelin sheath prevents the nerve action potential from being propagated continuously along the axon, and the action potential travels by jumping from node to node. This mode of conduction, known as ***saltatory conduction***, greatly enhances the conduction velocity of axons. The internodal length is related to the diameter of the axon and may be up to 1.5 mm in the largest fibres.

Fig. 7.7e illustrates the ultrastructure of a node of Ranvier **R**. The axon **A** is characterised by numerous neurofilaments, microtubules and elongated mitochondria. A myelin sheath **M** can be identified at each end of the field, the myelin becoming progressively thinner as it approaches the node. This is because, as it approaches the node, each compact major dense line expands to form a small membrane loop **L** containing Schwann cell cytoplasm, the loops directly abutting the axonal plasma membrane. Externally, a broader layer of Schwann cell cytoplasm **S** containing mitochondria envelops the nodal area. Note the external lamina **EL** of the Schwann cell and collagen fibrils **C** in surrounding endoneurium. Several non-myelinated axons **NMA** are seen nearby.

At certain points within the internodal myelin sheath, narrow channels of cytoplasm are retained and connect the main bulk of the Schwann cell cytoplasm peripherally to the narrow zone of Schwann cell cytoplasm adjacent to the axon. These uncompacted regions are known as ***Schmidt–Lanterman incisures*** or clefts; in longitudinal section, as in electron micrograph (Fig. 7.7d), the incisure passes obliquely across the width of the compact sheath. The axon is marked **A**, the peripheral Schwann cell cytoplasm S_1 and the periaxonal Schwann cell cytoplasm S_2.

The layers of cell membrane that form myelin are bound together by special proteins that differ between the central and peripheral nervous systems (CNS and PNS). In the CNS, proteolipid protein links the exoplasmic surfaces, while cytoplasmic surfaces are linked by myelin basic protein. In the PNS, P0 protein associates with myelin basic protein to form the major dense line. PNS myelin also contains peripheral myelin protein-22.

A axon **C** collagen fibrils **EL** external lamina **L** membrane loop **M** myelin sheath **N** Schwann cell nucleus **NMA** non-myelinated axon **R** node of Ranvier **S** Schwann cell cytoplasm S_1 peripheral Schwann cell cytoplasm S_2 periaxonal Schwann cell cytoplasm

SYNAPSES AND NEUROMUSCULAR JUNCTIONS

Synapses are highly specialised intercellular junctions which allow communication by linking neurones to neurones. Individual neurones communicate via a widely variable number of synapses, depending on their location and function. Classically, the axon of one neurone synapses with the dendrite of another neurone (***axodendritic synapse***), but axons may synapse with the cell bodies of other neurones (***axosomatic synapses***) or with other axons (***axoaxonic synapses***); dendrite-to-dendrite and cell body–to–cell body synapses have also been described.

The mechanism of conduction of the nerve impulse involves the release from one neurone of a chemical ***neurotransmitter*** which then diffuses across the narrow intercellular space in the synapse to induce excitation or inhibition in the target neurone or effector cell of that synapse. This is achieved via specific receptors for the neurotransmitter incorporated in the opposing plasma membrane. Neurotransmitter is cleared from the synaptic cleft by specific enzymatic degradation or reuptake by the axon or both, freeing the synapse for further signals.

The chemical nature of neurotransmitters varies and the morphology of synapses are highly variable in different parts of the nervous system, but the principle of synaptic transmission and the basic structure of synapses are similar throughout. For a given synapse, the signal transmission is unidirectional, but the response on the target cell may be either excitatory or inhibitory, depending on the specific synapse and its location.

Similar intercellular junctions link neurones to their effector cells, such as muscle fibres; where neurones synapse with skeletal muscle, the specialised synapses are referred to as ***neuromuscular junctions*** or ***motor end plates***.

FIG. 7.8 Synapse

Fig. 7.8 illustrates the general structure of the synapse. The axon responsible for propagating the stimulus terminates at a bulbous swelling or ***terminal bouton***; this is separated from the plasma membrane of the opposed neurone or effector cell by a narrow intercellular gap of uniform width (20–30 nm) called the ***synaptic cleft***. The terminal boutons are not myelinated. The boutons contain mitochondria and membrane-bound vesicles of neurotransmitter substance known as ***synaptic vesicles*** which are approximately 50 nm in diameter.

There are many different types of neurotransmitter substance which are different in CNS and PNS, e.g. acetylcholine, noradrenaline (norepinephrine), glutamate or dopamine. Synaptic vesicles are transported into the synaptic bouton down the axon from the cell body. Vesicles can also be formed in the synaptic bouton by recycling of vesicle membrane. Protein synthesis can also occur in the synaptic bouton.

Synaptic vesicles aggregate towards the ***presynaptic membrane*** and, on arrival of an action potential, dock with the membrane and release their contents into the synaptic cleft by exocytosis (see Ch. 1). The neurotransmitter diffuses across the synaptic cleft to stimulate receptors in the ***postsynaptic membrane***. Associated with synapses are a variety of biochemical mechanisms such as hydrolytic and oxidative enzymes which inactivate the released neurotransmitter between successive nerve impulses. Transmitter may also be taken up back into the terminal bouton and be recycled into new synaptic vesicles. The cytoplasm beneath the postsynaptic membrane often contains a feltwork of fine fibrils, the ***postsynaptic web***, which may be associated with desmosome-like structures in maintaining the integrity of the synapse.

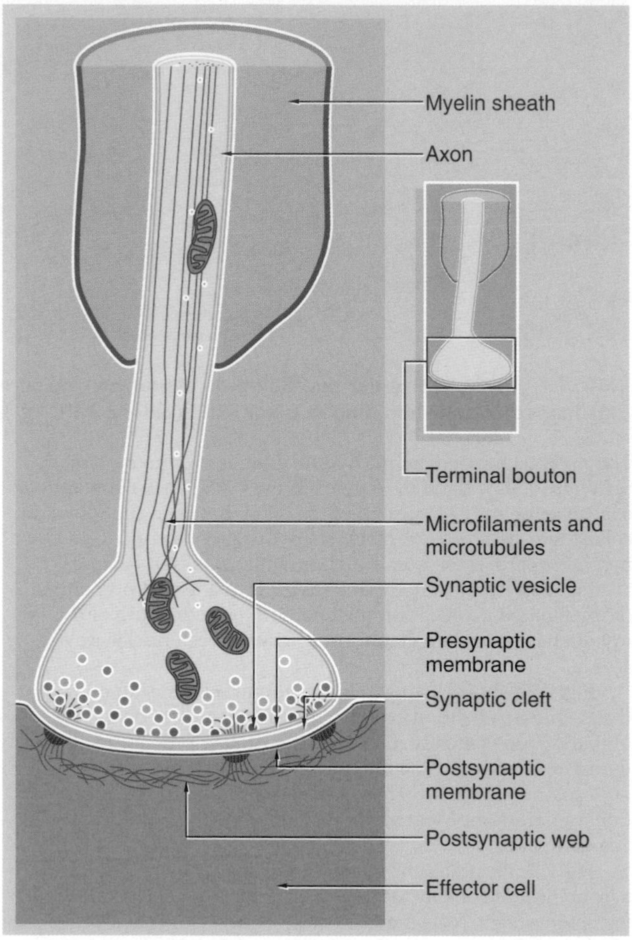

Synaptic loss and Alzheimer's disease

Alzheimer's disease, the commonest cause of dementia, is characterised histologically by accumulation of abnormal proteins (beta amyloid and tau) and neuronal loss (e-Fig. 7.1). An early feature is synaptic dysfunction in the hippocampus and the cerebral cortex. The synapses mediating neurotransmission by acetylcholine (***cholinergic system***) are particularly affected. Identification of this transmitter deficit has led to development of drugs to maximise the concentration of acetylcholine in the remaining synapses. Once secreted into the synaptic cleft, acetylcholine is rapidly destroyed by the action of cholinesterases. Cholinesterase inhibitor drugs are now given to patients with Alzheimer's disease to compensate for the synaptic loss by maximising the impact of remaining cholinergic synaptic activity.

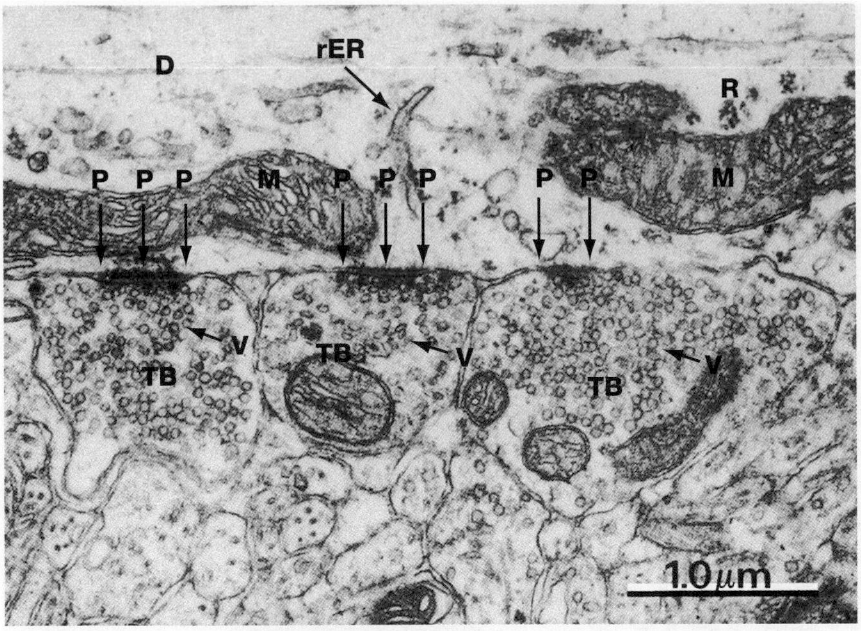

FIG. 7.9 Axodendritic synapse EM ×22 000

Fig. 7.9 from the CNS illustrates three terminal boutons **TB** (probably from different axons) forming synapses with a dendrite **D**. The dendrite can be identified as such by its content of ribosomes **R** and rough endoplasmic reticulum **rER** (which are not present in axons). Note the presence of numerous uniform-sized synaptic vesicles **V** and a few mitochondria **M** within the terminal boutons. The postsynaptic density **P** contributes to the structural stability of the closely apposed pre- and postsynaptic membranes.

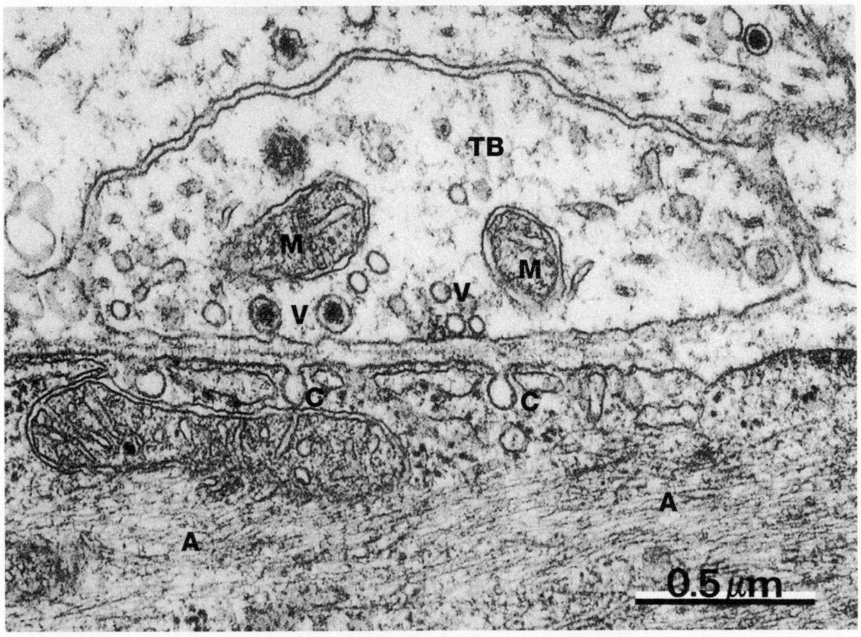

FIG. 7.10 Autonomic synapse EM ×42 000

Fig. 7.10 illustrates a synapse between an axon of the autonomic nervous system and a smooth muscle cell in the intestine. The terminal bouton **TB** contains mitochondria **M** and a number of synaptic vesicles **V**, some of which contain a dense central core, probably representing an electron-dense carrier protein; such ***dense core vesicles*** are a feature of autonomic synapses. Frequently more than one neurotransmitter substance is present in individual autonomic neurones.

The postsynaptic membrane exhibits flask-like invaginations **C** which may represent caveolae. Note the uniform width of the synaptic cleft between the pre- and postsynaptic membranes. The smooth muscle cell contains numerous fine actin microfilaments **A**.

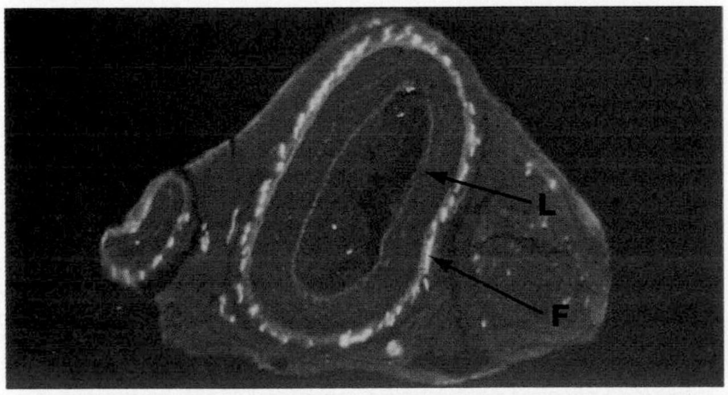

FIG. 7.11 Sympathetic nerve endings Formalin-induced fluorescence (MP)

Noradrenaline (norepinephrine) is the main postganglionic neurotransmitter in the sympathetic nervous system. When noradrenaline combines with formalin (and some other compounds) it becomes fluorescent and can be visualised by fluorescence microscopy.

Fig. 7.11 illustrates formalin-induced fluorescence **F** in the outer layer of large and small arteries, corresponding to the presence of sympathetic noradrenergic nerve endings. Weak background autofluorescence outlines the general structure; note that the internal elastic lamina **L** (see Fig. 8.10) of the large artery in midfield is particularly autofluorescent.

A actin filaments **C** caveola **D** dendrite **F** fluorescent sympathetic nerves **L** internal elastic lamina **M** mitochondrion **P** postsynaptic density **R** ribosomes **rER** rough endoplasmic reticulum **TB** terminal bouton **V** synaptic vesicles

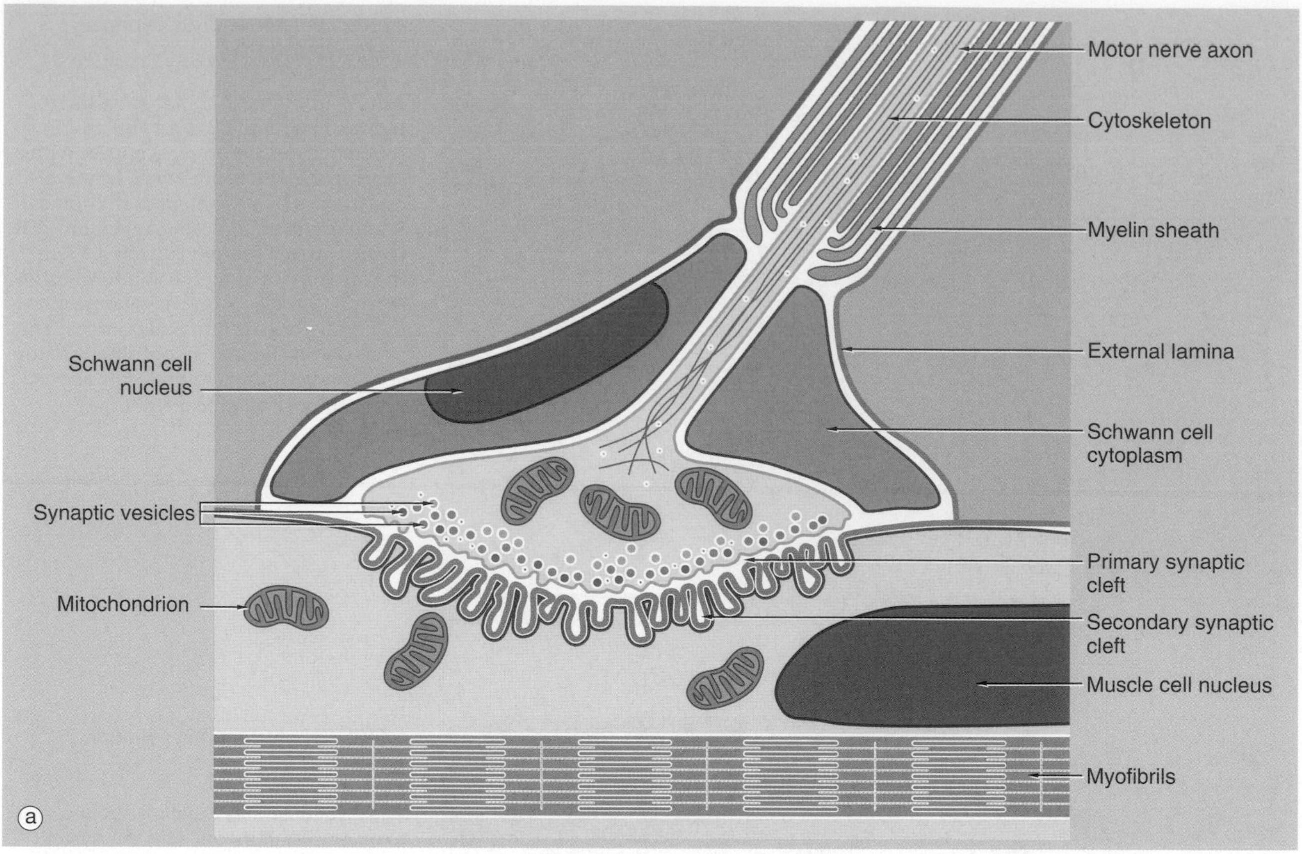

FIG. 7.12 Motor end plates *(illustrations (b) to (e) opposite)*
(a) Schematic diagram (b) Teased preparation, gold method (MP) (c) Teased preparation, gold method (HP) (d) Histochemical method for acetylcholinesterase (MP) (e) EM ×26 000

The motor end plates of skeletal muscle have the same basic structure as other synapses, with the addition of several important features. Firstly, one motor neurone may innervate from a few to more than a thousand muscle fibres depending on the precision of movement of the muscle; the motor neurone and the muscle fibres which it supplies together constitute a ***motor unit***.

At low magnification in Fig. 7.12b, the terminal part of the axon of a motor neurone is seen dividing into several branches, each terminating as a motor end plate on a different skeletal muscle fibre near to its midpoint. Fig. 7.12c shows the lowermost of these motor end plates at higher magnification. The axonal branch is seen to lose its myelin sheath and divides to form a cluster of small bulbous swellings (***terminal boutons***) on the muscle fibre surface.

As seen in Fig. 7.12a, the motor end plate occupies a recess in the muscle cell surface, described as the ***sole plate***, and is covered by an extension of the cytoplasm of the last Schwann cell surrounding the axon. The external lamina (basement membrane) of the Schwann cell merges with that of the muscle fibre and the delicate collagenous tissue investing the nerve (***endoneurium***) becomes continuous with the ***endomysium*** of the muscle fibre (not illustrated).

Each of the terminal swellings of the cluster making up the motor end plate has the same basic structure as the synapse shown in Fig. 7.8, but the postsynaptic membrane of the neuromuscular junction is deeply folded to form ***secondary synaptic clefts*** perpendicular to the primary synaptic cleft. The overlying presynaptic membrane is also irregular, and the cytoplasm immediately adjacent contains numerous synaptic vesicles. The remaining cytoplasm of the terminal bulb contains many mitochondria and a membrane compartment for recycling secretory vesicles. The sole plate of the muscle fibre also contains a concentration of mitochondria and an aggregation of muscle cell nuclei.

The neurotransmitter of somatic neuromuscular junctions is ***acetylcholine***, the receptors for which are concentrated at the margins of the secondary synaptic clefts. The hydrolytic enzyme ***acetylcholinesterase*** is present deeper in the clefts, associated with the external lamina, and is involved in deactivation of the neurotransmitter between successive nerve impulses. The histochemical technique illustrated in Fig. 7.12d defines the location of motor end plates by an insoluble brown deposit produced by the enzyme.

Fig. 7.12e demonstrates the ultrastructure of a motor end plate, the terminal bouton **TB** typically lying in a depression in the skeletal muscle surface and invested externally by Schwann cell cytoplasm **S** and its external laminan **L**. Note the uniform width of the primary synaptic cleft $\mathbf{C_1}$ and the branching nature of the numerous secondary synaptic clefts $\mathbf{C_2}$. The underlying cytoplasm is packed with mitochondria **M**. Myofibrils **Mf** are seen in transverse section at the lower right of the field. The terminal bouton contains numerous synaptic vesicles **V** of uniform size; other membranous elements represent parts of the endoplasmic reticulum and a few mitochondria.

Myasthenia gravis: An autoimmune disease affecting the motor end plate

Myasthenia gravis is the most common primary disorder of neuromuscular transmission. Patients develop fatigue and muscle weakness. Normally, the motor end plate releases acetylcholine (ACh) which binds to receptors on the muscle surface to cause depolarisation and muscle contraction. In myasthenia gravis, ACh is released normally but its effect on the postsynaptic membrane is reduced because acetylcholine receptors (AChR) have been depleted by binding to autoantibodies specific for the receptor. Detection of serum antibodies that bind human AChR is used to help diagnose the condition. Treatment with cholinesterase inhibitors temporarily prolongs the effects of the ACh signal and leads to improved muscle strength.

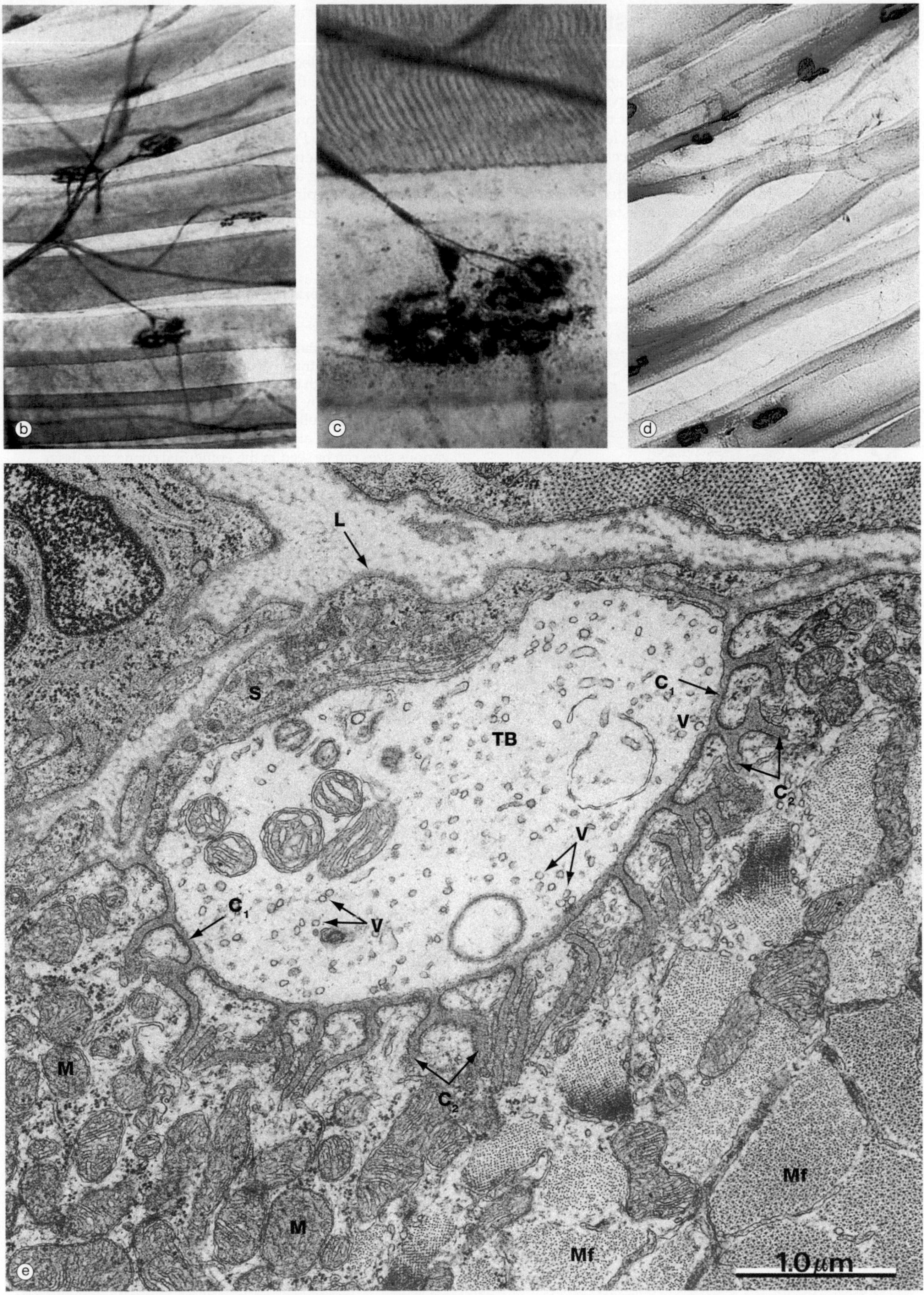

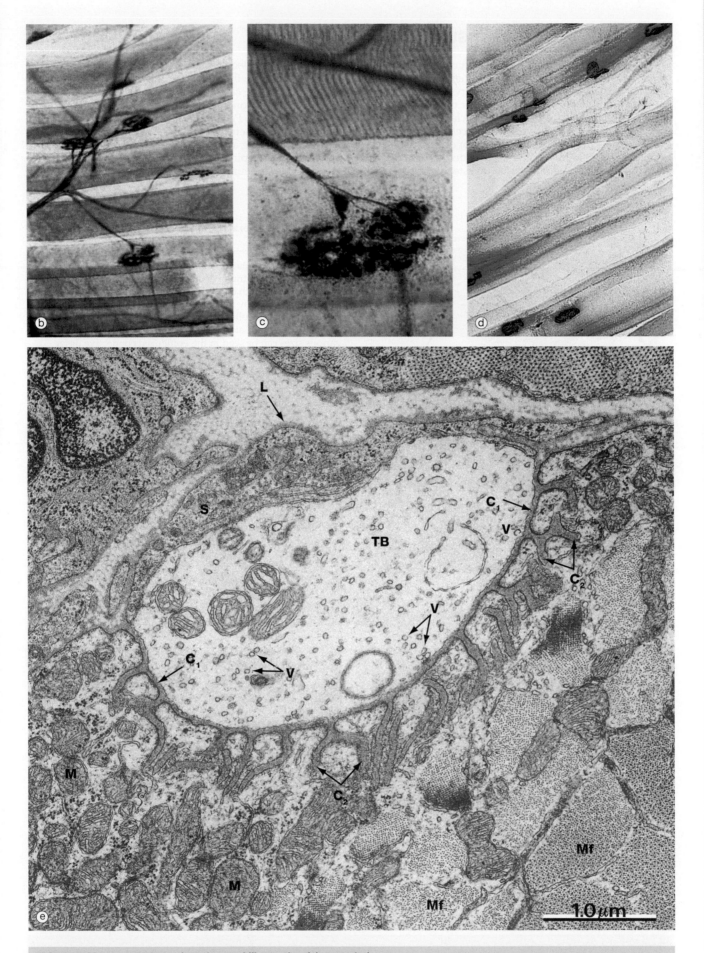

FIG. 7.12 Motor end plates *(caption and illustration (a) opposite)*
(a) Schematic diagram (b) Teased preparation, gold method (MP) (c) Teased preparation, gold method (HP) (d) Histochemical method for acetylcholinesterase (MP) (e) EM ×26 000

C_1 primary synaptic cleft **C_2** secondary synaptic cleft **L** external lamina **M** mitochondrion **Mf** myofibrils **S** Schwann cell cytoplasm **TB** terminal bouton **V** synaptic vesicles

PERIPHERAL NERVOUS TISSUES

Peripheral nerves are anatomical structures which may contain any combination of ***afferent*** or ***efferent*** nerve fibres, of either the somatic or autonomic nervous systems. Each peripheral nerve is composed of one or more bundles (***fascicles***) of nerve fibres. Within the fascicles, each individual nerve fibre with its investing Schwann cell is surrounded by a delicate packing of loose vascular supporting tissue called ***endoneurium***. Each fascicle is surrounded by a condensed layer of robust collagenous tissue invested by a layer of flat epithelial cells called the ***perineurium***. In peripheral nerves consisting of more than one fascicle, a further layer of loose collagenous tissue called the ***epineurium*** binds the fascicles together and is condensed peripherally to form a strong cylindrical sheath. Peripheral nerves receive a blood supply via numerous penetrating vessels from surrounding tissues and accompanying arteries. Larger vessels course longitudinally within the epineurium, with a capillary network penetrating the perineurium into endoneurium.

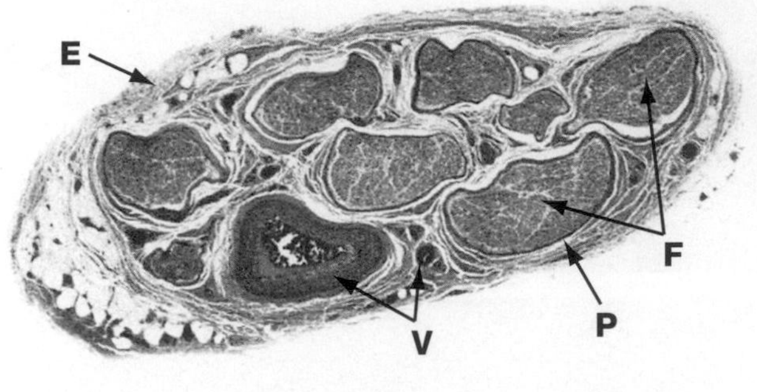

FIG. 7.13 Peripheral nerve
H&E (LP)

Fig. 7.13 illustrates the typical appearance of a medium-sized peripheral nerve in transverse section. This specimen consists of eight fascicles **F**, each of which contains many nerve fibres. Each fascicle is invested by perineurium **P** and the nerve as a whole is encased in a loose collagenous tissue sheath, the epineurium **E**, which is condensed at its outermost aspect. Blood vessels **V** of various sizes can be seen in the epineurial connective tissue.

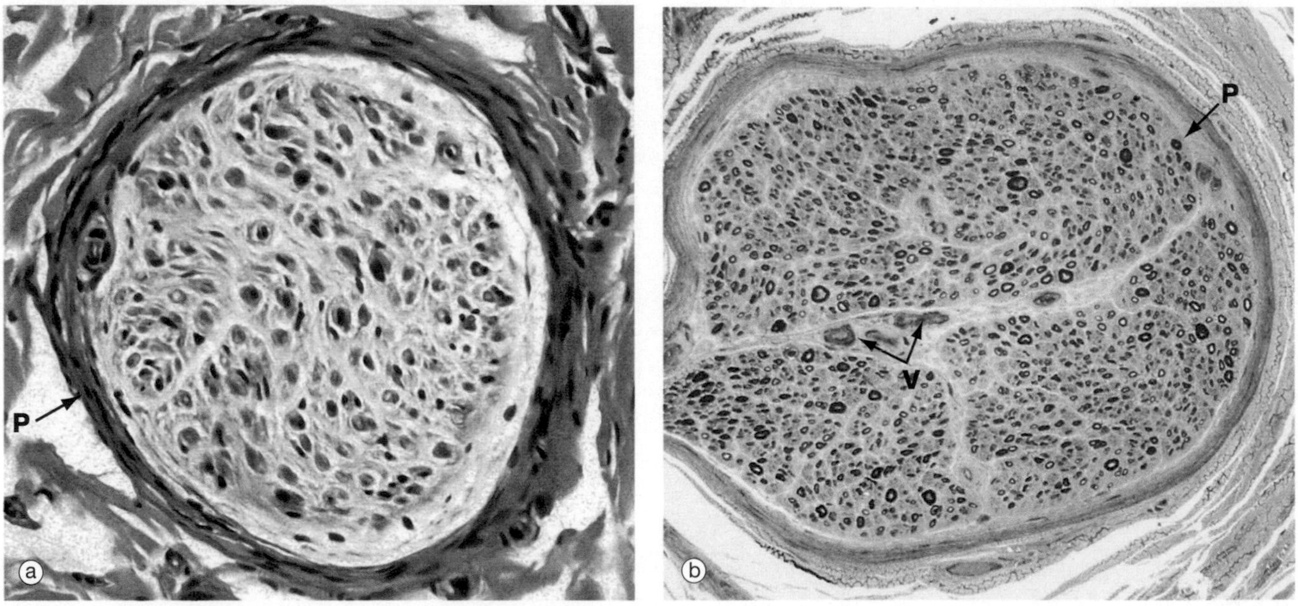

FIG. 7.14 Peripheral nerve
(a) H&E (MP) (b) Resin toluidine blue (MP)

The peripheral nerves shown in transverse section in Fig. 7.14a and b each consists of a single fascicle, invested by the perineurium **P** composed of several layers of flattened cells with elongated nuclei.

In Fig. 7.14a individual myelin sheaths are just visible as small circular structures, formed of myelin sheath proteins left after removal of lipid by tissue processing. Most of the nuclei seen within the fascicle are those of Schwann cells which mark the course of individual axons. Fibroblasts of the endoneurium are scattered amongst the much more numerous Schwann cells. It is possible to distinguish a minority of the large myelinated axons in this paraffin-embedded material stained with H&E. Around the outside of the perineurium are bundles of pink-staining epineurial collagen.

Fig. 7.14b is a preparation of nerve embedded in epoxy resin and stained with toluidine blue. The myelin sheaths are stained dark blue and can be seen as small circular structures. Axons run down the centre of each myelin sheath but are not resolved at this magnification. In the centre of the fascicle are small endoneurial blood vessels **V**. The perineurium **P** runs around the fascicle.

Peripheral nerve diseases

There are two main types of ***peripheral neuropathy*** which result in sensory loss and weakness. In ***demyelinating neuropathy***, there is damage to the Schwann cells and myelin, causing reduced conduction velocity in nerves. In ***axonal neuropathy*** there is damage to the axons. After injury, Schwann cells can remyelinate axons. Axons can also regenerate providing the neuronal cell body is not damaged.

Tumours can also arise in the PNS, the majority of which are benign and slow growing. Examples include ***schwannomas***, derived from Schwann cells (e-Fig. 7.6), ***neurofibromas*** derived from a mixture of cell types (e-Fig. 7.7), and ***perineuriomas*** derived from perineurial cells. Malignant tumours known as malignant peripheral nerve sheath tumours are rare and often are associated with underlying inherited conditions such as ***neurofibromatosis***.

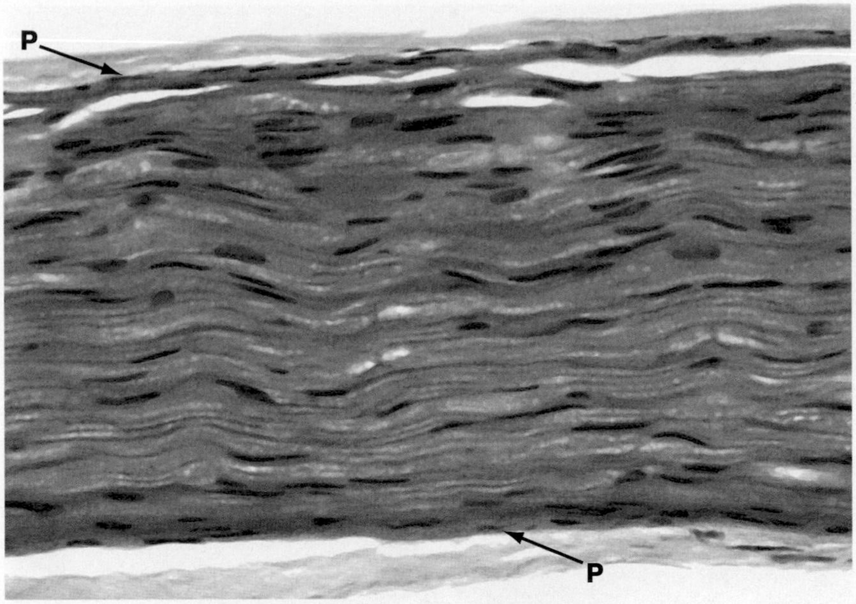

FIG. 7.15 Peripheral nerve H&E (HP)

Fig. 7.15 illustrates the typical appearance of a single nerve fascicle in longitudinal section. It contains many nerve fibres. The perineurium **P** is seen on each side. The elongated nuclei are mainly those of Schwann cells, but some will also be those of endoneurial fibroblasts. It is not easy to discriminate between these cells in this type of preparation. Nerve fibres often follow an undulating or zigzag pattern in longitudinal section, as shown here.

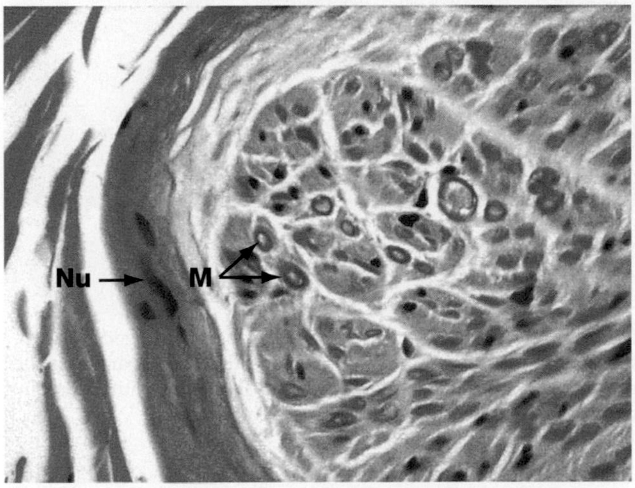

FIG. 7.16 Peripheral nerve H&E (HP)

In routinely fixed and stained preparations, myelin is poorly preserved because it is largely composed of lipid material. Schwann cell cytoplasm and structural proteins in the myelin are, however, well-preserved and have eosinophilic staining properties. Fig. 7.16 shows the edge of a peripheral nerve cut transversely; the nerve contains axons of different types and calibre, some of which are myelinated. Heavily myelinated fibres **M** can be identified by a pink ring formed by the protein remnants of the myelin sheath, with a pale centrally located axon. Small non-myelinated fibres cannot easily be identified. Several flattened nuclei **Nu** of perineurial cells are also seen in the perineurium.

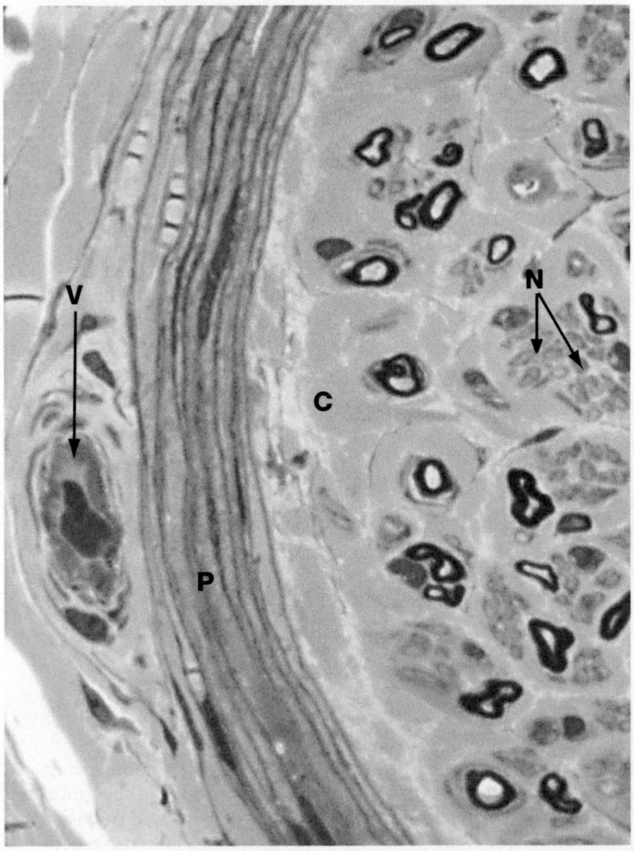

FIG. 7.17 Peripheral nerves in section Toluidine blue (HP)

In tissue which has been fixed in glutaraldehyde and embedded in epoxy resin, myelin is well preserved and stains darkly with toluidine blue. A mixture of large and small myelinated fibres can be seen in Fig. 7.17 as dark-staining ring-like structures. These are often collapsed or elliptical in profile in sections, as here. The axon contained within each myelin sheath is seen as a pale structure, but no detail can be resolved at this magnification.

Schwann cell cytoplasm stains a paler shade of blue than the myelin and can be seen surrounding small clusters of small, non-myelinated axons **N**. In between bundles of nerve fibres is the paler-staining endoneurial collagen **C**.

The perineurium **P** is well shown in this type of preparation and resolves into several layers of flattened cells separated by thin layers of collagen. The elongated nuclei of perineurial cells are well seen. Outside the perineurium are bundles of epineurial collagen and a small blood vessel **V**.

C collagen **E** epineurium **F** fascicle **M** myelin **N** non-myelinated fibres **Nu** nucleus of perineurial cell **P** perineurium **V** vessel

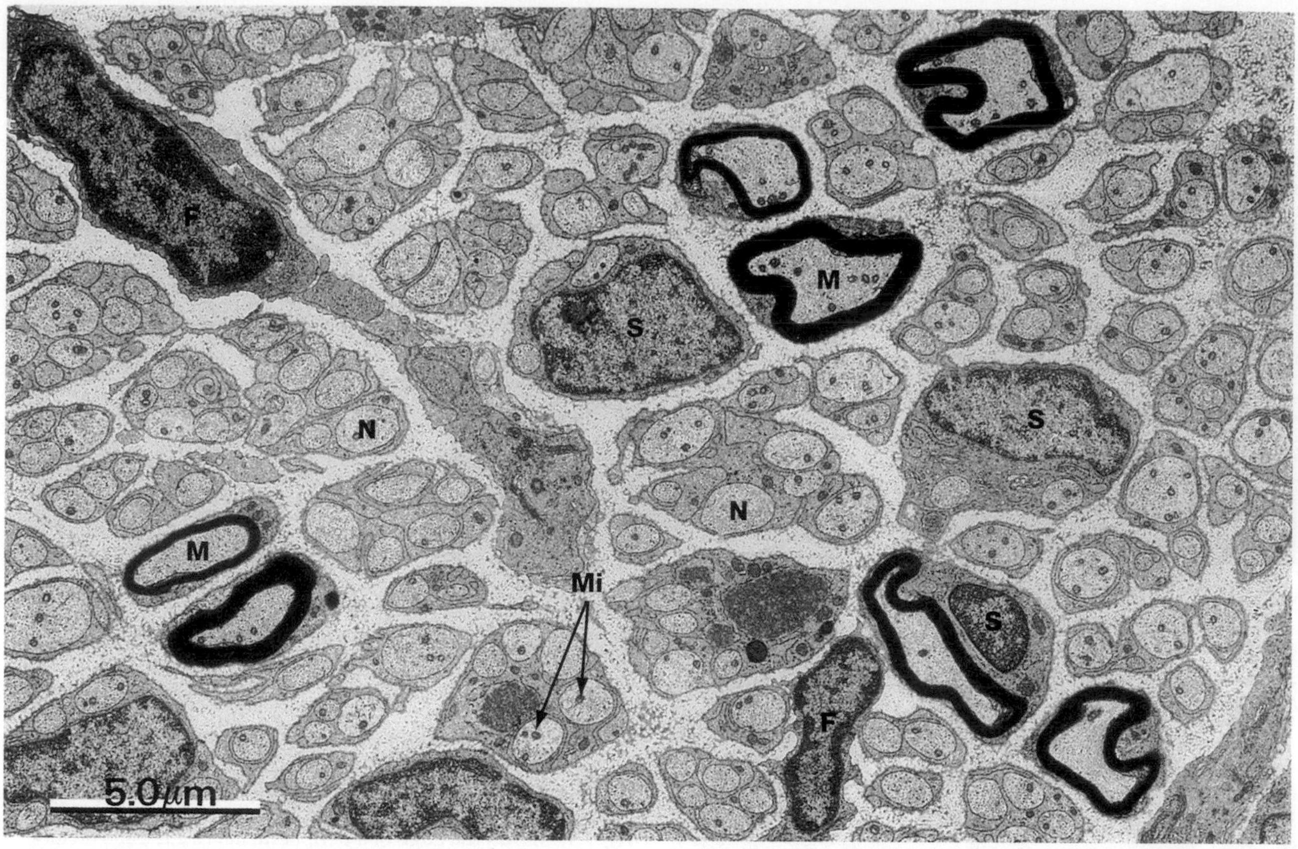

FIG. 7.18 Peripheral nerve
EM ×5000

The ultrastructural features of a typical peripheral nerve are shown in Fig. 7.18. Both myelinated axons **M** and more numerous non-myelinated axons **N** are present, both ensheathed by Schwann cells **S**. The axons contain dot-like structures which are mitochondria **Mi**. The endoneurium mainly consists of loosely arranged collagen fibrils (difficult to identify at this magnification) lying parallel to the nerve fibres. The nuclei of two fibroblasts **F** can be identified and fibroblast processes extend through the endoneurium.

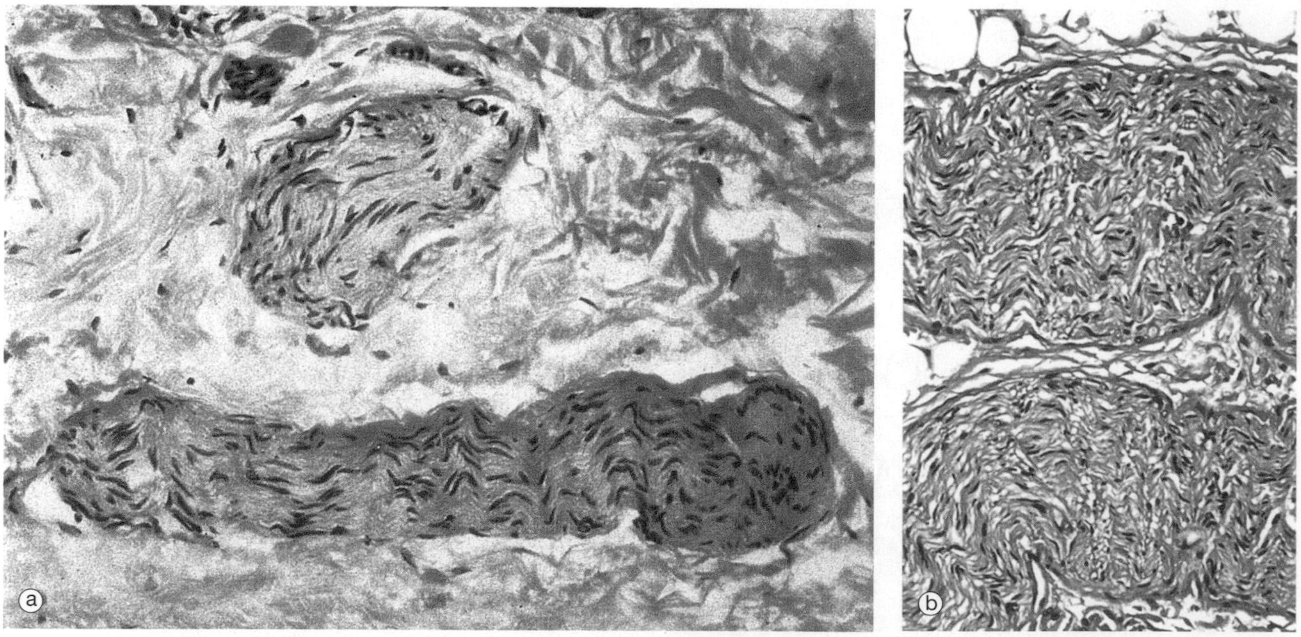

FIG. 7.19 Small peripheral nerves
(a) H&E (HP) (b) H&E (HP)

These micrographs illustrate the appearance of small peripheral nerves in the tissues. Fig. 7.19a shows two small nerves in the dermis of the skin, each nerve consisting of a single fascicle of fibres. The nerve at the bottom of the field is cut in longitudinal section; the wavy shape of the Schwann cell nuclei reflects the course of the axons, which are thereby protected from damage when the skin is stretched. The nerve in the upper part of the field is cut in oblique section. Note the dense irregular collagenous dermal tissue surrounding the nerves in this specimen. Fig. 7.19b shows a small peripheral nerve in the submucosa of the large bowel. This nerve runs a zigzag course in the tissue and the plane of section has cut it in the long axis as it folds. This allows the nerve to stretch as the bowel moves with peristalsis.

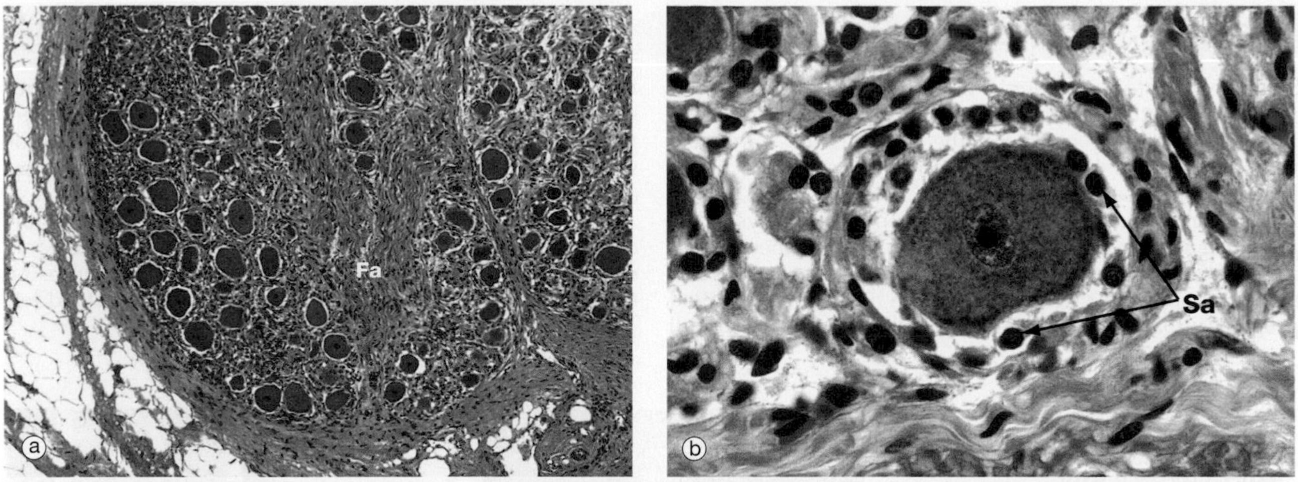

FIG. 7.20 Spinal ganglion
(a) H&E (MP) (b) H&E (HP)

Ganglia are discrete aggregations of neurone cell bodies located outside the CNS. The spinal ganglia are located on the posterior nerve roots of the spinal cord as they pass through the intervertebral foramina; they contain the cell bodies of the primary sensory neurones which are of the pseudo-unipolar form (see Fig. 7.2).

At low magnification in Fig. 7.20a, note the fascicle **Fa** of nerve fibres passing to the centre of the ganglion, the ganglion cells being located peripherally. At high magnification in Fig. 7.20b, a nerve cell body is seen to be surrounded by a layer of rounded ***satellite cells*** **Sa** which provide structural and metabolic support and have similar embryological origin to the Schwann cells (neural crest). The whole ganglion is encapsulated by condensed supporting tissue which is continuous with the perineurial and epineurial sheaths of the associated peripheral nerve.

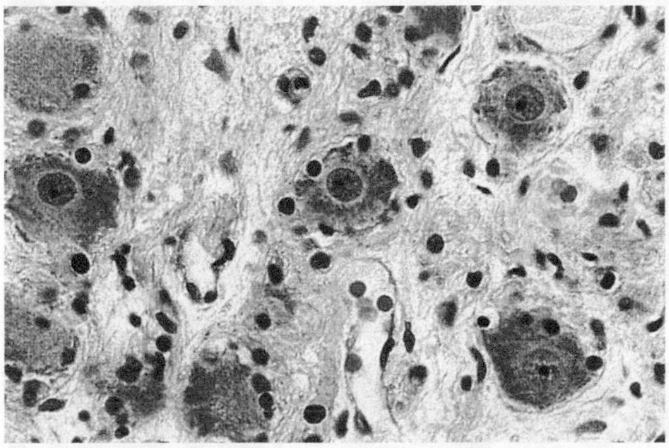

FIG. 7.21 Sympathetic ganglion
H&E (HP)

Sympathetic ganglia are found adjacent to the vertebral column. They have a similar structure to that of somatic sensory ganglia, with a few minor differences. The ganglion cells are multipolar and thus more widely spaced, being separated by numerous axons and dendrites, many of which pass through the ganglion without being involved in synapses. As seen in Fig. 7.21, the nuclei of the ganglion cells tend to be eccentrically located and the peripheral cytoplasm contains a variable quantity of brown-stained ***lipofuscin*** granules, representing cellular debris sequestered in residual bodies. The satellite cells are smaller in number and irregularly placed due to the numerous dendritic processes of the ganglion cells.

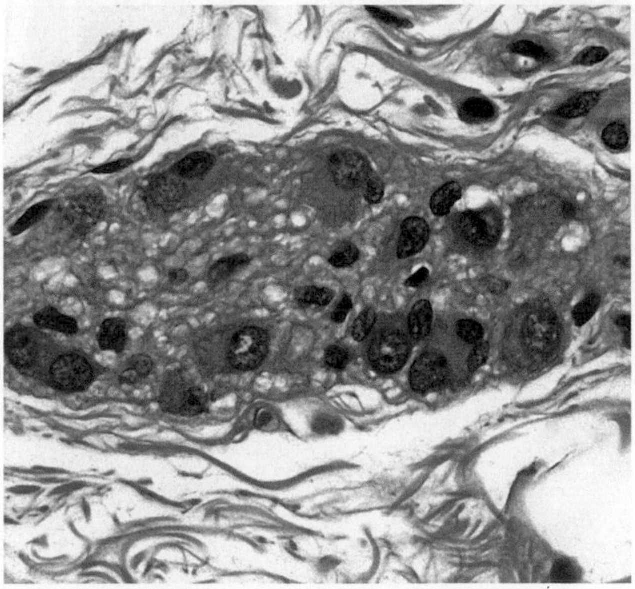

FIG. 7.22 Parasympathetic ganglion
H&E (HP)

In the parasympathetic nervous system, the cell bodies of the terminal effector neurones are usually located within or near the organ concerned. Commonly, a few neurone cell bodies are clumped together with supporting cells to form tiny ganglia scattered in the supporting tissue.

Fig. 7.22 shows a minute ganglion from the wall of the gastrointestinal tract. Like all neurones, the ganglion cells are recognised by their large nuclei, dispersed chromatin, prominent nucleoli, and extensive basophilic cytoplasm. As in other ganglia, the neurones are surrounded by small Schwann cells and afferent and efferent nerve fibres.

F fibroblast **Fa** fascicle **M** myelinated axon **Mi** mitochondrion **N** non-myelinated axon **S** Schwann cell **Sa** satellite cell

SENSORY RECEPTORS

Sensory receptors are nerve endings or specialised cells which convert (***transduce***) stimuli from the environment into afferent nerve impulses; the impulses pass into the CNS where they initiate appropriate voluntary or involuntary responses. ***Muscle spindles***, along with the ***Golgi tendon apparatus*** (not described), are part of the system of ***proprioception*** which provides conscious and unconscious information about orientation, skeletal position, muscle tension and movement. The receptors can be generically called ***proprioceptors***. Receptors which respond to external stimuli including touch, pressure, cutaneous pain, temperature, smell, taste, sight and hearing have been called ***exteroceptors***. By tradition, the eye, ear and receptors for the senses of smell and taste are described as organs of special sense; they are the subject of Ch. 21.

There are also receptors sensing aspects of body physiology and the functioning of viscera, such as blood ***chemoreceptors***, vascular (pressure) ***baroreceptors***, and receptors for the distension of hollow viscera such as the urinary bladder. These have been called ***interoceptors***.

FIG. 7.23 Neuromuscular spindle (a) Schematic diagram (b) H&E, TS (MP) (c) H&E, LS (MP)

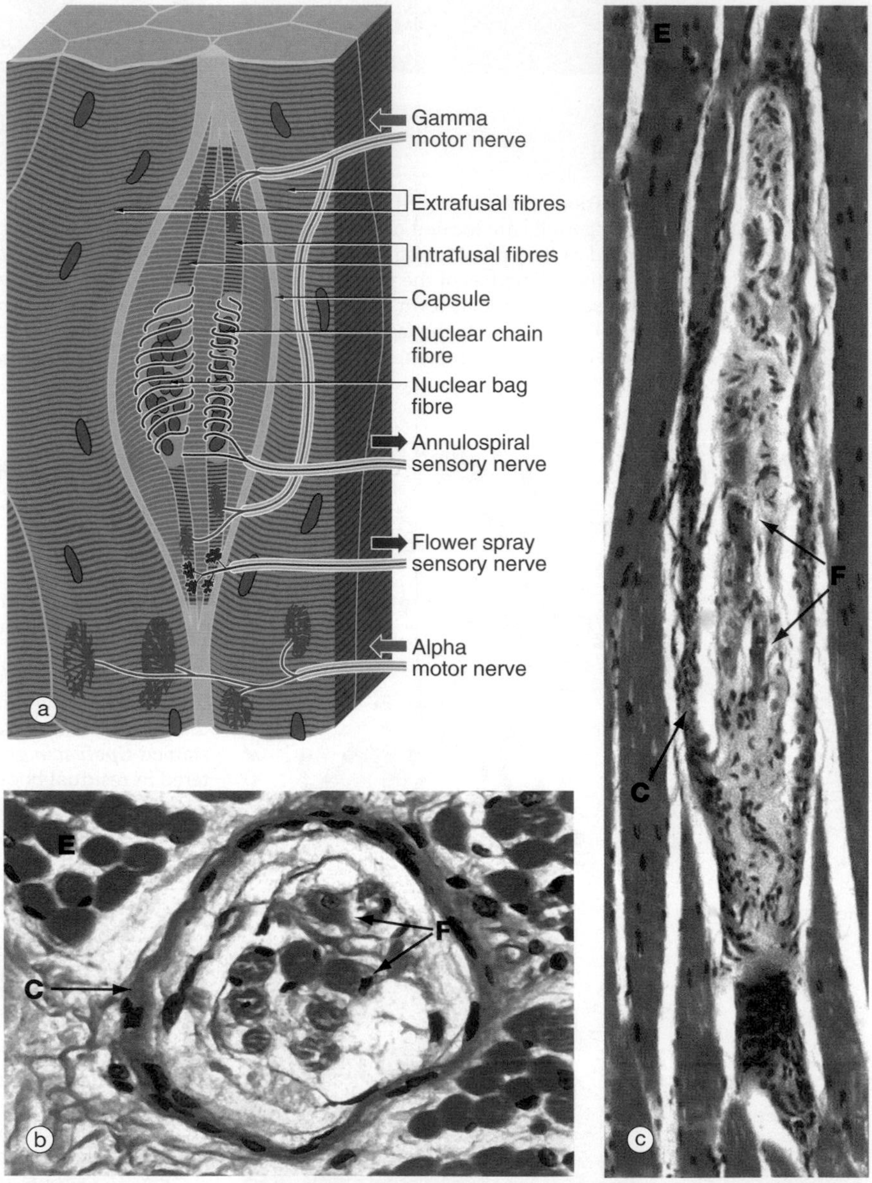

Neuromuscular spindles are stretch receptor organs within skeletal muscles which are responsible for the regulation of muscle tone via the ***spinal stretch reflex***. Neuromuscular spindles are encapsulated fusiform structures up to 6 mm long but less than 1 mm in diameter. They lie parallel to the muscle fibres, embedded in endomysium or perimysium. Each spindle contains 2 to 10 modified skeletal muscle fibres called ***intrafusal fibres*** **F**, which are much smaller than skeletal muscle fibres proper **E** (extrafusal). The intrafusal fibres have a central non-striated area in which their nuclei tend to be concentrated. Two types of intrafusal fibres are recognised. In one type, the central nuclear area is dilated, these fibres being known as ***nuclear bag fibres***. In the other type, there is no dilatation and the nuclei are arranged in a single row, giving rise to the name ***nuclear chain fibres***.

Associated with the intrafusal fibres are branched non-myelinated endings of large myelinated sensory fibres which wrap around the central non-striated area, forming ***annulospiral endings***.

Additionally, ***flower-spray endings*** of smaller myelinated sensory nerves are located on the striated portions of the intrafusal fibres. These sensory receptors are stimulated by stretching of the intrafusal fibres, which occurs when the (extrafusal) muscle mass is stretched.

This stimulus evokes a simple two-neurone spinal cord reflex, causing contraction of the extrafusal muscle mass. This removes the stretch stimulus from the spindle and equilibrium is restored (tap a tendon and see).

The sensitivity of the neuromuscular spindle is modulated via small (gamma) motor neurones controlled by the ***extra-pyramidal motor system***. These gamma motor neurones innervate the striated portions of the intrafusal fibres; contraction of the intrafusal fibres increases the stretch on the fibres and thus the sensitivity of the receptors to stretching of the extrafusal muscle mass. Many of the features of the spindle organ are shown in Figs 7.23a to c. The most easily recognisable features are the discrete capsule **C**, which is continuous with the endomysium of the surrounding muscle, and the small size of the intrafusal muscle fibres **F**, best seen in longitudinal section in Fig. 7.23c.

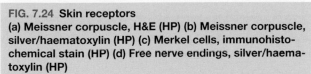

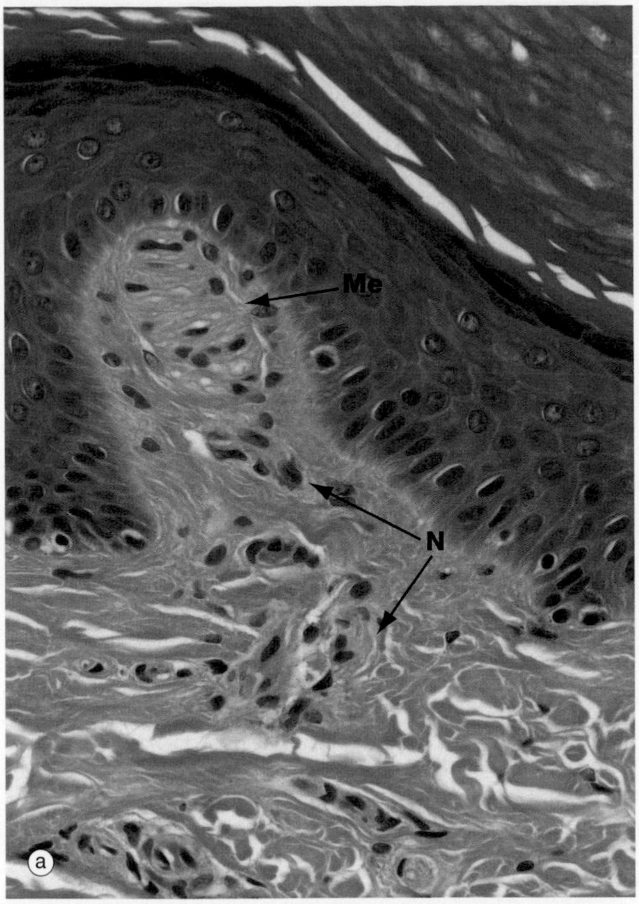

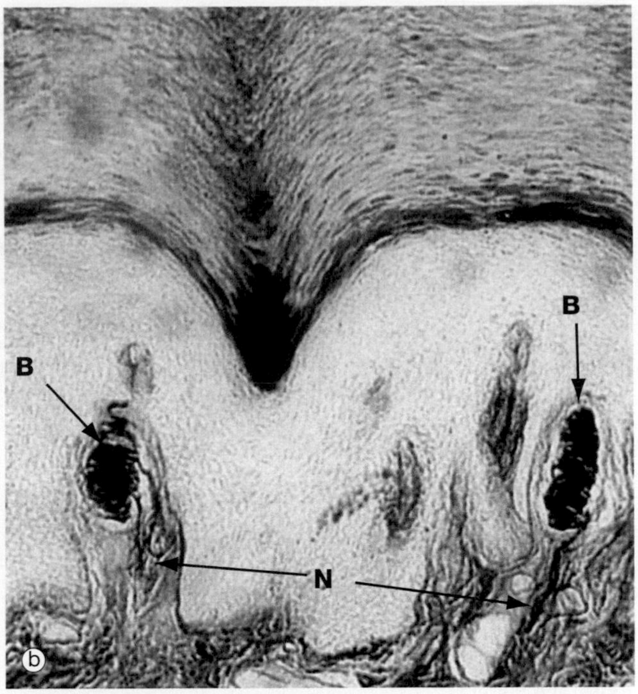

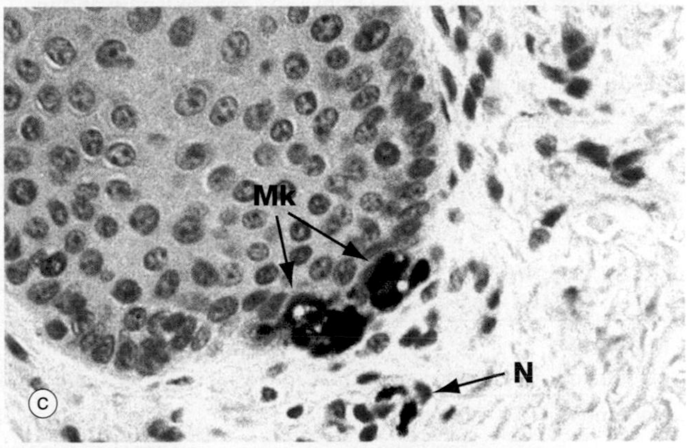

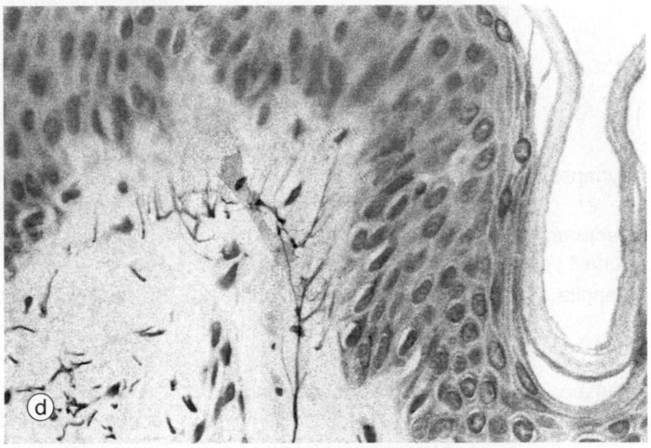

FIG. 7.24 Skin receptors
(a) Meissner corpuscle, H&E (HP) (b) Meissner corpuscle, silver/haematoxylin (HP) (c) Merkel cells, immunohistochemical stain (HP) (d) Free nerve endings, silver/haematoxylin (HP)

Fig. 7.24a shows a ***Meissner corpuscle*** **Me**. These are small, encapsulated receptors found in the papillary dermis of fingertips, soles of the feet, nipples, eyelids, lips and genitalia. They are fast-adapting mechanoreceptors which detect changes in texture and vibration (10–50 Hz). They are ovoid with a delicate collagenous tissue capsule surrounding a mass of plump oval cells arranged transversely; these are probably specialised Schwann cells. Non-myelinated branches from a large myelinated sensory nerve **N** ramify throughout the cell mass of the Meissner corpuscle as seen in Fig. 7.24b in which the nerve processes **B** are stained black.

Merkel cells **Mk** are located in the basal layers of the epidermis and are illustrated in Fig. 7.24c (see also Fig. 9.8). Merkel cell cytoplasm contains dense core vesicles with ultrastructural features similar to those found in synapses. An adjacent free nerve ending, served by large-diameter myelinated fibres **N**, forms a *Merkel cell–neurite complex*.

These are slow-adapting mechanoreceptors, sensitive to sustained touch and pressure. Merkel cell–based receptor arrays provide information about prolonged pressure, while Meissner corpuscle–based arrays provide information about changes in pressure and vibrations; together these provide the sense of fine discriminatory touch as in finger tips, lips, etc. Free nerve endings, Fig. 7.24d, provide mainly general light touch, stretching, temperature and pain sensations.

There are other skin receptors of note. These include the free nerve endings associated with hair follicles which sense hair position or movement (think cats' whiskers!). ***Ruffini corpuscles*** are robust spindle-shaped structures found in deep skin, particularly in the soles of the feet; these detect tension. ***Krause end bulbs*** are delicate encapsulated receptors found in the lining of the oropharynx and in the conjunctiva of the eye.

B nerve processes **C** capsule **E** extrafusal muscle fibres **F** intrafusal fibres **Me** Meissner corpuscle **Mk** Merkel cell **N** nerve fibre

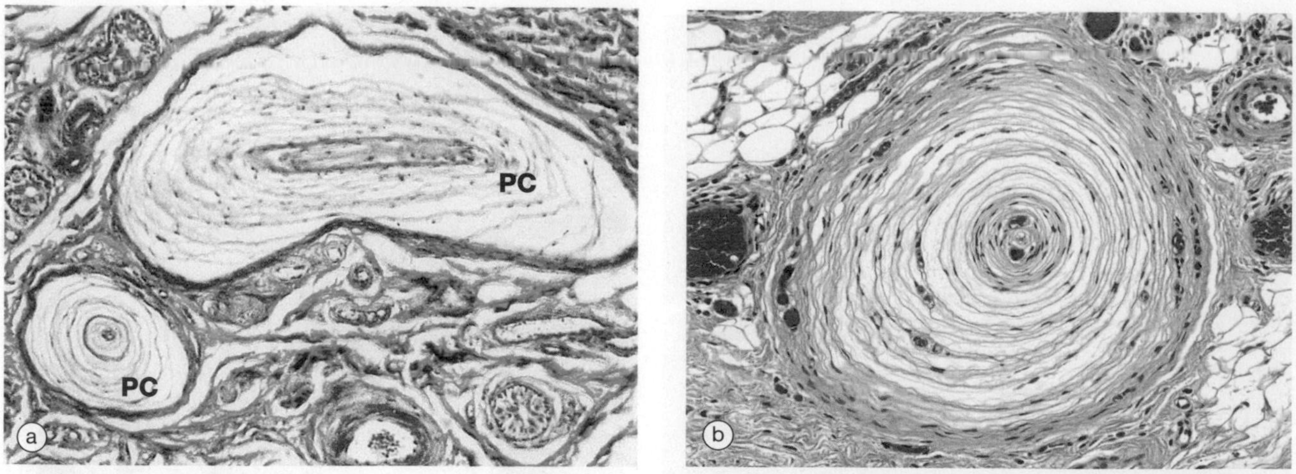

FIG. 7.25 Pacinian corpuscles
(a) Masson trichrome (MP) (b) H&E (MP)

Pacinian corpuscles are large, encapsulated sensory receptors responsive to pressure, coarse touch and rapid vibration (200–300 Hz); they are found in the deeper layers of the skin, ligaments and joint capsules, in some serous membranes, mesenteries, and viscera.

Pacinian corpuscles range from 1 to 4 mm in length and in section have the appearance of an onion (Figs 7.25a and b). These organs consist of a delicate capsule enclosing many concentric lamellae of flattened cells (probably modified Schwann cells) separated by interstitial fluid spaces and delicate collagen fibres. Towards the centre of the corpuscle the lamellae become closely packed and the core contains a single, large, unbranched, non-myelinated nerve fibre with several club-like terminals. The nerve fibre becomes myelinated on leaving the corpuscle.

Distortion of the Pacinian corpuscle produces an amplified mechanical stimulus in its core which is transduced into an action potential in the sensory neurone. It is a rapidly adapting mechanoreceptor.

REVIEW

TABLE 7.1 Review of nervous tissues

Major structures	Main structures/cells	Further description	Figure
Neurones	Cell body	Cells specialised in carrying electrical signals as communication	7.1–7.4
	Dendrites	Branched processes receiving incoming signals from synapses and at sensory receptors	7.1–7.4
	Axons	Often long, always solitary outgoing process; may branch at destination • Non-myelinated: no myelin wrapping layer; slower • Myelinated: Schwann cells wrap cell membrane around protecting and insulating the axon and speeding transmission (oligodendrocytes in CNS)	7.5–7.6
Synapses	Motor end plate	Axon endings at which neurotransmitter chemicals are released to pass the signal to the next cell or end organ	7.8
Peripheral nerves	Neuronal processes	Supporting cells in a wrapped protected structure traversing tissue	7.14–7.19
Ganglia	Nerve cell bodies and support cells external to CNS	Spinal; cell body of sensory nerves, dorsal spinal	7.20
		Sympathetic; along vertebral column	7.21
		Parasympathetic; in end organs, such as wall of bowel	7.22
Sensory receptors	Neuromuscular spindles	Complex encapsulated structure; monitors tension in muscles; receptors for tendon reflex	7.23
	Meissner corpuscles	Encapsulated body in papillary dermis; fast-adapting discriminatory touch and vibration (10–50 Hz) receptor	7.24
	Merkel cell–neurite	Merkel cell in basal epidermis and adjacent nerve ending; slow-adapting discriminatory touch and pressure receptor	7.24
	Free nerve endings	Common sensory receptors for pain, temperature, touch, pressure and other	7.24
	Pacinian corpuscle	Encapsulated bodies in deep skin; fast adapting for rapid vibration (200 Hz)	7.25
	Others	Ruffini corpuscles, Krause end bulbs, etc.	

PC Pacinian corpuscle

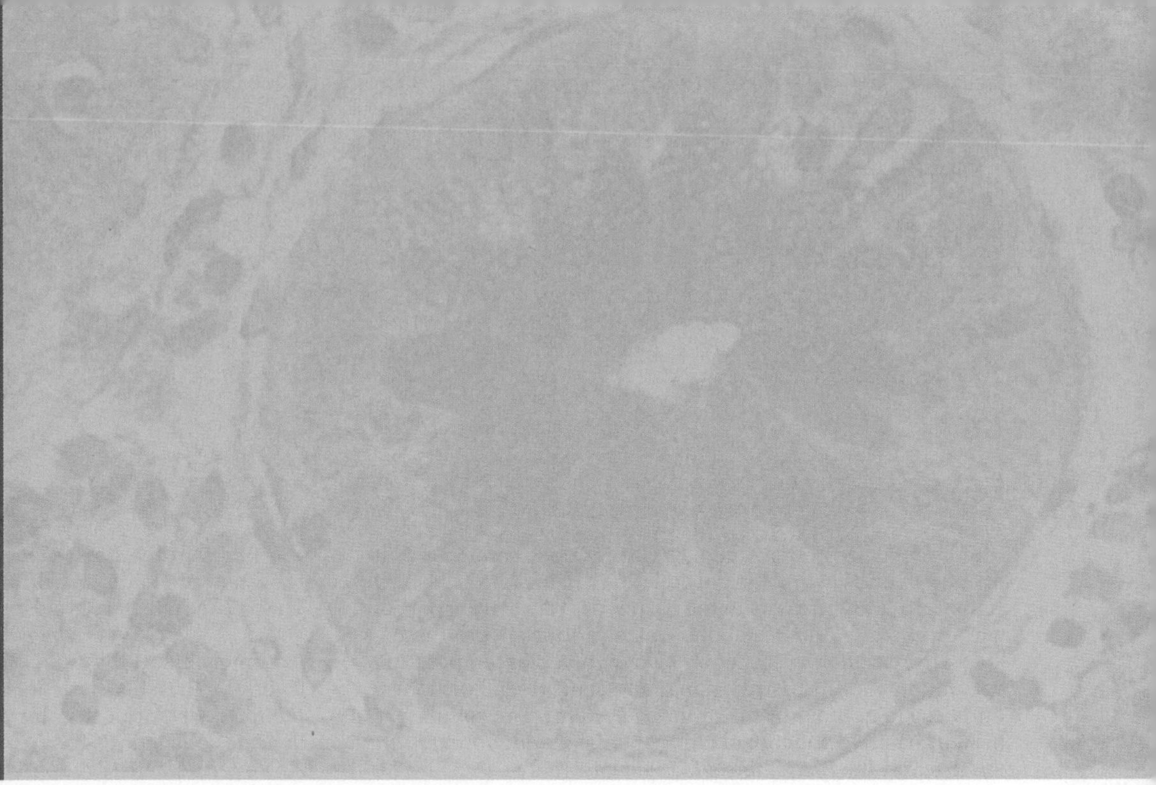

PART III

ORGAN SYSTEMS

8 Circulatory system

INTRODUCTION

The circulatory system mediates continuous movement of all body fluids, its principal functions being the transport of oxygen and nutrients to the tissues as well as transport of carbon dioxide and metabolic waste products from the tissues. The circulatory system is also involved in temperature regulation and the distribution of molecules (e.g. hormones) and cells (e.g. those of the immune system). The circulatory system has two functional components: the ***blood vascular system*** and the ***lymph vascular system***.

The blood circulatory system comprises a circuit of vessels through which blood flow is initiated by continuous action of a central muscular pump, the ***heart***. The ***arterial system*** provides a distribution network to the peripheral ***microcirculation***, the ***capillaries*** and ***postcapillary venules***, the main sites of interchange of gas and metabolite molecules between the tissues and the blood. The ***venous system*** carries blood from the capillary system back to the heart.

The lymph vascular system is a network of drainage vessels for returning excess extravascular fluid, the ***lymph***, to the blood circulatory system and for transporting lymph to the lymph nodes for immunological screening (see Ch. 11). The lymphatic system has no central pump but there is an intrinsic pumping system effected by contractile smooth muscle fibres in the lymph vessel walls, combined with a valve system preventing backflow.

The whole circulatory system has a common basic structure:

- An inner lining, the ***tunica intima***, comprising a single layer of extremely flattened epithelial cells called ***endothelial cells*** supported by a basement membrane and delicate collagenous tissue.
- An intermediate predominantly muscular layer, the ***tunica media***.
- An outer supporting tissue layer called the ***tunica adventitia***.

The tissues of the thick walls of large vessels (e.g. aorta) cannot be sustained by diffusion of oxygen and nutrients from their lumina, and are supplied by small arteries (***vasa vasorum***) which run in the tunica adventitia and send arterioles and capillaries into the tunica media.

The muscular content exhibits the greatest variation from one part of the system to another. For example, it is totally absent in capillaries but comprises almost the whole mass of the heart. Blood flow is predominantly influenced by variation in activity of the muscular tissue.

THE HEART

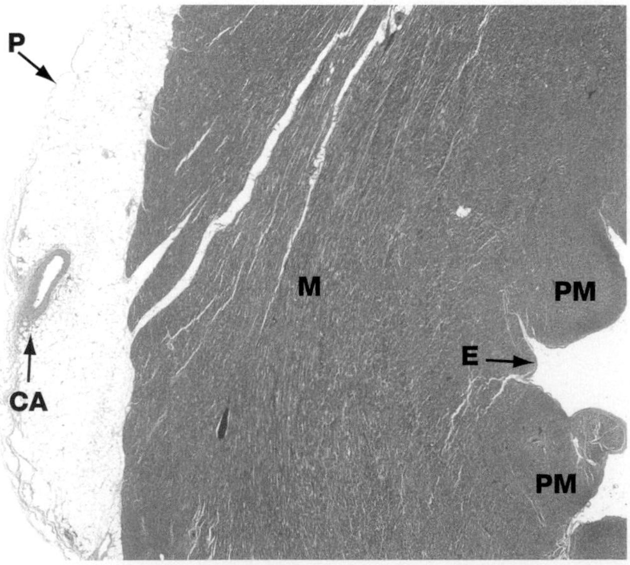

FIG. 8.1 Heart: left ventricular wall H&E (LP)

Fig. 8.1 is a low-power micrograph showing the three basic layers of the heart wall, in this case the *left ventricle*.

The tunica intima equivalent of the heart is the ***endocardium*** **E**, normally a thin layer in a ventricle. This is lined by a single layer of flattened endothelial cells, as is the case elsewhere in the circulatory system.

The tunica media equivalent is the ***myocardium*** **M**, made up of cardiac-type muscle (see Ch. 6). In the left ventricle, this layer is very prominent due to its role in pumping oxygenated blood throughout the systemic circulation, but it is less thick in the right ventricle and in the atria which operate at much lower pressures. Note the origins of the ***papillary muscles*** **PM**, extensions of the myocardium which protrude into the left ventricular cavity and provide attachment points of the ***chordae tendinae*** which tether the cusps of the atrio-ventricular valves.

The equivalent of the tunica adventitia is the ***epicardium*** or ***visceral pericardium*** **P**, usually a thin layer but, in some areas, as shown here, containing adipose tissue (see Fig. 8.2a). The ***coronary arteries*** **CA**, run within the epicardial fat.

The myocardium: changes in health and disease

The segment of left ventricular wall illustrated above is composed almost entirely of cardiac muscle. As indicated, the thickness of the myocardium differs in the different chambers of the heart, reflecting differences in their functional requirements. Myocardial thickness also differs between individuals, both in health and in various disease states.

Hypertrophy of the heart muscle may occur due to the effects of long-standing physical exertion and training, as in athletes, or it may occur in pathological states. High blood pressure (***hypertension***) leads to the heart muscle pumping against increased resistance and this commonly causes marked thickening of the left ventricular wall. Less commonly but importantly, there are inherited forms of cardiac hypertrophy such as hypertrophic cardiomyopathy (see e-Fig. 8.1). This disorder is an important cause of sudden unexpected cardiac death, especially in young athletes.

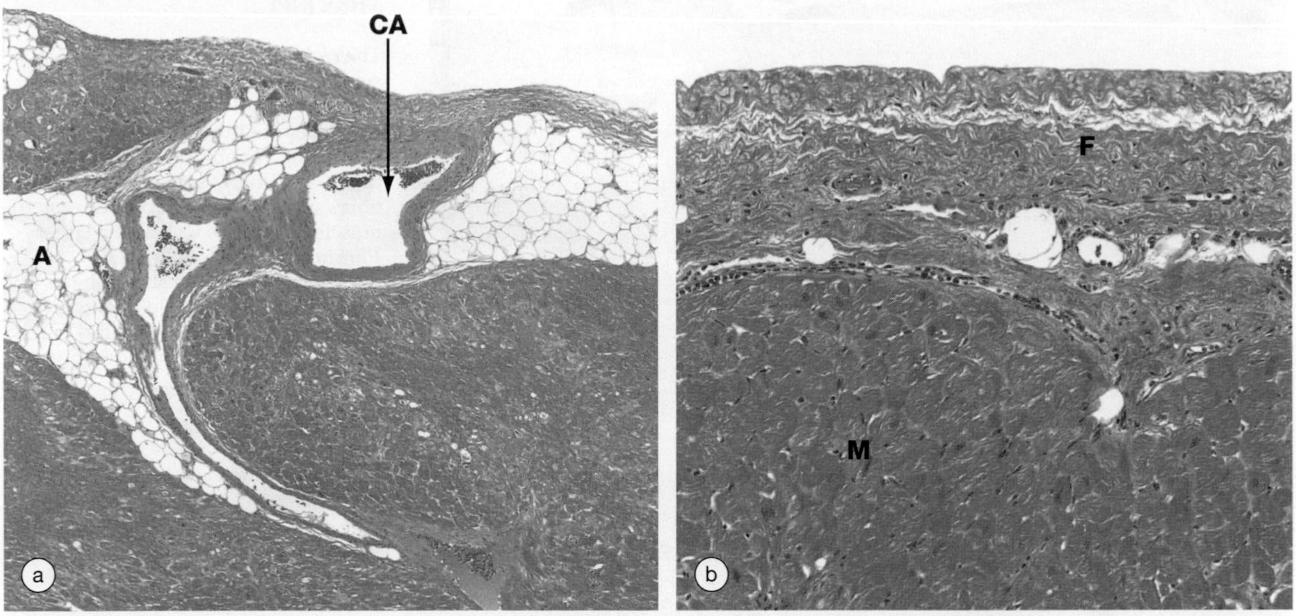

FIG. 8.2 Heart: epicardium (visceral pericardium)
(a) H&E (MP) (b) H&E (HP)

The constant layer of the epicardium is a dense sheet of fibrocollagenous tissue **F** which also contains elastic fibres. On its outer surface, there is a flat monolayer of mesothelial cells (not clearly seen here). These cells are responsible for secretion of lubricating fluid. Fig. 8.2a shows an area where the epicardium contains a large branch of the ***coronary artery*** **CA**, with a smaller branch penetrating the myocardium **M**. Note that in areas containing artery branches, there is a variable layer of adipose tissue **A**. Fig. 8.2b shows the appearance of the epicardium over most of the heart surface, where the fibrocollagenous layer **F** lies directly on the myocardium **M** without significant intervening adipose tissue.

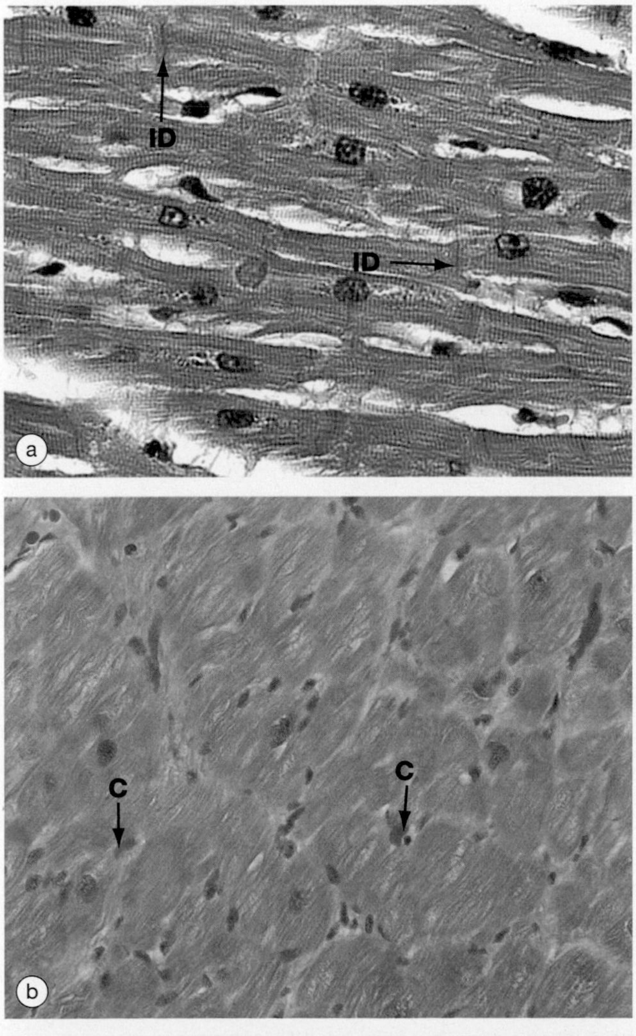

FIG. 8.3 Myocardium
(a) H&E, LS (HP) (b) H&E, TS (HP)

In longitudinal section (Fig. 8.3a), cardiac muscle fibres form an interconnecting network, joined to each other by ***intercalated discs*** **ID**. These specialised intercellular junctions provide both mechanical and electrophysiological coupling, allowing the cardiac myocytes to act as a functional syncytium. The cells possess central nuclei and regular cytoplasmic cross-striations. The intercalated discs and cross-striations can be clearly seen using special methods such as the immunohistochemical technique for α-B crystallin and in thin resin sections stained with toluidine blue (see Fig. 6.24).

In transverse section in Fig. 8.3b, the extensive and intimate capillary network **C** between the myocardial fibres is easily seen. The vessels in this section are distended with red blood cells (see also Fig. 6.21). This high level of vascularity is a reflection of the high and constant oxygen demand of the myocardium, particularly in the left ventricle which is shown in these two pictures. Further structural details of the cardiac muscle of the myocardium are given in Ch. 6.

Myocarditis

Myocarditis is an uncommon inflammatory disorder affecting the cardiac muscle. Its causes are diverse, but viral forms are the most frequent. The diagnosis requires the combination of interstitial inflammation (inflammation between myocytes) and myocyte damage (known as the ***Dallas criteria***). Myocarditis can be classified by the predominance of inflammatory cells seen on microscopy. A lymphocytic myocarditis is the typical pattern seen in viral myocarditis (see e-Fig. 8.2a). An eosinophilic myocarditis can be seen in the setting of hypersensitivity. Other rarer types of myocarditis include giant cell myocarditis (see e-Fig. 8.2b). Sarcoidosis, a systemic granulomatous condition, is a cause of granulomatous myocarditis (see e-Fig. 8.2c).

A adipose tissue **C** capillary **CA** coronary artery **E** endocardium **F** fibrocollagenous pericardium **ID** intercalated disc
M myocardium **P** pericardium **PM** papillary muscle

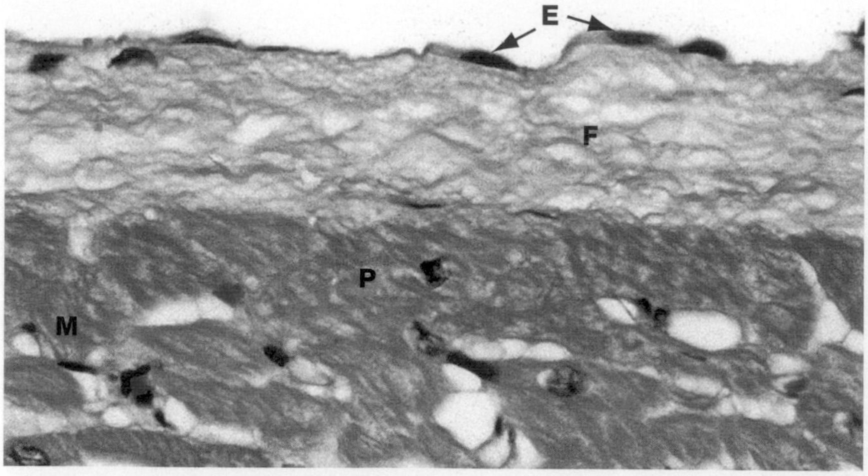

FIG. 8.4 Endocardium H&E (HP)

The *endocardium* (Fig. 8.4) has a surface layer of flattened endothelial cells **E**. The endothelium is supported by a layer of fibrous connective tissue **F** containing variable amounts of elastic tissue. This merges into the collagen fibres surrounding adjacent cardiac muscle cells **M**, as well as the larger *Purkinje fibres* **P** (see Fig. 8.6).

The endocardium shown here is from the wall of the left ventricle. The endocardium of the atria is much thicker than this and includes more elastic fibres.

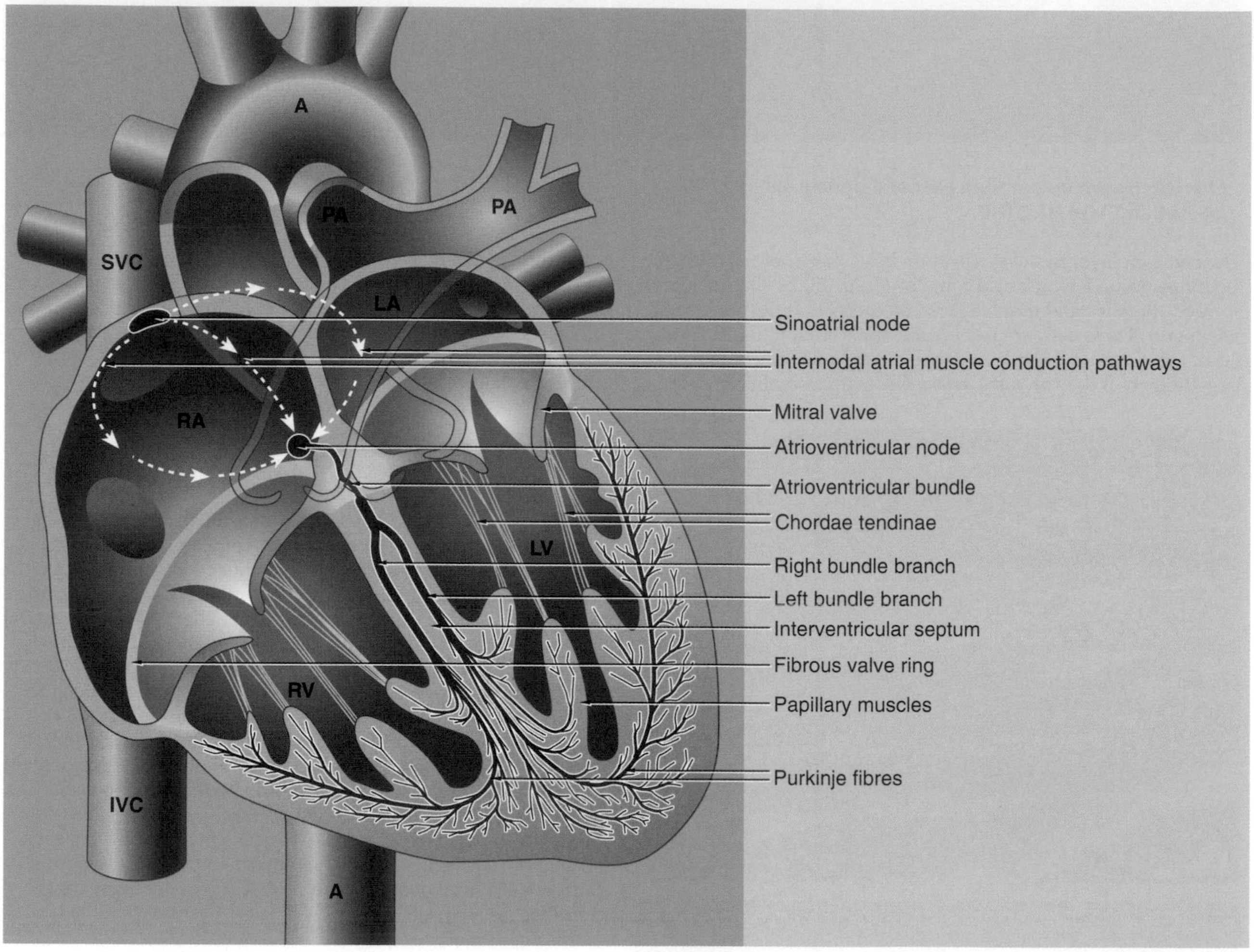

FIG. 8.5 The conducting system of the heart

The co-ordinated contraction of the heart is largely effected by a specialised *conducting system* of modified cardiac muscle fibres (Fig. 8.5). The initial impulse originates spontaneously in the *sinoatrial node*, situated in the right atrial wall near the entry of the superior vena cava **SVC**. The impulse rate is controlled by the autonomic nervous system.

The impulse passes through the muscle of the atria **RA** and **LA**, causing them to contract, and reaches the *atrioventricular node* in the medial wall of the right atrium just above the tricuspid valve ring at the base of the interatrial septum. Both the sinoatrial and atrioventricular nodes are irregular meshworks of very small specialised myocardial fibres, with electrochemical stimuli being transmitted via *gap junctions*. The nodal fibres are embedded in collagenous fibrous tissue which contains blood vessels and many autonomic nerve fibres.

From the atrioventricular node, the impulse is passed along a specialised bundle of conducting fibres, the *atrioventricular bundle (of His)*, which initially divides into right and left bundle branches that then (halfway down the interventricular septum) become *Purkinje fibres* which run immediately beneath the endocardium before penetrating the myocardium (see Figs 8.4 and 8.6).

A aorta **BB** bundle branch **E** endothelial cell **En** endocardium **F** fibrous connective tissue **IVC** inferior vena cava **LA** left atrium **LF** lamina fibrosa **LV** left ventricle **M** cardiac myocytes **P** Purkinje fibre **PA** pulmonary artery **RA** right atrium **RV** right ventricle **SVC** superior vena cava **VR** valve ring

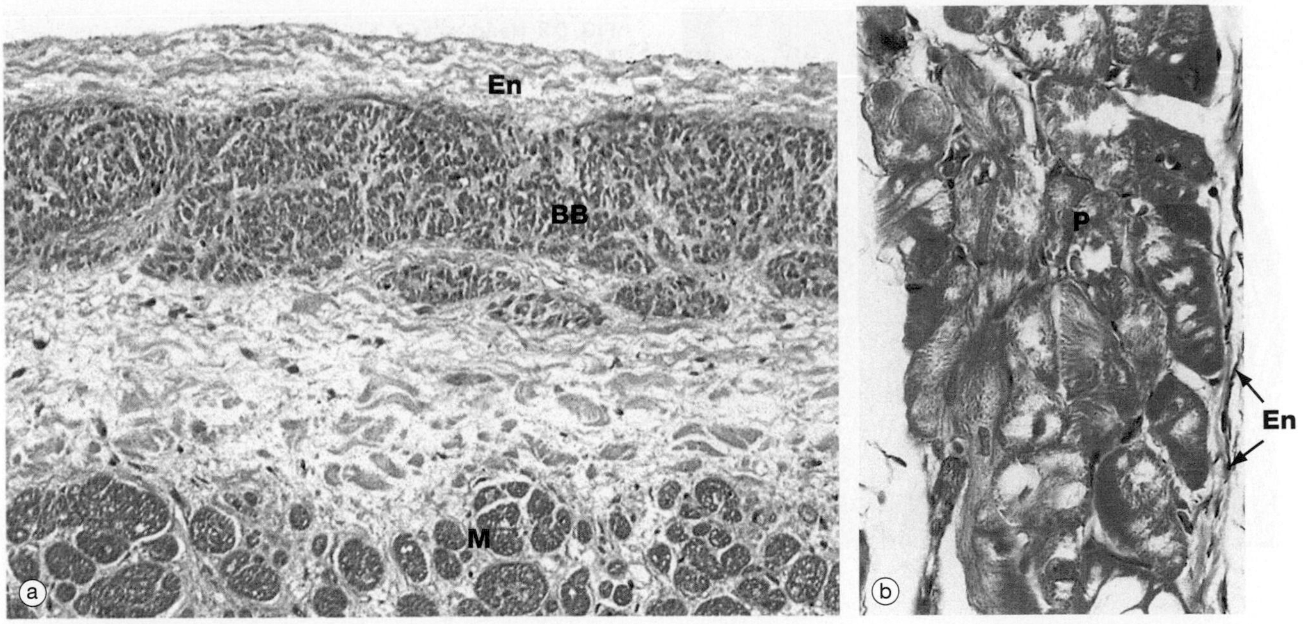

FIG. 8.6 Heart
(a) Bundle branch, H&E (MP) (b) Purkinje fibres, H&E (HP)

Fig. 8.6a shows the left branch bundle of conducting fibres **BB** running in the interventricular septum, just beneath the endocardium **En** lining the left ventricular cavity. At this level, the conducting fibres are separated from the myocardial fibres **M** of the septum by a layer of fibrous tissue. The conducting fibres are specialised cardiac muscle fibres and contain comparatively few myofibrils, which are mainly located beneath the cell membrane, but abundant glycogen granules and mitochondria. This makes these fibres paler staining than normal myocardial fibres by most stains.

Fig. 8.6b shows the distal extension of the branch bundle, with the ***Purkinje fibres*** **P** beneath the thin endocardium **En**. These fibres are larger than cardiac muscle fibres and have a pale-staining central area with most of the red-staining myofibrils around the periphery of the cell. Unlike myocardial fibres, Purkinje and other conducting fibres have no T tubule system and connect with each other by desmosomes and gap junctions, rather than intercalated discs.

Common disorders of the myocardium

The myocardial cells have a high energy demand and therefore a high and constant oxygen requirement. When there is a reduction of blood flow to the myocardium caused by ***atherosclerosis*** of the epicardial coronary arteries (e-Fig. 8.3a), the cardiac myocytes supplied by the artery can die (***necrosis***). The patient develops ***angina*** (a characteristic crushing central chest pain on exertion, disappearing on rest). With increasingly severe ischaemia of the myocardium, the angina symptoms appear with minimal or no exertion.

Histologically, the dead muscle fibres are replaced by collagenous fibrous tissue (***replacement fibrosis***) (e-Fig. 8.3b) and remaining muscle fibres enlarge and increase their work rate (***hypertrophy***) to compensate (e-Fig. 8.3c).

When a coronary artery suddenly becomes completely occluded (e.g. by ***thrombosis***), a substantial mass of the heart muscle cells dies. For example, the muscle comprising the entire anterior wall of the left ventricle and the anterior part of the interventricular septum dies if the left anterior descending coronary artery is blocked. This is called ***myocardial infarction***, commonly referred to as a 'heart attack'. Death of some of the conducting bundles of Purkinje fibres can also lead to potentially fatal abnormalities of cardiac rhythm (***arrhythmia***). When the area of infarction heals, the large areas of replacement fibrosis are strong but not contractile, so the patient may suffer from persistent left ***heart failure*** as the heart cannot adequately pump blood from the left ventricle to the systemic circulation.

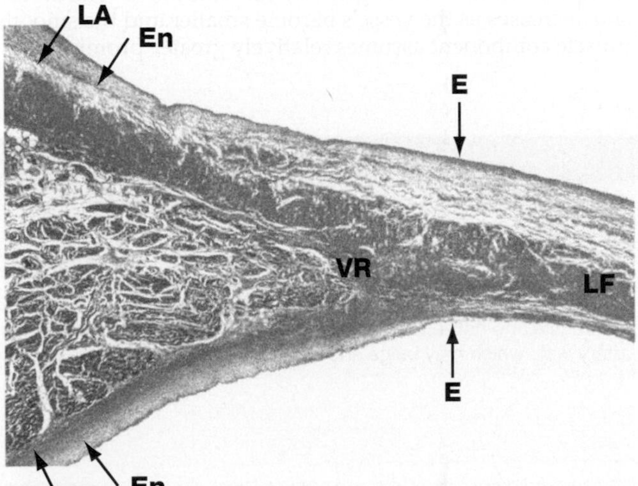

FIG. 8.7 Heart valve
H&E (LP)

The heart valves consist of leaflets of fibroelastic tissue. The surfaces are covered by a thin layer of endothelium **E** which is continuous with that lining the heart chambers and great vessels. This low-power image in Fig. 8.7 shows the left atrioventricular valve (the ***mitral valve***), arising at the junction of the walls of the left atrium **LA** and left ventricle **LV**.

The fibroelastic layer of the endocardium **En** condenses to form the ***valve ring*** **VR**, and from this arises the central fibroelastic sheet of the valve, the ***lamina fibrosa*** **LF**.

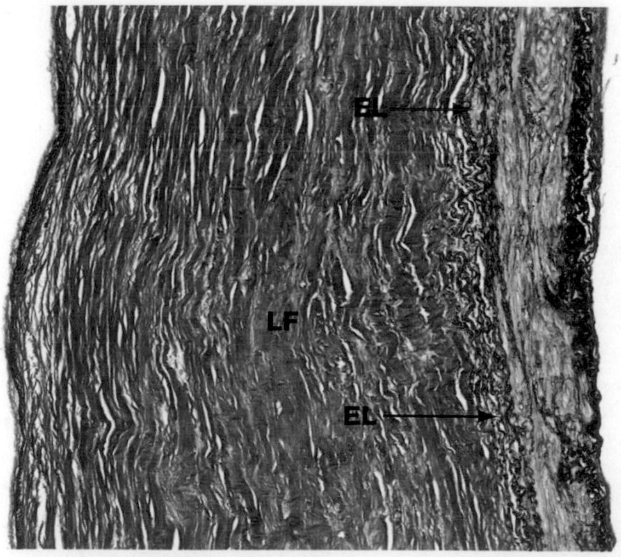

FIG. 8.8 Heart valve
Elastic van Gieson (LP)

The valves are sheets of fibroelastic tissue covered on both sides by endocardium (Fig. 8.8). There is a dense central plate of collagen (the ***lamina fibrosa*** **LF**) containing scattered elastic fibres (black in this stain) as shown in the micrograph at low magnification. In the left atrioventricular valves (as here), there is a distinct elastic lamina (**EL**) towards the atrial surface and the collagen (red staining here) is particularly prominent on the ventricular surface where the chordae tendinae are attached.

Common disorders of heart valves

The aortic valve normally has three cusps, but occasionally there are only two (bicuspid) due to a developmental anomaly. Bicuspid aortic valves are particularly prone to develop fibrous thickening, within which calcium salts are deposited to make fibrocalcific nodules. These severely distort the cusps, which also tend to fuse. This disease, called ***calcific aortic valve disease*** (see e-Fig. 8.4a), interferes with valve function, reducing flow of blood through the valve during systole (***aortic stenosis***) and allowing blood to leak back from the aorta into the left ventricle during diastole (***aortic regurgitation***).

Thrombosis may occur on the free edges of heart valves and, if there is subsequent ***bacteraemia***, they may become infected (***valvitis*** or ***endocarditis***) (see e-Fig. 8.4b). Depending on the bacterium involved, the infected thrombus may erode the valve, leading to severe valve failure, or fragments of the thrombus may break off and pass in the circulation to distant sites where they may block arteries (***embolism***).

THE ARTERIAL SYSTEM

The function of the arterial system is to distribute blood from the heart to capillary beds throughout the body. The cyclical pumping action of the heart produces a pulsatile blood flow in the arterial system. With each contraction of the ventricles (***systole***), blood is forced into the arterial system causing expansion of the arterial walls; subsequent recoil of the arterial walls assists in maintenance of arterial blood pressure between ventricular beats (***diastole***). This expansion and recoil is a function of elastic tissue within the walls of the arteries.

The flow of blood to various organs and tissues may be regulated by varying the diameter of the distributing vessels. This function is performed by the circumferentially disposed smooth muscle of vessel walls and is principally under the control of the sympathetic nervous system and adrenal medullary hormones.

The walls of the arterial vessels conform to the general three-layered structure of the circulatory system but are characterised by the presence of considerable elastin and the smooth muscle wall is thick relative to the diameter of the lumen. There are three main types of vessel in the arterial system:

- **Elastic arteries**. These comprise the major distribution vessels and include the aorta, the innominate (brachiocephalic trunk), common carotid and subclavian arteries and most of the large pulmonary arterial vessels.
- **Muscular arteries**. These are the main distributing branches of the arterial tree, such as the radial, femoral, coronary and cerebral arteries.
- **Arterioles**. These are the terminal branches of the arterial tree which supply the capillary beds.

There is a gradual transition in structure and function between the three types of arterial vessel rather than an abrupt demarcation. In general, the amount of elastic tissue decreases as the vessels become smaller and the smooth muscle component assumes relatively greater prominence.

Common disorders of arteries

Elastic and muscular arteries develop ***atherosclerosis*** in which lipid material infiltrates the tunica intima and accumulates in macrophages. This stimulates the proliferation of intimal fibroblasts and myointimal cells, with collagen deposition to produce a ***plaque*** which thickens the intima. If severe and in a small-diameter artery, this intimal thickening can severely reduce the artery lumen and limit the blood flow. These plaques commonly rupture, leading to aggregation of platelets and fibrin. This forms a ***thrombus*** (see e-Fig. 8.5) which narrows the vessel lumen leading to infarction.

A further consequence of severe atheroma in elastic arteries is that the muscle cells in the tunica media are replaced by non-contractile and non-elastic collagen, leading to a weakness in the artery wall, which may bulge and rupture (***aneurysm***).

A tunica adventitia **EEL** external elastic lamina **EL** elastic lamina **I** tunica intima **IEL** internal elastic lamina **LF** lamina fibrosa **M** tunica media **VV** vasa vasorum

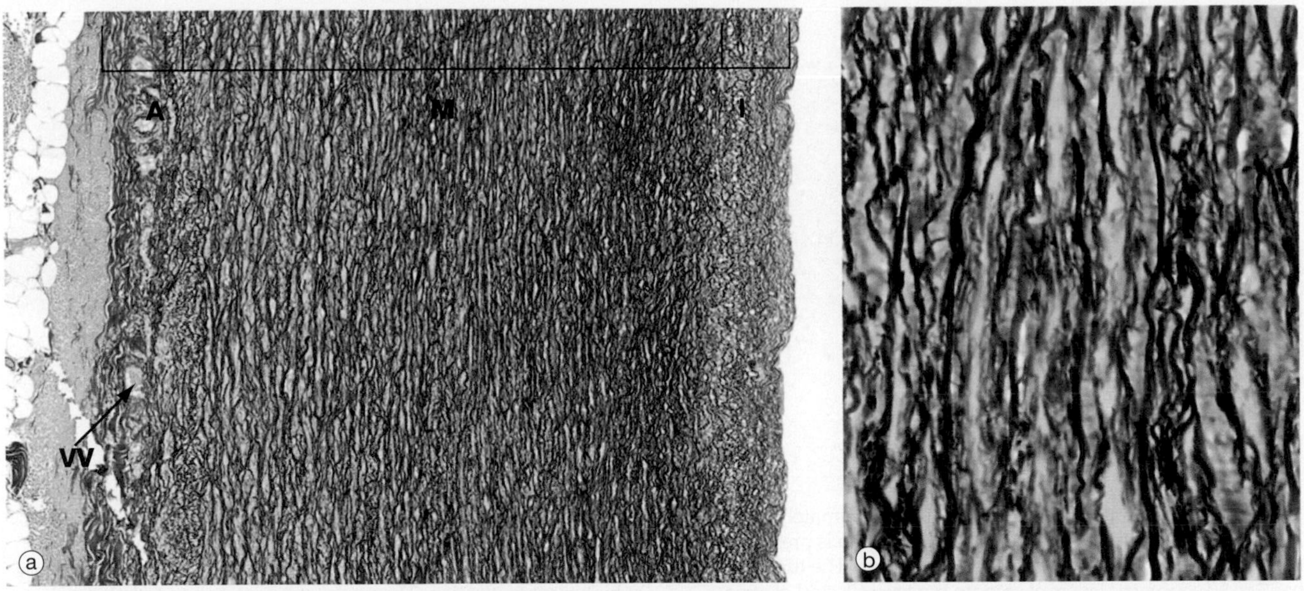

FIG. 8.9 Elastic artery: aorta
(a) Elastic van Gieson (LP) (b) Elastic van Gieson (HP)

The highly elastic nature of the aortic wall is demonstrated in these preparations in which the elastic fibres are stained brownish-black. In Fig. 8.9a, the three basic layers of the wall can be seen: the narrow ***tunica intima*** **I**, the broad ***tunica media*** **M** and the ***tunica adventitia*** **A**.

The tunica intima consists of a single layer of flattened endothelial cells (not seen at this magnification) supported by a layer of collagenous tissue rich in elastin disposed in the form of both fibres and discontinuous sheets. The subendothelial supporting tissue contains scattered fibroblasts and other cells with ultrastructural features akin to smooth muscle cells and known as ***myointimal cells***. Both cell types are probably involved in elaboration of the extracellular constituents. The myointimal cells are not invested by basement membrane and are thus not epithelial (myoepithelial) in nature. With increasing age, the myointimal cells accumulate lipid and the intima progressively thickens. If this process continues, ***atherosclerosis*** will develop.

The tunica media is particularly broad and extremely elastic. At high magnification in Fig. 8.9b, it is seen to consist of concentric fenestrated sheets of elastin (stained black) separated by collagenous tissue and smooth muscle fibres. As seen in Fig. 8.9a, the collagenous tunica adventitia (stained red) contains small ***vasa vasorum*** **VV** which also penetrate the outer half of the tunica media.

Blood flow within elastic arteries is highly pulsatile. With advancing age, the arterial system becomes less elastic, thereby increasing peripheral resistance and thus arterial blood pressure.

Aneurysms

An ***aneurysm*** is an abnormal and permanent dilatation of the wall of an artery. Various types of aneurysm can occur, and these can be classified in several different ways: according to morphology (shape) into ***saccular*** and ***fusiform*** types, according to aetiology (cause) into congenital, acquired, atherosclerotic, mycotic, etc., or by the nature of the aneurysmal wall into true or false aneurysms. The wall of a true aneurysm includes all of the normal layers of the vessel wall, whilst a false aneurysm is deficient in one or more of these layers and essentially represents a protrusion at a site of weakness or deficiency in the vessel wall.

Atherosclerotic aneurysms are common in developed cultures and most often affect the abdominal aorta (see e-Fig. 8.6a). These aneurysms are acquired and are usually fusiform in shape.

Rupture of such aneurysms can occur when the wall becomes attenuated due to increasing dilatation. Catastrophic and rapidly fatal haemorrhage can occur unless immediate treatment is available. If such aneurysms are identified before acute presentation with haemorrhage, planned operative repair can be performed. This approach dramatically reduces morbidity and mortality when compared against attempted repair after bleeding has occurred. Some patients can be treated by minimally invasive radiological techniques instead of open surgery.

An ***aortic dissection*** (see e-Fig. 8.6b) can be caused by weakening of the aortic wall due to longstanding hypertension or inherited connective tissue disease affecting the aorta, such as Marfan syndrome.

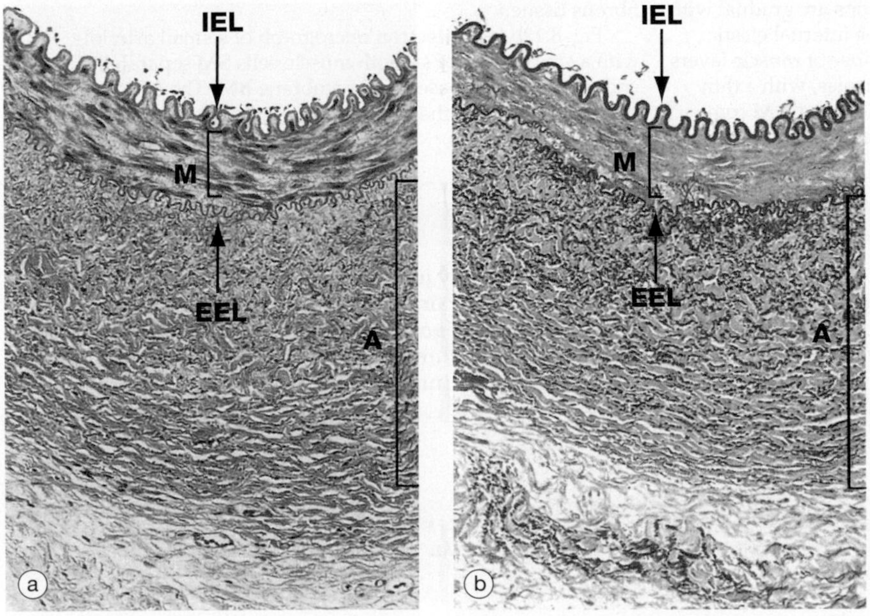

FIG. 8.10 Muscular artery
(a) H&E (MP) (b) Elastic van Gieson (MP)

In muscular arteries, as shown in Figs 8.10a and b, the elastic tissue is largely concentrated as two well-defined elastic sheets. One sheet is the ***internal elastic lamina*** **IEL** between the tunica intima and the tunica media. The less prominent and more variable ***external elastic lamina*** **EEL** lies between the tunica media **M** and the adventitia. The tunica intima is usually a very thin layer, not visible at low magnification, and the tunica media **M** is composed of concentrically arranged smooth muscle fibres with scanty elastic fibres between them. The tunica adventitia **A** is of variable thickness and is composed of collagen and a variable amount of elastic tissue. In larger muscular arteries, this layer may contain prominent vasa vasorum.

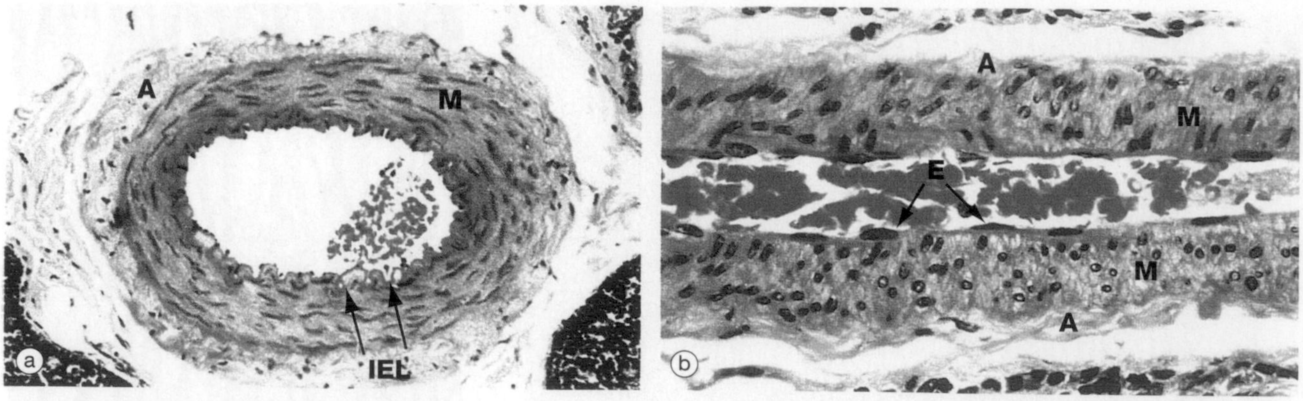

FIG. 8.11 Small muscular artery
(a) H&E, TS (MP) (b) H&E, LS (HP)

The diameter of a small muscular artery is approximately 0.5 to 2 mm and a thin but distinct internal elastic lamina is present, but there is usually little or no external elastic lamina. The tunica media has 3 to 10 concentric layers of smooth muscle cells and contains almost no elastic fibres. Fig. 8.11a shows an artery in transverse section. The distinction between the tunica media **M** and adventitia **A** is obvious. The internal elastic lamina **IEL** can just be distinguished as a densely staining wavy line. Fig. 8.11b is a smaller artery at higher magnification. The nuclei of the intimal endothelial cells **E** are visible, but the elastic lamina has largely disappeared.

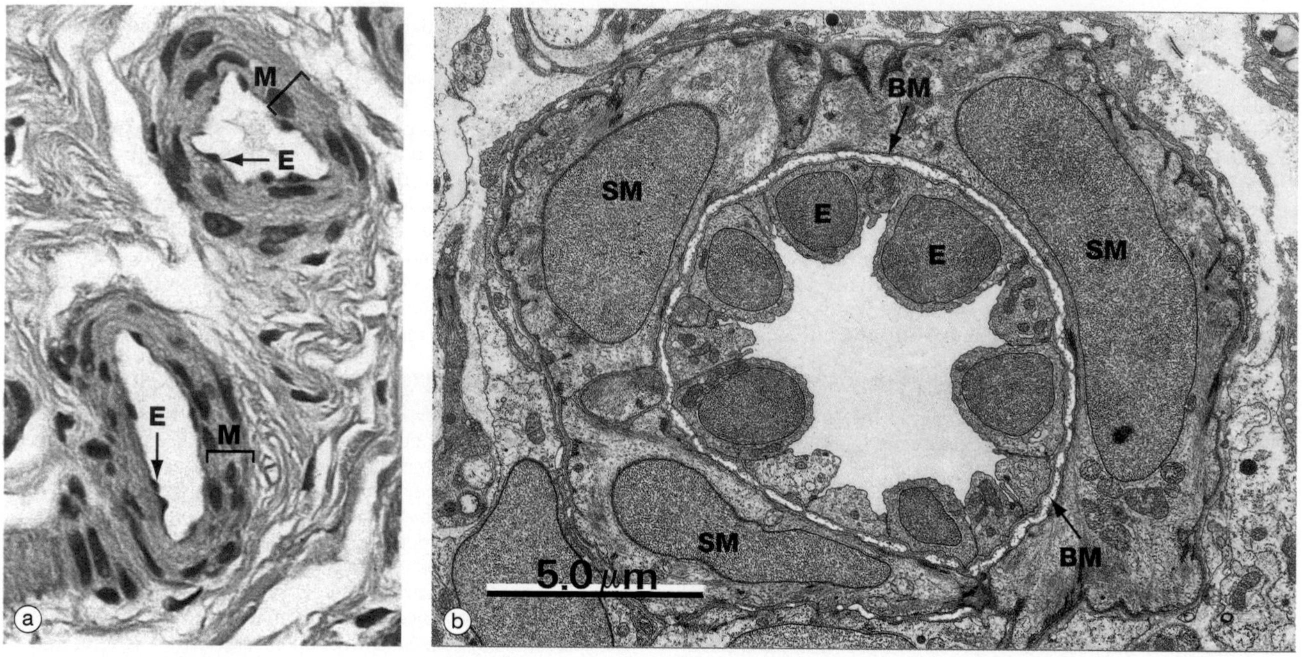

FIG. 8.12 Arterioles
(a) Large arteriole H&E, TS (MP) (b) Small arteriole, EM ×5250, TS

Small muscular arteries merge into large arterioles, which eventually become small arterioles. These transitions are gradual with no sharp demarcations and involve loss of the internal elastic lamina and progressive reduction of the number of muscle layers in the media. Fig. 8.12a shows two large arterioles, with a thin intima lined by endothelial cells **E** and a tunica media **M** comprising only 2 to 3 layers of muscle. The adventitia is thin and merges imperceptibly with surrounding supporting collagenous fibrous tissue.

Fig. 8.12b is an electron micrograph of a small arteriole, with a single layer of smooth muscle cells **SM** separated from endothelium **E** by basement membrane **BM**. The endothelium is prominent because the arteriole is constricted.

THE MICROCIRCULATION

The ***microcirculation*** is that part of the circulatory system concerned with the exchange of gases, fluids, nutrients and metabolic waste products. Exchange occurs mainly within the capillaries, extremely thin-walled vessels forming an interconnected network. Blood flow within the capillary bed is controlled by the ***arterioles*** and muscular sphincters at the arteriolar–capillary junctions called ***precapillary sphincters***. The capillaries drain into a series of vessels of increasing diameter, namely ***postcapillary venules***, ***collecting venules*** and ***small muscular venules*** which make up the venous component of the microcirculation.

A tunica adventitia **At** arteriole **BM** basement membrane **BMp** pericyte basement membrane **C** capillary
E endothelial cell **F** collagen fibrils **IEL** internal elastic lamina **M** tunica media **Ma** metarteriole **MF** marginal fold
P pericyte **S** arteriovenous shunt **SM** smooth muscle cell **V** venule

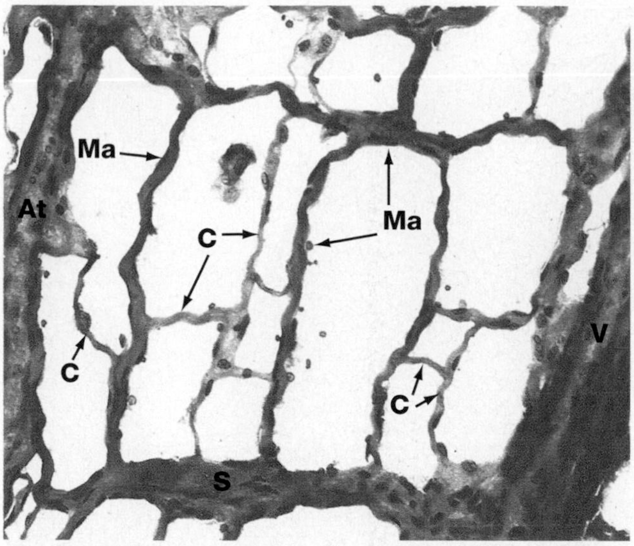

FIG. 8.13 The microcirculation, mesenteric spread H&E (MP)

Fig. 8.13 demonstrates a network of anastomosing capillaries between an arteriole **At** and a venule **V**. The capillary network comprises small-diameter capillaries **C** with a single layer of endothelial cells and basement membrane, as well as larger-diameter capillaries known as ***metarterioles*** **Ma**. These are characterised by a discontinuous outer layer of smooth muscle cells. Small capillaries arise from both arterioles and metarterioles.

At the origin of each capillary, there is a sphincter mechanism, the ***precapillary sphincter***, which is involved in regulation of blood flow. There is also a direct wide-diameter link between the arteriole and venule, an ***arteriovenous shunt*** **S**. Metarterioles also form direct communications between arterioles and venules. Contraction of the smooth muscle of shunts and metarterioles directs blood through the network of small capillaries. Thus arterioles, metarterioles, precapillary sphincters and arteriovenous shunts regulate blood flow in the microcirculation. The smooth muscle activity of these vessels is modulated by the autonomic nervous system and by circulating hormones (e.g. adrenal catecholamines).

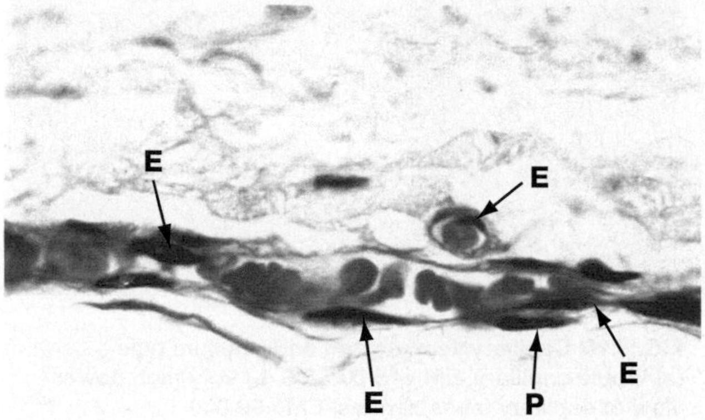

FIG. 8.14 Capillaries H&E (HP)

The vessels seen in Fig. 8.14 in longitudinal and transverse section illustrate the characteristic features of capillaries. A single layer of flattened endothelial cells lines the capillary lumen. The thin layer of cytoplasm is difficult to resolve by light microscopy.

The flattened endothelial cell nuclei **E** bulge into the capillary lumen. In longitudinal section, the nuclei appear elongated, whereas in transverse section they appear more rounded.

Muscular and adventitial layers are absent. Occasional flattened cells called ***pericytes*** **P** embrace the capillary endothelial cells and may have a contractile function. Note that the diameter of capillaries is similar to that of the red blood cells contained within them.

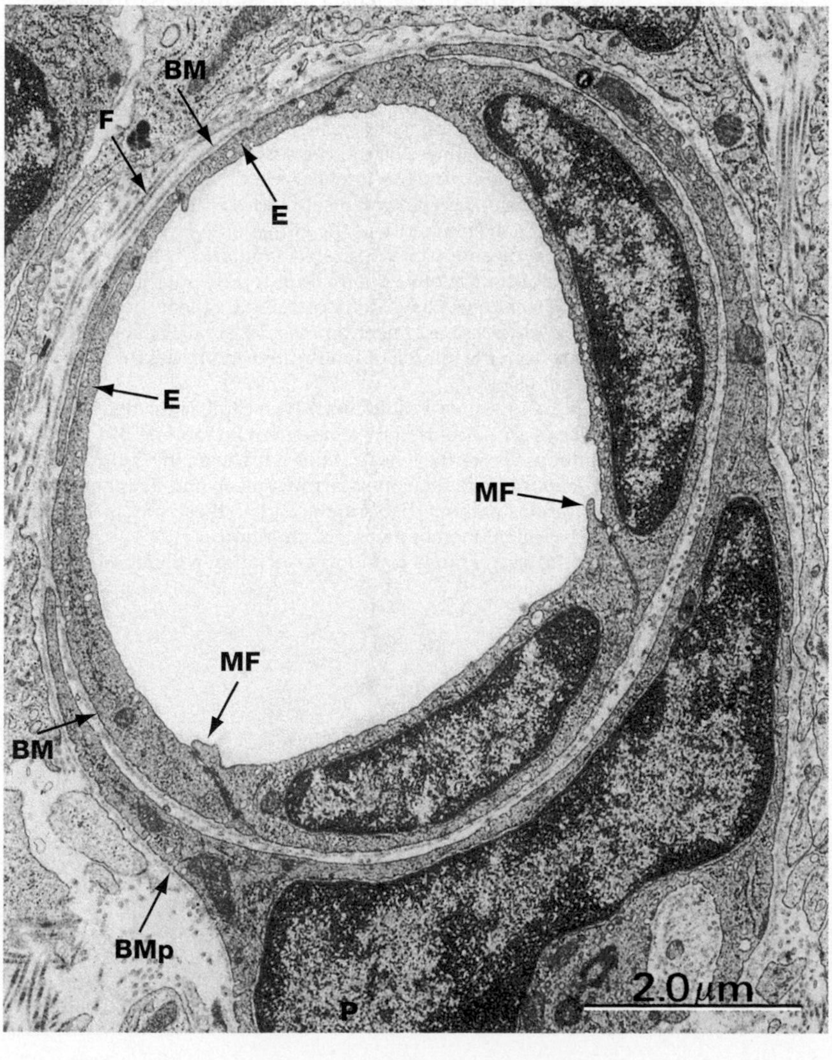

FIG. 8.15 Capillary, continuous endothelium type EM ×12 000

This electron micrograph (Fig. 8.15) illustrates the ultrastructure of capillaries of the continuous endothelium type, the type found in most tissues. Endothelial cells **E** encircle the capillary lumen, their plasma membranes approximating one another very closely and bound together by scattered tight junctions of the fascia occludens type (see Fig. 5.11). Small cytoplasmic flaps called ***marginal folds*** **MF** extend across the intercellular junctions at the luminal surface. The capillary endothelium is supported by a thin ***basement membrane*** **BM** and adjacent collagen fibrils **F**. A pericyte **P** embraces the capillary and is supported by its own basement membrane **BMp**.

Exchange between the lumen of the continuous-type capillary and the surrounding tissues is believed to occur in three ways. ***Passive diffusion*** through the endothelial cell cytoplasm mediates exchange of gases, ions and low molecular weight metabolites. Proteins and some lipids are transported by ***pinocytotic vesicles*** (see Ch. 1). White blood cells pass through the intercellular space between the endothelial cells, in some way negotiating the endothelial intercellular junctions. Some researchers maintain that the intercellular spaces also permit molecular transport. In capillaries of the continuous endothelial type, the basement membrane is thought to present little barrier to exchange between capillaries and surrounding tissues.

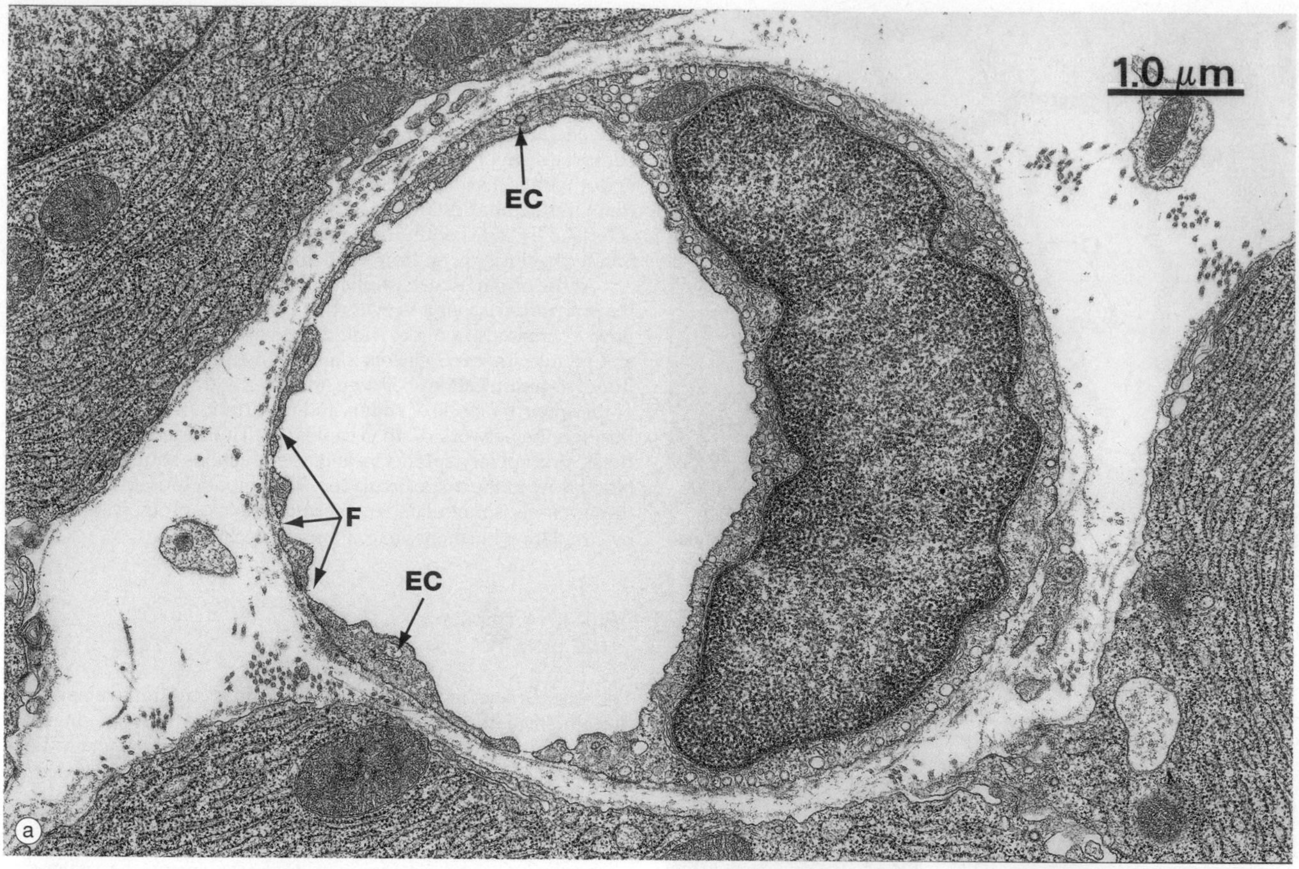

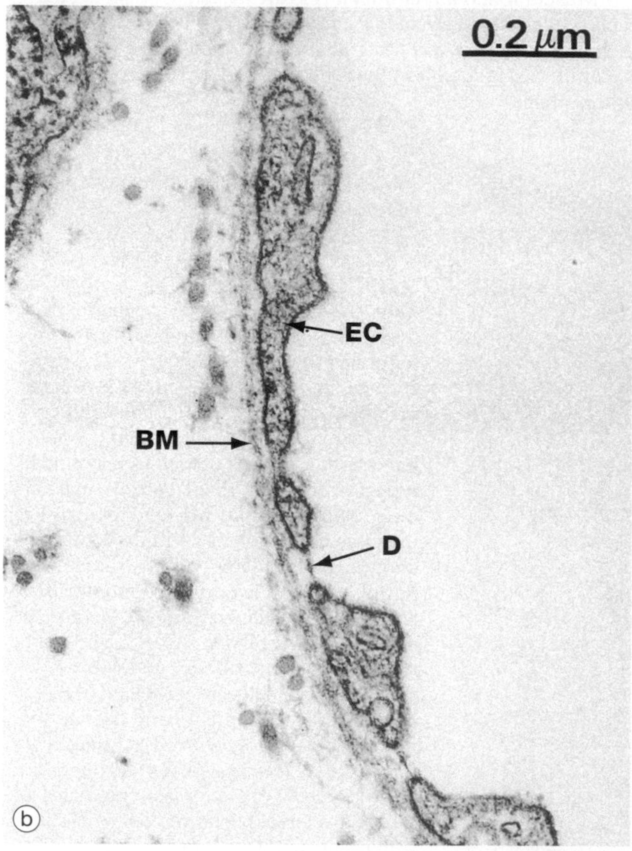

FIG. 8.16 Capillary, fenestrated endothelium type (a) Whole capillary, EM ×15 000, TS (b) Very high power view of capillary fenestrations, EM ×60 000

Fenestrated capillaries are found in some tissues where there is extensive molecular exchange with the blood. Such tissues include the small intestine, endocrine glands and kidney.

At low magnification in Fig. 8.16a, fenestrations **F** appear as pores through attenuated areas of the endothelial cytoplasm **EC**; however, only a small proportion of these areas are fenestrated. At high magnification in Fig. 8.16b, the fenestrations appear to be traversed by a thin electron-dense line **D** which may constitute a diaphragm. The biochemical and functional nature of this is not understood. Fenestrated capillaries without a diaphragm are found in the glomeruli of the kidney (see Fig. 16.14).

The permeability of fenestrated capillaries is much greater than that of continuous endothelium-type capillaries. Molecular labelling techniques have demonstrated that fenestrations permit rapid passage of macromolecules smaller than plasma proteins from the lumina of fenestrated capillaries into surrounding tissues.

Like continuous endothelium-type capillaries, all fenestrated capillaries are supported by a basement membrane **BM** which is continuous across the fenestrations. However, the endothelium of the ***sinusoids*** in the bone marrow, spleen and liver has large fenestrations without diaphragms and, in these sites, the underlying basement membrane is discontinuous.

Pericytes are rarely found in association with fenestrated capillaries.

BM basement membrane **D** diaphragm **EC** endothelial cell cytoplasm **F** fenestration **MF** marginal fold **Ps** pseudopodium **V** pinocytotic vesicle **WP** Weibel–Palade body

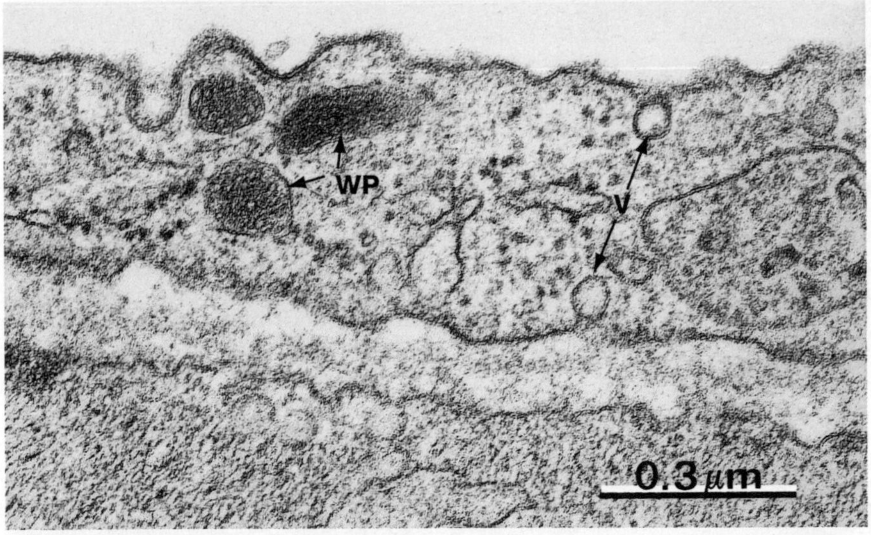

FIG. 8.17 Endothelial cell EM ×68 000

Endothelial cells are flat polygonal cells which are connected to each other by junctional complexes (Fig. 8.17). They have numerous pinocytotic vesicles **V** and specialised membrane-bound organelles called ***Weibel–Palade bodies*** **WP** which store von Willebrand factor.

Endothelial cells have a range of metabolic functions (see textbox 'Summary of functions of endothelial cells'), many concerned with the fine control of blood coagulation and thrombosis, as well as regulating local control of blood vessel constriction/dilatation and changes in vessel wall permeability. Endothelial cell damage may lead to pathological thrombosis or haemorrhage, or exudation of some components of blood into the extravascular tissues.

Summary of functions of endothelial cells

- Act as a permeability barrier
- Synthesise collagen and proteoglycans for basement membrane maintenance
- Synthesise and secrete molecules which minimise pathological thrombus formation e.g. prostacyclin, thrombomodulin, nitric oxide (which inhibits platelet adhesion and aggregation)

When damaged, endothelial cells:

- Secrete vasoactive factors controlling blood flow e.g. nitric oxide, prostacyclin and vasoactive peptides such as endothelin
- Synthesise and secrete molecules which promote protective thrombus formation e.g. von Willebrand factor (factor VIII)

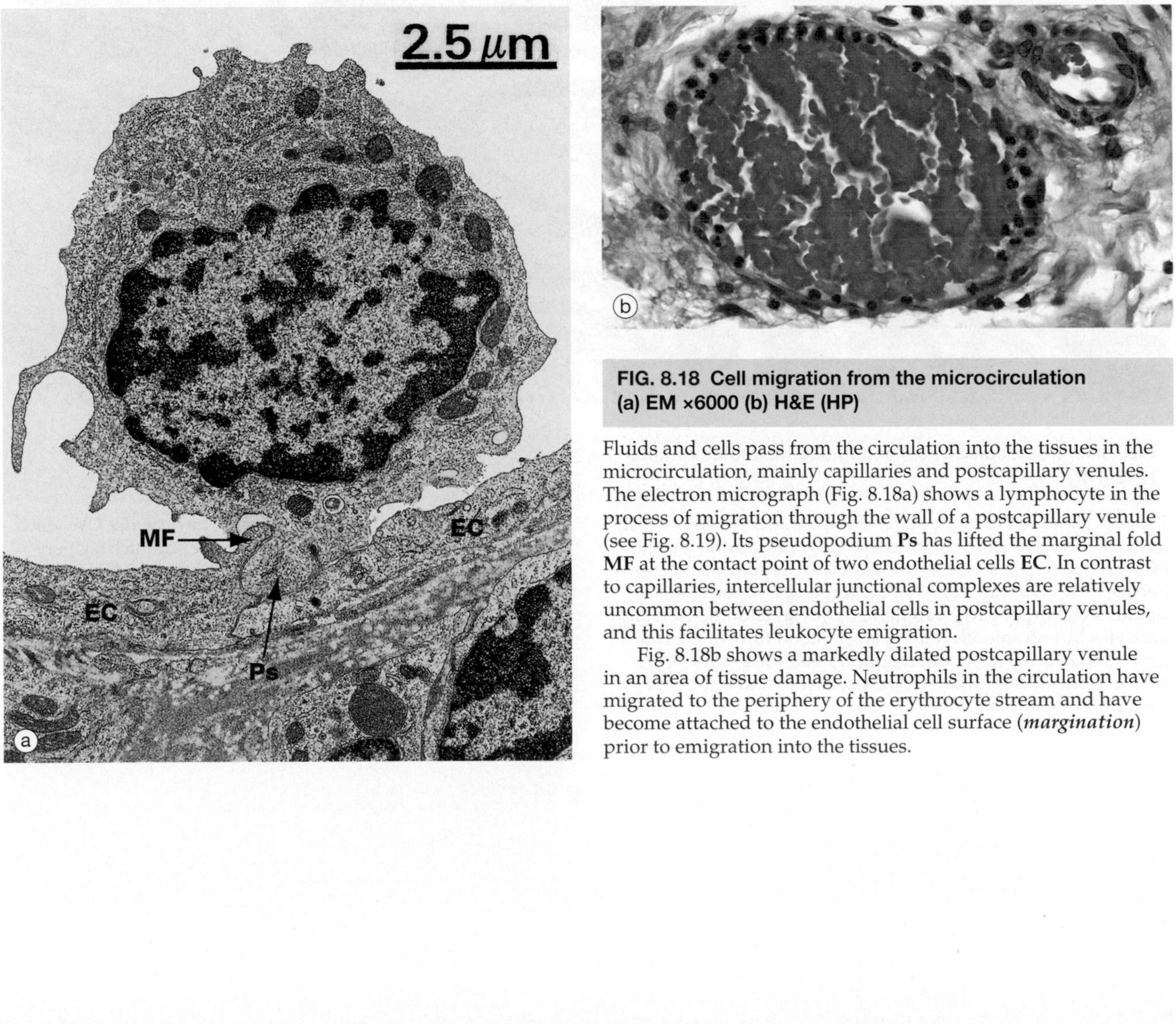

FIG. 8.18 Cell migration from the microcirculation (a) EM ×6000 (b) H&E (HP)

Fluids and cells pass from the circulation into the tissues in the microcirculation, mainly capillaries and postcapillary venules. The electron micrograph (Fig. 8.18a) shows a lymphocyte in the process of migration through the wall of a postcapillary venule (see Fig. 8.19). Its pseudopodium **Ps** has lifted the marginal fold **MF** at the contact point of two endothelial cells **EC**. In contrast to capillaries, intercellular junctional complexes are relatively uncommon between endothelial cells in postcapillary venules, and this facilitates leukocyte emigration.

Fig. 8.18b shows a markedly dilated postcapillary venule in an area of tissue damage. Neutrophils in the circulation have migrated to the periphery of the erythrocyte stream and have become attached to the endothelial cell surface (***margination***) prior to emigration into the tissues.

THE VENOUS SYSTEM

The systemic venous system is a low-pressure component of the blood circulatory system which is responsible for carrying blood from the capillary networks back to the right atrium of the heart.

The force impelling the blood towards the heart, often against gravity, is a combination of contraction of the smooth muscle of the vein wall and external compression of veins by contraction of skeletal muscles, particularly in the lower limbs. Backflow of blood is prevented by ***valves***, particularly in small and medium-sized veins. These valves are derived from the intima of the vessel. Valve failure in the veins of the legs is the basis for the development of the common condition known as varicose veins.

The structure of the venous system conforms to the general three-layered arrangement elsewhere in the circulatory system, but the elastic and muscular components are much less prominent features. A major part of the total blood volume is contained within the venous system.

Variations in relative blood volume, for example due to dilation of capillary beds or haemorrhage, may be compensated for by changes in the capacity of the venous system. These changes are mediated by contraction or relaxation of the smooth muscle in the tunica media. This controls the luminal diameter of muscular venules and veins.

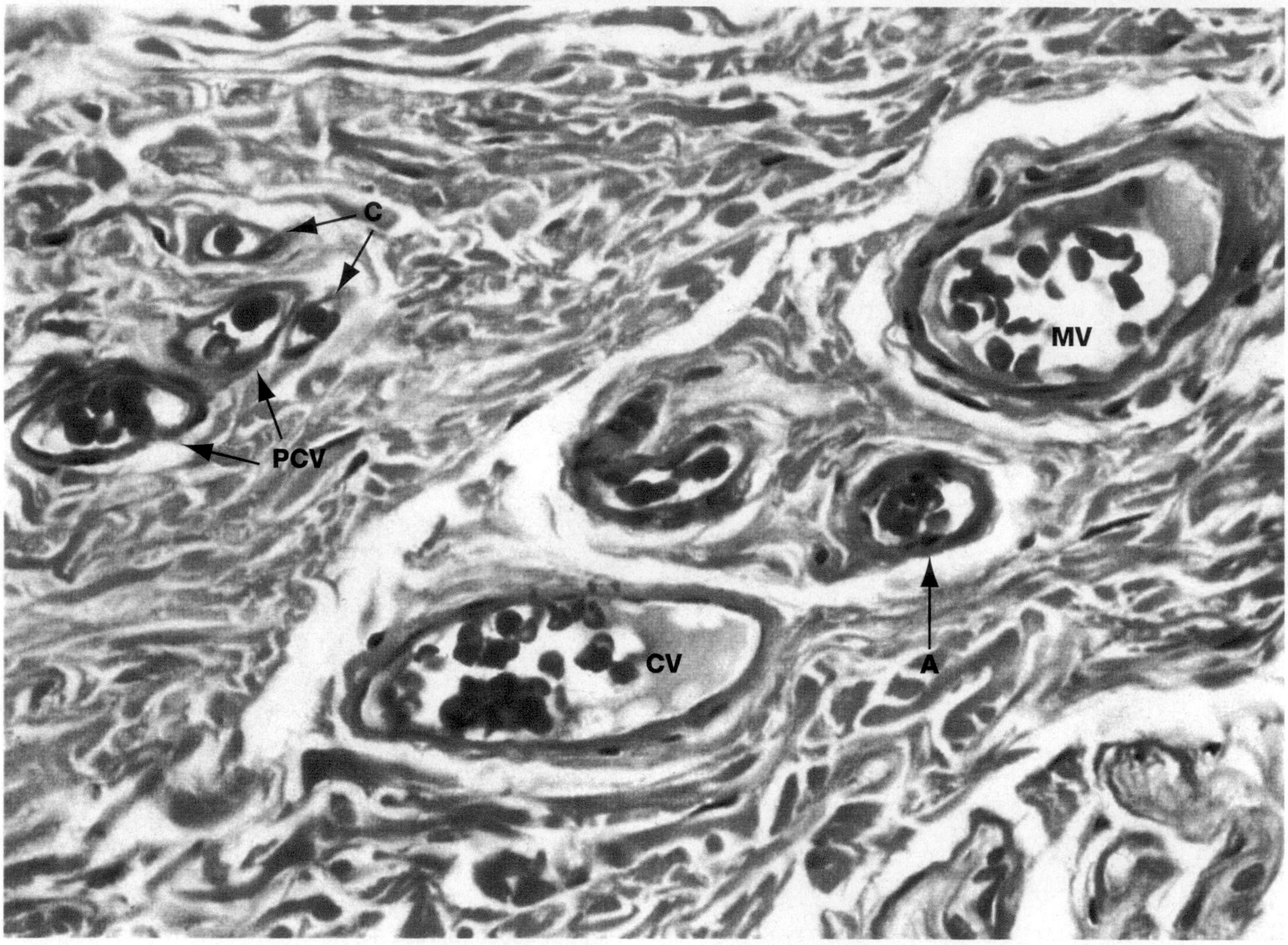

FIG. 8.19 Postcapillary, collecting and muscular venules H&E (HP)

The capillaries drain into a series of thin-walled vessels which form the first part of the venous system. ***Postcapillary venules*** **PCV** are the smallest of these vessels and are formed by confluence of several capillaries **C**. Postcapillary venules have a similar structure to large capillaries, with an endothelium and pericytes but no smooth muscle layer. Blood flow in postcapillary venules is sluggish and it appears that these vessels are the main site of migration of white cells into and out of the circulation.

Postcapillary venules drain into ***collecting venules*** **CV** which are structurally similar but larger, with more surrounding pericytes. Collecting venules drain into vessels of increasing diameter which eventually acquire a wall of smooth muscle cells two or three layers thick; at this stage the vessels are called ***muscular venules*** **MV**. This micrograph also shows a small arteriole **A** with only a single layer of smooth muscle cells in the wall. Its wall structure is similar to that of muscular venules, but the lumen is considerably smaller.

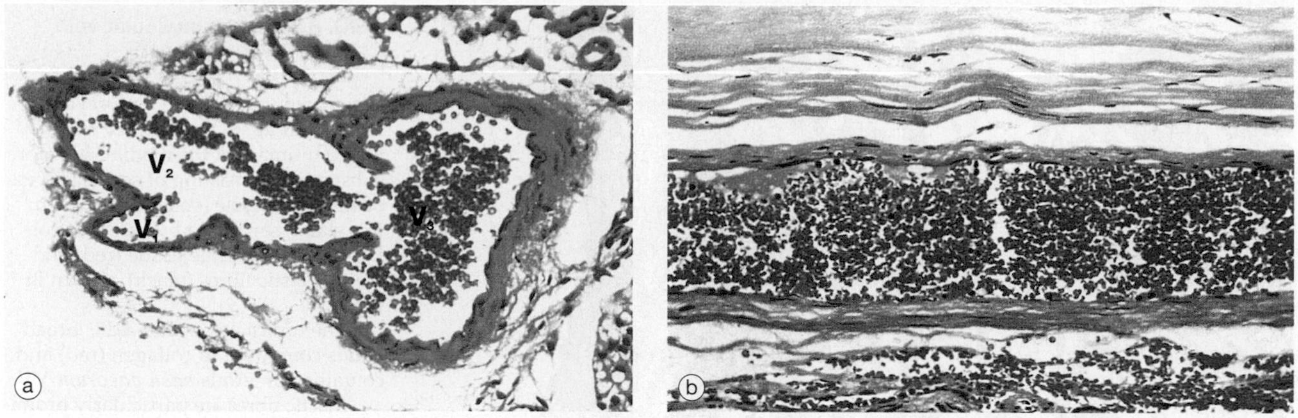

FIG. 8.20 Muscular venules and small veins
(a) H&E (MP) (b) H&E (MP)

Fig. 8.20a illustrates the confluence of a small muscular venule $\mathbf{V_1}$ with a larger muscular venule $\mathbf{V_2}$ which then joins a small vein $\mathbf{V_3}$ cut in transverse section. Note the valve at the junction of the large venule and vein. ***Muscular venules*** are characterised by a clearly defined intimal layer devoid of elastic fibres and a tunica media consisting of one or two layers of smooth muscle fibres. ***Veins*** are characterised by a thicker muscular wall and a poorly developed internal elastic lamina. Note that the tunica adventitia of these vessels is continuous with the surrounding collagenous supporting tissue.

Fig. 8.20b shows a small vein cut in longitudinal section and fixed whilst still distended with blood. The wall of the vein consists of two to three layers of smooth muscle fibres. Note the wide diameter of the lumen relative to the thickness of the wall.

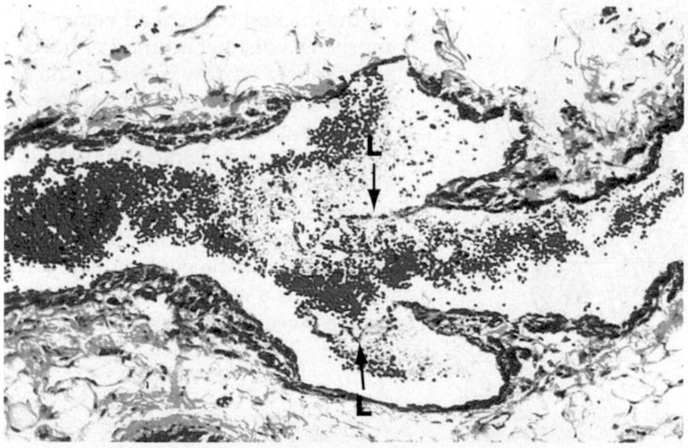

FIG. 8.21 Vein with valve
Masson trichrome (MP)

Fig. 8.21 demonstrates a valve in a small vein. The valve consists of delicate semilunar projections of the tunica intima of the vein wall. These projections are composed of a layer of fibroelastic tissue which is lined on both sides by endothelium.

Each valve usually consists of two ***leaflets*** **L**, the free edges of which project in the direction of blood flow. These serve to prevent backflow of blood due to the effects of gravity. Valves only occur in veins which are more than 2 mm in diameter, particularly those draining the extremities.

Varicose veins are abnormal dilatations of superficial veins which typically occur in the lower legs. These form due to incompetence of valves in the leg veins.

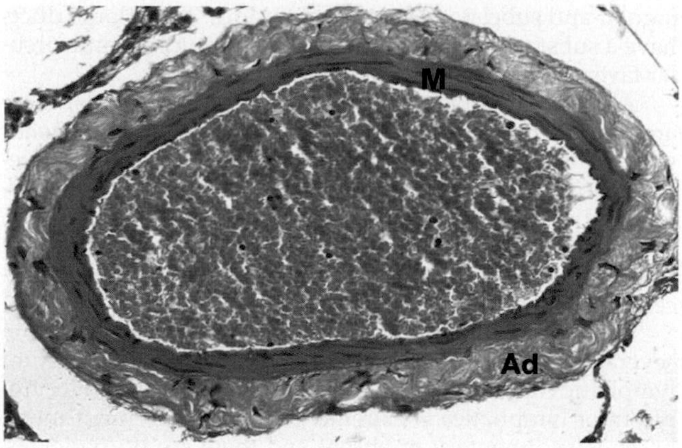

FIG. 8.22 Medium-sized vein
H&E (MP)

Fig. 8.22 shows a medium-sized vein which is distended with red blood cells. The tunica intima consists of little more than the endothelial cell layer supported by a very narrow band of supporting intimal fibrous tissue. The intima is difficult to discern in this micrograph. The tunica media **M** is thin when compared with that of an equivalent-sized artery (compare with Fig. 8.11a) and consists of only 2 to 4 layers of smooth muscle fibres. These are arranged in a circumferential fashion.

In veins, the tunica adventitia **Ad** is usually the thickest layer of the vessel wall. The adventitia is composed of collagenous fibrous tissue and the collagen fibres usually run in a predominantly longitudinal direction.

A arteriole **Ad** adventitia **C** capillary **CV** collecting venule **L** valve leaflet **M** media **MV** muscular venule **PCV** postcapillary venule **V** venule

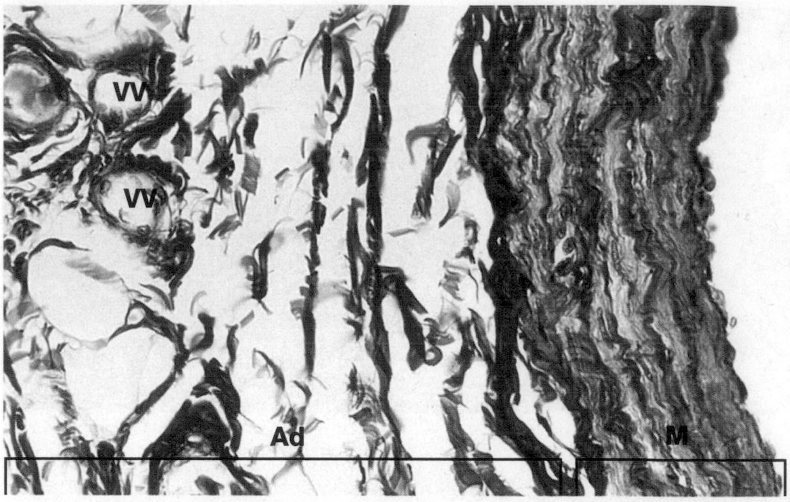

FIG. 8.23 Large muscular vein
Elastic van Gieson (HP)

Large veins such as the femoral and renal veins again have a very narrow tunica intima, but the media **M** is more substantial, consisting of several layers of smooth muscle (stained yellow in this stain), separated by layers of collagenous connective tissue (red) and scanty elastic fibres (black), shown in Fig. 8.23.

The tunica adventitia **Ad** is broad and is composed of collagen (red) and contains numerous ***vasa vasorum*** **VV**.

Elastic fibres are particularly prominent at the junction between media and adventitia, but there are no distinct elastic laminae as there are in arteries.

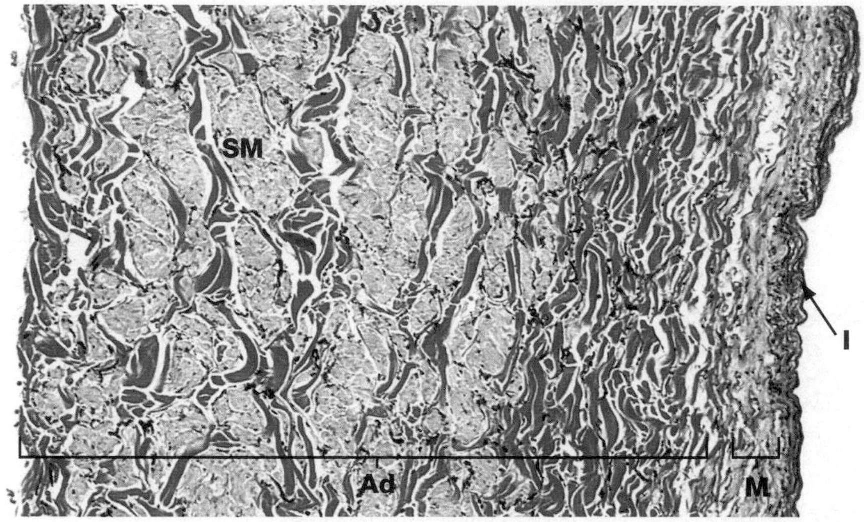

FIG. 8.24 Inferior vena cava
Elastic van Gieson (MP)

The ***superior*** and ***inferior venae cavae*** are the largest veins in the body and return deoxygenated blood from all areas of the body (except the lungs) to the right atrium of the heart. They have the thickest walls of all veins, comprising a distinct intima **I** of fibroelastic tissue, a narrow tunica media **M** composed of mainly circular smooth muscle, beneath which is a thick adventitia **Ad** composed of collagen (red) and thick bundles of longitudinally arranged smooth muscle fibres (yellow) **SM**. There are elastic fibres (black) scattered throughout the wall and, in some areas, there is a variable internal elastic lamina between intima and media.

THE LYMPH VASCULAR SYSTEM

The lymph vascular system drains excess fluid, the ***lymph***, from extracellular spaces and returns it to the blood vascular system. Lymph is formed in the following manner. At the arterial end of blood capillaries, the hydrostatic pressure of blood exceeds the colloidal osmotic pressure exerted by plasma proteins. Water and electrolytes therefore move out of capillaries and into the extracellular space. Some plasma proteins also leak out through the endothelial wall. At the venous end of blood capillaries, the pressure relationships are reversed and fluid tends to be drawn back into the blood vascular system. In this way, about 2% of plasma passing through the capillary bed is exchanged with the extracellular tissue fluid. The rate of tissue fluid formation at the arterial end of capillaries generally exceeds the re-uptake of fluid at the venous end. The excess fluid, lymph, is drained by a system of lymph capillaries which converge to form progressively larger-diameter lymphatic vessels.

As lymphatics get larger, they acquire smooth muscle cells in their walls and these contribute to the movement of lymph by pumping it onwards, the valves preventing backflow. Lymph eventually passes into much larger ducts (the ***thoracic*** and ***right lymphatic ducts***) which empty lymph into the blood circulation at the confluence of the internal jugular and subclavian veins of both sides. These large ducts have a substantial muscle layer with longitudinal and circular layers, but the layers are poorly demarcated.

Along the course of the larger lymphatic vessels, there are aggregations of lymphoid tissues called ***lymph nodes*** where lymph is sampled for the presence of foreign material (***antigen***) and where activated cells of the immune system and antibodies join the general circulation (see Ch. 11). Lymphatic vessels are found in all tissues except the central nervous system, cartilage, bone, bone marrow, thymus, placenta, cornea and teeth.

Lymphatic capillaries differ from blood capillaries in several respects which reflect the greater permeability of lymphatic capillaries. In particular, the endothelial cell cytoplasm of lymphatics is extremely thin, the basement membrane is rudimentary or absent and there are no pericytes. Fine collagenous filaments known as ***anchoring filaments*** link the endothelium to the surrounding supporting tissue, preventing collapse of the lymphatic lumen.

Ad adventitia **F** follicle **I** intima **M** media **ML** muscle layer **P** paracortex **S** subcapsular sinus **SM** smooth muscle **V** lymphatic valve **VV** vasa vasorum

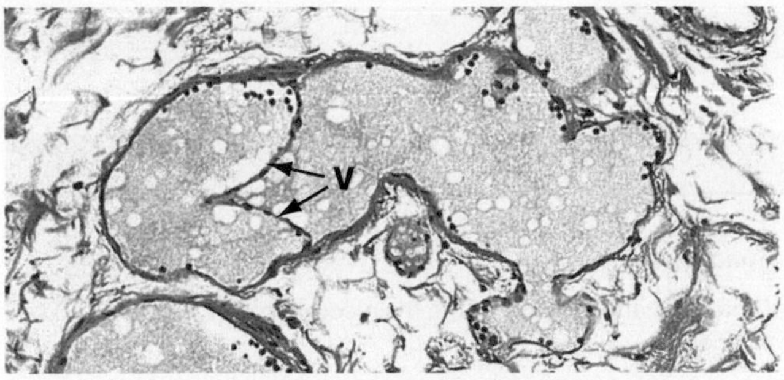

FIG. 8.25 Valve of a lymphatic vessel
H&E (LP)

A characteristic feature of the lymphatic system is the presence of numerous delicate valves within small and medium-sized vessels.

The structure of these valves **V** (Fig. 8.25) is similar to that of valves in the venous system, but the supporting tissue core includes only some reticulin fibres and a little ground substance. Note the presence of light pink–stained proteinaceous lymph fluid in the channels, with scattered lymphocytes around the periphery.

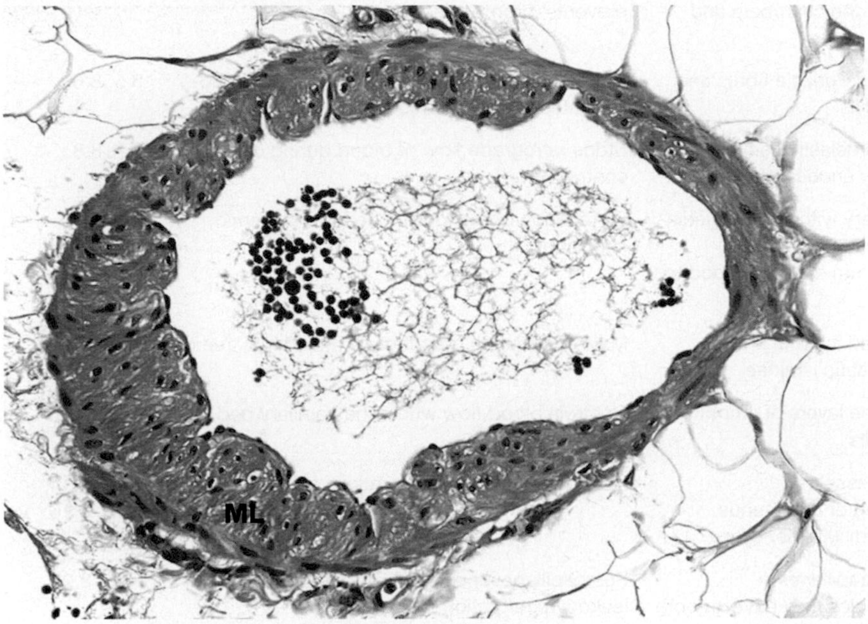

FIG. 8.26 Medium-sized lymphatic vessel
H&E (MP)

Fig. 8.26 shows small lymphatic vessels containing only a very small amount of smooth muscle in their walls. As lymphatic channels become larger, the muscle layer **ML** becomes thicker and its contraction makes a greater contribution to the movement of lymph along the vessel. Backflow of lymph fluid is prevented by valves (not illustrated here).

The muscle layers are most prominent in the largest lymphatic vessels which drain into the venous system (the thoracic duct and right lymphatic duct).

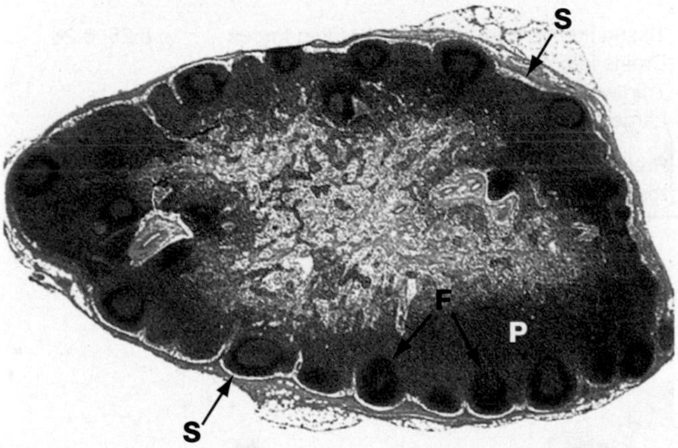

FIG. 8.27 Normal lymph node
H&E (LP)

Fig. 8.27 illustrates a normal lymph node (see also Ch. 11), the site of filtration of lymph fluid.

Afferent lymphatic channels enter the convexity of the lymph node, and fluid drains into the peripheral ***subcapsular sinus*** **S**. The sinuses of the lymph node are lined by macrophages, and these cells filter out any particulate debris from the fluid. The fluid percolates through the sinuses and emerges via an efferent lymphatic channel at the hilum of the node (not shown here).

Note the presence of ***follicles*** **F** in the cortex of the lymph node, the site of B-cell activation. The intervening ***paracortical area*** **P** is the main site of T cells within the lymph node.

The importance of lymphatic channels and lymph nodes in cancer patients

Lymphatic channels normally drain away excess tissue fluid and return this to the blood stream. In patients with cancer, malignant cells can enter into lymphatic channels and spread to the local and regional lymph nodes. Eventually, malignant cells can reach the blood stream in this way. Examination of lymph nodes draining many malignant tumours is a routine part of the pathological assessment of tumour ***stage*** (the extent of disease spread). This is important in planning treatment and in predicting likely prognosis. The surgeon will usually excise not only the main tumour mass for examination, but also any associated groups of regional lymph nodes which drain the site of the primary mass (e.g. axillary lymph nodes in breast carcinoma, hilar and mediastinal nodes in lung cancer).

On occasion, the pathologist may receive a lymph node which contains metastatic tumour from a patient who is not already known to have pre-existing malignant disease. In this setting, examination of the metastatic deposit, often with use of special staining techniques such as immunohistochemistry, may allow the pathologist to suggest a likely site of origin of the tumour and so to guide further investigation and management of the patient.

REVIEW

TABLE 8.1 Review of the circulatory system

Organ/ structure	Structure	Key features	Functional attributes	Figure
Heart	Epicardium	Adventitial fat with vessels and mesothelial surface	Protection and support of the main coronary arteries	8.2
	Myocardium	Functional syncytium of cardiac myocytes	Propagates cardiac contraction, producing blood circulation	8.3
	Endocardium	Flattened layer of endothelial cells lining the chambers and valves	Reduces sheer stress within the heart and prevents thrombosis	8.4
	Conducting system	Specialised Purkinje fibres and bundle of His	Conducts the cardiac action potential and co-ordinates cardiac conduction	8.5, 8.6
	Valves	Core of fibroelastic tissue covered by endocardium	Stops retrograde flow of blood during cardiac contraction	8.7, 8.8
Vascular system	Aorta	Elastic artery with intima, media and adventitia Vaso vasorum supplies blood to adventitia	Distribution of blood from heart to systemic circulation	8.9
	Muscular artery	Well-defined internal and external elastic laminae	Main distributing branches of the arterial tree	8.10, 8.11
	Arteriole	Two to three layers of smooth muscle cells	Controls blood flow within the capillary bed	8.12
	Capillary	Smallest vessel Fenestrated or continuous endothelium with pericytes	Permits cell and fluid migration	8.13, 8.14, 8.15, 8.16
	Venule	Similar to capillaries Larger venules may have smooth muscle in the wall	Postcapillary venules offer the main site of leukocyte migration	8.19, 8.20
	Vein	Thin muscular wall Ill-defined elastic layers	Valves allow return of blood to the heart	8.21, 8.22 8.23, 8.24
Lymphatic system	Lymphatic vessels	Vessels responsible for returning fluid to the vascular system	Tissue fluid is formed due to Starling forces Drains into great veins via the thoracic duct Thin walled channels with valves, lack pericytes Larger vessels have smooth muscle in the wall	8.25, 8.26
	Lymph nodes	Filter lymph fluid	Presentation of antigens to B and T cells within the lymph node	8.27, Ch. 11

9 Skin

INTRODUCTION

The skin is the largest organ in the body, both in weight and surface area. It shows significant regional variation, with the thickest skin being found on the soles of the feet while the thinnest is the delicate skin on the upper and lower eyelids; some of these variations are illustrated and discussed later in this chapter.

The skin is the external body surface and provides ***protection*** against a wide variety of external threats, including mechanical, water loss, biological, ultraviolet light and chemical. The most frequent mechanical insult is the frictional and shearing forces experienced by the soles and ventral aspect of the toes in walking and, to a lesser extent the palms and ventral aspects of the fingers during use of the hands. In these areas, skin structure is adapted to resist these shearing forces (see Fig. 9.20).

The skin provides ***moisture control***, providing a barrier against both excessive water loss and wetting. It resists bacterial and fungal invasion; bacteria and fungi do live on the skin surface but cannot penetrate into underlying tissues unless the skin is breached. It is rich in antigen-presenting cells (***Langerhans cells***) and, when breached, an immune response against any foreign antigen is readily initiated.

Skin pigmentation from ***melanin*** provides protection against ultraviolet (UV) radiation, and exposure induces increased pigmentation (tanning). Skin has a metabolic function, namely the synthesis of vitamin D_3 (cholecalciferol) by the action of UV light on the precursor, 7-dehydrocholesterol. Cholecalciferol is further processed in the liver and kidney to produce the active agent 1,25-dihydroxycholecalciferol, which is important in Ca^{2+} metabolism and bone formation. Adequate levels of UV exposure are needed to ensure that enough vitamin D is synthesised. Individuals with darker skin (more melanin pigment) require more UV exposure to ensure adequate vitamin D levels.

Skin is important in ***thermoregulation***. Adjustments to blood circulation through skin, particularly extremities (hands, feet and ears), provides for both heat conservation and heat loss. The production of a watery secretion by skin eccrine glands, known as ***sweat***, and its subsequent evaporation, is a major heat-loss mechanism. In humans, body hair is scanty and so provides only minimal heat conservation; however, subcutaneous adipose tissue can provide some heat conservation.

The skin is the largest ***sensory*** organ in the body, containing a range of different receptors for touch, pressure, pain and temperature (see Ch. 7). As a regional variation in structure, sensory receptors are most numerous in skin which has the most physical contact with solid objects in the environment, such as soles and palms, fingers and toes (see Fig. 7.24), or with specialised sexual functions.

Hair and nails are specialised components of skin. In humans, hair mostly defines sexual differences, sexual maturity and age; in most other mammals, it provides protection against cold in the form of fur. Nails provide physical support for finger tips and toes and can serve as tools.

The overall appearance of the skin (condition, pigmentation, hair and nails) cannot be underestimated, both clinically as an important indicator of health and in human behaviour.

Rapid repair of injuries to the skin such as lacerations (cuts and tears) and other wounds is critical to minimise infection risks and, while this happens in all tissues, this can rightly be seen as a critical skin function.

SKIN STRUCTURE

The skin has three main layers:

- The **epidermis** is a continuously proliferating stratified squamous epithelium which produces a non-living surface layer of the protein ***keratin***, with associated lipid which is in direct contact with the external environment and is constantly shed.
- The **dermis** consists of fibrous and fibroadipose tissue which supports the epidermis, both physically and metabolically. It contains blood vessels, nerves and sensory receptors.
- The **subcutis** or **hypodermis** or **panniculus** is the layer beneath the dermis and usually consists of adipose tissue with supporting fibrous bands (***septa***). This layer contains the larger vessels which supply and drain the dermal blood vasculature.

In addition, there are the specialised skin structures and ***adnexae*** (***appendages***) such as ***nails***, ***hair follicles***, ***sebaceous glands***, ***eccrine (sweat) glands*** and ***apocrine glands***. The adnexae mainly occupy the dermis and variably the superficial subcutis. They arise as downgrowths from the epidermis into the dermis during embryological development.

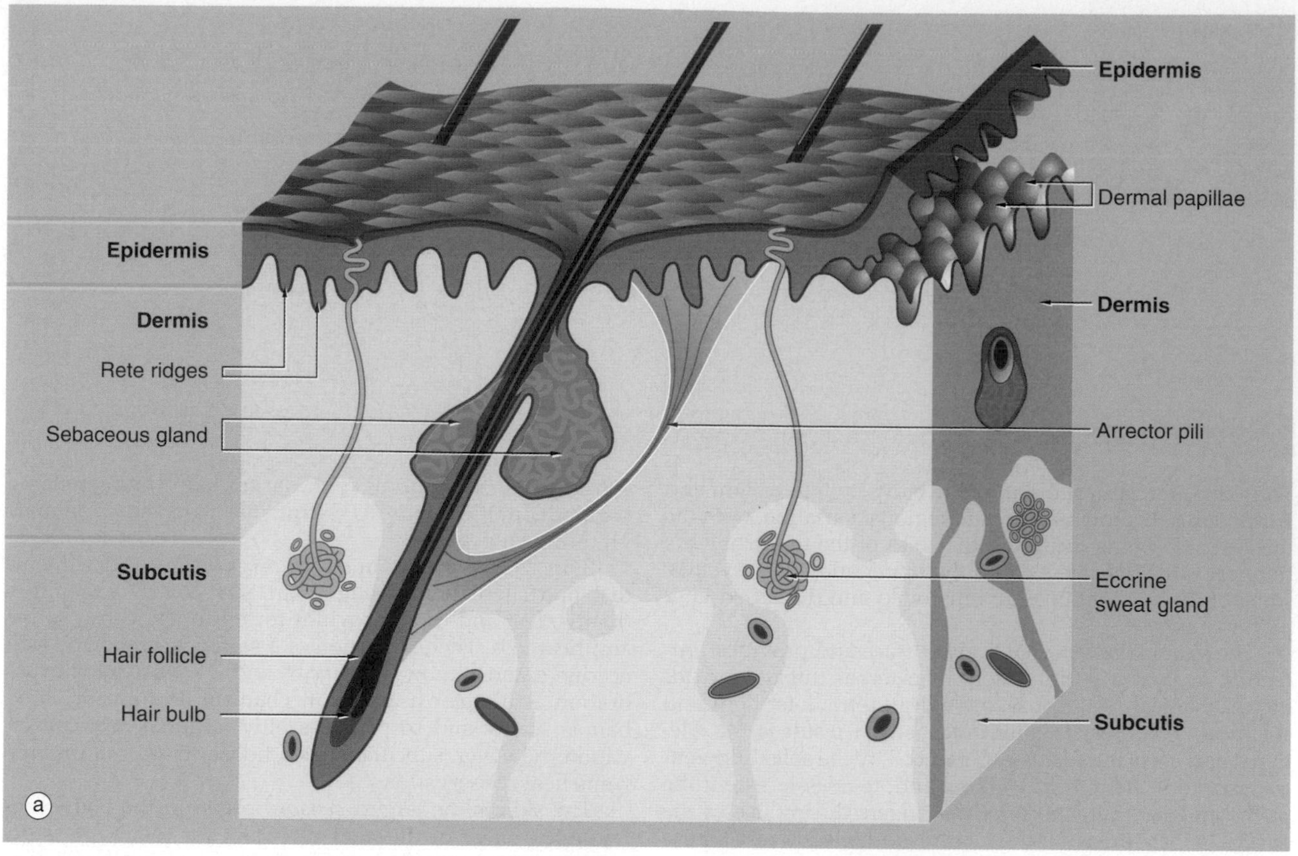

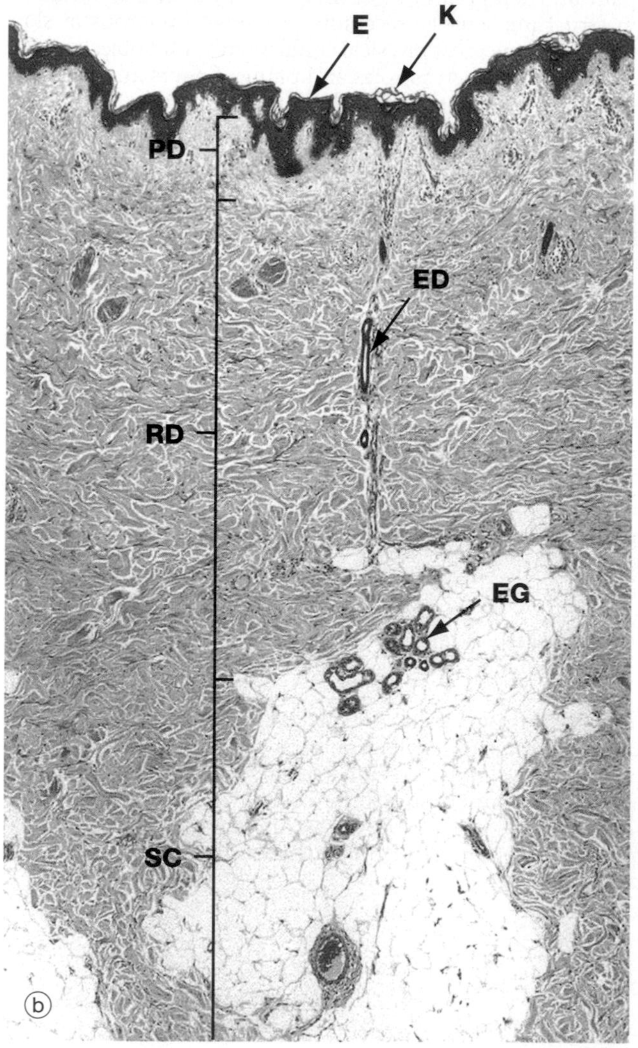

FIG. 9.1 Skin architecture
(a) Diagram (b) H&E (LP)

These illustrations show the basic structure of the skin, with the three component layers: ***epidermis, dermis*** and ***subcutis***.

The surface layer in contact with the exterior is the epidermis **E**, a highly specialised self-regenerating stratified squamous epithelium which produces a non-living surface rich in a protein, ***keratin*** **K**, that is tough and protective and is also partially water resistant (see Ch. 5). The epidermis also contains non-epithelial cells: ***melanocytes*** produce melanin pigment to protect against UV light, ***Langerhans cells*** act as antigen-presenting cells and induce immune responses to new antigens and ***Merkel cells*** act as touch receptors. The epidermis is tightly bound to the underlying dermis by a specialised basement membrane. Additional resistance to frictional shearing force is provided by a series of epidermal downgrowths (***rete ridges***) which extend into the superficial dermis, with their papillary dermal mirror images projecting upwards (***dermal papillae***) to provide stronger tethering. These are most developed where exposure to shearing forces is almost constant (e.g. sole, palm).

The dermis immediately adjacent to the epidermis is called the ***papillary dermis*** **PD**; it has relatively fine collagen fibres and contains numerous small blood vessels, sensory nerve endings and sensory structures. The ***reticular dermis*** **RD** is the deeper tough layer of horizontally arranged collagen and elastin fibres with fibroblasts.

The deepest layer is the subcutis **SC**, also called the ***panniculus*** or ***hypodermis***. It is a layer of adipose tissue often compartmentalised by fibrous septa, extending downwards from dermis to the underlying structural connective tissue fascia. The subcutis acts as a shock absorber and thermal insulator as well as a fat store.

The dermis and subcutis contain an assortment of skin ***adnexae (appendages)*** such as ***hair follicles, sebaceous glands, eccrine (sweat) glands*** **EG** and ducts **ED** and, in some areas, ***apocrine glands***.

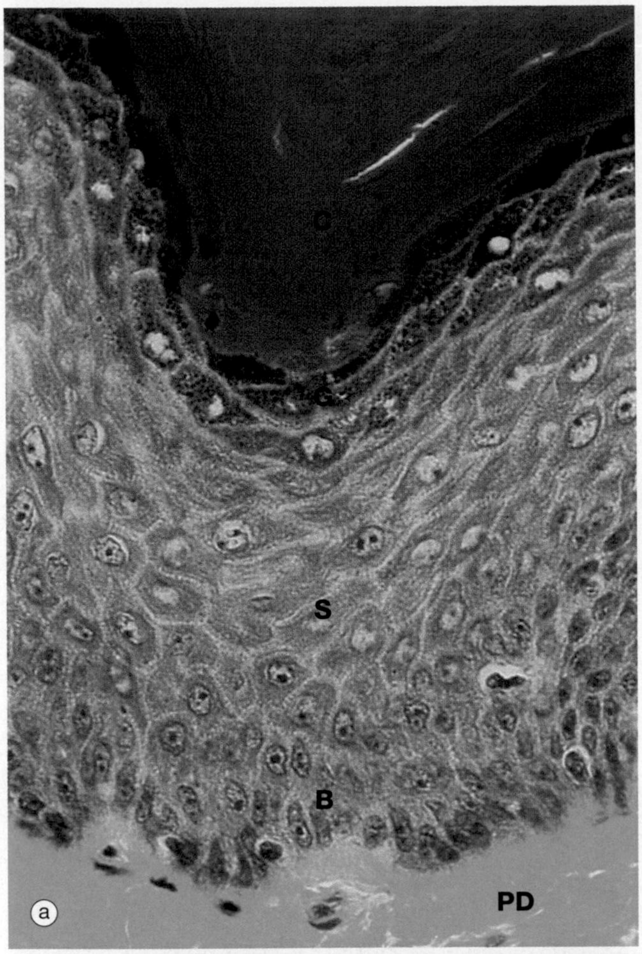

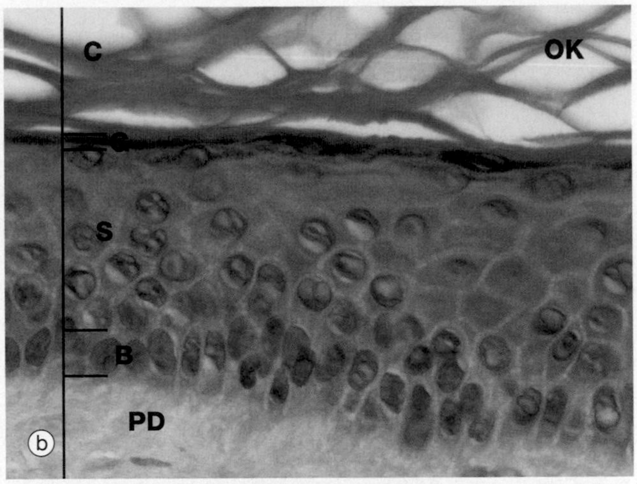

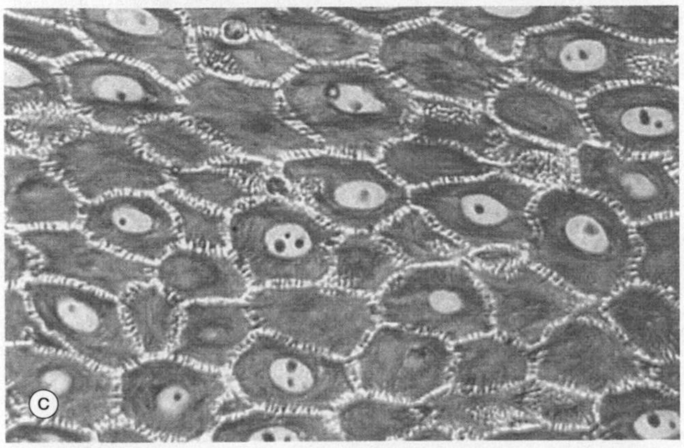

FIG. 9.2 Epidermis
(a) Masson trichrome (HP) (b) H&E (HP) (c) Epoxy resin section, toluidine blue (HP)

Fig. 9.2a and b show epidermis. The cells of the epidermis are called ***keratinocytes***. The ***basal layer*** of keratinocytes (***stratum basale***) **B** proliferates continuously with repeated mitotic divisions. This provides cells for a progressive process of displacement towards the surface (upward migration), with associated ***maturation*** to renew the other layers. The basal cells are arranged as a single layer of cuboidal or low columnar cells. They are attached to the basement membrane (not seen in these preparations) on their dermal (basal) surface. This basal surface is irregular; the basal cells have a highly indented and folded basal cell membrane with numerous hemidesmosomes.

Superficially, the basal cells are attached to and mature into the cells of the ***stratum spinosum*** **S** which forms the majority of the epidermis. The stratum spinosum is also known as the ***prickle cell layer***. It is multilayered and composed of polyhedral-shaped keratinocytes with round-oval nuclei, prominent nucleoli and cytoplasm, forming a pavement-like pattern. These cells synthesise cytoplasmic intermediate filaments called ***cytokeratins*** (see Ch. 5 textbox 'Keratins') which accumulate in aggregates called ***tonofibrils*** made up of bundles of ***tonofilaments***. These tonofibrils bind to the numerous ***desmosomes*** that form strong contacts between adjacent keratinocytes. In appropriate preparations as in Fig. 9.2c, the desmosome junctions are seen as ***prickles*** or ***spines*** between the cells, hence the name for this layer.

The keratinocytes mature into the ***stratum granulosum*** **G** or ***granular layer***. Here they acquire dense basophilic, ***keratohyaline granules*** which contain proteins rich in sulphur-containing amino acids (cysteine) and proteins such as ***involucrin*** which interact with the cytokeratin tonofibrils in the final maturation. The combination of tonofibrils with keratohyaline granule proteins produces keratin, in a process called ***keratinisation***. Progressing towards the surface, the cells lose their nuclei and cytoplasm, becoming flattened interconnected ***keratin squames*** (plates/flakes of keratin) which comprise the surface coating of the skin, the ***stratum corneum*** **C**.

These keratin squames connect at their edges, and in transverse sections form a folded basket-weave pattern called ***orthokeratosis*** **OK**. The squames are water repellent, in part because they are coated with lipid-containing anti-wetting agents synthesised during maturation in the granular layer.

Fig. 9.2a illustrates skin from a friction-prone area (sole of foot) where keratin production is enhanced. The stratum spinosum has more layers, the granular layer **G** is thicker and more prominent and the stratum corneum **C** is thick with dense compact keratin. These changes are a non-specific response to friction.

B basal layer (stratum basale) **C** keratin layer (stratum corneum) **E** epidermis **ED** eccrine duct **EG** eccrine gland
G granular layer (stratum granulosum) **K** keratin **OK** orthokeratosis **RD** reticular dermis **PD** papillary dermis
S prickle cell layer (stratum spinosum) **SC** subcutis

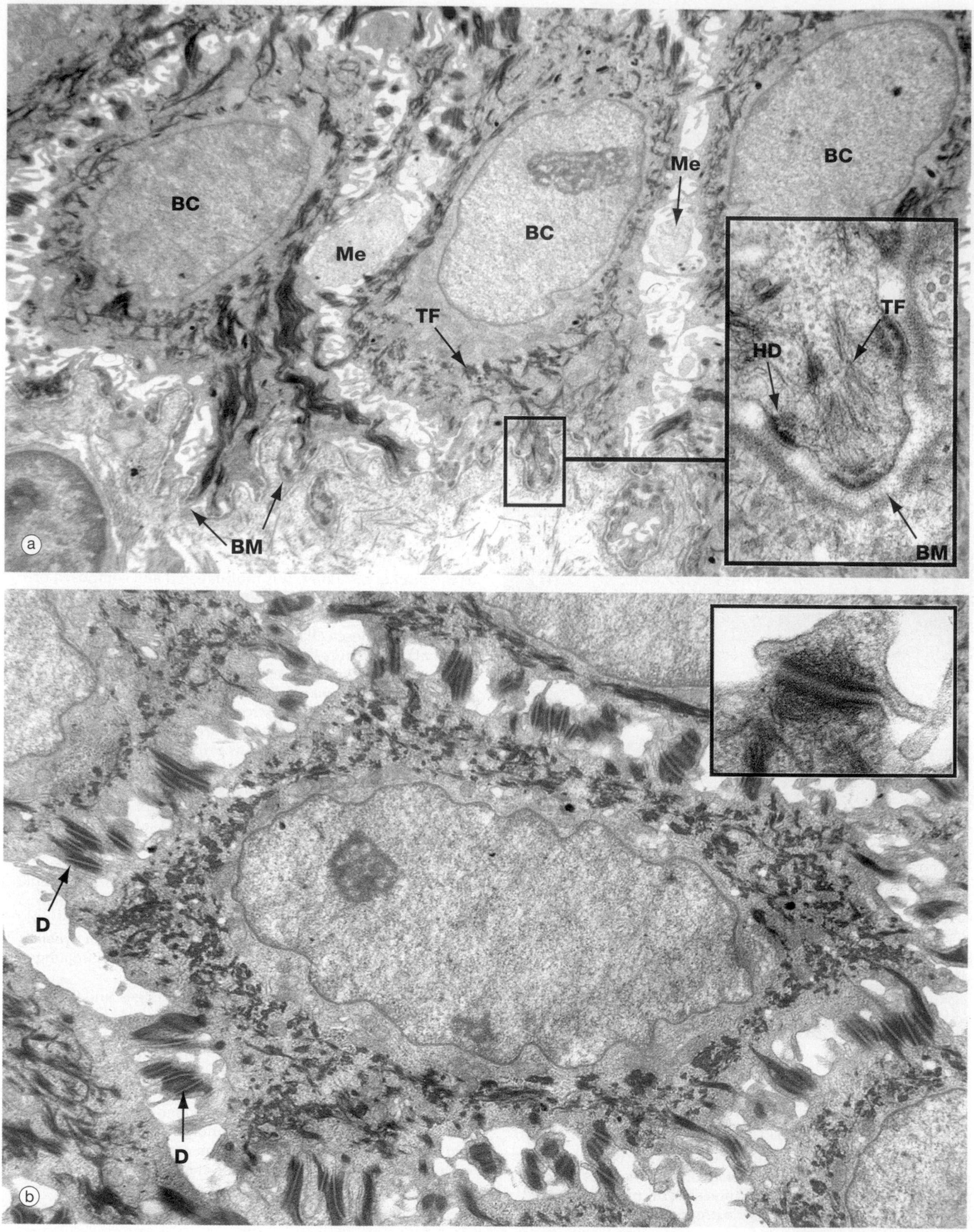

FIG. 9.3 Keratinocytes ***(caption and illustration (c) opposite)***
(a) Basal keratinocytes, EM ×10 000, inset ×30 000 (b) Keratinocyte from prickle cell layer, EM ×15 000, inset ×40 000
(c) Keratinocyte from granular layer, EM ×12 000, inset ×50 000

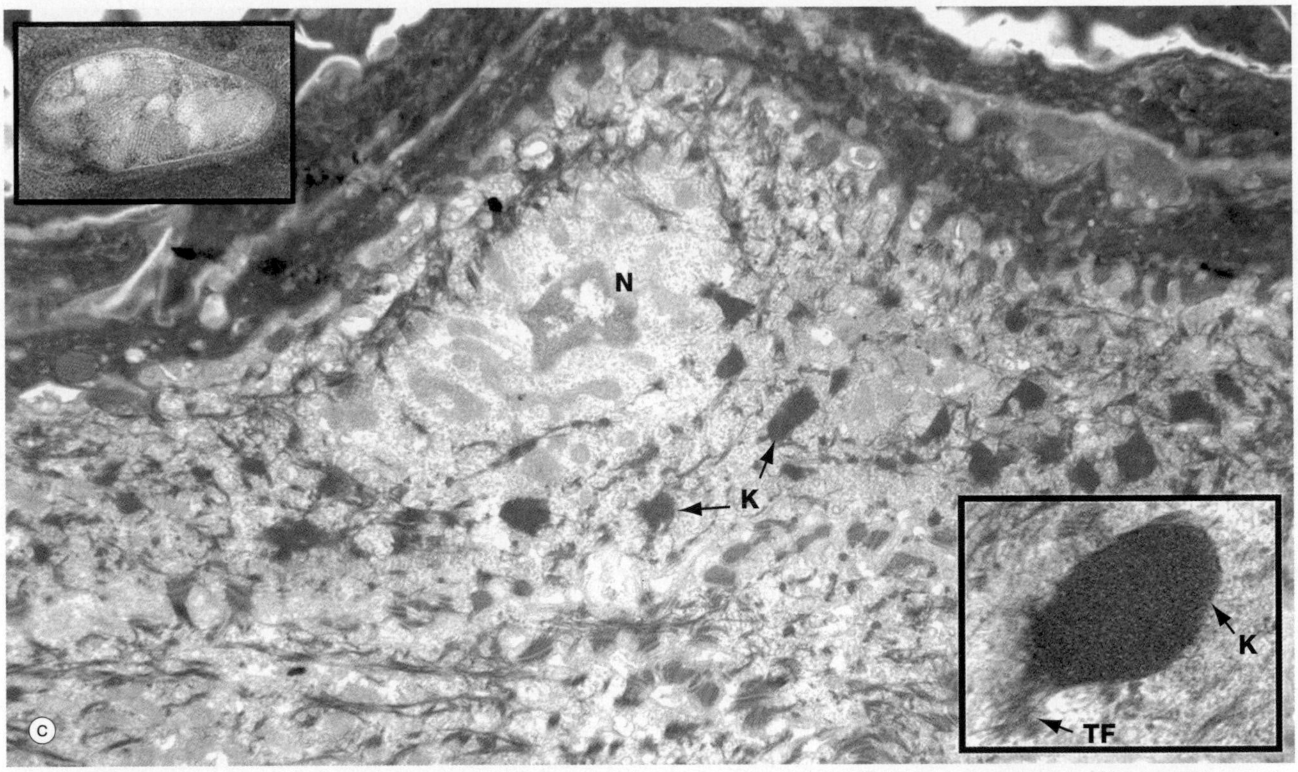

FIG. 9.3 Keratinocytes *(illustrations (a) and (b) opposite)*
(a) Basal keratinocytes, EM ×10 000, inset ×30 000 (b) Keratinocyte from prickle cell layer, EM ×15 000, inset ×40 000
(c) Keratinocyte from granular layer, EM ×12 000, inset ×50 000

Fig. 9.3a shows a row of three ***basal cells*** **BC** sitting on the epidermal ***basement membrane*** **BM**, which can only just be discerned as a convoluted line in the low-magnification main picture. The basal cells are cuboidal with prominent nuclei, nucleoli, and a perinuclear zone containing ribosomes and mitochondria. ***Tonofibrils*** **TF** are present towards the periphery of the cell.

The inset shows the linkage of the basal surface of the cell to the basement membrane **BM** by hemidesmosomes **HD** into which tonofibrils **TF** are inserted. Basal cells link to each other and to overlying keratinocytes of the prickle cell layer by desmosomes. The pale processes in the spaces between basal cells are cytoplasmic melanocyte processes **Me**.

Fig. 9.3b shows a single keratinocyte from the ***prickle cell layer***. It has abundant electron-dense tonofibrils which extend into the many ***desmosomes*** **D** that link it firmly to adjacent keratinocytes. The inset shows a desmosome linking the cytoplasmic processes of two keratinocytes. Electron-dense tonofibrils from each cell attach to the desmosome.

Fig. 9.3c shows a flattening keratinocyte in the ***granular layer*** immediately beneath the keratin layer. The cell is keratinising with an ill-defined remnant of the nucleus **N**. The cytoplasm contains both linear cytokeratin tonofibrils and electron-dense ovoid ***keratohyaline granules*** **K**, one of which is shown merging with tonofibrils **TF** at higher magnification in the inset bottom right. Also present but not clearly visible in the low-magnification micrograph are lamellated pale-staining ovoid bodies (about 500 nm long) called ***keratinosomes*** or ***Odland*** bodies; one is shown at higher magnification in the inset top left. They contain a hydrophobic glycolipid which, when released, coats and binds together the keratin flakes, rendering them relatively water repellent.

Psoriasis

The transition of keratinocytes from replicating basal cells, through the prickle cell layer, to the flattened degenerating granular layer cells packed with tonofibrils and keratohyaline granules is a well-ordered maturation sequence, culminating in the production of a tough, water-resistant keratin layer on the surface of the skin. The normal transit time from basal cell to formed keratin is 50 to 60 days.

Psoriasis (see e-Fig. 9.1) is a common skin condition, in part manifesting as epidermal hyperplasia with accelerated maturation to as short as 7 days. The maturation process is so rushed that there is insufficient time for full development of tonofibrils and keratohyaline in the prickle cell layers and for nuclear degeneration. The granular layer does not form normally, with only scant keratohyaline visible in H&E sections. Nuclei, while small and condensed, remain in the keratin squames, a condition called ***parakeratosis*** (see e-Fig. 9.2). Clinically, the skin has a surface of opaque, flaky, white scale overlying thickened red epidermis.

BC basal cell **BM** basement membrane **D** desmosome **HD** hemidesmosome **K** keratohyaline granule
Me melanocyte cytoplasmic process **N** nucleus **TF** tonofibrils

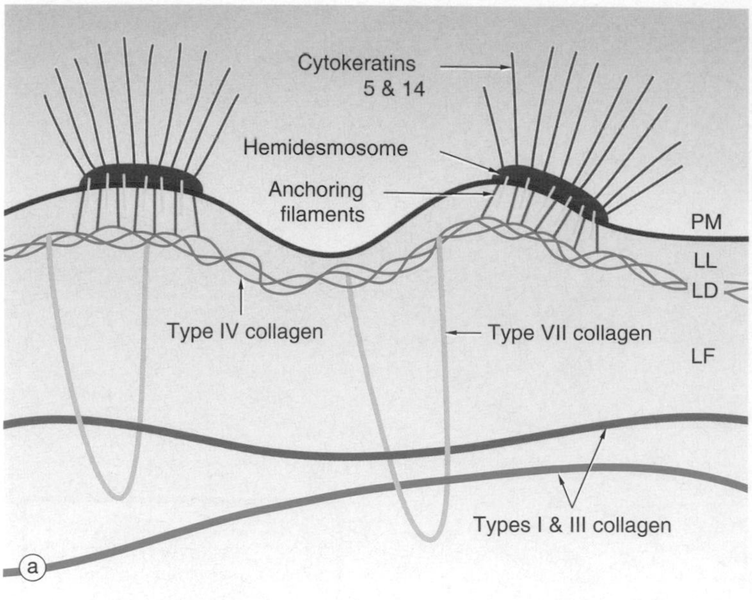

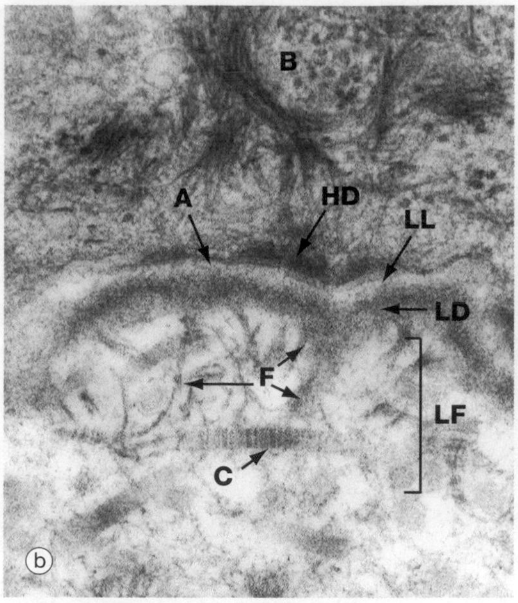

FIG. 9.4 Dermo-epidermal junction
(a) Diagram (b) EM ×64 000

The ***basement membrane*** at the junction of epidermis and dermis, known as the ***dermo-epidermal junction***, is a specialised structure which binds epidermis to dermis. The major components are illustrated in Fig. 9.4a.

Cytoplasmic tonofibrils, consisting of ***cytokeratins 5*** and ***14***, bind to hemidesmosomes in the plasma membrane **PM** at the base of the basal cells of the epidermis. The ***hemidesmosomes*** contain multiple transmembrane and binding proteins including type XVII collagen and integrins. Binding to these on the outside of the plasma membrane are the ***anchoring filaments***, including ***nidogen-1*** and ***laminins***. These correspond to an electron-lucent layer on electron microscopy called the ***lamina lucida*** **LL**. This appears to be the most easily disrupted of the basement membrane layers.

These anchoring filament proteins bind to a type IV collagen layer, type IV collagen being a specialised network/mesh-forming basement membrane collagen. On EM, this corresponds to the ***lamina densa*** **LD**, an electron-dense layer.

Type VII collagen is a basement membrane specialised collagen which forms loops extending from the type IV collagen layer around fibres of structural types I and III collagens in the dermis, thereby tethering the basement membrane to the dermis; these are the ***anchoring fibrils***. These form the ***lamina fibroreticularis*** **LF**, a poorly defined layer on EM.

The electron micrograph (Fig. 9.4b) shows part of a basal cell **B**, basement membrane layers of lamina lucida **LL**, lamina densa **LD** and lamina fibroreticularis **LF**, in addition to fibrils of type VII collagen **F** which tie to the type I collagen fibres **C** in the dermis. There are also finer fibrillin microfilaments which link to dermal elastic fibres. Basal cell hemidesmosomes **HD** can be seen at the plasma membrane with their fine anchoring protein filaments **A** which cross the lamina lucida.

Disorders of the dermo-epidermal junction/epidermal basement membrane

Any disease which damages the dermo-epidermal junction can lead to separation of epidermis from dermis. Initially the space formed between the layers fills with fluid, leading to blisters, also called ***vesicles*** or ***bullae*** depending on their size. In two groups of disorders, the abnormality in the basement membrane is at a molecular level.

In bullous pemphigoid and related disorders, the affected patient has antibodies which react against specific antigens located in the hemidesmosomes or lamina lucida. An antigen–antibody reaction occurs, triggering damage to the basement membrane and leading to separation of the epidermis and dermis with blistering (see e-Fig. 9.3).

Epidermolysis bullosa is a group term for hereditary defects involving basement membrane or epidermal adhesion to dermis (although an antibody-mediated acquired form exists). There are several genetic forms, each with a different molecular abnormality. In one, there are mutations in the type VII collagen gene leading to deficiency in the anchoring fibrils. In another, mutations in the genes for cytokeratins 5 or 14 affect the binding of the tonofibrils to the hemidesmosomes; here separation occurs within the cytoplasm near the basal surface of the basal cells.

The basement membrane of oral and oesophageal squamous epithelium is similar to skin and various diseases affect these sites in addition to skin.

A anchoring filaments **B** basal keratinocyte **C** type I collagen fibres **CP** Langerhans cell cytoplasmic process **F** anchoring fibrils (type VII collagen) **HD** hemidesmosome **L** Langerhans cell **LD** lamina densa **LF** lamina fibroreticularis **LL** lamina lucida **PM** plasma membrane

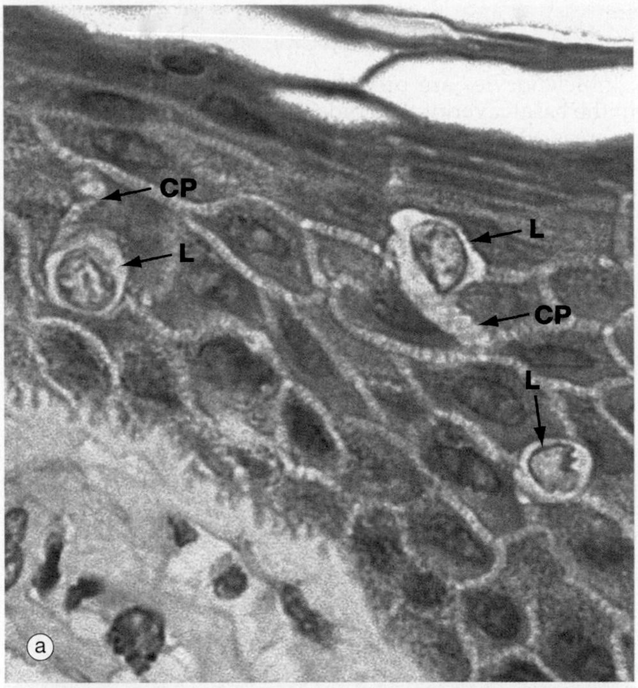

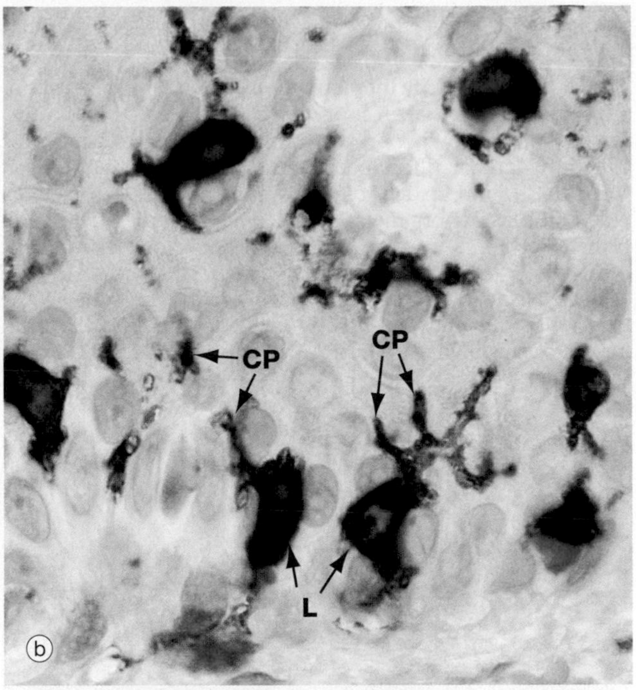

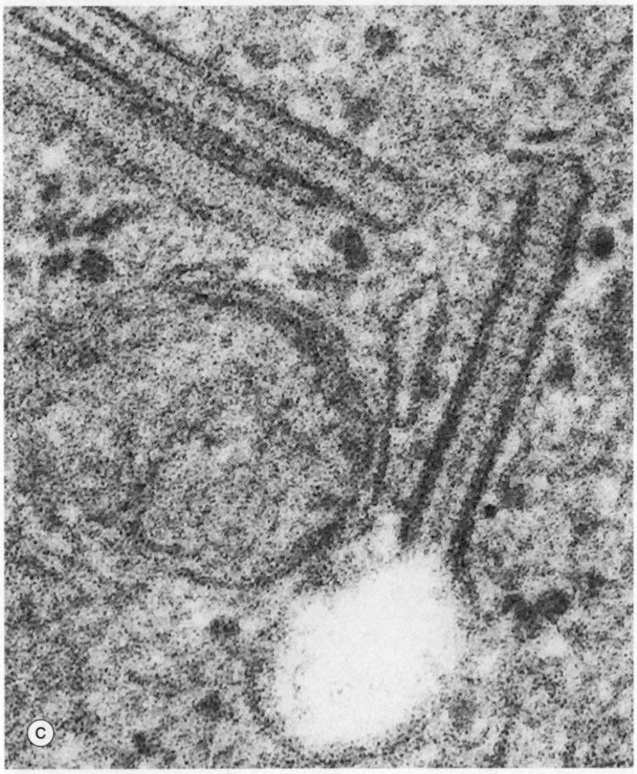

FIG. 9.5 Langerhans cells
(a) H&E (HP) (b) Immunohistochemistry for CD1a (HP)
(c) Birbeck granule, EM ×100 000

Langerhans cells are intra-epidermal antigen-presenting cells, historically referred to as histiocytes. They are present in all layers of the epidermis but are most easily recognised in the prickle cell layer. They are also present in the upper dermis, particularly around small blood vessels. When stimulated, they migrate to dermis and then via lymphatics to lymph nodes.

Fig. 9.5a shows pale-staining Langerhans cells **L** in the epidermis; they have irregularly lobulated nuclei and almost clear cytoplasm. Cytoplasmic processes **CP** extend from the cells and insinuate between keratinocytes of all layers. The extensive network of cytoplasmic processes is highlighted in the immunohistochemical preparation shown in Fig. 9.5b.

Fig. 9.5c is an electron micrograph illustrating the characteristic cytoplasmic organelle of Langerhans cells, the ***Birbeck granule***, a rod-like structure with regular cross-striations, one end of which frequently distends in a vesicle so that they resemble a tennis racket. They are part of the endosome system. Their exact function is not known.

Langerhans cells and skin disease

Langerhans cells are antigen-presenting cells (APC), the skin's antigen recognition and processing cells. They express a large number of lymphocyte and macrophage surface markers (see Ch. 11). They constantly monitor the environment on the epidermal surface and in the spaces between epidermal cells with their dendritic cytoplasmic processes. When activated, they are potent stimulators of cell-mediated immunological responses. They are present in increased numbers in epidermis and upper dermis in many inflammatory skin diseases, particularly allergic contact dermatitis. Langerhans cells play an important role in rejection mechanisms in skin allografts, and it has been suggested that their activity may have a protective effect against the development of epidermal tumours. Some chemical carcinogens, immunosuppressive agents and excessive ultraviolet light have been shown to reduce the number and effectiveness of Langerhans cells, and these are all factors which predispose to the development of epidermal tumours.

Technology for intra-epidermal vaccination with minimal antigen doses, as compared to intramuscular, is under development to take advantage of these large APC populations.

MELANOCYTES

Melanocytes produce the pigment ***melanin*** which is responsible for skin and hair colour. The pigment exists in various forms from yellowish brown to black and has a protective function against ultraviolet light. Melanin is synthesised from the amino acid tyrosine by melanocytes within specific cytoplasmic organelles called ***melanosomes***. These are transferred to the keratinocytes through a complex network of melanocyte cytoplasmic processes; these processes can be seen in electron micrographs of epidermis, running in the narrow spaces between keratinocytes (see Fig. 9.3). Within keratinocytes, melanosomes usually form a cap sitting over the nucleus.

Melanocytes are present as separated individual cells in the basal layer of the epidermis and are more numerous in areas which are more exposed to light. There is no great difference in numbers of melanocytes between white- and dark-skinned people, but they are considerably more synthetically active in darker-skinned people. Melanocytes can be stimulated into producing more melanin by increasing exposure to UV light. This may produce a socially desirable suntan, but forced stimulation of melanocytes has its draw-backs and can be associated with the development of malignant tumours (see textbox 'Disorders of melanocytes').

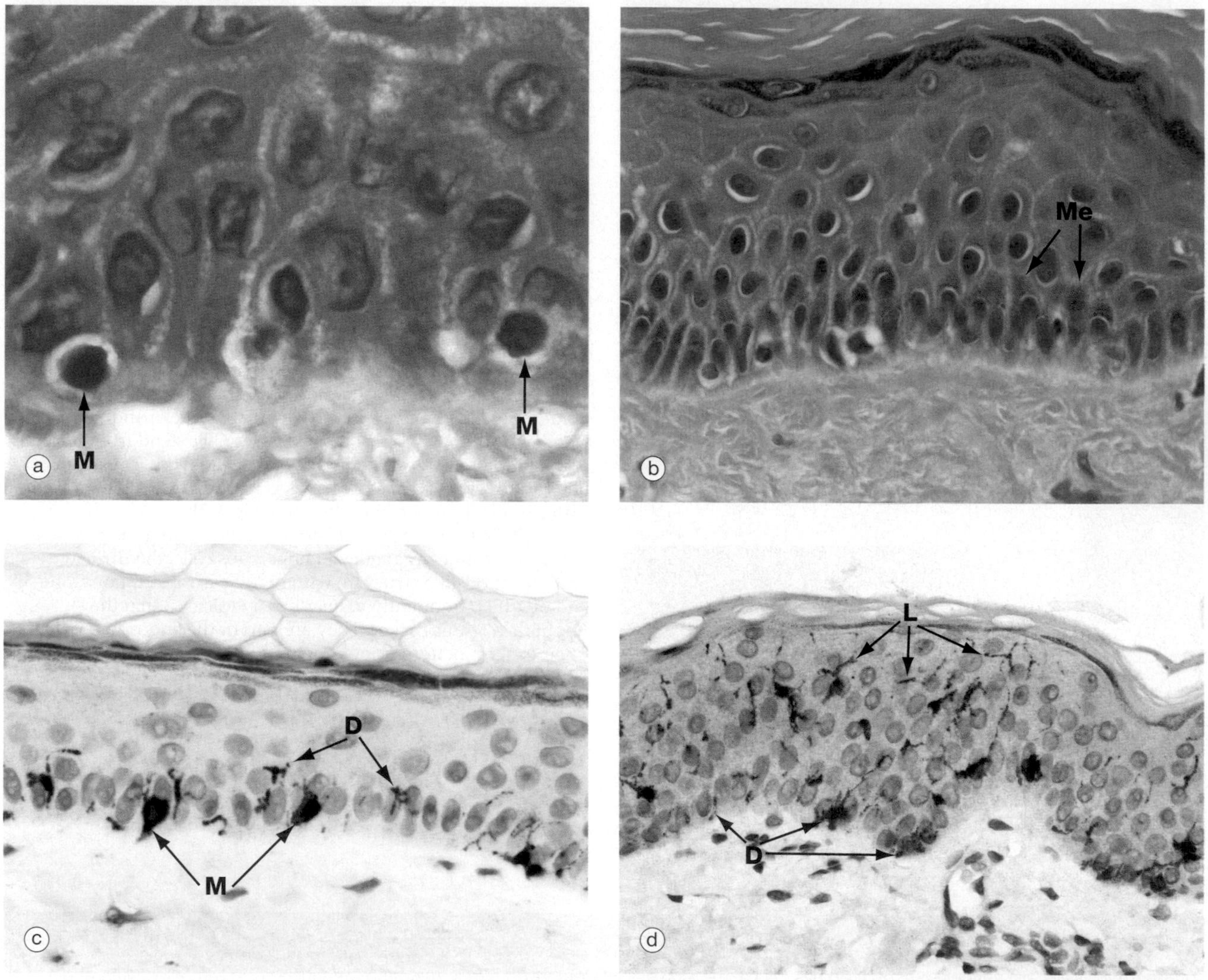

FIG. 9.6 Melanocytes
(a) H&E (HP) (b) H&E, pigmented skin (MP) (c) Immunohistochemistry for melanA (MP) (d) Dual immunohistochemistry for melanA (red) and langerin (brown) (MP)

Fig. 9.6a shows normal epidermis with scattered melanocytes **M** in the basal layer. They appear to have rounded cell bodies with clear cytoplasm, but in fact have multiple fine, branching dendritic processes not seen in the H&E stains.

Fig. 9.6b demonstrates basal brown melanin pigment **Me** in dark-coloured skin.

Fig. 9.6c is an immunohistochemical stain against a melanocyte antigen (melanA); it shows the globular cell bodies **M** situated in the basal layer and their branching dendritic processes **D** extending between keratinocytes. Because of the tortuous routes of these processes between the keratinocytes, their full length is rarely seen, often only short segments in any section. Melanocytes transfer melanosomes to the keratinocytes. These dendritic processes extend the numbers of keratinocytes serviced by each melanocyte.

Fig. 9.6d is a dual immunohistochemical stain with melanocytes (red) and Langerhans cells (brown), showing both cell types and the dendritic processes of melanocytes **D** and Langerhans cells **L**.

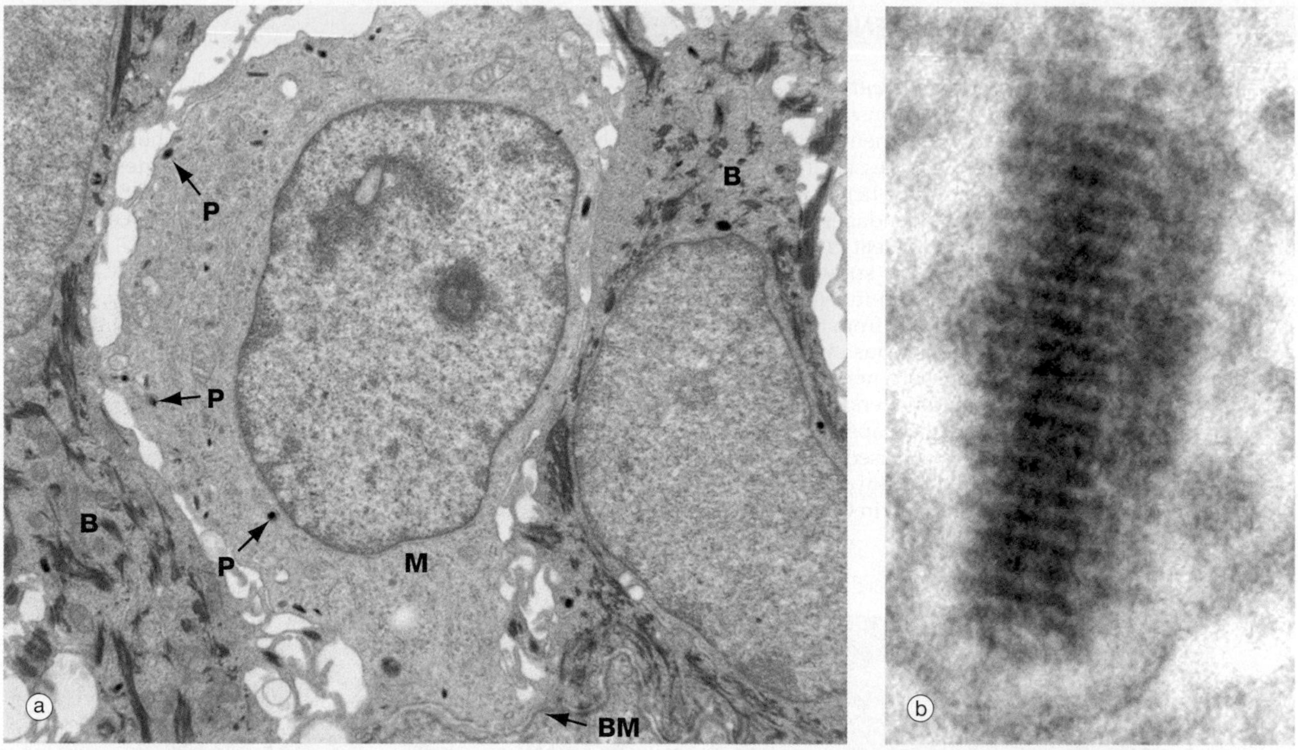

FIG. 9.7 Melanocytes
(a) EM ×15 000 (b) EM ×300 000

At low-power, Fig. 9.7a shows a pale-staining melanocyte **M** between two tonofibril-containing basal keratinocytes **B**; all are sitting on an indistinct basement membrane **BM**. The cytoplasm of the melanocyte has no tonofibrils but contains scanty tiny round or oval dark-staining ***premelanosomes*** and ***melanosomes*** **P**, responsible for the synthesis of melanin. Tyrosine is converted into dihydroxyphenylalanine (DOPA) and then polymerised into melanin, which later links to protein to form ***melanoprotein***.

The high magnification, Fig. 9.7b, shows the ultrastructural features of a premelanosome. It is a round or cylindrical electron-dense structure with distinct transverse striations and sometimes faint longitudinal striations. Sometimes, an indistinct surrounding membrane can be seen.

Disorders of melanocytes

Vitiligo is a common disease in which symmetrical areas of depigmentation of the skin occur, often on the hands, fingers and face. The disease destroys all the melanocytes in the affected skin and the skin becomes glaringly white; the keratinocytes are not affected. Vitiligo is due to an autoimmune destruction of melanocytes and is associated with other autoimmune diseases, such as thyroiditis, pernicious anaemia, type I diabetes mellitus and Addison's disease.

'Moles' or naevi (see e-Fig. 9.4) are common benign accumulations of melanocytes in the dermis (intradermal naevus), epidermis (junctional naevus) or both (compound naevus).

Malignant melanoma (see e-Fig. 9.5) is a dangerous malignant tumour of melanocytes, particularly affecting pale-skinned people who are exposed to excessive UV light, especially in childhood, but can also occur in non-sun-exposed areas such as soles of feet in darkly pigmented people.

B basal keratinocyte **BM** basement membrane **D** melanocyte dendritic process **L** Langerhans cell **M** melanocyte **Me** melanin pigment **P** melanosomes or pre-melanosomes

INNERVATION AND NERVE ENDINGS OF THE SKIN

The skin has both an *efferent* and an *afferent* nerve supply. The efferent (outgoing from brain) supply consists of non-myelinated fibres from the sympathetic component of the autonomic nervous system. It supplies the blood vessels in the skin and is responsible for vessel diameter and hence blood flow. It also provides a supply to the skin appendages, particularly to arrector pili muscles and the eccrine sweat glands. The afferent nervous system (ingoing to brain) subserves sensation and comprises both myelinated and non-myelinated fibres. It is responsible for transmitting impulses from the various sensory nerve endings to the central nervous system, and with them cutaneous sensation. The sensory nerve endings in the skin are in the form of both free nerve endings and specialised encapsulated nerve endings, the 'capsules' being modifications of Schwann cells; these specialised nerve endings in the skin are Meissner, Pacinian and Ruffini corpuscles and are illustrated and discussed in more detail in Ch. 7.

Free nerve endings (see Fig. 7.24) may be myelinated or non-myelinated and are mainly responsible for pain and itch sensations and detecting temperature. They occupy the papillary dermis and send twigs into the epidermis where some of them associate with ***Merkel cells*** (Fig. 9.8); this combination acts as a slowly adapting mechanoreceptor. Free nerve endings also ramify around hair follicles.

Meissner corpuscles (see Fig. 7.24) are rapidly adapting mechanoreceptors responsible for touch sensation. They are particularly prominent in the papillary dermis of the pulps of the fingers and toes and soles and palms.

Pacinian corpuscles (see Fig. 7.25) are responsible for detection of deep pressure and vibration. In the skin, they are usually found deep in the subcutis, singly or in small clusters, being particularly numerous in the palms and soles.

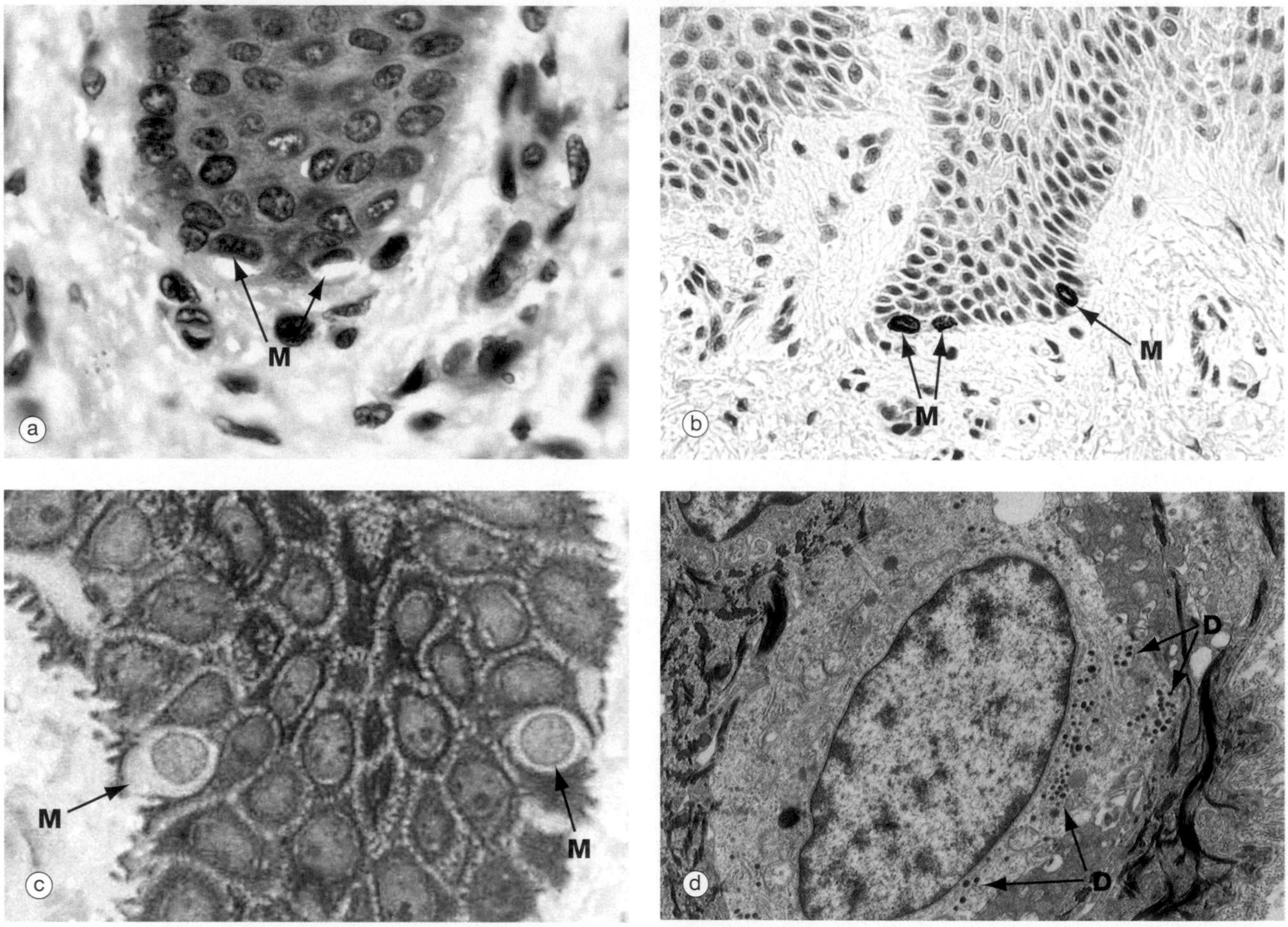

FIG. 9.8 Merkel cells
(a) H&E (MP) (b) Immunohistochemistry for CK20 (MP) (c) Epoxy resin thin section, toluidine blue ×1000 (d) EM ×10 000

Merkel cells are intra-epidermal touch receptors and contain neuroendocrine-type membrane-bound vesicles (dense core granules) in their cytoplasm, particularly near their base where they make synaptic junctions with myelinated sensory nerve twigs in the upper dermis. They are difficult to detect in routine H&E sections.

Fig. 9.8a shows two Merkel cells **M** in the basal layer of epidermis. They are rounded cells with pale-staining cytoplasm. The immunohistochemical preparation in Fig. 9.8b illustrates three Merkel cells **M**. Fig. 9.8c shows Merkel cells with pale nuclei and cytoplasm, while in the electron micrograph, Fig. 9.8d, the dense core granules **D** can be seen.

HAIR AND NAILS

Skin appendages first develop in the second trimester of intrauterine development as simple downgrowths of the surface epithelium (epidermis) into the developing subepithelial layers of mesoderm which will eventually become dermis and subcutis. The skin appendages include ***hair follicles, sebaceous glands, eccrine glands, apocrine glands*** and ***nails*** (fingers and toes).

Hair is produced in follicles in association with sebaceous glands and a smooth muscle bundle (***arrector pili***); these can be called ***pilosebaceous follicles*** or ***units***. Hairs are long, thin, cylindrical shafts composed of keratin; hair shafts have a surface cuticle composed of a single layer of flattened keratin scales. This covers a cortex of keratin forming the bulk of the hair. Large hairs may have a central medulla.

In mammals, the function of hair and fur is thermoregulation, particularly heat conservation. Hair also serves a display function, providing colour and shape. The structure of the hair follicle is complex (Fig. 9.10). Hair growth is cyclical, with three phases: a long phase of active growth (***anagen***), a short phase of involution (***catagen***) and a short inactive involuted phase (***telogen***). The growth cycle of hairs varies from site to site: scalp hair follicles have an anagen growth phase of more than 2 years and a short telogen resting phase of a few months; correspondingly, scalp hair can grow to a great length. Pubic hair, coarse trunk hair, eyelashes and eyebrows have a short growth phase (anagen) and a relatively long resting phase (telogen), thereby limiting hair length at these sites.

In infancy, childhood and in adult females, body hair is fine and soft and is known as ***vellus***, in contrast to the coarser hair of the scalp, which is known as ***terminal hair***. Male sex hormone production at puberty stimulates development of terminal pubic and axillary hair in both sexes and the replacement of vellus hair with terminal hair on the mature male body.

The structure of hair follicles depends on the type of hair being produced: follicles of the scalp and other terminal hairs tend to be long and straight, whereas those which produce fine, downy vellus hairs are relatively short. Curly hair may be produced by curved follicles or follicles in which the hair bulb lies at an angle to the hair shaft.

Contraction of the arrector pili smooth muscle makes the hair stand up, a response called 'goose flesh', in a thermoregulation-related response.

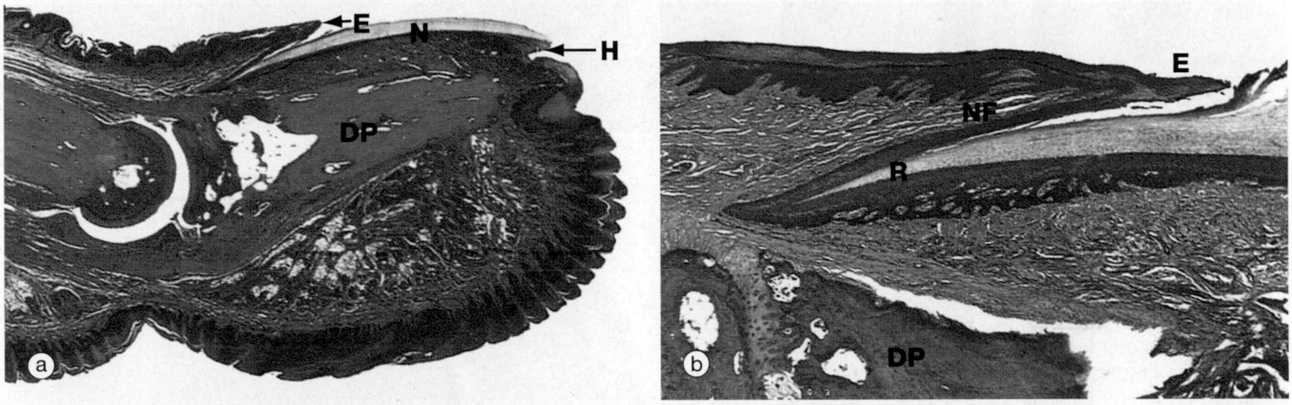

FIG. 9.9 Fingernail, monkey
(a) H&E (LP) (b) H&E (LP)

The dorsal skin surface of the tip of each finger and toe (Fig. 9.9a) forms a highly specialised appendage, the nail, consisting of a dense keratinised plate, the ***nail plate* N**, which rests on a stratified squamous epithelium, the ***nail bed***. The proximal end of the nail, the ***nail root* R**, and the underlying nail bed extend deep into the dermis to lie in close apposition to the distal interphalangeal joint. The dermis beneath the nail plate is firmly attached to the periosteum of the ***distal phalanx* DP**.

Nail growth occurs by proliferation and differentiation of the epithelium underlying the nail root (known as the ***nail matrix***). The nail plate slides distally over the rest of the nail bed, which does not actively contribute to nail growth.

Reflecting its proliferative activity, the nail matrix is thicker than the epithelium of the rest of the nail bed and exhibits pronounced epidermal ridges as seen in Fig. 9.9b; on the surface, the distal part of the nail matrix is marked by the white crescent-shaped ***lunula*** at the base of the nail.

The skin overlying the root of the nail is known as the ***nail fold* NF** and its highly keratinised free edge is known as the ***eponychium* E**. The skin beneath the free end of the nail is known as the ***hyponychium* H**.

D dense core granules **DP** distal phalanx **E** eponychium **H** hyponychium **M** Merkel cells **N** nail plate **NF** nail fold
R nail root

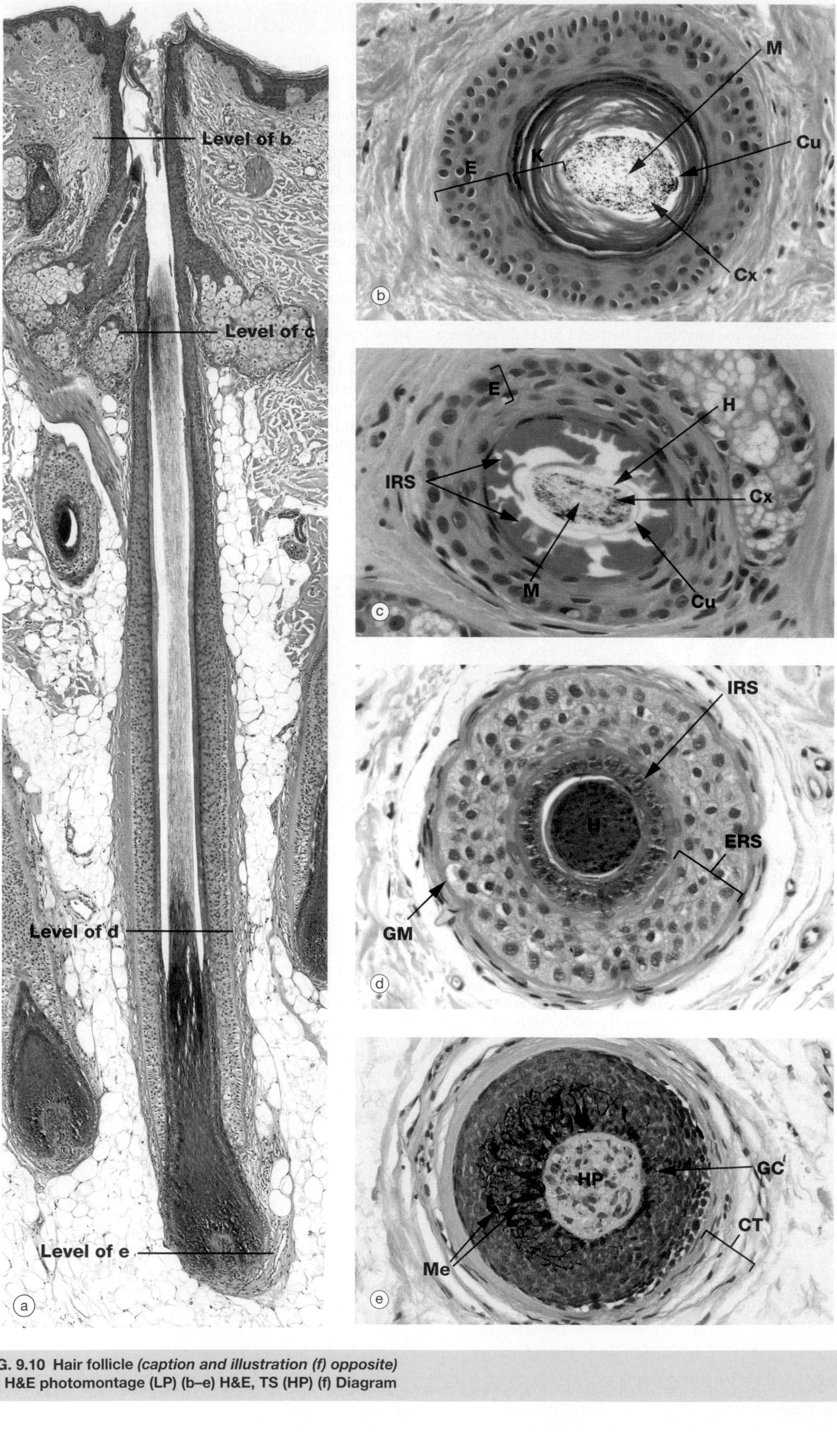

FIG. 9.10 Hair follicle ***(caption and illustration (f) opposite)***
(a) H&E photomontage (LP) (b–e) H&E, TS (HP) (f) Diagram

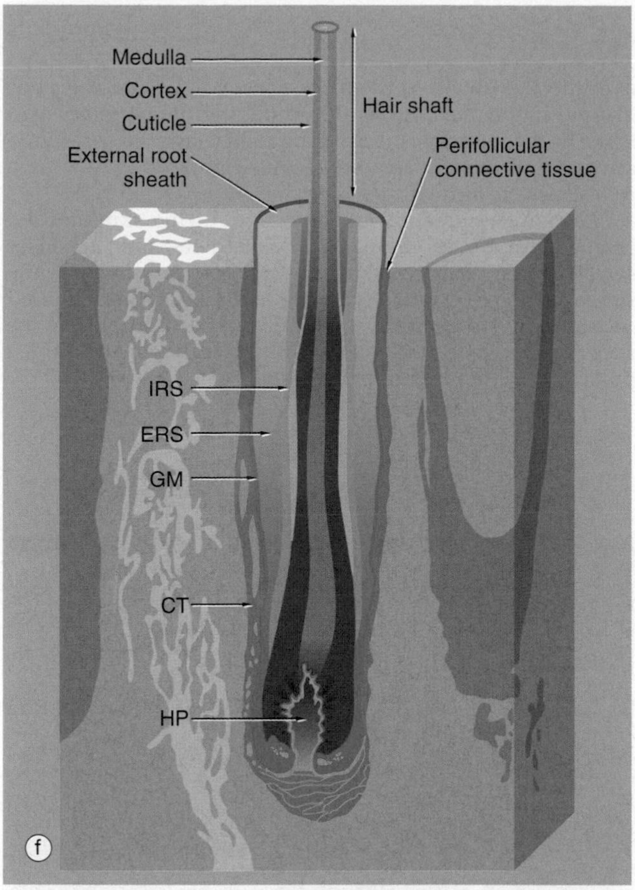

FIG. 9.10 Hair follicle *(illustrations (a) to (e) opposite)* (a) H&E photomontage (LP) (b–e) H&E, TS (HP) (f) Diagram

The hair follicle is a tubular structure formed of specialised peri-follicular connective tissue and epithelium. Fig. 9.10a is a full-length image of a terminal scalp hair. At the base, there is a bulbous expansion, the hair bulb, enclosing the ***hair papilla* HP**.

During active hair growth, the epithelial cells around the hair papilla proliferate to form the layers of the follicle. In the hair bulb, all the layers start as an indistinguishable proliferative cell mass known as the *hair matrix*. As they grow, they are pushed towards the skin surface from the hair bulb, and five epithelial layers form. The inner three epithelial layers undergo keratinisation to form the ***hair shaft*** (the hair) whilst the outer two layers form an internal and external sheath.

The cells of the innermost layer of the follicle undergo keratinisation to form the ***medulla* M** or core of the hair shaft; the medullary layer may not be distinguishable, especially in fine hairs. The medulla is surrounded by a broad, highly keratinised layer, the ***cortex* Cx**, which forms the bulk of the hair shaft. A third cell surface layer keratinises to form a hard, thin ***cuticle* Cu** on the surface of the hair, consisting of overlapping keratin plates, an arrangement which is said to prevent matting of the hair.

The outer fourth layer of the follicle constitutes the ***internal root sheath* IRS**; the cells of this layer become only lightly keratinised and lock with the developing cuticle, keeping the developing hair as a solid unit as it matures. After keratinisation, this layer fractures and fragments, leaving the hair shaft free in the follicle lumen, forming a space into which sebum is secreted around the maturing hair.

The outermost layer, the ***external root sheath* ERS**, is the external epithelial layer and merges with epidermis at the sebaceous glands. There is a thick, specialised basement membrane known as the ***glassy membrane* GM** and a surrounding specialised ***perifollicular connective tissue sheath* CT**.

Fig. 9.10e shows a transverse section of the hair bulb, the distended base of the hair follicle, with an invaginated core of connective tissue, the hair papilla **HP**, containing small blood vessels and myelinated and non-myelinated nerve twigs. This is surrounded by a basal layer of palisaded active ***germinative cells* GC**. This germinative epithelium forms the follicle. In active (anagen) growth, the hair bulbs are prominent, with a well-formed hair papilla, and are located in subcutis.

In people with dark-coloured hair, melanocytes **Me** (see Fig. 9.6) are scattered amongst the proliferating cells of the hair bulb, with melanin being incorporated in the cells which will form the hair shaft. Black, brown and yellow forms of melanin are produced in various combinations and determine final hair colour.

Fig. 9.10d is a transverse section through the hair follicle at the level shown by the line. The external root sheath **ERS** is separated from the connective tissue sheath **CT** by the glassy membrane **GM**. Passing inwards, the outermost cells, the external root sheath, have a homogeneous appearance. The internal root sheath **IRS** is recognised by its prominent, coarse, eosinophilic (***keratohyaline***) granules. Centrally is the hair shaft **H**.

In Fig. 9.10c at the level of sebaceous glands, the hair shaft is mature with a thin, pale-stained cuticle layer **Cu** which surrounds the pigmented cortex **Cx** and pale medulla **M**. The internal root sheath **IRS** has now keratinised and is fragmenting as it is no longer required to support the developing hair shaft **H**, while the external root sheath is replaced by epidermis **E**.

Fig. 9.10b is above the sebaceous glands. This part of the follicle is called the ***follicular infundibulum***. It shows the hair shaft surrounded by epidermal-type keratin **K** and epidermis. Note that the hair shaft is out of the plane of section in Fig. 9.10a at this level.

Each pilosebaceous follicle has an attached small smooth muscle called an ***arrector pili muscle*** (Fig. 9.11).

CT connective tissue sheath **Cu** cuticle **Cx** cortex **E** epidermis **ERS** external root sheath **GC** germinative cells **GM** glassy membrane **H** hair shaft **HP** hair papilla **IRS** internal root sheath **K** keratin **M** medulla **Me** melanocytes

SKIN GLANDS

The skin has a range of different glands including sebaceous, eccrine and apocrine glands. ***Sebaceous glands*** occur in two forms. The majority are associated with hair follicles and develop as lateral protrusions from the hair follicle near the junction between its upper third (***follicular infundibulum***) and lower two thirds. Sebaceous glands secrete a mixture of lipids called ***sebum*** which may provide some waterproofing of the skin surface and hair shafts; the sebum is secreted into the hair follicle (Fig. 9.11). At some sites in the skin (areolae and nipples, labia minora of vulva, eyelids), the sebaceous glands are independent of hair follicles and open directly onto the skin or mucosal surface.

Each hair follicle has an ***arrector pili muscle*** consisting of a bundle of smooth muscle fibres. These insert at one end into the sheath of the follicle just below the sebaceous glands, and at the other end into the dermal papillary area beneath the epidermis. Each hair follicle and its associated arrector pili muscle and sebaceous glands is known as a ***pilosebaceous unit***.

Eccrine glands are found throughout the skin and are essential for thermoregulation through the production of sweat, opening onto the skin surface. ***Apocrine glands***, while similar in architecture to eccrine glands, have a very limited distribution and connect to the follicular infundibulum, the superficial part of pilosebaceous (hair) follicles, and have a possible function in producing odour.

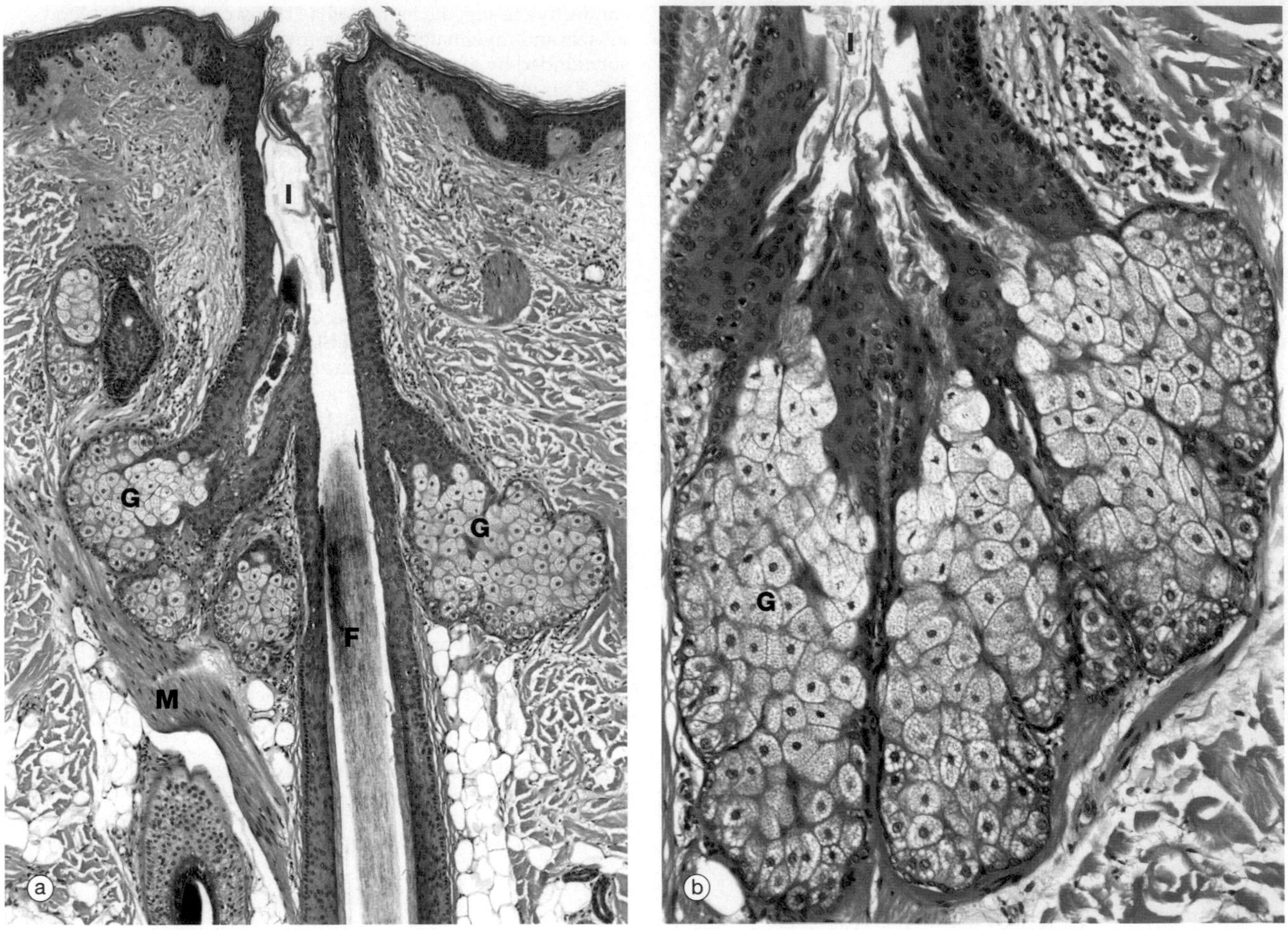

FIG. 9.11 Sebaceous glands and arrector pili
(a) H&E (LP) (b) H&E (MP)

Fig. 9.11a illustrates the relationship of a sebaceous gland **G** and an ***arrector pili muscle*** **M** to a hair follicle **F**. At about mid-dermis, each hair follicle is surrounded by sebaceous glands which discharge their secretions onto the hair follicle and thence onto the skin surface. The superficial part of the follicle is called the ***infundibulum*** **I**. Sebaceous glands lie within the fibrous sheath surrounding the hair follicle and the glandular epithelium represents an outgrowth of the external root sheath. Arrector pili bind to the follicle just below the sebaceous glands.

More detail of sebaceous gland structure can be seen in Fig. 9.11b. Each sebaceous gland has a branched acinar form, the acini converging upon a short duct which empties into the hair follicle beside the hair shaft. Each acinus consists of a mass of rounded cells packed with lipid-filled vacuoles; during tissue preparation, the lipid is largely removed, leaving clear spaces in the cytoplasm of these cells. Towards the duct, the lipid content of the acinar cells increases and the distended cells degenerate, releasing their contents, sebum, into the duct. This process is known as ***holocrine secretion*** (see Ch. 5). Cells lost by holocrine secretion are replaced by mitosis in the basal layer of the acinus.

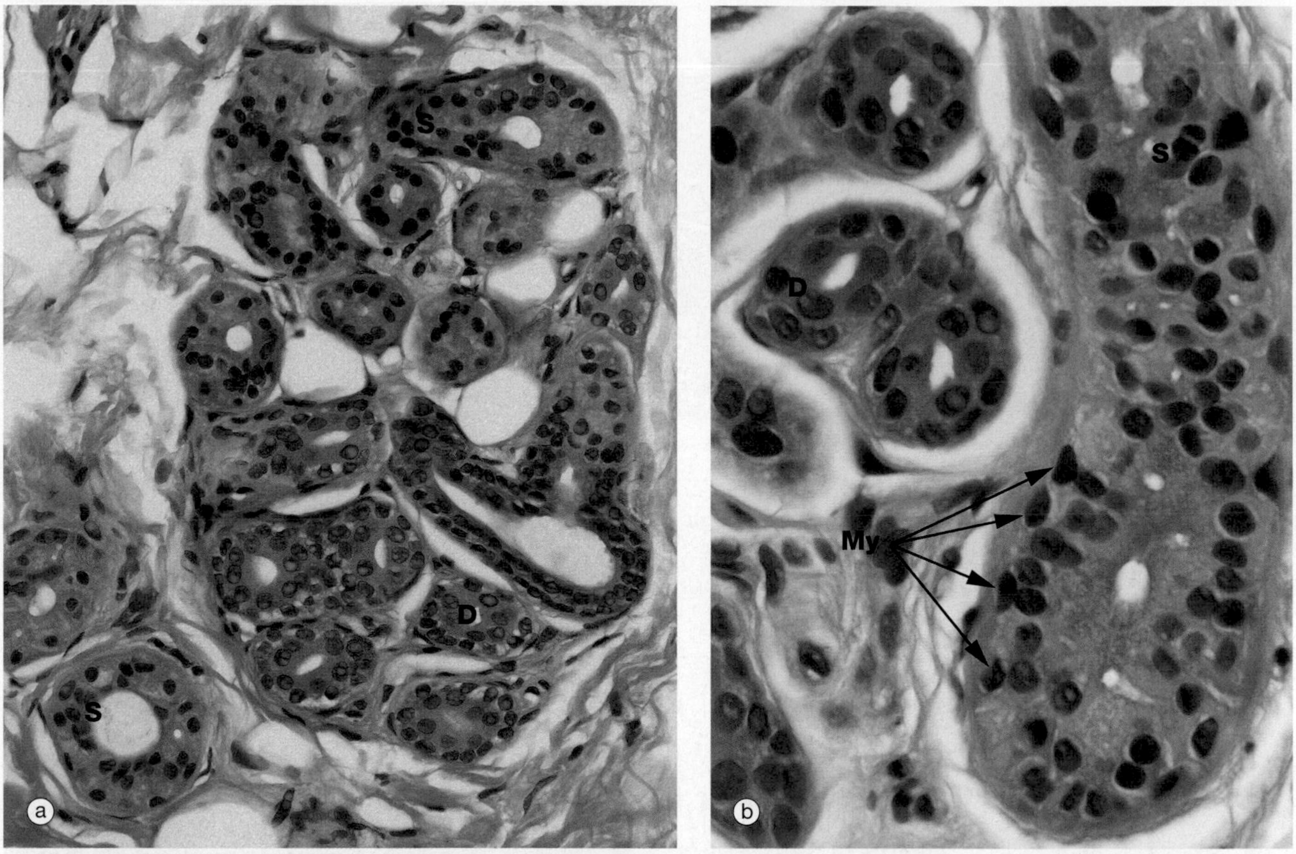

FIG. 9.12 Eccrine sweat glands and ducts
(a) H&E (MP) (b) H&E (HP)

Eccrine glands occur everywhere in the skin and are particularly frequent on the palms, soles, forehead and axillae. They arise as downgrowths from the epidermis during the second trimester of intrauterine life and their function is to secrete sweat. The evaporation of sweat provides a means of lowering body temperature and is an important component of the thermoregulatory system. In addition to water, sweat contains significant quantities of sodium and chloride ions, some other ions, urea and some low molecular weight metabolites.

Histologically, an eccrine gland has two main components. The ***secretory component*** is a coiled secretory gland situated in the deep reticular dermis; the secretions formed there are passed into a coiled ***eccrine duct*** close to the secretory gland. The duct then becomes straight as it ascends vertically through the dermis towards the skin surface.

The secretory gland component **S** has an inner layer of large columnar or pyramidal cells with central oval nuclei and pale eosinophilic cytoplasm, interspersed with smaller, rarer, darker-staining cells best identified by a specific stain for mucopolysaccharides such as the PAS reaction. The clear cells secrete the bulk of the watery sweat and the smaller cells secrete a glycoprotein. The lateral walls of the secretory cells show prominent interdigitations which separate in places to form canaliculi that open into the gland lumen (not illustrated). These interdigitations greatly expand the area of the lateral plasma membrane, facilitating ion exchange.

The glands have an attenuated outer layer of contractile ***myoepithelial cells*** **My**, which form a discontinuous layer between the secretory cells and the basement membrane. They are spindle shaped and are arranged with their long axes tangential to the long axis of the coiled tubular gland.

The eccrine ducts **D** appear darker staining and have an obvious double layer of epithelial cells, the inner layer being larger and more cuboidal with microvilli lining the lumen. The luminal aspect often has a characteristic eosinophilic appearance (sometimes called the cuticle). This is partly due to the presence of a compact layer of circumferentially arranged tonofibrils in the cuboidal duct epithelial cells at the base of the abundant microvilli. The duct epithelium is biochemically active and modifies the composition of sweat, reabsorbing sodium ions.

D eccrine ducts **F** hair follicle **G** sebaceous gland **I** infundibulum **M** arrector pili muscle **My** myoepithelial cells **S** eccrine secretory gland

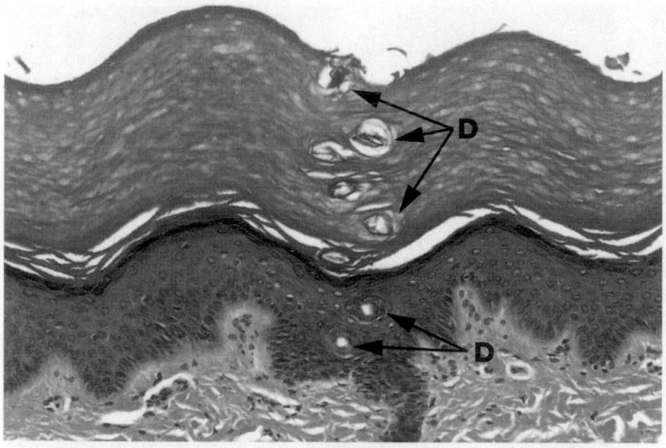

FIG. 9.13 Acrosyringium
H&E (MP)

As it passes through the epidermis, the eccrine duct (here called the ***acrosyringium***) becomes coiled, a feature which is particularly apparent as it passes through the thick epidermis and the overlying keratin of the sole of the foot. Multiple cross-sections of the coiled duct **D** can be seen in the epidermis, continuing as a structure formed of keratin through the overlying stratum corneum.

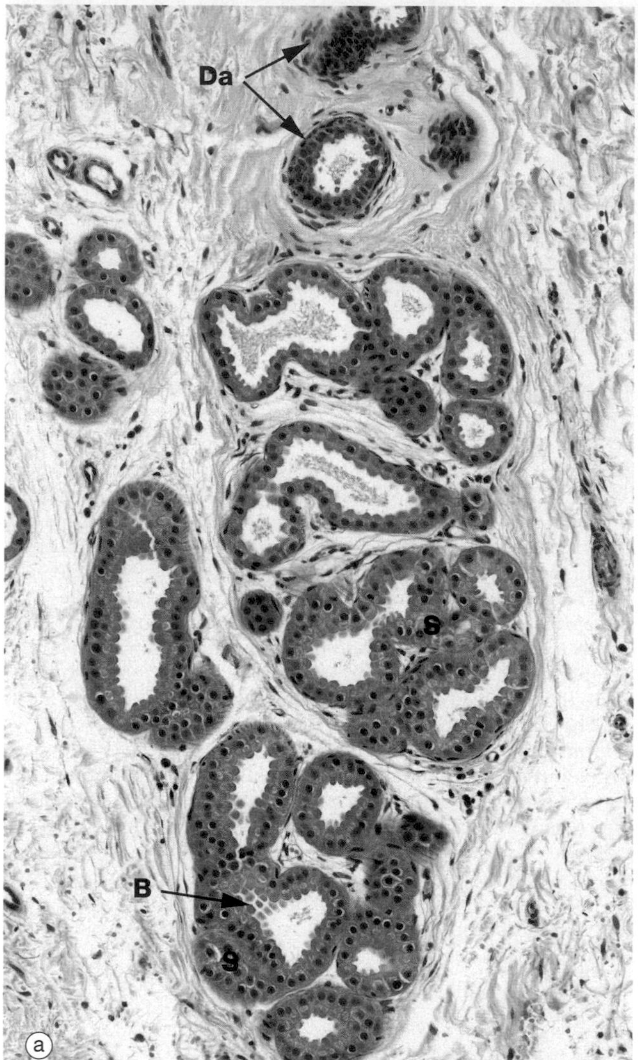

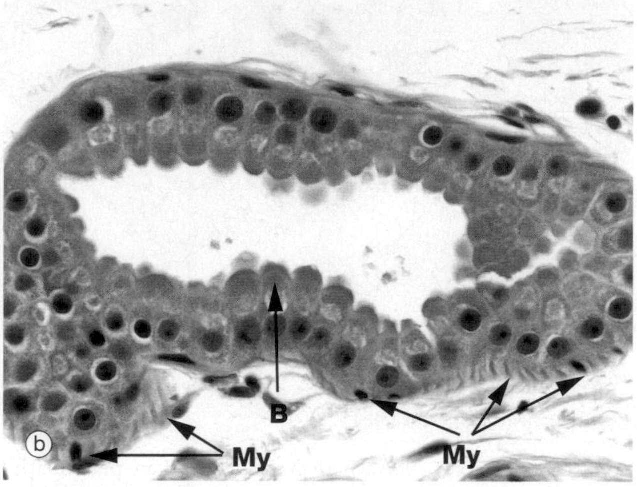

FIG. 9.14 Apocrine glands
(a) H&E (MP) (b) H&E (HP)

Apocrine glands are confined to a few localised areas, mainly in the axilla and groin. The secretory component is located in deep reticular dermis or subcutis and a duct system carries the secretion to be discharged into the upper part of the hair follicle above the sebaceous duct.

Apocrine gland secretions in humans have no defined function but, in other mammals, they are responsible for scent production, used in territory marking and as a sexual attractant. The secretory portion of the gland **S** is of the coiled tubular type with a widely dilated lumen. The secretory cells are usually low cuboidal with eosinophilic cytoplasm. The budding appearance **B** of the apical cytoplasm of some cells gave rise to the belief that the mode of secretion was of the apocrine type, but recent evidence suggests that this appearance may be due to a fixation artefact and that the original interpretations were erroneous. Like eccrine sweat glands, apocrine glands have a discontinuous layer of myoepithelial cells **My** between the base of the secretory cells and the prominent basement membrane. Their duct **Da** is histologically similar to that of eccrine sweat glands.

Apocrine glands do not become functional until puberty and, in women, undergo cyclical changes under the influence of the hormones of the menstrual cycle.

B budding apocrine apical cytoplasm **D** acrosyringium **Da** apocrine duct **My** myoepithelial cell **P** papillary dermis **R** reticular dermis **S** secretory apocrine gland

DERMIS AND SUBCUTIS

The ***dermis*** and the ***subcutis*** (also known as the ***hypodermis*** or ***panniculus***) are the layers beneath the epidermis. The overall thickness of skin is dependent on the thickness of the dermal and subcutaneous layers; in the eyelids, both layers are very thin and the skin is consequently thin and highly flexible whereas, in the back and buttocks, the dermis is thick and the subcutis variable but usually thick.

The dermis is composed of collagen and elastin fibres and is responsible for the tone and texture of the skin. In the young, the skin is tight because of the quality of the collagen and elastin but, with increasing age, the collagen and elastin in upper dermis progressively degenerate and the skin loses some of its texture and may wrinkle. The dermis also contains the skin appendages, the vascular supply to the skin, and nerves and sensory nerve endings.

The subcutis is predominately composed of adipose tissue, in many areas compartmentalised by vertical fibrous septa running from the deep reticular dermis to the fascial fibrous tissue layer which frequently underlies the subcutis. In areas with terminal hairs, the subcutis contains the deeper parts of anagen hair follicles (e.g. scalp), apocrine glands (e.g. axilla and groin) and eccrine glands (e.g. palms and soles). In parts of the face, the subcutis also contains sheets of skeletal muscle, the muscles of facial expression.

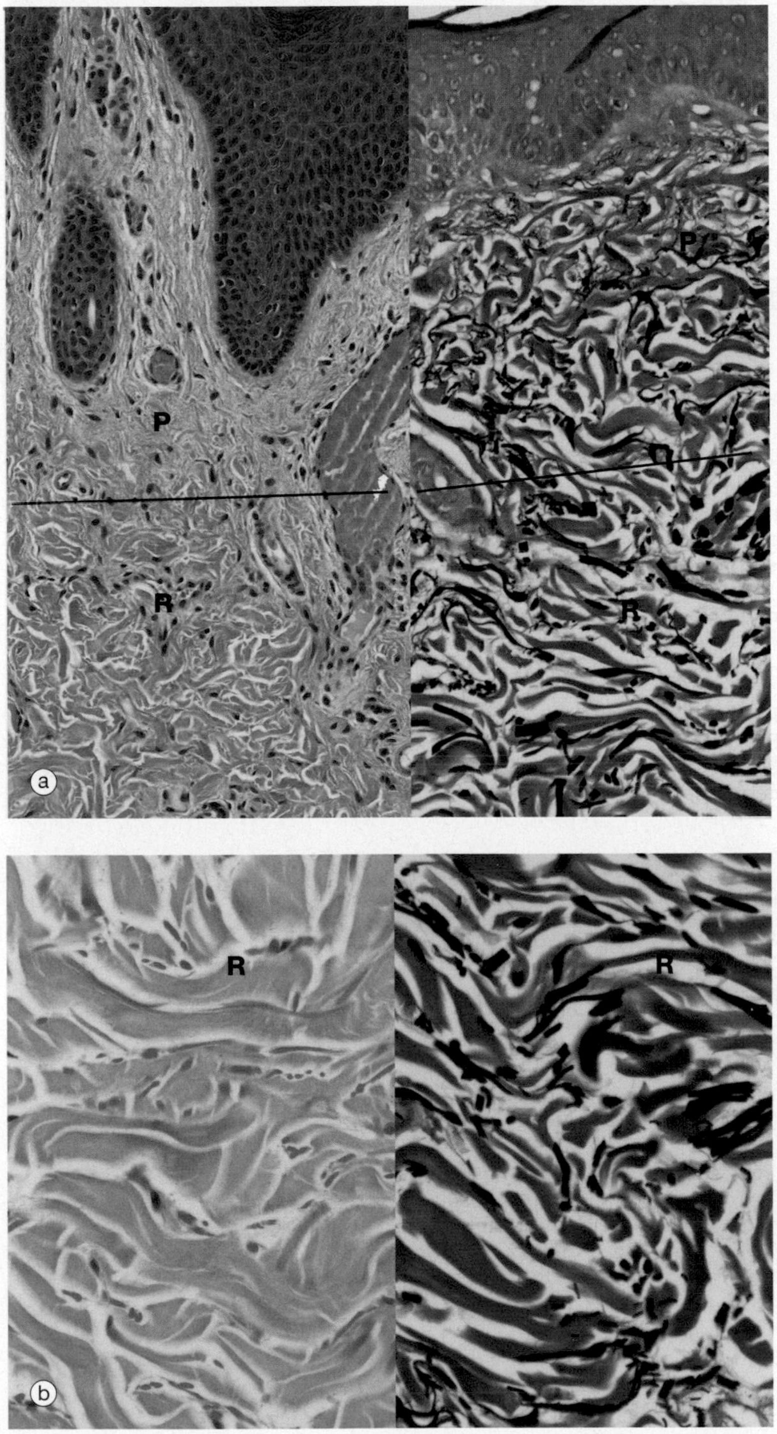

FIG. 9.15 Dermis
(a) Papillary and reticular dermis, H&E and EVG (LP) (b) Reticular dermis, H&E and EVG (HP)

The dermis is composed of bundles of collagen fibres and strands of elastic fibres embedded in scanty amounts of acellular ground substance, together with occasional fibroblasts which synthesise the collagen, elastic fibres and matrix. The dermis contains the vascular supply (see Fig. 9.16) and innervation of the skin and has two layers, a superficial ***papillary dermis*** beneath the epidermis and a deeper ***reticular dermis*** which borders the subcutis. Fig. 9.15a shows the papillary dermis **P**, which is loose and contains very fine, interlacing collagen and elastic fibres that stain red and black, respectively, in the EVG stain. It contains arterioles, capillary loops and venules, as well as lymphatics and fine nerve twigs from the sensory nerve endings, such as Meissner corpuscles. Beneath the narrow papillary dermis is the reticular dermis **R**, generally a much thicker layer. The interface may be poorly defined as in these micrographs and has been marked by a line drawn across the images.

High-power micrograph (Fig. 9.15b) shows the reticular dermis. The collagen bundles and elastic fibres are much thicker than in the papillary dermis. The reticular dermis also contains blood vessels and nerves and the skin appendages.

Lymphocytes, mast cells and macrophages are present but are scarce in normal dermis, but increase in number in many skin diseases. The reticular dermis varies greatly in thickness at different sites; it is thickest on the back and thinnest in the eyelids.

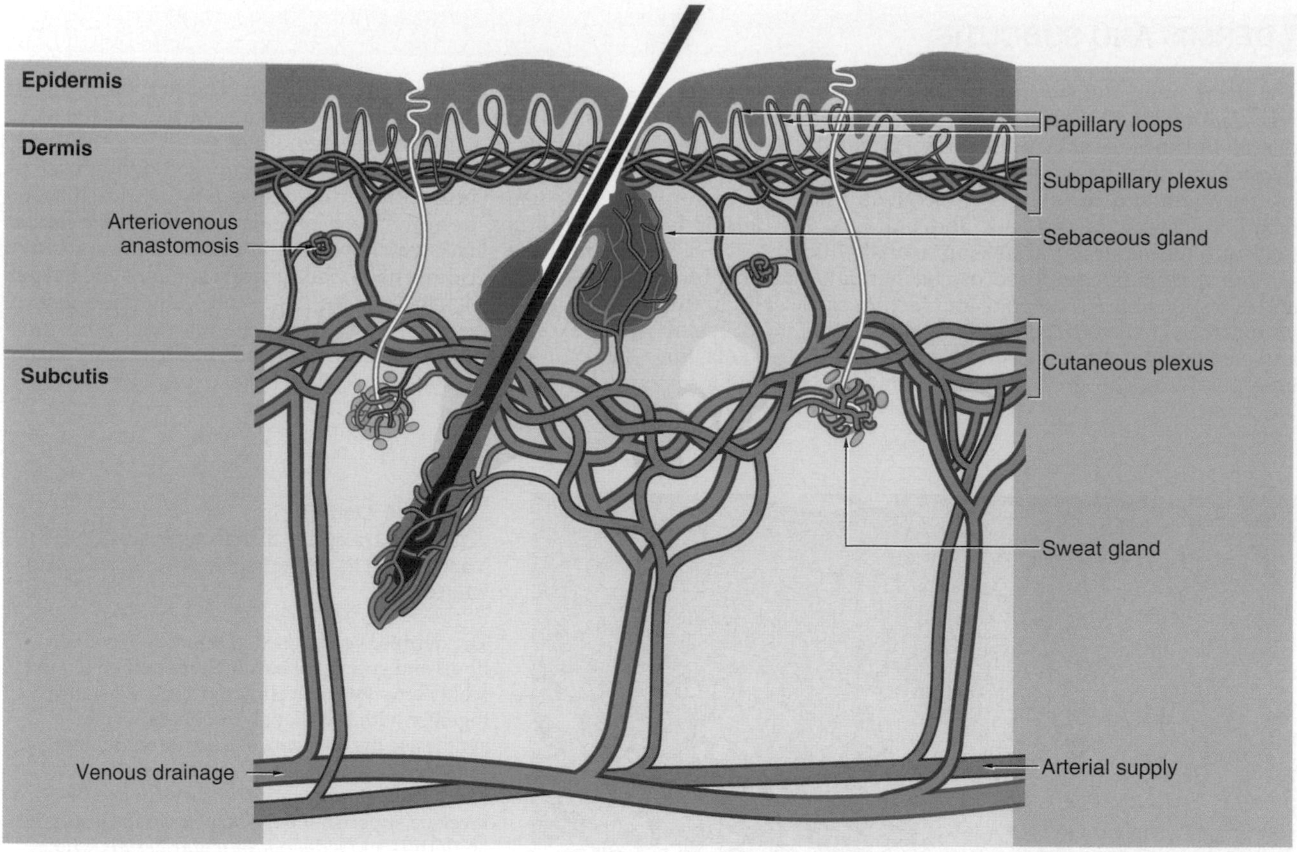

FIG. 9.16 The skin circulation

The circulation of the skin accommodates several different, sometimes conflicting, functional requirements: nutrition of the skin and appendages, increased blood flow to facilitate heat loss in hot conditions and decreased blood flow to minimise heat loss in cold conditions, whilst nevertheless maintaining adequate nutritional flow.

The arteries supplying the skin are located deep in the subcutis, from which they give rise to branches passing upwards to form two plexuses of anastomosing vessels. The deeper plexus lies at the junction of the subcutis and dermis and is known as the ***cutaneous plexus***; the more superficial plexus lies at the junction between papillary and reticular dermis (see Fig. 9.15) and is known as the ***subpapillary*** or ***superficial plexus***. This subpapillary plexus supplies the upper aspect of the dermis and gives rise to a capillary loop in each dermal papilla. The cutaneous (deep) plexus supplies the fatty tissue of the subcutis, the deeper aspect of the dermis and the capillary networks which envelop the hair follicles, deep sebaceous glands and sweat glands.

The venous drainage of the skin is arranged into plexuses broadly corresponding to the arterial supply. The skin has a rich lymphatic drainage which forms plexuses corresponding to those of the blood vascular system.

Special shunts called ***glomus bodies***, under nerve control, provide direct arterial-to-venous diversion of blood, particularly in the extremities. This diversion plays an important role in thermoregulation by controlling blood flow to the appropriate parts of the dermis.

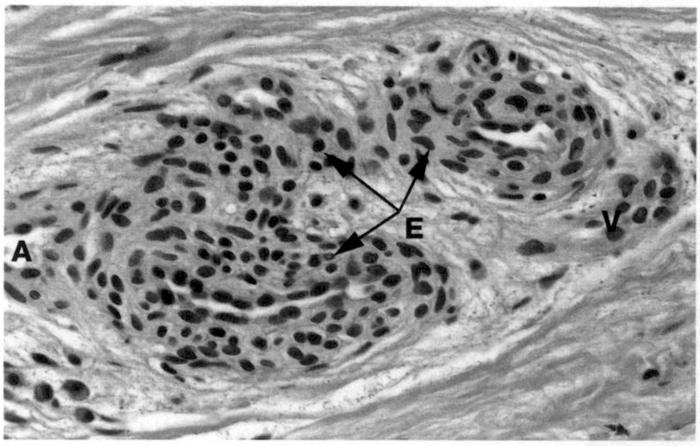

FIG. 9.17 Glomus body H&E (MP)

In the dermis of the fingertips and other peripheral sites prone to excessive cold, such as the feet and external ear, the skin blood flow is controlled by structures called glomus bodies. The glomus consists of a highly convoluted segment of muscular vessel forming an arteriovenous shunt enveloped by condensed collagenous tissue. In histological section, one or more convolutions of the arterial **A** and venous **V** elements of the shunt are usually seen (Fig. 9.17). The wall of the glomus vessel is greatly thickened by numerous smooth muscle cells assuming an epithelioid appearance **E**. This muscular structure enables controlled diversion of blood from small arteries to veins while dissipating the arterial pressure, thereby protecting the veins from excess pressure.

A arterial glomus **As** acrosyringium **AT** adipose tissue **B** hair bulbs **D** dermis **E** epithelioid smooth muscle glomus **Ep** epidermis **F** fibrous septum **Fg** galea **G** granular layer **K** keratin (stratum corneum) **RR** rete ridge **S** sebaceous gland **V** venous glomus

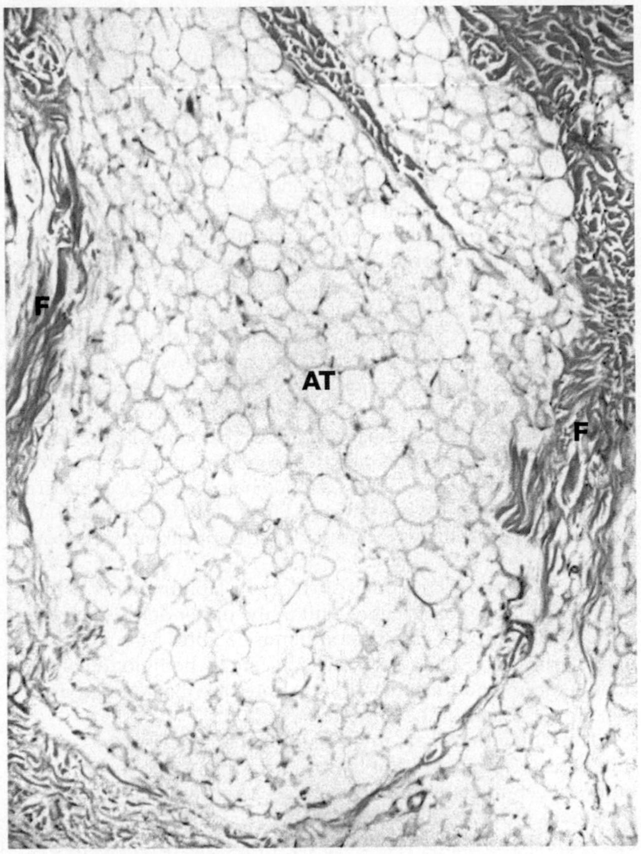

FIG. 9.18 Subcutis
H&E (LP)

This photomicrograph shows the subcutis from the skin of the upper thigh. It is composed of mature adipose tissue **AT**, partially compartmentalised by collagenous fibrous septa **F** which pass vertically from the lower reticular dermis.

The thickness of the subcutis and the degree of compartmentalisation by fibrous septa varies from site to site. At this site, the subcutis normally contains no hair follicles or apocrine glands.

EXAMPLES OF REGIONAL VARIATIONS

As already mentioned, the skin shows regional variations in different areas of the body. The typical appearances of scalp, sole of foot, and vulval skin are illustrated in the following micrographs.

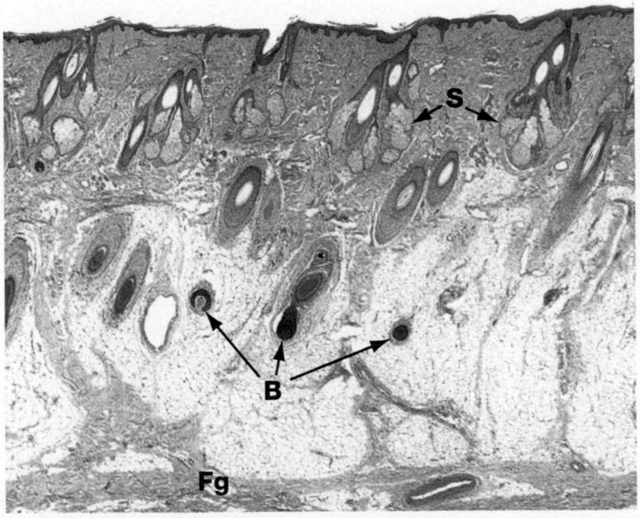

FIG. 9.19 Scalp
H&E (LP)

Fig. 9.19 shows the full thickness of the skin of the scalp. The dermis is a broad layer containing the upper parts of the abundant hair follicles with their associated sebaceous glands **S**. The subcutis is similarly broad and contains the deeper parts of the hair follicles, particularly the hair bulbs **B**. The section does not contain complete pilosebaceous units because they are arranged obliquely; the owner has curly hair. The fibrous tissue layer **Fg** deep to the subcutis is a layer of fascia, the ***galea***, which slides over the periosteum of the skull.

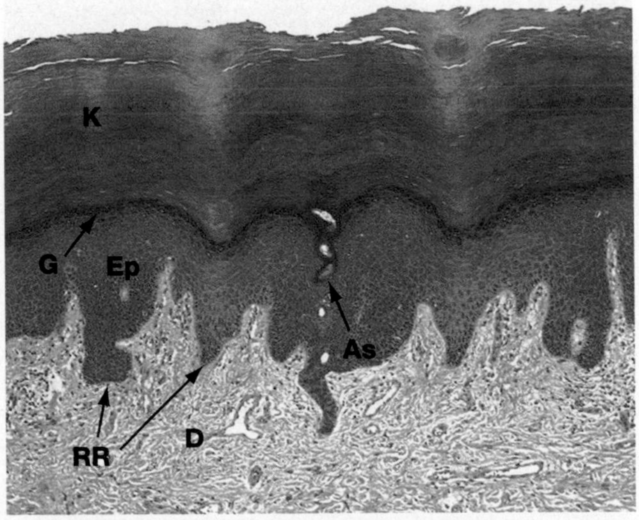

FIG. 9.20 Sole
H&E (LP)

The skin of the soles and palms is ***glabrous***, i.e. completely devoid of hair and hair follicles. Because both are areas subject to regular shearing and frictional forces, the skin is structurally modified to resist these forces (Fig. 9.20). The epidermis **Ep** is thick, with a prominent granular layer **G** producing a thick layer of compact keratin **K**, the stratum corneum. Elongated epidermal rete ridges **RR** extend into dermis, providing an increased area for attachment of epidermis to dermis **D** to minimise the risk of separation due to shearing forces during walking. Note the intraepidermal part of a sweat duct, the acrosyringium **As**, spiralling through epidermis. Sweat glands and nerve endings are numerous at both sites.

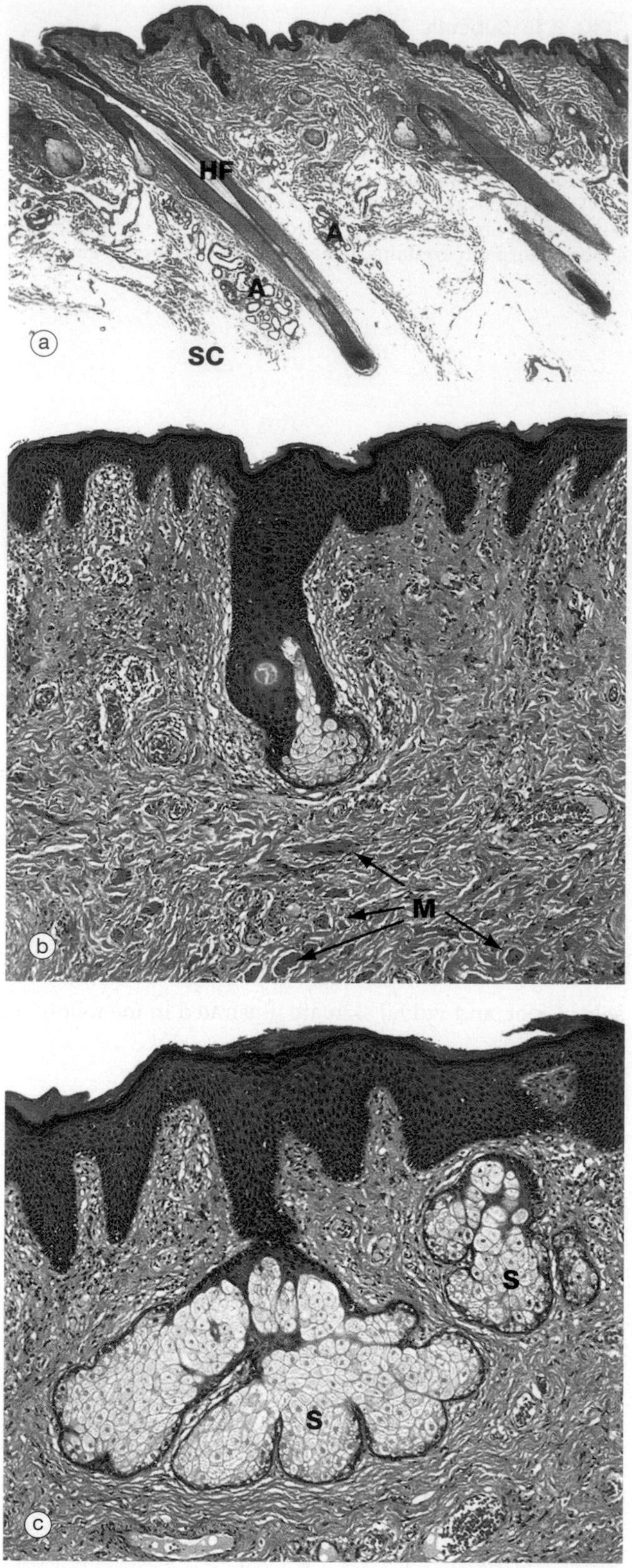

FIG. 9.21 Vulva
(a) Mons pubis, H&E (LP) (b) Labium majus, H&E (LP)
(c) Labium minus, H&E (MP)

The vulva comprises the ***mons pubis***, ***labia majora*** (singular is labium majus), ***labia minora*** (singular is labium minus), and the ***vestibule*** with its vestibular glands which mark the junction between vulva and vaginal canal. The vulva is also the site of the opening of the female urethra and the location of the erectile ***clitoris***, the female homologue of the penis. The squamous epithelium of the labia minora is continuous with the squamous epithelium of the lower vagina.

Fig. 9.21a shows the mons pubis skin with abundant oblique hair follicles **HF** (producing curly hair) and some apocrine glands **A**. This area has a thick pad of subcutaneous adipose tissue **SC**. The labia majora are longitudinal folds of skin which extend posteriorly from the mons pubis; the outer surface of the fold has the same type of skin as the mons pubis, i.e. with abundant pilosebaceous units, oblique hair follicles and apocrine glands in the subcutis, as shown in Fig. 9.21a. On the inner surface, the hair follicles progressively disappear but sebaceous glands persist.

Fig. 9.21b shows the inner surface of a labium majus, with the residue of a pilosebaceous unit in the upper dermis and numerous clumps of small smooth muscle fibres **M** in mid and deep dermis. The labia majora are the female homologue of the male scrotum and the labial muscle fibres are the homologue of the dartos muscle of the scrotum (see Ch. 18).

The labia minora are internal to the labia majora and are thin flaps of skin devoid of hair follicles. Fig. 9.21c shows the outer aspect of a labium minus. It has a keratinising stratified squamous epidermis and scattered sebaceous glands **S** which open directly onto the skin surface, rather than into the necks of hair follicles as they do in hair-bearing skin (see Fig. 9.11). On the inner aspect, the labia minora have a thinner epidermis and keratin layer. The vaginal orifice is one of the sites of a muco-cutaneous junction, where the skin of the labia minora of the vulva meets the mucosa of the vaginal canal (see Ch. 19); similar mucocutaneous junctions exist at the oral, nasal and anal orifices.

A apocrine gland **HF** hair follicle **M** smooth muscle fibres **S** sebaceous gland **SC** subcutaneous adipose tissue

REVIEW

TABLE 9.1 Review of skin

Major structures	Main structures or cells	Brief description/ function	Figures
Epidermis	Keratinocytes	Proliferate from base, move upward and keratinise to form a non-living protective, abrasion-resistant waterproofing keratin layer, the stratum corneum	9.2, 9.3
	Melanocytes	Basally located; produce melanin pigment and pass this to keratinocytes; provide UV light protection	9.6, 9.7
	Langerhans cells	Antigen-presenting cells throughout epidermis (and superficial dermis)	9.5
	Merkel cells	Basally located sensory neuroendocrine cells	9.8
	Basement membrane (dermo-epidermal junction)	Specialised structure produced by epidermis and dermis in combination; ties the epidermis to dermis	9.4
Dermis	Collagen and elastin	Provide strength and elasticity	9.15
	Vessels • Papillary/superficial plexus • Cutaneous plexus	 • Supplies dermal papillae and thus epidermis with superficial dermis • Supplies deep dermis and subcutis	9.16
	Glomus bodies	AV shunts; divert blood from skin to conserve heat; found mainly in hands, feet, ears	9.17
Adnexae	Nails	Keratin plates; strengthen tips of fingers and toes	9.9
	Pilosebaceous units • Hair follicles • Sebaceous glands • Arrector pili muscles	 • Produce hair • Sebum (oil) producing holocrine glands • Follicle associated smooth muscle bundles	9.10, 9.11
	Eccrine glands	Produce sweat, a critical means of body cooling	9.12, 9.13
	Apocrine glands	Glands of groin and axilla; produce odour	9.14
Subcutis	Adipose tissue	Triglyceride (fat) store; provides insulation and structural padding	9.18
	Fibrous tissue septa	Strengthen adipose tissue and tie subcutis to both dermis and underlying structures such as fascia	9.18, 9.19
Nerves	Meissner corpuscles	Papillary dermal touch receptors, concentrated in hands and feet	7.24
	Merkel cell neurites	Papillary dermal touch receptors, concentrated in hands and feet	7.24
	Free nerve endings	Pain and temperature receptors	7.24
	Pacinian corpuscles	Deep in subcutis, concentrated in palms and soles; deep pressure and vibration sense	7.25

10 Skeletal tissues

INTRODUCTION

The skeletal system is formed from highly specialised types of supporting/connective tissue. The tissues are made up of collagen and acellular matrix, as well as the cells which synthesise them. ***Bone*** provides a rigid protective and supporting framework, the rigidity resulting from the deposition of calcium salts within the collagen and matrix. ***Cartilage*** occurs in different forms and provides a smooth articular surface at bone ends, as well as structural support in special areas (e.g. trachea, pinna). It is also important in one form of new bone formation.

Joints are composite structures which join the bones of the skeleton and, depending on the function and structure of individual joints, permit varying degrees of movement.

Ligaments are robust but flexible bands of collagenous tissue which contribute to the stability of joints. ***Tendons*** provide strong, pliable connections between muscles and their points of insertion into bones.

The functional differences between the various tissues of the skeletal system relate principally to the different nature and proportion of the ground substance and fibrous elements of the extracellular matrix. The cells of all the skeletal tissues, like the cells of the less specialised supporting/connective tissues, have close structural and functional relationships and a common origin from primitive mesenchymal cells (see Ch. 4).

CARTILAGE

The semi-rigid nature of cartilage stems from the predominance of proteoglycan ground substance in the extracellular matrix.

Proteoglycans (see Ch. 4), disposed in ***proteoglycan aggregates*** of 100 or more molecules, make up the ground substance and account for the solid, yet flexible, consistency of cartilage. Sulphated glycosaminoglycans (GAGs, chondroitin sulphate and keratan sulphate) predominate in the proteoglycan aggregates, with molecules of the non-sulphated GAG ***hyaluronic acid*** forming the central back-bone of the complex. The different types of cartilage vary in the amount and nature of fibres in the ground substance: ***hyaline cartilage*** contains few fibres, ***fibrocartilage*** contains abundant collagen fibres and ***elastic cartilage*** contains elastin fibres.

Cartilage formation commences with the differentiation of stellate shaped primitive mesenchymal cells (see Fig. 4.2) to form rounded cartilage precursor cells called ***chondroblasts***. Subsequent mitotic divisions give rise to aggregations of closely packed chondroblasts which grow and begin synthesis of ground substance and fibrous extracellular material. Secretion of extracellular material traps each chondroblast within the cartilaginous matrix, thereby separating the chondroblasts from one another. Each chondroblast then undergoes one or two further mitotic divisions to form a small cluster of mature cells separated by a small amount of extracellular material.

Mature cartilage cells, known as ***chondrocytes***, maintain the integrity of the cartilage matrix. Most mature cartilage masses acquire a surrounding layer called the ***perichondrium***, composed of collagen fibres and spindle-shaped cells which resemble fibroblasts. These have the capacity to transform into chondroblasts and form new cartilage by ***appositional growth***. There is also very limited capacity in mature cartilage masses for ***interstitial growth***. This occurs by further division of chondrocytes trapped within the previously formed matrix and subsequent deposition of more matrix material. The hyaline cartilage of the articular surfaces of joints does not have perichondrium on the surface and has no capacity to regenerate new cartilage after damage. In general, mature cartilage has a very limited capacity to repair and regenerate, partly because of its poor blood supply.

Most cartilage is devoid of blood vessels and, consequently, the exchange of metabolites between chondrocytes and surrounding tissues depends on diffusion through the water of the ground substance. This limits the thickness to which cartilage may develop while maintaining viability of the innermost cells. In sites where cartilage is particularly thick (e.g. costal cartilage), ***cartilage canals*** convey small vessels into the centre of the cartilage mass.

The role of cartilage in bone formation is discussed in Figs 10.18 to 10.21.

Cartilage

The various different forms of cartilage are specialised to perform distinct functions. The nature of the extracellular matrix differs in these subtypes.

Hyaline cartilage is found on the articular surfaces of many joints, lying over the surface of the bone ends and forming a smooth, firm, but slightly flexible surface. Hyaline cartilage has very abundant gel-like ground substance.

Fibrocartilage is found in the intervertebral discs as well as in sites such as the pubic symphysis. Fibrocartilage resembles dense connective tissue and has very abundant collagen fibres but with intervening bands of extracellular matrix.

Elastic cartilage is important in the structure of the external ear and the larynx, being firm but very flexible due to the presence of many elastin fibres within an extracellular matrix which is similar to that of hyaline cartilage.

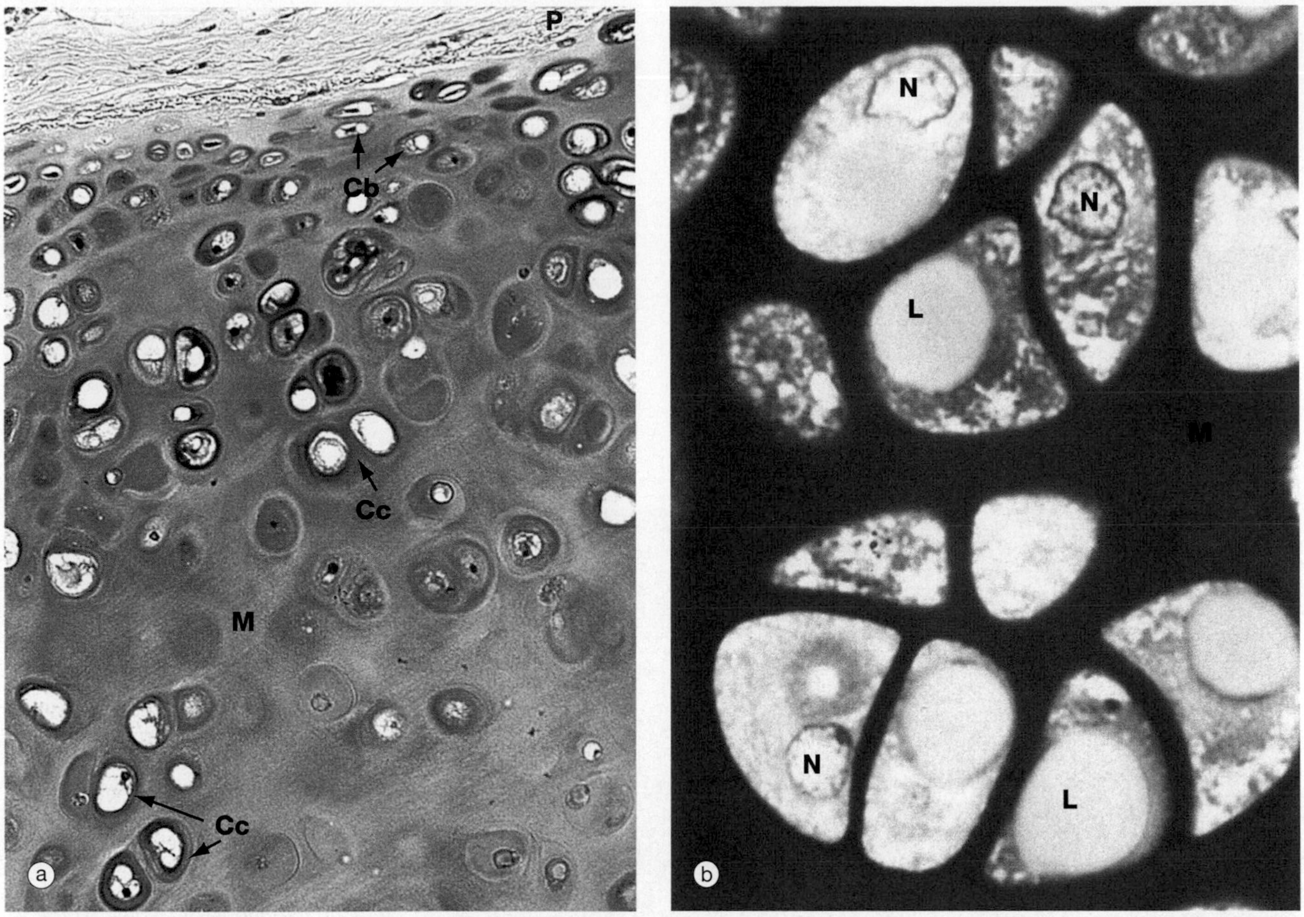

FIG. 10.1 Hyaline cartilage
(a) H&E (MP) (b) Thin epoxy resin section, toluidine blue (HP)

Hyaline cartilage is the most common type of cartilage. It is found in the nasal septum, larynx, tracheal rings, most articular surfaces and the sternal ends of the ribs. It also forms the precursor of bone in the developing skeleton. Mature hyaline cartilage is characterised by small aggregates of chondrocytes embedded in an amorphous matrix of ground substance, reinforced by collagen fibres.

Fig. 10.1a shows a hyaline cartilage mass with its outer ***perichondrium*** **P**. The ***chondrocytes*** of the formed cartilage **Cc** are arranged in clusters, usually of 2 to 4 cells, each cluster being separated from its neighbours by amorphous cartilage matrix **M**. The perichondrium is composed of parallel collagen fibres containing a few spindle-shaped nuclei of inactive fibrocytes but, on its inner surface, these cells are transforming into small ***chondroblasts*** **Cb** which are in the process of enlarging, dividing and synthesising new cartilage matrix.

The matrix of hyaline cartilage appears fairly amorphous, since the ground substance and collagen have similar refractive properties. With the exception of articular cartilage, the collagen of hyaline cartilage, designated as type II collagen (see Ch. 4), is not cross-banded and is arranged in an interlacing network of fine fibrils. This collagen cannot be demonstrated by light microscopy.

The thin epoxy resin section of hyaline cartilage in Fig. 10.1b shows the cellular details of mature chondrocytes. Note that the chondrocytes fully occupy the spaces in the matrix **M**, each space containing a single chondrocyte. Mature chondrocytes are characterised by small nuclei **N** with dispersed chromatin and basophilic granular cytoplasm, reflecting a well-developed rough endoplasmic reticulum. Lipid droplets **L**, often larger than the nuclei, are a prominent feature of larger chondrocytes. The cytoplasm is also rich in glycogen. These characteristics reflect the active role of chondrocytes in synthesis of both the ground substance and fibrous elements of the cartilage matrix. In fully formed cartilage, the constituents of the extracellular matrix are continuously turned over, the integrity of the matrix being thus absolutely dependent on the viability of the chondrocytes.

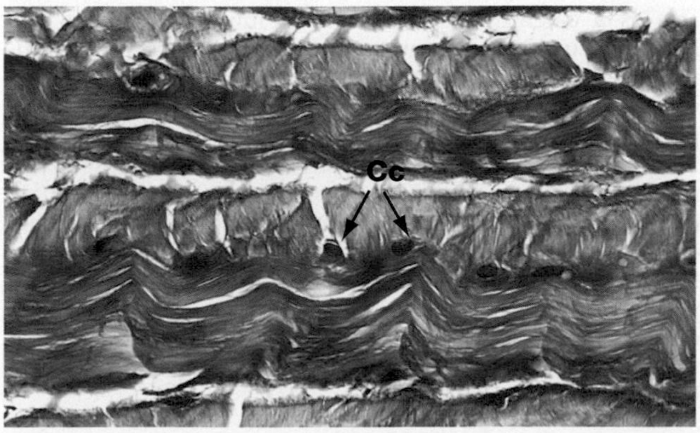

FIG. 10.2 Fibrocartilage
H&E/Alcian blue (HP)

Fibrocartilage has features intermediate between cartilage and dense fibrous supporting tissue. It is found in intervertebral discs, some articular cartilages, the pubic symphysis, in association with dense collagenous tissue in joint capsules, in ligaments and in the connections of some tendons to bone. It consists of alternating layers of hyaline cartilage matrix with thick layers of dense collagen fibres, orientated in the direction of the functional stresses.

Fig. 10.2 is taken from the same specimen of intervertebral disc illustrated in Fig. 10.30. Pink-stained collagen characteristically permeates the blue-stained cartilage ground substance. Chondrocytes **Cc** are arranged in rows between the dense collagen layers within lacunae in the glycoprotein matrix.

Cb chondroblast **Cc** chondrocyte **L** lipid droplet **M** cartilage matrix **N** nucleus **P** perichondrium

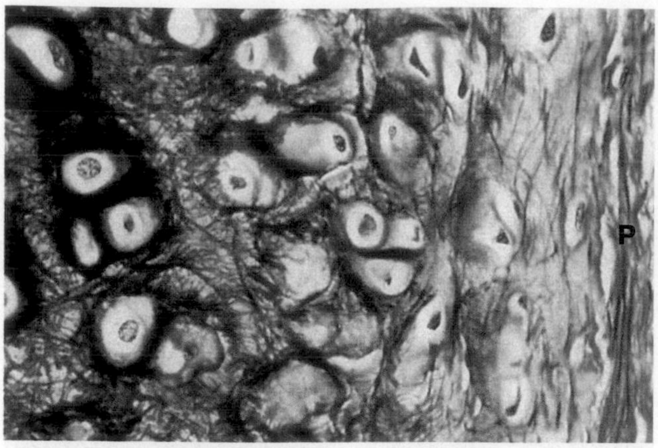

FIG. 10.3 Elastic cartilage
Elastic van Gieson (HP)

Elastic cartilage occurs in the external ear and external auditory canal, the epiglottis, parts of the laryngeal cartilages and in the walls of the Eustachian tubes.

The histological structure of elastic cartilage is similar to that of hyaline cartilage. Its elasticity is derived from the presence of numerous bundles of branching elastin fibres in the cartilage matrix. This network of elastin fibres (stained black in this preparation) is particularly dense in the immediate vicinity of the chondrocytes. Collagen (stained red) is also a major constituent of the cartilage matrix and makes up the bulk of the perichondrium **P**, intermingled with a few elastic fibres.

Development and growth of elastic cartilage occurs by both interstitial and appositional growth, in the same manner as for hyaline cartilage.

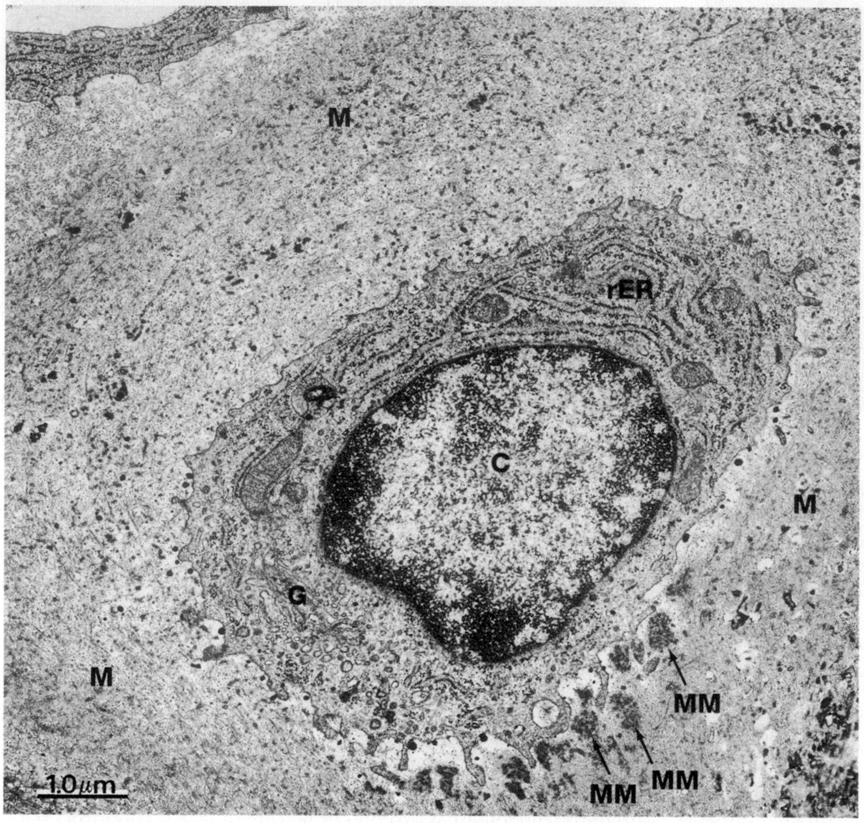

FIG. 10.4 Chondrocyte
EM ×16 000

This electron micrograph illustrates a single chondrocyte **C** lying within its lacuna and surrounded by abundant cartilaginous matrix material **M**. As is typical of cells active in protein synthesis (in this case matrix turnover), chondrocytes have very prominent rough endoplasmic reticulum **rER** which is distended with secretory material. A well-developed Golgi apparatus **G** is present.

Some glycogen granules are scattered in the cytoplasm. Note that the chondrocyte completely fills its lacuna within the matrix. Small cytoplasmic extensions mediate the constant interaction between chondrocytes and the surrounding extracellular matrix material.

At this magnification, the fibrous elements of the extracellular matrix can just be discerned. The deposits of electron-dense material which can be seen lying adjacent to the deep aspect of the cell represent some recently secreted extracellular matrix material **MM**.

BONE

Bone is composed of cells and a predominantly collagenous extracellular matrix (type I collagen) called ***osteoid*** which becomes mineralised by the deposition of ***calcium hydroxyapatite***, thus giving the bone considerable rigidity and strength. The cells of bone are:

- **Osteoblasts** which synthesise osteoid and mediate its mineralisation. These are found lined up along bone surfaces.
- **Osteocytes** which represent largely inactive osteoblasts trapped within formed bone. These may assist in the nutrition of bone.
- **Osteoclasts** are phagocytic cells which are capable of eroding bone. These are important, along with osteoblasts, in the constant turnover and refashioning of bone.

Osteoblasts and osteocytes are derived from a primitive mesenchymal (stem) cell called the ***osteoprogenitor cell***.

Osteoclasts are multinucleate phagocytic cells derived from the macrophage–monocyte cell line.

Bone forms the strong and rigid endoskeleton to which skeletal muscles are attached to permit movement. It also acts as a calcium reservoir and is important in calcium homeostasis. Bone is heavy and its architecture is optimally arranged to provide maximum strength for the least weight. Most bones have a dense, rigid outer shell of compact bone, the ***cortex***, and a central ***medullary*** or ***cancellous*** zone of thin, interconnecting narrow bone trabeculae. The number, thickness and orientation of these bone trabeculae is dependent upon the stresses to which the particular bone is exposed. For example, there are many thick intersecting trabeculae in the constantly weight-bearing vertebrae, but very few in the centre of the ribs, which are not subjected to constant stress. The space in the medullary bone between trabeculae is occupied by ***haematopoietic bone marrow*** (see Fig. 3.3).

C chondrocyte **G** Golgi apparatus **H** Howship lacuna **M** matrix material **MM** extracellular matrix material **O** osteoclast **Ob** osteoblast **Oc** osteocyte **Os** osteoid **P** perichondrium **rER** rough endoplasmic reticulum

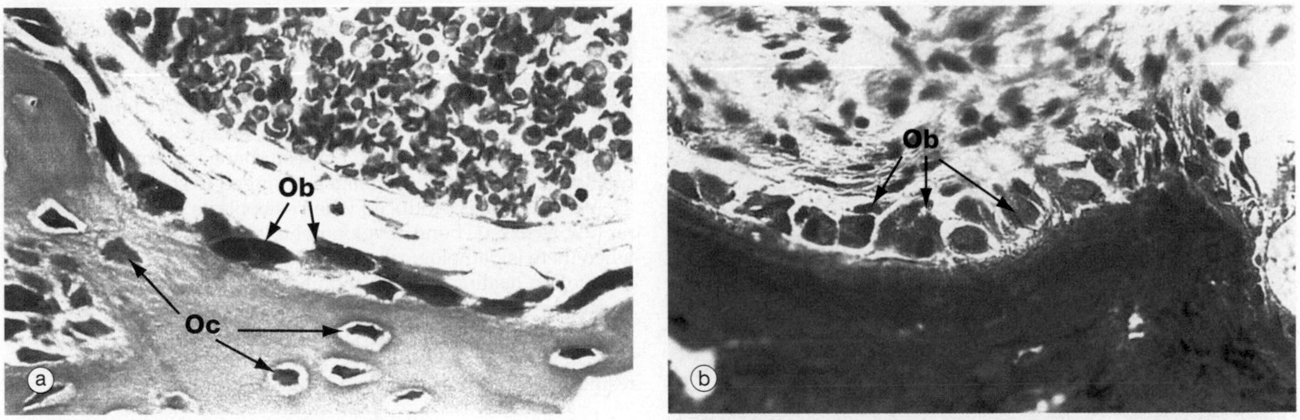

FIG. 10.5 Active osteoblasts and osteoid
(a) H&E (HP) (b) Undecalcified resin section, Goldner trichrome stain (HP)

Fig. 10.5a and b illustrate ***osteoblasts*** actively depositing new osteoid on a bone surface. When active, the osteoblasts **Ob** are large, broad, spindle-shaped or cuboidal cells with abundant basophilic cytoplasm containing much rough endoplasmic reticulum and a large Golgi apparatus. These features reflect a high rate of protein (type I collagen) and proteoglycan synthesis.

In Fig. 10.5a, the tissue has been decalcified before sectioning and staining, so the distinction between mineralised bone and the newly formed unmineralised osteoid cannot be seen. In Fig. 10.5b, which has not been decalcified, the mineralised bone (blue) can easily be distinguished from the new osteoid (red) which is being produced by the row of cuboidal osteoblasts. There is always a short delay between osteoid production and its mineralisation.

When inactive, osteoblasts are narrow, attenuated, spindle-shaped cells lying on the bone surface. In Fig. 10.5a, the burst of new bone formation is nearly over and the osteoblasts are becoming spindle-shaped again and will soon become virtually undetectable, only the long, narrow nucleus being visible histologically. A few cells are being incorporated in the newly formed bone as ***osteocytes*** **Oc**.

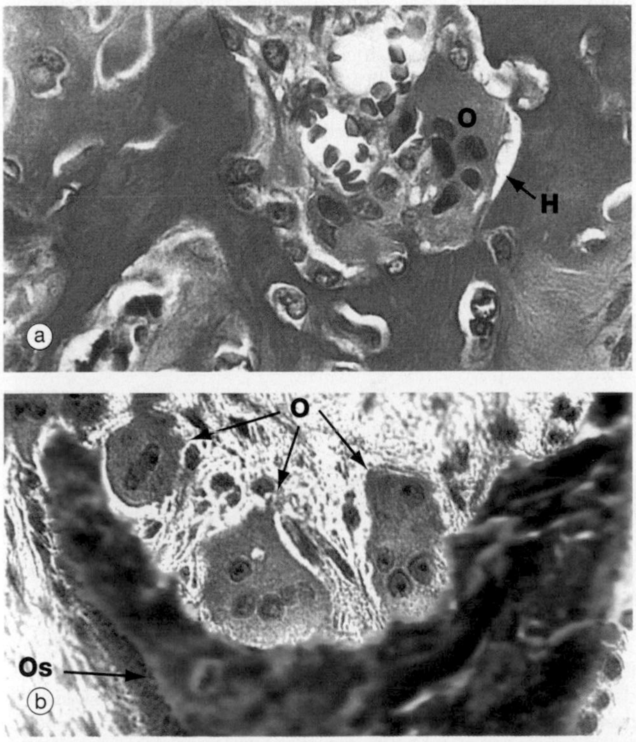

FIG. 10.6 Osteoclasts
(a) H&E (HP) (b) Undecalcified resin section, Goldner trichrome (HP)

Resorption of bone is performed by large multinucleate cells called ***osteoclasts*** **O**, which are often seen lying in depressions resorbed from the bone surface called ***Howship lacunae*** **H**. The aspect of the osteoclast in apposition to bone is characterised by fine microvilli which form a ***ruffled border*** that is readily visible with the electron microscope. The ruffled border secretes several organic acids which dissolve the mineral component, while lysosomal proteolytic enzymes are employed to destroy the organic osteoid matrix.

Osteoclastic resorption contributes to bone ***remodelling*** in response to growth or due to changing mechanical stresses upon the skeleton. Osteoclasts also participate in the long-term maintenance of blood calcium homeostasis by their response to ***parathyroid hormone*** and ***calcitonin*** (see Ch. 17). Parathyroid hormone stimulates osteoclastic resorption and so increases the release of calcium ions from bone, whereas calcitonin inhibits osteoclastic activity.

Fig. 10.6a and b are taken from bone showing excessive osteoclastic activity due to the effects of Paget disease of bone, a disorder characterised by continuous disorganised bone resorption and associated new bone formation (see textbox). Fig. 10.6b shows uncoordinated new osteoid formation **Os** by a row of cuboidal osteoblasts.

Disorders of osteoblasts and osteoclasts

The normal maintenance and refashioning of bone is the result of coordinated activity of osteoblasts depositing new bone and osteoclasts eroding redundant bone. Some diseases are the result of excessive unbalanced activity of one or other of the cell types, commonly osteoclasts.

In hyperparathyroidism, excessive uncontrolled secretion of parathyroid hormone by the parathyroid gland (see Fig. 17.11) stimulates an increase in numbers and erosive activity of osteoclasts. This leads to diffuse destruction of bone, producing radiological areas of lucency ('brown tumours') and predisposition to fracture. A serious side effect of excessive bone erosion is the release of large amounts of ionic calcium into the bloodstream, producing severe symptoms of ***hypercalcaemia***.

Paget disease is a disease of unknown cause in which there is random and haphazard excessive osteoclastic erosion of bone occurring in waves, followed by increased osteoblastic activity attempting to replace eroded bone (Fig. 10.6 and e-Fig. 10.1).

However, the new osteoid and bone formation does not always occur where bone has previously been eroded, so the architecture of the bone is grossly distorted (usually with ***woven bone***, Fig. 10.7) and the bone is structurally weak.

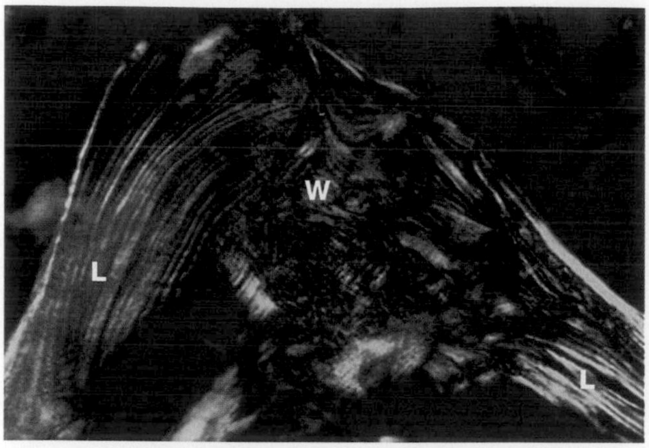

FIG. 10.7 Woven and lamellar bone, polarising microscopy H&E (MP)

Bone exists in two main forms, ***woven bone*** **W** and ***lamellar bone*** **L**. Woven bone is an immature form with randomly arranged collagen fibres in the osteoid. Lamellar bone is composed of regular parallel bands of collagen arranged in sheets.

Woven bone is produced when osteoblasts synthesise osteoid rapidly, as in fetal bone development. It can also occur in adults when there is pathological rapid new bone formation e.g. at the site of a healing fracture and in Paget disease (see textbox 'Fractures' and e-Fig. 10.1).

The rapidly formed woven bone is eventually ***remodelled*** to form lamellar bone, which is physically stronger and more resilient. Virtually all bone in a healthy adult is lamellar.

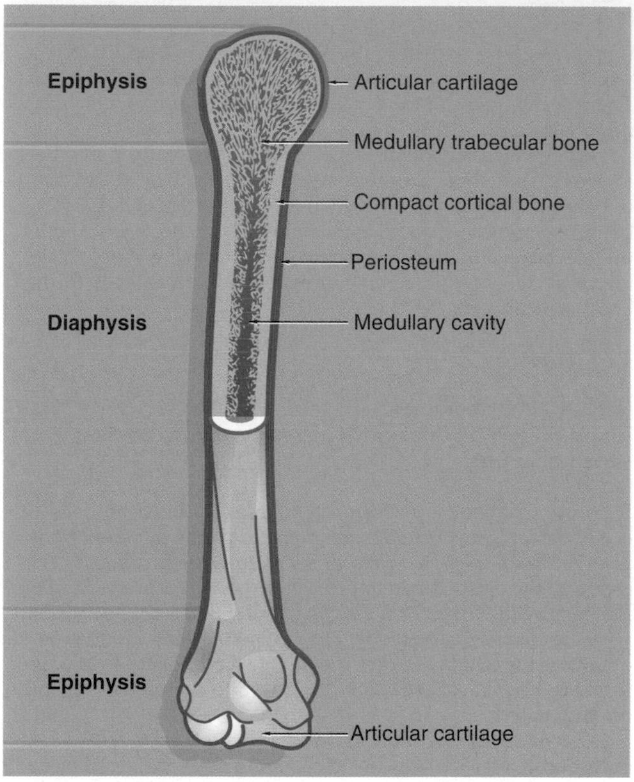

FIG. 10.8 Long bone

This diagram illustrates the general structure of long bones in the mature skeleton and the gross morphological appearance of the two types of lamellar bone found in the mature skeleton, i.e. ***compact*** (cortical) bone and ***cancellous*** (medullary) bone.

Compact bone forms the dense walls of the shaft or diaphysis, while cancellous bone occupies part of the large central medullary cavity. Cancellous bone consists of a network of fine, irregular plates called ***trabeculae*** separated by intercommunicating spaces.

The ***articular*** (joint) surfaces of the expanded ends, or epiphyses, of long bones are protected by a layer of specialised hyaline cartilage called ***articular cartilage***. The external surface of the bone is invested in a dense fibrous layer called the ***periosteum***, into which are inserted muscles, tendons and ligaments. The inner surfaces of the bone, including the trabeculae of cancellous bone, are invested by a delicate layer called the ***endosteum***. The endosteum and periosteum contain cells of the osteogenic series which are responsible for growth, continuous remodelling and repair of bone fractures (see textbox).

Prior to the attainment of skeletal maturity, the long bones grow in length by the process of ***endochondral ossification*** which occurs at a ***growth*** or ***epiphysial plate*** situated at each end of the bone at the junction of the ***diaphysis*** (shaft) and ***epiphysis***.

Fractures

Bone fractures (broken bones) are common and usually occur due to trauma. Sometimes fractures occur in abnormal or weakened bone, termed ***pathological fractures***, and may be due to a wide range of underlying disorders, including osteoporosis (see e-Fig. 10.2), Paget disease and metastatic cancer.

Fractures can be described as ***closed*** or ***simple*** (with no damage to the overlying skin) versus ***open*** or ***compound*** (where there is an overlying skin wound exposing the broken bone). In ***comminuted*** fractures, the bone is broken into a number of pieces.

Healing and repair of fractures is a specialised process which involves the formation of ***callus*** between the damaged bone ends (Figs 10.9 and 10.23). Bleeding occurs immediately at the fracture site to form a ***haematoma***.

Fibroblasts and blood vessels then grow into this haematoma to form ***granulation tissue***. The fibroblasts and other cells then develop into osteoblasts and chondroblasts, which produce ***woven bone*** and hyaline cartilage. This callus acts to temporarily unite the bone ends, and over time there is ***remodelling*** into mature lamellar bone.

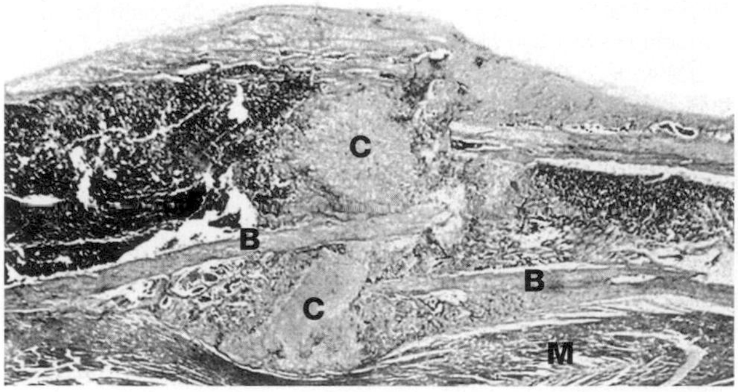

FIG. 10.9 Fracture callus H&E (LP)

This image shows fracture callus **C** around the site of a rib fracture. This mass of healing tissue acts to stabilise the broken ends of the bone **B** so that repair can occur. There is new bone formation within the callus and, over time, this will become organised into mature lamellar bone. Striated muscle **M** is present at the lower border of the bone.

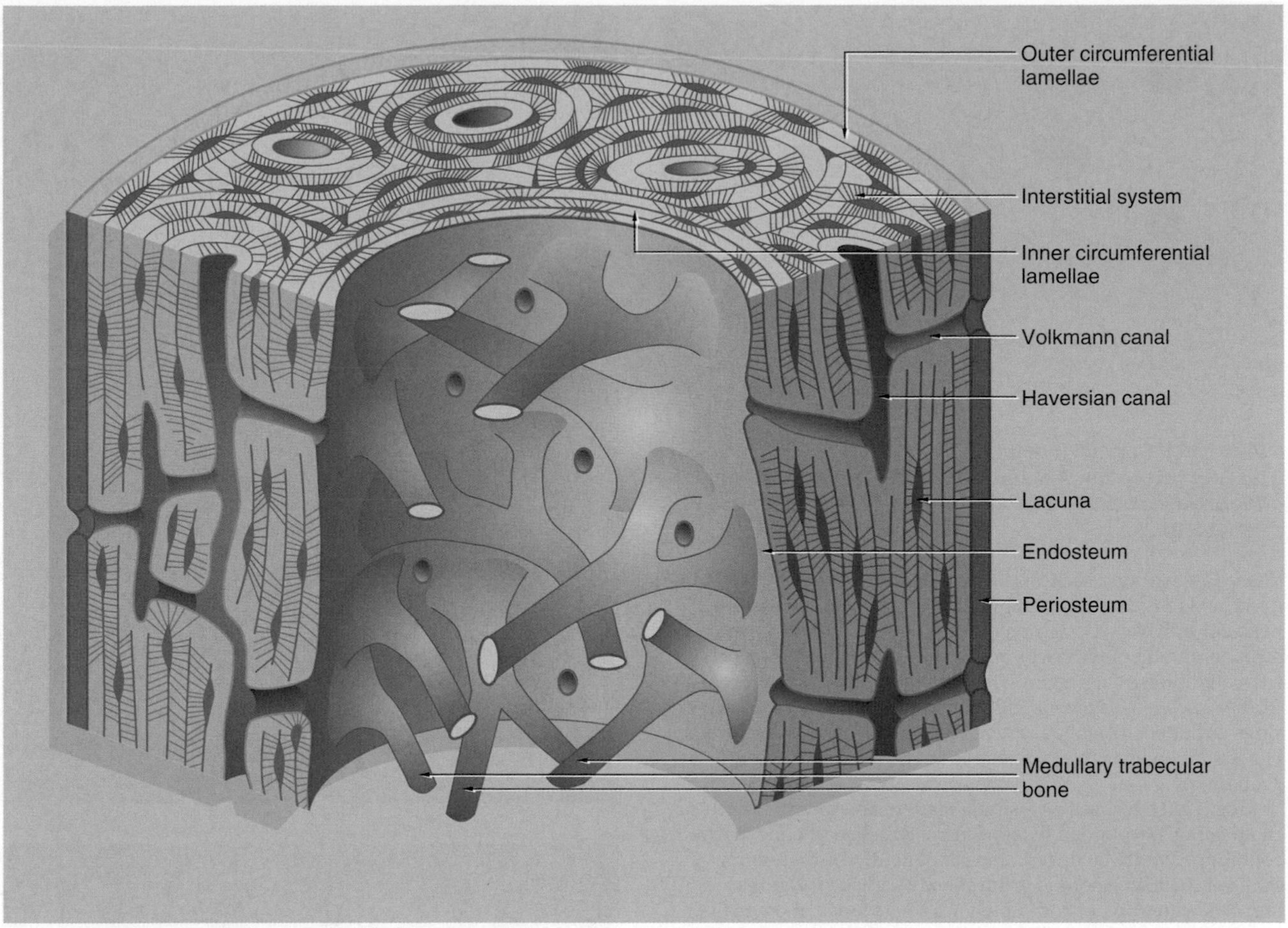

FIG. 10.10 Cortical (compact) bone

Compact bone is made up of parallel bony columns which, in long bones, are disposed parallel to the long axis, i.e. in the line of stress exerted on the bone. Each column is made up of concentric bony layers or ***lamellae*** arranged around a central channel containing blood vessels, lymphatics and nerves. These neurovascular channels are known as ***canals of Havers*** or ***Haversian canals*** and, with their concentric lamellae, form ***Haversian systems***. The neurovascular bundles interconnect with one another and with the endosteum and periosteum via ***Volkmann canals*** which pierce the columns at right angles (or obliquely) to the Haversian canals.

Each Haversian system (***osteon***) develops by osteoclastic tunnelling of a mass of compact bone to form a broad channel into which blood vessels and nerves grow, after which it becomes lined internally by active osteoblasts which lay down concentric lamellae of bone.

With the deposition of successive lamellae, the diameter of the Haversian canal decreases and ***osteoblasts*** are trapped as ***osteocytes*** in spaces called ***lacunae*** in the matrix. The osteocytes are thus arranged in concentric rings within the lamellae. Between adjacent lacunae and the central canal, there are numerous minute interconnecting canals called ***canaliculi*** which contain fine cytoplasmic extensions of the entrapped osteocytes.

As a result of the continuous resorption and redeposition of bone, complete newly formed Haversian systems are disposed between partly resorbed systems formed earlier. The remnants of lamellae no longer surrounding Haversian canals form irregular ***interstitial systems*** between intact Haversian systems.

At the outermost aspect of compact bone, Haversian systems give way to concentric lamellae of dense cortical bone, laid down partly by the osteoblasts of the periosteum (***outer circumferential lamellae***). Similar circumferential lamellae line the inside of the cortical bone (***inner circumferential lamellae***) where it abuts the marrow cavity.

The inner surface of cortical bone (***endosteum***) is composed of the innermost layer of the inner circumferential lamellae, with a layer of inactive flat osteoblasts on its surface. When activated, these cells enlarge to become active cuboidal osteoblasts and synthesise new lamellar osteoid which, on mineralisation, forms another layer of inner circumferential lamella. This occurs regularly as part of the constant dynamic refashioning of bone and is particularly prominent during bone growth. It is also seen in response to increased or altered stress on the cortical bone, for example in the leg bones during periods of increased physical training for running and other sports.

An interconnecting network of ***trabecular*** or ***cancellous*** bone occupies the central marrow cavity of the bone, and the ends of these bony trabeculae are attached to the inner circumferential lamellae of the cortical bone (Fig. 10.13). The inactive osteoblasts of the endosteum also extend onto the surface of the trabecular bone and similarly deposit new osteoid when required for strengthening or remodelling.

Small blood vessels and nerves enter the cortical bone from the marrow space through defects in the endosteum and inner circumferential lamellae. These connect with the Volkmann canals, which in turn connect with Haversian canals.

B bone **C** callus **L** lamellar bone **M** striated muscle **W** woven bone

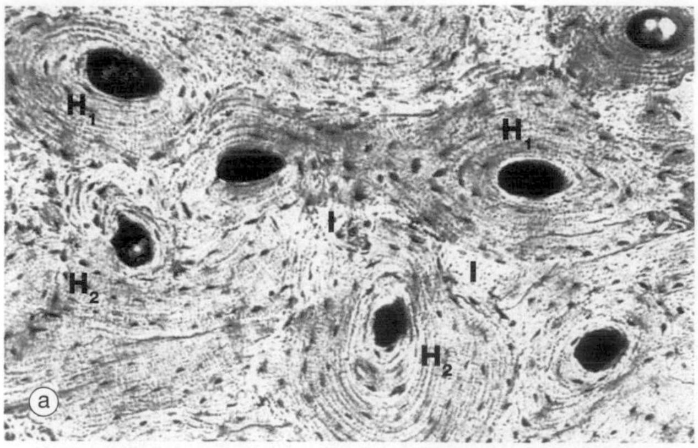

FIG. 10.11 Cortical (compact) bone
(a) Ground section, TS, unstained (LP) (b) Ground section, TS, unstained (HP) (c) Ground section, LS, unstained (LP) (d) H&E (MP)

These three ground sections illustrate many of the features described in the preceding figure. In Fig. 10.11a, the bone has been cut transversely, demonstrating newly formed Haversian systems $\mathbf{H_1}$ and older, partly resorbed Haversian systems $\mathbf{H_2}$. Irregular interstitial systems **I**, representing the remnants of former Haversian systems, fill the intervening spaces. Concentric rings of flattened lacunae can be seen to surround the central Haversian canals, which appear as very dark areas in this preparation.

Fig. 10.11b focuses on a single Haversian system, the central canal being surrounded by concentric lamellae of bone matrix containing empty lacunae **L**. Fine canaliculi **C** radiate from each lacuna to anastomose with those of adjacent lacunae. In life, osteocytes do not completely fill the lacunae, the remaining narrow space being filled with extracellular bone fluid. Fine cytoplasmic processes of the osteocytes pass in the canaliculi to communicate via ***gap junctions*** with the processes of osteocytes in adjacent lamellae. These canaliculi provide passages for circulation of extracellular fluid and for diffusion of metabolites between the lacunae and vessels of the Haversian canals.

Osteocytes maintain the structural integrity of the mineralised matrix and mediate release or deposition of calcium for the purpose of calcium homeostasis in the body as a whole. The activity of osteocytes in calcium regulation is controlled directly by plasma calcium concentration and indirectly by ***parathyroid hormone*** and ***calcitonin***, secreted by the parathyroid and thyroid glands, respectively (see Ch. 17). Osteoblasts and osteocytes also appear to respond to minute piezo-electric currents induced by bone deformation, increasing or decreasing local bone formation as appropriate and inducing complementary activity in local osteoclasts via the secretion of local humoral factors. Thus bone is remodelled to adapt to mechanical stresses.

Fig. 10.11c shows compact bone cut in longitudinal section, the plane of section including some Haversian canals **HC** and traces of the interconnecting Volkmann canal system **V**. These appear dark in colour as in Fig. 10.11a due to an optical artefact related to air trapped in the section. For the same reason, the tiny osteocyte lacunae appear as brown elongated specks which are arranged in concentric layers around the Haversian canals.

Fig. 10.11d is an H&E-stained section of decalcified bone. It shows compact cortical bone with ***periosteum*** **P** on its outer surface. The outer circumferential lamellae **OCL** lie between the periosteum and three Haversian systems **H**, seen here in transverse section. At the centre of each Haversian system is a canal containing blood vessels. Between adjacent systems, there are irregular interstitial lamellae **I**. The lamellae of the Haversian systems are not clearly seen in this section, but fine basophilic cement lines **CL**, rich in proteoglycan ground substance, can be seen in the outer circumferential lamellae and defining the outer limits of each Haversian system. Osteocytes **Oc** have dark-staining nuclei.

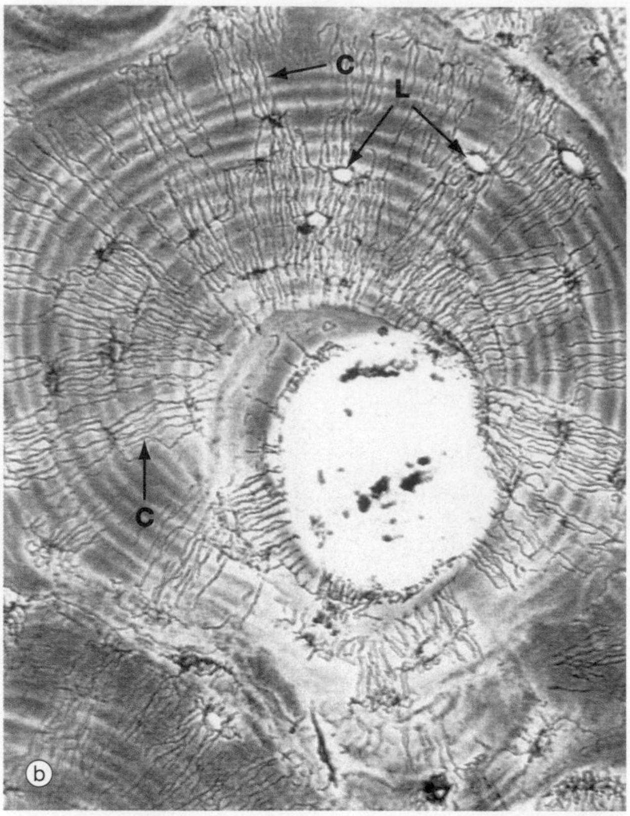

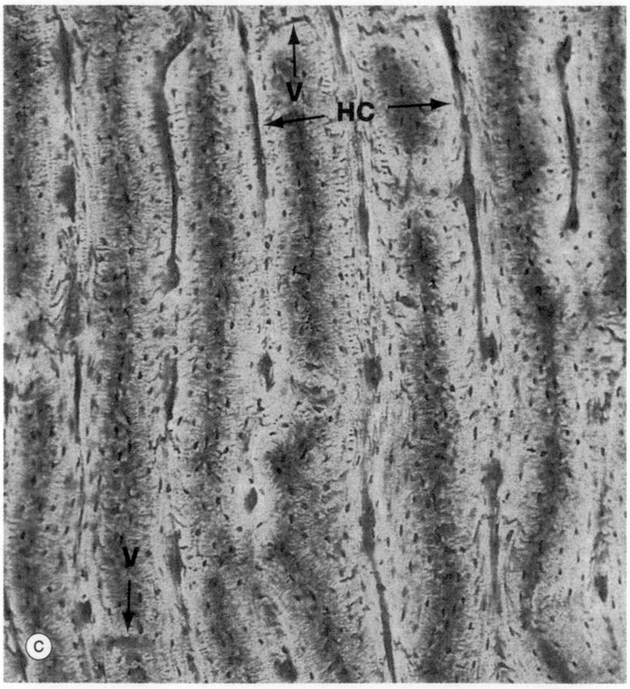

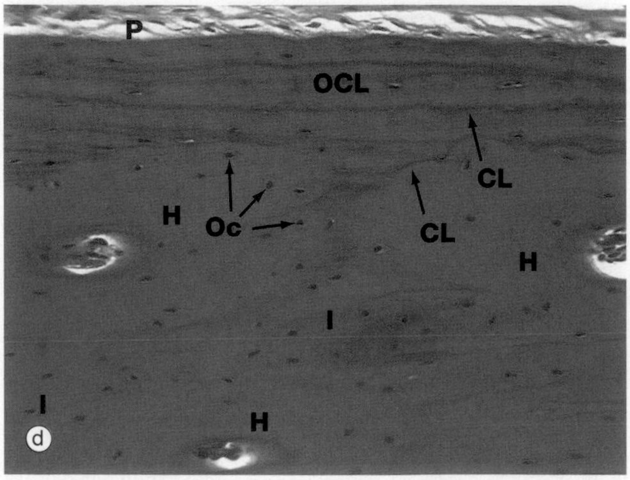

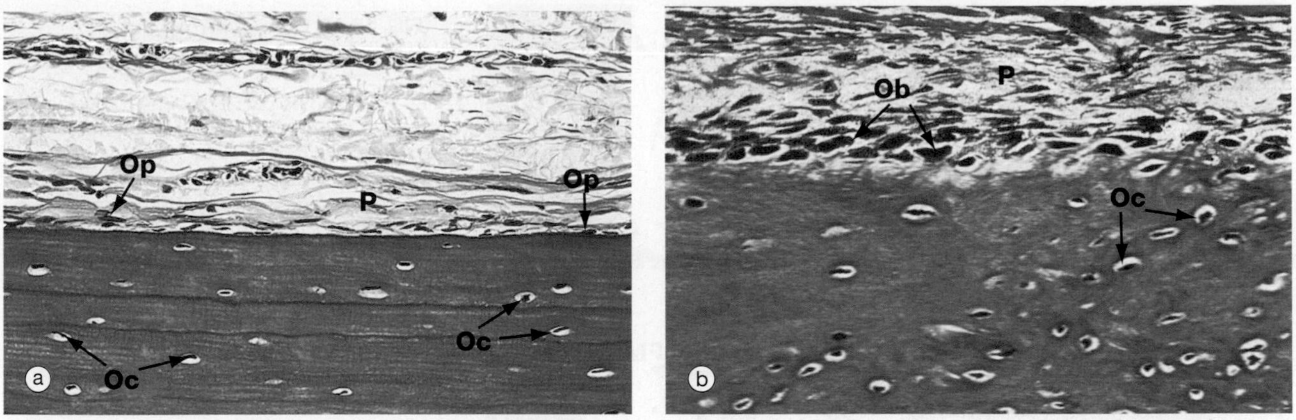

FIG. 10.12 Periosteum
(a) Inactive, H&E (MP) (b) Active, H&E (HP)

The outer surface of most bone is covered by a layer of condensed fibrous tissue, the ***periosteum*** **P**, which contains cells capable of converting into ***osteoprogenitor cells*** and osteoblasts. When no new bone is being formed on the bone surface, these cells are insignificant flattened cells with spindle-shaped nuclei but, when there is active new bone formation at the periosteal surface, these cells proliferate and increase in size to become ***osteoblasts***. Fig. 10.12a shows inactive periosteum with barely detectable inactive osteoprogenitor cells **Op** and mature formed bone containing established osteocytes **Oc**. Fig. 10.12b shows active periosteum with new bone being formed by active periosteal osteoblasts **Ob**, some of which are being incorporated into newly formed bone to become osteocytes **Oc**.

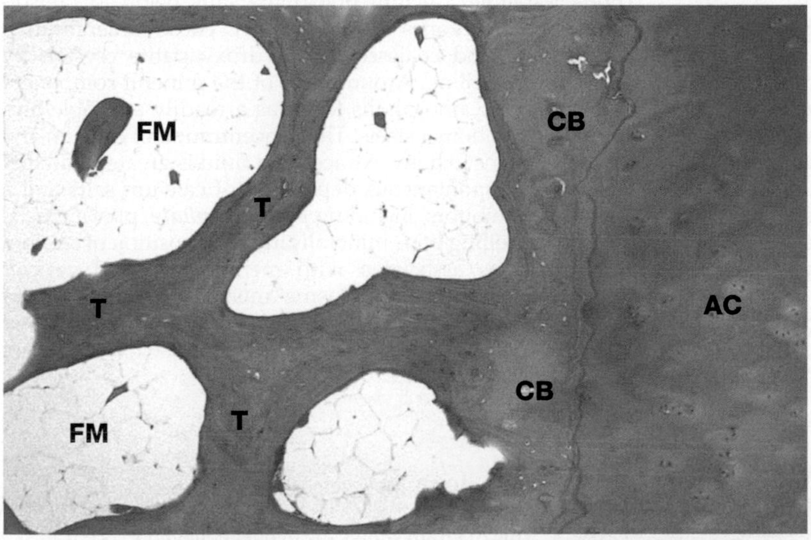

FIG. 10.13 Bone, cortical and trabecular H&E (LP)

Fig. 10.13 shows bone from the head of the femur. It illustrates the origin of the trabecular (cancellous) bone **T** from the compact cortical bone **CB**. As this end of the bone forms part of a synovial joint (see Fig. 10.25), the outer cortical plate consists of articular hyaline cartilage **AC**. On the shaft of this long bone, the outer layer would be formed from fibrous periosteum. Between the bony trabeculae, there are intervening spaces. Note that these marrow spaces **FM** are filled with adipose tissue (fatty or yellow marrow).

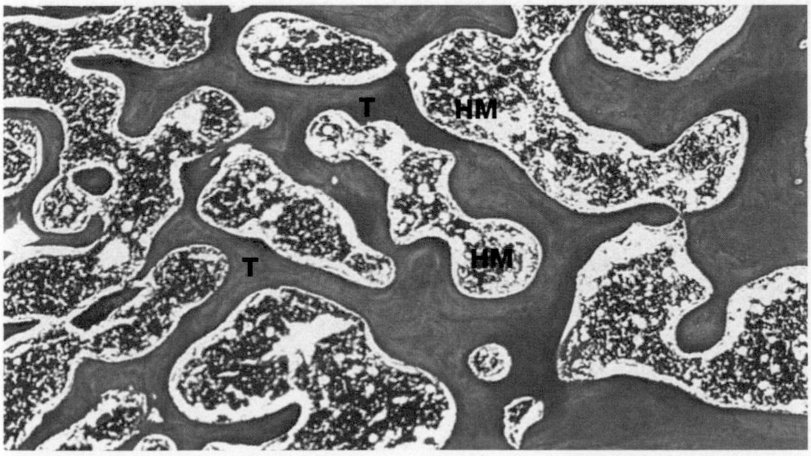

FIG. 10.14 Bone, trabecular H&E (LP)

Trabecular (cancellous) bone consists of a network of interconnecting struts which are orientated in positions that provide the maximum strength for the minimum mass. They are composed of lamellar bone with scanty lacunae containing osteocytes. These exchange metabolites via canaliculi which communicate with each other and with blood sinusoids in the haematopoietic (red) marrow spaces **HM**. The trabeculae **T** have a thin external coating of endosteum with flat inactive osteoblasts.

AC articular cartilage **C** canaliculus **CB** cortical bone **CL** cement line **FM** fatty marrow **H** Haversian system **HC** Haversian canal **HM** haematopoietic marrow **I** interstitial system **L** lacuna **Ob** osteoblast **Oc** osteocyte **Op** osteoprogenitor cell **OCL** outer circumferential lamellae **P** periosteum **T** trabecular bone **V** Volkman canal

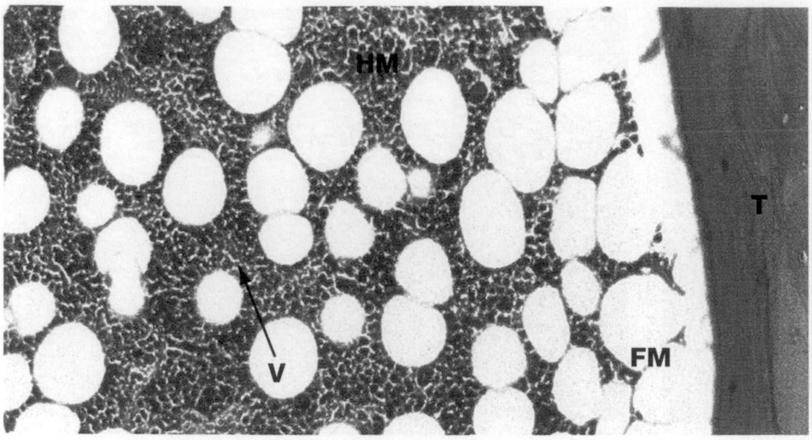

FIG. 10.15 Bone marrow
H&E (HP)

Fig. 10.15 shows part of a bone trabecula **T** of lamellar bone and the adjacent marrow space. In this figure, as in Fig. 10.14, the marrow space contains a mixture of fatty marrow **FM**, composed of adipose tissue, and haematopoietic ('red') marrow **HM**, composed of red and white blood cell precursors. These haematopoietic cells lie in intimate contact with numerous thin-walled blood vessels (sinusoids) **V**.

The various cell types and processes involved in haematopoiesis are described in Ch. 3.

BONE MATRIX AND MINERALISATION

Mature compact bone is made up of about 70% inorganic salts and 30% organic matrix by weight. Collagen makes up over 90% of the organic component, the remainder being ground substance proteoglycans and non-collagen molecules which appear to regulate bone mineralisation. The collagen of bone is almost exclusively in the form of type I fibres. Spaces within this three-dimensional structure, called ***hole zones***, are the initial site of mineralisation.

Ground substance proteoglycans contribute a much smaller proportion of the matrix than in cartilage and mainly consist of chondroitin sulphate and hyaluronic acid in the form of proteoglycan aggregates. As well as controlling the water content of bones, ground substance is probably involved in regulating formation of collagen fibres. The remaining non-collagen organic material includes ***osteocalcin*** (***Gla protein***), involved in binding calcium during the mineralisation process, ***osteonectin***, which may serve some bridging function between collagen and the mineral component, and ***sialoproteins***.

The mineral component of bone mainly consists of calcium and phosphate in the form of ***hydroxyapatite*** crystals. These are conjugated to a small proportion of magnesium carbonate, sodium and potassium ions but also have affinity for heavy metals and radioactive pollutants.

Collagen and the other organic matrix constituents are synthesised by the rough endoplasmic reticulum of osteoblasts, packaged by the Golgi apparatus and then secreted from the cell surface, resulting in the production of ***osteoid***. After a maturation phase lasting several days, amorphous (non-crystalline) calcium phosphate salts begin to precipitate in the hole zones of the collagen. These mineralisation foci expand and coalesce into hydroxyapatite crystals by further remodelling. Around 20% of the mineral component remains in the amorphous form, as a readily available buffer in calcium homeostasis. The concentration of calcium and phosphate ions in bony extracellular fluid is greater than that required for spontaneous deposition of calcium salts and a variety of inhibitors, including ***pyrophosphate***, play a crucial role in controlling bone mineralisation. Deposition of calcium appears to be associated with membrane-bound vesicles derived from osteoblast plasma membrane called ***matrix vesicles***. These contain the enzyme ***alkaline phosphatase*** and other phosphatases which may neutralise the inhibitory effect of pyrophosphate.

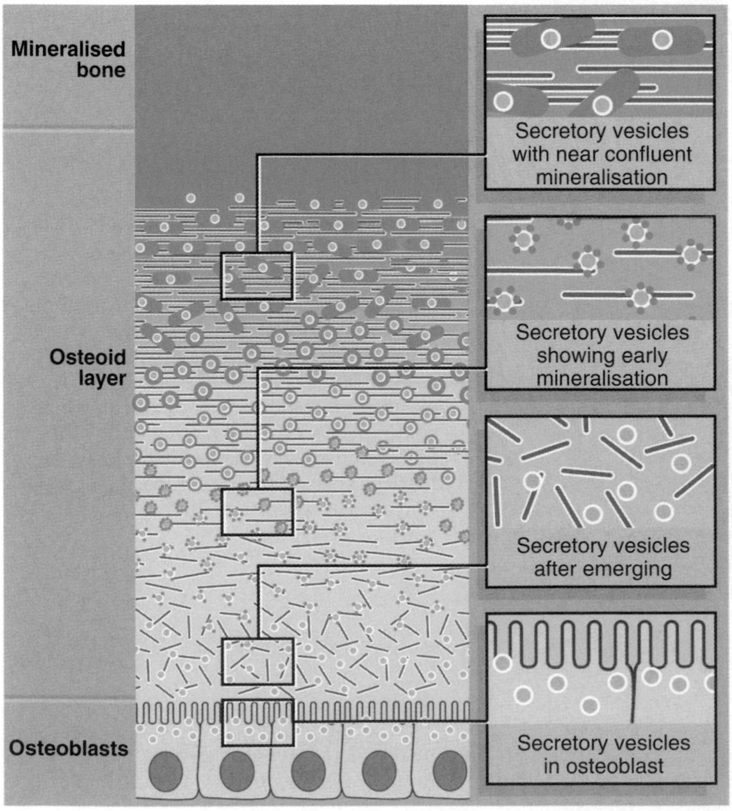

FIG. 10.16 Mineralisation of bone

This diagram shows the events believed to occur in the mineralisation of osteoid to form mineralised bone. The active cuboidal osteoblasts secrete osteoid collagen (red) but also matrix vesicles (yellow). The matrix vesicles are the focus for deposition of hydroxyapatite crystals (green), the first step in mineralisation. Continued accretion of mineral on these early foci leads eventually to confluent mineralisation of the osteoid collagen and supporting glycosaminoglycan matrix.

The matrix vesicles are rich in the enzymes alkaline phosphatase and pyrophosphatase, which can both produce phosphate ions from a range of molecules. The phosphate ions accumulate in the matrix vesicles with calcium ions and form the raw material for production of hydroxyapatite.

Osteomalacia

Osteomalacia is a disease which results from failure of normal mineralisation of newly formed osteoid (see e-Fig. 10.3). Successful mineralisation requires adequate concentrations of calcium and phosphate ions. If there is deficiency (e.g. due to poor diet, malabsorption, etc.), mineralisation of osteoid cannot take place and osteomalacia develops. Severe osteomalacia produces bone trabeculae which are only mineralised at their centre, the bulk being soft non-rigid osteoid. The bone is soft and prone to fracture.

BONE DEVELOPMENT AND GROWTH

The fetal development of bone occurs in two ways, both of which involve replacement of primitive collagenous supporting tissue by bone. The resulting ***woven bone*** is then extensively remodelled by ***resorption*** and ***appositional growth*** to form the mature adult skeleton, which is made up of ***lamellar bone***. Thereafter, resorption and deposition of bone occur at a much reduced rate to accommodate changing functional stresses and to effect calcium homeostasis.

The long bones, vertebrae, pelvis and bones of the base of the skull are preceded by the formation of a continuously growing cartilage model which is progressively replaced by bone. This process is called ***endochondral ossification*** and the bones so formed are called ***cartilage bones***.

In contrast, the bones of the vault of the skull, the maxilla and most of the mandible are formed by the deposition of bone within primitive mesenchymal tissue. This process of direct replacement of mesenchyme by bone is known as ***intramembranous ossification*** and the bones so formed are called ***membrane bones***. Bone development is controlled by growth hormone, thyroid hormone and the sex hormones.

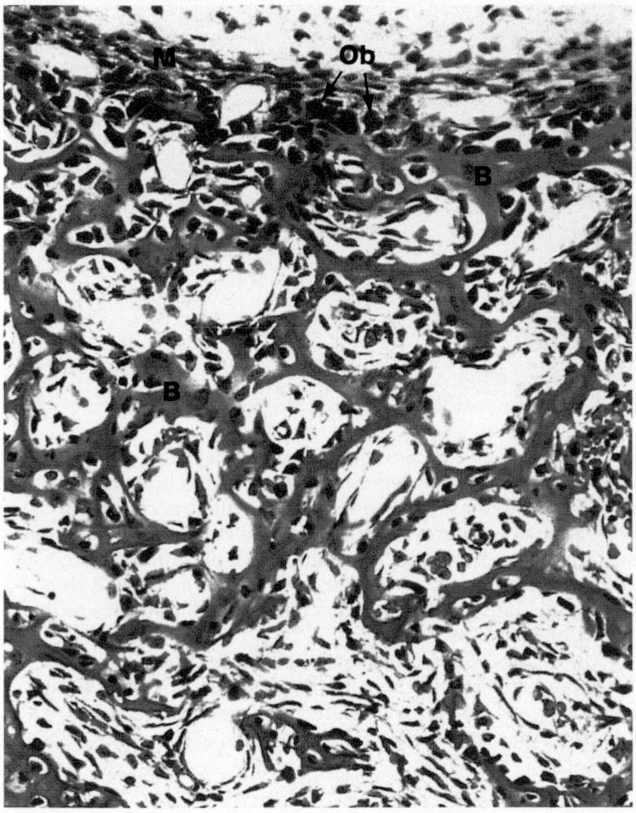

FIG. 10.17 Intramembranous ossification H&E (HP)

Intramembranous bone formation occurs within 'membranes' of condensed primitive mesenchymal tissue. Mesenchymal cells differentiate into osteoblasts **Ob** which begin synthesis and secretion of osteoid at multiple ***centres of ossification***.

Mineralisation of osteoid follows closely. As osteoid is laid down, osteoblasts are trapped in lacunae to become osteocytes and their fine cytoplasmic extensions shrink to form the fine processes contained within the canaliculi. Osteoprogenitor cells at the surface of the centres of ossification undergo mitotic division to produce further osteoblasts which then lay down more bone. This progressive bone formation results in the eventual fusion of adjacent ossification centres to form bone which is spongy in gross appearance.

The collagen fibres of developing bone are randomly arranged in interlacing bundles, giving rise to the term woven bone. The woven bone then undergoes progressive remodelling into lamellar bone by osteoclastic resorption and osteoblastic deposition to form mature ***compact*** or ***trabecular bone***. The primitive mesenchyme remaining in the network of developing bone differentiates into bone marrow.

This preparation from the developing skull vault of a cat fetus illustrates spicules of woven bone **B** separated by primitive mesenchymal tissue. Note the condensed primitive mesenchyme **M** which delineates the outer margin of the developing bone. This will eventually develop into the periosteum.

Inherited defects of bone development: achondroplasia

Achondroplasia is a common cause of dwarfism. Patients with achondroplasia have short stature, mainly due to a marked reduction in the lengths of the long bones of the limbs. The trunk and skull bones tend to be of more normal size. This reflects differences in bone development in these different parts of the skeleton.

The primary defect in achondroplasia affects the process of endochondral ossification, the type of bone development necessary for normal long bone growth. The processes of intramembranous and periosteal ossification are normal in achondroplastic individuals. As a result, those parts of the skeleton such as the skull which develop by intramembranous ossification are of normal size. Similarly, whilst limb bones tend to be short they are also broad, since growth in the diameter of long bones usually occurs via the process of subperiosteal new bone formation.

B woven bone **FM** fatty marrow **HM** haematopoietic marrow **M** primitive mesenchyme **Ob** osteoblast **T** bone trabecula **V** sinusoidal blood vessels

FIG. 10.18 Endochondral ossification

Endochondral ossification is a method of bone formation that permits functional stresses to be sustained during skeletal growth. It is well demonstrated in the development of the long bones.

A small model of the long bone is first formed in solid hyaline cartilage. This undergoes mainly appositional growth to form an elongated dumbbell-shaped mass of cartilage consisting of a shaft (***diaphysis***) and future articular portions (***epiphyses***), surrounded by perichondrium.

Within the shaft of the cartilage model, the chondrocytes enlarge greatly, resorbing the surrounding cartilage so as to leave only slender, perforated trabeculae of cartilaginous matrix.
This cartilage matrix then becomes calcified and the chondrocytes degenerate, leaving large interconnecting spaces. During this period, the perichondrium of the shaft develops osteogenic potential and assumes the role of periosteum. The periosteum then lays down a thin layer of bone around the surface of the shaft.

At the same time, primitive mesenchymal cells and blood vessels invade the spaces left within the shaft after degeneration of the chondrocytes. These primitive mesenchymal cells differentiate into osteoblasts and blood-forming cells of the bone marrow. The osteoblasts form a layer of cells on the surface of the calcified remnants of the cartilage matrix and commence the formation of irregular woven bone.

A large site of primary ossification in the shaft has by now separated the ends of the original cartilage model. The cartilaginous ends of the model, however, continue to grow in diameter. Meanwhile, the cartilage at the ends of the shaft continues to undergo regressive changes followed by ossification, so that the developing bone now consists of an elongated bony diaphysial shaft with a semilunar cartilage epiphysis at each end. The interface between the shaft and each epiphysis constitutes a ***growth*** or ***epiphysial plate***. Within the growth plate, the cartilage proliferates continuously, resulting in progressive elongation of the bone. At the diaphysial aspect of each growth plate, the chondrocytes mature and then die, the degenerating zone of cartilage being replaced by bone. Thus the bony diaphysis lengthens and the growth plates are pushed further and further apart.

On reaching maturity, hormonal changes inhibit further cartilage proliferation and the growth plates are replaced by bone, causing fusion of the diaphysis and epiphyses. In the meantime, in the centre of the mass of cartilage of each developing epiphysis, regressive changes and bone formation similar to that in the diaphysial cartilage occur, along with appositional growth of cartilage over the whole external surface of the epiphysis. This conversion of central epiphysial cartilage to bone is known as ***secondary ossification***. A thin zone of hyaline cartilage always remains at the surface as the ***articular cartilage***.

Under the influence of functional stresses, the calcified cartilage remnants and the surrounding irregular woven bone are completely remodelled so that the bone ultimately consists of a compact outer layer with a central medulla of cancellous bone.

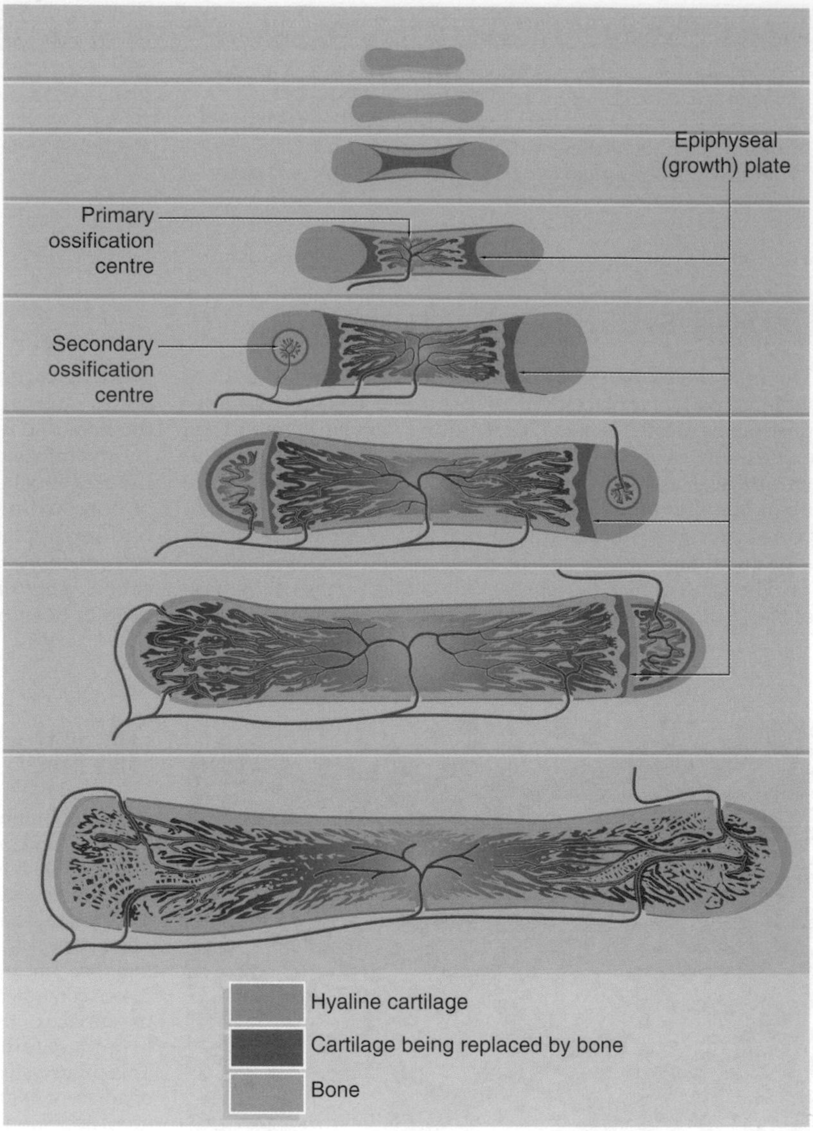

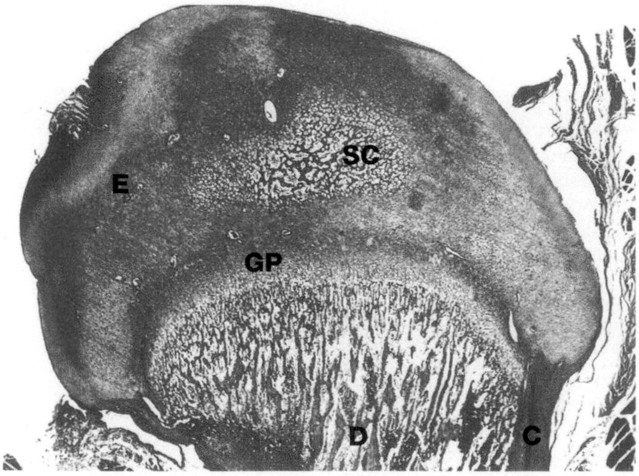

FIG. 10.19 Epiphysis H&E/Alcian blue (LP)

Fig. 10.19 illustrates the head of a kitten femur at an advanced stage of development. The cartilaginous epiphysis **E** is separated from the diaphysis **D** by the epiphysial growth plate **GP**. Note the thickening cortical bone **C** at the outer aspect of the diaphysis and the network of trabecular bone in the medulla of the diaphysis. Note also the centre of secondary ossification **SC** in the epiphysial cartilage.

Epiphysial growth plates provide for growth in length of long bones while accommodating functional stresses in the growing skeleton. Figs 10.20 to 10.22 illustrate particular areas of the epiphyseal plate at higher magnification.

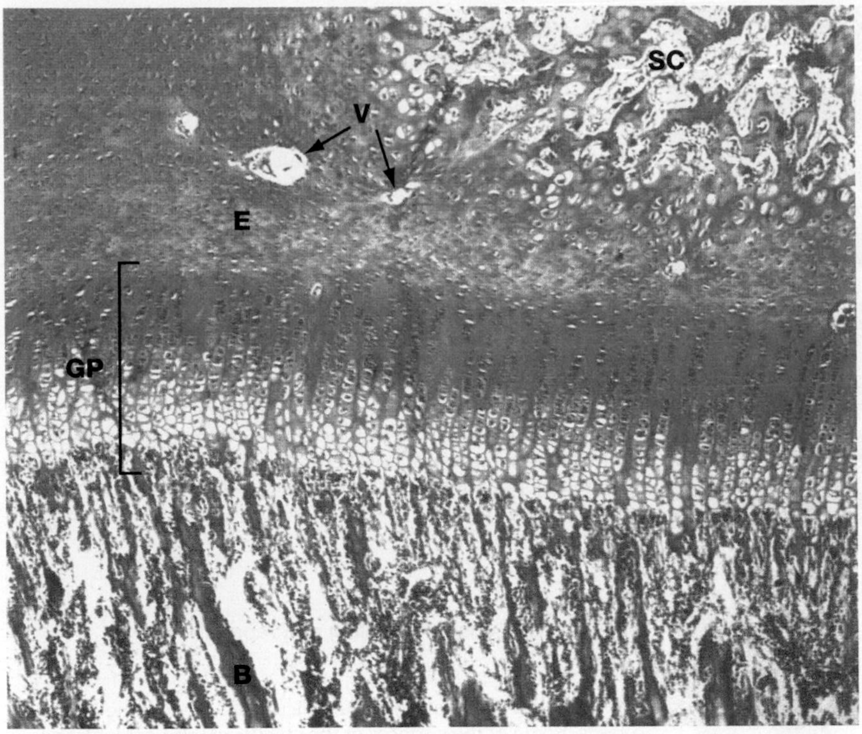

FIG. 10.20 Epiphyseal growth plate H&E/Alcian blue (MP)

At higher magnification in Fig. 10.20, the epiphysial growth plate **GP** shows a distinct progression of morphological changes between the epiphysial cartilage **E** and the newly forming bone **B** of the diaphysis. Similar but less stratified morphological changes are seen between the epiphysial cartilage and the centre of secondary ossification **SC** within the epiphysis, although this does not represent a growth plate. The Alcian blue counter-stain has been employed here as it has particular affinity for the ground substance of cartilage. Note the presence of blood vessels **V** which are cut in transverse section, passing into the secondary ossification centre of the epiphysis via cartilage canals.

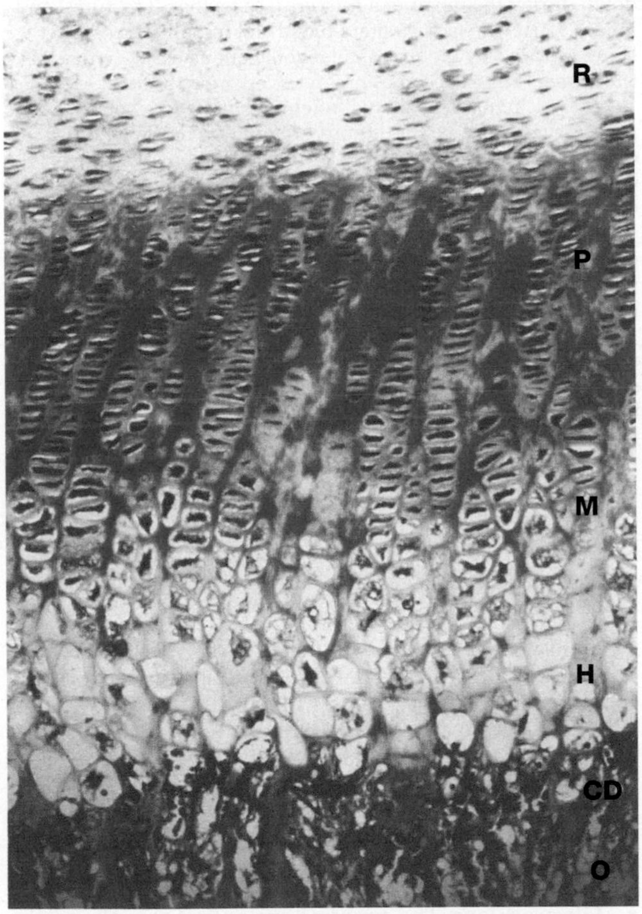

FIG. 10.21 Epiphyseal growth plate H&E/Alcian blue (HP)

The dynamic process of endochondral ossification is summarised in this micrograph of the epiphysial growth plate at high magnification (Fig. 10.21). The transition between epiphysial cartilage and new bone occurs in six functional and morphological stages:

- **Zone of reserve cartilage R**. This consists of typical hyaline cartilage (see Fig. 10.1) with the chondrocytes arranged in small clusters surrounded by a large amount of moderately stained matrix.
- **Zone of proliferation P**. The clusters of cartilage cells undergo successive mitotic divisions to form columns of chondrocytes separated by strongly stained matrix, rich in proteoglycans.
- **Zone of maturation M**. Cell division has ceased and the chondrocytes increase in size.
- **Zone of hypertrophy and calcification H**. The chondrocytes become greatly enlarged and vacuolated and the matrix becomes calcified.
- **Zone of cartilage degeneration CD**. The chondrocytes degenerate and the lacunae of the calcified matrix are invaded by osteogenic cells and capillaries from the marrow cavity of the diaphysis.
- **Osteogenic zone O**. The osteogenic cells differentiate into osteoblasts which congregate on the surface of the spicules of calcified cartilage matrix where they commence bone formation. This transitional zone is known as the ***metaphysis***.

B newly forming bone **C** cortical bone **CD** zone of cartilage degeneration **D** diaphysis **E** epiphysis **GP** growth plate
H zone of hypertrophy and calcification **M** zone of maturation **O** osteogenic zone **P** zone of proliferation
R zone of reserve cartilage **SC** secondary ossification centre **V** blood vessels

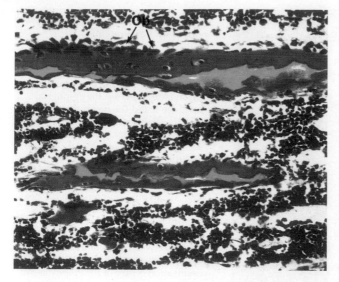

FIG. 10.22 Endochondral ossification, metaphysis H&E/Alcian blue (HP)

The ***metaphysis*** is the name given to the area where the shaft of a long bone joins the epiphyseal growth plate (Fig. 10.22). Here, the blue-stained spicules of calcified cartilage matrix are surrounded by active osteoblasts **Ob** and newly formed woven bone, stained pink. Further growth of metaphyseal woven bone is followed by extensive remodelling to produce mature trabecular bone.

At physical maturity, endochondral ossification ceases and the diaphysis fuses with the epiphysis, obliterating the growth plates. From this point, no further endochondral ossification or bone lengthening are possible. Although bones grow in length by endochondral ossification, growth in diameter of the shaft occurs by appositional growth at the periosteal surface and complementary osteoclastic resorption at the endosteal (medullary) aspect. Note that the marrow spaces between the developing trabeculae are already populated by numerous small haematopoietic cells (red marrow).

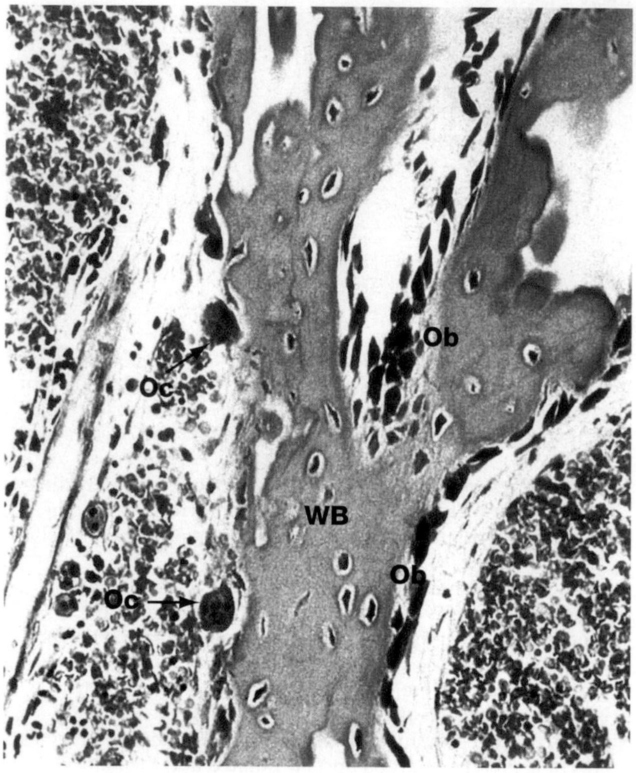

FIG. 10.23 Bone remodelling and repair H&E (HP)

Fig. 10.23 illustrates an irregular spicule of woven bone **WB** from a fetus. Some of the surfaces of the spicule exhibit osteoblastic proliferation and activity **Ob**, whereas other surfaces are in the process of being resorbed by osteoclasts **Oc**.

Woven bone is not only the first type of bone to be formed during skeletal development but is also the first bone to be laid down during the repair of a ***fracture*** (see textbox 'Fractures' and Fig. 10.9). At the fracture site, a blood clot initially forms, later being replaced by highly vascular collagenous tissue (***granulation tissue***) which becomes progressively more fibrous.

Mesenchymal cells then differentiate into chondroblasts and progressively replace this fibrous granulation tissue with hyaline cartilage. This firm but still flexible bridge is known as the ***provisional callus***. The provisional callus is then strengthened by deposition of calcium salts within the cartilage matrix.

Meanwhile, osteoprogenitor cells in the endosteum and periosteum are activated and lay down a meshwork of ***woven bone*** within and around the provisional callus. The provisional callus thus becomes transformed into the ***bony callus***.

Bony union is achieved when the fracture site is completely bridged by woven bone. Under the influence of functional stresses, the bony callus is then slowly remodelled to form mature lamellar bone.

JOINTS

Joints may be classified into two main functional groups, ***synovial*** and ***non-synovial***, both of which may show wide morphological variations.

Synovial joints

In this type of joint, there is extensive movement of the bones upon one another at the ***articular surfaces***. The articular surfaces are maintained in apposition by a ***fibrous capsule*** and ***ligaments*** and the surfaces are lubricated by ***synovial fluid***. Synovial joints are known as ***diarthroses***.

In some diarthroses such as the temporomandibular and knee joints, plates of fibrocartilage may be completely or partially interposed between the articular surfaces but remain unattached to the articular surfaces.

Non-synovial joints

These joints have limited movement, the articulating bones having no free articular surfaces, instead being joined by dense collagenous tissue. This may be of three types:

- **Dense fibrous tissue**. This forms the sutures between the bones of the skull and permits moulding of the fetal skull during its passage through the birth canal. The sutures are progressively replaced by bone with advancing age. Such fibrous tissue joints are called ***syndesmoses***, and, when replaced by bone, are called ***synostoses***.
- **Hyaline cartilage**. This type of joint, called a ***synchondrosis*** or ***primary cartilaginous joint***, unites the first rib with the sternum and is the only synchondrosis found in the human adult.
- **Fibrocartilage**. The opposing surfaces of some bones are covered by hyaline cartilage but, instead of a synovial space, are directly connected to each other by a plate of fibrocartilage. Such fibrocartilaginous joints are called ***symphyses*** or ***secondary cartilaginous joints*** and occur in the pubic symphysis and at the intervertebral discs. The fibrocartilage disc of the pubic symphysis develops a central cavity and the intervertebral discs have a fluid-filled central cavity.

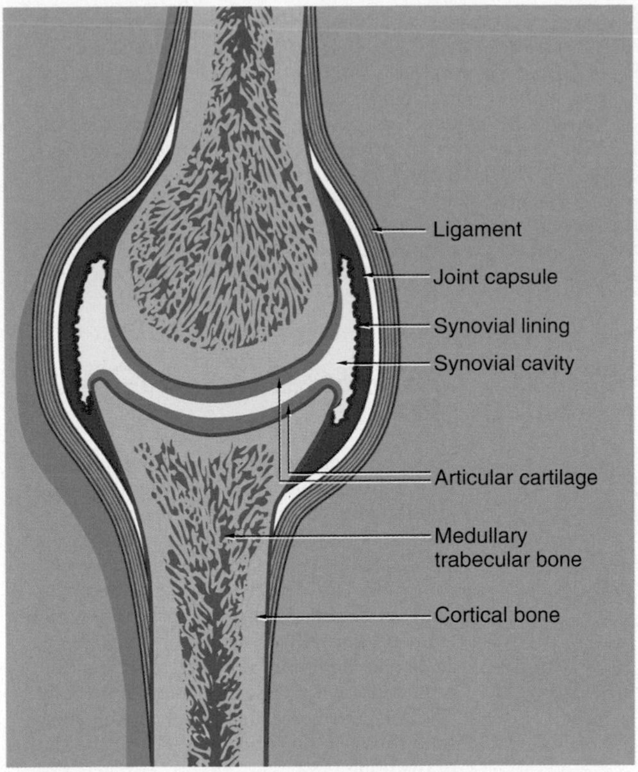

FIG. 10.24 Typical synovial joint

In synovial joints, the articulating bone surfaces are covered by a thick layer of ***hyaline cartilage*** (***articular cartilage***). This provides smooth, low-friction surfaces and also offers a degree of resistance to compressive forces, acting act as shock-absorbers in weight-bearing joints.

The joint is enclosed within a fibrocollagenous joint ***capsule*** which is lined internally by a specialised secretory cell layer, the ***synovium***. The synovium secretes a small amount of lubricant fluid into the synovial cavity, aiding the smooth articulation of the cartilage-covered bone surfaces.

Excessive movement at the joint is limited by the fibrous joint capsule and by external fibro-elastic ***ligaments*** which prevent over-flexion and over-extension. In some joints such as the knee, there are internal ligaments (the ***cruciate ligaments***) which prevent excessive joint movement, particularly excessive twisting rotation. Damage to these ligaments may occur, often during sporting pursuits, and this can lead to instability of the knee joint.

Muscles attach to bones via ***tendons*** (Fig. 10.32b), and these may also play a role in stabilising synovial joints.

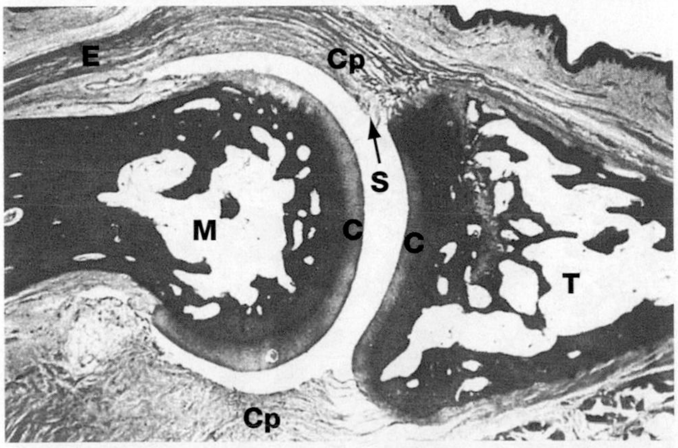

FIG. 10.25 Synovial joint H&E, monkey (LP)

Fig. 10.25 illustrates a typical synovial joint, in this case a distal interphalangeal joint from a monkey. The articular surfaces of the terminal phalanx **T** and the middle phalanx **M** are covered by hyaline cartilage **C**. The joint space is artefactually widened. In vivo, the articular surfaces are maintained in close contact by a fibrous capsule **Cp** which is inserted into the articulating bones at some distance beyond the articular cartilages. The synovium **S** is a specialised layer of collagenous tissue which lines the inner aspect of the capsule. Note the extensor tendon **E** which inserts into the base of terminal phalanx.

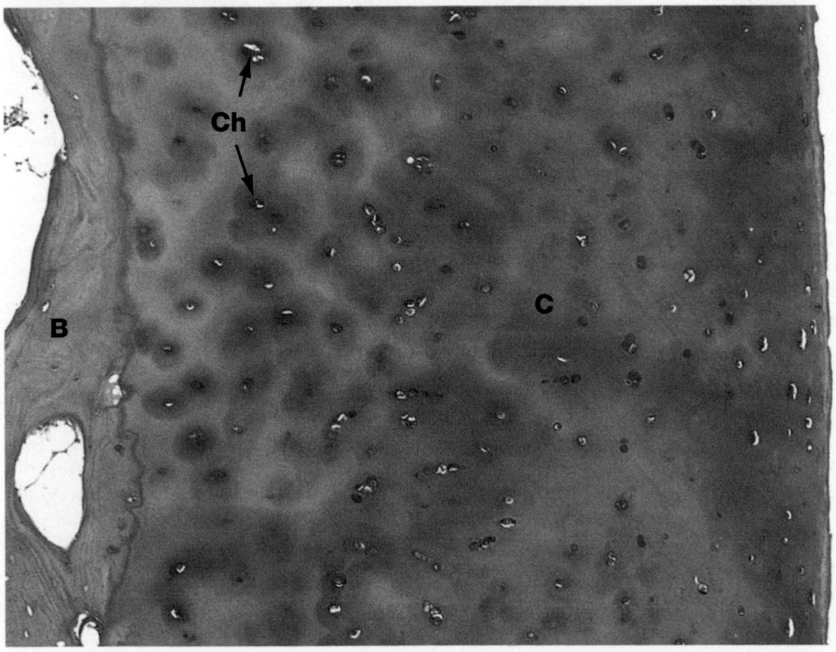

FIG. 10.26 Articular cartilage H&E (LP)

Fig. 10.26 shows the articular cartilage on the surface of the head of the femur of a young adult. It is composed of hyaline cartilage **C** and is attached to the cortical bone **B** of the head of the femur. The bluish colour of the cartilage on H&E staining is due to the presence of glycosaminoglycans in the matrix. It is these, together with the collagen of the matrix, which provides the resistance to compression that is such an important property of hyaline cartilage. Both the glycosaminoglycans and collagen are synthesised and maintained by the chondrocytes **Ch** (see Fig. 10.1).

In this young person, the articular cartilage layer is thick and healthy. In older people, the cartilage near the surface undergoes degenerative changes as a result of wear and tear, eventually leading to arthritis (see textbox).

B bone **C** hyaline cartilage **Ch** chondrocyte **Cp** joint capsule **E** extensor tendon **M** middle phalanx **Ob** osteoblast **Oc** osteoclast **S** synovium **T** terminal phalanx **WB** woven bone

Arthritis

Osteoarthritis is a degenerative disease of synovial joints due to excessive wear and tear, leading initially to degenerative change in the articular cartilages of both opposing bone ends which participate in the joint (see e-Fig. 10.4). Eventually the cartilage is eroded completely and the cortical bone of one bone end is in frictional contact with the cortical bone of the opposing bone. Both areas of cortical bone undergo refashioning to become thick layers with hard surfaces (***eburnation***), and continued use of the joint may produce tiny eroded bone fragments which float in the fluid of the joint cavity and are eventually deposited in the synovium of the joint capsule.

Rheumatoid arthritis is a destructive disease of synovial joints in which the synovium lining the joint capsule becomes thickened and heavily infiltrated with lymphocytes and plasma cells (see e-Fig. 10.5). The articular cartilage is destroyed and replaced by fibrovascular tissue (***pannus***). There are many other causes of arthritis, including bacterial infection (septic arthritis) and deposition of crystals in the joint (crystal arthropathy, e.g. gout, see e-Fig. 10.6).

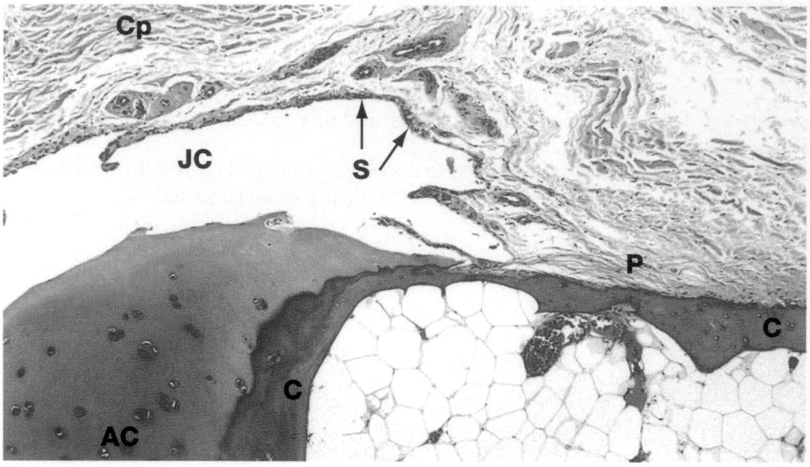

FIG. 10.27 Joint capsule and synovium H&E (LP)

This photomicrograph shows the relationship between the articular surfaces of bone and the joint capsule. The bone end is cortical bone **C**, covered by a cap of articular cartilage **AC**. This protrudes into the joint cavity **JC**. The joint cavity is contained by a dense collagenous fibrous capsule **Cp** which is lined internally by a layer of synovium **S**. The synovial lining cells secrete serous fluid which lubricates the articulation of the joint. The collagen fibres of the joint capsule merge with those of the periosteum **P** over the shaft of the bone.

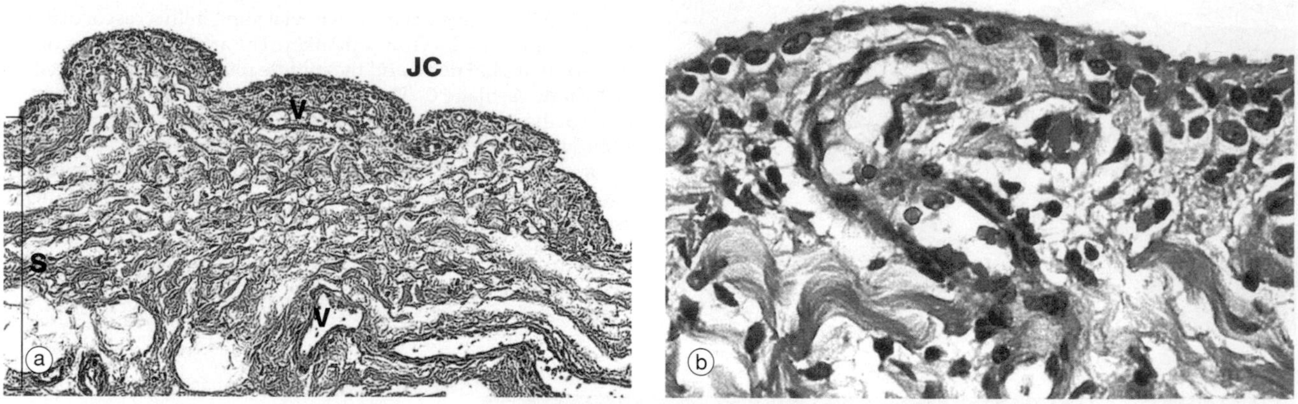

FIG. 10.28 Synovium
(a) H&E (LP) (b) H&E (HP)

The inner surface of the capsule of synovial joints and tendon sheaths is lined by a specialised collagenous tissue, the ***synovium***, which is responsible for the elaboration of the ***synovial fluid*** that lubricates the movement of articular surfaces. Depending on the location, the bulk of the synovial tissue may be of loose collagenous type (***areolar synovium***), of more dense collagenous type (***fibrous synovium***) or predominantly composed of fat (***adipose synovium***), as in the case of intra-articular fat pads.

As seen in Fig. 10.28a, the surface of the synovium **S** is thrown up into folds and small villi which may extend for some distance into the joint cavity **JC**. The synovial tissue contains numerous blood vessels **V**, lymphatics and nerves.

Fig. 10.28b illustrates the free surface of the synovium, which is characterised by a discontinuous layer of cells up to four cells deep. These ***synovial cells*** are not connected by junctional complexes and do not rest on a basement membrane. As a result, the synovial surface does not constitute an epithelium. The synovial cells are of mesenchymal origin. The majority are plump, with an extensive Golgi complex and numerous lysosomes, features suggestive of macrophages (***type A synoviocytes***). The remainder have profuse rough endoplasmic reticulum and represent fibroblasts (***type B synoviocytes***). Also in Fig. 10.28b, note the rich network of capillaries and the thick strands of collagen which would define this as fibrous synovium.

In the normal joint, the synovial fluid is little more than a thin film covering the articular surfaces. In that the articular space is not demarcated from the synovium by an epithelium, the synovial fluid represents a highly specialised fluid form of synovial extracellular matrix rather than a secretion in the usual sense. Its major constituents are ***hyaluronic acid*** and associated glycoproteins which are secreted by the type B synoviocytes. Its fluid component is a ***transudate*** from the synovial capillaries. This arrangement facilitates the continuous exchange of oxygen, carbon dioxide and metabolites between blood and synovial fluid, which is the major source of metabolic support for articular cartilage. Normal synovial fluid also contains a small number of leukocytes (<100/mL), predominantly monocytes.

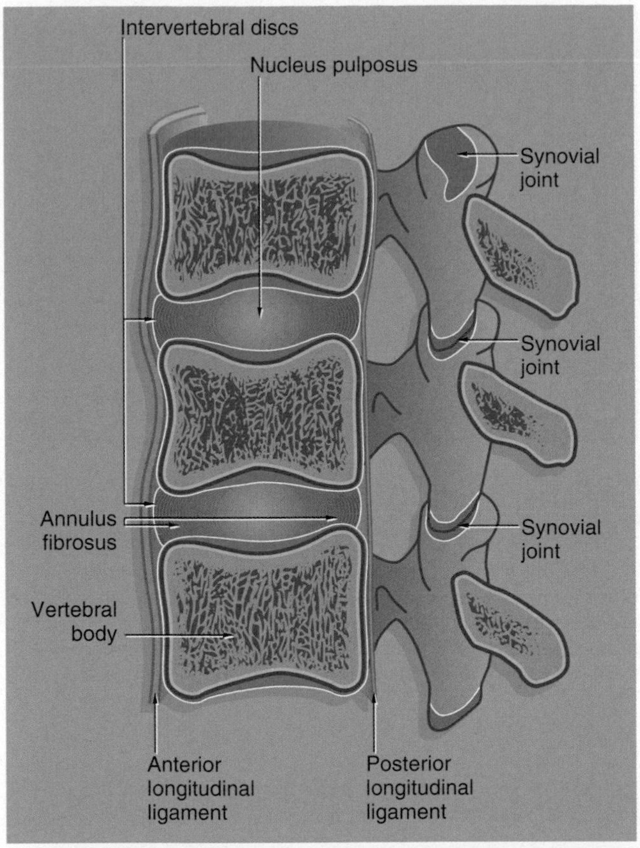

FIG. 10.29 The intervertebral joints

The vertebrae articulate by means of two different types of joints:

- The vertebral bodies are united by ***symphysial joints***, the ***intervertebral discs***, which permit movement between the vertebral bodies while maintaining a union of great strength. The fibrocartilage of each intervertebral disc is arranged in concentric rings, forming the ***annulus fibrosus***. Within the disc, there is a central cavity containing a viscous fluid, the ***nucleus pulposus***, which acts as a shock absorber. The annulus fibrosus is reinforced peripherally by ***circumferential ligaments***. A thick ligament extending down the anterior aspect of the spinal column merges with and further reinforces the annulus fibrosus and a similar but thinner ligament reinforces the posterior aspect.
- The vertebral arches articulate with each other by pairs of ***synovial joints*** known as ***facet*** or ***zygapophyseal joints***. Strong elastic ligaments connecting the bony processes of the vertebral arches contribute to the stability of the spinal column.

Disc degeneration and prolapse

The intervertebral discs act as shock absorbers, supporting and springing the vertebral column. In bipeds (like humans) they are particularly vulnerable to damage because of the weight they have to support and the rotational and flexional/extensional forces they are subjected to in daily activities.

These can lead to weakening of the annulus fibrosus, which may give way, allowing the soft central nucleus pulposus to extrude (***disc prolapse***) through into the spaces beneath the ligaments (Fig. 10.29). This leads to soft tissue swelling around the protrusion which may involve the spinal nerve roots emerging from the spinal column. Nerve damage may produce severe pain symptoms in the leg (e.g. ***sciatica***).

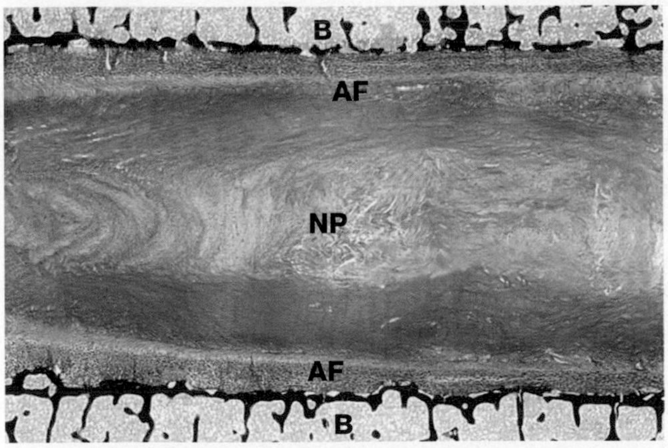

FIG. 10.30 Intervertebral disc
Haematoxylin–von Kossa (LP)

The intervertebral disc (Fig. 10.30) lies between the surfaces of adjacent vertebral bodies **B** and acts as a shock absorber. The disc is composed of an outer compact region of dense fibrocollagenous tissue containing occasional chondrocytes, the ***annulus fibrosus*** **AF**, with a variable thin layer of hyaline cartilage between this and the bone. The annulus fibrosus surrounds a central area of semi-fluid gelatinous matrix material known as the ***nucleus pulposus*** **NP**.

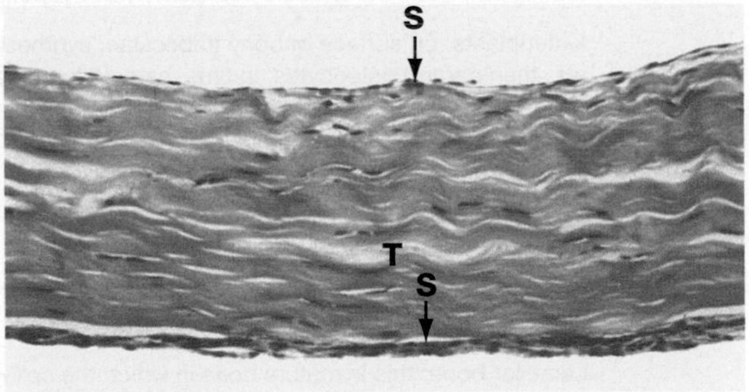

FIG. 10.31 Tendon
H&E (MP)

Tendons are tough, flexible straps or cords which connect muscles to bone (Fig. 10.31). They are composed of compact linear collagen fibres with the compressed nuclei of inactive fibroblasts (***tenocytes***) between the collagen bundles. Tendon **T** is poorly vascularised and heals slowly when damaged. It also contains tiny nerve fibres and tendon stretch receptors. Some tendons have a thin outer layer of synovium **S**. These tendons run for part of their course through a cylindrical fibrous sheath which is lined internally by synovium. The synovia secrete lubricating fluid.

AC articular cartilage **AF** annulus fibrosus **B** vertebral body **C** cortical bone **Cp** joint capsule **JC** joint cavity
NP nucleus pulposus **P** periosteum **S** synovium **T** tendon **V** blood vessel

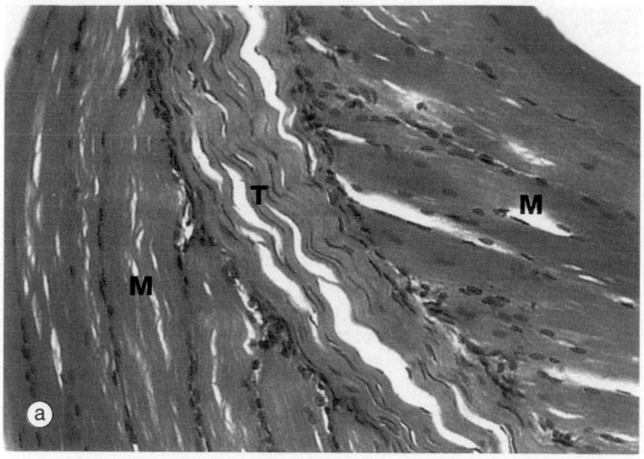

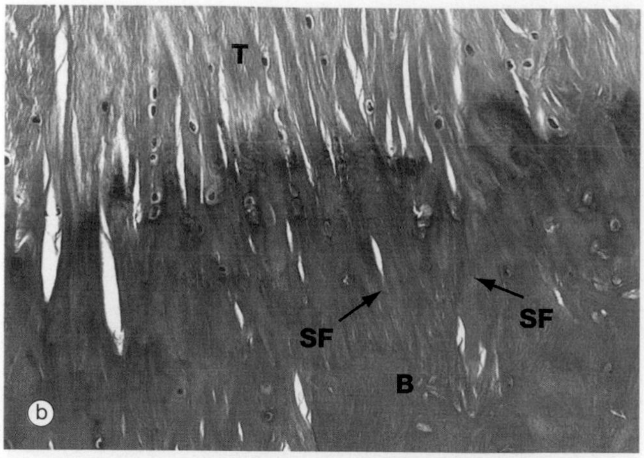

FIG. 10.32 Tendon insertions
(a) Muscle insertion, H&E (MP) (b) Insertion into bone, H&E (MP)

Fig. 10.32a shows two masses of skeletal muscle **M** which are inserted into a common tendon **T**. Within the muscle close to the tendon, some of the muscle fibres show splitting of their ends. In addition, some of the collagen fibres from the tendon penetrate the muscle to form a complex interdigitation with the split muscle fibres (***myotendinous junction***), thus increasing the surface area for anchorage and so improving the overall strength of the attachment.

Tendons sometimes attach to bone by the tendon collagen fibres intermingling with the collagen of the periosteum, a few of the fibres penetrating into the bone. At other sites, the collagen fibres of the tendon **T** penetrate directly into the bone **B** in the form of ***Sharpey fibres*** **SF**. This is illustrated in Fig. 10.32b.

REVIEW

TABLE 10.1 Review of skeletal tissues

Structure	Key components and features	Figures
Cartilage	Hyaline cartilage: most common type, forms articular surfaces of synovial joints, role in development of bony skeleton. Abundant ground substance.	10.1, 10.4
	Fibrocartilage: found in intervertebral discs and symphyses. Features intermediate between hyaline cartilage and dense regular connective tissue. Abundant collagen.	10.2
	Elastic cartilage: forms parts of larynx and external ear. Resembles hyaline cartilage, but abundant elastic fibres.	10.3
Bone	Major supporting tissue of the skeleton, composed of cells surrounded by collagenous osteoid matrix which is mineralised by calcium hydroxyapatite deposition.	
	Osteoblasts: on surface of bony trabeculae, synthesise new osteoid, becoming entrapped by this and then named osteocytes. In time, osteoid becomes mineralised.	10.5
	Osteocytes: inactive osteoblasts trapped within the bone matrix. Fine canaliculi within the bone contain interconnecting cytoplasmic processes from the cells.	10.5, 10.11
	Osteoclasts: large multinucleate cells, lie in small depressions called Howship lacunae, involved in resorption and remodelling of bone.	10.6
	Woven bone: this is immature bone with randomly orientated collagen fibres, found during development, associated with healing and repair, remodelled into lamellar bone.	10.7, 10.23
	Lamellar bone: this is mature bone in which the collagen fibres are orientated in parallel arrays, aligned to withstand stresses on the skeleton.	10.7
	Cortical bone: parallel columns of bone (osteons) with concentric lamellae around central Haversian canals containing neurovascular bundles.	10.10, 10.11
	Cancellous bone: interconnecting network of bony struts with intervening bone marrow.	10.14, 10.15
	Two forms of bone development: intramembranous ossification (mainly skull bones) and endochondral ossification (bone forms on a template of hyaline cartilage).	10.17–10.22
Joints	Synovial joints (diarthroses): permit extensive movement between articular surfaces. Surfaces lined by hyaline cartilage, fibrous capsule lined by synovium, lubricated by synovial fluid.	10.24–10.28
	Non-synovial joints: limited movement, bones united by dense collagenous tissues, including dense fibrous tissue (syndesmosis), hyaline cartilage (synchronosis) or fibrocartilage (symphysis).	10.29, 10.30
Tendons	Bands of dense regular connective tissue originating from muscle and inserting into bone to transmit the force of muscle contraction so that movement of joints may occur.	10.31, 10.32

B bone **M** skeletal muscle **SF** Sharpey fibres **T** tendon

11 Immune system

INTRODUCTION

All living tissues are subject to the constant threat of invasion by disease-producing foreign agents and microorganisms (pathogens), i.e. bacteria, viruses, fungi, protozoa and multicellular parasites such as worms. These organisms may invade the body, multiply and destroy functional tissue, causing illness and potentially death. Three main lines of defense have consequently evolved:

- Protective surface mechanisms
- The innate immune system
- The adaptive immune system

Protective surface mechanisms

These provide the first line of defense and, while intact, provide excellent protection from many disease-causing organisms. However, pathogens may enter the body via breaches in the skin or mucosal linings of the gut, respiratory and genitourinary tracts. The skin, with its surface layer of keratin, constitutes an impenetrable barrier to most microorganisms, unless breached by injury such as abrasion or burning. The mucous surfaces of the body, such as the conjunctiva and oral cavity, are protected by a variety of antibacterial substances including ***defensins***, short antimicrobial peptides that are found in surface mucus, and the enzyme ***lysozyme***, which is secreted in tears and saliva. The respiratory tract is protected by a layer of surface mucus that is continuously removed by ciliary action and replaced by ***goblet cells***. Maintenance of an acidic environment in the stomach, vagina and, to a lesser extent, the skin, inhibits the growth of pathogens in these sites. When such defenses fail and an infection takes hold, the two other main types of defense mechanism are activated.

The innate immune system

The ***innate immune response*** provides a rapid reaction to infections and, characteristically, the same magnitude of response each time the same pathogen is encountered (i.e. there is no learning in the innate system). The cells, proteins and peptides involved circulate in the blood of healthy individuals in sufficient amounts to overcome many trivial infections and contain more serious infections until an ***adaptive immune response*** can develop. The cellular components include ***neutrophils***, ***eosinophils***, ***basophils*** and ***macrophages***, as well as tissue resident cells such as ***histiocytes*** and ***mast cells***. The proteins and peptides of the innate response include ***complement***, ***acute-phase proteins***, ***chemokines*** and ***interleukins***. The major functions of the most important components of the innate immune system are outlined in Table 11.1. The innate immune response causes a pathological condition known as ***inflammation***, familiar to anyone who has ever had a cut finger. ***Acute inflammation*** is characterised by vascular changes including dilatation, enhanced permeability of capillaries and increased blood flow, resulting in the production of a fibrin-rich inflammatory exudate, thus bringing the proteins and cells required for early defence to the site of infection. Many of the cells and signalling molecules of the innate immune system are vital to the functioning of the adaptive immune system.

TABLE 11.1 Major components of innate immunity

Component	Actions
Neutrophil polymorphs	Phagocytosis and killing of pathogenic organisms Secretion of cytokines and extracellular antimicrobial molecules, including neutrophil extracellular traps (NETs) and pattern recognition receptors (PRRs)
Macrophages	Phagocytosis and killing of pathogenic organisms, removal of foreign material and dead cells Secretion of a wide range of cytokines and interleukins Present antigen to lymphocytes (adaptive immune system)
Eosinophils	Destroy larger multicellular pathogens Modulate allergic responses
Natural killer (NK) cells	Recognise and kill virus-infected and cancerous cells
Complement	Opsonises organisms to facilitate phagocytosis Chemoattractant for various cells Membrane attack complex (MAC) kills cells by puncturing plasma membrane
Acute-phase proteins	Plasma proteins which are increased during inflammation e.g. C-reactive protein (CRP) Wide range of actions that promote defense against pathogens
Chemokines	Recruit cells to specific sites and activate cells of innate and adaptive immune systems Induce differentiation of cells to more active and effective subtypes Wound healing and angiogenesis
Interleukins	Signalling molecules produced by many cell types, including macrophages, dendritic cells, lymphocytes Regulate the immune system

The adaptive immune system

The ***adaptive immune system*** is characterised by the ability to learn, so that second and subsequent encounters with a pathogen elicit a greater, more specific and faster response. This is the basis of lifelong immunity to certain infections after an initial infection or vaccination. The adaptive system builds on and is intimately associated with the innate immune system. Adaptive immunity depends on cell division to produce large numbers of ***lymphocytes*** with specificity for a particular pathogen (or ***antigen***) and thus takes 3 to 5 days to develop a significant response. Lymphocytes are able to kill or disable pathogens either by a ***cellular response*** (***T lymphocytes*** or ***T cells***) or a ***humoral response*** (***B lymphocytes*** or ***B cells***) or, commonly, a combination of both. Adaptive immunity amplifies some of the mechanisms of the innate response. For instance, ***antibody***, produced by B cells, coats bacteria (***opsonisation***) to facilitate phagocytosis by neutrophils and also directly activates the ***complement cascade***. The adaptive immune response is also controlled by the innate response, as T lymphocytes require the services of ***antigen-presenting cells*** (***APCs***) such as ***macrophages*** and ***dendritic cells*** for activation.

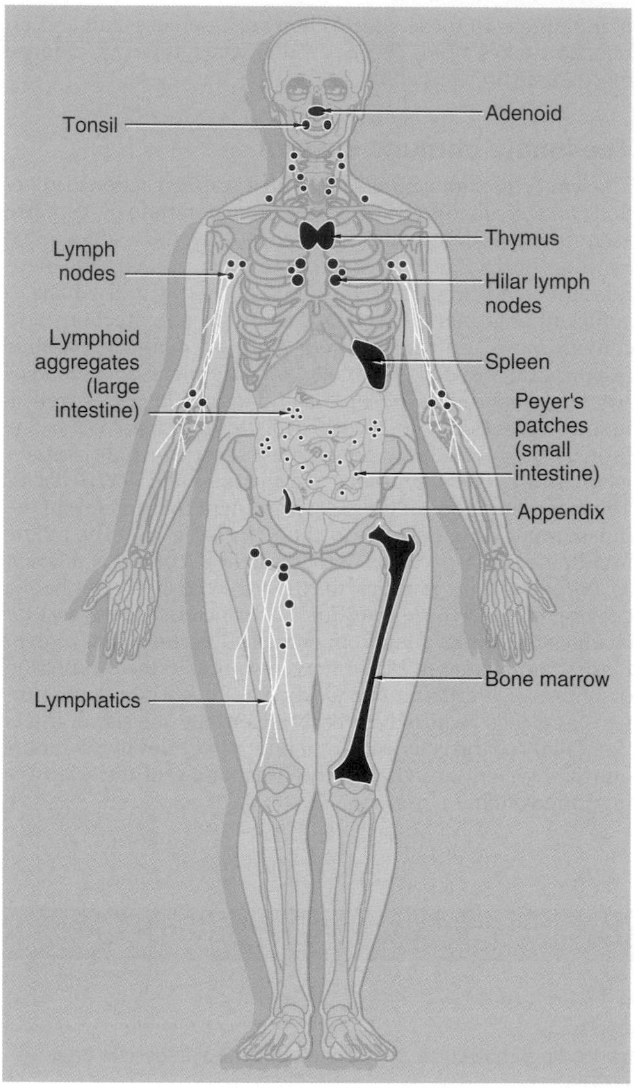

FIG. 11.1 The organs of the immune system

The components of both the innate and adaptive systems are found throughout the body (Fig. 11.1). The lymphocytes of the adaptive immune system are produced in the bone marrow from haematopoietic stem cells along with the cells of the innate system (see Ch. 3). As well as circulating in the blood, the cells of the adaptive immune system form specialised lymphoid tissues and also constitute a significant component of other tissues such as the gastrointestinal tract. The major lymphoid organs include:

- The ***thymus***, situated in the anterior mediastinum, is the site of maturation of immature T lymphocytes.
- The ***bone marrow*** is not only the home of lymphocyte stem cells but is also the site of B lymphocyte maturation.
- The ***lymph nodes***, found at the junctions of major lymphatic vessels, are the sites where both T and B lymphocytes may interact with antigen and APCs from the circulating lymph, leading to lymphocyte activation and cell division.
- The ***spleen***, situated in the left upper quadrant of the abdomen, is the location where T and B lymphocytes may interact with blood-borne antigen and undergo stimulation and cell division.
- ***Mucosa-associated lymphoid tissue*** (***MALT***) includes the ***tonsils*** (see Fig. 11.15) and ***adenoids*** in the oropharynx, ***Peyer's patches*** and ***lymphoid aggregates*** of the small and large intestines, respectively (see Fig. 11.16), and a diffuse population of lymphocytes and plasma cells in the mucosae of the gastrointestinal, respiratory and genitourinary tracts. These specialised lymphoid tissues respond to antigens entering the body through these mucosae.

The thymus and bone marrow, where immature lymphocytes acquire the receptors to recognise antigen, are known as ***primary lymphoid organs***. The spleen, lymph nodes and organised lymphoid tissues of MALT, where lymphocytes are activated in response to antigen, are the ***secondary lymphoid organs***.

LYMPHOCYTES

Lymphocytes comprise some 20% to 50% of white cells in the circulation. Most circulating lymphocytes measure 6 to 9 μm (i.e. about the same size as erythrocytes) and are called ***small lymphocytes***. About 3% are ***large lymphocytes***, measuring 9 to 20 μm. The light and electron microscopic features of lymphocytes are described in Fig. 3.17. Briefly, small lymphocytes have a round to ovoid nucleus occupying about 90% of the cell volume, with a thin rim of basophilic (bluish) cytoplasm.

Lymphocytes constantly patrol the body, circulating in the blood, lymph and other extracellular fluids and pausing in the organised lymphoid tissues. Secondary lymphoid organs are arranged to optimise the chances of an ***antigen*** meeting a potentially reactive lymphocyte and facilitating lymphocyte activation. If an antigen binds to a lymphocyte ***surface receptor***, the lymphocyte will be activated and a specific response to that antigen is triggered. Obviously, the immune response must be tightly controlled so as to be active when there is a potentially serious infection, but not react against harmless components of everyday life such as food proteins or even against normal components of the body (***autoimmunity***).

The effectiveness of the adaptive immune system in recognising the huge range of pathogenic organisms found in nature depends upon the unique ability of lymphocytes to produce an equally huge range of antigen receptors, i.e. the ***B cell receptor*** (***BCR***), comprising ***surface immunoglobulin*** (***sIg***) plus accessory molecules for B cells and the ***T cell receptor*** (***TCR***) for T cells. The ability of antibody to bind to antigen is determined by the physico-chemical properties of the antibody. Put simply, the shape and electrical charge of the binding site of the antibody must be complementary to the antigen, and the closer the fit of binding site to antigen, the stronger the bond formed and the greater the likelihood of the lymphocyte being stimulated. The TCR binds to antigen by similar reciprocity of shape and charge but it must also bind to the ***major histocompatibility complex*** (***MHC***) (see Figs 11.2 and 11.3). During maturation of lymphocytes, alternate components of the antigen-binding part of the antigen receptor genes are spliced together (***rearranged***) in a random fashion. Thus a huge range of possible antigen specificities are generated before the lymphocytes have a chance to meet external antigen.

The role of T lymphocytes

T cells have a number of effector and regulatory functions. Immature T lymphocytes migrate from the bone marrow to the ***thymus*** where they develop into mature T lymphocytes. The process of maturation includes proliferation, rearrangement of TCR genes, and acquisition of the surface receptors and accessory molecules of the mature T cell. At this stage, T cells with the ability to react with 'self-antigens' (normal body components) are removed by ***apoptosis***, creating a state of ***self-tolerance***. Mature T cells then populate the secondary lymphoid organs and, from there, continuously recirculate via the bloodstream in the quest for antigen.

T lymphocytes may develop into one of the functional subsets detailed below. These subsets develop from naïve T cells, depending on the mixture of cytokines and interleukins to which they are exposed, and can be identified in the laboratory by means of their surface receptors and accessory molecules.

The best known subsets of T cells include:

- **T helper cells (T_H cells)**. These T lymphocytes 'help' other cells to perform their effector functions by secreting a variety of mediators known as ***interleukins***. T_H cells thus provide 'help' to B cells, cytotoxic T cells (see below) and macrophages. T_H cells can be subdivided into subgroups with different functions. T_H1 cells tend to promote a ***cell-mediated reaction***, important for defence against viruses and intracellular pathogens. T_H2 cells are important for ***humoral*** (antibody mediated) responses and T_H17 cells modify and augment certain types of acute inflammation. T_H cells express the surface markers CD2, CD3 and CD4.
- **Cytotoxic T cells (T_C cells)**. These lymphocytes are able to kill virus-infected and some cancer cells. They require interaction with T_H cells to become activated and proliferate to form clones of effector cells. T_C cells express CD2, CD3 and CD8.
- **Regulatory T cells (T_{REG})**. These cells suppress immune responsiveness to self-antigens (autoimmunity) and switch off the response when antigen is removed. These cells usually express CD4, CD25 and FOXP3.
- **Memory T cells** develop from activated T cells to provide a 'rapid reaction force' for a subsequent encounter with the same antigen. This is the basis of persisting immunity after infection with some organisms and also the basis of vaccination.
- **γδ T cells** are a subset of T cells where the TCR is a heterodimer consisting of one γ chain and one δ chain, rather than the usual heterodimer of one α and one β chain. These cells populate the epithelium of the gastrointestinal tract and are CD8 positive.

The role of B lymphocytes

B lymphocytes are derived from precursors in the bone marrow and also mature there. Stimulated B cells mature into ***plasma cells*** that synthesise large amounts of ***antibody*** (***immunoglobulin***). Immunoglobulins fall into five different structural classes (IgG, IgA, IgD, IgM and IgE) and are secreted into and circulate in the blood. Immunoglobulin molecules are also anchored in the plasma membrane of B cells, with the antigen-binding region exposed to the external environment. This surface immunoglobulin is the antigen receptor for B lymphocytes (part of the BCR), and when it binds antigen the B cell is activated, generally with the 'help' of a T_H cell responding to the same antigen.

Once activated, the B cell undergoes mitotic division to produce a ***clone*** of cells able to synthesise immunoglobulin of the same antigen specificity. Most of the B cells of such a clone mature into plasma cells. When an antigen is encountered for the first time, this is described as the ***primary immune response***. A few cells from the same clone mature to become ***memory B cells***, small long-lived circulating lymphocytes that are able to respond quickly to any subsequent challenge with the same antigen. Antibody production during this ***secondary immune response*** occurs much more rapidly, is of much greater magnitude and produces IgG rather than IgM. This phenomenon explains the lifetime immunity that follows many common infections; it is also the general principle on which vaccination is based. Antibodies neutralise or destroy invading organisms by a number of methods (see Fig. 11.2).

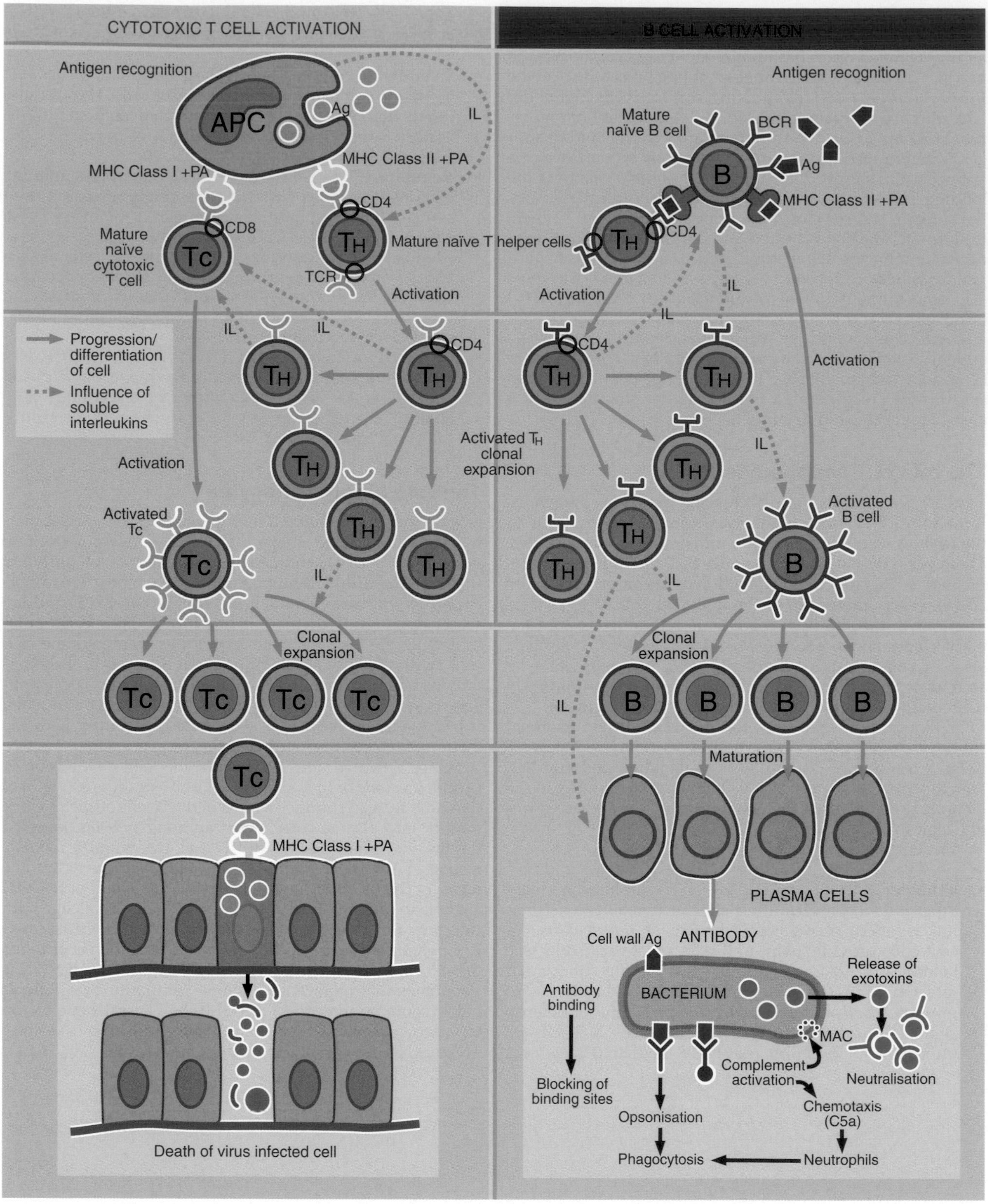

FIG. 11.2 The basics of the immune response *(caption opposite)*

Ag antigen **APC** antigen-presenting cell **B** B lymphocyte **BCR** B cell receptor **CD4** cluster of differentiation 4 **IL** interleukins **MAC** membrane attack complex **MHC** major histocompatibility complex **PA** processed antigen **T_C** cytotoxic T lymphocyte **TCR** T cell receptor **T_H** helper T lymphocyte

FIG. 11.2 The basics of the immune response *(illustration opposite)*

This diagram outlines the key steps in the adaptive immune response, i.e. recognition of antigen, activation of the response, generation of effector mechanism and destruction or inactivation of the antigen.

Recognition of antigen

T and B cells carry antigen receptors on their surface, the ***T cell receptor*** (**TCR**) and ***B cell receptor*** (**BCR**). The BCR consists of surface immunoglobulin plus certain accessory molecules.

Random rearrangement of the genes for the ***variable region*** of the receptor molecules gives rise to receptors with a truly staggering range of antigen binding sites. Each individual T or B cell has specificity for only one antigen, but the entire population is very varied.

Activation of the immune system

Initiation of an immune response first requires contact between ***antigen*** **Ag** and surface receptors on mature lymphocytes. There are several mechanisms of activation:

1. Activation of T cells is dependent on ***antigen-presenting cells*** **APC**. The antigen is taken up by an APC (e.g. macrophage, B lymphocyte, dendritic cell, Langerhans cell of skin) and broken down to short peptides (see Fig. 11.3). ***Processed antigen*** **PA** is then bound to a ***major histocompatibility complex molecule*** **MHC**, and the MHC–peptide complex is incorporated into the cell membrane so that the bound antigenic peptide is exposed to the extracellular fluid. Contact with a mature T cell bearing a T cell receptor with appropriate specificity activates the T cell. The type of response depends on whether the peptide is presented bound to MHC class I or II. Antigenic peptides bound to class II MHC molecules induce a T helper cell $\mathbf{T_H}$ response needed to activate B cells **B** and cytotoxic T cells $\mathbf{T_C}$. B cell receptors (sIg) or T_C receptors must also bind to the antigen for activation to occur. T_H cells secrete a variety of ***interleukins*** **IL** that mediate activation, clonal expansion and maturation of the B or cytotoxic T cell response.
2. Antigen synthesised within a body cell (e.g. tumour cell, virus-infected cell) is presented on the APC plasma membrane bound to a class I MHC protein where it is recognised by cytotoxic T cells $\mathbf{T_C}$. The T_H response is facilitated by a T cell expressing **CD4** protein on its surface. CD4 forms part of the T cell receptor on T_H cells. Cytotoxic T cells are able to kill the abnormal cells directly. T_H activation is also required for a T_C response to be mounted.
3. B lymphocytes interact with unprocessed antigens. They recognise antigen by means of the BCR (surface immunoglobulin, sIg). In most cases, the unprocessed antigen is presented to the B cell on the surface of an APC such as a ***follicular dendritic cell*** in a lymphoid follicle. The majority of antigens can only activate a B cell if there is 'help' from an activated T helper cell $\mathbf{T_H}$. Activation without T cell help will occur if sIg binds to a protein or polysaccharide antigen with a repeating chemical structure (e.g. the polysaccharide coat of the bacterium **Pneumococcus**). Such antigens are often known as ***T cell–independent antigens***. Few naturally occurring antigens are of this type (not illustrated).

Generation of effector mechanisms

1. Production of ***antibodies***. Antibody blocks the entry of organisms (such as viruses) into cells by binding to viral surface antigens.
   - Antigen–antibody complexes (***immune complexes***) activate complement to produce (among other factors) the ***membrane attack complex*** **MAC**, which punctures the outer membrane of the attacking organism.
   - Bound antibody with or without complement ***opsonises*** organisms and facilitates phagocytosis by ***neutrophils*** and ***macrophages***.
   - Antibody is essential for ***antibody-dependent cell cytotoxicity*** (***ADCC***) (see below).
   - Antibody bound to toxins inactivates them and facilitates their removal by phagocytic cells.
2. ***Cell-mediated cytotoxicity*** is the destruction by apoptosis of abnormal cells by cytotoxic T cells, natural killer (NK) cells or antibody-dependent cytotoxic cells.
3. Certain types of organism, such as *Mycobacterium tuberculosis*, the cause of tuberculosis, activate T helper cells (T_H1) to secrete cytokines that in turn activate macrophages. Activated macrophages are more effective at killing phagocytosed organisms. This is the mechanism of ***type IV hypersensitivity*** (***chronic granulomatous inflammation***) (not illustrated).

Termination of the immune response

There are a number of mechanisms for switching off the immune response when the need for it has been removed. These include removal of antigen, the short life span of plasma cells, the activities of regulatory T cells and a variety of other mechanisms that downregulate the activity of T and B cells. It is vital that the immune response is terminated when no longer needed to prevent damage to normal tissue from an overenthusiastic immune response. These mechanisms are also important in the prevention of autoimmunity.

Immunological memory

When activated lymphocytes undergo clonal expansion during an immune response, some of the cells so generated mature to become ***memory T*** and ***B cells***. These lymphocytes have a similar appearance to naïve lymphocytes but are able to produce a faster and more effective response to a smaller quantity of antigen. This is known as a ***secondary immune response*** and is the basis of lifelong immunity after certain infections and of vaccination.

FIG. 11.3 Lymphocytes and antigen presenting cells *(illustration (b) opposite)*
(a) Schematic diagram (b) EM ×18 000

Antigen-presenting cells **APC** are vital for the activation of lymphocytes to produce an adaptive immune response. They include ***macrophages, dendritic cells*** and ***B lymphocytes.***

Dendritic cells patrol the body surfaces and phagocytose invading pathogens. Dendritic cells are versatile and potent APCs. Some appear to be resident in the lymph node while others, carrying antigen from peripheral tissues, migrate in the lymph to the regional lymph nodes. Dendritic cells are found in the paracortical area of lymph nodes. This group of cells also includes ***interdigitating cells*** of the thymus and ***Langerhans cells*** of the skin. ***Follicular dendritic cells*** are accessible to B cells in the germinal centres of lymph nodes. They are similar cells which are able to bind antibody–antigen complexes to their surface without prior processing.

APC function is shown on the right side of Fig. 11.3a. Antigen (e.g. a bacterium **B**) is taken up by APCs into an early endosome **EE** that fuses with a lysosome containing ***major histocompatibility complex class II*** molecules **MHC II**. The antigen is broken down into short antigenic peptides **AP** that bind to MHC II and the peptide–MHC II complex is transported to the plasma membrane. After fusion of the phagolysosome **PL** with the plasma membrane **PM**, the MHC II–peptide complex is exposed on the cell surface where it may come into contact with helper T cells $\mathbf{T_H}$. If the T cell receptor **TCR** on the T_H cell can bind to that particular peptide–MHC II complex, activation will occur and the adaptive immune response will proceed.

Obviously, processing of a bacterium will generate many different antigenic peptides, but only one peptide and one T_H cell is shown here for simplicity.

In general, T_H cells recognise peptide bound to MHC II and cytotoxic T cells $\mathbf{T_C}$ recognise antigen bound to MHC class I **MHC I**. On the left of Fig. 11.3a, processing of intrinsic viral antigen in a virus-infected cell is shown. The viral protein **VPr** is chopped into short peptides **VP** by a ***proteasome*** (an organelle that breaks down abnormal proteins). The peptides are translocated to the endoplasmic reticulum **ER**, bind to MHC I and are presented on the cell surface for interaction with a T_C. Almost all body cells express MHC I but usually only APCs express MHC II.

Fig. 11.3b illustrates several lymphocytes and an APC in a lymph node. Lymphocytes and APCs exhibit similar features in other lymphoid tissues. The lymphocytes **L** are relatively small with round nuclei and condensed chromatin that tends to be clumped around the periphery of the nucleus. Cell outlines are fairly regular with occasional surface projections. The scanty cytoplasm contains plentiful free ribosomes and a few mitochondria but little endoplasmic reticulum, lysosomes or secretory granules.

The centre of the field is occupied by the large cell body of an antigen-presenting cell **APC**, in this case a dendritic cell. These have numerous long branched cytoplasmic extensions **CE** reaching out between the surrounding lymphocytes so that a single dendritic cell can be in contact with many different lymphocytes. Its nucleus is deeply indented with dispersed chromatin; in this example, the plane of section has resulted in a small nuclear extension appearing to be separate from the main part of the nucleus. Typically, the APC cytoplasm contains numerous small lysosomes **Ly** and larger phagosomes **P**.

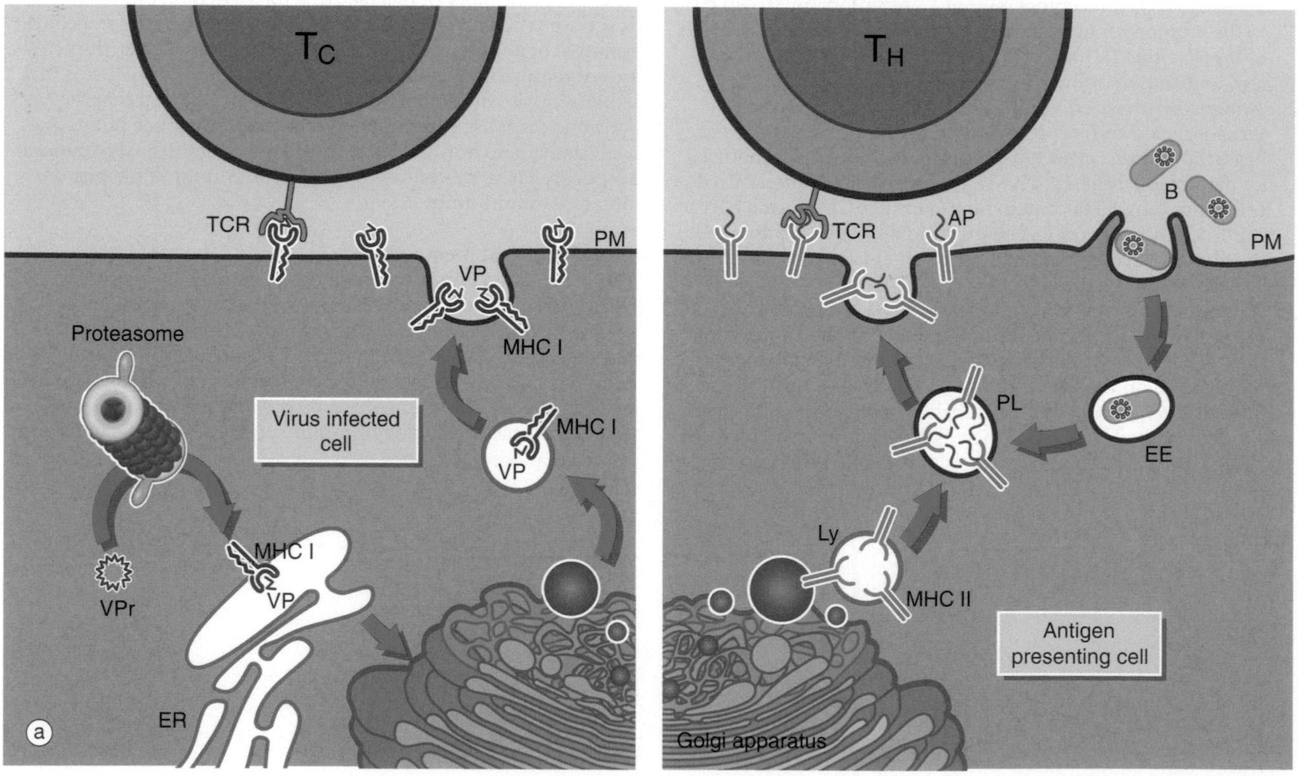

AP antigenic peptide **APC** antigen-presenting cell **B** bacterium **CE** cytoplasmic extension **EE** early endosome **ER** endoplasmic reticulum **L** lymphocyte **Ly** lysosome **MHC I** major histocompatibility complex class I **MHC II** major histocompatibility complex class II **P** phagosome **PL** phagolysosome **PM** plasma membrane $\mathbf{T_C}$ cytotoxic T cell **TCR** T cell receptor $\mathbf{T_H}$ T helper cell **VP** viral peptide **VPr** viral protein

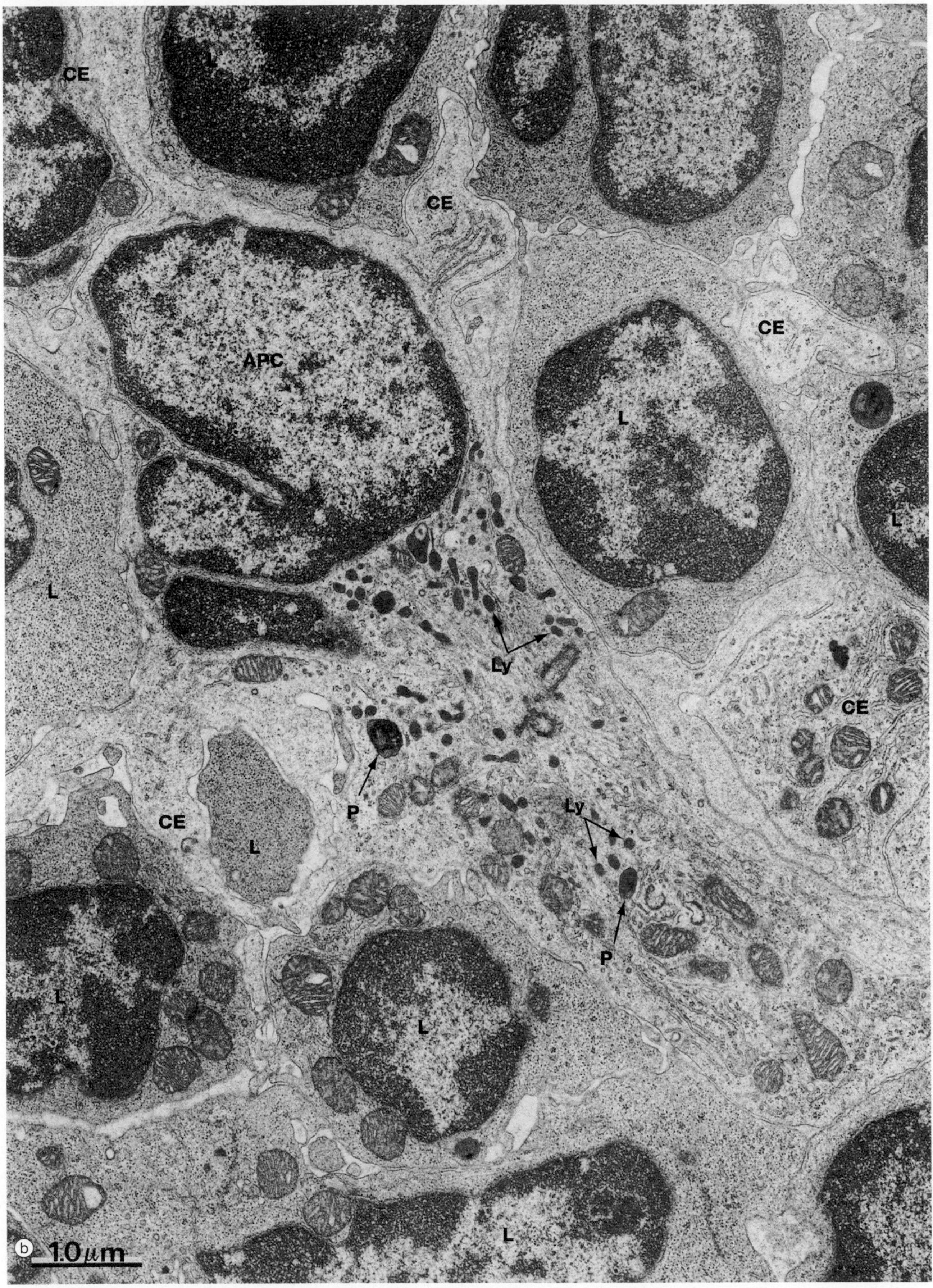

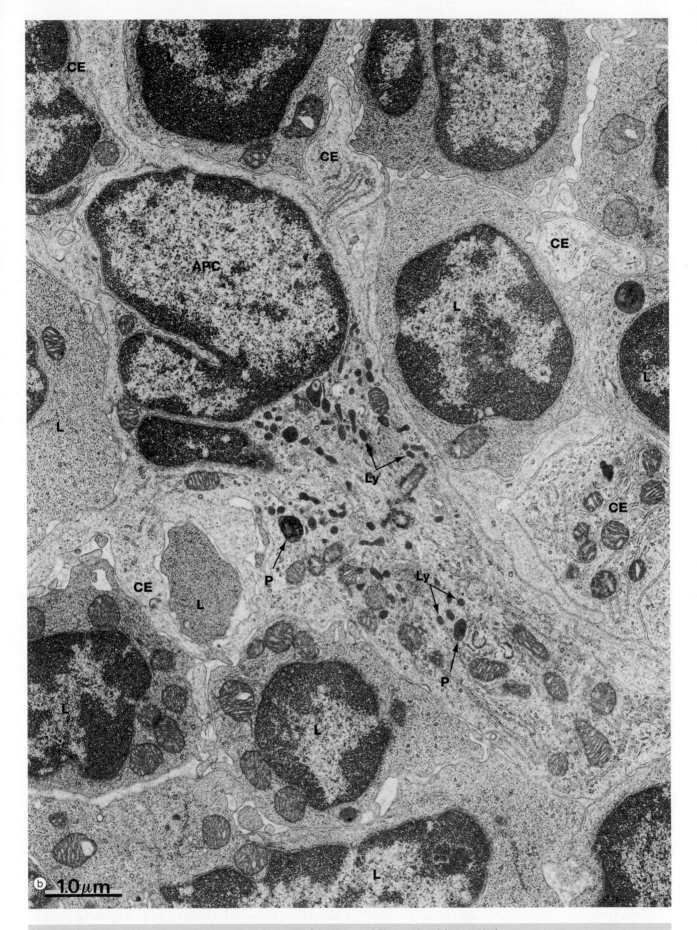

FIG. 11.3 Lymphocytes and antigen presenting cells ***(caption and illustration (a) opposite)***
(a) Schematic diagram (b) EM ×18 000

THYMUS

The thymus is a flattened lymphoid organ located in the upper anterior mediastinum and lower part of the neck. The thymus is most active during childhood, reaching a weight of about 30 to 40 g at puberty, after which it undergoes slow involution so that in the middle-aged or older adult it may be difficult to differentiate from adipose tissue macroscopically.

In the embryo, the thymus originates from epithelial outgrowths of the ventral wing of the third pharyngeal pouch on each side. These merge in the midline, forming a single organ subdivided into numerous fine lobules. The epithelium develops into a sponge-like structure containing a labyrinth of interconnecting spaces that become colonised by immature T lymphocytes derived from haematopoietic tissue elsewhere in the developing embryo. Towards the centre of the organ, the epithelial framework has a coarser structure with smaller interstices and a much smaller lymphocyte population, so that on microscopic examination, the gland has a highly cellular outer ***cortex*** and a less cellular central ***medulla***.

The epithelial cells of the thymus provide a mechanical supporting framework for the lymphocyte population. Cortical epithelial cells also promote T cell differentiation and proliferation. Furthermore, the epithelial cells secrete a number of different hormones that regulate T cell maturation and proliferation within the thymus and in other lymphoid organs and tissues. The inner surfaces of the thymic capsule and septa are invested by a continuous layer of thymic epithelial cells resting on a basement membrane. The epithelium also forms sheaths around the blood vessels, creating a barrier to the entry of antigenic material into the thymic parenchyma. This is known as the ***blood–thymus barrier***.

The functions of the thymus include:

- Development of immunocompetent T lymphocytes from bone marrow–derived T cell precursors to produce mature T_H and T_C cells.
- Proliferation of clones of mature naïve T cells to supply the circulating lymphocyte pool and peripheral tissues.
- Development of immunological self-tolerance. More than 98% of maturing cells die by apoptosis within the thymus, and many of these are self-reactive.
- The thymus secretes various polypeptides with hormonal characteristics, including ***thymulin***, ***thymopoietin*** and various ***thymosins***. These hormones regulate T cell maturation, proliferation and function within the thymus and peripheral lymphoid tissues. They also interact with other endocrine systems in the regulation of inflammation.

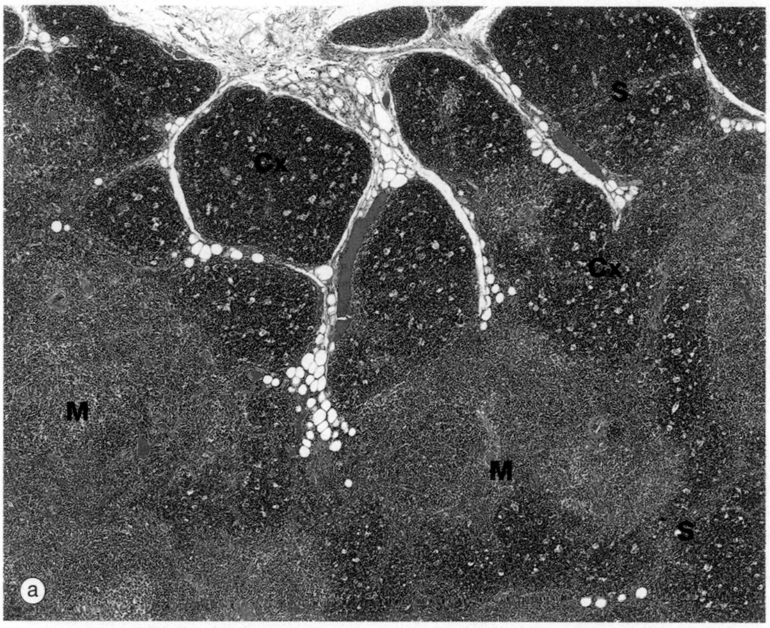

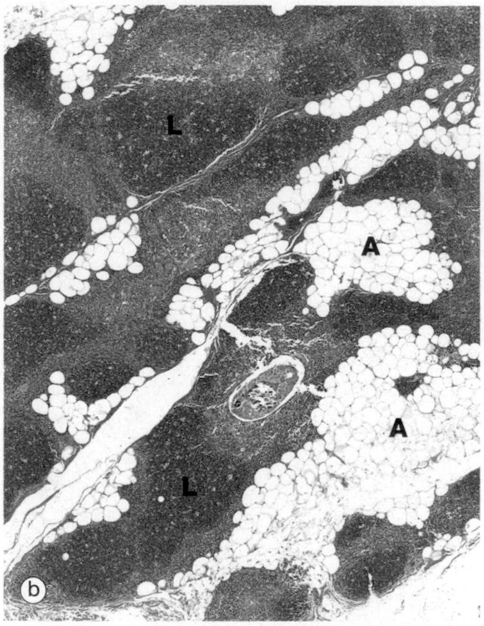

FIG. 11.4 Thymus *(caption continued opposite)*
(a) Infant, H&E (LP) (b) Adult, H&E (LP)

The infant thymus (Fig. 11.4a) is a lobulated organ invested by a loose collagenous ***capsule*** from which interlobular ***septa*** **S** containing blood vessels radiate into the substance of the organ. The thymic tissue is divided into two distinct zones, a deeply basophilic outer cortex **Cx** and an inner eosinophilic ***medulla*** **M**; distinction between the two is most marked in early childhood, as in this specimen.

In the adult (mid-30s in this case), the thymus (Fig. 11.4b) is already well into the process of involution, which involves two distinct processes, fatty infiltration and lymphocyte depletion. Fat cells (adipocytes) first begin to appear at birth, their numbers slowly rising until puberty when the rate of fatty infiltration increases markedly. Fatty infiltration of the interlobular septa occurs first, spreading out into the cortex and later the medulla. Thus, in the mature thymus islands of lymphoid tissue **L** are separated by areas of adipose tissue **A**. At this age, the cortex and medulla can still be differentiated. In the elderly, the thymus can be very difficult to detect both macroscopically and microscopically, with only small islands of lymphoid tissue lost in a sea of adipose tissue. Lymphocyte numbers begin to fall from about 1 year of age, the process continuing thereafter at a constant rate. Despite this, the thymus continues to provide a supply of mature T lymphocytes to the circulating pool and peripheral tissues. Lymphocyte depletion results in collapse of the epithelial framework. However, cords of epithelial cells persist and continue to secrete thymic hormones throughout life.

The normal process of slow thymic involution associated with aging should be distinguished from acute thymic involution, which may occur in response to severe disease and metabolic stress associated with pregnancy, lactation, infection, surgery, malnutrition, malignancy and other systemic insults.

FIG. 11.4 **Thymus** ***(illustrations (a) and (b) and start of caption opposite)***
(a) Infant, H&E (LP) (b) Adult, H&E (LP)

Stress involution is characterised by greatly increased lymphocyte death and is probably mediated by high levels of corticosteroids; thus the size and activity of the adult thymus are often underestimated if examined after prolonged illness.

Numerous small branches of the internal thoracic and inferior thyroid arteries enter the thymus via the interlobular septa, branching at the corticomedullary junction to supply the cortex and medulla. Postcapillary venules in the corticomedullary region have a specialised cuboidal endothelium similar to that of the ***high endothelial venules*** of the lymph node (see Fig. 11.11), which allows passage of lymphocytes into and out of the thymus. The venous and lymphatic drainage follow the course of the arterial supply; there are no afferent lymphatics. Sympathetic and parasympathetic nerve fibres derived from the sympathetic chain and phrenic nerves, respectively, accompany the blood vessels into the thymus.

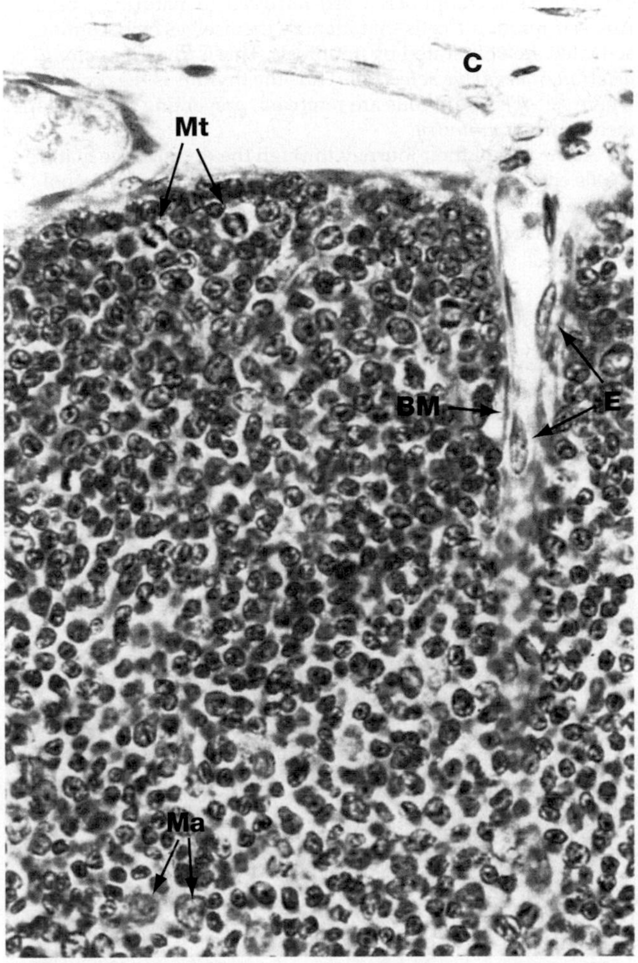

FIG. 11.5 Thymic cortex
H&E (HP)

Prothymocytes migrate in the blood from the bone marrow and enter the thymus at the corticomedullary junction. They move to the subcapsular area of the cortex to begin their maturation into mature naïve T cells. The thymic cortex is thus packed with immature and maturing T cells (***thymocytes***). In the outer cortex, large lymphocytes (***lymphoblasts***) divide by mitosis to produce clones of smaller mature T cells. These undergo further maturation as they move deeper into the cortex towards the medulla. This differentiation is promoted by interaction with the specialised epithelial cells known as ***thymic nurse cells***, which are found in the outer cortex. Each nurse cell envelops multiple lymphocytes and supports their progression through the early stages of maturation. It is during this process that the T cell receptor genes are rearranged and the cells acquire the surface markers or ***phenotype*** of mature helper and cytotoxic T cells. T cells in the cortex begin to express the TCR–CD3 complex and the co-receptors CD4 and CD8. Cells failing to make these adjustments successfully die by apoptosis and are taken up by pale-stained macrophages **Ma**. Several mitotic figures **Mt** can be seen in the outer cortex in this micrograph.

Note also in this micrograph a small capillary lined by flattened endothelial cells **E**, entering the cortex from the capsule **C**. Around the capillary, the basement membrane **BM** of epithelial cells can be discerned at the interface between the thymic framework and supporting tissue elements. The epithelial framework of the cortex is more delicate and finely branched than that of the medulla and the cells cannot be distinguished in this H&E-stained micrograph, being obscured by the mass of lymphocytes. However, immunostaining techniques can demonstrate these cells (see Fig. 11.7).

A adipose tissue **BM** basement membrane **C** capsule **Cx** cortex **E** endothelial cell **L** lymphoid tissue **M** medulla **Ma** macrophage **Mt** mitotic figure **S** septum

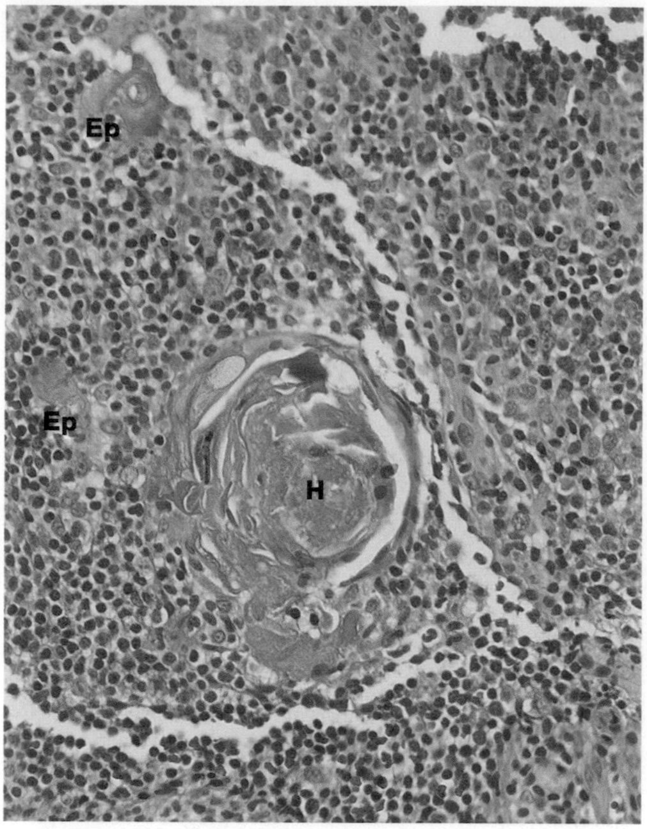

FIG. 11.6 Thymic medulla
H&E (HP)

Maturing ***thymocytes*** migrate from the cortex to the medulla. The dominant histological feature of the thymic medulla is the robust epithelial component **Ep**. The epithelial cells have large pale-stained nuclei, eosinophilic cytoplasm and prominent basement membranes. A particular feature in the medulla are the lamellated ***Hassall corpuscles*** **H** that first appear in fetal life and increase in number and size thereafter. These are formed from groups of keratinised epithelial cells, often with fragments of debris at their centre, and probably represent a degenerative phenomenon.

Also found in the medulla are ***dendritic cells***, also known as ***thymic interdigitating cells***, which express high levels of both class I and II MHC proteins. It appears that these cells present normal self-components, ***self-antigens***, to maturing T cells. Any self-reactive T cells that identify themselves by becoming activated are obliterated by apoptosis. This is known as ***clonal deletion*** or ***negative selection***. Thus the thymus is the organ where self-reactive T cells are removed, preventing the development of ***autoimmunity***.

At the end of their journey through the thymus, the mature T cells enter the blood vessels and lymphatics to join the pool of circulating T lymphocytes and populate the T lymphocyte domains of other lymphoid organs.

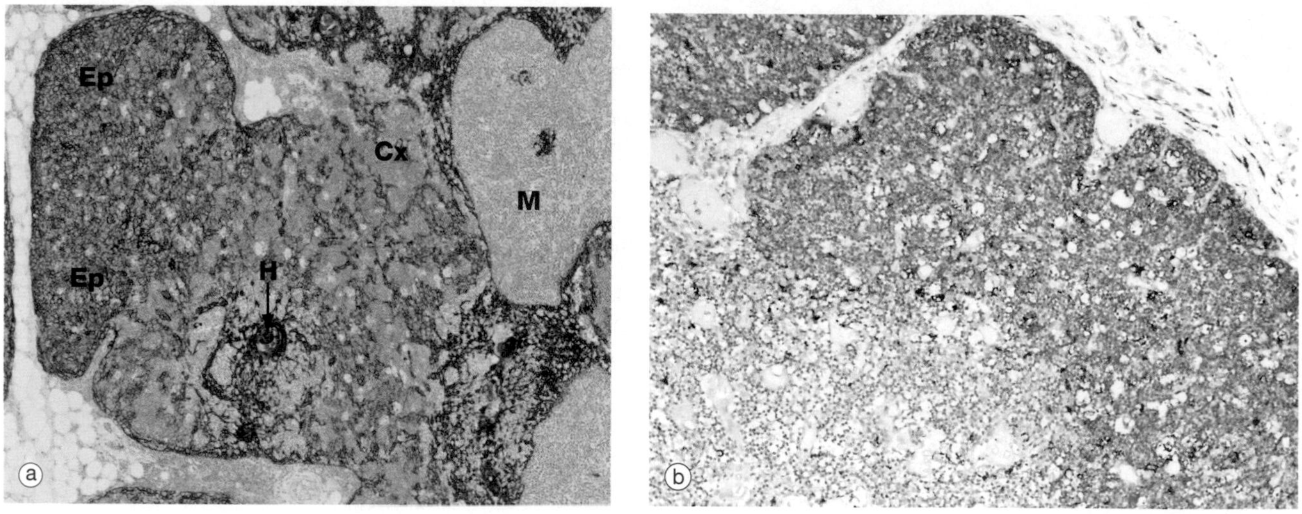

FIG 11.7 Thymus
(a) Immunohistochemical stain for cytokeratin (AE1/3) (MP) (b) Immunohistochemical stain for CD68 (MP)

The epithelial cells and macrophages of the thymus are generally difficult to visualise in a standard H&E section, as they are obscured by the dense population of lymphocytes. However, they may be highlighted by immunohistochemical techniques (see Appendix 2). Fig. 11.7a shows infant thymus tissue that has been stained using an antibody to cytokeratin. Many different cytokeratin antibodies are commercially available and are widely used in routine histopathology practice. This micrograph demonstrates the extensive delicate network of epithelial cells in the cortex **Cx**, as well as the more rugged epithelial framework of the medulla **M**. Individual epithelial cells **Ep** as well as Hassall corpuscles **H** are stained brown. In Fig. 11.7b the tissue has been stained with an antibody to CD68, which is strongly expressed by macrophages. Some dendritic cells also express CD68, so the brown-stained cells visible in both the cortex and medulla will include a mixture of both cell types, although predominantly macrophages. Macrophages phagocytose lymphocytes that have died by apoptosis, either because they have failed to go through the sequential steps of maturation properly or because having done so they have shown themselves to be self-reactive.

Dendritic cells (or thymic interdigitating cells) present self-antigens to developing T cells. Those T cells that declare themselves to be self-reactive are culled (clonal deletion) to maintain a state of self-tolerance.

Cx cortex **Ep** epithelial cells **H** Hassall corpuscle **M** medulla

LYMPH NODES

Lymph nodes are bean-shaped, encapsulated, highly organised structures that are interposed along the larger regional vessels of the lymph vascular system. The human body has about 450 lymph nodes, grouped mainly in areas where the lymphatics converge to form larger trunks as in the neck, axillae, groins, lung hila, mesentery of the bowel and para-aortic areas. Lymph nodes process antigen from the interstitial fluid that arrives at the node in the lymph.

Lymph nodes are the primary site to stimulate an immune response to antigens in the lymph. They are organised to bring together antigen, potentially reactive lymphocytes and APCs and to provide the best environment to stimulate an adaptive immune response. As described earlier, antigen-loaded dendritic cells from skin and mucosal sites, along with free antigen and cytokines, migrate in the lymph to the regional lymph nodes. The acute inflammatory process increases the flow of lymph by flooding the infected or damaged tissue with extracellular fluid. Mature naïve lymphocytes constantly traffic between the periphery and organised lymphoid tissues via the blood and lymph circulation to maximise their chances of encouraging appropriate antigen.

Thus within the lymph node, the necessary elements for stimulation of the adaptive immune response are brought together, and T and B cells undergo clonal expansion and maturation. B cells mature into antibody-secreting ***plasma cells***. Effector T lymphocytes and plasma cells leave the nodes in the ***efferent lymph*** and recirculate to the damaged or infected tissue. In addition, water and electrolytes from the lymph that percolate through the node are also returned to the blood circulation via the ***high endothelial venules***.

Lymph nodes can be considered as three functional compartments:

- The ***stromal compartment*** which is packed with lymphocytes and APCs
- The ***lymphatic/sinus compartment*** which acts as a sieve for antigen
- The ***vascular compartment*** which delivers lymphocytes to the lymph node along with the usual nutrients

Lymph node enlargement

Lymph nodes can become enlarged for a wide variety of reasons but by far the most common is infection. In most cases, the lymph nodes are not actively infected themselves but are responding to infection in the tissues they drain. Most readers will have experienced a sore throat at some point in their lives. This may be due either to a viral or a bacterial infection of the mucosa of the pharynx (pharyngitis) which may in turn lead to inflammation and enlargement of the tonsils (tonsillitis), large aggregates of lymphoid tissue in the throat (see Fig. 11.15). In addition, the regional lymph nodes in the neck are recruited with increased flow of antigen-bearing lymph and the triggering of an adaptive immune response. These lymph nodes become enlarged and tender and can easily be palpated in the neck, a situation known colloquially as 'swollen glands'. The end result of all this activity is recruitment of all the effector mechanisms of the adaptive and innate immune responses and clearance of the infection, with a return to normal good health.

In some situations, however, the infective organism can directly invade and grow in the lymph node. Such infections include *Mycobacterium tuberculosis* (TB), *Mycobacteria other than tuberculosis (MOTT)* or *non-tuberculous Mycobacteria (NTM)* and *Toxoplasma gondii*, all of which typically give rise to a ***granulomatous*** pattern of chronic inflammation (see e-Fig. 11.1).

Another common cause of lymph node enlargement is malignant tumours. Tumours of the immune system itself (lymphomas and leukaemias) are discussed briefly later (see also *Wheater's Pathology*, Ch. 6). However, it is common for lymph nodes draining a malignant epithelial tumour to become enlarged. This may simply be a reactive process caused by increased flow of lymph to the nodes, perhaps due to necrosis of the tumour. Much more sinister is the spread of tumour to the lymph nodes, a process known as ***metastasis***. This is so important for ***staging*** a tumour that, for many common carcinomas, the local lymph nodes are either sampled or removed in their entirety to assess the presence of tumour deposits in the lymph node. This is routine in the assessment of breast, colonic and head and neck cancers (see e-Fig. 11.2). The presence or absence of tumour in the lymph nodes allows a prediction to be made about whether that particular tumour is likely to spread elsewhere and allows informed planning of future treatment.

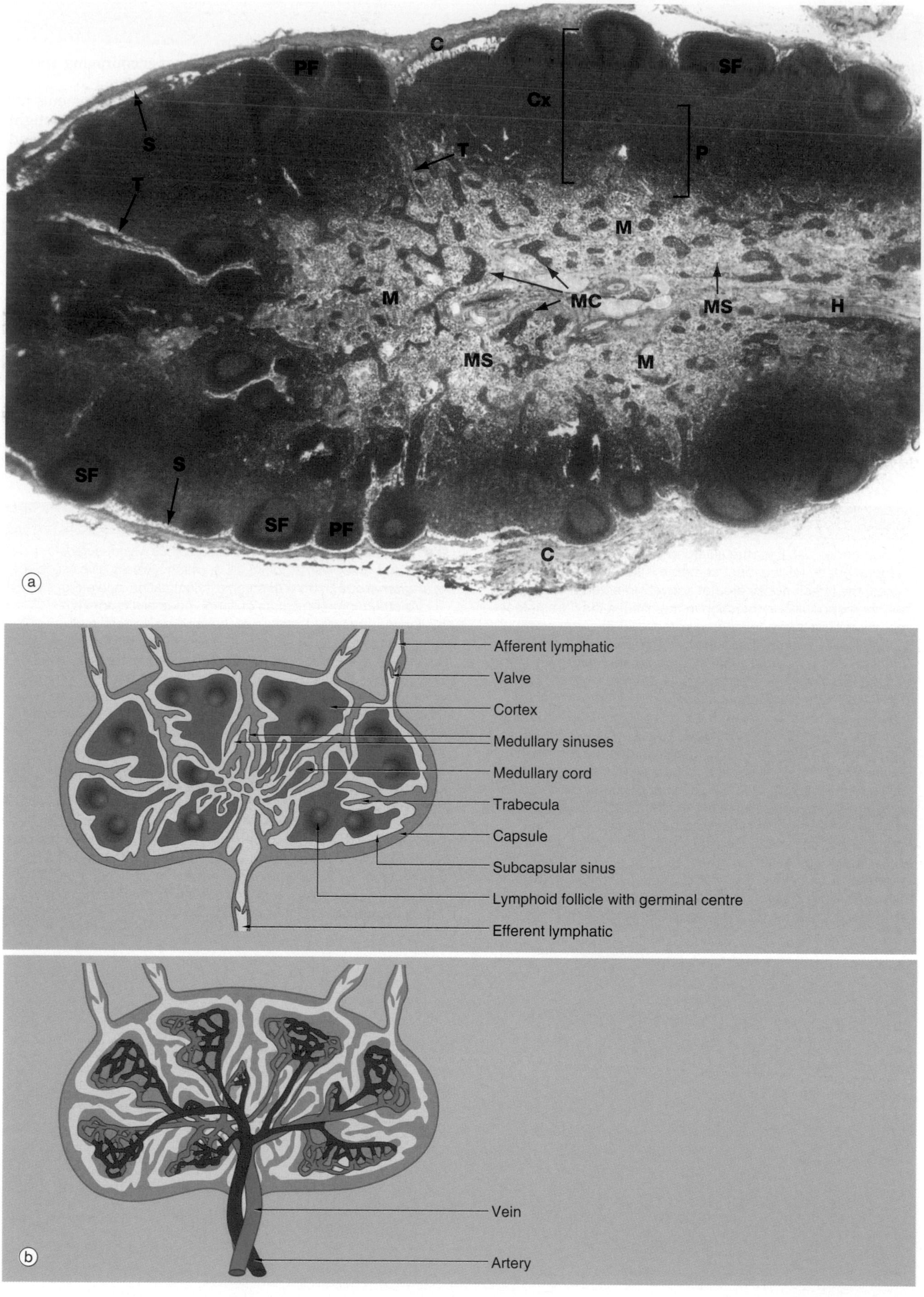

FIG. 11.8 Lymph node structure and vascular organisation *(caption opposite)*
(a) H&E (LP) (b) Schematic diagram

FIG. 11.8 Lymph node structure and vascular organisation *(illustrations (a) and (b) opposite)*
(a) H&E (LP) (b) Schematic diagram

Lymph nodes are small, bean-shaped organs situated in the course of lymphatic vessels such that lymph draining back to the bloodstream first passes through one or more lymph nodes. Inactive nodes are only a few millimetres long but may increase greatly in size when mounting an active immunological response. Most lymph nodes in the body show some degree of 'reactive change' in response to the constant barrage of antigen to which they are exposed. As shown in Fig. 11.8a, the outer part of the lymph node is highly cellular and is known as the ***cortex*** **Cx**, whilst the central area, the ***medulla*** **M**, is less cellular. At the ***hilum*** **H**, the ***efferent lymphatic*** drains efferent lymph from the lymph node. The hilum is also the site of entry of the artery bringing blood to the lymph node and the vein leaving the node. The lymph node is surrounded by a collagenous ***capsule*** **C** from which ***trabeculae*** **T** extend for a variable distance into the substance of the node.

Afferent lymphatic vessels, as shown in Fig. 11.8b, divide into several branches outside the node then pierce the capsule to drain into a narrow space called the ***subcapsular sinus*** **S** that encircles the node beneath the capsule. From here, a labyrinth of channels called ***cortical sinuses*** passes towards the medulla through the cortical cell mass; sinuses adjacent to the trabeculae (***trabecular sinuses***) pursue a more direct course towards the medulla, but nevertheless form part of the cortical sinus system. The cortical sinuses are generally difficult to visualise because of their highly convoluted shape and numerous fine extensions that penetrate the cellular mass of the cortex (see Fig. 11.9). The superficial cortex contains a number of dense cellular aggregations, the ***follicles***. Most of these in this particular example are ***secondary follicles*** **SF** with a pale-stained ***germinal centre***; others are inactive ***primary follicles*** **PF**. B cells respond to antigen in the cortex and undergo stimulation, clonal expansion and maturation in the follicles, the presence of germinal centres indicating that an active immune response is underway.

The deeper cortex or ***paracortex*** **P** is also densely cellular but has a more homogeneous staining appearance. T lymphocytes interact with antigen presenting cells in the paracortex and undergo a similar process of activation and clonal expansion. T helper cells migrate towards the cortex to provide 'help' to B cells while activated cytotoxic T cells leave the node to perform their functions in the periphery.

At the left of the field, some lymphoid follicles appear to be located deep in the paracortex; this is not the case but is a product of the plane of section, which passes at that point through the superficial cortex.

The dominant feature of the medulla is the network of broad interconnected lymphatic channels called ***medullary sinuses*** **MS** that converge upon the hilum in the concavity of the node. Lymph drains from the hilum in the ***efferent lymphatic*** into one or more additional nodes, which in turn drain into more proximal nodes before eventually joining the bloodstream via the ***thoracic duct*** or ***right lymphatic duct***. Thus the lymph is filtered through a number of lymph nodes to facilitate the exposure of large numbers of lymphocytes to antigens in the lymph. Extensions of the cortical cell mass extend into the medulla as ***medullary cords*** **MC**.

The blood supply of the lymph node, as shown in Fig. 11.8b, is derived from one or more small arteries which enter at the hilum and branch in the medulla, giving rise to extensive capillary networks supplying the cortical follicles, paracortical zone and medullary cords. The vascular system provides the main route of entry of lymphocytes into the node, as well as supplying its metabolic requirements. Within the paracortex, the postcapillary ***high endothelial venules*** (HEV) have a cuboidal endothelium specialised for the exit of lymphocytes. Recognition by lymphocytes of these exit sites requires the presence of specific complementary ***adhesion molecules*** on the surface of both the endothelial cells and lymphocytes. Different groups of lymphocytes home to different tissues. Thus lymphocytes from the mucosa of the gut migrate to mesenteric lymph nodes, then to the spleen and back to mucosal tissues. Lymphocytes from the skin travel to their regional lymph nodes and then return to the skin. This is made possible by the different adhesion molecules or ***vascular addressins*** in the HEV of the different lymph node groups and the corresponding binding molecules on the lymphocytes. The HEV drain into small veins that leave the node via the hilum.

C capsule **Cx** cortex **H** hilum **M** medulla **MC** medullary cords **MS** medullary sinus **P** paracortex **PF** primary follicle **S** subcapsular sinus **SF** secondary follicle **T** trabecula

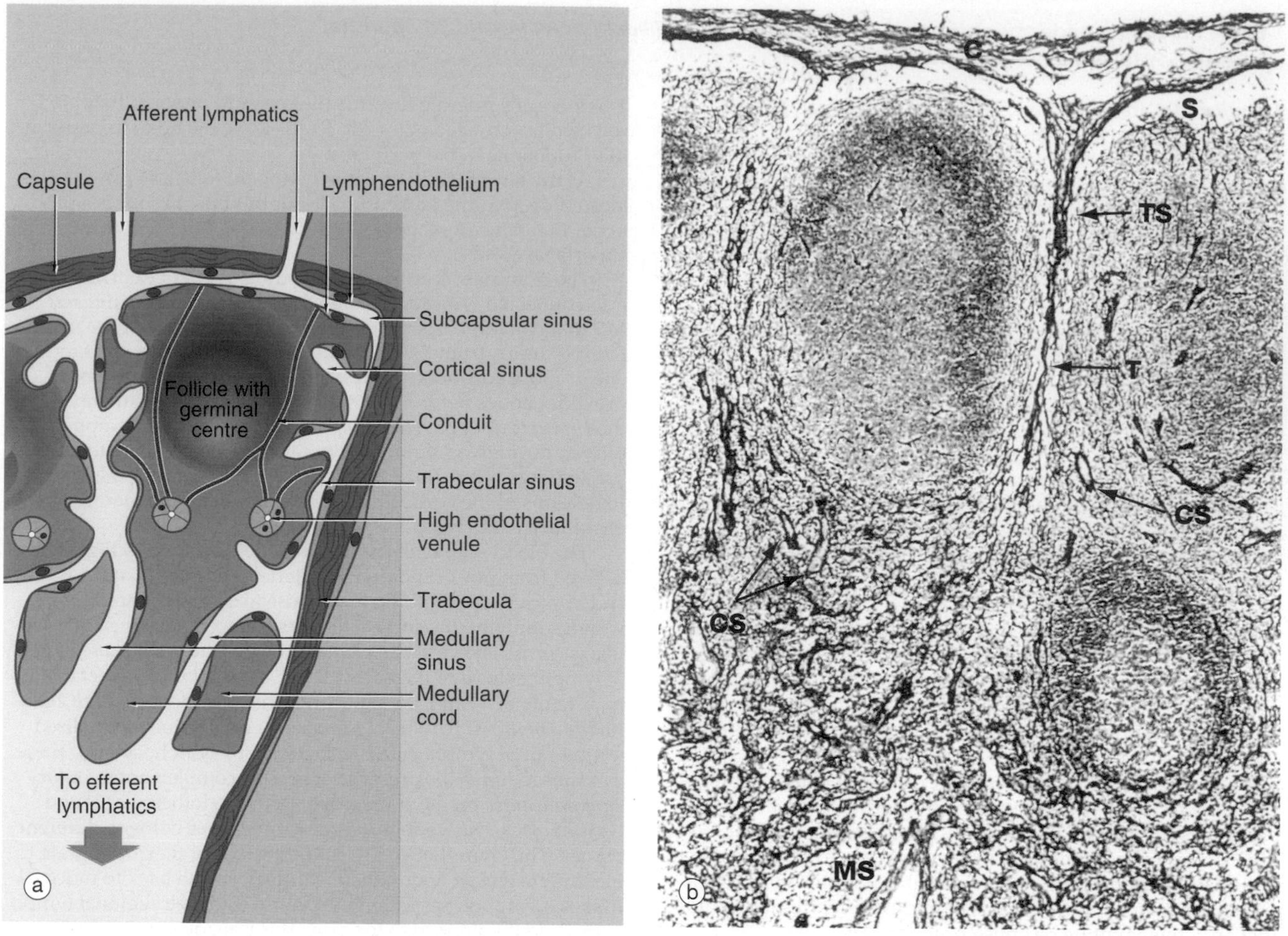

FIG. 11.9 Structure of the lymph node
(a) Schematic diagram (b) Reticulin method (LP)

Fig. 11.9a illustrates the three functional compartments within the lymph node: the ***lymphatic sinuses***, the ***blood vessels*** and the ***stromal compartment***. A network of lymphatic sinuses permeates the node and is continuous with the lumen of the ***afferent*** and ***efferent lymphatic vessels***. The sinuses are lined by lymphatic endothelial cells and contain a population of macrophages (see Fig. 11.14). Sinuses carry lymph, lymphocytes, antigen, dendritic cells and macrophages into the node. Blood vessels form a microvascular network in the node; of particular note are the high endothelial venules (HEV) that are the major site of entry of circulating lymphocytes into the node. The interstitial compartment is packed with lymphocytes. Lymphocytes that do not recognise antigen while in the node leave in approximately 12 to 18 hours in the efferent lymph to circulate through other lymph nodes. The lymphatic and blood vessel endothelia thus define the boundaries of the three compartments and control passage of cells and molecules between the different compartments.

Fig. 11.9b shows the fine reticular architecture of the lymph node; reticulin fibres are stained blackish-brown and lymphocyte nuclei appear lighter brown. The main structural support for the lymph node is derived from the collagenous ***capsule*** **C** and ***trabeculae*** **T**, which extend into the node. From these, a fine meshwork of reticulin fibres extends throughout the node, providing a supporting framework for the mass of lymphocytes and accessory cells within the stroma. The reticular network is particularly dense in the cortex, except for the follicular areas where it is relatively sparse. This network is draped in specialised stromal cells, ***fibroblastic reticular cells*** (***FRC***), which form a structural skeleton similar to a sponge. The spaces of the sponge are filled with lymphocytes and dendritic cells. The subcapsular sinus **S**, trabecular sinuses **TS**, other cortical sinuses **CS** and medullary sinuses **MS** are kept patent by a fine skeleton of reticulin fibres which traverse the sinuses.

Another component of the collagenous skeleton of the paracortex is the ***conduit system***. Conduits are bundles of specialised collagen fibres that run from the subcapsular sinus to the HEV; they are too small to be identified in Fig. 11.9b. The conduits are wrapped in a basement membrane which is in turn covered by fibroblastic reticular cells. FRC are the cells that produce the collagen framework of the node but also have a role in bringing together dendritic cells and T cells to facilitate antigen presentation. Conduits are thought to carry soluble antigens (small molecules) and cytokines into the lymph node parenchyma. They also carry fluid from the lymph back to the bloodstream, i.e. from the subcapsular sinus to the HEV, so that the lymph leaving the node is more concentrated than the lymph entering it.

Antigen may enter the subcapsular sinus either as soluble or particulate antigen or as antigen carried by dendritic cells. Soluble antigen that is smaller than 70 kDa is able to pass into the stromal compartment via pores in the floor of the subcapsular sinus. These small antigens are transported in the conduits into the stroma where they may interact with APCs and lymphocytes. Larger particles are phagocytosed by the sinus macrophages and processed before presentation to T cells; thus intact bacteria and virus cannot pass rapidly through the lymph node to enter the blood.

C capsule **CS** cortical sinus **GC** germinal centre **MS** medullary sinus **MZ** mantle zone **P** paracortex **S** subcapsular sinus **SF** secondary follicle **T** trabecula **TC** T cells **TS** trabecular sinus **V** high endothelial venule

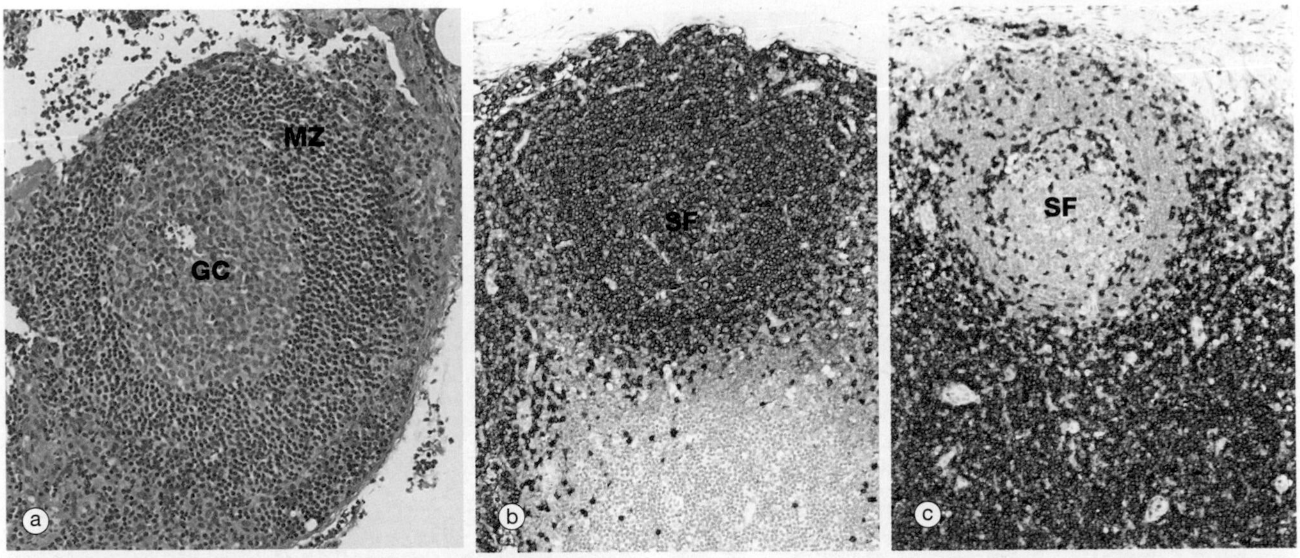

FIG. 11.10 Lymph node distribution of T and B lymphocytes
(a) H&E (MP) (b) Immunohistochemical method CD20 (MP) (c) Immunohistochemical method CD3 (MP)

The outer part of the lymph node cortex is characterised by ***lymphoid follicles***. These are aggregates of B cells which may be in a resting state as in a ***primary follicle***. However, once B cells have encountered a suitable antigen and become stimulated, the follicle undergoes a change as shown in the ***secondary follicle*** in Fig. 11.10a. Secondary follicles consist of a pale centre, the ***germinal centre*** **GC** surrounded by a darker zone known as the ***mantle zone*** **MZ**. The mantle zone is made up of small resting B cells, the condensed nuclear chromatin giving the dark blue colour. The mantle zone is usually asymmetrical, with the wider side towards the capsule. The germinal centre is the site of B cell activation, clonal expansion and differentiation and consists of dividing B cells which are larger and paler than the small inactive lymphocytes of the marginal zone.

Fig. 11.10b and c employ the immunohistochemical method with markers for B lymphocytes (CD20) and T lymphocytes (CD3), respectively. It is obvious that the bulk of the cells in the secondary follicle **SF** illustrated are B lymphocytes, which are stained dark brown in Fig. 11.10b, while the paracortex contains very rare B cells. However, using antibody to CD3 shows that the paracortex is densely packed with T cells, with only a few T cells found within the secondary follicle. CD3 is found on both T_H and T_C cells, but use of other markers such as CD4, characteristic of T_H cells, would demonstrate that these are T_H which are present in the germinal centre to provide 'help' for B cells undergoing activation.

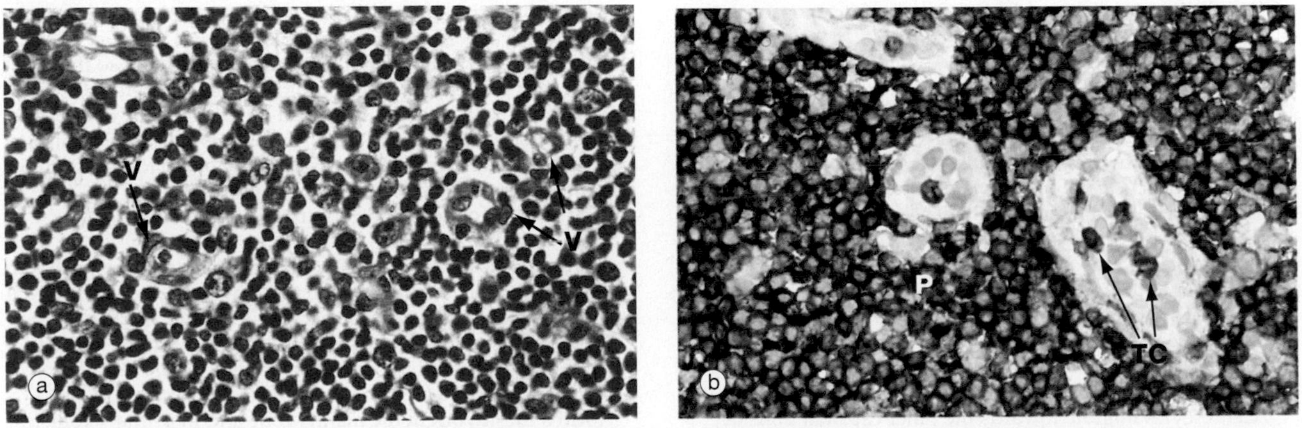

FIG. 11.11 Paracortical zone
(a) H&E (HP) (b) Immunohistochemical method CD3 (HP)

T lymphocytes are the main cell type in the paracortical zone. Circulating T cells enter the lymph node through the walls of high endothelial venules **V** into the paracortical zone; they rejoin the circulation some 12 to 18 hours later in the efferent lymph.

When activated, T lymphocytes enlarge to form immunoblasts, histologically similar to their B cell counterparts, and divide to produce clones of activated T lymphocytes.

Indeed, in a T cell–dominated immunological response, the paracortical zone may be greatly expanded, a pattern known as the ***paracortical reaction***. Activated T cells are then disseminated via the circulation to peripheral sites where much of their activity occurs.

The main antigen presenting cells in the paracortex are the ***dendritic cells***, which are in close contact with the naïve T cells circulating through this zone. These cells are derived from macrophage precursors including the Langerhans cells of the skin. Fig. 11.11b illustrates two high endothelial venules V which are lined by tall cuboidal rather than the usual flattened endothelial cells. The endothelial cell nuclei are stained pale blue. T cells **TC** are seen passing through the endothelium to enter the paracortex **P**, which is packed with further T cells.

These endothelial cells express on their surface specific lymphocyte-binding molecules known as ***addressins*** that allow lymphocytes to bind to the endothelium as the first step of migration into the tissue.

Approximately 90% of lymphocytes enter the parenchyma of the node via the HEV, while the rest arrive in the afferent lymph. While in the lymph node, lymphocytes are highly motile, moving through the parenchyma to come into contact with a large number of APCs to optimise their chances to encounter cognate antigen.

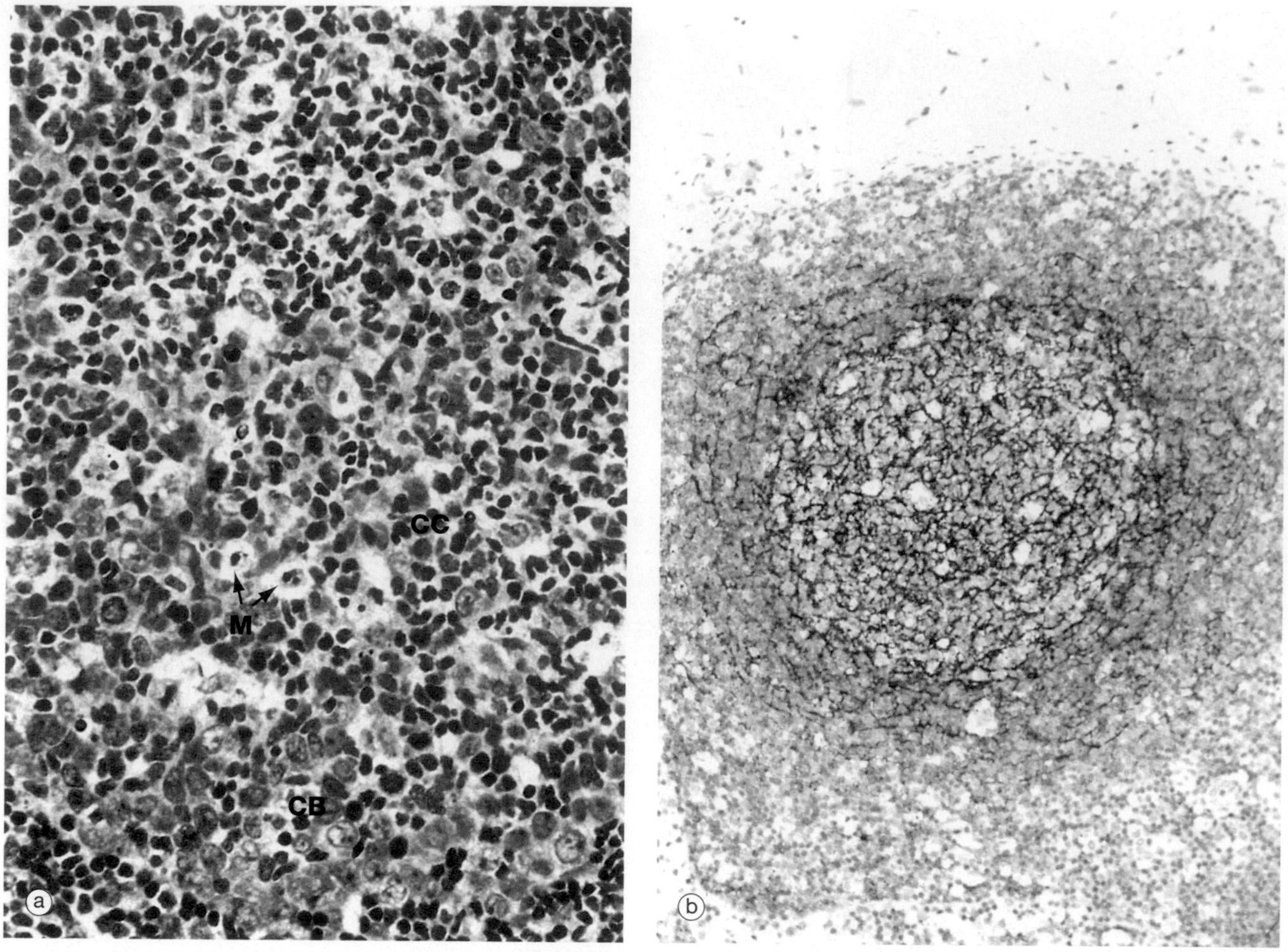

FIG. 11.12 Lymphoid follicle and germinal centre
(a) H&E (HP) (b) Immunohistochemical method CD21 (HP)

Fig. 11.12a shows the ***germinal centre*** of a ***secondary lymphoid follicle***. Primary follicles which are unstimulated consist entirely of the same cell types as the mantle zone.

The cells of the germinal centre are mainly actively dividing B cells. The germinal centre is not uniform in colour but is darker towards the medulla, reflecting the organisation of the different cell types within it. Resting B cells enter the lymph node via the HEV and, if they encounter an antigen with which they can react, enter the cycle of ***blast transformation*** to produce clones of plasma cells and B memory cells. The first step is activation to give rise to ***centroblasts*** **CB**, large mitotically active cells with round nuclei that are found in the darker zone of the germinal centre closer to the medulla. These differentiate into ***centrocytes*** **CC**, found in the paler zone of the germinal centre towards the lymph node capsule. These cells are of variable size and have folded, irregular ('cleaved') nuclei. Mitotic figures are absent in this area.

Centrocytes migrate towards the paler capsular zone of the germinal centre where they go through further cycles of division to produce either ***immunoblasts*** or memory B cells. Immunoblasts move to the medullary cords where they complete their differentiation into plasma cells, capable of secreting large amounts of antibody. In the germinal centre, a further ingenious device ensures even greater diversity of antibody specificity. Centroblasts undergo increased mutation of the immunoglobulin genes (***somatic hypermutation***), thus creating further variations in immunoglobulin structure.

Those centroblasts with the antibody structure that binds most tightly to the antigen (***high-affinity antibody***) are then stimulated to differentiate into plasma cells and memory cells. At this stage, ***class switch recombination*** also occurs so that the plasma cells produced by the germinal centres secrete IgG or IgA antibody rather than IgM, which is characteristic of the early immune response. Memory cells, which resemble small lymphocytes, take up residence in the mantle zone of the follicle or may join the recirculating pool of small lymphocytes.

Other cells found in the germinal centres include:

- ***Follicular dendritic cells*** (***FDC***) are the major antigen-presenting cells of the follicles and are thought to be of mesenchymal cell origin. These are difficult to see in routine H&E stains, but their dendritic processes can be demonstrated (stained brown) as in Fig. 11.12b using an antibody to CD21. These cells are found in all areas of the germinal centre and also form a meshwork in the mantle zone and in primary follicles. They can retain antigen on their surface for many months and present this unprocessed antigen to B cells. FDCs may have a role in maintaining the activity of memory cells, as well as stimulating a primary immune response.
- The interestingly named ***tingible body macrophages*** **M** are easily seen in routine sections in active germinal centres. They contain within their cytoplasm numerous ***apoptotic bodies*** derived from B lymphocytes that have not been successful in generating a high-affinity antibody.

CB centroblasts **CC** centrocytes **M** macrophages **MC** medullary cord **MS** medullary sinus **P** plasma cell **T** trabecula

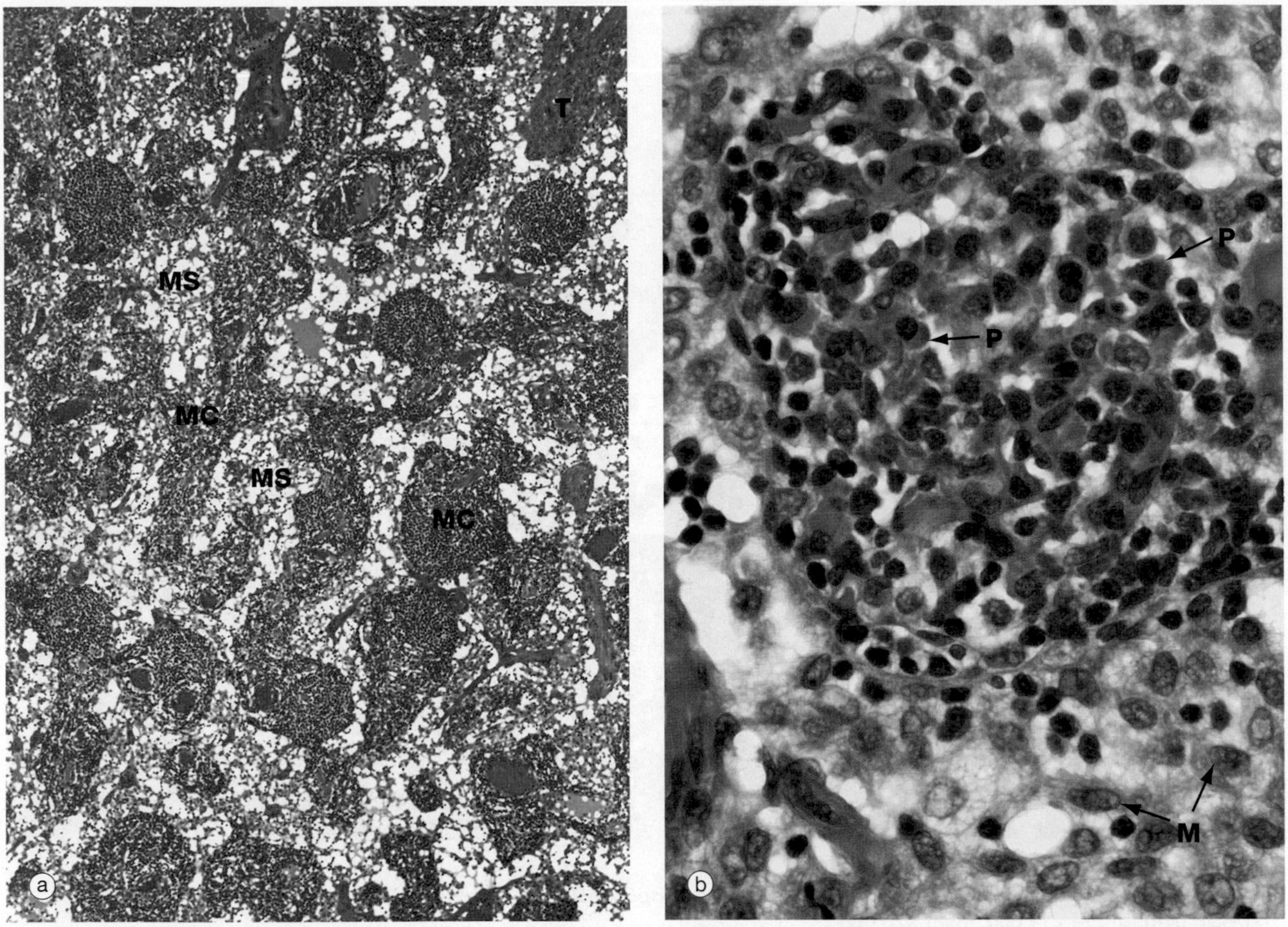

FIG. 11.13 Medullary cords and sinuses
(a) H&E (LP) (b) H&E (HP)

Fig. 11.13a illustrates the structure of the lymph node medulla, with branching ***medullary cords*** **MC** separated by irregular ***medullary sinuses*** **MS**. Throughout the medulla are trabeculae **T** extending from the collagenous supporting tissue of the capsule. Plasma cells and their precursors, ***plasmablasts*** which have migrated from the germinal centres, are the major cell types in the medullary cords. Here, B lymphocytes complete the final stages of maturation to form plasma cells. Plasma cells synthesise antibody that is carried to the general circulation in efferent lymph; some plasmablasts also migrate from the node in efferent lymph to take up residence in peripheral tissues.

Fig. 11.13b shows a higher magnification view of the medullary cords and sinuses. In the right and central part of the micrograph, there is a medullary cord packed with plasmablasts and plasma cells **P**. In contrast, the sinus, which contains mainly ***sinus macrophages*** **M**, is paler stained. As in the subcapsular and trabecular sinuses, fine reticular strands traverse the medullary sinuses, providing support for sinus macrophages.

Plasma cells are differentiated B lymphocytes which are specialised for the production of large quantities of antibody. Plasma cells are not usually detectable in the circulating blood but are found in the tissues, in particular the medullary cords of lymph nodes, the white pulp of the spleen, the supporting tissues of mucosal surfaces (e.g. lamina propria of intestine) and the bone marrow.

Transplantation

Transplantation of organs such as heart (see e-Fig.11.3), liver and kidneys has transformed the lives of many patients with chronic organ failure, but it is fraught with difficulties due to ***rejection*** of the transplanted organ. The immune system of the recipient reacts mainly against the MHC complexes (known as the ***h***uman ***l***eukocyte ***a***ntigens (**HLA**) in humans). Indeed, these antigens were first discovered in the context of organ transplantation, and it was many years before their function became known. Each class of HLA antigens includes a number of different proteins, each of which may be coded by a number of different alleles.

Thus an individual will have two different variants of each HLA type. The overall HLA makeup is called the ***HLA phenotype***, and no two individuals (except identical twins) have the exact same HLA phenotype. Tissue matching is used to find the closest match possible, but most transplants occur between individuals with some degree of ***HLA mismatch***.

Immunosuppressive drugs of various types are used to suppress the immune response against the foreign antigens in the donor organ. Unfortunately, these drugs also suppress desirable immune responses to pathogens, putting the patient at risk of life-threatening infections; a careful balance is needed between loss of the grafted organ through rejection and danger of infection. The search continues for more specific drugs to control rejection.

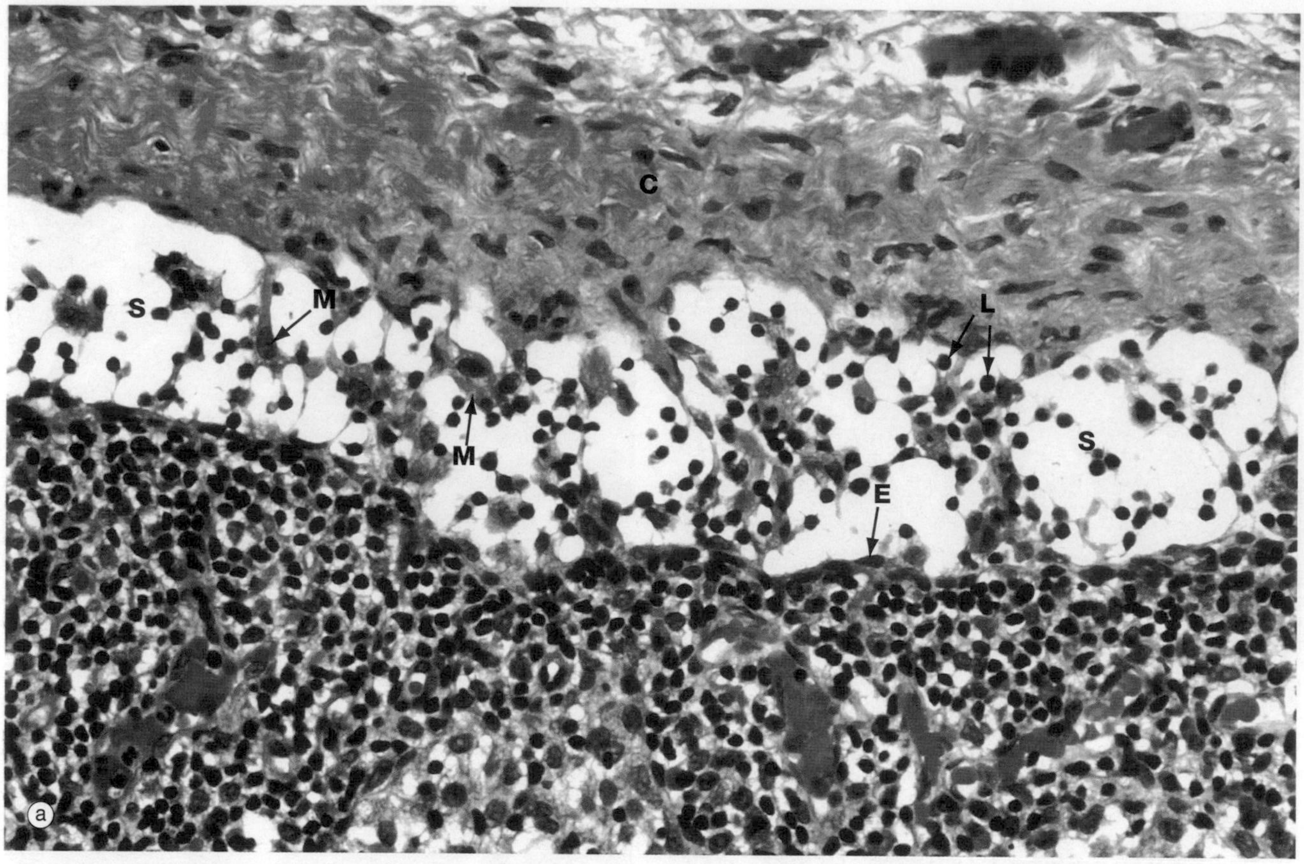

FIG. 11.14 Capsule and subcapsular sinus *(illustration (b) opposite)*
(a) H&E (HP) (b) EM ×11 000, inset ×20 000

The fibrous capsule **C** of the lymph node is pierced by branches of afferent lymphatic vessels with valves to ensure one-way flow. The afferent lymphatics bring lymphocytes, antigen-carrying dendritic cells, macrophages and particulate antigen into the node. Fig. 11.14a illustrates the subcapsular sinus **S** at high magnification. Endothelial cells **E** lining the sinus can just be identified at this magnification but are much better seen in Fig. 11.14b. The lymph node sinuses are traversed by fine reticulin strands that provide support for large eosinophilic ***sinus macrophages*** **M**. These macrophages filter antigen and other debris from afferent lymph. Large molecules and particulate antigen are retained within the sinus, but small antigenic molecules percolate through the parenchyma of the lymph node via the ***conduit system***, a system of bundles of collagenous fibres that form a transport route for fluid and small molecules between the sinus system and the high endothelial venules via the paracortex. The macrophages and dendritic cells in the sinus process larger antigens and carry them into the node to present them to lymphocytes within the node. Lymphocytes **L** arriving in the afferent lymph also are found within the subcapsular sinus.

In Fig. 11.14b, the structures of the subcapsular sinus are seen in much more detail. Endothelial cells **E** line the sinus. Reticular fibres **RF** are surrounded by the cytoplasmic projections (or ***dendrites***) of dendritic cells **DC** that wrap all the way around the reticular fibres and form junctions **J** with themselves (see inset, which is an enlargement of the area outlined). A sinus macrophage **M** is draped between the two reticular fibres and, within its cytoplasm, the machinery for antigen processing is readily apparent, i.e. plentiful lysosomes **Ly** and endocytotic vacuoles **V**. The macrophage also has plentiful cell processes **P** to increase the surface area. Thus the subcapsular sinus of the lymph node acts as a 'strainer' for antigen entering the node.

C capsule **DC** dendritic cell **E** endothelial cell **J** cell junction **L** lymphocytes **Ly** lysosomes **M** macrophage **P** cell process **RF** reticular fibre **S** subcapsular sinus **V** endocytotic vacuole

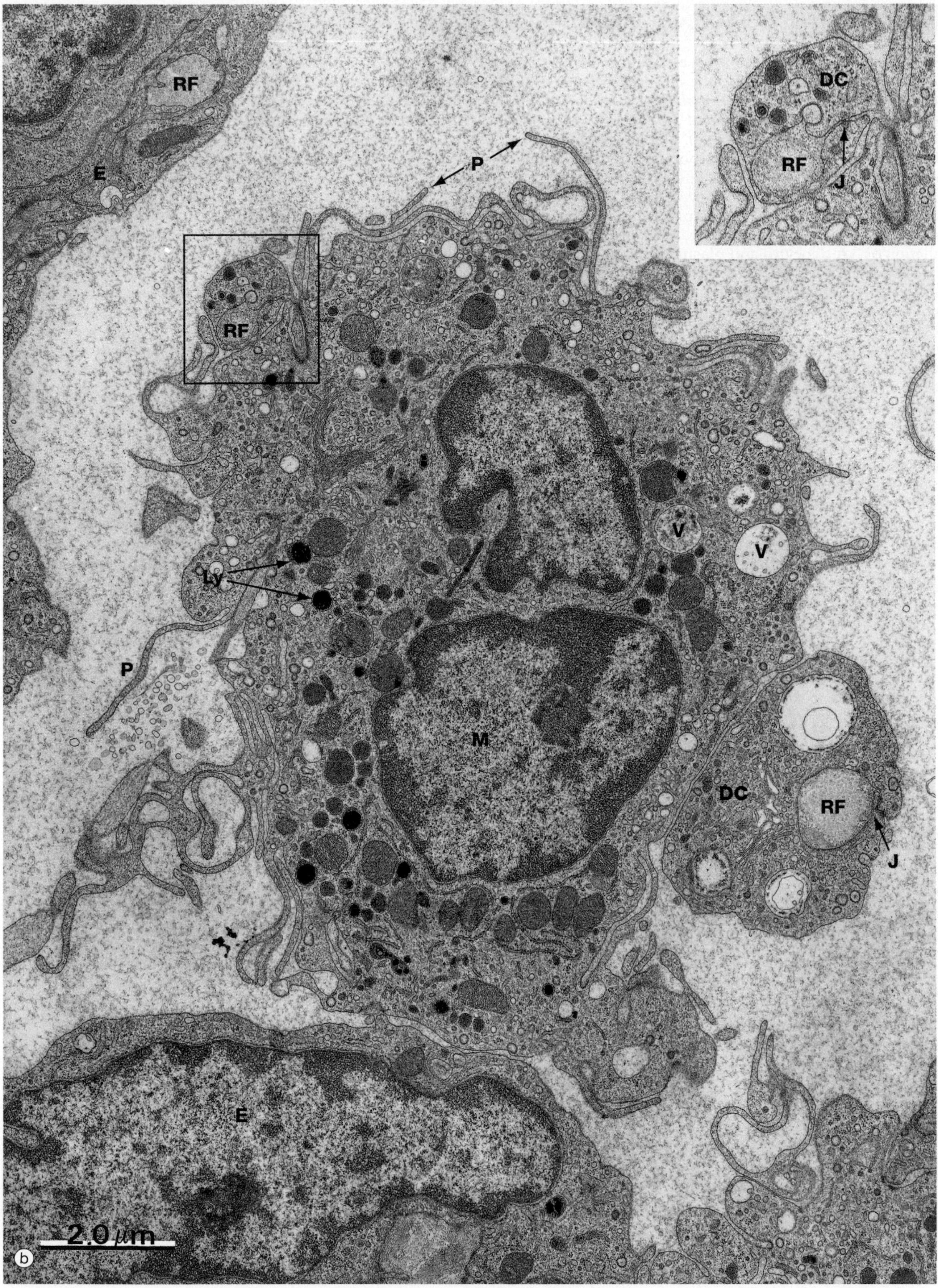

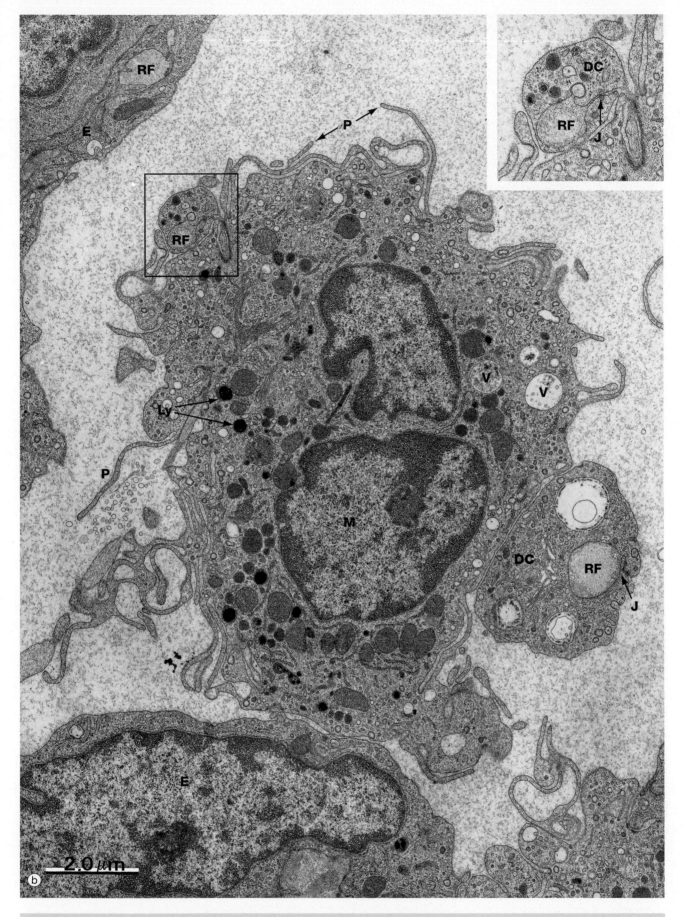

FIG. 11.14 Capsule and subcapsular sinus ***(caption and illustration (a) opposite)***
(a) H&E (HP) (b) EM ×11 000, inset ×20 000

MUCOSA-ASSOCIATED LYMPHOID TISSUE (MALT)

Lymphoid tissue is distributed at many mucosal surfaces throughout the body, important sites being the gastrointestinal tract (***gut-associated lymphoid tissue, GALT***), bronchial tree (***bronchial-associated lymphoid tissue, BALT***), and oropharynx (***Waldeyer ring***). The lymphoid tissue may be arranged either as a diffuse population or as non-encapsulated organised aggregations, such as the ***tonsils*** or the ***Peyer's patches*** of the small bowel. Follicles with germinal centres, similar to those of lymph nodes, are found in the organised lymphoid tissues. The breast also contains a population of lymphocytes and plasma cells.

The total mass of lymphoid tissue in the gastrointestinal, respiratory and genitourinary tracts is enormous and is collectively known as ***mucosa-associated lymphoid tissue*** (***MALT***). The larger aggregations function in a manner analogous to lymph nodes, sampling antigenic material entering the tracts and initiating both antibody-mediated and cytotoxic immune responses where appropriate; they contain discrete B and T cell zones as well as antigen-processing accessory cells.

The diffusely scattered lymphocytes seen in the lamina propria of the gut and respiratory tree are mainly T lymphocytes. Smaller numbers of B cells are also present, as well as plasma cells. All classes of antibody are produced, with IgA predominating. IgA is secreted into the gut lumen bound to a carbohydrate moiety, ***secretory piece***, which is synthesised in the epithelium and renders IgA resistant to proteolytic enzymes. This ***secretory IgA*** protects against pathogens in the gut lumen before they breach the tissues. IgA also reaches the gut in bile, being taken up from blood and secreted into bile in a similar fashion. IgG and IgM are secreted into the lamina propria to deal with organisms that elude the surface protective mechanisms. IgE is also produced and triggers release of histamine from mast cells that are present in large numbers in the lamina propria.

Considerable numbers of lymphocytes are found within the epithelium of the small and large intestines and are present in particularly large numbers in the epithelium overlying Peyer's patches. These lymphocytes are almost exclusively CD8 positive $\gamma\delta$ T cells.

The epithelium overlying all MALT aggregations is specialised for the sampling of luminal contents for antigen and acts as the equivalent of the afferent lymphatics of the lymph node. The lymphatics associated with MALT are all efferent from the MALT and pass to regional lymph nodes (e.g. cervical, mesenteric, hilar).

MALT acts as an integrated unit with a separate route of lymphocyte circulation in parallel with the peripheral lymphoid circulation. When antigen is encountered, it is carried to local MALT tissue. Stimulated lymphocytes migrate to regional lymph nodes where clonal expansion takes place. Effector cells then pass via the thoracic duct and general circulation to the gastrointestinal and respiratory mucosae. MALT lymphocytes carry surface binding molecules that attach to the addressins on high endothelial venules in MALT tissue but not in peripheral tissue.

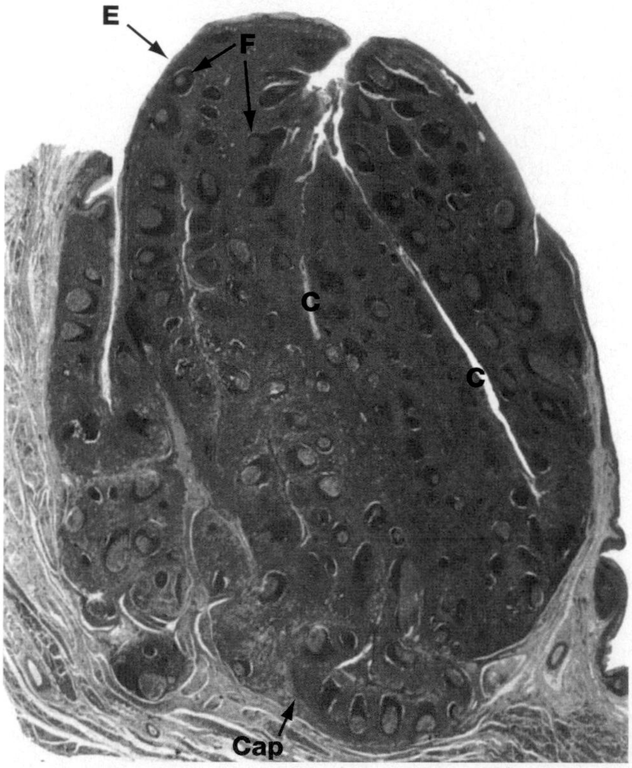

FIG. 11.15 Palatine tonsil
(a) H&E (LP) (b) H&E (HP)

The ***palatine tonsils*** (Fig. 11.5) are organised masses of lymphoid tissue which along with the ***lingual, pharyngeal*** and ***tubal tonsils*** (***adenoids***) form Waldeyer ring.

The luminal surface is covered by stratified squamous epithelium **E** that deeply invaginates the tonsil, forming blind-ended ***tonsillar crypts*** **C**. The base of the tonsil is separated from underlying muscle by a dense collagenous ***hemicapsule*** **Cap**. The tonsillar parenchyma contains numerous lymphoid follicles **F** with germinal centres similar to those found in lymph nodes. Particulate matter or bacteria entering the crypts from the oropharynx are passed to the follicles by transcytosis by the epithelial cells of the crypt lining and an immune response is initiated. Efferent lymphatics pass to the deep cervical chain of lymph nodes, and activated lymphocytes migrate to the lamina propria of the oral mucosa and nasopharynx and other mucosae.

Antigen uptake occurs in a similar manner in the lingual, pharyngeal and tubal tonsils, the latter being covered with respiratory-type epithelium rather than stratified squamous epithelium.

C tonsillar crypt **Cap** hemicapsule **E** epithelium **F** lymphoid follicle **GC** germinal centre

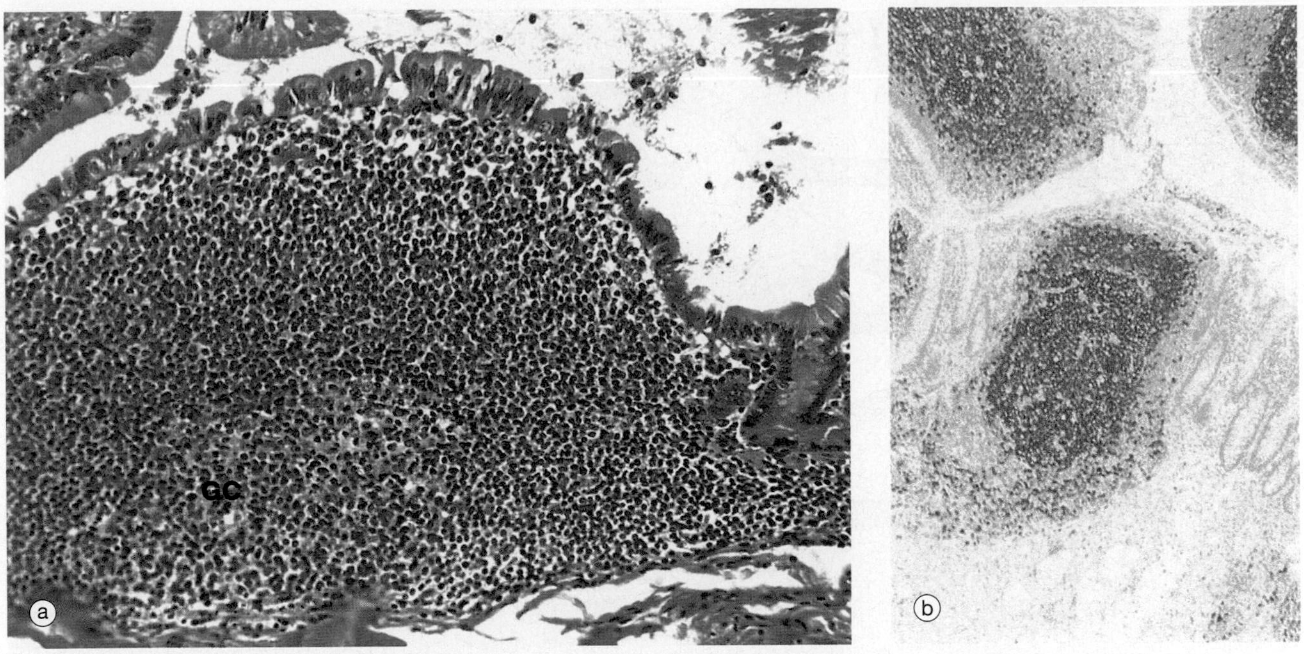

FIG. 11.16 Gut-associated lymphoid tissue
(a) Peyer's patch, H&E (MP) (b) Appendix, immunohistochemical stain for CD20 (LP)

Organised lymphoid tissue is found in all parts of the normal gastrointestinal system except the stomach. This is often called ***gut-associated lymphoid tissue*** (GALT). The largest lymphoid aggregates are the Peyer's patches of the small intestine, which are groups of lymphoid follicles located in the mucosa, where they bulge dome-like into the gut lumen. Usually there are few villi overlying Peyer's patches. They are least numerous in the duodenum and most prominent in the terminal ileum.

Fig. 11.16a illustrates part of a Peyer's patch in the ileum, showing only a single lymphoid follicle. The follicle is similar to those in lymph nodes, consisting of a ***germinal centre*** **GC** composed of proliferating and maturing B cells (centroblasts and centrocytes) surrounded by a mantle of small, resting lymphocytes. Immediately beneath the epithelium is a zone of mixed lymphocytes and macrophages. The area between follicles is occupied by T lymphocytes and, like its lymph node equivalent the ***paracortex***, contains high endothelial venules.

The epithelium overlying these dome areas is specialised for antigen uptake. Scattered among the epithelial cells are low cuboidal M cells, epithelial cells with numerous surface microfolds instead of the usual microvilli. These cells are specialised for transcytosis and take up antigen from the lumen of the gut and transport it into the underlying Peyer's patch.

Goblet cells are scanty in these areas.

Antigen entering the Peyer's patch is taken up by antigen-presenting cells and presented to T lymphocytes. IgA-committed B cells responding to the antigen migrate via afferent lymphatics to mesenteric lymph nodes where the immunological response is greatly amplified. Activated lymphocytes enter the circulation via the thoracic duct and home to the lamina propria of the gut where they undergo final maturation into plasma cells. During lactation, GALT B cells migrate to the breast, mature into plasma cells and secrete IgA into the milk to protect the newborn.

Fig. 11.16b shows lymphoid tissue in the wall of the appendix. The immunohistochemical method used here stains the B cells brown and confirms that, as in lymph nodes, lymphoid follicles consist mainly of B cells with intervening T cell areas.

SPLEEN

The spleen is a large lymphoid organ situated in the left upper part of the abdomen. It receives a rich blood supply via a single artery, the splenic artery, and is drained by the splenic vein into the hepatic portal system. The splenic parenchyma is basically dark red, the ***red pulp***, with small macroscopically visible white nodules, the ***white pulp***, scattered throughout its substance.

In humans, the spleen has four main functions:

- Production of immunological responses against blood-borne antigens
- Removal of particulate matter and aged or defective blood cells, particularly erythrocytes, from the circulation
- Recycling iron to the bone marrow
- Haematopoiesis in the normal fetus and in adults with certain diseases

Removal of the spleen in childhood or adolescence renders the individual susceptible to infection by certain pyogenic bacteria, but in adults splenectomy has less effect. Presumably adults have been naturally immunised against these organisms.

The spleen performs the same function for blood that lymph nodes perform for lymph. The structure of the spleen allows intimate contacts to be made between blood and lymphocytes, just as the structure of the lymph node facilitates the interaction of afferent lymph and lymphocytes. The histology of the spleen varies according to the animal models used. This description is specific to the human spleen.

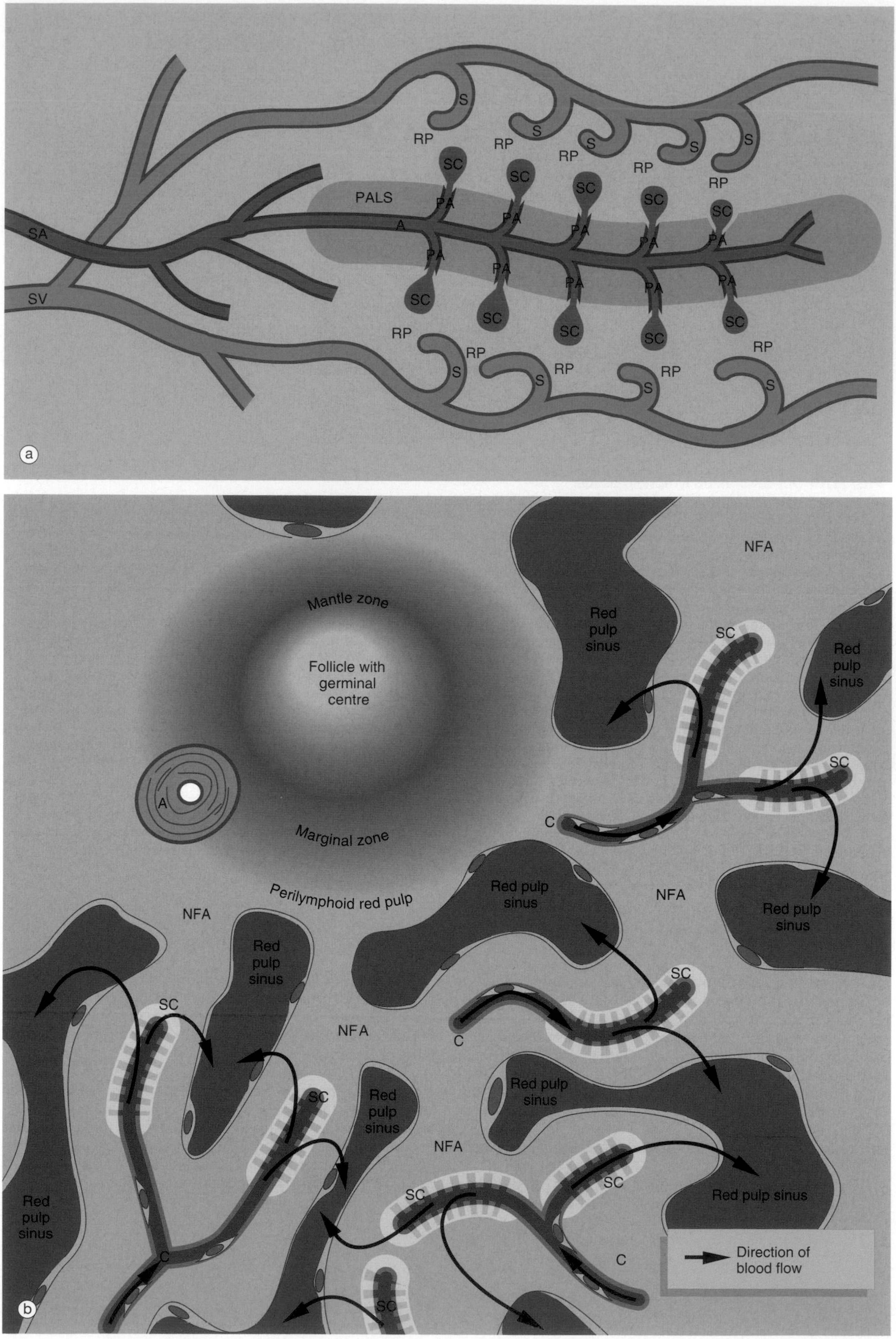

FIG. 11.17 Splenic vasculature and red pulp *(caption opposite)*

FIG. 11.17 Splenic vasculature and red pulp *(illustrations (a) and (b) opposite)*

An overview of the splenic circulation is shown in Fig. 11.17a and a more detailed view of the red pulp in Fig. 11.17b. Blood enters the spleen in the splenic artery **SA**, which branches repeatedly within the parenchyma (only a few branches are shown for simplicity). The larger arteries are surrounded by a fibrocollagenous sheath that disappears in the smaller branches. These ***central arteries*** **A** are so named because they have a cylindrical cuff of lymphoid tissue around them, the ***periarteriolar lymphoid sheath*** **PALS**, consisting mainly of T_H cells. The central artery gives off a number of short branches at right angles, the ***penicilliary arteries*** **PA**, and these terminate in two to three ***sheathed capillaries*** **SC** (only one is shown for each penicilliary artery). These unique vessels are small blind-ending capillaries with no endothelial lining but surrounded instead by an aggregate of macrophages. Thus the blood arriving in a sheathed capillary must traverse this wall of macrophages before entering the red pulp **RP**. The sheathed capillaries therefore form the first part of the filtering mechanism of the spleen.

Splenic red pulp

The splenic parenchyma is permeated by an interconnected network of ***sinuses*** **S** that drain in turn into larger sinuses, tributaries of the splenic vein **SV** and finally the hepatic portal vein. The sinuses are lined by endothelial cells resting upon a basement membrane with numerous narrow slits. The reticulin fibres of the sinusoidal basement membrane are arranged in a circular fashion and are continuous with the reticulin meshwork of the parenchyma (see Fig. 11.19b).

Blood cells entering the parenchyma from the sheathed capillaries squeeze through the walls of the sinuses to drain out of the organ via the splenic vein, an arrangement known as the ***open circulation***. The rate of flow in this system approximates the rate through capillaries elsewhere in the body.

Most of the red pulp parenchyma in Fig. 11.17b consists of loose tissue supported by reticulin fibres permeated by capillaries **C**, terminating as sheathed capillaries **SC**. The parenchyma removes particulate matter and aged or abnormal erythrocytes from the blood, the defective cells being less deformable and thus unable to negotiate the narrow slits in the sinusoidal basement membrane. Trapped cells are removed by the macrophages of the sheathed capillaries and the parenchyma. The mechanism of recognition of effete red cells is probably based on diminished deformability, but immunological mechanisms may also be involved.

Numerous small patches of the red pulp parenchyma (comprising in total a volume comparable to that of the white pulp) are devoid of capillaries and contain mainly T and B lymphocytes and macrophages. Adjacent sinuses are blind-ended and bulb-shaped and their endothelial lining cells have been shown to have characteristics similar to high endothelial venules of lymph nodes. Lymphocytes probably exit these sinuses to enter these ***non-filtering areas*** **NFA** of the red pulp parenchyma, and these areas should be considered as a functional part of the splenic lymphoid tissue.

Perilymphoid (perifollicular) zones

The zone of red pulp immediately surrounding the white pulp differs from the rest of the red pulp, being devoid of sinuses, having only a sparse reticulin meshwork and containing a large number of red and white blood cells in the same proportion as that of blood. About 10% of blood entering the spleen is believed to pass into this perilymphoid parenchyma, from which it passes much more slowly into the surrounding more widely spaced sinuses than in the rest of the red pulp. The function of these ***perilymphoid*** (***perifollicular***) ***zones*** is unclear, but the sluggish blood flow may be a means of enhancing the interaction of blood cells, antigens and antibodies.

Tumours of the immune system

Malignant tumours occur in the immune system just as in all other systems of the body. As a group they are called ***lymphomas*** (involving solid organs) and ***leukaemias*** (involving the blood) and exist in many forms with many characteristic clinical presentations, occurring in virtually all age groups.

Lymphomas may be systemic or may be localised to a particular lymphoid organ or to non-lymphoid organs such as the skin or brain. They may occur in otherwise healthy individuals, in immunosuppressed people such as AIDS patients or organ transplant recipients or in certain infections.

For instance, patients with lymphoma of the stomach (MALT lymphoma or MALToma) almost always have infection of the stomach with *Helicobacter pylori*, a bacterium also associated with gastritis (e-Fig. 11.4), peptic ulcer and gastric adenocarcinoma. Interestingly, eradication of the infection may bring about resolution of the lymphoma, at least in the early stages.

Common clinical presentations include enlargement of some or all lymph nodes (***lymphadenopathy***), enlargement of the spleen (***splenomegaly***) and liver (***hepatomegaly***), as well as fever, weight loss and malaise. Lymphomas of lymphoid tissues are generally divided into Hodgkin and non-Hodgkin lymphomas. Non-Hodgkin lymphomas composed of malignant B lymphocytes may have a follicular (nodular) architecture, recapitulating normal lymphoid follicle formation. Lymphomas are also generally classified as high and low grade, but interestingly, there are no truly benign tumours of lymphoid tissues.

A central artery **C** capillary **NFA** non-filtering area **PA** penicilliary artery **PALS** periarteriolar lymphoid sheath **RP** red pulp **S** sinus **SA** splenic artery **SC** sheathed capillary **SV** splenic vein

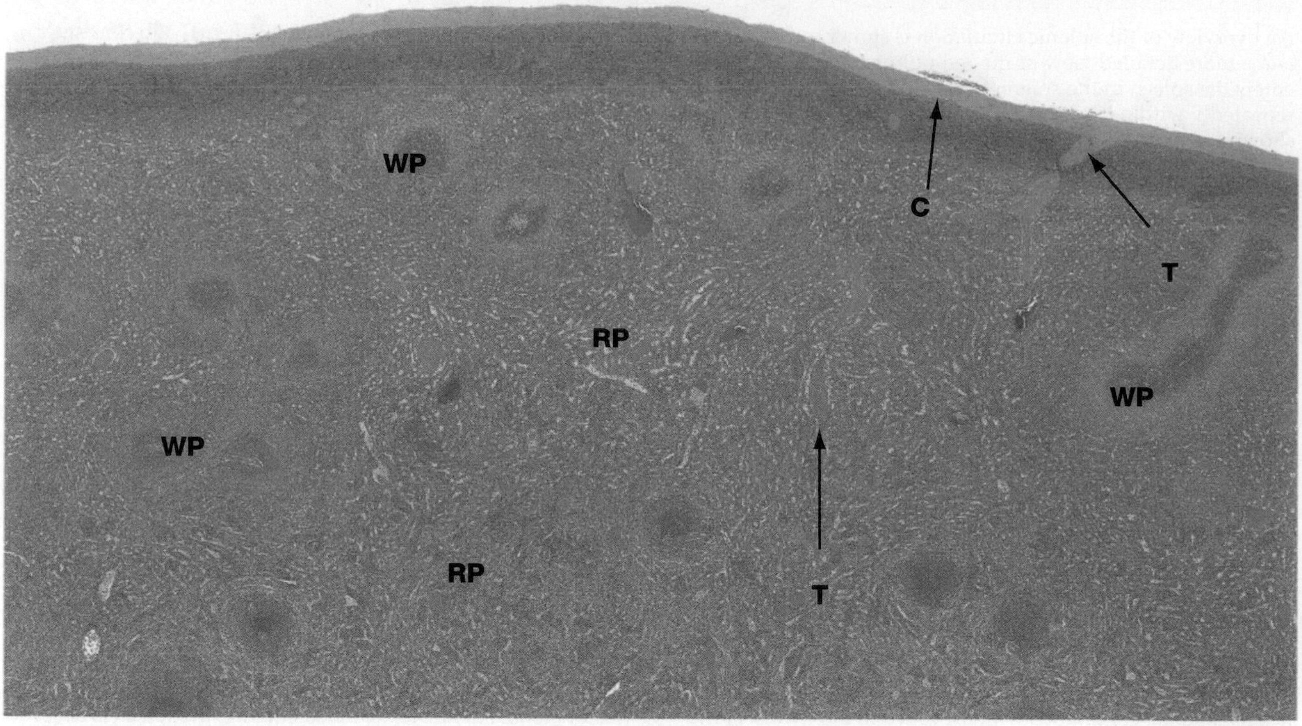

FIG. 11.18 Spleen
H&E (LP)

Macroscopically the spleen appears to consist of discrete 0.5 to 1.0 mm white nodules called the ***white pulp***, embedded in a red matrix called the ***red pulp***. Microscopically, as shown here, the white pulp **WP** consists of lymphoid aggregations and the red pulp **RP**, making up the bulk of the organ, is a highly vascular tissue.

The spleen has a thin fibroelastic capsule **C** which has an outer surface covering of mesothelium (the peritoneum) from which short ***trabeculae*** **T** extend into the parenchyma. The capsule is thickened at the hilum and is continuous with supporting tissues that sheath the larger blood vessels entering and leaving the organ. The spleen has no afferent lymphatics, but efferent lymphatics also exit the spleen at the hilum.

In dogs and horses the spleen is also a reservoir of blood, and these supporting tissues contain smooth muscle to pump blood out; in humans only a few smooth muscle cells persist. The splenic artery divides into several major branches which enter the hilum and branch to form numerous arterioles.

In the white pulp, the T cell areas surround the central arteries, forming the ***periarteriolar lymphoid sheath*** (***PALS***). In humans this lymphoid tissue is less well organised than in other animals, but the term PALS persists.

Immunodeficiency

Immunodeficiency syndromes may be either primary or acquired. There are many well-characterised but rare types of primary immunodeficiency. In severe combined immunodeficiency, both T and B lymphocytes are severely deficient and patients are subject to a wide range of infections; the most severe forms are fatal in infancy. Di George syndrome, where T cells are deficient, is due to thymic aplasia. Patients suffer from severe viral and fungal infections, as the cell-mediated arm of their immune system is defective.

Patients with IgA deficiency are more prone to infections of the respiratory and gastrointestinal tracts. Common variable immunodeficiency is characterised by hypogammaglobulinaemia and frequent bacterial infection. X-linked agammaglobulinaemia (Bruton's agammaglobulinaemia), where there is failure to rearrange immunoglobulin light chain genes, leads to overwhelming bacterial infections.

Acquired immunodeficiency disorders are much more common and range from the mild immunodeficiency that comes with old age to severe forms where the white blood cells are wiped out by tumour growing in the bone marrow (most often leukaemias and lymphomas). Many patients on chemotherapy for malignant tumours have drug-induced immunodeficiency, as have those who are deliberately immunosuppressed to avoid rejection of a transplanted organ. Possibly the most common form of all is the mild immunodeficiency that is common in patients with chronic diseases such as diabetes mellitus or who are taking low-dose corticosteroids for conditions such as asthma.

C capsule **E** endothelium **P** parenchyma **RP** red pulp **T** trabecula **VS** venous sinus **WP** white pulp

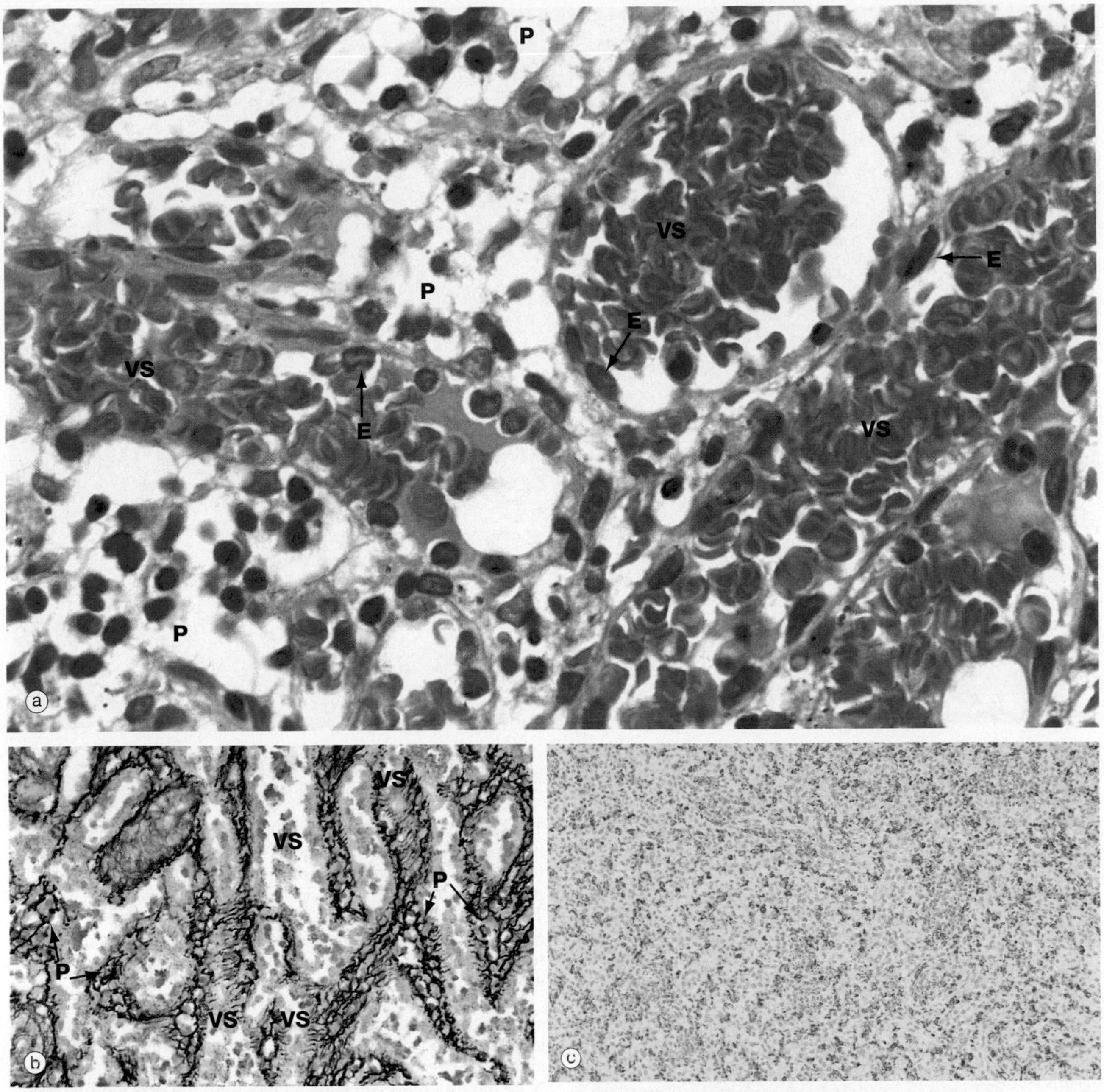

FIG. 11.19 Red pulp
(a) H&E (HP) (b) Reticulin method (MP) (c) Immunohistochemistry for CD68 (MP)

Fig. 11.19a illustrates the red pulp, consisting of the ***parenchyma*** **P** permeated by broad interconnected ***venous sinuses*** **VS**. Seen in section, the parenchymal tissue between the sinusoids is considerably narrower than the diameter of the sinusoids and the area occupied by sinuses is greater than that of the parenchyma; in three-dimensional terms, however, the parenchyma makes up 70% of the volume and the sinuses only 30%. The two-dimensional view gave rise to the misleading term ***cords*** (***of Billroth***) to describe the parenchymal tissue. The three-dimensional structure of the red pulp is analogous to a Swiss cheese, with the holes representing the sinuses and the cheese representing the parenchyma.

The parenchyma is composed of the macrophages of sheathed capillaries, other macrophages and blood cells in transit. Non-filtering areas are devoid of sheathed capillaries and contain a greater proportion of lymphocytes. The macrophages are responsible for destruction of aged or damaged blood cells. The different nucleated cell types of the parenchyma cannot be reliably distinguished in this type of preparation.

The venous sinuses are lined by elongated, spindle-shaped endothelial cells **E** lying parallel to the long axes of the sinuses. The venous sinuses have thus been likened to tall wooden barrels with both ends open, with the endothelial cells represented by the wooden staves and hence described as ***stave cells***. Slits occur between the endothelial cells, the endothelial basement membrane being discontinuous over the slits. Blood cells, particularly viable erythrocytes, squeeze between the stave cells to reach the venous sinuses; these drain into progressively larger vessels that converge to form the splenic vein. Fig. 11.19b shows red pulp stained by the reticulin method to demonstrate the supporting framework of the parenchyma **P**. The basement membranes of the venous sinuses **VS** show the greatest concentration of reticulin fibres, encircling the endothelium in a manner reminiscent of the steel bands holding together a wooden barrel. Fine reticular strands traverse the parenchyma, linking the whole structure together and providing support for parenchymal macrophages and a small number of fibroblasts responsible for elaboration of the reticulin. In some sinuses, the plane of section is such that the parallel bands of reticulin can be seen encircling the sinuses.

Other sinuses are cut in such a way that only the erythrocytes in the lumina are visible. The parenchymal macrophages are demonstrated in Fig. 11.19c, stained brown by the immunohistochemical method. The meshwork structure of the splenic parenchyma is easily seen in this micrograph.

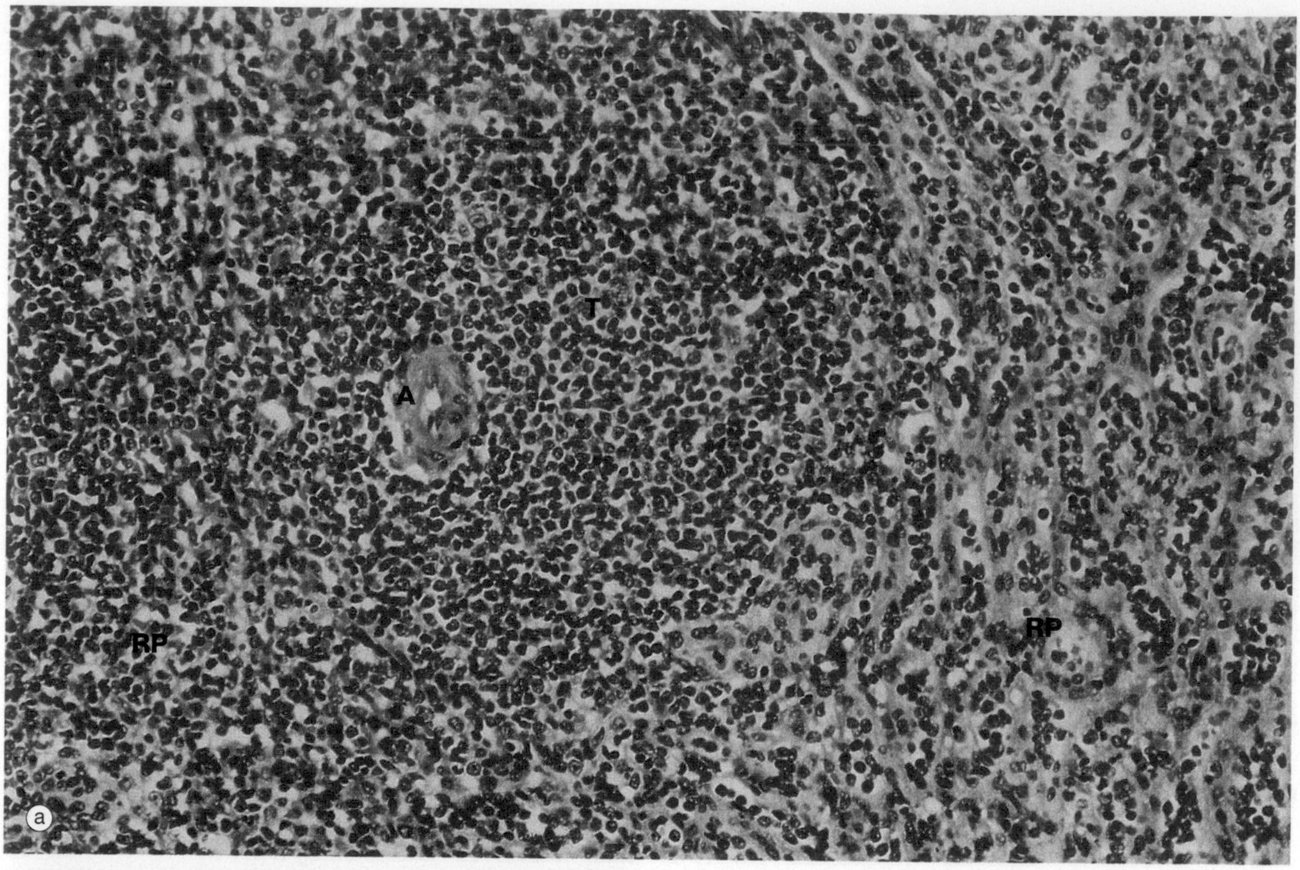

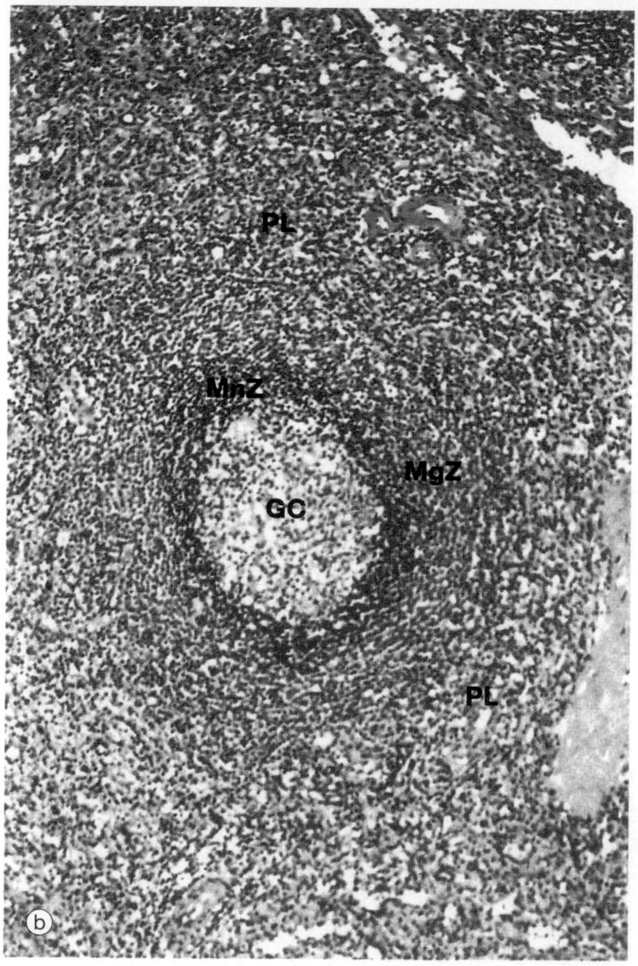

FIG. 11.20 Splenic lymphoid tissue
(a) H&E (HP) (b) H&E (HP)

The splenic white pulp is of two types, T cell and B cell, together making up 5% to 20% of the total mass of the spleen. The functions of these areas appear to be similar to those of the paracortex and superficial cortex of lymph nodes, respectively. The non-filtering areas of red pulp parenchyma (see Fig. 11.17) should probably be considered part of the splenic lymphoid tissue mass also, but its immunological function remains to be elucidated.

Fig. 11.20a shows a T cell area typically forming an eccentric cylindrical sheath **T** around a central artery **A** and containing small lymphocytes, mainly of the T helper subset. This is equivalent to the periarteriolar lymphoid sheath (PALS) in animals. Note the way the T cell mass merges with the surrounding red pulp parenchyma **RP**. Small lymphatics arise in the T lymphocyte areas, forming a network around the arterioles and then continuing with the larger arteries to the hilum to drain into a group of adjacent lymph nodes.

B cells form follicles, usually located at the edge of the PALS, as illustrated in Fig. 11.20b. In young people, many of the follicles exhibit ***germinal centres*** **GC** similar to those of the lymph node, although the proportion of follicles with germinal centres diminishes with age. At the follicle periphery is a narrow zone of small lymphocytes called the ***mantle zone*** **MnZ** beyond which is a broader ***marginal zone*** **MgZ** of less densely packed medium-sized lymphocytes, supported by a framework of reticulin fibres. The marginal zone contains unique subsets of B cells and macrophages. The red pulp around the marginal zone, the ***perilymphoid red pulp*** **PL**, also contains lymphocytes which may simply be migrating from the sinuses to the white pulp.

A central artery **GC** germinal centre **MgZ** marginal zone **MnZ** mantle zone **PF** primary follicle **PL** perilymphoid red pulp **RP** red pulp **T** T cell zone

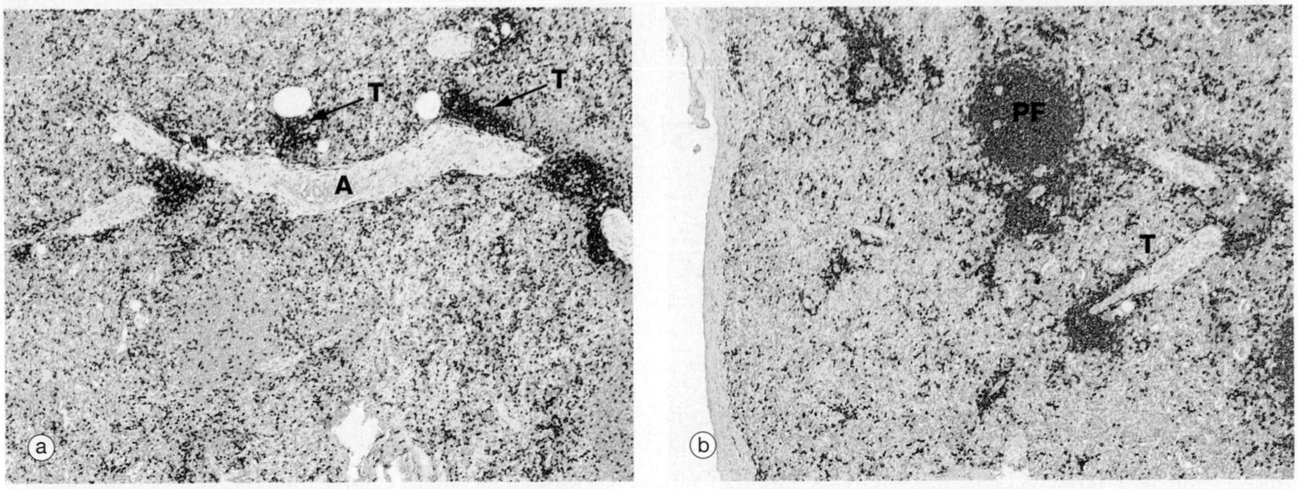

FIG 11.21 Splenic lymphoid tissue
(a) Immunohistochemistry for CD3 (MP) (b) Immunohistochemistry for CD20 (MP)

The distribution of T and B cells in the white pulp of the spleen can be demonstrated using immunostains for T and B cell markers. The section of spleen in Fig. 11.21a is stained using the T cell marker CD3. Thus the congregation of T cells **T** around the central artery **A** is easily identified. As mentioned above, in humans the periarteriolar lymphoid sheath is much less prominent than it is in many other species. A largely unstained primary lymphoid follicle is also noted.

In Fig. 11.21b the antibody CD20 highlights the B cell follicles. As in lymph nodes, unstimulated follicles consist of homogeneous lymphoid aggregates as shown here **PF** with no germinal centers, in contrast to the stimulated lymphoid follicle in Fig. 11.20b. The unstained T cell zone **T** is also easily identified.

REVIEW

TABLE 11.2 Review of the immune system

Organ/tissue	Basic structural components	Component functions	Figure
Bone marrow	Red marrow	Production of all circulating and tissue resident blood cells, including immature T and B lymphocytes Site of B lymphocyte maturation	3.2, 3.3
	Yellow marrow	Resting bone marrow with little haematopoietic activity	3.2b
Thymus	Cortex	Maturation of immature T lymphocytes	11.5
	Medulla	Development of self-tolerance by deletion of self-reactive clones of T cells	11.6
Lymph node	Cortex	B cell activation and clonal expansion to produce large numbers of T lymphocytes reactive to specific antigens Production of memory T lymphocytes	11.9, 11.10, 11.12
	Paracortex	T cell activation and clonal expansion to produce large numbers of T lymphocytes reactive to specific antigens Production of memory T lymphocytes	11.11
	Medulla	Plasma cell maturation and secretion of antibody	11.13
Mucosal associated lymphoid tissue (MALT)	Tonsils Bronchial-associated lymphoid tissue (BALT) Gut-associated lymphoid tissue (GALT)	All components of MALT function in the same fashion as lymph nodes to protect the body from infective organisms presenting at mucosal surfaces	11.15, 11.16
Spleen	White pulp	Mounts an adaptive immune response against blood-borne infective agents	11.20, 11.21
	Red pulp	Filtering the blood to remove particulate matter Removing damaged and aged erythrocytes Recycling of iron to the bone marrow	11.19

12 Respiratory system

INTRODUCTION

Respiration is a term used to describe two different but interrelated processes: ***cellular respiration*** and ***mechanical respiration***. Cellular respiration is the series of intracellular biochemical processes by which the cell produces energy by metabolism of organic molecules (see Ch. 1). This chapter is concerned with mechanical respiration, which involves the following steps:

- Air is drawn into the body (to the ***lungs***) from the atmosphere by ***inhalation***.
- Before it reaches the furthest parts of the lungs, the air is cleaned by removal of particulate matter, warmed so that its temperature equals that of the body and is also moistened.
- In the lung parenchyma, oxygen is extracted from the air and transferred into the blood vascular system where it bonds tightly with ***haemoglobin*** in the red cells for transport in the systemic arterial circulation.
- At the same time that oxygen is passing from air into the blood, carbon dioxide (a by-product of cellular metabolic activity) is transferred from the blood to the air.
- After gaseous exchange, the air is returned to the atmosphere by ***exhalation***.

Inhalation and exhalation are achieved by expanding and contracting the thoracic cavity using the ***intercostal muscles*** and the ***diaphragm***, drawing air in when the thoracic cavity expands and driving air out when it contracts. The respiratory system has two main functional elements: a conducting/cleaning system and a gaseous interchange mechanism. The ***conducting system*** begins as a system of cavities (***nasal cavity, paranasal sinuses*** and ***nasopharynx***) which begin the cleansing, warming and moistening of air drawn in through the ***anterior nares*** (nostrils). These cavities are lined by respiratory epithelium with two cell types, one of which secretes mucus which traps particulate matter, whilst the other bears surface cilia which move the thin layer of mucus. Abundant blood vessels beneath the epithelium warm the air and seromucous glands in the submucosa secrete both mucus and a watery fluid which moistens the air. Lymphoid tissue in the nasopharynx provides immunological surveillance against inhaled antigens. Some air is also taken in through the mouth and therefore bypasses these early cavities.

The air then enters a single tube (the ***trachea***) that divides repeatedly to form airways of ever-decreasing diameter (***primary*** or ***main bronchi***, ***secondary*** or ***lobar bronchi*** and ***tertiary*** or ***segmental bronchi***). In the larger airways, the epithelium has a similar structure and function to the upper respiratory tract. The wall of the trachea is held open by hyaline cartilage rings, which become irregular cartilage plates in smaller branches. ***Smooth muscle*** is also an important component of the wall, which contracts and relaxes to modify the diameter of the airway and therefore the flow of air, particularly in those air passages with less cartilage. The tertiary bronchi ramify into numerous orders of progressively smaller airways called ***bronchioles;*** these have muscle but no cartilage in their walls. The smallest bronchioles are called ***terminal bronchioles***. These are the last of the purely conducting tubes.

The gaseous interchange system is a vast number of blind-ending sacs called ***alveoli***, the walls of the sacs containing an extensive network of thin-walled blood vessels, the ***pulmonary capillaries***. Gaseous exchange occurs between the air in the alveoli and the blood in the capillaries. This arrangement provides a huge surface area where blood and air are separated by a very thin barrier, facilitating gaseous exchange. The continuous process of gaseous diffusion requires appropriate gaseous pressure gradients to be maintained across the alveolar/capillary walls. This is achieved by rapid and continuous perfusion of the pulmonary capillaries by deoxygenated venous blood from the right side of the heart and regular replacement of alveolar gases by breathing. Between the end of the purely conducting part of the system (terminal bronchioles) and the alveoli is a series of transitional airways, the ***respiratory bronchioles*** and ***alveolar ducts***, which become increasingly involved in gas exchange. These passages terminate in dilated air spaces called ***alveolar sacs*** which open into the alveoli.

The respiratory tract also contains two further elements with separate functions:

- The roof of the nasal cavity contains areas of highly specialised mucosa, the ***olfactory mucosa***, responsible for the detection of smell and the more complex aspects of taste (see Fig. 21.2).
- The ***larynx*** is a specialised structure located at the upper end of the trachea. This utilises forcibly expired air from the respiratory tract below it to generate sound by vibrating the true vocal cords.

Disorders of the tracheobronchial tree

The tracheobronchial mucosa is subjected to many forms of damaging agent, including inhaled chemical toxins, viruses and bacteria. Prolonged or repeated damage to the respiratory epithelial cells leads to their death and replacement by squamous epithelium (***squamous metaplasia***).

Viral infections kill epithelial cells and lead to vulnerability to secondary bacterial infection (purulent tracheobronchitis).

Repeated damage to the mucosa leads to a state called chronic bronchitis in which the bronchial wall is thickened due to an increase in numbers and activity of seromucous glands as well as thickening of the muscle layers. It is commonly associated with asthma (a combination of severe ***bronchoconstriction*** due to bronchial smooth muscle contraction and the production of particularly viscid mucus) and ***emphysema*** (in which alveolar walls are destroyed). The combination of all three is called chronic obstructive pulmonary disease (COPD).

The bronchial tree is an important site for the development of malignant tumours (***bronchial carcinoma***), often originating in areas of squamous metaplasia in the bronchial mucosa in heavy smokers. One particularly aggressive type of bronchial carcinoma is derived from the neuroendocrine cells of the bronchial mucosa.

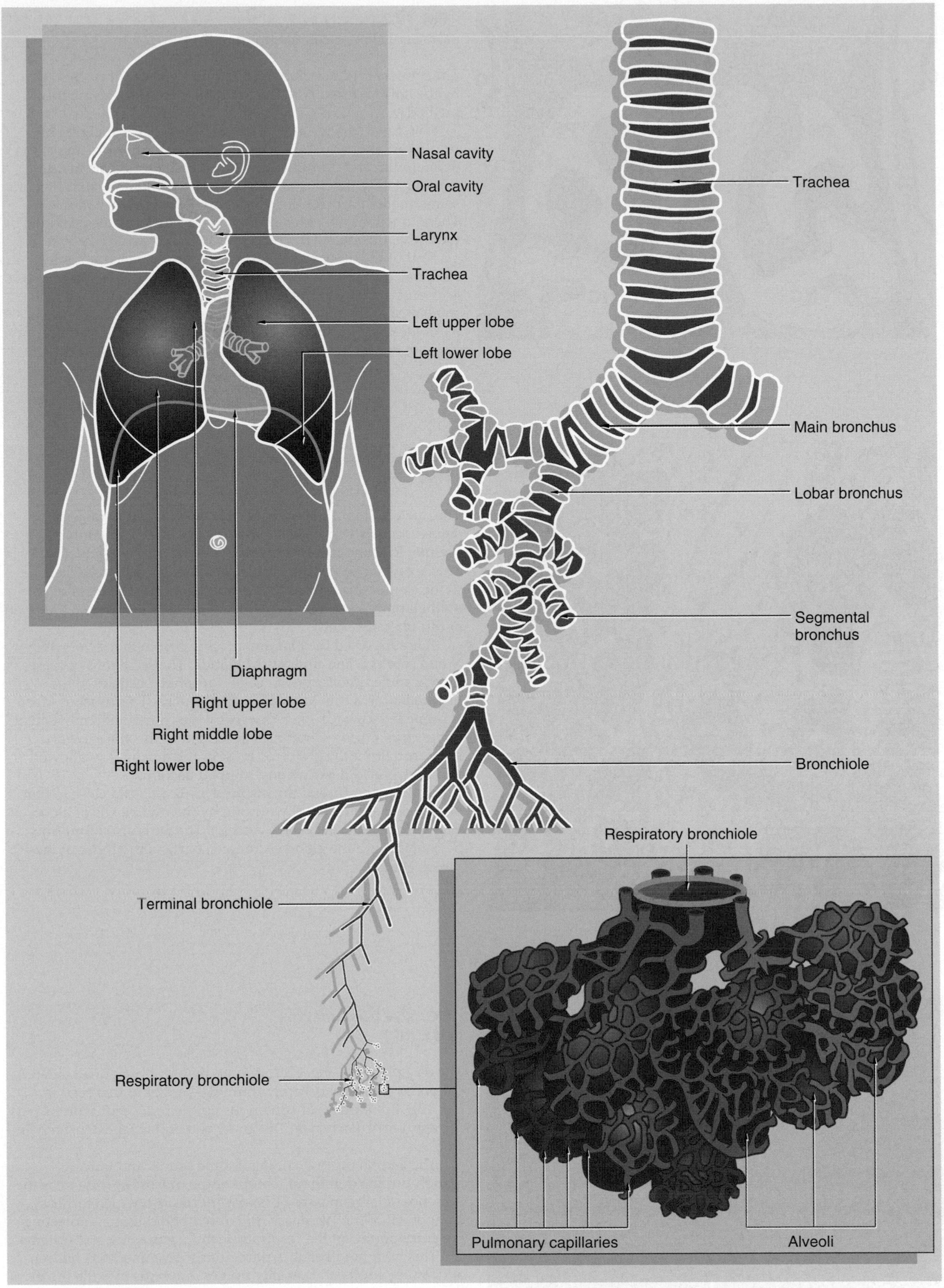

FIG. 12.1 Structure of the respiratory system

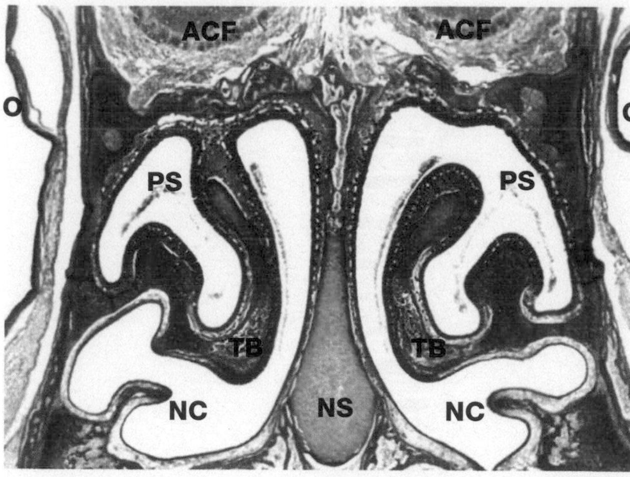

FIG. 12.2 Nasal cavity, kitten
Coronal slice, H&E/Alcian blue (LP)

The nose (Fig. 12.2) is subdivided into two ***nasal cavities*** **NC** by the ***nasal septum*** **NS**. The cartilage stains blue using this method.

The nasal cavities and ***paranasal sinuses*** **PS** are lined by respiratory mucosa, the major function of which is to adjust the temperature and humidity of inspired air. Particulate matter entering the nares is usually trapped by the hairs at that site, but some smaller particles are caught on the respiratory mucosa. These functions are enhanced by a large surface area provided by the ***turbinate bones*** **TB** which project into the nasal cavities.

Part of the nasal mucosa, the ***olfactory mucosa***, contains receptors for the sense of smell (see Fig. 21.2). Olfactory mucosa is extensive in lower mammals, but in man it is confined to a small area in the roof of the nasal cavity. Note the close proximity of the nasal cavities to the orbital cavities **O** and the anterior cranial fossa **ACF**.

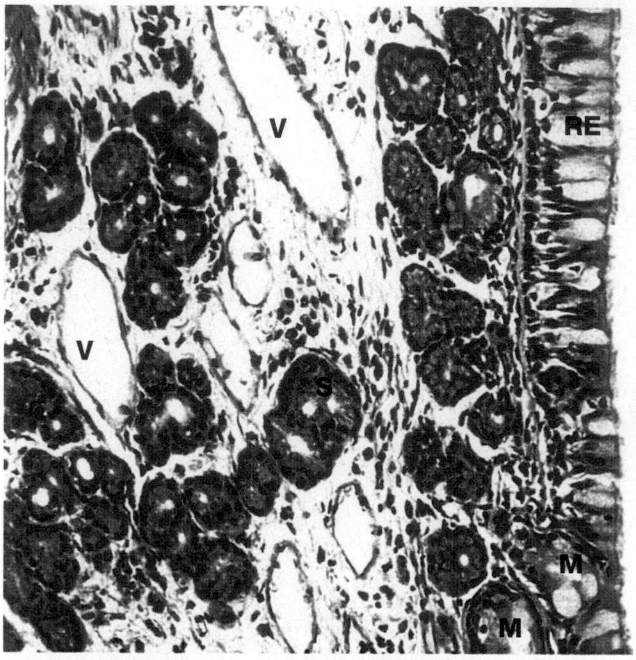

FIG. 12.3 Nasal mucosa
H&E (HP)

The mucosa (Fig. 12.3) of the nasal cavities (and paranasal sinuses) consists of a ***pseudostratified ciliated columnar epithelium*** **RE** containing numerous mucin-secreting ***goblet cells***. This is called ***respiratory epithelium*** and is found elsewhere in the conducting part of the respiratory tract. The respiratory epithelium has an unusually thick basement membrane (not seen at this magnification).

It is supported by a lamina propria rich in blood vessels **V** and serous **S** and mucous **M** glands. The secretions of these glands and epithelial goblet cells trap small particles in the inspired air in a thin layer of surface mucus. This mucous layer is propelled towards the pharynx by the coordinated movement of the ***cilia***. This is sometimes described as the ***muco-ciliary escalator***. From the pharynx, most of the mucus is swallowed and gastric acid destroys any trapped bacteria.

The temperature of the inspired air is adjusted close to that of the body as a result of warming by the rich plexus of blood vessels (mainly thin-walled vessels). The air is also humidified by contact with the gland secretions, particularly those of the serous glands.

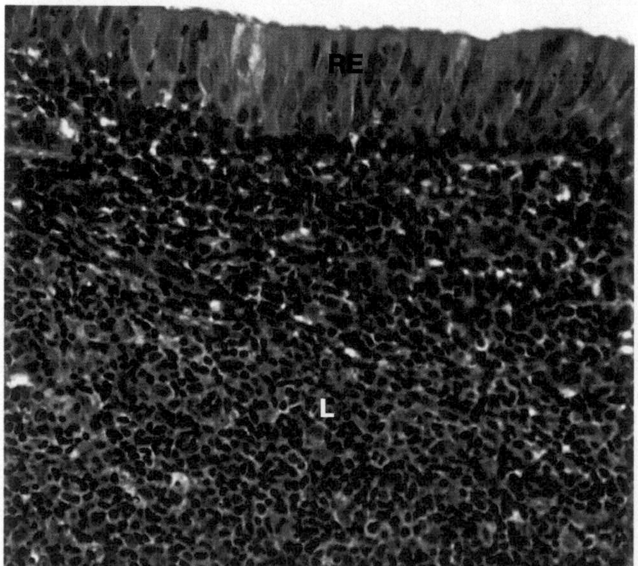

FIG. 12.4 Nasopharynx
H&E (HP)

The nasopharynx (Fig. 12.4) is lined by pseudostratified ciliated columnar (respiratory) epithelium **RE** similar to that seen in Fig. 12.3, but patches of squamous epithelium occur with increasing age, particularly near the lower end and most extensively in smokers.

The lamina propria contains some serous and mucous glands, but the dominant feature of the mucosa at this site is the presence of large masses of ***lymphoid tissue*** **L** which forms a component of the ***Waldeyer ring*** of lymphoid tissue, protecting the entry portals of the respiratory and gastrointestinal systems.

This lymphoid tissue is particularly prominent in children and young adults and usually bulges outwards into the lumen of the nasopharynx, producing an appearance similar to that seen in the ***lingual tonsil*** (see Fig. 13.13) with epithelial crypts. This is called the ***nasopharyngeal tonsil*** or ***adenoid***.

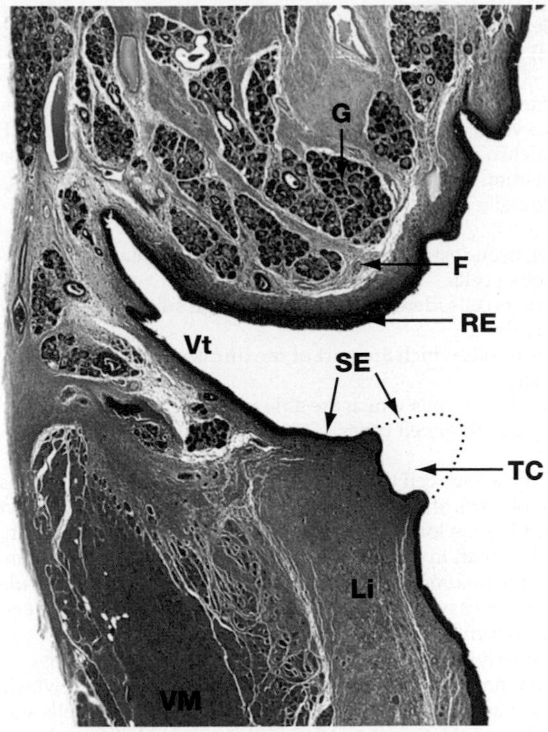

FIG. 12.5 Larynx
H&E (LP)

Fig. 12.5 shows the constituents of one half of the *larynx*. It comprises two folds which protrude into the airway. The upper fold is the ***false vocal cord*** **F** which is covered by columnar ciliated respiratory-type epithelium **RE** and contains seromucous glands **G**.

The lower fold is the ***true vocal cord*** **TC**. In this surgically removed human larynx, the sharp tip of the true cord has been removed by diathermy in the distant past and a dotted line shows its normal outline. The true cord contains the ***vocalis muscle*** **VM** and ***vocalis ligament*** **Li** which are responsible for moving the true cord so that it moves towards or away from the true cord on the other side, thus controlling the pitch of the sound made. The true cords are covered by stratified squamous epithelium **SE** which is more resistant to the effects of physical trauma caused by the free margins of the true cords contacting each other during speech.

Between the true and false cords, there is a narrow cleft, the ***ventricle*** **Vt**, which terminates in a blind-ending ***saccule*** (not shown). The ventricle and saccule are lined by respiratory-type columnar epithelium and also contain seromucous glands.

Common disorders of the nose, nasopharynx and larynx

Viral infections (coryza, the common cold) and allergic inflammation (allergic rhinitis, hay fever) very commonly affect the nose, nasal sinuses and nasopharynx.

Nasal polyps (e-Fig. 12.1) are oedematous protrusions of the respiratory mucosa and are a common consequence of prolonged or recurrent inflammation, particularly allergic inflammation. Patients typically complain of nasal blockage or snoring because these lesions can occupy much of the space in the nasal cavity.

Malignant tumours of the nasal passages and sinuses are rare but nasopharyngeal carcinoma (e-Fig. 12.2) is of special interest because it is associated with Epstein–Barr virus (EBV) infection. This virus is also linked to some other malignant tumours, including lymphomas.

The stratified squamous epithelium of the larynx may undergo hyperplastic or dysplastic change to form benign squamous papillomas or invasive squamous cell carcinoma (e-Fig. 12.3). Cigarette smoking and alcohol consumption predispose to the development of carcinoma of the larynx.

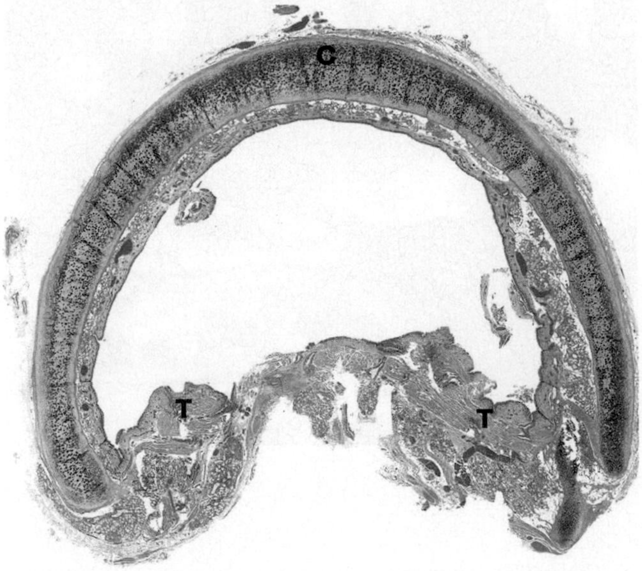

FIG. 12.6 Trachea
H&E (LP)

Fig. 12.6 shows the general structure of the trachea. This is a flexible tube of fibroelastic tissue and cartilage which permits expansion in diameter and extension in length during inspiration, and passive recoil during expiration. A series of C-shaped rings of hyaline cartilage **C** (stained blue) support the tracheal mucosa and prevent its collapse during inspiration.

Bands of smooth muscle called the ***trachealis muscle*** **T** join the free ends of the rings posteriorly. Contraction of the trachealis reduces tracheal diameter and thereby assists in raising intrathoracic pressure during coughing. A few strands of longitudinal muscle can sometimes be seen disposed behind the trachealis muscle.

ACF anterior cranial fossa **C** hyaline cartilage **F** false cord **G** seromucinous glands **L** lymphoid tissue **Li** vocalis ligament **M** mucous gland **NC** nasal cavity **NS** nasal septum **O** orbital cavity **PS** paranasal sinus **RE** respiratory epithelium **S** serous gland **SE** stratified squamous epithelium **T** trachealis muscle **TB** turbinate bone **TC** true cord **V** blood vessel **VM** vocalis muscle **Vt** ventricle

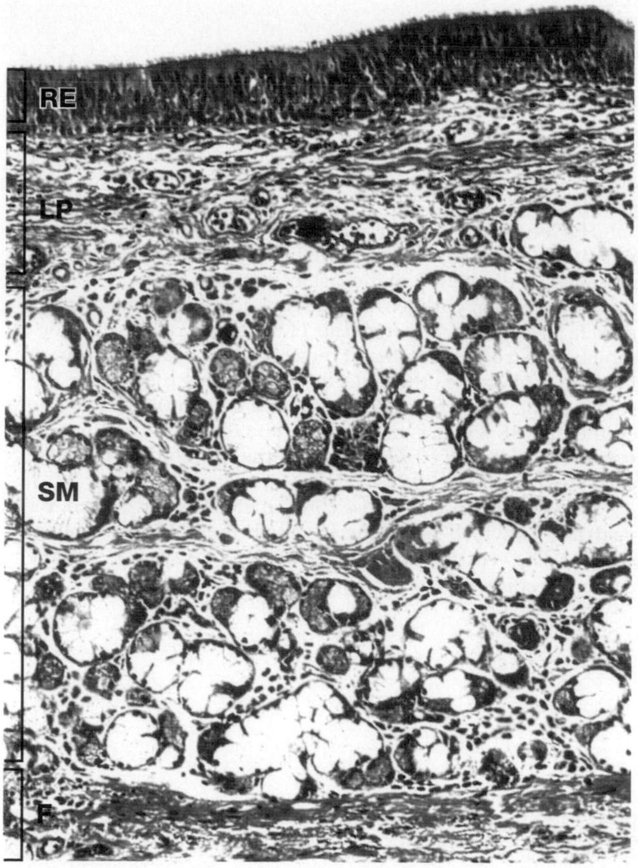

FIG. 12.7 Trachea
H&E (MP)

The inner layers of the tracheal wall are shown in this specimen from a young adult (Fig. 12.7). The respiratory epithelium **RE** of the trachea is similar to the rest of the bronchial tree and nasal epithelium. A variety of cell types is found in the epithelium, including:

- Tall pseudostratified columnar cells with cilia
- Goblet cells
- Serous cells identical to the cells of the submucosal serous glands
- Basal cells which are part of the diffuse neuroendocrine system
- Basal stem cells which are able to divide and differentiate to replace other cell types

The various cell types are present in different proportions in different parts of the trachea. Ciliated columnar cells are more plentiful in the lower trachea whilst goblet and basal cells are more common in the upper trachea. Beneath the basement membrane, the ***lamina propria*** **LP** consists of loose, highly vascular supporting tissue which becomes more condensed at its deeper aspect to form a band of fibroelastic tissue.

Underlying the lamina propria is the loose submucosa **SM** containing numerous mixed seromucinous glands which decrease in number in the lower trachea. The serous cells stain strongly and the mucous cells poorly with H&E. The submucosa merges with the perichondrium of the underlying hyaline cartilage rings (not seen here) or, as here, with the dense fibroelastic tissue **F** between the cartilage rings.

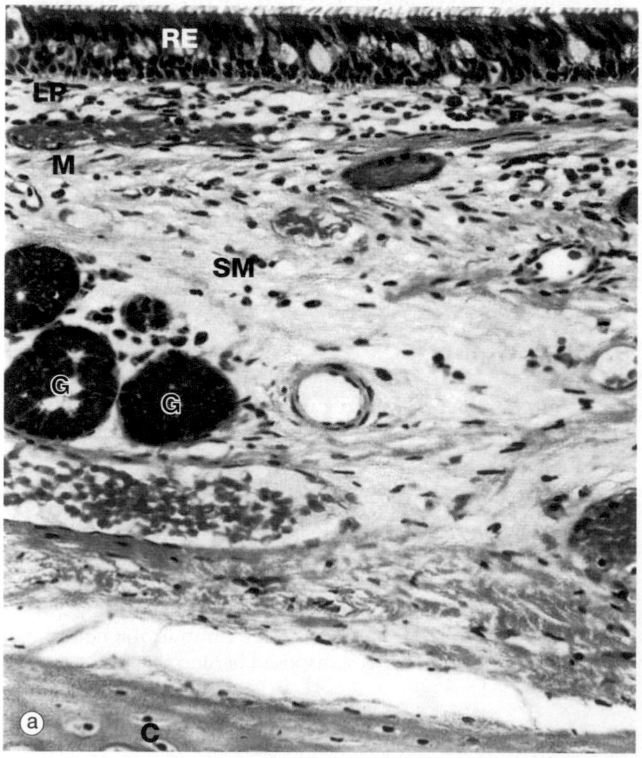

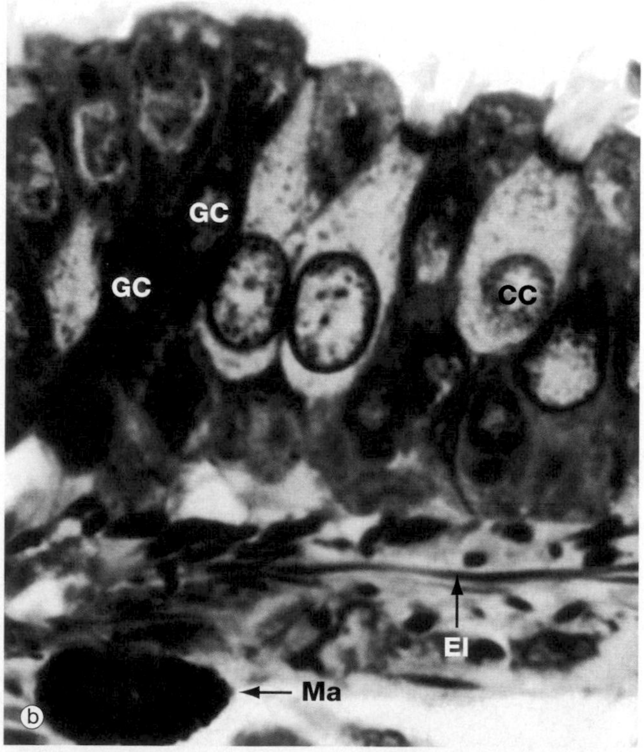

FIG. 12.8 Primary bronchus
(a) H&E (MP) (b) Thin resin section, toluidine blue (HP)

The basic structure of the wall of a main bronchus (Fig. 12.8a) is similar to that of the trachea but differs in several details:

- The respiratory epithelium **RE** is less tall and contains fewer goblet cells.
- The upper lamina propria **LP** contains more elastin.
- The lamina propria is separated from the submucosa **SM** by a layer of smooth muscle **M** which becomes more prominent in more distal bronchi.
- The submucosa contains fewer seromucinous glands **G**.
- The cartilage support **C** is in flattened interconnected plates rather than distinct rings.

Fig. 12.8b shows the epithelial layer at very high magnification. The cells are ***pseudostratified***, the bases of all the cells contacting the basement membrane but not all the cells reaching the luminal surface. The ciliated **CC** and goblet **GC** cells can be easily distinguished. The underlying lamina propria contains elastic fibres **El** and occasional mast cells **Ma**.

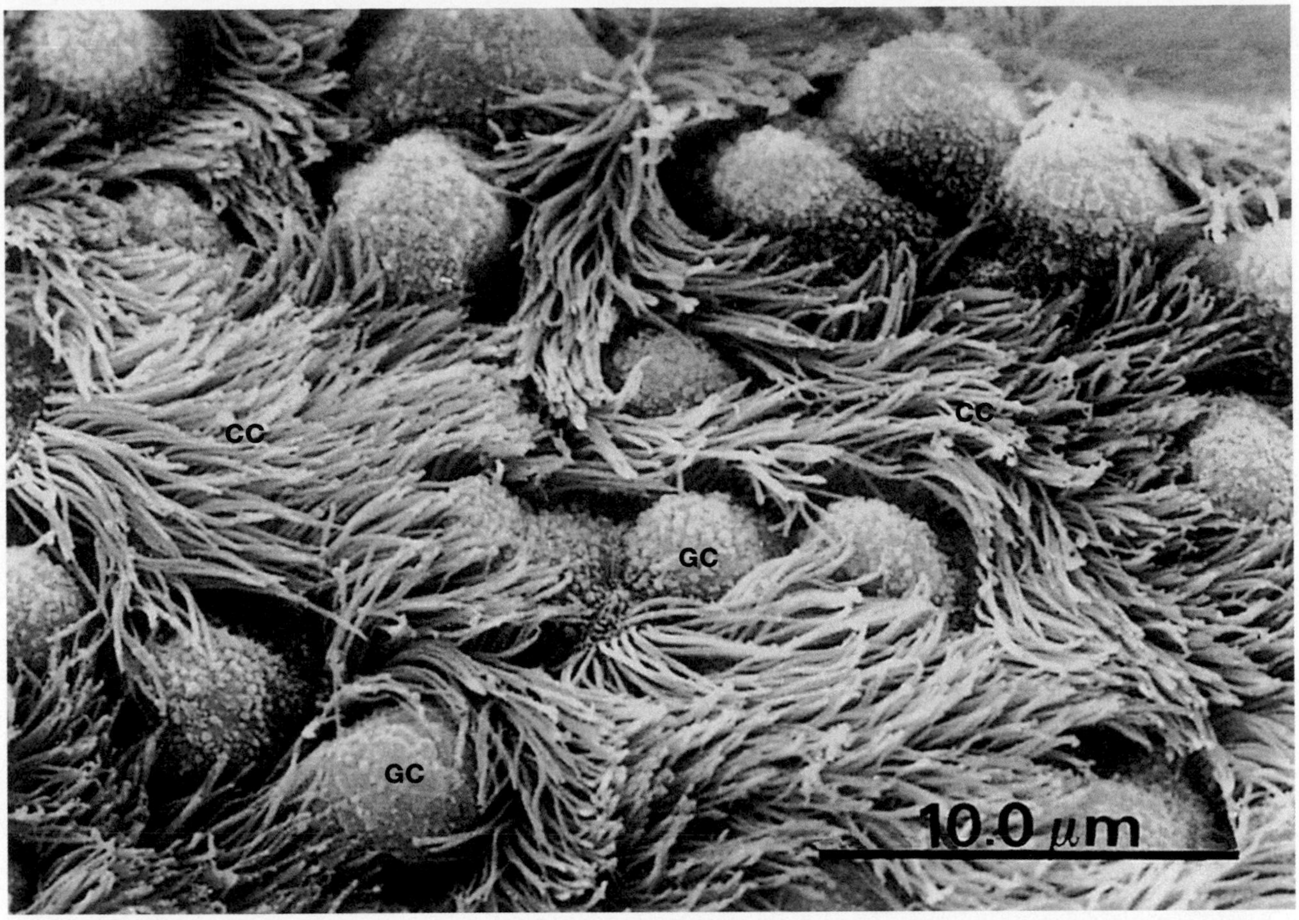

FIG. 12.9 Primary bronchus
SEM ×2000

This scanning electron micrograph (Fig. 12.9) illustrates the surface of a primary bronchus. The film of surface mucus has been removed.

The ciliated epithelial cells **CC** have numerous surface cilia, each several microns long, that move in a coordinated fashion in order to sweep mucus up the bronchus.

Scattered goblet cells **GC** are recognisable by their bulbous surface outline, lack of cilia and the presence of small surface projections associated with mucus secretion. The fragile cilia are particularly vulnerable to damage and destruction by inhaled toxic chemicals (cigarette smoke, car exhaust fumes) and by bacterial and viral infections.

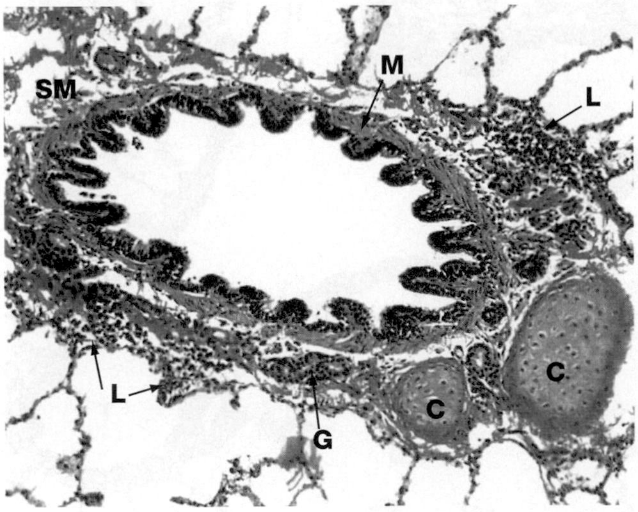

FIG. 12.10 Tertiary (segmental) bronchus
Elastic van Gieson (MP)

As bronchi diminish in diameter, the structure progressively changes to resemble more closely that of large bronchioles. The epithelium, just visible in Fig. 12.10, is tall and columnar with little pseudostratification. Goblet cell numbers are greatly diminished.

The lamina propria is thin, elastic and completely encircled by smooth muscle **M** which is disposed in a spiral manner. This arrangement permits contraction of the bronchi in both length and diameter during expiration. Seromucinous glands **G** are sparse in the submucosa. These glands are rarely found within smaller airways. The cartilage framework **C** is reduced to a few irregular plates. Cartilage does not usually extend beyond tertiary bronchi.

Note that the submucosa **SM** merges with the surrounding adventitia and then with the lung parenchyma. Small aggregates of lymphocytes **L**, part of the mucosa-associated lymphoid tissue (MALT), are seen in the adventitia.

C cartilage **CC** ciliated cell **El** elastic fibre **F** fibroelastic tissue **G** seromucinous glands **GC** goblet cell **L** lymphoid tissue **LP** lamina propria **M** smooth muscle **Ma** mast cell **RE** respiratory epithelium **SM** submucosa

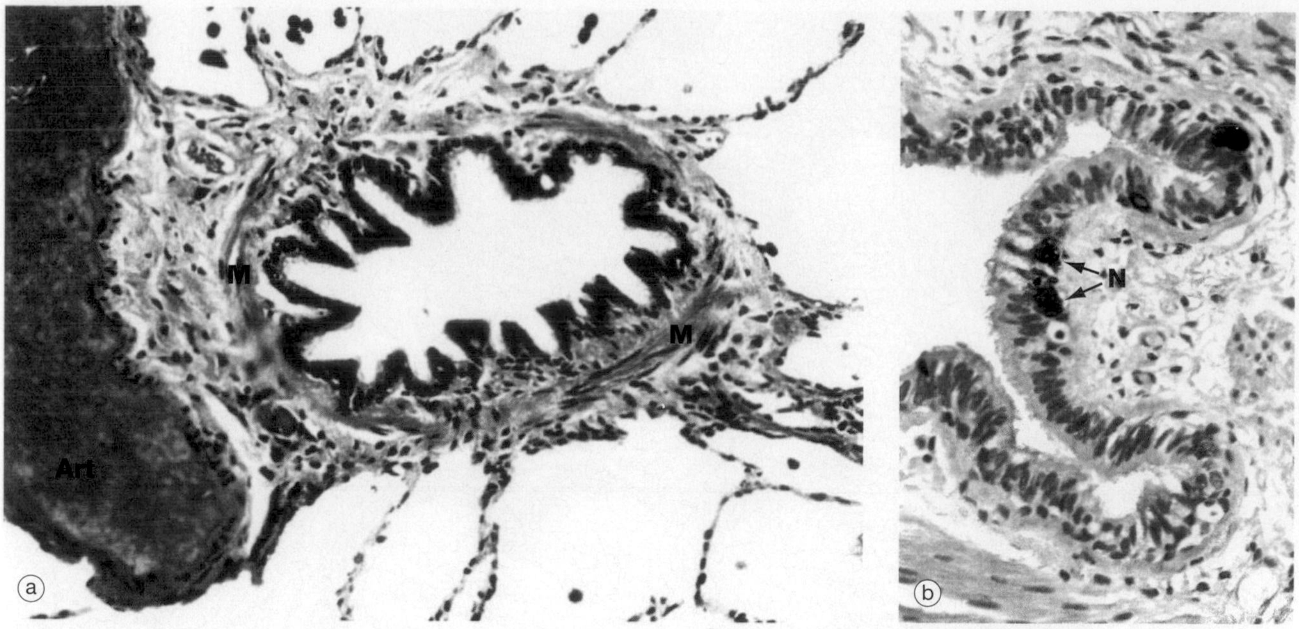

FIG. 12.11 Bronchiole
(a) H&E (MP) (b) Immunohistochemical staining for chromogranin (HP)

A *bronchiole* (Fig. 12.11a) is an airway of less than 1 mm diameter which has neither cartilage or submucosal glands in its wall. The epithelium is composed of ciliated columnar cells and few goblet cells. In the *terminal* and *respiratory bronchioles*, goblet cells are replaced by *Clara cells* (see Fig. 12.12), tall columnar cells with apical secretory granules. The wall is also composed of smooth muscle **M**, the tone of which controls the bore of the tube and therefore resistance to airflow within the lungs.

A distended thin-walled pulmonary artery branch **Art** lies next to the bronchiole.

Fig. 12.11b demonstrates the presence of neuroendocrine cells **N** using an immunohistochemical method. These cells form part of the *diffuse neuroendocrine system* (see Ch. 17), secreting a number of peptide hormones including 5-HT (serotonin) and bombesin which regulate muscle tone in bronchial and vessel walls.

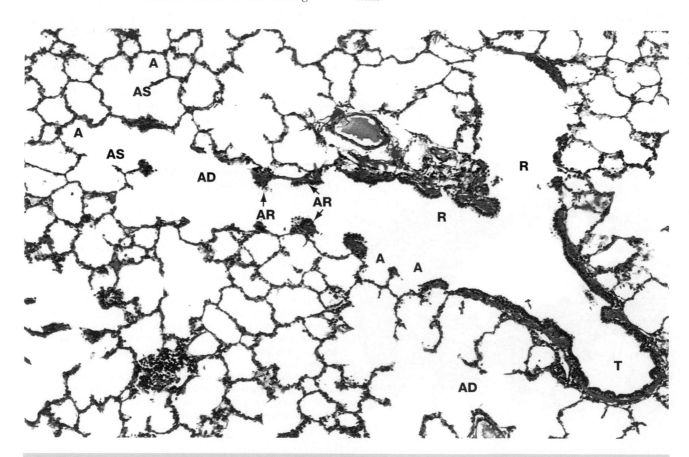

FIG. 12.12 Terminal portion of the respiratory tree ***(caption opposite)***
H&E (LP)

A alveolus **AD** alveolar duct **AM** alveolar macrophage **AR** alveolar ring **AS** alveolar sac **Art** artery **C** capillary **E** endothelial cell **M** smooth muscle **N** neuroendocrine cell **P_1** type I pneumocyte **P_2** type II pneumocyte **R** respiratory bronchiole **RBC** red blood cell **T** terminal bronchiole

FIG. 12.12 Terminal portion of the respiratory tree *(illustration opposite)*
H&E (LP)

Illustrated in Fig. 12.12, ***terminal bronchioles*** **T** are the smallest diameter passages of the purely conducting portion of the respiratory tree. Beyond this, branches become increasingly involved in gaseous exchange.

Each terminal bronchiole divides to form short, thinner walled branches called ***bronchioles*** **R** which contain a small number of single ***alveoli*** **A** in their walls. The epithelium of the respiratory bronchioles is devoid of goblet cells and largely consists of ciliated cuboidal cells and smaller numbers of non-ciliated cells called ***Clara cells***. In the most distal part of the respiratory bronchioles, Clara cells become the predominant cell type. Clara cells have three functions:

- They produce one of the components of ***surfactant***.
- They act as ***stem cells***, i.e. they are able to divide, differentiate and replace other damaged cell types.
- They contain enzyme systems which can detoxify noxious substances.

Each respiratory bronchiole divides further into several ***alveolar ducts*** **AD** which have numerous alveoli **A** opening along their length. The alveolar ducts end in an ***alveolar sac*** **AS**, which in turn opens into several alveoli.

In histological sections, all that can be seen of the walls of the alveolar ducts are small aggregations of smooth muscle cells, collagen and elastin fibres which form alveolar rings **AR** surrounding the alveolar ducts and the openings of the alveolar sacs and alveoli. The smooth muscle of the respiratory bronchioles and alveolar ducts regulates alveolar air movements.

Each alveolus consists of a pocket, open at one side, lined by flattened epithelial cells (***pneumocytes***). The alveolar septa contain occasional small openings about 8 µm diameter, the ***alveolar pores*** (of ***Kohn***), which allow some movement of air between adjacent alveoli. The collagen and elastic fibres of the septum condense around the openings of the alveoli and form a supporting meshwork for the lung parenchyma.

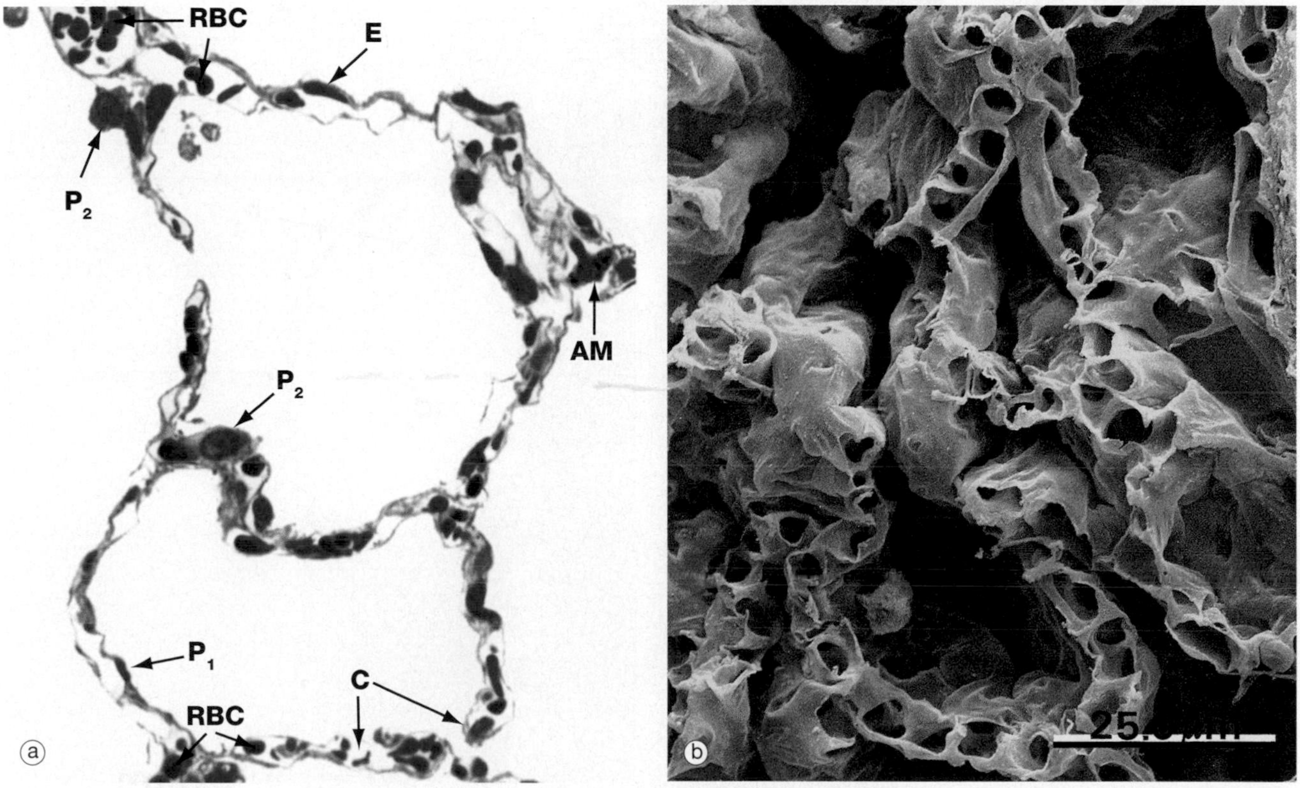

FIG. 12.13 Alveoli
(a) Thin resin section, toluidine blue (HP) (b) SEM ×500

The alveolar wall consists of three tissue components: ***surface epithelium, supporting tissue*** and ***blood vessels***.

The epithelium provides a continuous lining to each alveolus and consists of cells of two types. Most of the alveolar surface area is covered by large squamous cells called ***type I pneumocytes*** (***alveolar lining cells***). Because the cytoplasm of these cells covers such an extensive area, the characteristic densely stained nuclei of type I pneumocytes $\mathbf{P_1}$ are relatively infrequently seen in histological section. The ***type II pneumocyte*** $\mathbf{P_2}$ represents some 60% of cells in the lining epithelium, but is rounded in shape and thus occupies a much smaller proportion (about 5%) of the alveolar surface area.

Type II pneumocytes secrete a surface-active material called ***surfactant*** which reduces alveolar surface tension, preventing alveolar collapse during expiration. ***Clara cells*** of the respiratory bronchioles probably synthesise other components of surfactant. Type II pneumocytes retain the capacity for cell division and can differentiate into type I pneumocytes if required.

Supporting tissue forms an attenuated layer surrounding the blood vessels of the alveolar wall. This layer consists of reticular, collagenous and elastic fibres and occasional fibroblasts. Blood vessels, mainly capillaries **C**, form an extensive plexus around each alveolus. In most of the alveolar wall, the basement membrane of the capillary endothelium is directly applied to the basement membrane of the surface epithelium. In such sites, the two basement membranes are fused and supporting tissue is absent. This arrangement provides an interface of minimal thickness between alveolar air and blood.

In Fig. 12.13a, red blood cells within the capillary lamina are seen as densely stained round or elliptical structures **RBC**. Nuclei of the endothelial cells **E** lining the capillaries are elongated, flat and usually sparse. An alveolar macrophage **AM** is present in the alveolar wall. Fig. 12.13b is a low-magnification scanning electron micrograph of a group of alveoli, showing their three-dimensional architecture. The capillaries in the alveolar walls have been distended by injection. No cellular detail is visible.

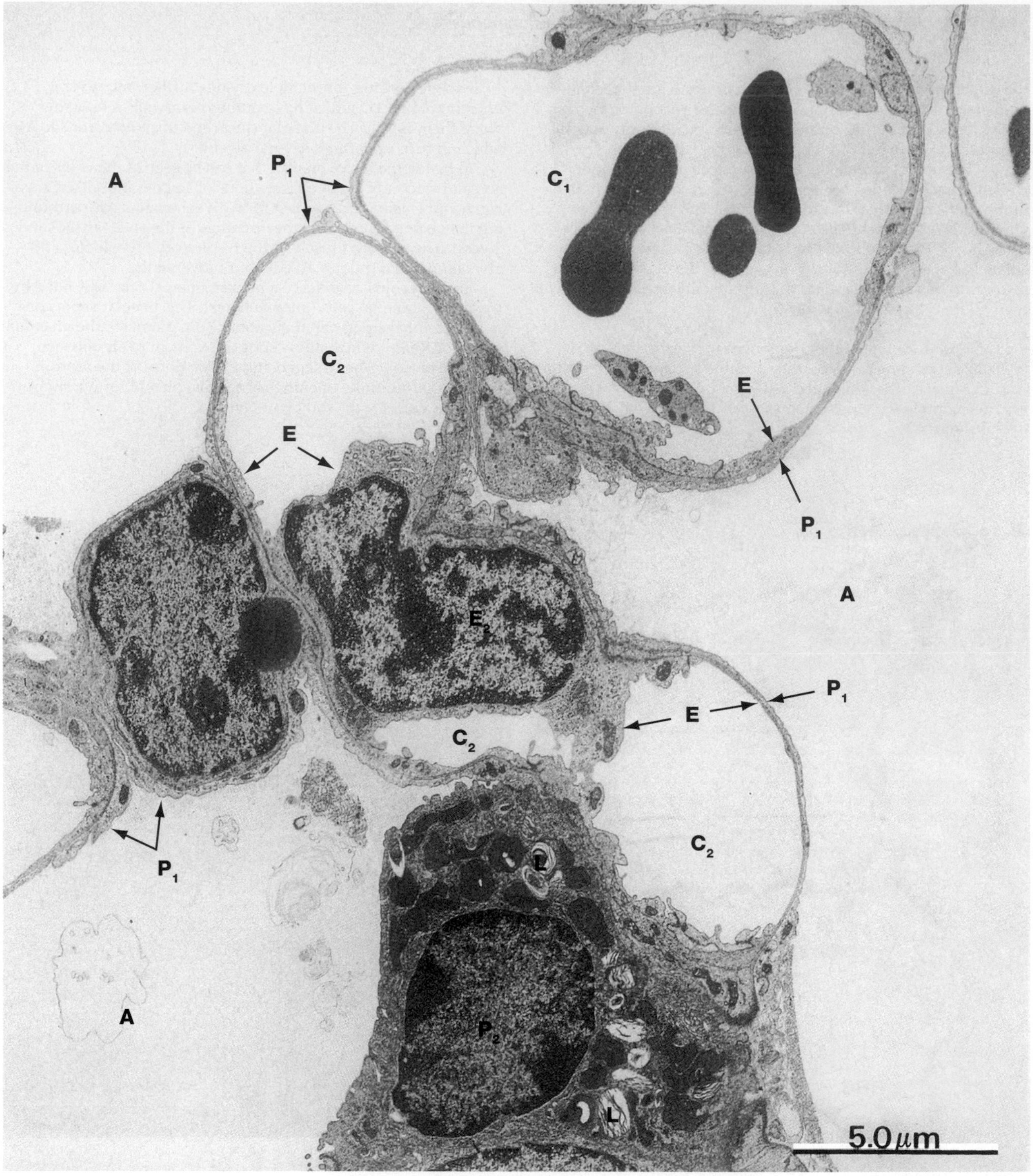

FIG. 12.14 Alveolar wall
EM ×6000

This electron micrograph (Fig. 12.14) shows the alveolar wall between three alveoli **A** at low magnification. Capillaries make up the bulk of the alveolar wall, branching and anastomosing to create a basket-like arrangement around each alveolus. This field shows parts of several capillaries, the uppermost $\mathbf{C_1}$ containing erythrocytes and a platelet. The plane of section has cut the lumen of a second capillary $\mathbf{C_2}$ in three places and includes the nucleus of one of its lining endothelial cells **E**. The cytoplasm of type I pneumocytes $\mathbf{P_1}$, which cover most of the alveolar surface, and capillary endothelial cells **E** are both extremely attenuated, and distinction between them is best made by tracing their basement membranes. Alveolar lining cells lie on the convex side of the basement membrane, whilst endothelial cells are on the concave side and adjacent to any erythrocytes within the capillary.

A type II pneumocyte $\mathbf{P_2}$ is also seen, typically located at a branching point of the alveolar septum. The cytoplasm is filled with vesicles containing phospholipid in the form of ***lamellar bodies*** **L**. These bodies are discharged into the alveolar air space where they contribute to a surfactant layer at the epithelium/air interface.

A alveolus **BM_2** basement membrane **C** capillary **E** endothelial cell **F** fibroblast **L** lamellar body **Mv** microvilli **NE** endothelial cell nucleus **P_1** type I pneumocyte **P_2** type II pneumocyte **S** supporting tissue **TJ** tight junction

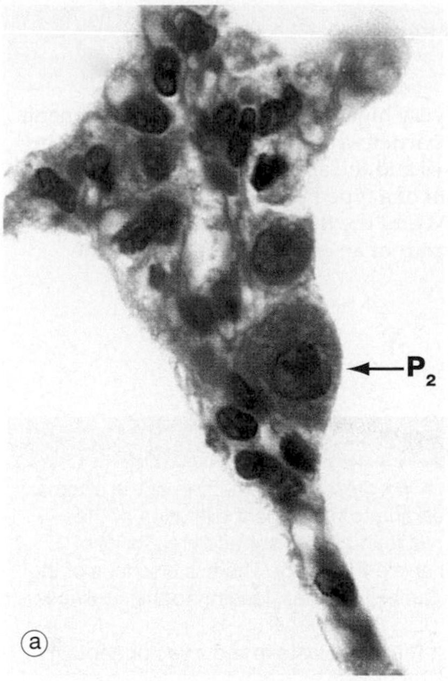

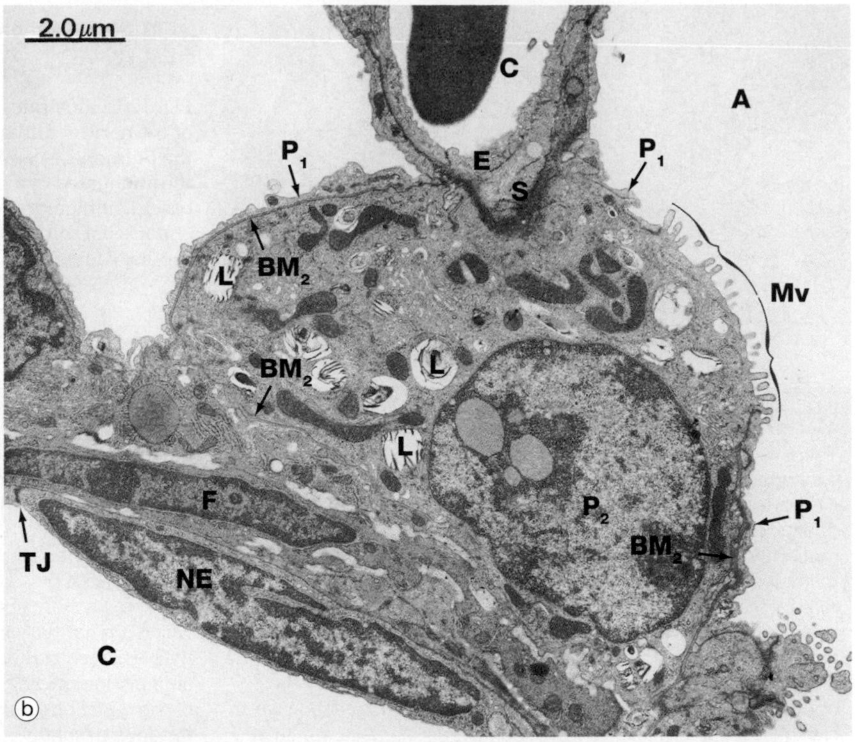

FIG. 12.15 Type II pneumocytes
(a) H&E (HP) (b) EM ×9000
(c) EM ×35 000

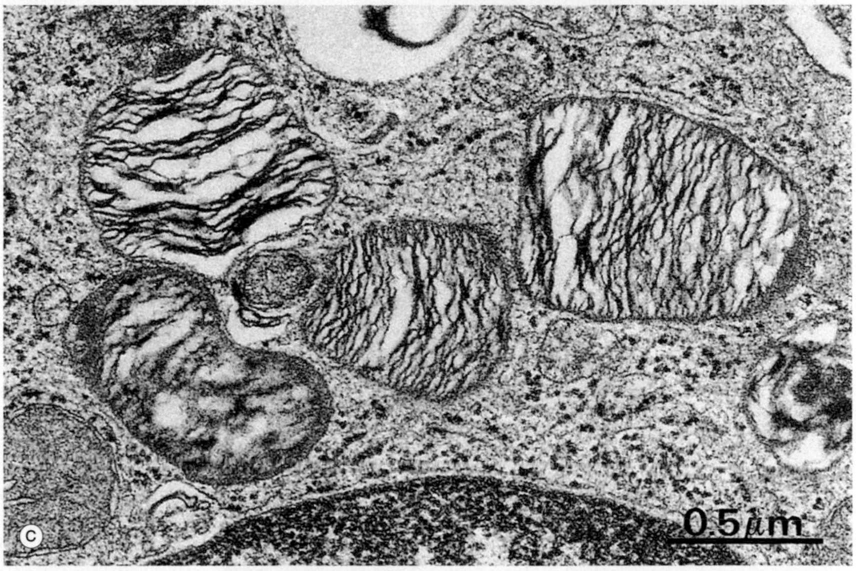

Fig. 12.15a shows the light microscopic appearance of type II pneumocytes $\mathbf{P_2}$ or ***surfactant cells***, which are responsible for surfactant production. Their nuclei are large and plump with dispersed chromatin and prominent nucleoli. The plentiful eosinophilic cytoplasm is filled with fine unstained vacuoles representing lamellar bodies, the phospholipid of which is dissolved out during tissue preparation. In comparison, the nuclei of ***type I pneumocytes*** (***alveolar lining cells***) and capillary endothelial cells are small, dense and flattened.

Fig. 12.15b shows a branch point in an alveolar wall, typically containing a type II pneumocyte $\mathbf{P_2}$, recognisable by its ***lamellar bodies*** **L**. Most of the type II pneumocyte is surrounded by basement membrane $\mathbf{BM_2}$, and only a small proportion of its surface is exposed directly to the alveolar space **A**, where it exhibits numerous small microvilli **Mv** associated with surfactant secretion. Elsewhere, the alveolar aspect of the type II pneumocyte is invested by a thin layer of cytoplasm of type I pneumocytes $\mathbf{P_1}$ but separated by a common basement membrane. At the top of the field, the type II pneumocyte abuts a capillary **C**, its cytoplasm being separated from that of the capillary endothelium **E** by the basement membranes of each cell and a little intervening supporting tissue **S**. At the lower left of the field, the type II cell rests upon a thin layer of septal supporting tissue containing a fibroblast **F**. Beyond this lies the flattened nucleus of a capillary endothelial cell **NE**, its attenuated cytoplasm spreading out to line the capillary lumen **C**. A tight junction **TJ** is seen where this endothelial cell abuts an adjacent cell. Basement membranes can be traced on both aspects of this alveolar supporting tissue. The surfactant cell contains rough endoplasmic reticulum, free ribosomes and moderate numbers of elongated mitochondria.

Fig. 12.15c shows lamellar bodies at high magnification. These are membrane bound and the lamellae within them are composed mainly of phospholipids, particularly ***palmitoyl phosphatidylcholine***. Phospholipid is released by exocytosis, spreading out over the alveolar surface where it combines with other carbohydrate- and protein-containing secretory products (some of which are derived from bronchiolar Clara cells) to form a tubular lattice of lipoprotein described as ***tubular myelin***. In the event of two alveolar surfaces coming together, this overcomes the effects of surface tension which would otherwise cause them to adhere. This allows for normal inflation of the alveoli at birth (see textbox) and for the reinflation of alveoli which collapse after airway obstruction.

Surfactant deficiency in newborn infants

Normally, the lungs of newborn infants are able to inflate easily at birth because of the presence of surfactant which overcomes the surface tension of the collapsed fetal lungs.

Surfactant production occurs late in gestation and, if the infant is born prematurely, there is often insufficient surfactant to allow normal breathing after delivery. This can result in severe acute breathing difficulties as well as persistent chronic lung disease in surviving infants. The disorder is known as respiratory distress syndrome of the newborn.

If premature delivery is anticipated during pregnancy, administering corticosteroids to the mother induces surfactant production in the fetal lung and reduces the risk of neonatal lung disease.

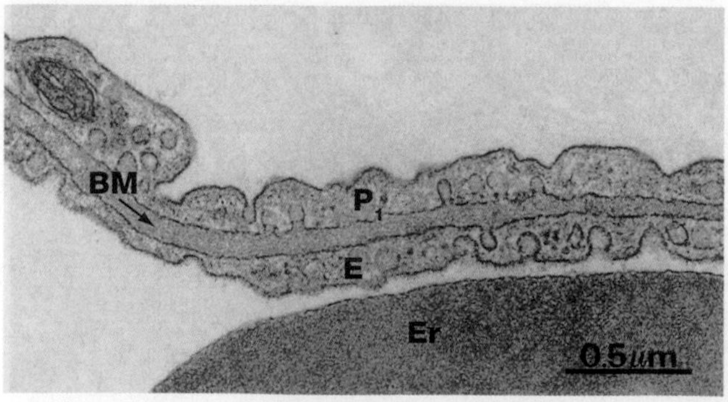

FIG. 12.16 Air–blood barrier EM ×34 000

Fig. 12.16 illustrates, at very high magnification, the components of the narrow diffusion barrier which lies between the blood in the pulmonary capillaries and the alveolar air. This consists of the attenuated cytoplasm of a type I pneumocyte P_1, the fused basement membrane **BM** and the thin cytoplasm of a capillary endothelial cell **E**. Note part of an erythrocyte **Er** within the capillary lumen.

Disorders of the alveoli

The alveolar walls provide an enormous surface area for exchange of gases between the air in the alveoli and the blood in capillaries of the septal wall. Any diseases that reduce the amount of air in the alveoli, or reduce the surface area of the alveoli, or render the alveolar walls thick and impermeable to gases will lead to inadequate oxygenation of blood (***hypoxia***), carbon dioxide retention and breathlessness. All three patterns of disease occur.

In lobar pneumonia, bacteria (usually streptococci) gain access to the alveoli and proliferate rapidly, spreading to all the alveoli in the lobe very rapidly through the alveolar pores. The body responds by mounting an acute inflammatory reaction which fills the alveolar cavities with a mixed fluid/cellular exudate, thus preventing the entry of air into the alveoli of an entire lung lobe, greatly reducing the capacity for adequate oxygenation (see Fig. 12.19 and e-Fig. 12.4).

In emphysema, there is progressive destruction of the alveolar ducts, sacs and alveoli, leading to permanent dilatation of the air spaces but a marked reduction in the surface area for gas exchange (see Fig. 12.19 and e-Fig. 12.5). There is also loss of the elastic tissue support for the bronchioles, leading to their collapse and air trapping.

In pulmonary fibrosis, the fibroblasts in the alveolar septa, which are normally scanty, increase in number and increase their collagen and elastin production. This thickens the alveolar septum, interposing layers of collagen between the cytoplasm of the type I pneumocyte and alveolar capillaries, thus impeding gaseous exchange. This is a diffuse change throughout the lung parenchyma and leads to slowly progressive hypoxia and breathlessness (see e-Fig. 12.6).

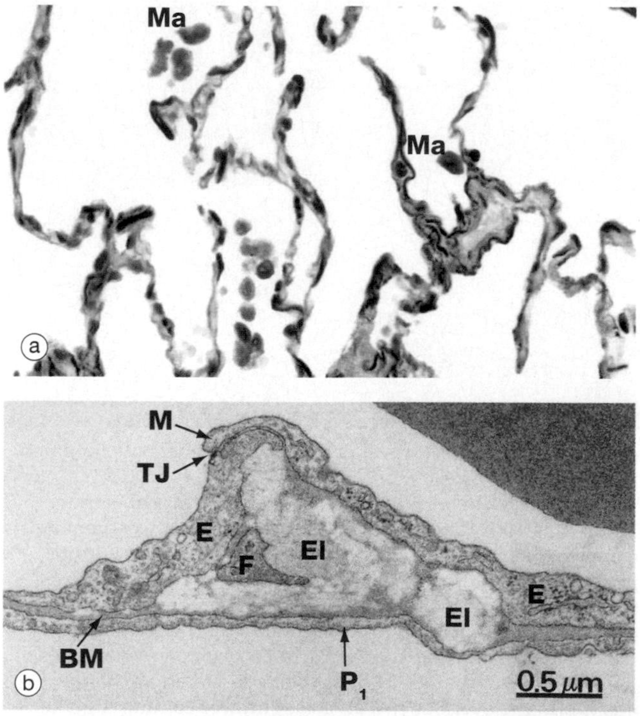

FIG. 12.17 Pulmonary elastic tissue (a) Elastic van Gieson (HP) (b) EM ×26 000

The staining method used in Fig. 12.17a demonstrates the large amount of elastin (stained black) in the alveolar walls. At the margins of the openings into the alveoli, the elastin is condensed to form a supporting ring. The elastin and septal collagen of the alveolar wall are continuous with those of adjacent alveoli, forming a fibroelastic supporting framework for the lung parenchyma as a whole. Occasional alveolar macrophages **Ma** can be seen within the lumen of the alveoli.

Fig. 12.17b shows part of an alveolar septum containing elements of the elastin meshwork. The septum consists of the thin cytoplasmic layers of a type I pneumocyte P_1 and two capillary endothelial cells **E** separated by a common basement membrane **BM**. Note the marginal fold **M** of one endothelial cell overlapping the other, creating a seal and reinforced by a tight junction **TJ**.

The elastin **El** is an amorphous, moderately electron-dense mass which is insinuated between the two cell layers. This space also contains a fine cytoplasmic extension from a fibroblast **F**.

Industrial lung disease

Silicosis of the lungs (see e-Fig. 12.7) varies depending on the particulate which is inhaled. In coal miners the silica is a component of the fine coal dust that is inhaled during mining and in haematite miners is a component of iron ore dust. Silica is inhaled into the alveoli and phagocytosed by macrophages. Particles which are not expectorated (coughed up) may remain in the alveolar septa for years where the silica is converted into silicic acid. This stimulates the proliferation of fibroblasts and subsequent collagen deposition. Eventually, lung fibrosis becomes extensive. Asbestos is a silicate which exists in the form of long crystalline needles. When inhaled, these also stimulate lung fibrosis, known as ***asbestosis*** (see e-Fig. 12.8). In contrast to silicosis, which requires prolonged inhalation, asbestos need only be inhaled in small quantities on a few occasions to stimulate the development (usually decades later) of a malignant tumour of the pleura (***mesothelioma***).

AP alveolar pore **B** bullae **BM** basement membrane **C** capillary **E** endothelial cell **El** elastin **Er** erythrocyte **Ex** neutrophil-rich exudate **F** fibroblast **L** lipid droplet **Ly** lysosome **M** marginal fold **Ma** macrophage P_1 type I pneumocyte P_2 type II pneumocyte **TJ** tight junction **W** air space widening

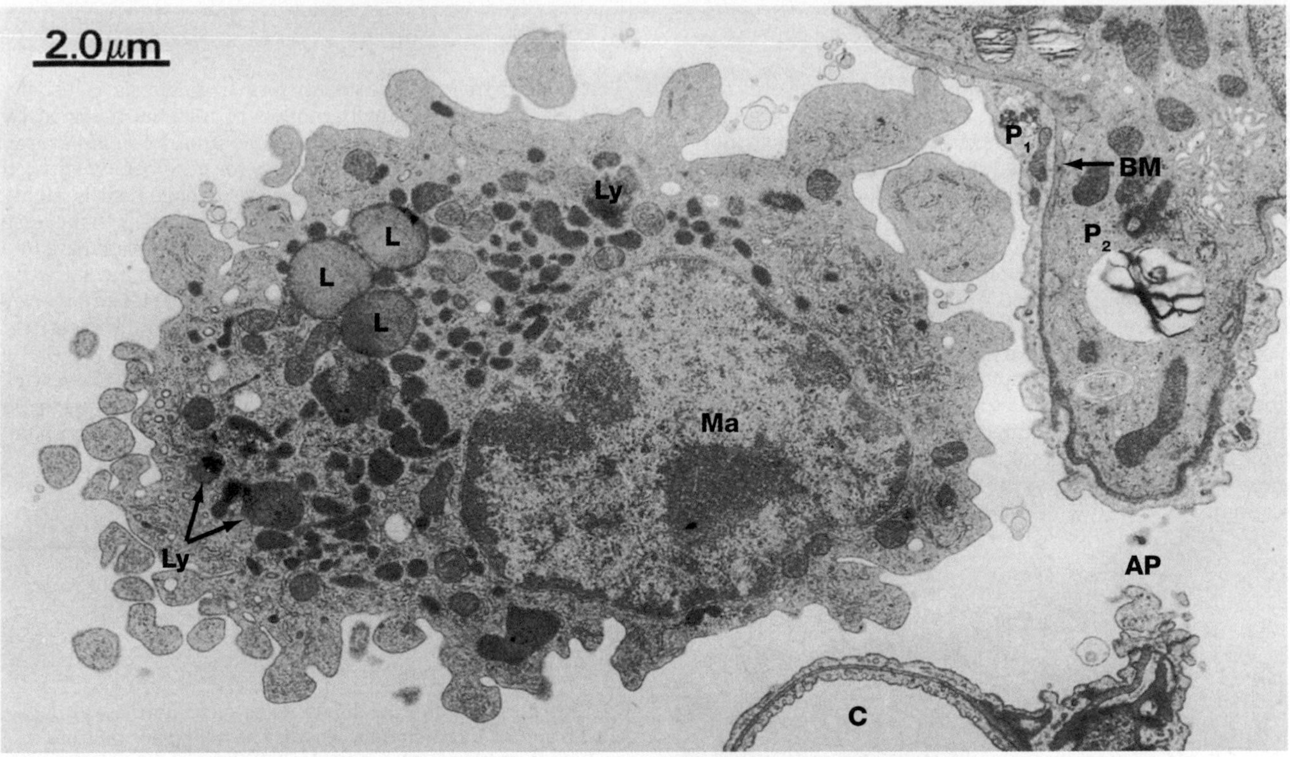

FIG. 12.18 Alveolar macrophage
EM ×9000

The lung contains macrophages, both free within the alveolar spaces and in the alveolar septa. They are derived from circulating blood monocytes, although some may arise by mitotic division of macrophages already present in the lung. Their function is the phagocytosis and removal of unwanted material which gains access to the air spaces, such as inhaled particulate matter and bacteria. The most common particles are carbon. In city dwellers, these are derived from car exhaust fumes and industrial smoke. Numerous carbon particles are typically seen in cigarette smokers. After phagocytosing the particles, most macrophages pass into the airways to become trapped in mucus and coughed up as sputum. Others stay in the septa whilst some gain access to the lymphatic system and pass with their phagocytosed material to the hilar lymph nodes.

The macrophage **Ma** in Fig. 12.18 lies within an alveolus adjacent to a septal capillary **C** and a type II pneumocyte $\mathbf{P_2}$. Between these, there is an alveolar pore **AP**. The aspect of the type II pneumocyte seen here is typically invested by the thin cytoplasm of a type I pneumocyte $\mathbf{P_1}$, the two being separated by a common basement membrane **BM** (see Fig. 12.16). The alveolar macrophage exhibits the typical features of macrophages elsewhere in the body (see Fig. 4.19), but in particular contains numerous secondary lysosomes **Ly** and lipid droplets **L**.

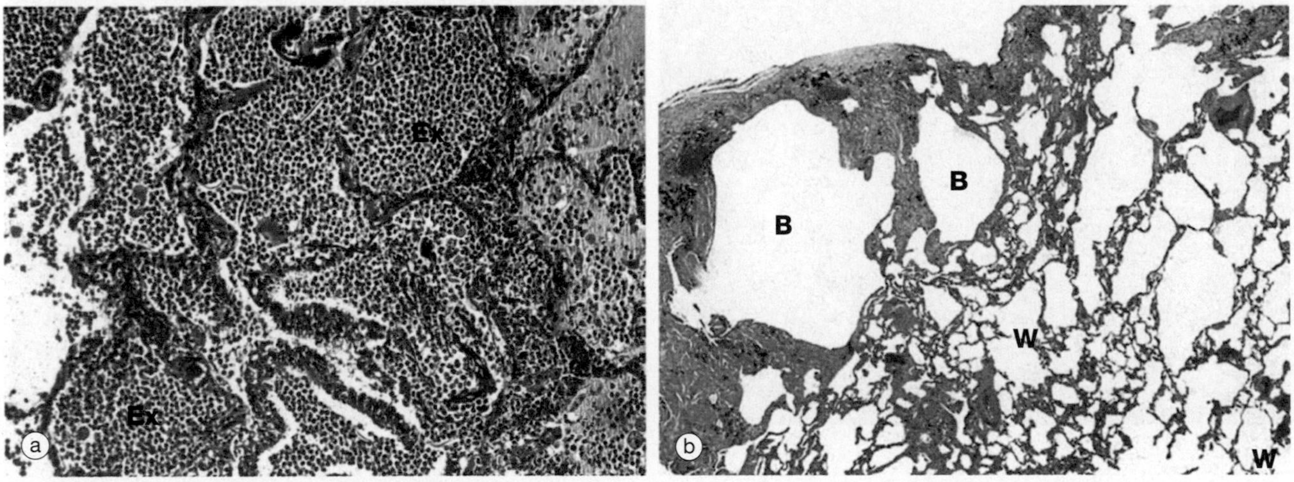

FIG. 12.19 Common lung pathology
(a) Bronchopneumonia, H&E (MP) (b) Emphysema, H&E (LP)

In bronchopneumonia (Fig. 12.19a, see also e-Fig. 12.4), an acute inflammatory exudate **Ex** including numerous neutrophils fill and expand the alveolar air spaces resulting in consolidation. Emphysema (Fig. 12.19b, see also e-Fig. 12.5), most commonly seen in smokers, results in irreversible destruction of the alveolar walls with resultant air space widening **W** and bullae formation at the periphery of the lungs **B**.

LUNG CANCER

The majority of malignant tumours of the lungs are carcinomas that arise in the bronchi. Lung carcinomas are broadly classified into small cell carcinoma and non-small carcinomas. Non-small carcinomas are further divided into squamous cell carcinomas, adenocarcinomas and large cell carcinomas which have distinctive histological appearances and treatment options. A few of these tumour types are illustrated below.

Risk factors for the development of lung cancer include cigarette smoking, exposure to radiation and asbestos. Air pollution, lung scarring and genetic predispositions may also be important causative agents.

The diagnosis of lung carcinoma is usually first suspected due to weight loss, breathlessness and ***haemoptysis*** (coughing up blood), often in cigarette smokers. Initial investigation typically involves obtaining a chest radiograph, followed by more detailed imaging such as computed tomography (CT) scanning.

If a lung mass is identified, formal diagnosis is usually made on the basis of small amounts of material obtained by minimally invasive techniques such as ***bronchoscopic biopsy*** or ***radiologically guided needle biopsy*** for peripherally situated lung masses. This is necessary because management is highly dependent upon classification. Most lung cancers actually arise within the epithelium of the bronchi and spread from there into the surrounding lung tissue. Thus, they are often accessible by bronchoscopy where cytological samples may be taken either by washings or brushings of a lesion. More peripheral lesions may be accessed by the technique of fine needle aspiration (FNA), by passing a long needle into the tumour through the chest wall. Least invasive of all is the examination of sputum coughed up by the patient. All of these specimens may be examined by cytological techniques (see Fig. 12.20).

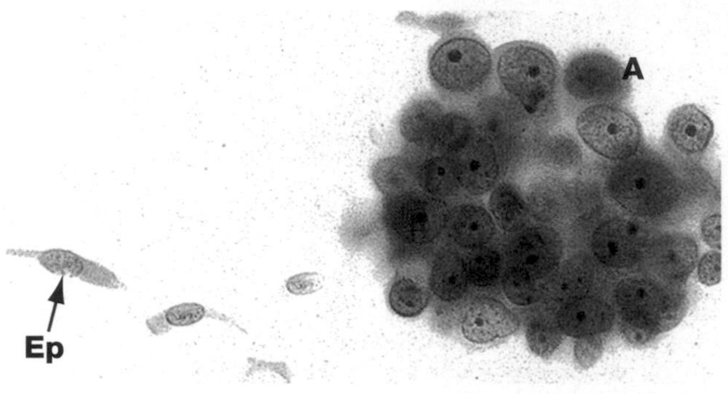

FIG. 12.20 Lung cancer cytology FNA sample Giemsa (HP)

Fig. 12.20 demonstrates the difference between normal epithelial cells **Ep** and adenocarcinoma cells **A**. The malignant cells are much larger with prominent nucleoli, large nuclei and increased nuclear to cytoplasmic (N:C) ratio. In contrast, the normal epithelial cells exhibit the expected columnar shape and have much smaller nuclei with inconspicuous nucleoli. Cilia can just be discerned on the luminal surface of the normal cells in this image.

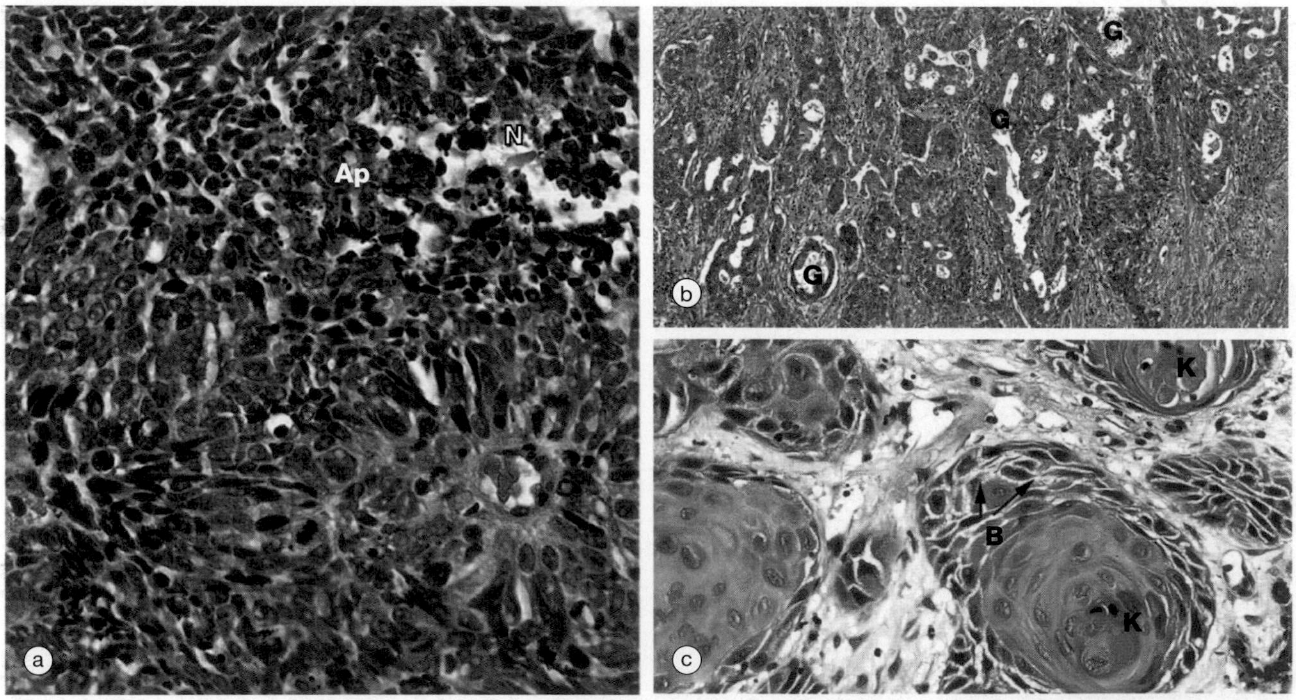

FIG. 12.21 Types of lung cancer
(a) Small cell carcinoma, H&E (HP) (b) Adenocarcinoma (c) Squamous cell carcinoma

Lung cancer can be broadly subtyped into small cell carcinoma and non–small cell carcinoma. Small cell carcinoma (Fig. 12.21a) is a highly malignant tumour composed of small, tightly packed, darkly stained cells with limited cytoplasm (e-Fig. 12.9). There is often necrosis **N**, prominent apoptosis **Ap** and brisk mitotic activity. These tumours are often aggressive with early lymphatic and blood-borne spread. Non–small cell carcinomas comprise a number of different types which are histologically distinct from small cell carcinoma and include adenocarcinoma (AC; Fig. 12.21b) and squamous cell carcinoma (SCC; Fig. 12.21c). ACs (e-Fig. 12.10) are malignant gland **G** forming tumours which often arise in the periphery of the lung. SCCs (e-Fig. 12.11) usually arise more centrally. These tumours show evidence of keratinisation **K** or intercellular bridge formation **B**. Immunohistochemistry is often used for final diagnosis.

PULMONARY VASCULATURE

The lungs have a double blood supply from the pulmonary vascular system, the major supplier, and the bronchial vascular system. Deoxygenated blood is carried by the systemic veins to the right atrium and into the right ventricle. The right ventricle pumps the blood through the ***pulmonary valve*** into the main ***pulmonary arterial trunk*** and then into the ***right*** and ***left pulmonary arteries***. The main right and left pulmonary arteries enter the lungs at the lung hila alongside the main bronchi and follow the course of the bronchi into the lungs, dividing into progressively smaller branches as the bronchi divide. With each division, the arteries become smaller and the structure of their wall changes. The proximal pulmonary arteries, the main pulmonary trunk and large pulmonary arteries, are elastic arteries similar to the aorta (see Fig. 8.9) but thinner walled, with elastic fibres an important component of the tunica media. Beyond the point where the bronchi lose their cartilage plates to become bronchioles, the pulmonary arteries become muscular arteries with distinct elastic laminae and a tunica media that is almost completely composed of smooth muscle. The transition from elastic to muscular arteries is gradual. The distal pulmonary arteries continue to follow the distribution of bronchioles and become progressively smaller as the tunica media becomes thinner, eventually becoming discontinuous in the pulmonary arterioles. The small pulmonary arterioles transfer blood into the pulmonary capillaries (see Figs 12.13 and 12.14) where it becomes oxygenated and it is then passed through pulmonary venules (indistinguishable from arterioles) into a series of gradually enlarging venules and veins. Some of these run in the fibrocollagenous septa of the lung before becoming medium-sized veins with a distinct tunica media and ill-formed elastic laminae. The largest pulmonary veins, that leave the lungs at the hilar regions and pass to the left atrium, show elastic fibres scattered in the media, rather than in distinct elastic laminae.

The ***bronchial vascular system*** is minor and provides lung structures such as bronchi with oxygenated blood at systemic pressure. The bronchial arteries are lateral branches of the thoracic aorta and run with the bronchial tree as far as respiratory bronchiole level where they anastomose with the pulmonary vascular system. The small bronchial veins and venules also anastomose freely with pulmonary veins and venules. The main bronchial veins drain into the ***azygos*** and ***hemiazygos veins***.

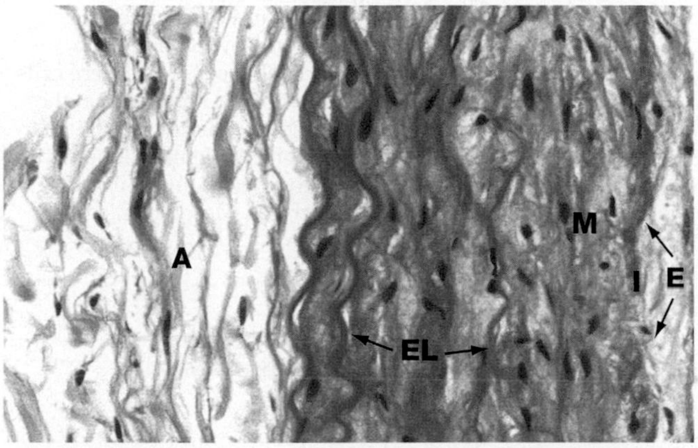

FIG. 12.22 Large pulmonary artery H&E (HP)

The pulmonary trunk, main right and left pulmonary arteries and their major lobar branches have a structure similar to that of the aorta (see Fig. 8.9), i.e. an elastic artery with prominent elastic lamellae as an important component of the tunica media. However, because the intravascular pressures are so much less in the pulmonary vascular system, the layers are thinner and less substantial than their equivalents in the aorta. In Fig. 12.22, the tunica intima **I** has surface endothelial cells **E**, and the tunica media **M** is composed of smooth muscle cells, collagen and prominent elastic lamellae **EL**. The adventitia **A** comprises loose fibrocollagenous tissue.

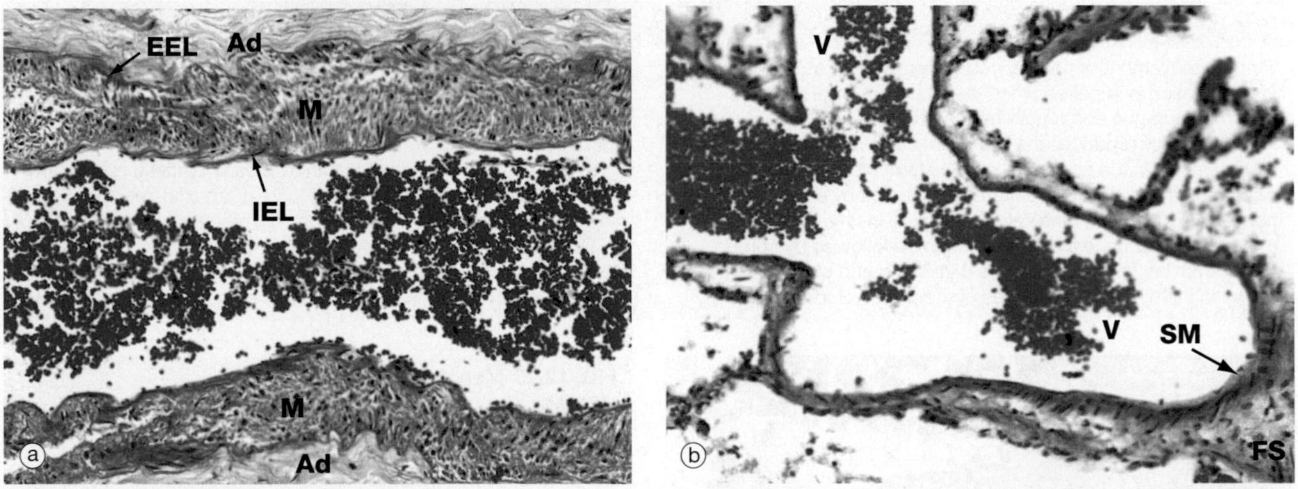

FIG. 12.23 Smaller pulmonary vessels (a) Muscular pulmonary artery, H&E (MP) (b) Small pulmonary vein, H&E (MP)

More distally, the elastic pulmonary artery progressively loses most of the elastic fibres in the media. A muscular pulmonary artery is illustrated in Fig. 12.23a. Most of the remaining elastic is in the form of internal **IEL** and external **EEL** elastic laminae so that the media **M** is largely composed of smooth muscle and collagen.

The intima is thin and indistinct, and the fibrocollagenous tunica adventitia **Ad** merges with the fibrocollagenous support tissue of the lung septa and peribronchial areas.

Pulmonary capillaries and venules empty oxygenated blood into thin-walled pulmonary veins **V**, as illustrated in Fig. 12.23b. The amount of smooth muscle media **SM** in the vein wall increases progressively along the venous network, and the largest pulmonary veins have a distinct muscular tunica media containing elastin fibres. Small pulmonary veins of the size shown here run in the fibrous septa **FS** of the lungs.

A adenocarcinoma cells **Ad** tunica adventitia **Ap** apoptosis **B** intercellular bridges **E** endothelial cell **Ep** Epithelial cells **EEL** external elastic lamina **EL** elastic lamellae **FS** fibrous septum **G** Malignant glands **I** tunica intima **IEL** internal elastic lamina **K** keratinisation **M** tunica media **N** necrosis **SM** smooth muscle **V** vein

THE PLEURA

The two cavities in the thorax which house the right and left lungs, the ***pleural cavities***, are lined internally by a thin smooth layer, the ***pleura***, which is also reflected over the external surfaces of the lungs. The part of the pleura which forms the internal lining of the chest cavities is called the ***parietal pleura*** and that which externally coats the lungs, the ***visceral pleura***. The parietal and visceral pleurae are normally in contact but separated by a potential space containing a small amount of ***serous fluid*** that lubricates the movement of visceral upon parietal pleura during breathing.

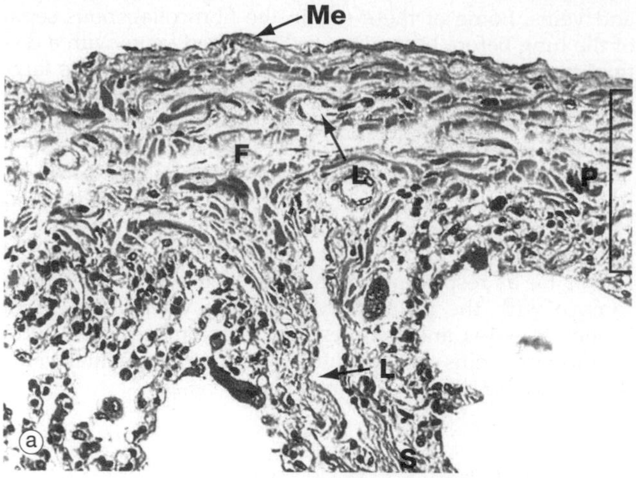

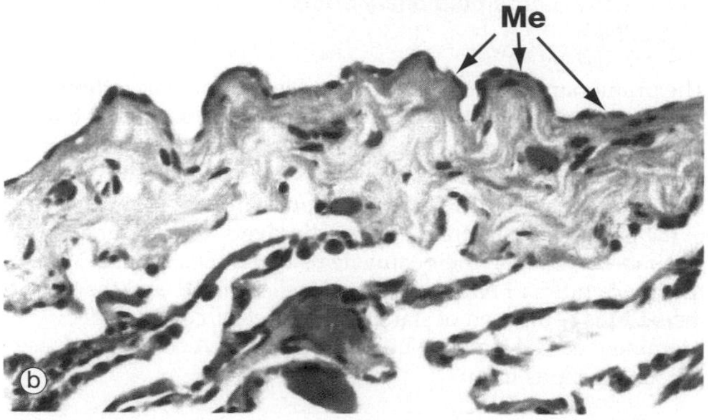

FIG. 12.24 Visceral pleura
(a) H&E (b) H&E (HP)

Fig. 12.24a illustrates visceral pleura **P**. The outer surface is lined by a layer of flattened ***mesothelium*** **Me**, supported by a thin basement membrane. The underlying fibrous supporting tissue **F** consists primarily of collagen and elastin fibres. The fibrous layer of visceral pleura extends into the lung as fibrous septa **S** which are continuous with the fibroelastic framework of the lung parenchyma.

The visceral pleura contains a superficial plexus of lymph vessels which drain via the septa into a deep plexus surrounding the pulmonary blood vessels and airways. Lymph from the deep plexuses drains into the thoracic duct via lymph nodes in the hilar region. Lymphatic capillaries are not found in alveolar walls, but they are present in the walls of respiratory bronchioles and in all larger airways. Several lymphatic vessels **L** can be seen in the pleura in this micrograph. The visceral pleura also contains numerous small blood vessels and capillaries.

Fig. 12.24b is a higher magnification view of the pleura showing the flattened cuboidal mesothelial cells **Me**. These cells stretch to accommodate the movement of the lungs so that the height of the cells varies from flattened to columnar.

Ultrastructurally, mesothelial cells have plentiful long surface microvilli which serve to trap hyaluronic acid, thus enhancing the lubrication of the two pleural surfaces. Mesothelial cells contain keratin intermediate filaments.

Disorders of the pleura

Smooth movement of parietal and visceral pleura during inspiration and expiration is impaired when the smooth pleural surfaces become damaged and roughened, particularly during bacterial infections. This produces the symptom called ***pleurisy***, a severe stabbing pain in the chest wall at the site of pleural damage during inspiration and expiration, often accompanied by a scratching noise on auscultation (***pleural friction rub***) in time with respiratory movements. Damage to the pleura can be followed by fibrous scar formation, leading to fibrous thickening and often adhesions between the two facing surfaces of the pleura. Some of the pulmonary lymphatics run in fibrous septa and empty their contents into the pleural cavity. If the lungs become severely waterlogged (e.g. due to heart failure), these lymphatics can disgorge large quantities of fluid into the pleural cavity (pleural effusion). Unfortunately, these lymphatics can also carry bacteria and tumour cells into the pleural cavity from the lung, producing infected pleural effusions and malignant pleural effusions, respectively.

Only one form of primary cancer occurs in the pleura, malignant mesothelioma, which is known to be associated with the inhalation of some forms of asbestos fibre and is illustrated below.

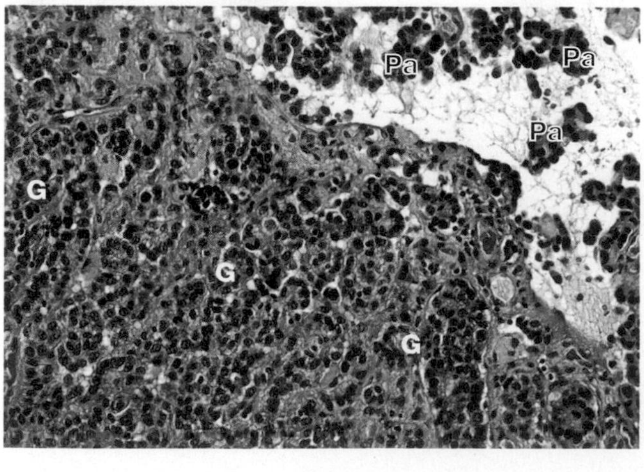

FIG. 12.25 Malignant mesothelioma
H&E MP

Malignant mesothelioma (see e-Fig. 12.12) is a primary malignant tumour of mesothelial surfaces, most commonly occuring in the pleural space. Tumours typically give rise to pleural effusions which can be sampled for cytological analysis.

Mesothelioma is often associated with a history of asbestos exposure. Mesotheliomas typically surround the lung(s) forming a 'rind like' shell and can infiltrate into the chest wall. Metastatic spread is rare.

Fig. 12.25 shows a typical epithelioid mesothelioma composed of infiltrating glandular **G** and papillary elements **Pa**. This can be difficult to distinguish from lung adenocarcinoma (Fig. 12.21b) and therefore immunohistochemistry is often performed to confirm mesothelial origin. This would include markers such as calretinin which would be positive in mesothelioma and negative in lung adenocarcinoma and TTF1 which would be negative in mesotheloma and positive in lung adenocarcinoma.

F fibrous tissue **G** glandular elements **L** lymphatic space **Me** mesothelium **P** pleura **Pa** papillary elements
S Fibrous septum

REVIEW

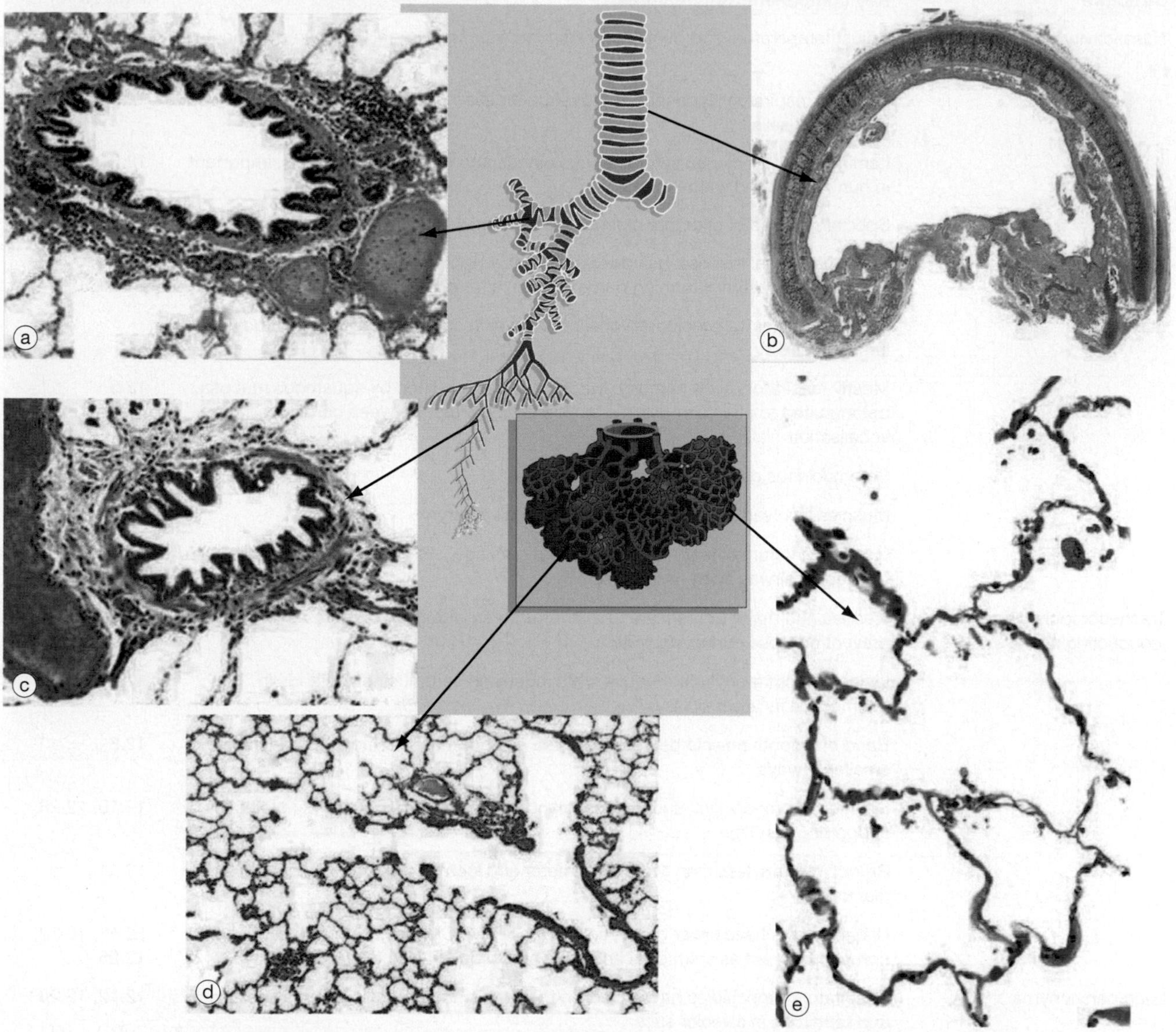

FIG. 12.26 Histological features throughout the respiratory tract
(a) Tertiary bronchus H&E (LP) (b) Trachea H&E (LP) (c) Bronchiole H&E (MP) (d) Terminal respiratory tree (terminal bronchiole and alveoli) H&E (MP) (e) Alveolar spaces H&E (HP)

TABLE 12.1 Review of the respiratory system

Structure	Key components and features	Figures
Nasal cavity and sinuses	Adjust temperature and humidity of inspired air, role in trapping inspired particulate debris	12.2
	Lined by respiratory-type mucosa (pseudostratified ciliated columnar epithelium with goblet cells)	12.3
	Lamina propria includes seromucinous glands and many blood vessels, important in humidifying and warming air	12.3
	Specialised area of olfactory mucosa in roof of nasal cavity	21.2
	Nasopharyngeal mucosa includes prominent lymphoid tissue, the adenoid or nasopharyngeal tonsil forming part of Waldeyer ring	12.4
Larynx	Part of upper airway; includes vocal cords, which are mucosal folds protruding into lumen of airway	
	Mostly respiratory-type mucosa, but vocal cords are lined by squamous mucosa, better suited to effects of chronic friction from contact between cords on vocalisation	12.5
	Seromucinous glands in submucosa	12.5
	Muscles involved in vocalisation lie within wall of larynx	12.5
	General structure of larynx is formed from cartilage, stiff but flexible and well suited to keeping airway open and protected	
Tracheobronchial tree (conducting airways)	Trachea and major bronchi are tubular structures with rings or plates of cartilage to prevent collapse during inspiration	12.6, 12.26
	Lining of respiratory type mucosa with underlying seromucinous glands in submucosa in larger airways	12.7
	Band of smooth muscle between mucosa and submucosa, more prominent in smaller airways	12.8
	Segmental bronchi lack submucosal glands and have only occasional plates of supporting cartilage	12.10, 12.26
	Bronchioles are less than 1mm in diameter and lack cartilage and submucosal glands	12.11
	Distal airways have fewer goblet cells but do have Clara cells (produce surfactant components, act as stem cells and have role in detoxifying noxious agents)	12.11, 12.12, 12.26
Lung parenchyma	Respiratory bronchioles have alveoli in their walls and branch to form alveolar ducts and terminate in alveolar sacs	12.12, 12.26
	Alveoli are small air-filled pouches with flattened pneumocytes and rich capillary network—site of gas exchange (thin blood–air barrier)	12.12–12.16
	Type I pneumocytes are very flat and attenuated, whilst type II pneumocytes are rounded cells which produce surfactant	12.15–12.16
Lung vasculature	Dual circulation: • Pulmonary circulation supplies deoxygenated blood • Bronchial circulation perfuses lung tissue with oxygenated blood from systemic circulation	12.22, 12.23
Pleura	Pleural cavities are lined by mesothelium and contain a small volume of serous fluid for lubrication during the movements of respiration	12.24
	Visceral and parietal layers are separated by a potential space	

13 Oral tissues

INTRODUCTION

The digestive process commences in the oral cavity with the ingestion, fragmentation and moistening of food but, in addition to its digestive role, the oral cavity is involved in speech, facial expression, sensory reception and breathing. The major structures of the oral cavity, the ***lips, teeth, tongue, oral mucosa*** and the associated salivary glands, participate in all these functions.

Mastication or chewing is the process by which ingested food is made suitable for swallowing. Chewing involves not only coordinated movements of the mandible and the cutting and grinding action of the teeth, but also activity of the lips and tongue, which continually redirect food between the occlusal surfaces of the teeth. The watery component of saliva moistens and lubricates the masticatory process, while salivary mucus helps to bind the food bolus ready for swallowing.

The entire oral cavity is lined by a protective mucous membrane, the ***oral mucosa,*** which contains many sensory receptors, including the taste receptors of the tongue. The epithelium of the oral mucosa is of the stratified squamous type, which tends to be keratinised in areas subject to considerable friction such as the palate. The oral epithelium is supported by dense collagenous tissue, the ***lamina propria.*** In highly mobile areas such as the soft palate and floor of the mouth, the lamina propria is connected to the underlying muscle by loose submucosal supporting tissue. In contrast, in areas where the oral mucosa overlies bone, such as the ***hard palate*** and tooth-bearing ridges, the lamina propria is tightly bound to the periosteum by a relatively dense fibrous submucosa. Throughout the oral mucosa, numerous small ***accessory salivary glands*** of both serous and mucous types are distributed in the submucosa.

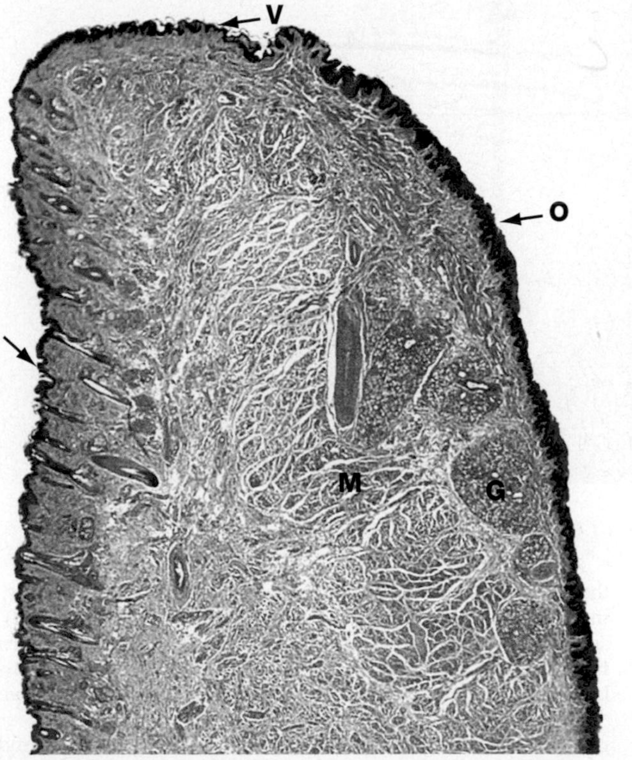

FIG. 13.1 Lip
H&E (LP)

Fig. 13.1 illustrates a midline section through a human lower lip, the bulk of which is made up of bundles of circumoral skeletal muscle **M** seen in transverse section. The external surface of the lip is covered by hair-bearing skin **S** which passes through a transition zone to merge with the oral mucosa **O** of the inner surface. The transition zone constitutes the free ***vermilion border*** of the lip **V**, and derives its colour from the richly vascular dermis, which here has only a thin, lightly keratinised epidermal covering. The free border is highly sensitive due to its rich sensory innervation. Since the vermilion border is devoid of sweat and sebaceous glands, it requires continuous moistening by saliva to prevent cracking. The oral mucosa covering the inner surface of the lip has a thick stratified squamous epithelium and the underlying submucosa contains numerous accessory salivary glands **G** of serous, mucous and mixed seromucous types.

Cancers of the mouth

Sunlight-induced damage and cancers such as squamous cell carcinoma are common on the exposed and unpigmented vermilion borders of the lips, particularly with increasing age.

Squamous cancers of the oral mucosa, including tongue (see e-Fig. 13.1), are strongly associated with tobacco use and with alcohol.

There are often preceding premalignant (dysplastic) changes in the epithelium (see e-Fig. 13.2). These are seen clinically as thickened white (leukoplakia) or red/white patches (erythroleukoplakia) in the mucosa.

G accessory salivary glands **M** skeletal muscle **O** oral mucosa **S** skin **V** vermilion border

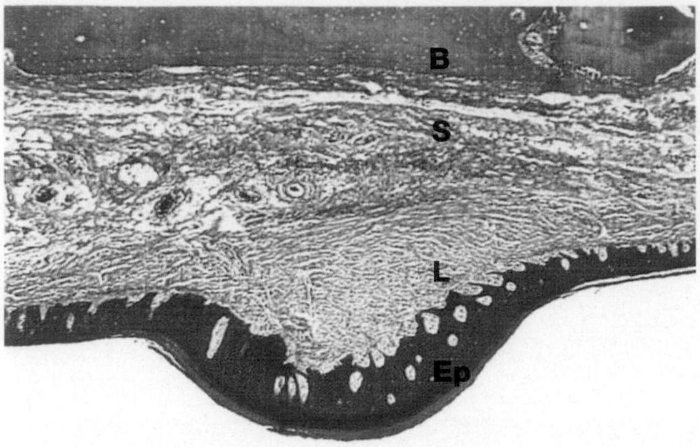

FIG. 13.2 Palatal mucosa, monkey H&E (LP)

Like the rest of the mouth, the ***palate*** (Fig. 13.2) is covered by a thick stratified squamous epithelium **Ep** supported by a tough, densely collagenous lamina propria **L**. To assist mastication, the palatal mucosa is thrown up into transverse folds or ***rugae***, one of which is shown in this micrograph. The mucosa of the hard palate is bound down to the underlying bone **B** by relatively dense submucosal tissue **S** containing a few accessory salivary glands.

In rodents and many other mammals with a coarse diet, the surface epithelium of particularly exposed areas is keratinised for extra protection, as in this specimen taken from a monkey.

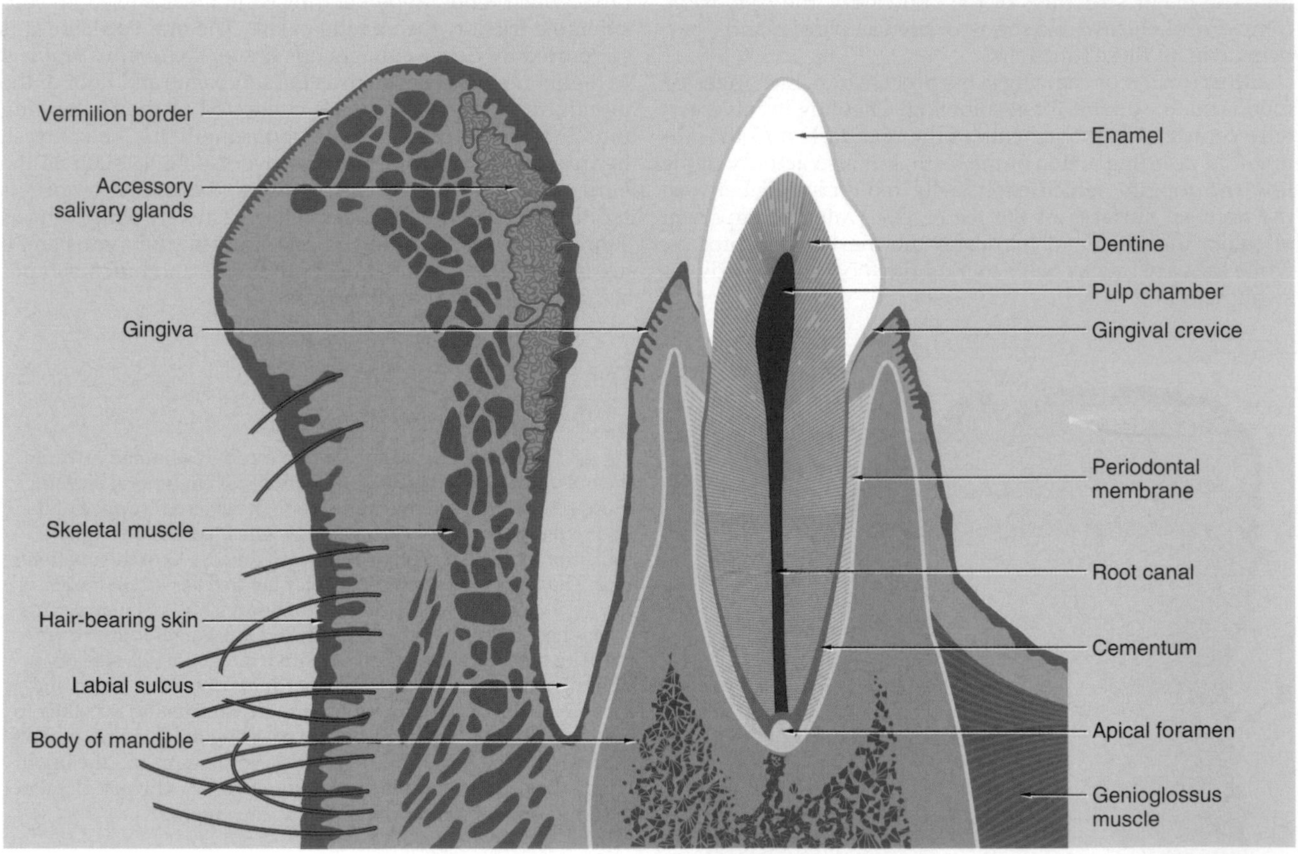

FIG. 13.3 Lip and tooth

Fig. 13.3 is a drawing of a section through the lower jaw near the midline and illustrates the general arrangement of the lip and a tooth with its supporting structures. Each tooth may be grossly divided into two segments, the ***crown*** and the ***root***; the crown is that portion which projects into the oral cavity and is protected by a layer of highly mineralised ***enamel*** which covers it entirely. The bulk of the tooth is made up of ***dentine***, a mineralised tissue which has a similar chemical composition to bone. The dentine has a central ***pulp cavity*** or ***chamber*** containing the ***dental pulp*** which consists of specialised supporting tissue containing many sensory nerve fibres. The tooth root is embedded in a bony ridge in the jaw called the ***alveolar ridge***; the tooth socket is known as the ***alveolus***. At the lip or cheek (***buccal***) aspect of the alveolus, the bony plate is generally thinner than at the tongue (***palatal***) aspect. The root of the tooth is invested by a thin layer of ***cementum*** which is connected to the bone of the socket by a thin fibrous layer called the ***periodontal ligament*** or ***periodontal membrane***.

The oral mucosa covering the upper part of the alveolar ridge is called the ***gingiva*** and, at the junction of the crown and root of the tooth (the neck of the tooth), the gingiva forms a tight protective cuff around the tooth. The potential space between the gingival cuff and the enamel of the crown is called the ***gingival crevice***. All of the tissues which surround and support the tooth are collectively known as the ***periodontium***.

B bone **C** cementum **D** dentine **E** enamel **Ep** epithelium **L** lamina propria **P** pulp cavity **S** submucosa

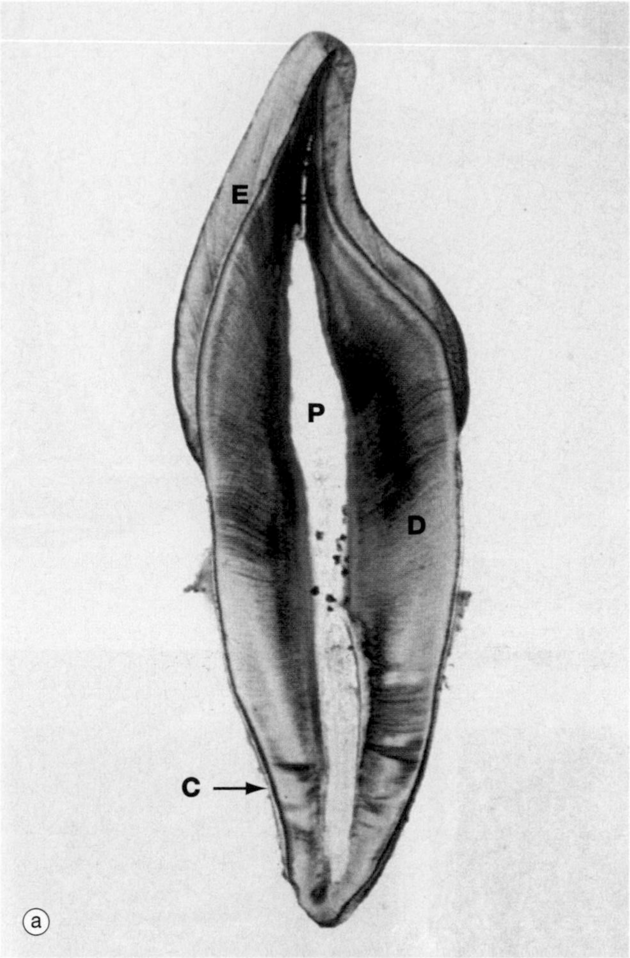

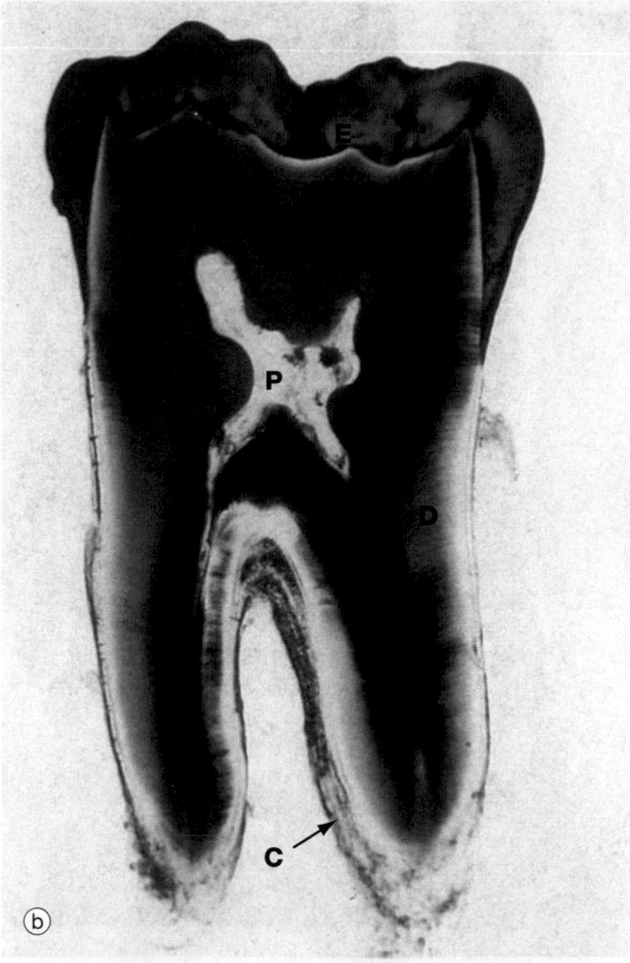

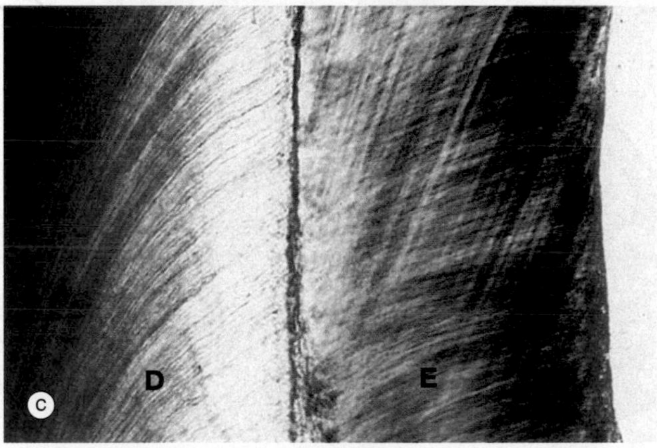

FIG. 13.4 Tooth structure
Undecalcified sections, unstained (a) LP (b) LP (c) (HP)

These undecalcified sections, cut with a diamond wheel, demonstrate the arrangement of the calcified tissues of an upper central incisor tooth (Fig. 13.4a), and a lower molar tooth (Fig. 13.4b). Fig. 13.4c demonstrates the tissues of the crown at high magnification.

The ***dentine*** **D**, which forms the bulk of the crown and root, is composed of a calcified organic matrix similar to that of bone.

The inorganic component constitutes a somewhat larger proportion of the matrix of dentine than that of bone and exists mainly in the form of ***hydroxyapatite crystals***. Teeth are thus harder than bone. From the pulp cavity **P**, minute parallel tubules called ***dentine tubules*** radiate to the periphery of the dentine.

The crown is covered by ***enamel*** **E**, a translucent substance composed of parallel ***enamel rods*** or ***prisms*** of highly calcified material, cemented together by an almost equally calcified ***interprismatic material***.

The root is invested by a thin layer of ***cementum*** **C** which is generally thicker towards the apex of the root. The cementum is an amorphous calcified tissue into which the fibres of the periodontal membrane are anchored.

The morphological form of the tooth crown and roots varies considerably in different parts of the mouth; nevertheless, the basic arrangement of the dental tissues is the same in all teeth.

In humans, the ***primary*** (***deciduous***) ***dentition*** consists of 20 teeth comprising two ***incisors***, one ***canine*** and two ***molars*** in each quadrant. These begin to be formed at the age of 6 weeks during fetal development and they erupt between the ages of 6 and 30 months after birth. Between the ages of 6 and 12 years, the deciduous teeth are succeeded by permanent teeth, namely two incisors, one canine and two ***premolars*** in each quadrant. Distal to these will develop three permanent molars which have no primary precursors; the first permanent molar erupts at age 6, the second at age 12 and the third (wisdom tooth) at age 17 to 21 years. The sharp points found on the posterior teeth are known as ***cusps***.

Tooth decay (caries)

Oral bacteria form ***plaque*** in crevices between teeth and indentations of the teeth. The bacteria metabolise sugar to organic acids which erode the adjacent enamel and then the dentine. Eventually, destruction extends into the pulp space, which becomes infected (***pulpitis***). There is pain and ultimately the tooth is lost.

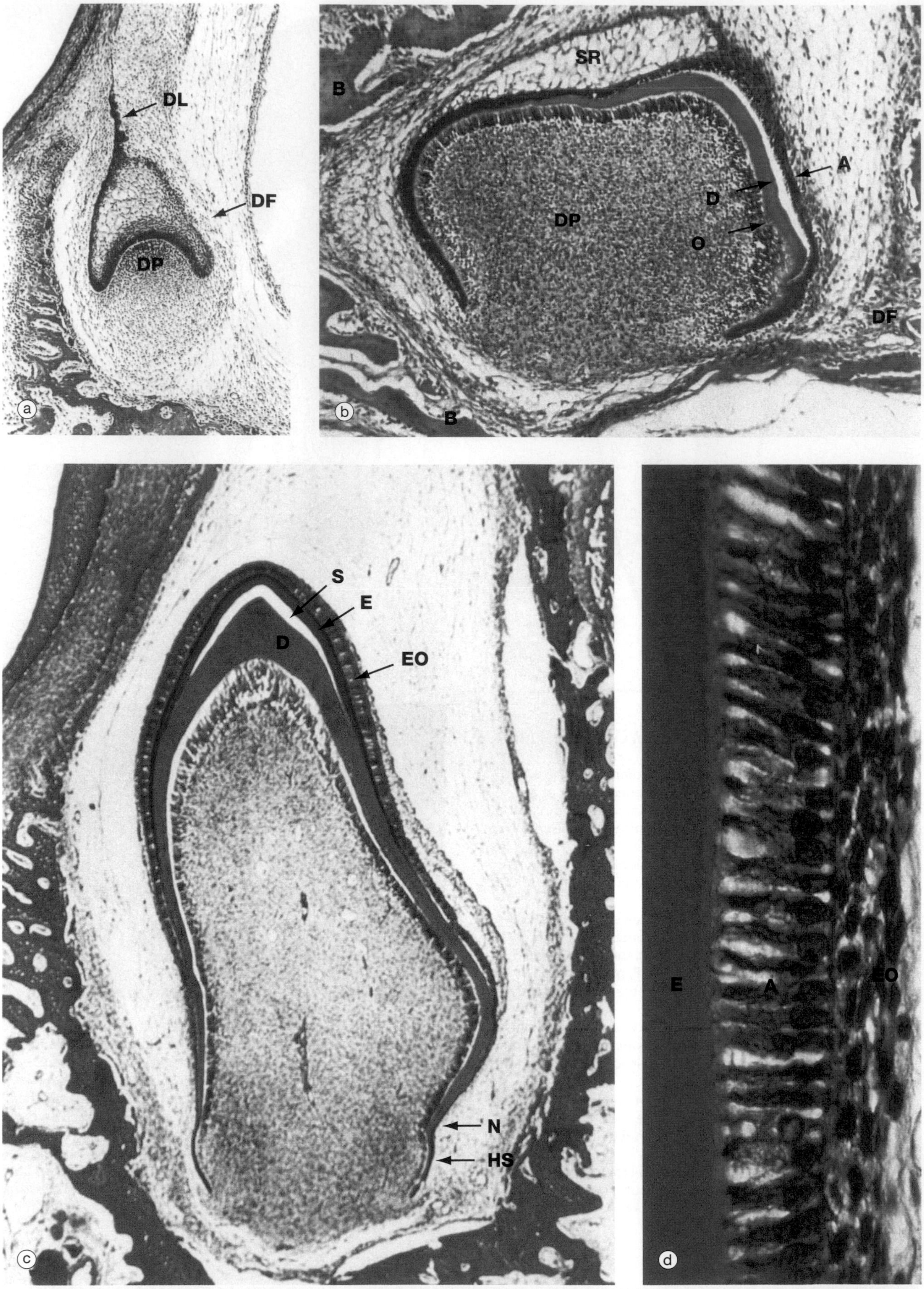

FIG. 13.5 Tooth development *(caption opposite)*
(a) H&E, cap stage (LP) (b) H&E, bell stage (MP) (c) H&E, onset of root development (LP) (d) H&E, ameloblasts (HP)

A ameloblasts **B** bone **D** dentine **DF** dental follicle **DL** dental lamina **DP** dental papilla **E** enamel **EO** enamel organ **HS** epithelial sheath of Hertwig **N** neck of tooth **O** odontoblasts **S** space (enamel) **SR** stellate reticulum

FIG. 13.5 Tooth development *(illustrations opposite)*
(a) H&E, cap stage (LP) (b) H&E, bell stage (MP) (c) H&E, onset of root development (LP) (d) H&E, ameloblasts (HP)

This series of micrographs illustrates the important stages of tooth development. The tissues of the teeth are derived from two embryological sources. The enamel is of epithelial (***ectodermal***) origin, while the dentine, cementum, pulp and periodontal ligament are of mesenchymal (***mesodermal***) origin. The first evidence of tooth development in humans occurs at 6 weeks of fetal life with the proliferation of a horseshoe-shaped epithelial ridge from the basal layer of the primitive oral epithelium into the underlying mesoderm in the position of the future jaws; this is known as the ***dental lamina***. In each quadrant of the mouth, the lamina then develops four globular swellings which will become the ***enamel organs*** of the future deciduous central and lateral incisors, canines and first molar teeth. Subsequently, the dental lamina proliferates backwards in each arch, successively giving rise to the enamel organs of the future second deciduous molar and the three permanent molars. The permanent successors of the deciduous teeth will later develop from enamel organs which bud off from the inner aspect of the enamel organs of their deciduous predecessors.

The primitive mesenchyme immediately subjacent to the developing enamel organ proliferates to form a cellular mass, the ***dental papilla* DP**. At the same time, the enamel organ becomes progressively cap-shaped, as seen in Fig. 13.5a, enveloping the dental papilla. During the cap stage, the cells lining the concave face of the enamel organ in contact with the dental papilla begin to differentiate into tall columnar cells, ***ameloblasts***, which will be responsible for the production of enamel. This, in turn, induces the differentiation of a layer of columnar ***odontoblasts***, the future dentine-producing cells, in the apical region of the dental papilla. The interface between the differentiating ameloblast and odontoblast layers marks the position and shape of the future junction between enamel and dentine.

As the enamel organ develops further, it assumes a characteristic bell shape as seen in Fig. 13.5b, the free edge of the 'bell' proliferating so as to determine the eventual shape of the tooth crown. Meanwhile, the cells of the main bulk of the enamel organ become large and star-shaped, forming the ***stellate reticulum* SR**, the extracellular matrix of which is rich in glycosaminoglycans. Between the stellate reticulum and ameloblast layer, two or three layers of flattened cells form the ***stratum intermedium***, while the outer surface of the enamel organ consists of a simple cuboidal epithelium called the ***external enamel epithelium***. By the cap stage of development, the dental lamina **DL** connecting the enamel organ with the oral mucosa has become fragmented and, around the whole developing bud, a condensation of mesenchyme forms the ***dental follicle* DF** which will eventually become the periodontal ligament.

As ameloblasts and odontoblasts differentiate at the tip of the crown, a layer of dentine matrix is progressively laid down between the ameloblast and odontoblast layers. As the odontoblasts retreat, each leaves a long cytoplasmic extension, the ***odontoblastic process***, embedded within the dentine matrix, thereby forming the ***dentine tubules***. Dentine matrix has a similar biochemical composition to that of bone and undergoes calcification in a similar fashion. Deposition of dentine induces the production of enamel by the adjacent ameloblasts. Each retreating ameloblast lays down a column of enamel matrix which then undergoes mineralisation, resulting in the formation of a dense prismatic structure as described below. With the deposition of dentine and enamel, the overlying stellate reticulum atrophies and the enamel organ is much reduced in thickness. These changes are well demonstrated in Fig. 13.5b. A thin layer of dentine **D** has been laid down by the underlying odontoblastic layer **O** of the highly cellular dental papilla **DP**. The ameloblastic layer **A** is about to lay down enamel in the space next to the dentine; note that in this area, the stellate reticulum has disappeared. Note also the surrounding dental follicle **DF** and early formation of cancellous bone **B**.

By the time dentine and enamel formation is well underway at the incisal edge or tips of the cusps (as the case may be), the enamel organ will have fully outlined the shape of the whole tooth crown. This is the case in Fig. 13.5c, the neck of the tooth **N** marking the junction of crown and root. A thin, densely stained layer of poorly mineralised enamel **E** can be seen, covered at its external surface by the now much thinner enamel organ **EO**. The unstained space **S** between this and the underlying dentine **D** represents fully mineralised enamel laid down earlier but dissolved away during tissue preparation.

Although enamel production is confined to the crown, the rim of the 'bell' of the enamel organ nevertheless continues to proliferate, inducing dentine formation and thereby determining the shape of the tooth root. This part of the enamel organ, known as the ***epithelial sheath of Hertwig* HS**, disintegrates once the outline of the root is completed. The cementum which later forms on the root surface is derived from the dental follicle. As the dentine of the crown and root are progressively laid down, the dental papilla shrinks and eventually becomes the dental pulp contained within the pulp chamber and root canals.

Growth of the tooth root is one of the principal mechanisms of tooth eruption and root formation is not completed until some time after the crown has fully erupted into the oral cavity.

Fig. 13.5d illustrates the characteristic appearance of ameloblasts. Active ameloblasts **A** are tall columnar epithelial cells which form a single layer apposed to the forming surface of the enamel **E**. Each ameloblast elaborates a column of organic enamel matrix which undergoes progressive mineralisation by the deposition of calcium phosphate, mainly in the form of hydroxyapatite crystals. Fully formed enamel contains less than 1% organic material and is the hardest and most dense tissue in the body.

Mature enamel consists of highly calcified ***enamel prisms*** separated by ***interprismatic enamel***, consisting of similar crystals orientated in a different direction. Each prism extends from the dentino-enamel junction to the enamel surface. The prisms are made up of groups of long, thin, parallel crystallites of hydroxyapatite, covered by a surface layer of organic material. Underlying the ameloblast layer are several layers of cells, also of epithelial origin, which constitute the remainder of the enamel organ **EO**. As enamel formation progresses, the enamel organ becomes much reduced in thickness compared with earlier stages of its development. At tooth eruption, the enamel organ, including the ameloblasts, degenerates leaving the enamel exposed to the hostile oral environment, completely incapable of regeneration.

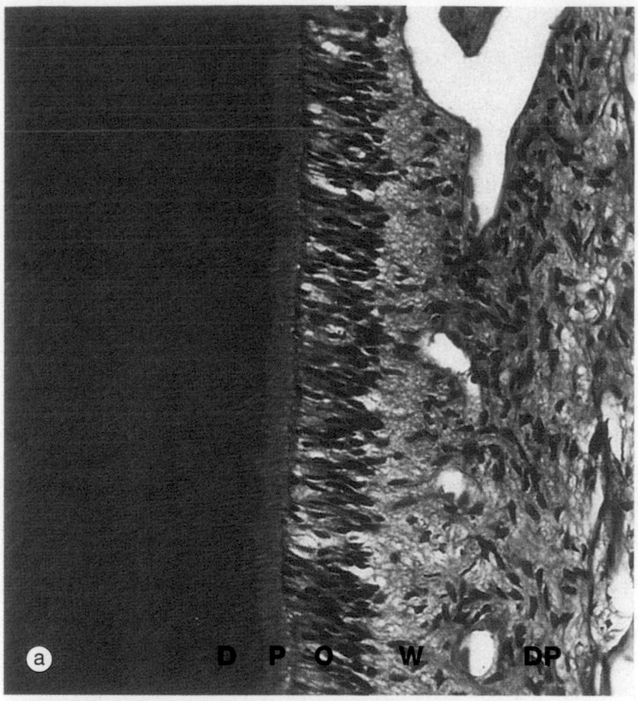

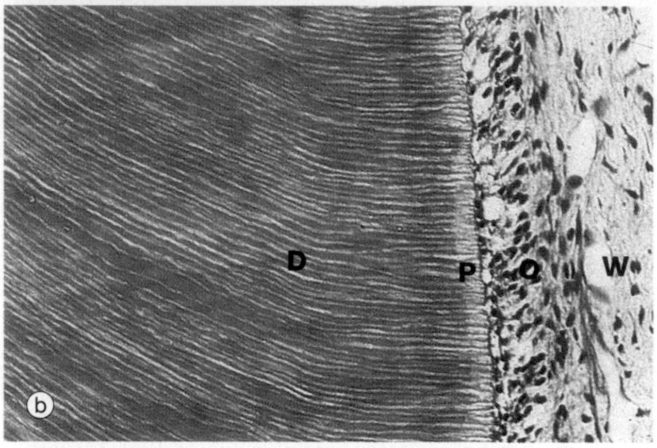

FIG. 13.6 Odontoblasts and dentine
Decalcified sections (a) H&E (MP) (b) H&E (MP)

Dentine, the dense calcified tissue which forms the bulk of the tooth, is broadly similar to bone in composition but is more highly mineralised and thus much harder than bone. The cells responsible for dentine formation, the ***odontoblasts***, differentiate as a single layer of tall columnar cells on the surface of the ***dental papilla***, apposed to the ***ameloblast*** layer of the ***enamel organ***. The odontoblasts initiate tooth formation by deposition of organic dentine matrix between the odontoblastic and ameloblastic layers; calcification of this dentine matrix then induces enamel formation by ameloblasts (see Fig. 13.5). Odontoblasts continue to produce dentine which subsequently calcifies. Unlike ameloblasts, each odontoblast leaves behind a slender cytoplasmic extension, the ***odontoblastic process***, within a fine dentine tubule. When dentine formation is complete, the dentine is thus pervaded by parallel odontoblastic processes radiating from the odontoblast layer on the dentinal surface of the reduced dental papilla which now constitutes the ***dental pulp***. After tooth formation is complete, a small amount of less organised ***secondary dentine*** continues to be laid down, resulting in the progressive obliteration of the pulp cavity with advancing age.

Figs 13.6a and b illustrate active odontoblasts **O** forming a pseudostratified layer of columnar cells at the dentine surface. Parallel dentine tubules containing odontoblastic processes extend through a narrow pale-stained zone of uncalcified dentine matrix called ***predentine*** **P** into the mature dentine **D**; the dentine tubules are best seen in Fig. 13.6b. Underlying the odontoblastic layer, a relatively acellular layer called the ***cell-free zone of Weil*** **W** gives way to the highly cellular dental pulp **DP**.

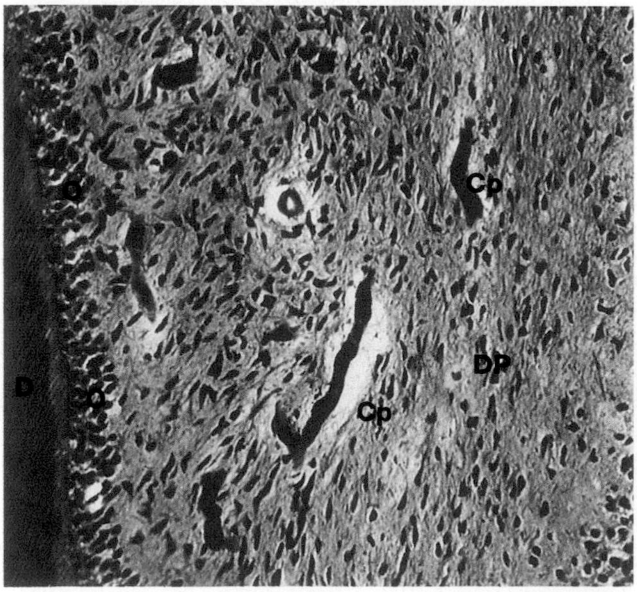

FIG. 13.7 Dental pulp
Decalcified section, H&E (MP)

The dental pulp **DP** (Fig. 13.7) consists of a delicate supporting/connective tissue resembling primitive mesenchyme (see Fig. 4.2); it contains numerous ***stellate fibroblasts***, reticulin fibres, fine collagen fibres and plentiful ground substance. The pulp contains a rich network of thin-walled capillaries **Cp** supplied by arterioles which enter the pulp canal from the ***periodontal membrane***, usually via one foramen at each root apex. The pulp is also richly innervated by a plexus of myelinated nerve fibres from which fine, non-myelinated branches extend into the odontoblastic layer. Despite the acute sensitivity of dentine, nerve fibres are rarely demonstrable and the mechanism of sensory reception is unknown; it has been suggested that the odontoblastic processes may act as sensory receptors. Odontoblasts **O** and the edge of the dentine **D** can also be identified.

B bone **C** cementum **CE** crevicular epithelium **CEJ** cemento-enamel junction **Cp** capillary **D** dentine **Db** organic debris **DP** dental pulp **FG** free gingiva **M** Malassez rest **O** odontoblasts **P** predentine **PM** periodontal membrane **W** Weil zone

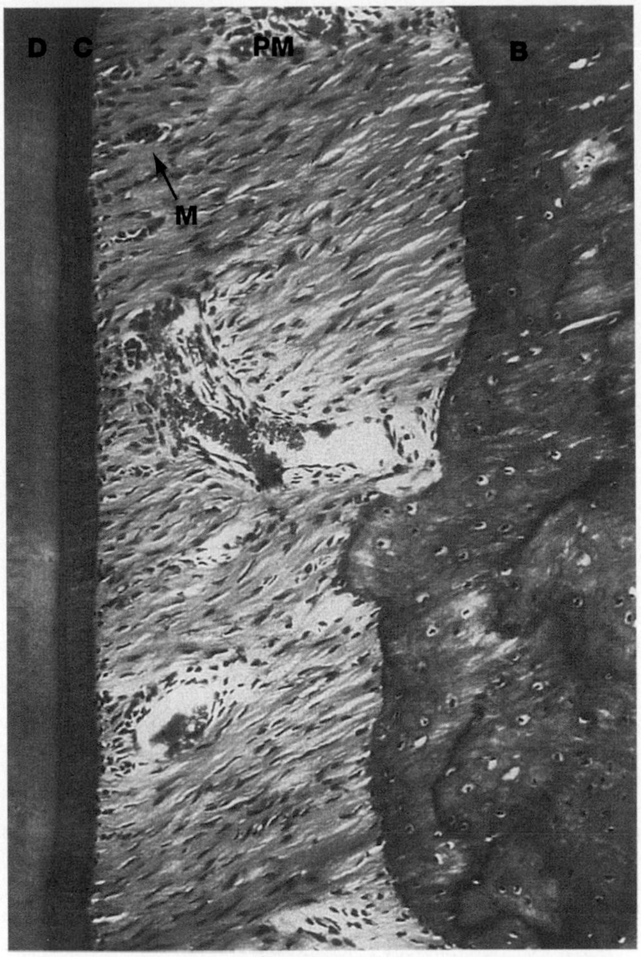

FIG. 13.8 Periodontal membrane and cementum
Decalcified section, H&E (MP)

The periodontal membrane **PM** (Fig. 13.8) forms a thin fibrous attachment between the tooth root and the alveolar bone. The dentine **D** comprising the root is covered by a thin layer of cementum **C** which is elaborated by cells called ***cementocytes***, lying on the surface of the cementum. Cementum consists of a dense, calcified organic material, similar to the matrix of bone, and is generally acellular. Towards the root apex, the cementum layer becomes progressively thicker and irregular and cementocytes are often entrapped in lacunae within the cementum.

The periodontal membrane consists of dense collagenous tissue. The collagen fibres, known as ***Sharpey's fibres***, run obliquely downwards from their attachment in the alveolar bone **B** to their anchorage in the cementum at a more apical position on the root surface. The periodontal membrane thus acts as a sling for the tooth within its socket, permitting slight movements which cushion the impact of chewing. The points of attachment of the collagen fibres in both cementum and bone are in a constant state of reorganisation to accommodate changing functional stresses upon the teeth. Osteoclastic resorption is often seen at one aspect of a tooth socket and complementary osteoblastic deposition at the opposite side, thus indicating bodily movement of the tooth through the bone; this is the mechanism which permits tooth movement during orthodontic treatment.

The periodontal membrane is richly supplied by blood vessels and nerves from the surrounding alveolar bone, the apical region and the gingiva. Small clumps of epithelial cells are often found scattered throughout the periodontal membrane; these cells are remnants of Hertwig's sheath (see Fig. 13.5) and are known as ***epithelial rests of Malassez*** **M**.

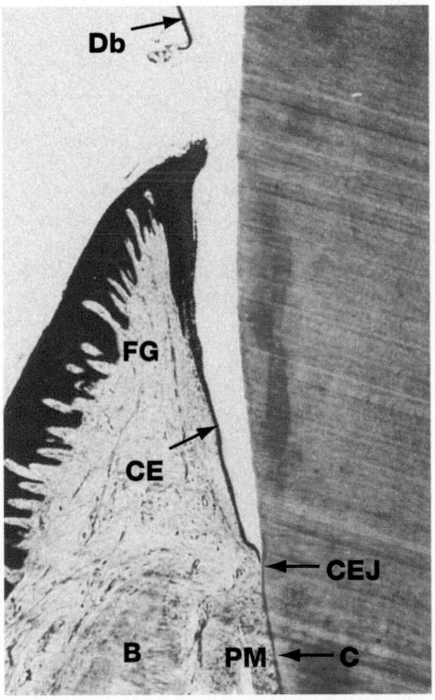

FIG. 13.9 Gingival attachment
Decalcified section, H&E (HP)

Fig. 13.9 shows the relationship of the gingiva (gum) to the neck of the tooth. During tissue preparation, the enamel has been completely dissolved from the surface of the crown, but the extent of the outer surface of the enamel can be visualised by shreds of remaining organic debris **Db** which had been adherent to the tooth surface.

The gingiva may be divided into the ***attached gingiva***, which provides a protective covering to the upper alveolar bone **B**, and the ***free gingiva*** **FG**, which forms a cuff around the enamel at the neck of the tooth. Between the enamel and the free gingiva is a potential space, the ***gingival crevice***, which extends from the tip of the free gingiva to the cemento-enamel junction **CEJ**.

The thick stratified squamous epithelium which constitutes the oral aspect of the gingiva undergoes abrupt transition at the tip of the free gingiva to form a thin layer of epithelial cells, tapering to only two or three cells thick at the base of the gingival crevice. This ***crevicular epithelium*** **CE** is easily breached by pathogenic organisms and the underlying supporting tissue is thus frequently infiltrated by lymphocytes and plasma cells. Collagen fibres of the ***periodontal membrane*** **PM** radiate from the cementum **C** near the cemento-enamel junction into the dense supporting tissue of the free gingiva; these fibres, together with circular fibres surrounding the neck of the tooth, maintain the role of the gingiva as a protective cuff.

Periodontitis and acquired odontogenic cysts

Bacterial colonisation of the crevice causes local inflammation called periodontitis. This damages the gingival attachment, which tends to migrate deeper into the alveolus (jaw), with permanent loss of gingiva and bone. This exposes dentine, causing tooth sensitivity and pain, especially upon temperature changes from cold drinks or ice. There is eventual loosening and tooth loss, a major cause of tooth loss in adults.

Inflammation can extend to the apex of the tooth. Here, the epithelial rests of Malassez can proliferate, becoming cystic and forming a ***periapical*** or ***radicular cyst*** (see e-Fig. 13.3).

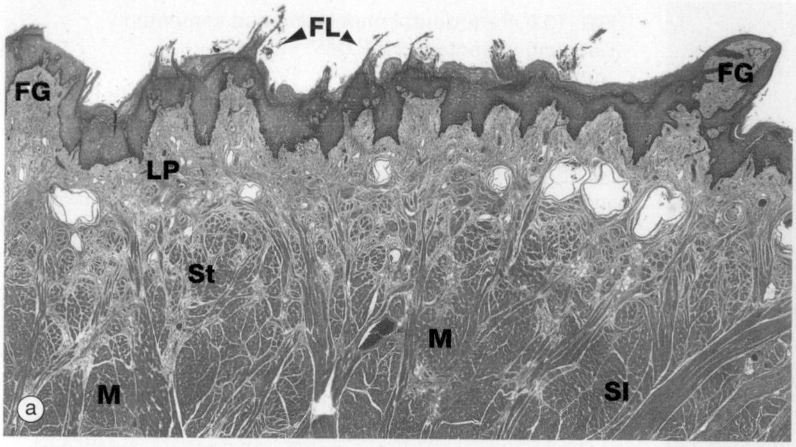

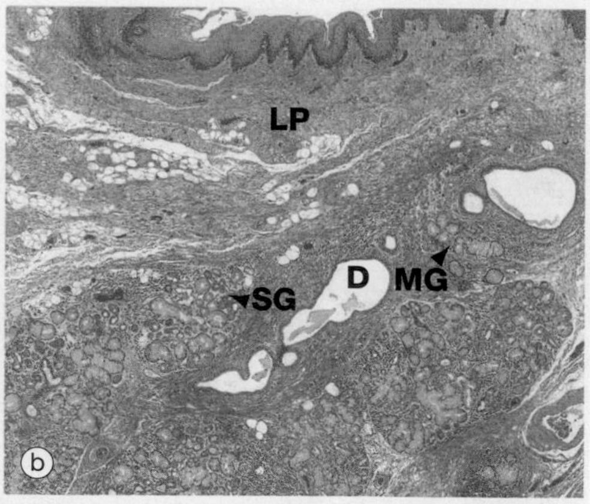

FIG. 13.10 Tongue, anterior two-thirds
(a) H&E (LP) (b) H&E (MP)

The tongue is a muscular organ covered by oral mucosa which is specialised for manipulating food, general sensory reception and the special sensory function of taste. The tongue is also vital for speech.

A V-shaped groove, the ***sulcus terminalis***, demarcates the anterior two-thirds of the tongue from the posterior one-third. The mucosa of the anterior two-thirds is formed into papillae of three types. The most numerous, the ***filiform papillae***, appear as short 'bristles' macroscopically. Among them are scattered the small red globular ***fungiform papillae***. Six to fourteen large ***circumvallate papillae*** form a row immediately anterior to the sulcus terminalis and these papillae contain most of the taste buds (see Figs 13.12 and 21.1); fungiform papillae **FG** and numerous filiform papillae **FL** are seen in Fig. 13.10a.

Foliate papillae, which are rudimentary in humans, are found in some animal species.

The body of the tongue consists of a mass of interlacing bundles of skeletal muscle fibres **M** which permit an extensive range of tongue movements. Note bundles of skeletal muscle cut in both transverse **St** and longitudinal **Sl** section. The mucous membrane covering the tongue is firmly bound to the underlying muscle by a dense, collagenous lamina propria **LP**, which is continuous with the epimysium of the tongue muscle.

Numerous small serous and mucous accessory salivary glands are scattered throughout the muscle and lamina propria of the tongue and are seen at higher magnification in Fig. 13.10b. In these preparations, the serous glands **SG** are stained strongly, whereas the mucous glands **MG** are pale and poorly stained.

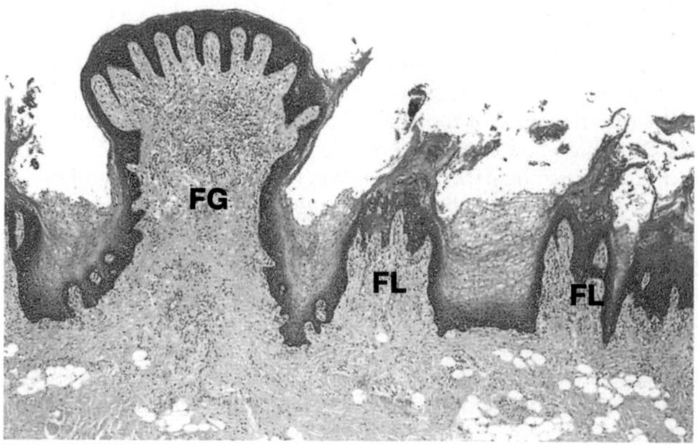

FIG. 13.11 Filiform and fungiform papillae
H&E (LP)

Fig. 13.11 illustrates several filiform papillae **FL** and a fungiform papilla **FG**. Filiform papillae are the most numerous type and consist of a dense supporting tissue core and a heavily keratinised surface projection. Fungiform papillae have a thin non-keratinised epithelium and a richly vascularised supporting tissue core, giving them a red appearance macroscopically among the more numerous whitish filiform papillae.

B taste bud **C** cleft **Cr** crypt **CV** circumvallate papilla **E** epithelium **F** lymphoid follicle **FG** fungiform papilla **FL** filiform papilla **L** lymphoid tissue **LP** lamina propria **M** skeletal muscle **MG** mucous gland **SG** serous gland **Sl** skeletal muscle in longitudinal section **St** skeletal muscle in transverse section **VE** von Ebner gland

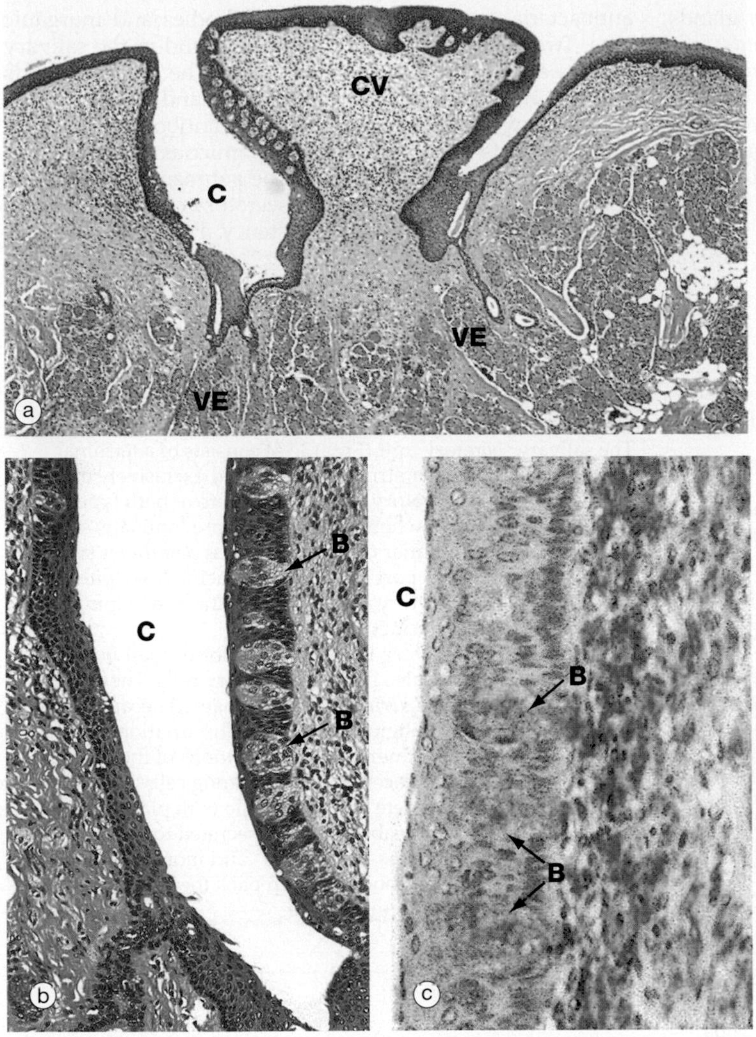

FIG. 13.12 Circumvallate papillae
(a) H&E (LP) (b) H&E (MP)
(c) Immunohistochemistry for NSE (MP)

Circumvallate papillae **CV** are the largest and least common type of papillae on the tongue. They are set into the tongue surface and encircled by a deep cleft **C**. Aggregations of serous glands called ***von Ebner glands*** **VE** open into the base of the circumvallate clefts (Fig. 13.12a), secreting a watery fluid which dissolves food constituents, thus facilitating taste reception. The stratified squamous epithelium lining the papillary wall of the cleft contains numerous ***taste buds*** **B** as shown in Fig. 13.12b (see also Fig. 21.1).

Fig. 13.12c is stained by the immunohistochemical method for the enzyme neurone-specific enolase (NSE). This demonstrates the neural nature of the taste buds **B** and the meshwork of fine axons (stained brown) in the lamina propria underlying the taste buds which subserve taste sensation.

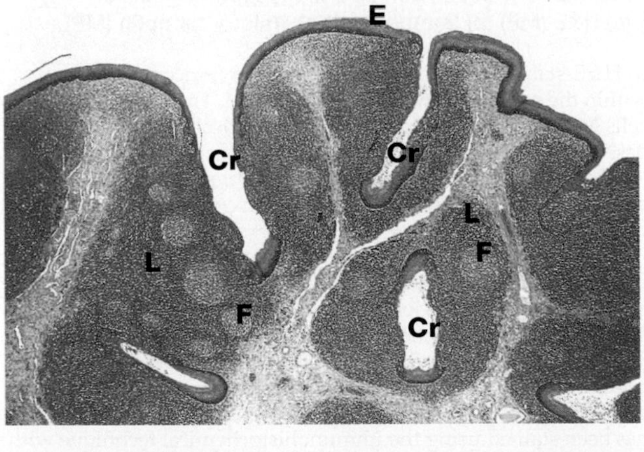

FIG. 13.13 Tongue, posterior third
H&E (LP)

The posterior surface of the tongue (Fig. 13.13) has a relatively smooth stratified squamous epithelium **E** overlying lymphoid tissue **L** containing lymphoid follicles **F**. This lymphoid tissue is the ***lingual tonsil*** and, with the palatine tonsils and adenoids, completes the ***Waldeyer*** ring of lymphoid tissue, guarding the entrance to the gastrointestinal and respiratory tracts. Like the palatine tonsils (see Fig. 11.15), epithelial crypts **Cr** penetrate the lingual tonsil.

Oropharyngeal carcinoma

A specific type of squamous cell carcinoma arises in the epithelial crypts of the tongue base and tonsil. This tumour is driven by high risk human papillomavirus subtypes, most commonly HPV16 and HPV18. p16 immunohistochemistry is used as a surrogate marker for HPV status within the tumours (see e-Figs 13.4a and b). A p16 positive squamous cell carcinoma of the oropharynx will, in general, have a better prognosis than a p16 negative squamous cell carcinoma of the oropharynx. p16 positive squamous cell carcinomas of the oropharynx tend to be treated with chemotherapy and radiotherapy rather than surgery.

SALIVARY GLANDS

Saliva is produced by three pairs of major salivary glands, the ***parotid***, ***submandibular*** and ***sublingual glands***, and numerous minor ***accessory glands*** scattered throughout the oral mucosa. The minor salivary glands secrete continuously and are in general under local control, whereas the major glands mainly secrete in response to parasympathetic activity which is induced by physical, chemical and psychological stimuli. Daily saliva production in humans is 600 to 1500 mL.

Saliva is a hypotonic watery secretion containing variable amounts of mucus, enzymes (principally ***amylase*** and the antibacterial enzyme ***lysozyme***), antibodies and inorganic ions. Two types of secretory cells are found in the salivary glands: ***serous cells*** and ***mucous cells***. The parotid glands consist almost exclusively of serous cells and produce a thin watery secretion rich in enzymes and antibodies. The sublingual glands have predominantly mucous secretory cells and produce a viscid secretion. The submandibular glands contain both serous and mucous secretory cells and produce a secretion of intermediate consistency. The overall composition of saliva varies according to the degree of activity of each of the major gland types.

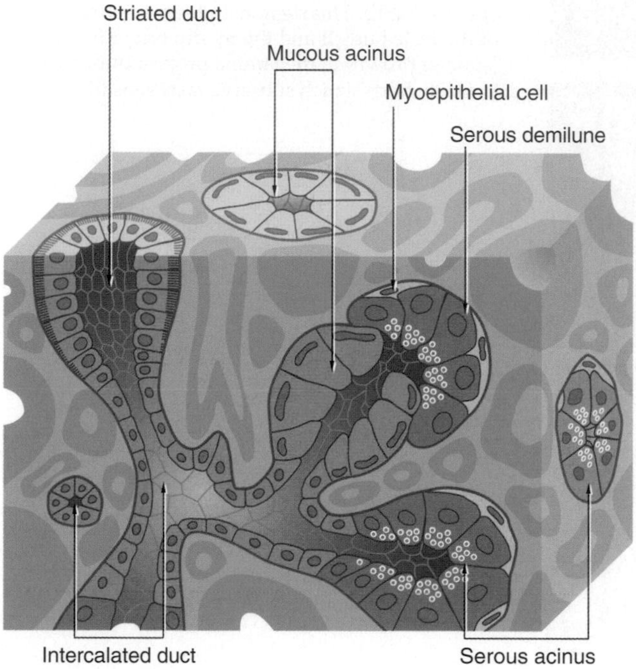

FIG. 13.14 Salivary secretory unit

The salivary secretory unit (Fig. 13.14) consists of a terminal branched tubulo-acinar structure composed exclusively of either serous or mucous secretory cells or a mixture of both types. In mixed secretory units where mucous cells predominate, serous cells often form semilunar caps called ***serous demilunes*** surrounding the terminal part of the mucous acini. Myoepithelial cells embrace the secretory units, their contraction helping to expel the secretory product.

The terminal secretory units merge to form small ***intercalated ducts*** which are also lined by secretory cells. They drain into larger ducts called ***striated ducts***, so named because of their striated appearance by light microscopy. The striations result from the presence of numerous interdigitations of the basal cytoplasmic processes of adjacent columnar lining cells.

The serous cells secrete a fluid isotonic with plasma. In the striated ducts, ions are reabsorbed and secreted to produce hypotonic saliva containing less Na^+ and Cl^- and more K^+ and HCO^- than plasma. The mitochondria which pack the basal processes provide the energy for ion transport.

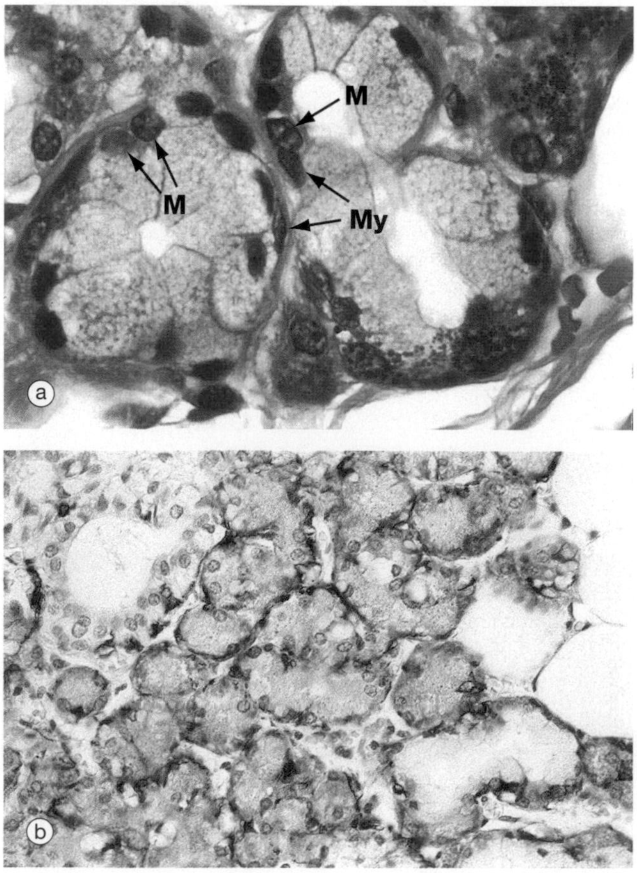

FIG. 13.15 Mucous acinus and myoepithelial cells (a) H&E (MP) (b) Immunohistochemistry for actin (MP)

In H&E-stained preparations, the ***mucigen*** (mucus) granules within the mucous acini are poorly stained. The nuclei of mucous cells **M** are condensed and are characteristically located at the base of the cell near the basement membrane.

Both serous and mucous acini are embraced by contractile cells called ***myoepithelial cells*** which, on contraction, force secretion from the acinar lumen into the duct system.

Myoepithelial cells are located between the basal plasma membranes of secretory cells and the basement membrane. These are flattened cells with long processes which extend around the secretory acinus; in section, they can only be recognised by their flattened nuclei lying within the basement membrane around the acinus. Fig. 13.15a shows the typical appearance of myoepithelial cells **My** embracing mucous acini. In Fig. 13.15b, a similar section has been stained using the immunohistochemical technique with an antibody specific for actin, a microfilament characteristic of muscle cells but not usually found in epithelial cells. The myoepithelial cells are stained brown. Myoepithelial cells also show characteristics of epithelial differentiation, including cytoplasmic cytokeratin intermediate filaments.

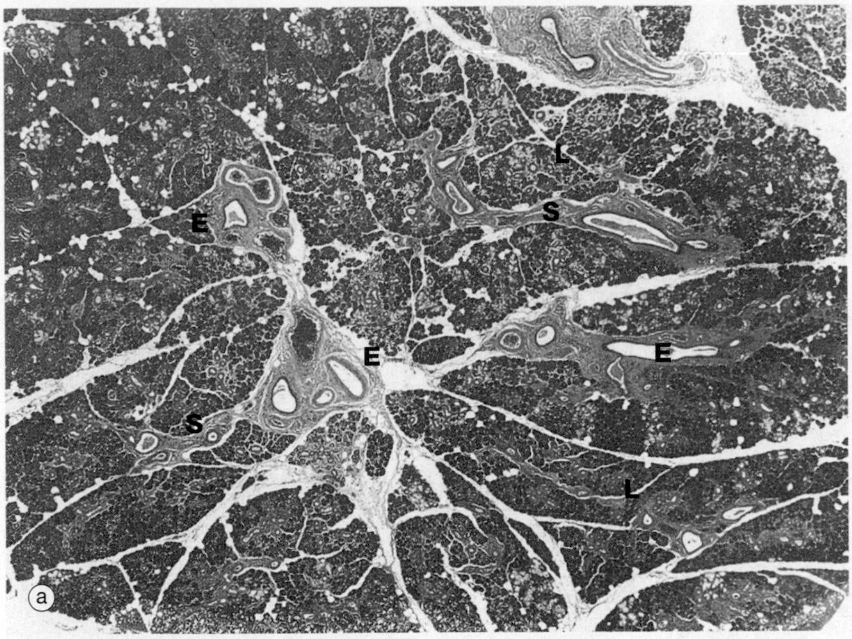

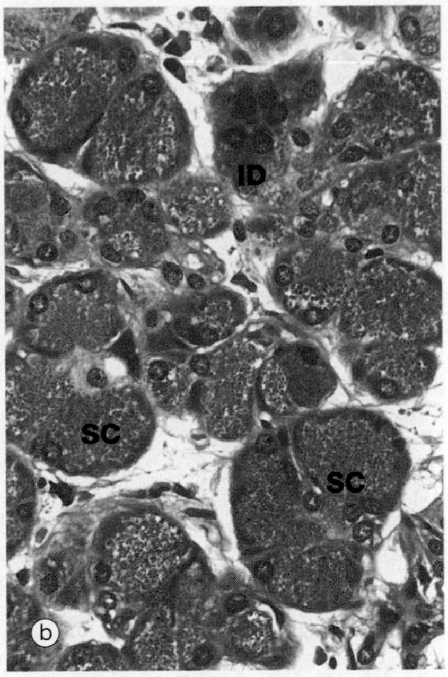

FIG. 13.16 Parotid gland
(a) H&E (LP) (b) Serous acinus and intercalated duct, H&E (MP)

The general architecture of the major salivary glands follows the pattern shown in Fig. 13.16a from the parotid gland. The gland is divided into numerous ***lobules*** **L**, each containing many secretory units. Connective tissue ***septa*** **S** radiate between the lobules from an outer capsule and convey blood vessels, nerves and large ***excretory ducts*** **E**. The parotid gland consists mainly of serous secretory units which are darkly stained in H&E preparations. Fig. 13.16b shows these serous secretory units at higher power. The serous cells **SC** have numerous ***zymogen*** granules. These are strongly stained cytoplasmic granules containing proteins. Their nuclei are rounded with dispersed chromatin and they usually occupy a more central position within the cell (compared to mucus-secreting cells; see Fig. 13.15). In EM sections (not illustrated), a large Golgi apparatus, prominent rough endoplasmic reticulum and mitochondria are found, in common with other protein-secreting cells (see Fig. 15.15, an EM of a pancreatic secretory cell which is ultrastructurally very similar).

An intercalated duct **ID** with a lining of cuboidal secretory cells can be seen.

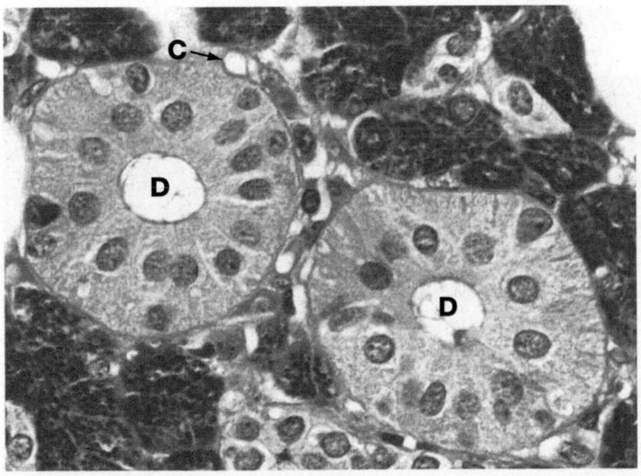

FIG. 13.17 Striated ducts
H&E (HP)

The striated ducts **D** are lined by tall columnar cells with large nuclei located towards the apex of the cell (Fig. 13.17). The basal cytoplasm appears striated, reflecting the presence of basal interdigitations of cytoplasmic processes of adjacent cells and associated columns of mitochondria. This feature greatly extends the area of membrane available for exchange of water and ions, in a similar fashion to the proximal convoluted tubule of the kidney (see Fig. 16.17). The duct epithelium also secretes lysozyme and immunoglobulin (Ig)A. In predominantly serous salivary glands, the striated ducts are larger than in predominantly mucous glands, a feature associated with the role of the striated duct in modifying isotonic basic saliva to produce hypotonic saliva. The sparse supporting tissue between the secretory acini contains a rich network of capillaries **C**.

Salivary gland pathology

Most neoplasms involving the parotid gland are benign. The commonest examples are pleomorphic adenoma (see e-Fig. 13.5) and Warthin's tumour (see e-Fig. 13.6). Most neoplasms involving the minor salivary glands are malignant. Examples include adenoid cystic carcinoma (see e-Fig. 13.7). In this tumour, the malignant cells are ***neurotropic***, meaning that they tend to grow along nerve fibres. This makes excision of these tumours very challenging and recurrence is common. Another common tumour type, most often occurring in the minor salivary glands of the upper lip, is the canalicular adenoma (see e-Fig.13.8).

A mucocoele is a collection of mucus that results from trauma to the minor salivary gland tissue, usually in the lip (see e-Fig 13.9).

C capillary **D** striated duct **ID** intercalated duct **E** excretory duct **L** lobule **M** mucous cell nucleus **My** myoepithelial cell **S** septum **SC** serous cells

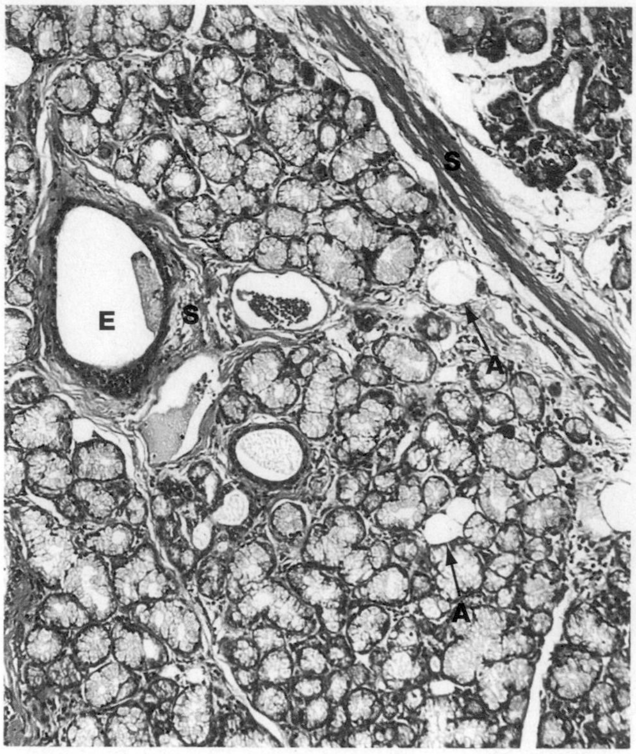

FIG. 13.18 Sublingual gland
H&E (LP)

Mucous acini predominate in the sublingual glands, making them stain very poorly with H&E (Fig. 13.18), in contrast to the serous acini shown in the parotid in Fig. 13.16. A large excretory duct **E** lined by a stratified cuboidal epithelium is present in the fibrous tissue septum **S**. The duct is accompanied by blood vessels and nerves. Note also that this gland contains occasional adipocytes **A**, a feature found in older individuals; the proportion of adipose tissue (fat) in the gland generally increases with increasing age.

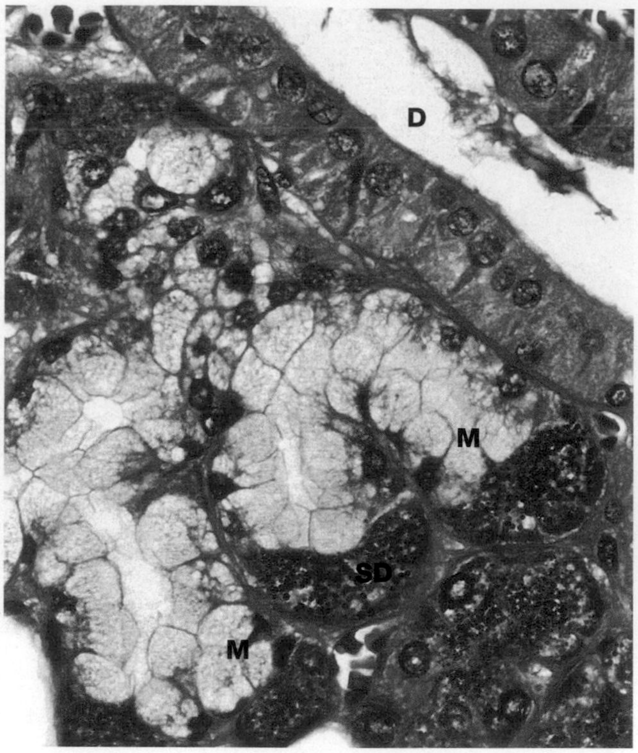

FIG. 13.19 Submandibular gland
H&E (HP)

The submandibular gland (Fig. 13.19) consists of a mixture of serous and mucous secretory units which are often found in the form of mixed seromucous secretory units as shown here. However, both pure serous and pure mucous secretory units are also found in the submandibular gland. The mixed secretory units consist of mucous acini **M** with ***serous demilunes*** **SD**. Running across the corner of the micrograph is a striated duct **D** cut in longitudinal section.

REVIEW

TABLE 13.1 Review of oral tissues

Specialised tissue type	Key features	Functional attributes	Figure
Oral mucosa	Stratified squamous epithelium	Variable site-dependent keratinisation Thicker keratin provides more protection	13.1, 13.2
Teeth	Enamel	Surface layer of closely packed calcium hydroxyapatite crystals formed by an external ameloblast layer; destroyed by tooth eruption	13.3–13.5
	Dentine	Deeper zone of calcified tissue containing numerous fine parallel tubules radiating from odontoblasts which line the pulp cavity and form dentine	13.6
	Pulp	Central core of loose tissue with nerves and vessels supplying odontoblasts	13.7
Tongue	Stratified squamous epithelium with underlying skeletal muscle Minor salivary glands Filiform, fungiform and circumvallate papillae	Skeletal muscle bundles are orientated perpendicular to each other Produce amylase and lubrication Sensory organs of taste	13.10, 13.13 13.10–13.12
Salivary glands	Serous and/or mucinous glands Parotid is the largest gland Others include submandibular, sublingual and minor salivary glands	Serous glands produce amylase Mucinous glands produce mucin to lubricate	13.14–13.19
Tonsillar tissue	Palatine tonsil Lingual tonsil	Located at the back of the mouth (fauces) Located in the base of tongue Lymphoid tissue part of mucosa associated lymphoid tissue (MALT)	11.15 13.13

A adipocyte **D** striated duct **E** excretory duct **M** mucous acinus **S** septum **SD** serous demilune

14 Gastrointestinal tract

INTRODUCTION

The function of the gastrointestinal (GI) system is to break down food for absorption into the body. This process occurs in five main phases: ***ingestion***, ***fragmentation***, ***digestion***, ***absorption*** and ***elimination*** of waste products. Digestion is the process by which food is enzymatically broken down into molecules that are small enough to be absorbed into the circulation. As an example, ingested proteins are first reduced to polypeptides and then further degraded to small peptides and amino acids that can be absorbed.

The gastrointestinal system is essentially a muscular tube lined by a mucous membrane that exhibits regional variations, reflecting the changing functions of the system from mouth to anus. The mucous membrane is protective, secretory, absorptive or a combination of these in different parts of the tract (see Fig. 14.3). The muscle gives strength to the wall of the tract as well as moving the food along. Muscle is arranged somewhat differently in different areas of the tract. Because of its continuity with the external environment, the gastrointestinal system is a potential portal of entry for pathogenic organisms. As a result, the system incorporates a number of defence mechanisms which include prominent aggregations of lymphoid tissue, known as the ***gut-associated lymphoid tissue*** (***GALT***), distributed throughout the tract (see Ch. 11).

FIG. 14.1 Parts of the gastrointestinal tract

Ingestion and initial fragmentation of food occur in the ***oral cavity***, resulting in the formation of a ***bolus*** of food. This is then conveyed to the ***oesophagus*** by the action of the tongue and pharyngeal muscles during swallowing. Secretion of saliva from major and minor ***salivary glands*** (see Ch. 13) aids fragmentation and lubricates the food for swallowing.

The oesophagus conducts food from the oral cavity to the ***stomach*** where fragmentation is completed and digestion begins. Initial digestion, accompanied by the intense muscular action of the stomach wall, converts the stomach contents to a semi-digested liquid called ***chyme***. Chyme is squirted through a muscular sphincter, the ***pylorus***, into the ***duodenum***, the short first part of the small intestine. Digestive enzymes from a large exocrine gland, the ***pancreas***, enter the duodenum together with bile from the liver via the ***common bile duct*** (see Ch. 15). ***Bile*** contains excretory products of liver metabolism, some of which act as emulsifying agents necessary for fat digestion. Duodenal contents pass along the rest of the ***small intestine*** where the process of digestion is completed and the main absorptive phase occurs. The middle segment of the small intestine is called the ***jejunum*** and the distal segment the ***ileum***. There is no distinct anatomical boundary between these parts of the small bowel.

The liquid residue from the small intestine passes through the ***ileocaecal valve*** into the ***large intestine***. Here, water is absorbed from the liquid residue, which becomes progressively more solid as it passes towards the ***anus***. The capacious first part of the large intestine is called the ***caecum***, from which projects a blind-ended sac, the ***appendix***. The next part of the large intestine, the ***colon***, is divided anatomically into ***ascending***, ***transverse***, ***descending*** and ***sigmoid*** segments, although histologically the segments are indistinguishable from one another. The terminal portion of the large intestine, the ***rectum***, is a holding chamber for faeces prior to defaecation via the ***anal canal***.

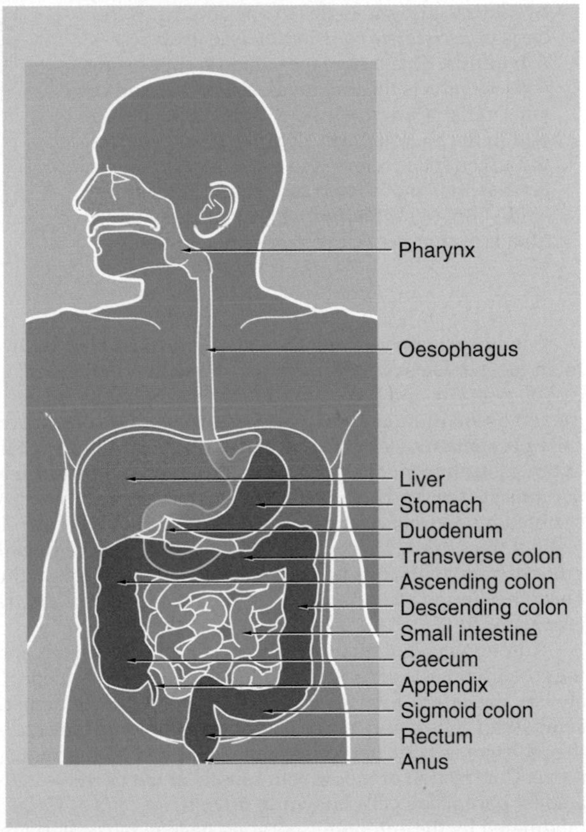

Development of the gastrointestinal tract

The GI tract is derived from ***endoderm***, the innermost of the three layers forming the developing embryo. During fetal life, it is divided into three segments described as the ***foregut*** (with blood supply derived from the coeliac trunk), ***midgut*** (supplied by the superior mesenteric artery) and ***hindgut*** (supplied by the inferior mesenteric artery). These parts develop into the parts of the definitive GI tract. The foregut extends from the oesophagus down to the second part of the duodenum where the common bile duct enters the GI tract. The midgut extends to the junction of the middle and distal thirds of the transverse colon (known as ***Cannon's point***), and the more distal structures are derived from the hindgut. An awareness of the embryological development of the GI tract often facilitates our understanding of disease. For example, visceral pain arising from the different parts of the gut typically localises in distinct parts of the abdomen due to the pattern of its innervation. As a result, foregut pain is typically felt in the ***epigastrium***, midgut pain in the ***periumbilical*** region and hindgut pain in the ***suprapubic*** area. This helps explains why the pain of acute appendicitis tends to begin in the periumbilical area (midgut origin) and only localises to the ***right iliac fossa*** later because of inflammation of the peritoneal surface.

FIG. 14.2 Structure of the gastrointestinal tract

The structure of the gastrointestinal tract (Fig. 14.2) conforms to a general plan that is clearly evident from the oesophagus to the anus. The tract is essentially a muscular tube lined by a mucous membrane. There are minor variations in the arrangement of the muscular component in different parts of the gut, but much more striking are the marked changes in the structure and therefore function of the mucosa in the different regions of the tract.

The gastrointestinal tract has four distinct functional layers: ***mucosa, submucosa, muscularis propria*** and ***adventitia***.

- **Mucosa**. The mucosa is made up of three components: the ***epithelium***, a supporting ***lamina propria*** and a thin smooth muscle layer, the ***muscularis mucosae***, which produces local movement and folding of the mucosa. At four points along the tract, the mucosa undergoes abrupt transition from one form to another: the gastro-oesophageal junction, the gastroduodenal junction, the ileocaecal junction and the rectoanal junction.
- **Submucosa**. This layer of loose collagenous connective tissue supports the mucosa and contains the larger blood vessels, lymphatics and nerves.
- **Muscularis propria**. The muscular wall proper consists of smooth muscle that is usually arranged as an inner circular layer and an outer longitudinal layer. In the stomach only, there is an inner oblique layer of muscle. The action of the two layers, at right angles to one another, is the basis of ***peristaltic contraction*** (see textbox).
- **Adventitia**. This outer layer of loose supporting tissue conducts the major vessels, nerves and contains variable adipose tissue. Where the gut lies within the abdominal cavity (***peritoneal cavity***), the adventitia is referred to as the ***serosa*** (***visceral peritoneum***) and is lined by a simple squamous epithelium (***mesothelium***). Elsewhere, the adventitial layer merges with retroperitoneal tissues.

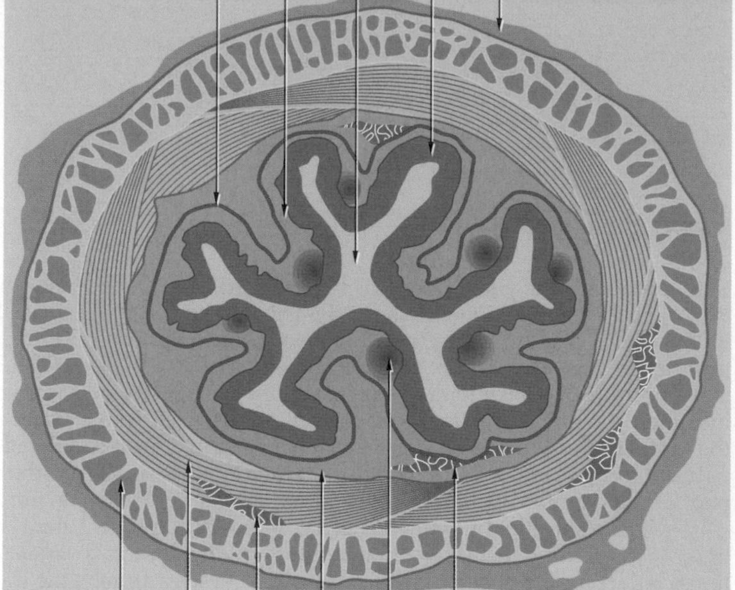

Food is propelled along the gastrointestinal tract by two main mechanisms: voluntary muscular action in the oral cavity, pharynx and upper third of the oesophagus is succeeded by involuntary waves of smooth muscle contraction called ***peristalsis***. Peristalsis and the secretory activity of the entire gastrointestinal system are modulated by the ***autonomic nervous system*** and a variety of hormones, some of which are secreted by neuroendocrine cells located within the gastrointestinal tract itself. These cells constitute a ***diffuse neuroendocrine system***, with cells producing a variety of locally acting hormones found scattered along the whole length of the tract (see also Ch. 17).

Autonomic regulation of certain glandular secretions and the smooth muscle of the gut and its blood vessels is mediated by the ***enteric nervous system***, comprising postganglionic sympathetic fibres and ganglia and postganglionic fibres of the parasympathetic nervous system, supplied by the vagus nerve. Contraction of the smooth muscle of the bowel is initiated by pacemaker cells known as ***interstitial cells of Cajal***, modulated by the autonomic nervous system, particularly the parasympathetic nervous system. As in other organs of the body, parasympathetic efferent fibres synapse with effector neurones in small ganglia located in or close to the organ involved. In the gastrointestinal tract, parasympathetic ganglia are concentrated in plexuses in the wall of the tract. In the submucosa, isolated or small clusters of parasympathetic ganglion cells give rise to postganglionic fibres which supply the mucosal glands and the smooth muscle of the muscularis mucosae. This ***submucosal plexus, Meissner plexus***, also contains postganglionic sympathetic fibres arising from the superior mesenteric plexus. Larger clusters of parasympathetic ganglion cells are found between the two layers of the muscularis propria, the postganglionic fibres mainly supplying the surrounding smooth muscle. This plexus is known as the ***myenteric plexus*** or ***Auerbach plexus***.

Glands are found throughout the tract at various levels in its wall. In some parts of the tract (i.e. stomach, small and large intestine), the mucosa is arranged into glands that secrete mucus for lubrication among other things. In the lower oesophagus and duodenum, glands penetrate the muscularis mucosae to lie in the submucosa. The ***pancreas*** and ***liver*** are large glands draining into the gastrointestinal lumen but lying entirely outside its wall (see Ch. 15).

Motility of the gastrointestinal tract: peristalsis

Peristalsis is the primary mechanism by which food is propelled along most of the length of the GI tract, with some voluntary muscular action involved at both extreme ends of the process. The particular anatomical arrangement of smooth muscle in the wall of the GI tract is specialised to allow constriction of the luminal diameter (via the circular layer of muscle) as well as shortening of its length (via action of the longitudinal muscle layer). The coordination of this very complex mechanism acts to progressively squeeze food along and, in certain sites such as the stomach, also facilitates churning and mixing of the food to aid digestion. The ***autonomic nervous system*** is responsible for the control of this involuntary process, primarily via parasympathetic innervation of the gut.

Disorders affecting peristalsis

Certain disease states and drug treatments can interfere with the normal process of peristalsis. One uncommon condition called Hirschsprung's disease is characterised by failure of migration of ganglion cells into the GI tract, usually in the rectum and distal colon. Patients with this disorder typically present with severe and chronic constipation and may develop progressive dilatation of the bowel. In its most extreme form, absolutely no ganglion cells are present in the bowel, and some patients develop aganglionic megacolon due to this failure of propulsion of food through the bowel.

A variety of drug treatments, including commonly using strong painkillers such as opiates, can produce severe constipation by interfering with normal peristaltic function.

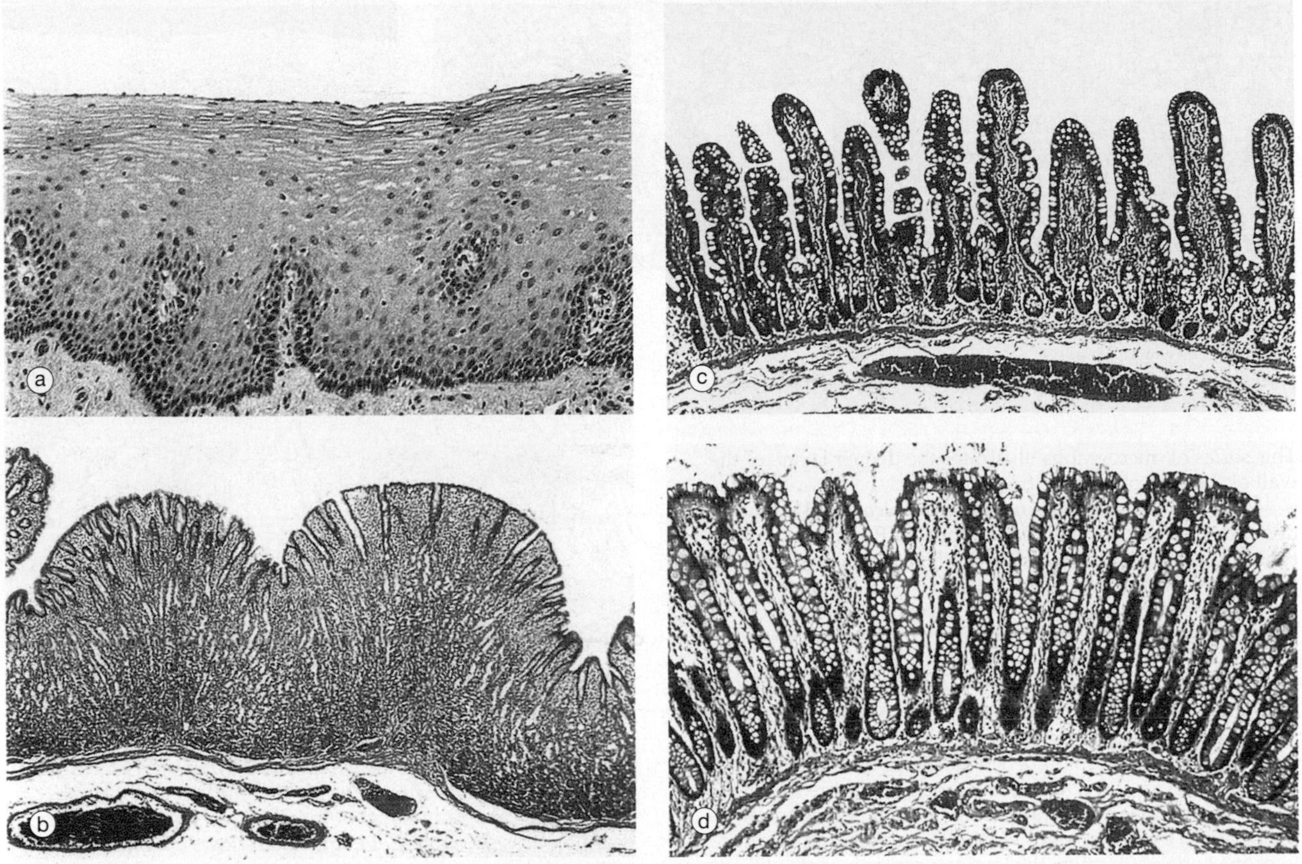

FIG. 14.3 Basic mucosal types in the gastrointestinal tract
(a) Squamous mucosa, H&E (MP) (b) Gastric type secretory mucosa, H&E (LP) (c) Intestinal type absorptive mucosa, H&E (MP) (d) Colorectal type absorptive/protective mucosa, H&E (MP)

Four basic mucosal types are found lining the gastrointestinal tract and these can be classified according to their main function:

- **Protective**. This type is found in the oral cavity, pharynx, oesophagus and anal canal and is illustrated in Fig. 14.3a. The surface epithelium is of stratified squamous type and, although not keratinised in humans, it may be keratinised in some animals that have a coarse diet (e.g. rodents, herbivores). A stratified mucosal lining of this type is well suited to sites of potential frictional trauma, such as that associated with the passage of food during mastication and swallowing, or during the passage of faeces through the anal canal.
- **Secretory**. This type of mucosa occurs only in the stomach and is illustrated in Fig. 14.3b. It consists of long, closely packed tubular glands that are simple or branched, depending on the region of the stomach. These glands act to produce various combinations of acid and digestive enzymes in order to facilitate digestion of food whilst also secreting mucus to protect the mucosa itself from injury.
- **Absorptive**. This mucosal form is typical of the entire small intestine and is illustrated in Fig. 14.3c. The mucosa is arranged into finger-like projections called ***villi*** which serve to dramatically increase surface area of the mucosa, with intervening short glands called ***crypts***. In the duodenum, some crypts extend through the muscularis mucosae to form submucosal glands called ***Brunner's glands***. This is the major histological feature that differentiates the duodenum from the jejunum and ileum.
- **Absorptive/protective**. This form lines the entire large intestine and is shown in Fig. 14.3d. The mucosa is arranged into closely packed, straight tubular glands consisting of cells specialised for water absorption, as well as mucus-secreting goblet cells to lubricate the passage of faeces.

Disorders of the gastrointestinal tract

A vast range of both neoplastic and non-neoplastic disorders can affect the GI tract. A 'surgical sieve' can be used to categorise all the potential differential diagnoses for a particular clinical presentation. For example: inflammation, infection, neoplastic (including dysplasia and invasive malignancy), metabolic, congenital, vascular, iatrogenic (including drug effects), autoimmune and trauma.

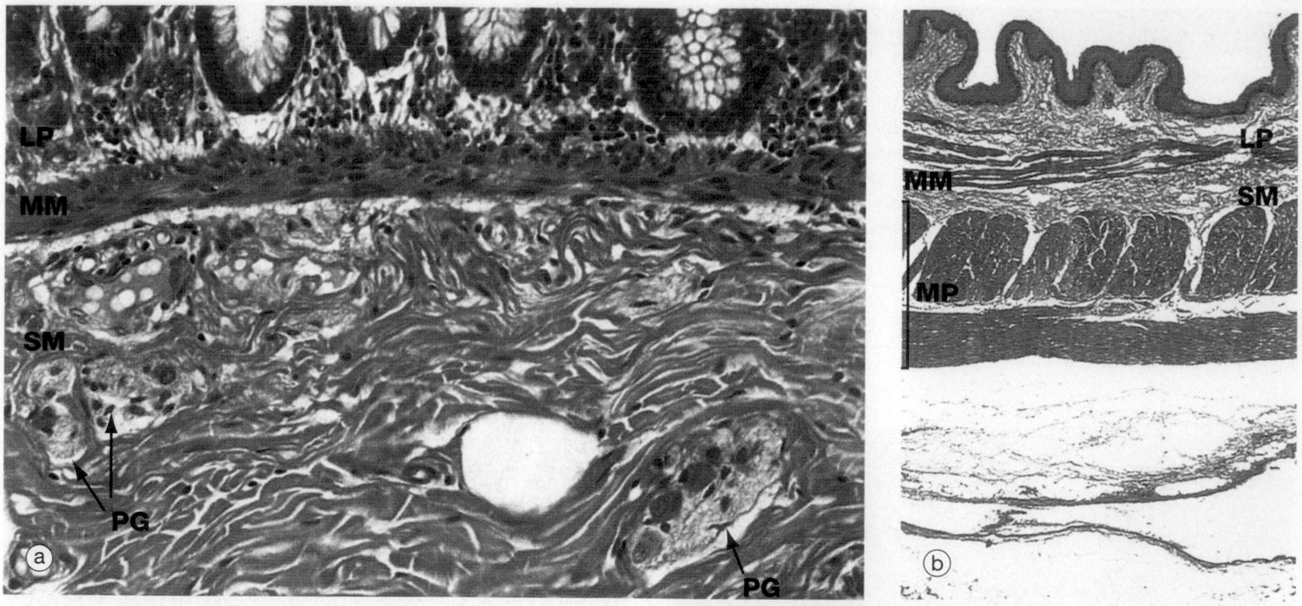

FIG. 14.4 Components of the wall of the gastrointestinal tract
(a) Colon, H&E (HP) (b) Oesophagus, H&E (LP) (c) Colon, H&E (HP)

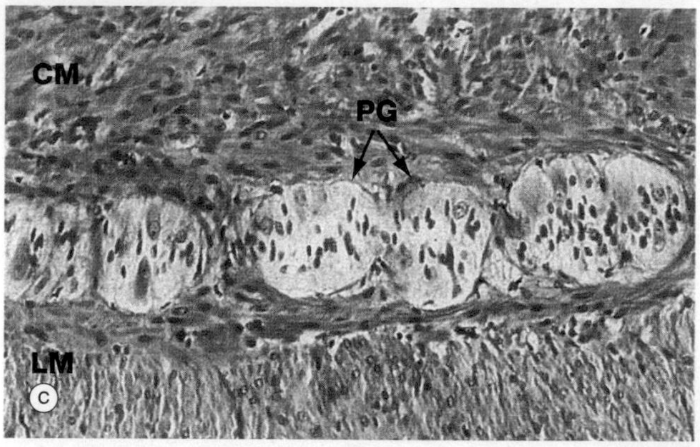

This series of micrographs illustrates the deeper layers of the wall of the gastrointestinal tract.

Fig. 14.4a illustrates the ***muscularis mucosae*** **MM**, clearly demarcating the delicate ***lamina propria*** **LP** from the more robust underlying ***submucosa*** **SM**. This arrangement is typical of the whole of the gastrointestinal tract.

In most of the gut, the lamina propria consists of loose supporting tissue with a diffuse population of lymphocytes and plasma cells. The exception is the stomach which normally has few, if any, resident lymphoid cells. At intervals throughout the oesophagus, small and large bowels and appendix, prominent aggregates of lymphocytes with lymphoid follicles are found. There are also smaller numbers of eosinophils and histiocytes (see Fig. 4.21) to deal with any microorganisms breaching the intestinal epithelium until a specific immune response can be mounted. In the oesophagus, where the function of the mucosa is to protect against friction, the lamina propria is more collagenous than elsewhere and the muscularis mucosae is more prominent. The lamina propria is also typically rich in blood and lymphatic capillaries necessary to support the secretory and absorptive functions of the mucosa.

The muscularis mucosae consists of several layers of smooth muscle fibres, those in the deeper layers orientated parallel to the luminal surface. The more superficial fibres are oriented at right angles to the surface; in the small intestine, the fibres extend up into the villi (see Fig. 14.22). The activity of the muscularis mucosae keeps the mucosal surface and glands in a constant state of gentle agitation which expels secretions from the deep glandular crypts, prevents clogging and enhances contact between epithelium and luminal contents for absorption.

The submucosa consists of collagenous and adipose connective tissue that binds the mucosa to the main bulk of the muscular wall. The submucosa contains the larger blood vessels and lymphatics, as well as the nerves supplying the mucosa.

Tiny ***parasympathetic ganglia*** **PG** are scattered throughout the submucosa, forming the ***submucosal (Meissner) plexus*** from which postganglionic fibres supply the muscularis mucosae.

The typical arrangement of the two layers of the muscular wall proper is seen in Fig. 14.4b, which shows a longitudinal section of the oesophagus. The ***muscularis propria*** **MP** is made up of an outer longitudinal layer and a somewhat broader inner circular layer. There has been some artefactual separation of the layers in this micrograph, making them easier to visualise. The submucosa **SM** is separated from the lamina propria **LP** by the muscularis mucosae **MM**.

Fig. 14.4c illustrates, at high magnification, the junction of outer longitudinal **LM** and inner circular **CM** layers of the muscularis propria in the large intestine. Between the layers, there are clumps of pale-stained parasympathetic ganglion cells of the ***myenteric (Auerbach) plexus***. The two layers of the muscularis propria undergo synchronised rhythmic contractions that pass in ***peristaltic waves*** down the tract, propelling the contents distally. Peristalsis is initiated by the pacemaker cells, the ***interstitial cells of Cajal***, but the level of activity is modulated by the autonomic nervous system, by locally produced gastrointestinal tract hormones and by other environmental factors. Parasympathetic activity enhances peristalsis while sympathetic activity slows gut motility.

CM circular muscle layer **E** stratified squamous epithelium **G** seromucous glands **LM** longitudinal muscle layer
LP lamina propria **Ly** lymphoid aggregate **MM** muscularis mucosae **MP** muscularis propria **Sk** skeletal muscle
Sm smooth muscle **SM** submucosa **PG** parasympathetic ganglion

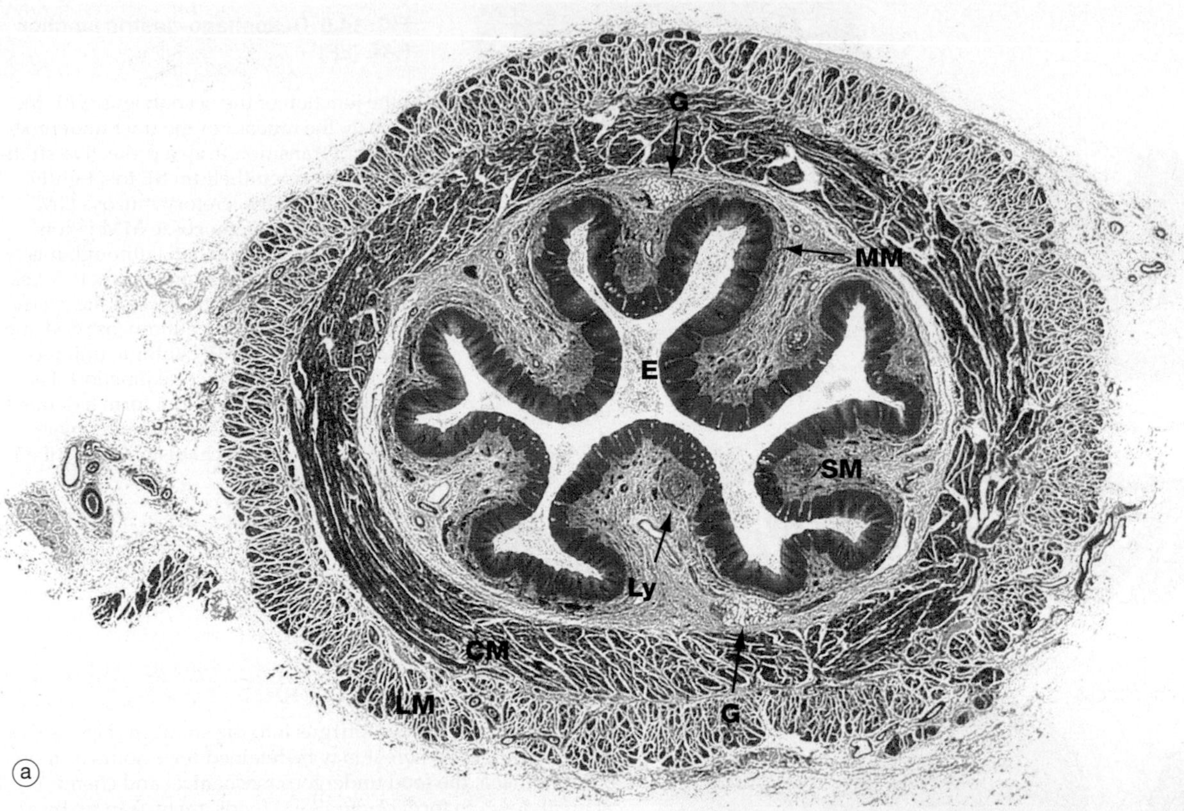

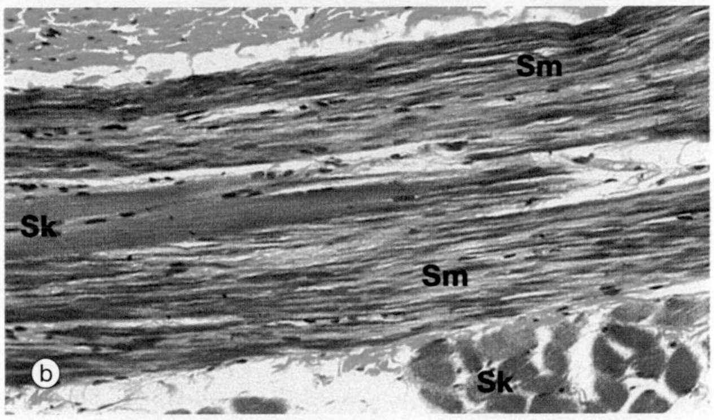

FIG. 14.5 Oesophagus
(a) Masson trichrome stain (LP) (b) Masson trichrome stain (HP)

The oesophagus is a strong muscular tube that conveys food from the oropharynx to the stomach. The initiation of swallowing is a voluntary act involving the skeletal muscles of the oropharynx. This is then succeeded by a strong peristaltic reflex that conveys the bolus of food or fluid to the stomach. Food and fluid do not normally remain in the oesophagus for more than a few seconds and reflux is usually prevented by a physiological sphincter at the gastro-oesophageal junction (see textbox 'Barrett's oesophagus').

Below the diaphragm, the oesophagus passes a centimetre or so into the abdominal cavity before joining the stomach at an acute angle. Sphincter control appears to involve four complementary factors: diaphragmatic contraction, greater intra-abdominal pressure than intragastric pressure being exerted upon the abdominal part of the oesophagus, unidirectional peristalsis and maintenance of correct anatomical arrangements of the structures.

Fig. 14.5a shows the lower third of the oesophagus. In the relaxed state, the oesophageal mucosa is deeply folded, an arrangement that allows marked distension during the passage of a food bolus. The lumen of the oesophagus is lined by a thick protective ***stratified squamous epithelium*** **E** (see Fig. 14.3). The underlying lamina propria is quite narrow and contains scattered lymphoid aggregates **Ly**. The muscularis mucosae **MM** is barely visible at this magnification.

The submucosa **SM** is quite loose with many elastin fibres, allowing for considerable distension during passage of a food bolus. The submucosa also contains small ***seromucous glands*** **G**, similar to salivary glands, which aid lubrication and are most prominent in the upper and lower thirds of the oesophagus.

The muscularis propria is thick, and inner circular **CM** and outer longitudinal **LM** layers of smooth muscle are clearly distinguishable. Since the first part of swallowing is under voluntary control, bundles of skeletal muscle predominate in the muscularis propria of the upper third of the oesophagus. In the middle third of the oesophagus, there is gradual transition from striated to smooth muscle and, in the lower oesophagus, the muscularis propria consists entirely of smooth muscle.

Fig. 14.5b shows part of the muscularis propria of the upper oesophagus at high magnification in the area of transition from skeletal to smooth muscle fibres. A bundle of smooth muscle fibres **Sm** is seen, with two skeletal muscle fibres **Sk** in their midst. Other skeletal muscle fibres are seen in transverse section in the lower right of the micrograph. The cross-striations of the skeletal muscle are just visible at this magnification. The collagen of the endomysial supporting tissue stains green with this method.

Barrett's oesophagus

The importance of the physiological sphincter at the gastro-oesophageal junction is apparent when the consequences of malfunction are considered. ***Reflux*** through the sphincter allows gastric acid into the lower oesophagus, causing the well-known symptom of 'heartburn'. With time, the epithelium of the lower oesophagus undergoes ***metaplasia***, i.e. it converts to a columnar mucus-secreting form, a reaction that may well be protective. Barrett's oesophagus (see e-Fig. 14.1) is the term given to this metaplastic columnar epithelium of the lower oesophagus. This metaplastic epithelium is at high risk of developing dysplasia and invasive adenocarcinoma. Oesophageal carcinoma generally has a poor prognosis.

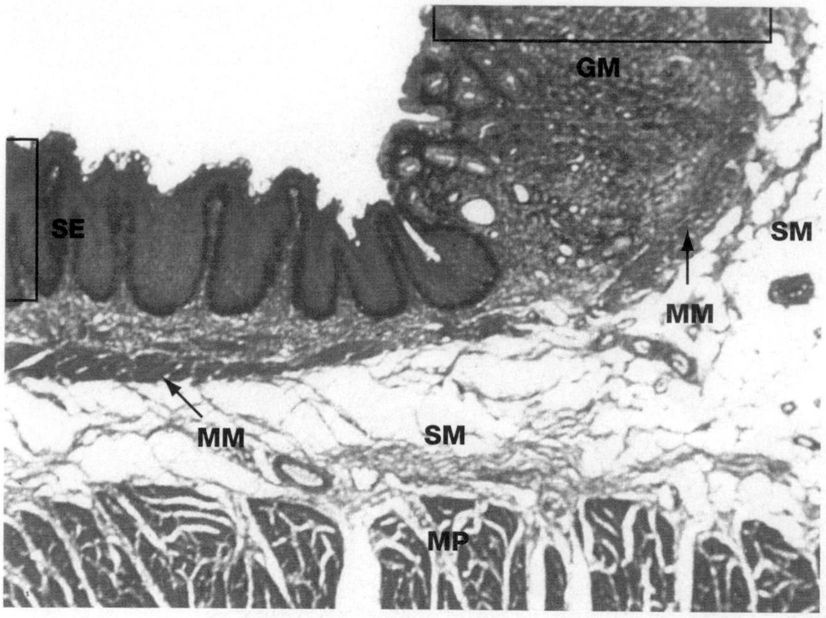

FIG. 14.6 Oesophago-gastric junction H&E (LP)

At the junction of the oesophagus with the stomach, the mucosa of the tract undergoes an abrupt transition from a protective stratified squamous epithelium **SE** to a tightly packed glandular secretory mucosa **GM**.

The muscularis mucosae **MM** is continuous across the junction, although it is less easily seen in the stomach where it lies immediately beneath the base of the gastric glands. The underlying submucosa **SM** and muscularis propria **MP** continue uninterrupted beneath the mucosal junction. The muscularis propria does not form a defined anatomical sphincter, but rather a physiological sphincter mechanism as described in Fig. 14.5.

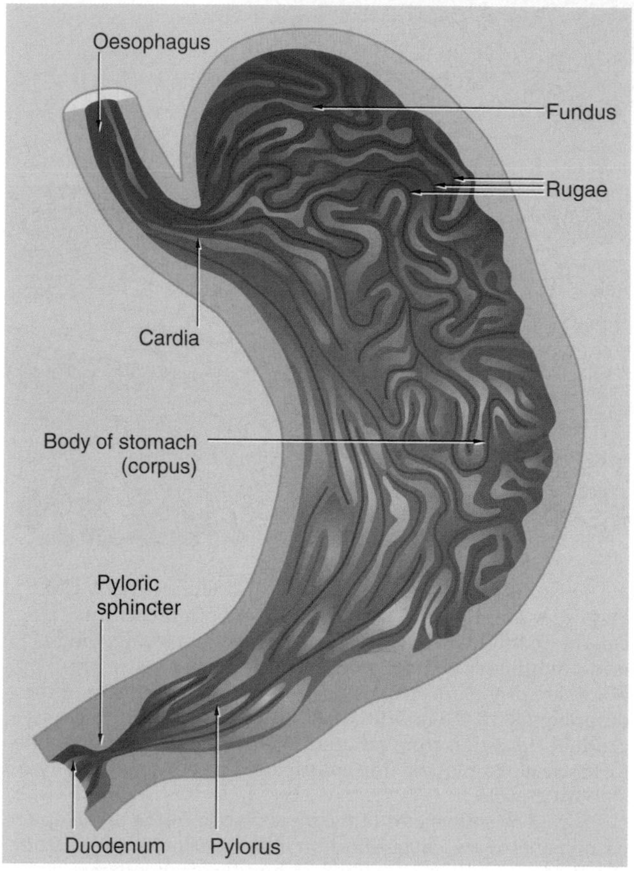

FIG. 14.7 Stomach

Food passes from the oesophagus into the stomach (Fig. 14.7), a distensible organ, where it may be retained for 2 hours or more. In the stomach, the food undergoes mechanical and chemical breakdown to form ***chyme***. Solid foods are broken up by a strong muscular churning action while chemical breakdown is produced by gastric juices secreted by the glands of the stomach mucosa.

There is little absorption from the stomach except for water, alcohol and some drugs. Once chyme formation is completed, the pyloric sphincter relaxes and allows the liquid chyme to be squirted into the duodenum.

In the non-distended state, the stomach mucosa is thrown into prominent longitudinal folds called ***rugae*** that allow distension after eating. Anatomically, the stomach is divided into four regions: the ***cardia***, ***fundus***, ***body*** (***corpus***) and ***pylorus*** (***pyloric antrum***). The pylorus terminates in a strong muscular ***sphincter*** at the gastroduodenal junction.

The mucosa of the entire stomach has a tubular glandular form, but there are three distinctly different histological zones:

- The cardia is a small area of mucus-secreting glands surrounding the entrance of the oesophagus. In some individuals the cardia measures only a few millimetres or may be incomplete or absent altogether.
- The mucosa of the fundus and body forms the major histological region and consists of glands that secrete acid-pepsin gastric juices as well as some protective mucus.
- The glands of the pylorus secrete mucus of two different types and there are associated endocrine cells which secrete the hormone *gastrin*.

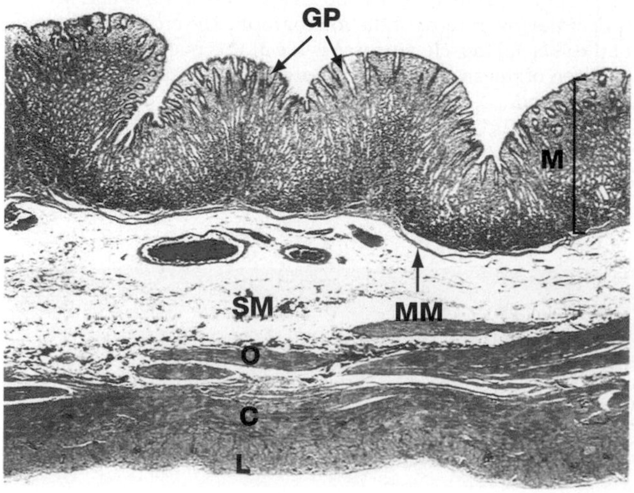

FIG. 14.8 Body of the stomach H&E (LP)

Fig. 14.8 illustrates the body of the stomach in the non-distended state. The mucosa **M** is thrown into prominent folds or rugae and consists of gastric glands that extend from the level of the muscularis mucosae **MM** to open into the stomach lumen via ***gastric pits*** or ***foveolae*** **GP**.

The muscularis propria comprises the usual ***inner circular*** **C** and ***outer longitudinal*** **L** layers, but the inner circular layer is reinforced by a further ***inner oblique layer*** **O**.

The submucosa **SM** is relatively loose and distensible and contains the larger blood vessels. The serosal layer, which covers the peritoneal surface, is thin and barely visible at this magnification.

The adipose tissue of the lesser and greater omentum is attached along the lesser and greater curvature of the stomach (not illustrated in this micrograph). Lymph nodes and large blood vessels lie within this omental fatty tissue.

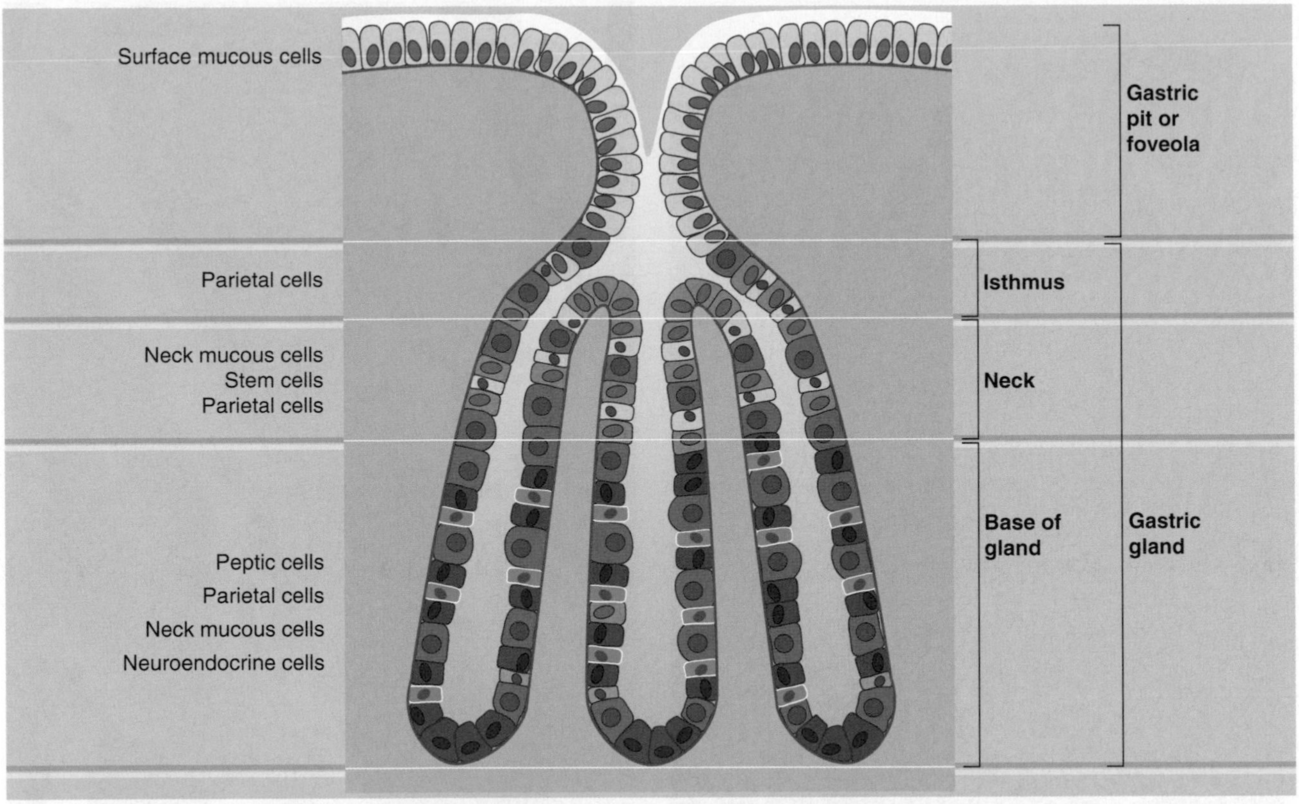

FIG. 14.9 Body of the stomach: structure of the gastric glands

The mucosa of the fundus and body of the stomach consists of straight tubular glands that synthesise and secrete gastric juice. The gastric pits occupy about one-quarter of the thickness of the gastric mucosa and each has between one and seven gastric glands opening into it. Gastric juice is a watery secretion containing ***hydrochloric acid*** (pH 0.9–1.5) and the digestive enzyme ***pepsin***, which hydrolyses proteins into polypeptide fragments. The stomach mucosa is protected from self-digestion by a thick surface covering of mucus, which is maintained at a higher pH than the gastric juice by the secretion of ***bicarbonate*** ions by the gastric surface mucous cells. The gastric glands contain a mixed population of cells:

- ***Surface mucous cells*** cover the luminal surface of the stomach and partly line the gastric pits. The cytoplasmic mucigen granules that pack these cells are stained poorly by the standard H&E stain. These cells have short surface microvilli and secrete protective bicarbonate ions directly into the deeper layers of the surface mucous coat.
- ***Neck mucous cells*** are squeezed between the parietal cells in the neck and base of the gastric glands. These cells have larger secretory granules and more polyribosomes than surface mucous cells.
- ***Parietal*** or ***oxyntic cells*** are distributed along the length of the glands but tend to be most numerous in the isthmus of the glands. These large, rounded cells have an extensive eosinophilic (oxyntic) cytoplasm and a centrally located nucleus. Parietal cells secrete gastric acid as well as ***intrinsic factor***, a glycoprotein necessary for the absorption of vitamin B_{12} in the terminal ileum.
- ***Chief, peptic*** or ***zymogenic cells*** are located towards the bases of the gastric glands. Peptic cells are recognised by their condensed, basally located nuclei and strongly basophilic granular cytoplasm. This reflects their large content of ribosomes. These are the pepsin-secreting cells.
- ***Neuroendocrine cells***, part of the diffuse neuroendocrine system, are also found in the base of the gastric glands. They secrete 5-HT (serotonin) and other hormones (see also Fig. 14.12).
- ***Stem cells*** are found mainly in the neck of the gastric glands. These undifferentiated cells divide continuously to replace all other types of cell in the glands. The maturing cells then migrate up or down as appropriate. These cells are not easily identified in sections of normal gastric mucosa but become very prominent with plentiful mitotic figures after damage to the mucosa has occurred, such as after an episode of gastritis (see textbox).

Gastritis and peptic ulceration

The stomach is a very unique environment due to the ability of its mucosa to secrete concentrated ***hydrochloric acid*** as well as digestive proteolytic enzymes. In order to avoid mucosal damage and digestion of the stomach itself, the normal stomach also secretes a protective alkaline mucus. The balance between potentially damaging and protective factors can be disrupted in various conditions, resulting in inflammation of the stomach or ***gastritis*** (see e-Fig. 14.2). More severe mucosal damage can occur, leading to development of an ***ulcer*** (complete loss of the mucosa) or ***erosion*** (loss of part of the thickness of the mucosa). When there is excessive secretion of acid and digestive enzymes, mucosal damage may not be limited to the stomach itself but often extends into the proximal duodenum. The underlying causes of such ***peptic ulceration*** are diverse (see e-Fig. 14.3). Agents such as alcohol and drugs can lead to mucosal damage, sometimes by direct toxic effects upon the mucosa and sometimes by interfering with normal protective mechanisms (e.g. non-steroidal anti-inflammatory drugs can cause damage by inhibiting synthesis of protective prostaglandins). Infection by the organism *Helicobacter pylori* is a very important cause of gastritis and peptic ulceration, and the mechanism by which it causes mucosal damage is discussed later.

C circular muscle **GM** glandular mucosa **GP** gastric pit **L** longitudinal muscle **M** mucosa **MM** muscularis mucosae **MP** muscularis propria **O** oblique muscle **SE** squamous epithelium **SM** submucosa

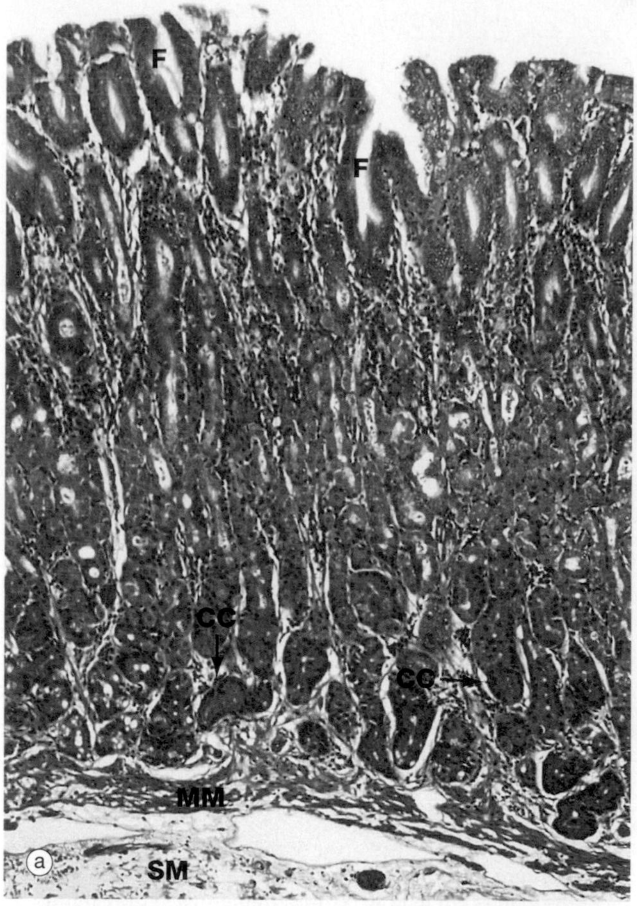

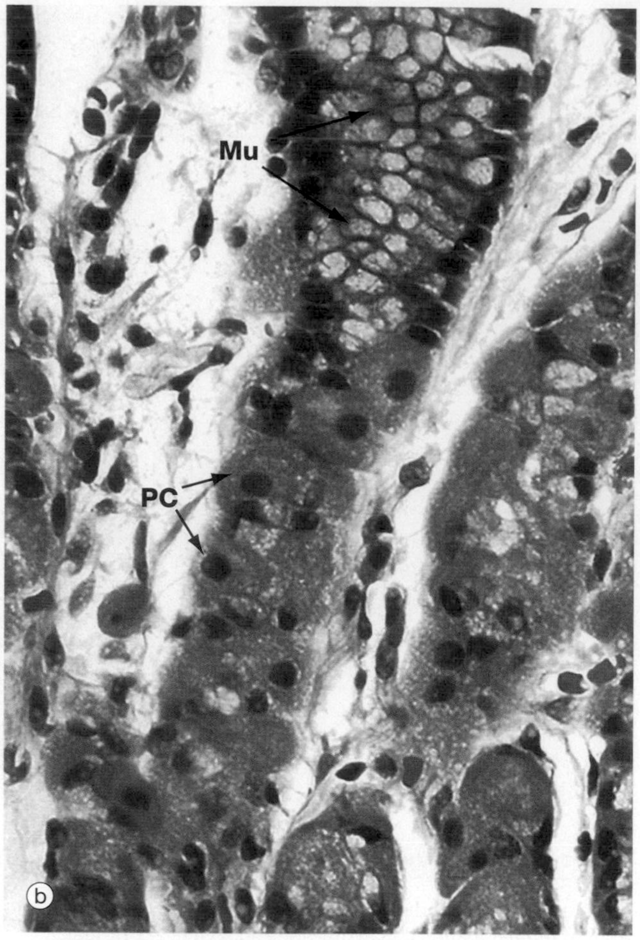

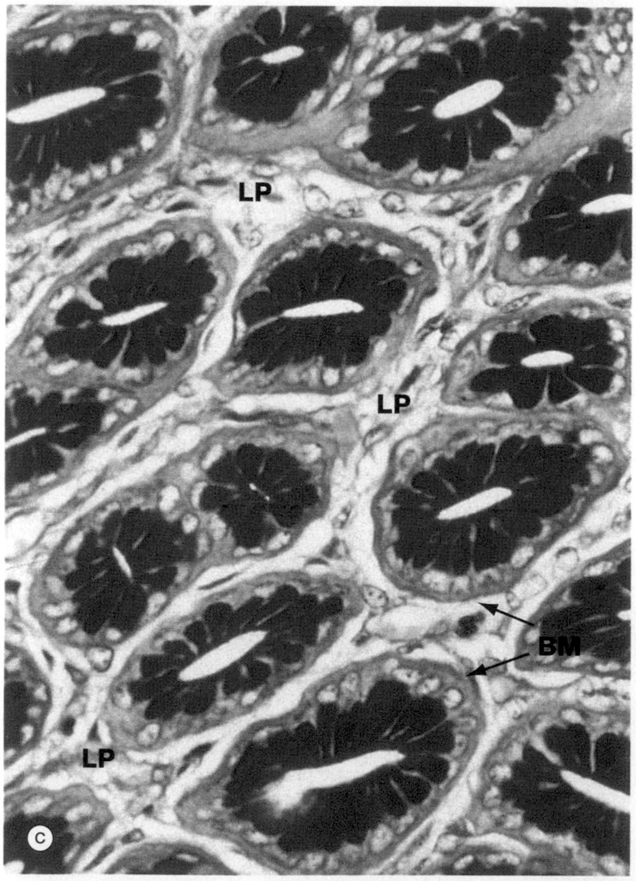

FIG. 14.10 Gastric body mucosa
(a) H&E (LP) (b) H&E (HP) (c) PAS/haematoxylin/ orange G (HP)

Fig. 14.10a shows the full thickness of the gastric body mucosa and includes a small amount of submucosa **SM**. The ***gastric pits*** or ***foveolae*** **F**, lined by pale-stained surface mucous cells, are easily identifiable. The isthmus and neck of the glands also appear pale due to the predominance of neck mucous cells and parietal cells **PC**. The base of the glands, where chief (zygomatic) cells **CC** predominate, are stained darker in this H&E preparation. The glands extend down to the muscularis mucosae **MM**. Normal gastric mucosa is virtually devoid of lymphoid cells.

Fig. 14.10b is a high-power view of the neck and isthmus of a gastric body gland. The neck mucous cells **Mu** and parietal cells **PC** are easily visualised at this magnification. The tall columnar mucus-secreting cells of the stomach are not of the goblet cell type which are found in small and large intestines. The mucus produced by these mucous cells protects the epithelium from autodigestion by acid gastric juice. The parietal cells are recognised by their copious eosinophilic cytoplasm and central nucleus, which is often described as a 'fried egg' appearance.

In transverse section, as in Fig. 14.10c, the tubular nature of the gastric pits is clearly evident. Between one and seven gastric glands may open into each gastric pit. Note the loose vascular but scanty lamina propria **LP** which supports the gastric pits and glands. The lightly PAS-positive basement membrane **BM** can be distinguished between the epithelium and lamina propria. The mucus of the neck mucous cells stains a strong magenta colour with this staining method.

Gastric cancer

Most gastric cancers (see e-Fig. 14.4) are adenocarcinomas which are of either intestinal type, characterised by glandular differentiation or diffuse type, characterised by infiltrating single tumour cells such as signet ring cells. The latter results in linitis plastica or the so-called 'leather bottle stomach' where the tumour diffusely infiltrates the stomach wall.

B bacterium **BM** basement membrane **C** canaliculus **CC** chief cells **E** neuroendocrine cells **F** foveola **LP** lamina propria **M** mitochondrion **MM** muscularis mucosae **Mu** mucous cell **PC** parietal cell **SM** submucosa

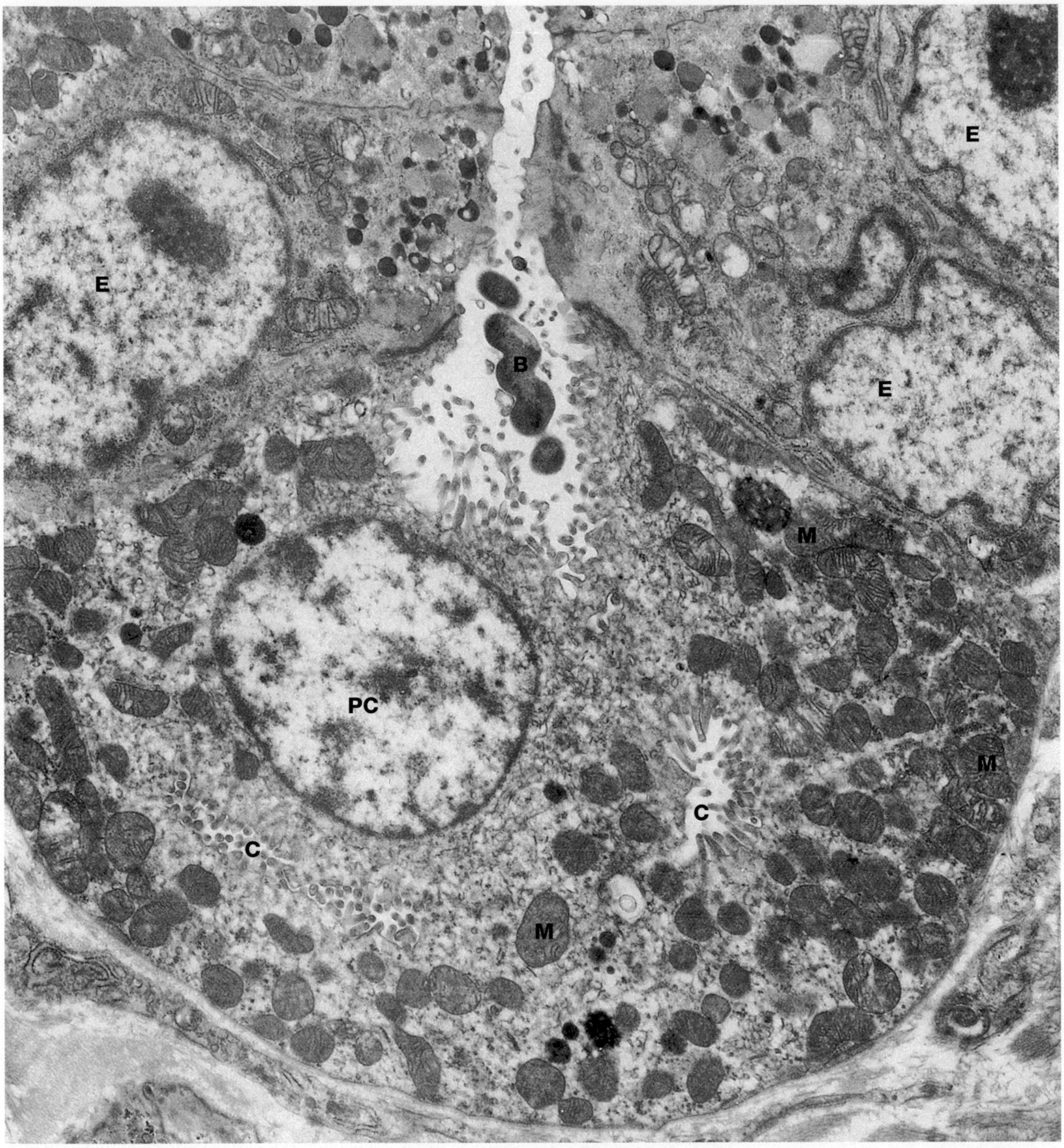

FIG. 14.11 Parietal cell, rat
EM ×9600

Fig. 14.11 shows a parietal cell **PC** within a gastric gland. The luminal plasma membrane of the parietal cell forms deep, branching ***canaliculi*** **C** that extend throughout the cytoplasm and between adjacent cells. Numerous short microvilli project into the lumina of the intracellular canaliculi, greatly increasing the surface area.

The canaliculi are closely related to a ***tubulovesicular membrane complex*** (not well seen in this micrograph). This system consists of numerous small, membrane-bound vesicles which include a transmembrane '***proton pump***' in the form of a H^+–K^+ ATPase. When there is a physiological increase in the demand for acid secretion, mediated via ***histamine***, ***acetylcholine*** and ***gastrin*** (see textbox), the vesicles of this tubulovesicular complex fuse with the canalicular membranes of the parietal cell to facilitate active secretion of hydrogen ions into the gastric lumen. In actively secreting cells, as in this case, the canalicular system becomes more prominent due to the large increase in its surface area from fusion with these pre-formed vesicles, whereas in resting parietal cells the canalicular system is inconspicuous and the complex is more prominent. This morphological change reflects altered functional demand and it is believed that when demand for acid secretion falls again, membrane-bound vesicles bearing proton pumps are endocytosed to re-form the tubulovesicular complex.

Secretion of hydrochloric acid begins with the production of ***carbonic acid*** in the cytoplasm of the parietal cell, catalyzed by the enzyme ***carbonic anhydrase***. Carbonic acid then dissociates into hydrogen and bicarbonate ions. The hydrogen ions are actively transported into the canalicular lumen and chloride ions follow passively. The end result is a hydrogen ion concentration in gastric juice about 1 million times that in plasma. This process is fuelled by the many mitochondria **M** of the parietal cells.

Parietal cells also secrete a glycoprotein called ***intrinsic factor*** which is essential for the absorption of vitamin B_{12} in the terminal ileum. Also seen in Fig. 14.11 are several neuroendocrine cells **E**, recognised by their small electron-dense secretory granules. Note the coiled bacterium **B** in the lumen of the gland; this is most likely *Helicobacter pylori*.

Physiological control of gastric acid secretion

Acid production by parietal cells is controlled via the autonomic nervous system and through the action of hormones. Parasympathetic innervation by branches of the ***vagus nerve*** results in release of ***acetylcholine***, which acts on muscarinic M3 receptors on parietal cells. The hormone ***gastrin*** is produced by G cells in the antrum in response to rising gastric pH, and it acts via CCK2 receptors on the parietal cells. ***Histamine*** also increases acid secretion, acting via H2 receptors.

Stimulation of these various receptors results in activation of protein kinases, either via an increase in the concentration of intracellular calcium (in the case of muscarinic and gastrin receptors) or by increasing levels of cAMP (in the case of histamine), leading to active secretion of acid (see Fig. 14.11). As acid production increases, the pH in the gastric antrum falls. In response to this, the ***D cells*** in the antrum produce another hormone, ***somatostatin***, and this acts on the antral G cells to reduce secretion of gastrin.

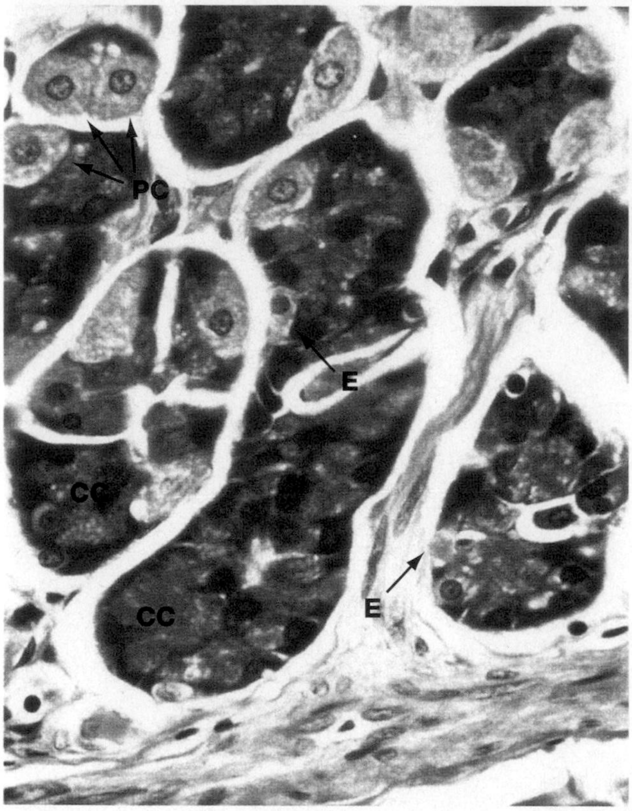

FIG. 14.12 Base of gastric gland H&E (HP)

Chief (*zymogen* or *peptic*) *cells* **CC**, which synthesise and secrete the proteolytic enzyme ***pepsin***, are the principal cell type in the basal third of the gastric glands, although some parietal cells **PC** are also found at this level (Fig. 14.12).

Chief cells have basally located nuclei and extensive granular cytoplasm packed with rough endoplasmic reticulum, the ribosomes accounting for the cytoplasmic basophilia. The inactive pepsin precursor, ***pepsinogen***, is synthesised by the ribosomes and stored in numerous secretory granules located towards the luminal surface. Pepsinogen remains inactive until it reaches the lumen of the stomach where it is activated by the low pH of the gastric juices. Secretion of an inactive precursor molecule prevents autodigestion of the gastric glands.

The much larger ***parietal cells*** are round with large, centrally located nuclei and eosinophilic (pink-stained) cytoplasm due to the numerous mitochondria that are a feature of highly metabolically active cells.

The secretory activity of both parietal and peptic cells is controlled by the autonomic nervous system and via the hormone ***gastrin***, which is secreted by neuroendocrine cells of the pyloric region (see textbox 'Physiological control of gastric acid secretion').

A variety of other neuroendocrine cells of the gastrointestinal endocrine system are also scattered in the gastric body mucosa and elsewhere in the gastrointestinal tract. Occasionally, the neuroendocrine cells **E** can be identified in sections fixed with chromium-containing fixatives, as in this example.

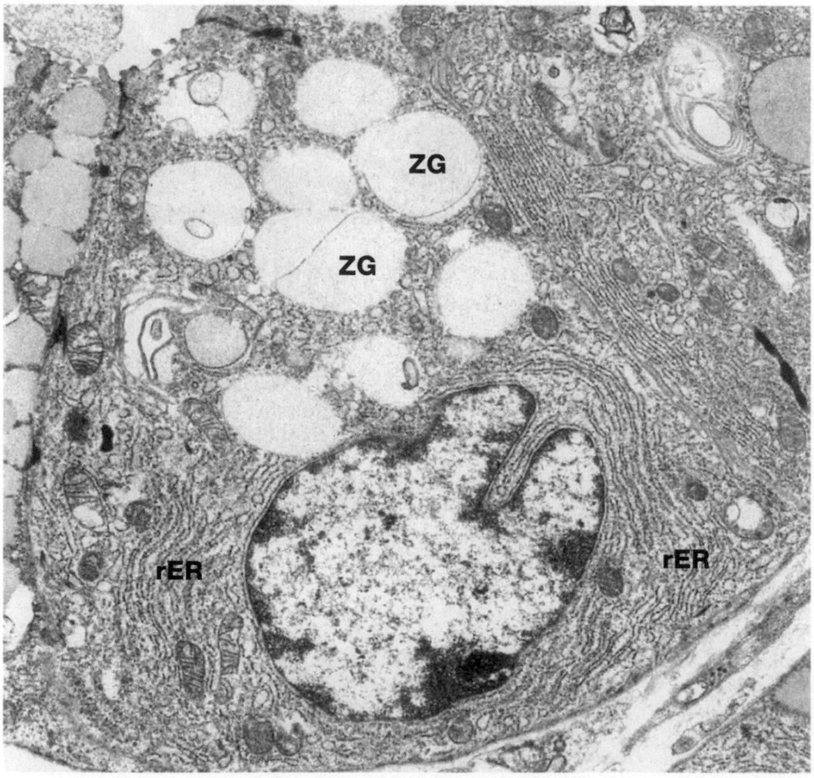

FIG. 14.13 Chief cell EM ×7200

Fig. 14.13 illustrates a chief (zymogen) cell at the base of a gastric gland. The typical ultrastructural features of chief cells are those of protein-secreting cells in general. These features include an extensive rough endoplasmic reticulum **rER** and membrane-bound secretory vesicles (***zymogen granules***) **ZG** containing pepsinogen. These are crowded in the apical cytoplasm, thus restricting the nucleus to the base of the cell. The extensive rough endoplasmic reticulum accounts for the basophilia of chief cells in H&E sections.

B Brunner's glands **CC** chief cells **CM** circular muscle **D** duodenum **E** neuroendocrine cell **G** G cells **LM** longitudinal muscle **MM** muscularis mucosae **P** gastric pit **PC** parietal cell **PS** pyloric sphincter **rER** rough endoplasmic reticulum **S** stomach **ZG** zymogen granule

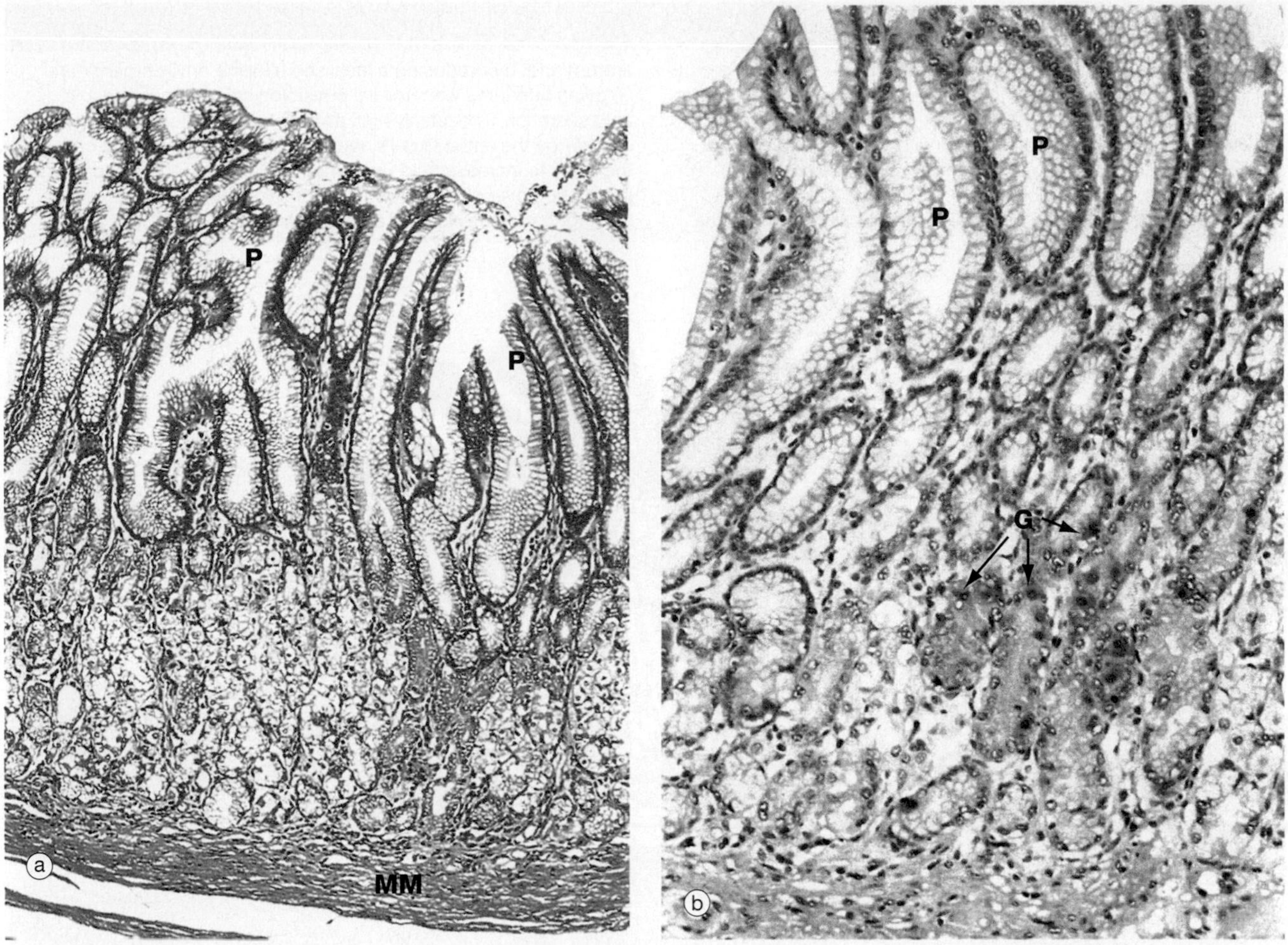

FIG. 14.14 Pyloric stomach
(a) H&E (LP) (b) Immunohistochemical staining for gastrin (MP)

In contrast to the simple tubular glands of the fundus and body, the pyloric glands are branched and coiled and the gastric pits **P** occupy about half the thickness of the pyloric mucosa (Fig. 14.14a). The glands are lined almost exclusively by mucus-secreting cells which are similar to the neck mucous cells of the gastric body and fundus. A small number of acid-secreting parietal cells are also scattered among the pyloric glands. Note the prominent muscularis mucosae **MM** separating the glands from the underlying submucosa. As in the body of the stomach, stem cells are found in the neck of the glands but cannot be easily identified by light microscopy.

Scattered among the pyloric mucous cells are neuroendocrine cells that secrete the peptide hormone ***gastrin*** and are thus called ***G cells***. In Fig. 14.14b, an antibody to gastrin has been used to highlight the G cells, which contain gastrin in secretory granules in their cytoplasm. The G cells are stained brown **G** and are found mainly in the neck of the glands. The presence of food in the stomach stimulates the secretion of gastrin into the bloodstream. Gastrin then promotes secretion of pepsin and acid by the gastric glands of the fundus and body, as well as enhancing gastric motility.

Other neuroendocrine cells in the pylorus secrete various other hormonal products, including somatostatin, which is involved in the regulation of insulin, glucagon, gastrin and growth hormone secretion.

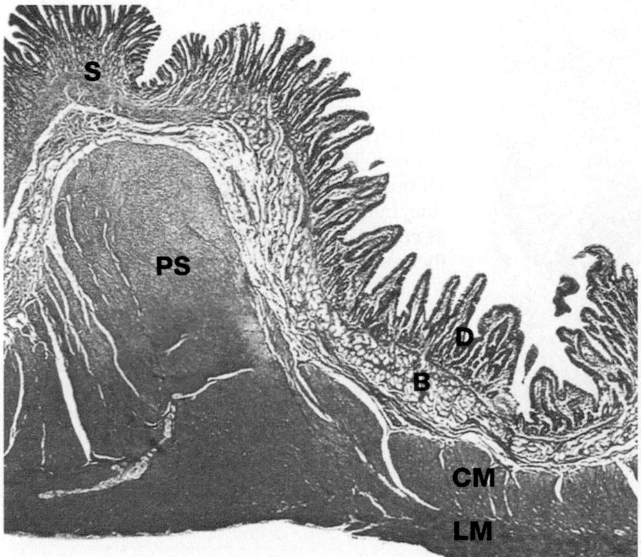

FIG. 14.15 Pyloric stomach
H&E (LP)

The ***pyloric sphincter*** **PS** marks a sharp transition from the glandular secretory type mucosa of the stomach **S** to the villous absorptive type mucosa of the duodenum **D** and the remainder of the small intestine (Fig. 14.15). In addition, the duodenum is distinguished from the jejunum and ileum by the presence of numerous mucus-secreting glands **B**. These glands, known as ***Brunner's glands***, are predominantly found in the submucosa but may extend into the mucosa. These glands secrete a thin, alkaline mucus. The pyloric sphincter consists of a marked thickening of the circular layer of the muscularis at the gastroduodenal junction. Note the continuity of both the circular **CM** and longitudinal **LM** layers of the muscularis between the pylorus and duodenum.

The inner oblique layer of the muscularis propria is found only in the body of the stomach.

Helicobacter pylori infection

H. pylori infection is a major cause of gastritis and peptic ulceration. The organism does not invade the tissues but inhabits the protective mucus layer which covers the surface of the mucosa. It has a unique ability to survive the acid environment of the stomach because of a bacterial enzyme, ***urease***. This allows it to produce ammonia by splitting urea, raising pH in the immediate vicinity of the organism. It typically colonises the antrum and, by producing a localised alkaline environment here, *H. pylori* interferes with normal physiological control of gastric acid secretion. The falsely high antral pH stimulates secretion of ***gastrin*** by the antral G cells, which acts upon the parietal cells in the body to increase acid production still further. This excess acid production overwhelms normal mucosal defence mechanisms, leading to the formation of an acute ulcer.

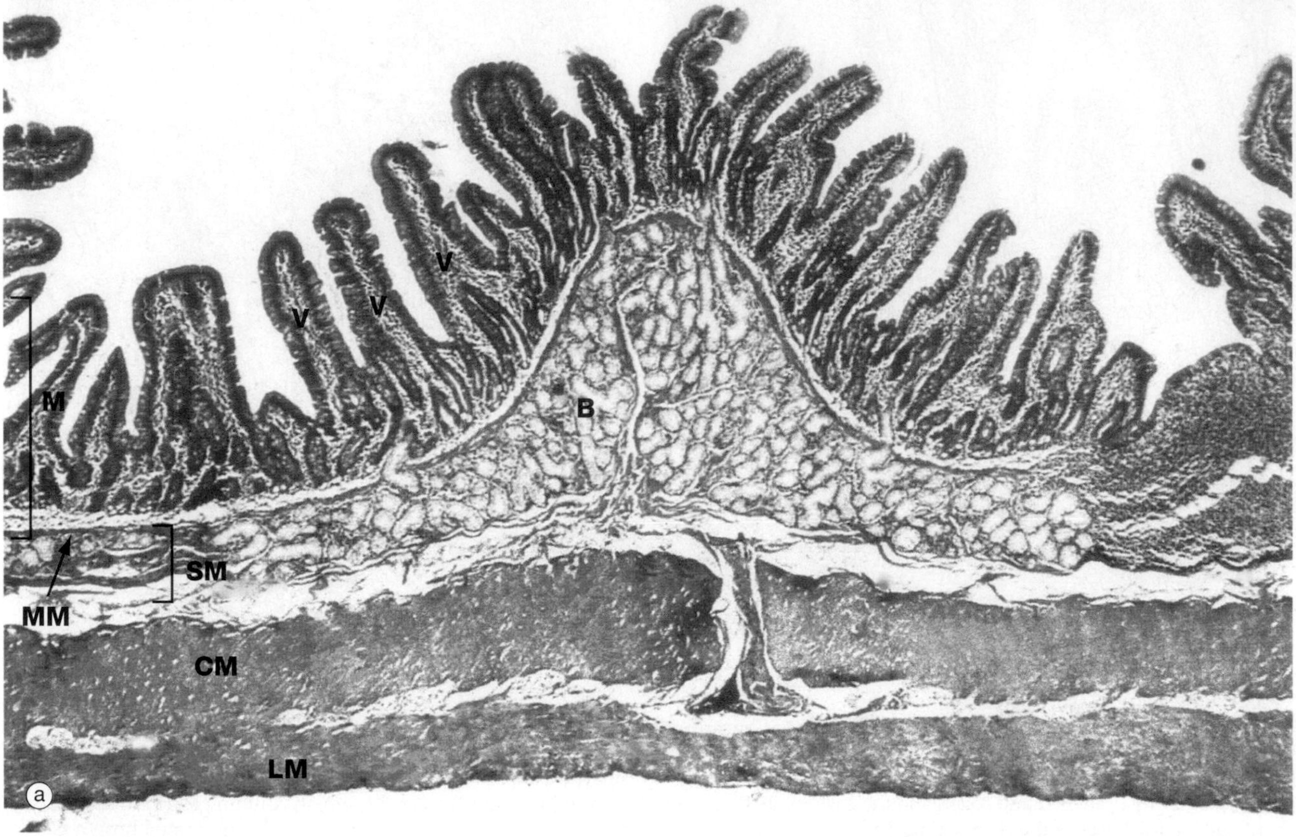

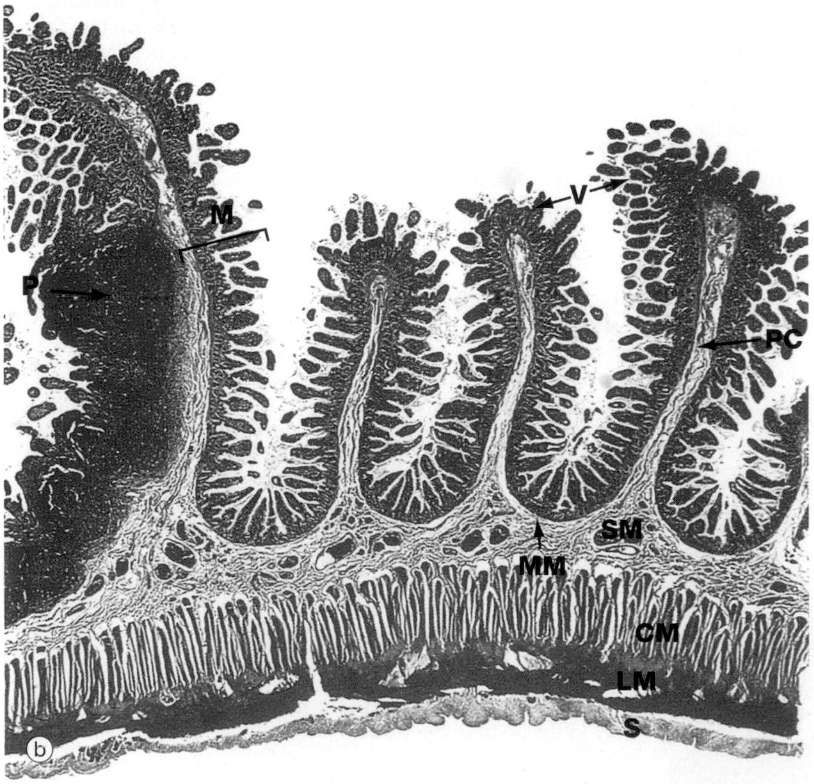

FIG. 14.16 Small intestine, monkey *(caption continues opposite)* (a) Duodenum, H&E (LP) (b) Ileum, H&E (MP)

The ***duodenum***, seen in Fig. 14.16a, represents the first part of the small intestine and receives partly digested food in the form of acidic chyme from the stomach via the pyloric canal. The main function of the duodenum is to neutralise gastric acid and pepsin and to initiate further digestive processes.

Fig. 14.16a illustrates monkey duodenum, the wall of the human duodenum being too thick to be photographed in its entirety. The mucosa **M** has the characteristic villous form of the whole of the small intestine, interspersed with short glands, known as ***crypts of Lieberkühn***, extending down to the muscularis mucosae **MM**.

The feature unique to the duodenum is the extensive mass of coiled branched tubular ***Brunner's glands*** **B**, found mainly in the submucosa **SM**. The ducts of the Brunner's glands pass through the muscularis mucosae to open into the crypts between the mucosal villi **V**. The muscularis propria of the duodenum consists of an inner circular layer **CM** and an outer longitudinal layer **LM**, as in the rest of the small intestine.

B Brunner's glands **C** crypt **CM** circular muscle **LM** longitudinal muscle **M** mucosa **MM** muscularis mucosae **P** Peyer's patch **PC** plica circularis **S** serosa **SM** submucosa **V** villus

FIG. 14.16 Small intestine, monkey *(illustrations (a) and (b) opposite)*
(a) Duodenum, H&E (LP) (b) Ileum, H&E (MP)

The tall columnar cells of Brunner's glands have extensive poorly stained mucin-filled cytoplasm and basally located nuclei. The presence of chyme in the duodenum stimulates Brunner's glands to secrete a thin, alkaline mucus that helps to neutralise the acidic chyme and protect the duodenal mucosa from autodigestion. Other products of Brunner's glands include ***lysozyme*** and ***epidermal growth factor***.

Chyme also stimulates the release of two peptide hormones, ***secretin*** and ***cholecystokinin–pancreozymin*** (***CCK***) from neuroendocrine cells scattered throughout the duodenal mucosa. Secretin and CCK promote pancreatic exocrine secretion into the duodenal lumen via the ***pancreatic duct***. CCK also stimulates contraction of the gallbladder, thus propelling bile into the ***common bile duct***. The pancreatic and common bile ducts merge to empty their contents into the duodenum via a single short duct that opens into the second part of the duodenum via the ***ampulla of Vater***.

Pancreatic juice is alkaline due to a high content of bicarbonate ions and thus helps to neutralise the acidic gastric contents entering the duodenum. The pancreas also secretes a variety of digestive enzymes, including the proteolytic enzymes ***trypsin*** and ***chymotrypsin***. Like pepsin in the stomach, these are secreted in an inactive pro-enzyme form. On entering the duodenal lumen, trypsin is activated by the enzyme ***enterokinase***, secreted by the duodenal mucosa. Activated trypsin in turn activates chymotrypsin. The pancreatic enzymes, which also include ***amylase*** and ***lipases***, initiate the processes of luminal digestion (see textbox overleaf). The biliary secretions contain ***bile acids*** which act as emulsifying agents and are particularly important in the absorption of lipids.

Fig. 14.16b shows a section of ileum at very low magnification. The mucosa **M** is thrown into transverse folds, the ***plicae circulares*** **PC** (also called ***valvulae conniventes*** or ***folds of Kerckring***), covered with villi **V**. The muscularis mucosae **MM** lies immediately beneath the crypts and is difficult to see at this magnification. The vascular submucosa **SM** extends into the plicae circulares. The inner circular **CM** and outer longitudinal **LM** layers of the muscularis propria lie deep to this and there is an outer layer of serosa **S**. ***Peyer's patches*** **P** (see Ch. 11) dominate the mucosa at the left of the field.

The small intestine has the same basic structure throughout, except for the following features:

- Brunner's glands are only found in the duodenum.
- The villi tend to be longest in the duodenum and become shorter towards the ileum.
- Lymphoid tissue becomes more prominent in the ileum and is fairly inconspicuous in the duodenum.
- The proportion of goblet cells in the epithelium increases distally.
- Plicae circulares are most prominent and numerous in the jejunum and proximal ileum and are generally absent in the proximal duodenum and distal ileum.

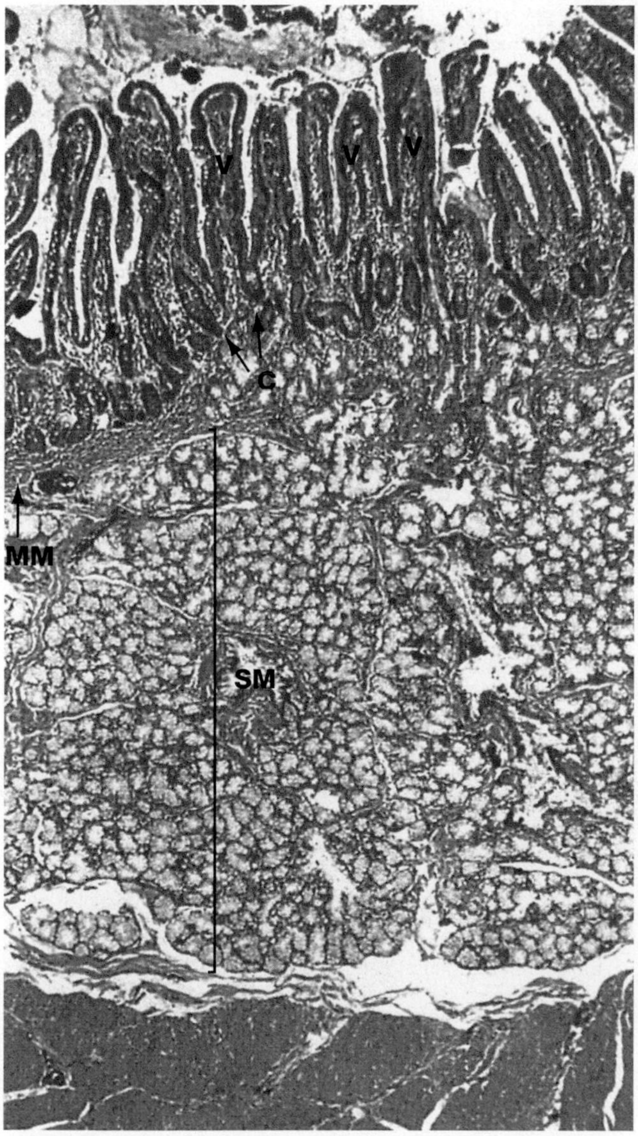

FIG. 14.17 Duodenum
H&E (LP)

Fig. 14.17 of the human duodenum is stained by the standard H&E method. The duodenal mucosa has the typical form found elsewhere in the small intestine, with numerous elongated villi **V**, between the bases of which are shorter crypts **C**. In the distal duodenum, the height of the villi is about four times the length of the crypts, while in the more distal small bowel the villus/crypt ratio is 2–3 : 1.

The pale-stained Brunner's glands occupy the entire submucosa **SM** deep to the muscularis mucosae **MM**. A small component of the Brunner's gland is sometimes found in the lamina propria where the duct of the gland empties into the base of a mucosal crypt. The Brunner's glands secrete alkaline mucins into the lumen of the small intestine.

Clinical management of peptic ulcer disease

Understanding of the role of *H. pylori* has revolutionised management of peptic ulceration. In the past, peptic ulcers were treated by surgical procedures which aimed to reduce acid production, such as partial gastrectomy (to remove the antral source of gastrin) or vagotomy and pyloroplasty (removing the vagal-driven pathway of acid secretion but requiring release of the pylorus, since the vagus nerve also controls gastric emptying). Such operations were associated with considerable morbidity.

Conventional medical management of peptic ulcer disease employed a range of drugs from simple alkalis to neutralise excess acid, through various drugs which interfere with normal physiological control of acid secretion (e.g. adrenergic antagonists and histamine (H_2) receptor blockers), to the more recent use of proton pump inhibitors (PPIs) which effectively block the final common pathway of acid production.

Although acid-blocking drugs were usually effective, treatment had to continue life-long. Now, treatment usually requires only a short course of *Helicobacter* eradication therapy, using a combination of two antibiotics with a proton pump inhibitor ('triple therapy').

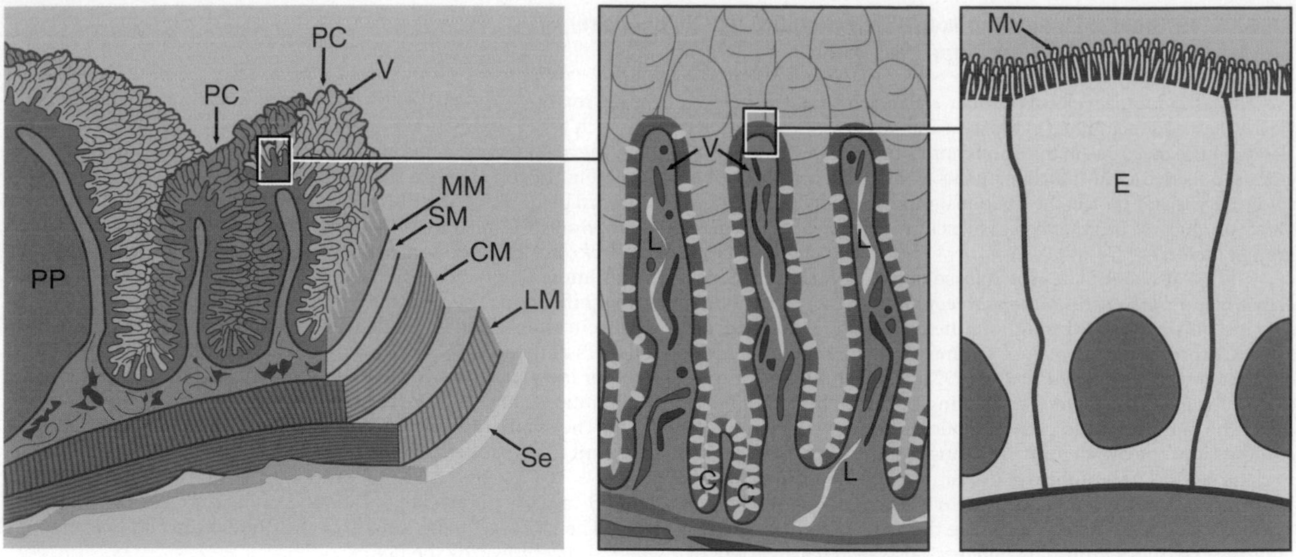

FIG. 14.18 Small intestine

The small intestine (Fig. 14.18), comprising the ***duodenum***, ***jejunum*** and ***ileum***, is the principal site for absorption of digestion products from the gastrointestinal tract. Digestion begins in the stomach and is completed in the small intestine in association with the absorptive process. Four factors combine to provide an enormous surface area:

- The small intestine is extremely long (4 to 6 m in humans).
- The mucosa and submucosa are thrown up into circularly arranged folds called ***plicae circulares*** **PC** or ***folds of Kerckring*** which are particularly numerous in the jejunum.
- The mucosal surface is made up of numerous finger-like projections called ***villi*** **V**.
- Thousands of microvilli **Mv** are present at the luminal surface of the enterocytes **E**, the columnar cells covering the villi. These cells are responsible for the process of absorption and some digestion.

The muscularis mucosae **MM** lies immediately beneath the mucosal crypts **C** and separates the mucosa from the submucosa **SM**. The vascular submucosa extends into, and forms the core of, the plicae circulares. Inner circular **CM** and outer longitudinal **LM** layers of the muscularis are responsible for continuous peristaltic activity of the small intestine. The peritoneal aspect of the muscularis is invested by the loose collagenous serosa **Se**, which is lined on its peritoneal surface by mesothelium identical in appearance to the mesothelial lining of the pleura (see Fig. 12.22).

Lymphoid aggregations known as ***Peyer's patches*** **PP** are a prominent feature within the lamina propria of the small intestine (see Fig. 11.16).

The products of protein and carbohydrate digestion (see textbox 'The mechanisms of digestion and absorption'), namely amino acids and monosaccharides, respectively, enter the intestinal capillaries and pass via the portal vein to the liver. In contrast, reconstituted triglycerides pass into intestinal lymphatics known as ***lacteals*** **L**, and thence via the thoracic duct to the general circulation, bypassing the liver. For lymphatic transport, the triglycerides become coated with phospholipids and proteins to form fine globules known as ***chylomicrons***. A minority of lipid digestion products, such as short-chain fatty acids and glycerol, pass in the portal system to the liver, along with almost all the bile acids which are reabsorbed and recirculated.

The mechanisms of digestion and absorption

Digestion occurs within the lumen or at the mucosal surface, where it is linked with the process of absorption.

Luminal digestion involves the mixing of chyme with pancreatic enzymes to break up foods into their component parts. The process is facilitated by adsorption of pancreatic enzymes onto the mucosal surface. ***Membrane digestion*** involves enzymes located in the luminal plasma membranes of the enterocytes. The principal means of digestion and absorption of the main food constituents are as follows:

- **Proteins** are first denatured by the gastric acid and then hydrolysed to polypeptide fragments by the enzyme pepsin. In the duodenum, pancreatic enzymes including ***trypsin***, ***chymotrypsin***, ***elastase*** and ***carboxypeptidases*** continue this process, producing small peptide fragments. Membrane-bound ***peptide hydrolases*** complete the digestion to amino acids that are then absorbed. Absorption is by active transport, with a different carrier system for each amino acid. In young infants, some proteins are absorbed without prior digestion by the process of endocytosis.
- **Carbohydrates** occur in the diet mainly in the form of starches and the disaccharides sucrose and lactose. ***Pancreatic amylase*** hydrolyses starch to glucose and the disaccharide maltose in the small intestinal lumen. This process is begun by ***salivary amylase*** in the mouth, although its contribution to digestion is probably minor. Membrane-bound disaccharidases and oligosaccharidases convert the sugars to monosaccharides, mainly glucose, galactose and fructose, which are absorbed by facilitated diffusion.
- **Lipids**, predominantly triglycerides, are converted by the mechanical action of the stomach into a coarse emulsion which is converted to a fine emulsion in the duodenum by ***bile acids***, synthesised in the liver. Each triglyceride molecule is broken down into a monoglyceride and two free fatty acids by pancreatic lipases, although some glycerol and diglycerides are also produced. These smaller lipid molecules are then absorbed and resynthesised back into triglycerides within the enterocytes.

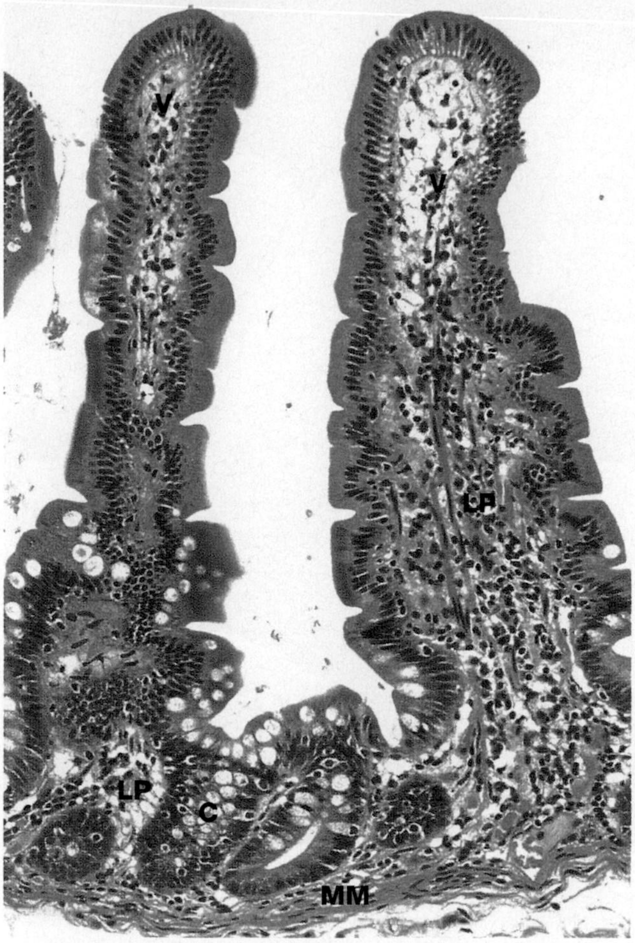

FIG. 14.19 Intestinal villi and crypts H&E (MP)

The intestinal ***villi*** **V**, shown in Fig. 14.19, are lined by a simple columnar epithelium which is continuous with that of the ***crypts*** **C**. As in other parts of the gastrointestinal tract, the epithelium includes a variety of cell types, each with its own specific function. Cell types in the small intestine epithelium include:

- **Enterocytes**, the most numerous cell type, are tall columnar cells with surface microvilli that are seen as a ***brush border*** in light micrographs. These cells are the main absorptive cells.
- **Goblet cells** are scattered among the enterocytes and produce mucin for lubrication of the intestinal contents and protection of the epithelium.
- **Paneth cells** are found at the base of the crypts and are distinguished by their prominent eosinophilic apical granules. These cells have a defensive function.
- **Neuroendocrine cells** produce locally acting hormones that regulate gastrointestinal motility and secretion.
- **Stem cells**, found at the base of the crypts, divide continuously to replenish all of the above four cell types.
- **Intraepithelial lymphocytes**, which are mostly T cells, provide defence against invasive organisms.

The lamina propria **LP** extends between the crypts and into the core of each villus and contains a rich vascular and lymphatic network into which digestive products are absorbed. The muscularis mucosae **MM** lies immediately beneath the base of the crypts.

Coeliac disease

Coeliac disease (see e-Fig. 14.5) (or coeliac sprue or gluten-sensitive enteropathy) is caused by an immunological response to ***gluten*** (***gliadin***), a component of wheat, oats, barley and rye. Individuals with this condition present with symptoms of malabsorption, including weight loss, diarrhoea, steatorrhoea, anaemia and vitamin deficiencies. The immune response damages the small bowel mucosa, resulting in loss of the surface villi and elongation of the crypts. Blood tests reveal characteristic ***anti-endomysial antibodies***, as well as specific antibodies against ***tissue transglutaminase***.

Endoscopic biopsy of the small intestine is usually performed for diagnosis. The typical histological changes are illustrated in Fig. 14.20. Although these histological appearances are very suggestive of coeliac disease, they are not specific and the diagnosis must be confirmed by resolution of the symptoms and histological changes after a period of time on a gluten-free diet.

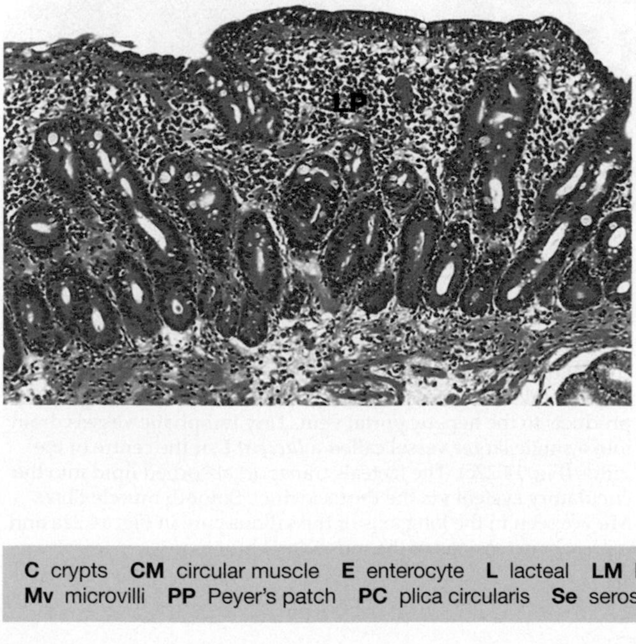

FIG. 14.20 Coeliac disease, atrophic small intestine H&E (MP)

Biopsies of the small bowel in coeliac disease (Fig. 14.20) typically reveal flattening or loss of the normal intestinal villi (compare Figs 14.17 and 14.19) as well as a marked increase in the number of lymphocytes and plasma cells in the lamina propria **LP**. In addition, there is usually a marked increase in the number of intraepithelial T lymphocytes in the surface epithelium, suggesting that the condition is at least partly due to a cell-mediated immune response against the small bowel enterocytes. In order to maintain the integrity of the mucosal surface in the face of this greatly increased enterocyte turnover, there must be increased proliferation of stem cells in the bases of the crypts and, as a result, the crypts appear greatly elongated.

C crypts **CM** circular muscle **E** enterocyte **L** lacteal **LM** longitudinal muscle **LP** lamina propria **MM** muscularis mucosae **Mv** microvilli **PP** Peyer's patch **PC** plica circularis **Se** serosa **SM** submucosa **V** villus

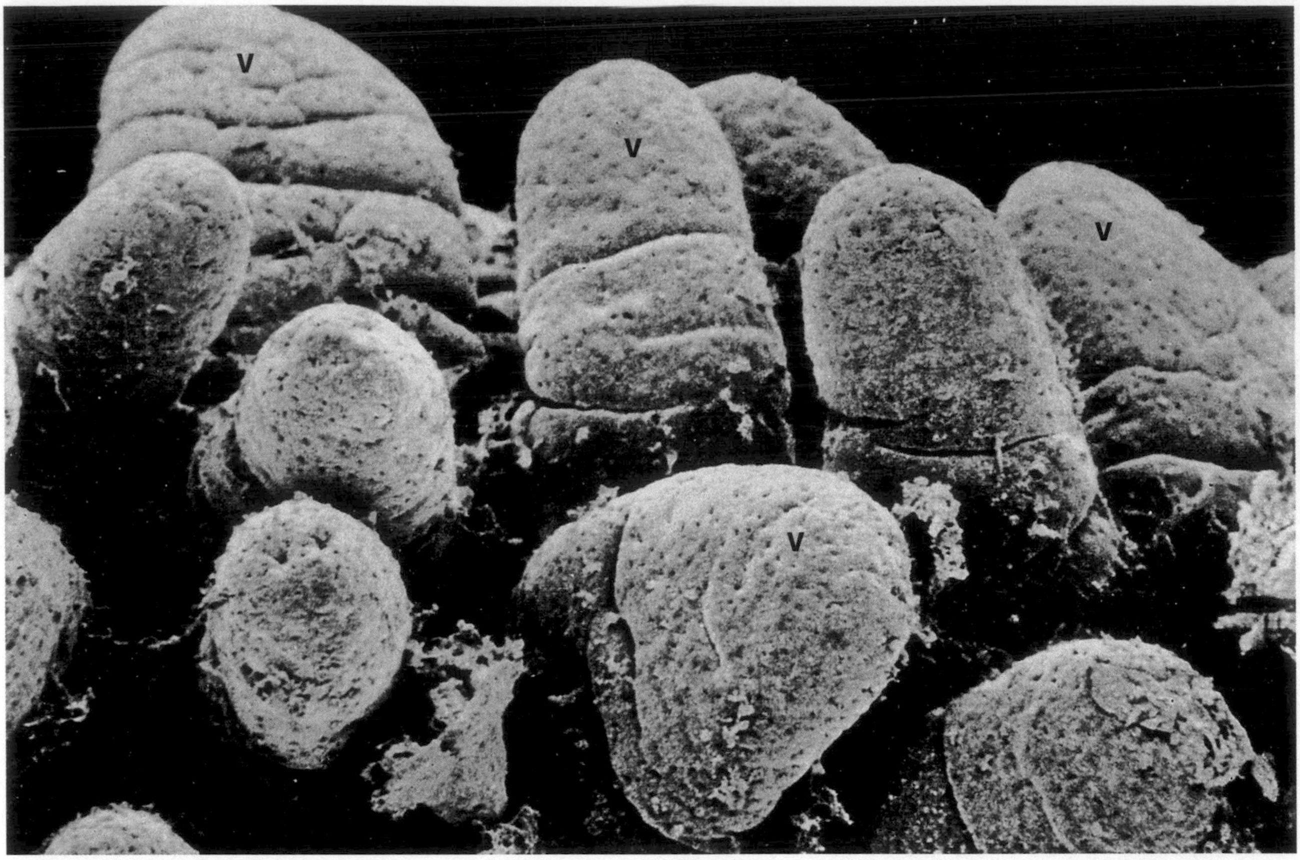

FIG. 14.21 Intestinal villi SEM ×100

This low-power scanning electron micrograph (Fig. 14.21) shows villi **V** along the crest of a plica circularis in the small intestine. Note the variability of the shape of the villi; some are finger-shaped while others have a broader leaf-like profile. Surface openings of scattered goblet cells stud the villous surface. Fragments of mucus can be seen trapped between the villi.

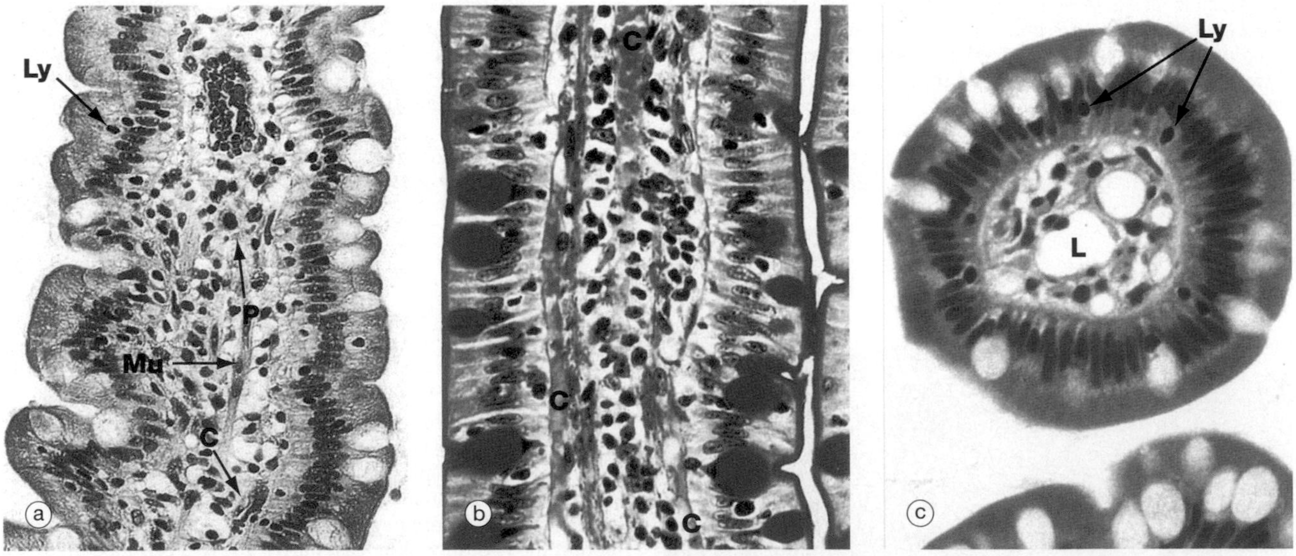

FIG. 14.22 Intestinal villi
(a) H&E, LS (MP) (b) PAS/iron-haematoxylin/orange G, LS (HP) (c) H&E, TS (HP)

These micrographs illustrate the tall columnar ***enterocytes*** that cover the intestinal villi, as well as the ***goblet cells*** scattered among them. The luminal surface of the enterocytes seen in Fig. 14.22b is strongly PAS-positive due to a particularly thick glycocalyx and a surface layer of goblet cell–derived mucus. Both features protect against autodigestion. The glycocalyx is also the site for adsorption of pancreatic digestive enzymes.

T lymphocytes **Ly** are scattered among the enterocytes (Fig. 14.22a). Plasma cells **P** in the villous core secrete IgA into the intestinal lumen by transcytosis across epithelial cells.

The cores of the villi are extensions of the lamina propria and consist of loose supporting tissue. Capillaries **C** lie immediately beneath the basement membrane and transport most digestive products to the hepatic portal vein. Tiny lymphatic vessels drain into a single larger vessel called a ***lacteal*** **L** at the centre of the villus (Fig. 14.22c). The lacteals transport absorbed lipid into the circulatory system via the thoracic duct. Smooth muscle fibres **Mu** are seen in the long axis of the villous core in Fig. 14.22a and represent extensions of the muscularis mucosae.

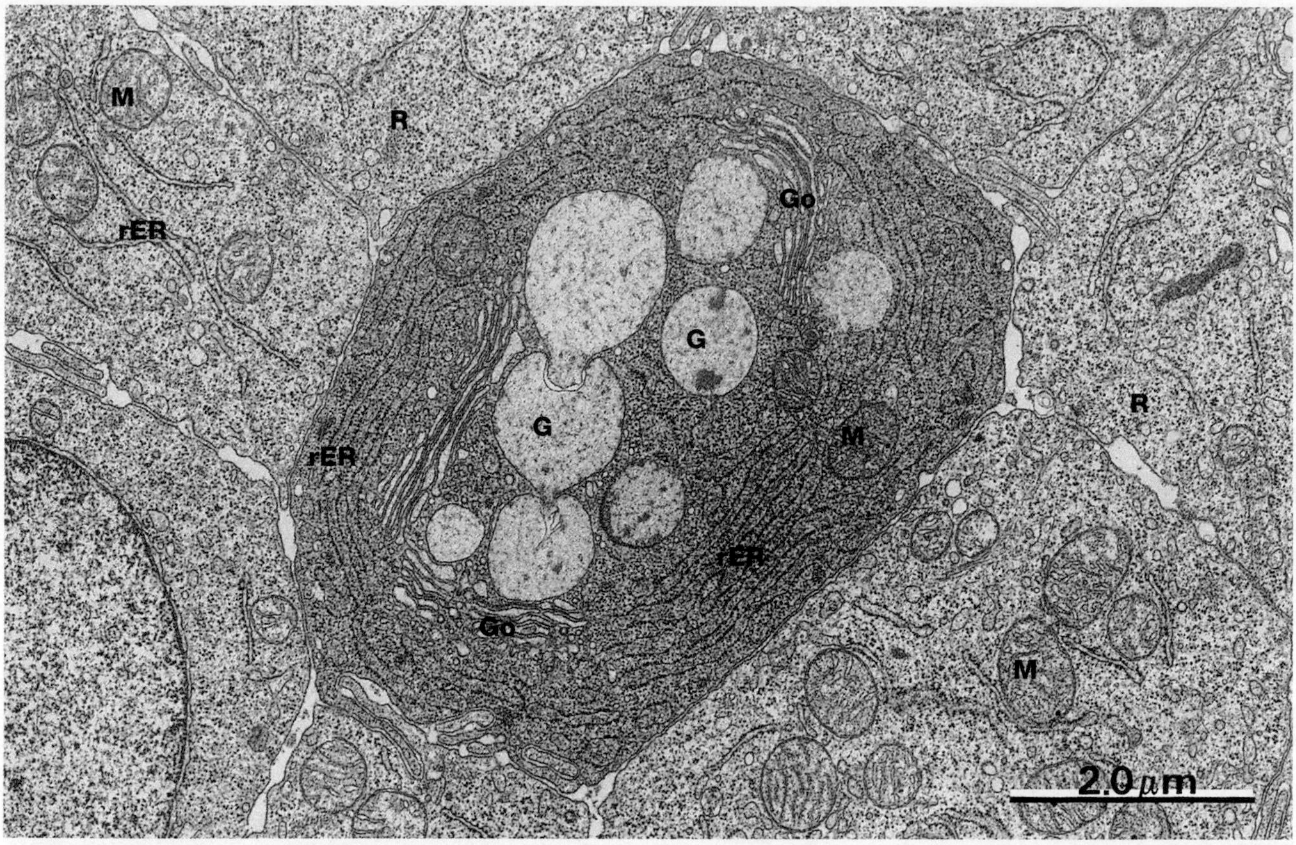

FIG. 14.23 Duodenal epithelium
EM ×14 500

This low-power electron micrograph of a horizontal section through the duodenal epithelium (Fig. 14.23) demonstrates several important features. In the central area, there is a goblet cell containing several mucin-containing granules **G**. The goblet cell appearance by conventional light microscopy is actually an artefact of preparation whereby water is taken up by the granules, causing them to expand and compress the surrounding cytoplasm. Adjacent to the mucin granules there are three Golgi apparatuses **Go** with plentiful rough endoplasmic reticulum **rER**, features typical of secretory cells. Occasional mitochondria **M** are also seen.

Surrounding the goblet cell are a number of enterocytes. These have much less prominent **rER** but contain large numbers of free ribosomes **R** and mitochondria **M** (see Fig. 14.25). This micrograph is of duodenal epithelium, but jejunal and ileal epithelium are identical.

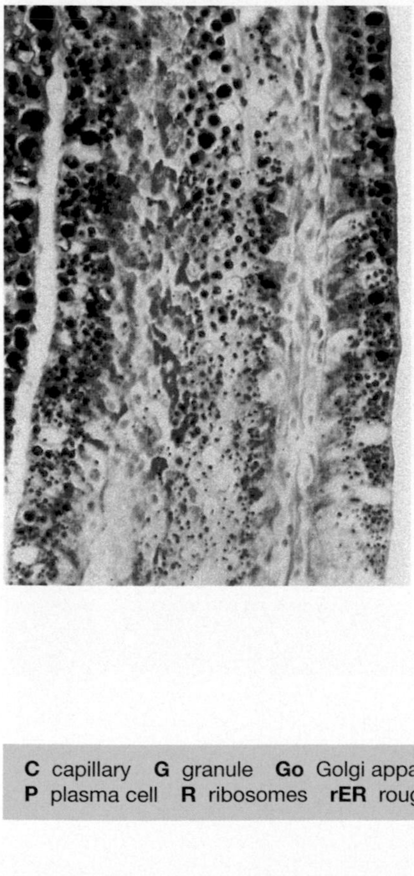

FIG. 14.24 Intestinal villus
Sudan black (HP)

Fig. 14.24 is a frozen section from the intestine of a rat fed with milk is stained to demonstrate the presence of absorbed lipids.

Ingested triglycerides are emulsified by bile and hydrolysed by the pancreatic enzyme ***lipase***. The degradation products, mainly free fatty acids and monoglycerides, are absorbed by enterocytes where they are resynthesised into triglycerides in the smooth endoplasmic reticulum. Here, the triglycerides are reconstituted into small globules and form a lipoprotein complex, incorporating protein, cholesterol and phospholipids. Membrane-bound vesicles containing multiple droplets bud from the smooth endoplasmic reticulum and pass towards the base of the cell where they are released by exocytosis into the intercellular clefts. From here, the small lipoprotein droplets known as ***chylomicrons*** pass into the lacteals and then into larger lymphatics, eventually entering the general circulation.

Note the high concentration of black-stained lipid in the enterocyte cytoplasm and in the chylomicrons within the central lacteal.

C capillary **G** granule **Go** Golgi apparatus **L** lacteal **Ly** lymphocyte **M** mitochondrion **Mu** smooth muscle fibres **P** plasma cell **R** ribosomes **rER** rough endoplasmic reticulum **V** villus

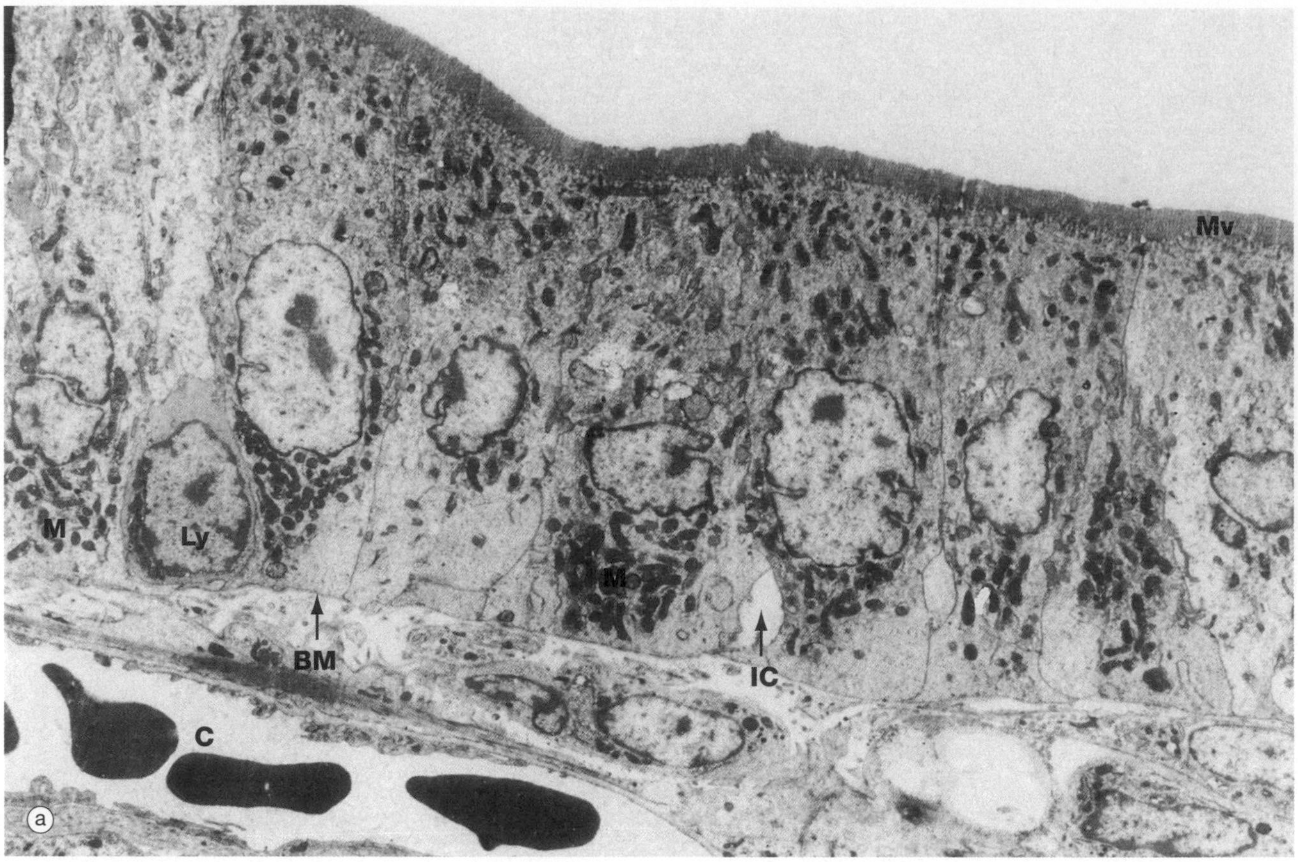

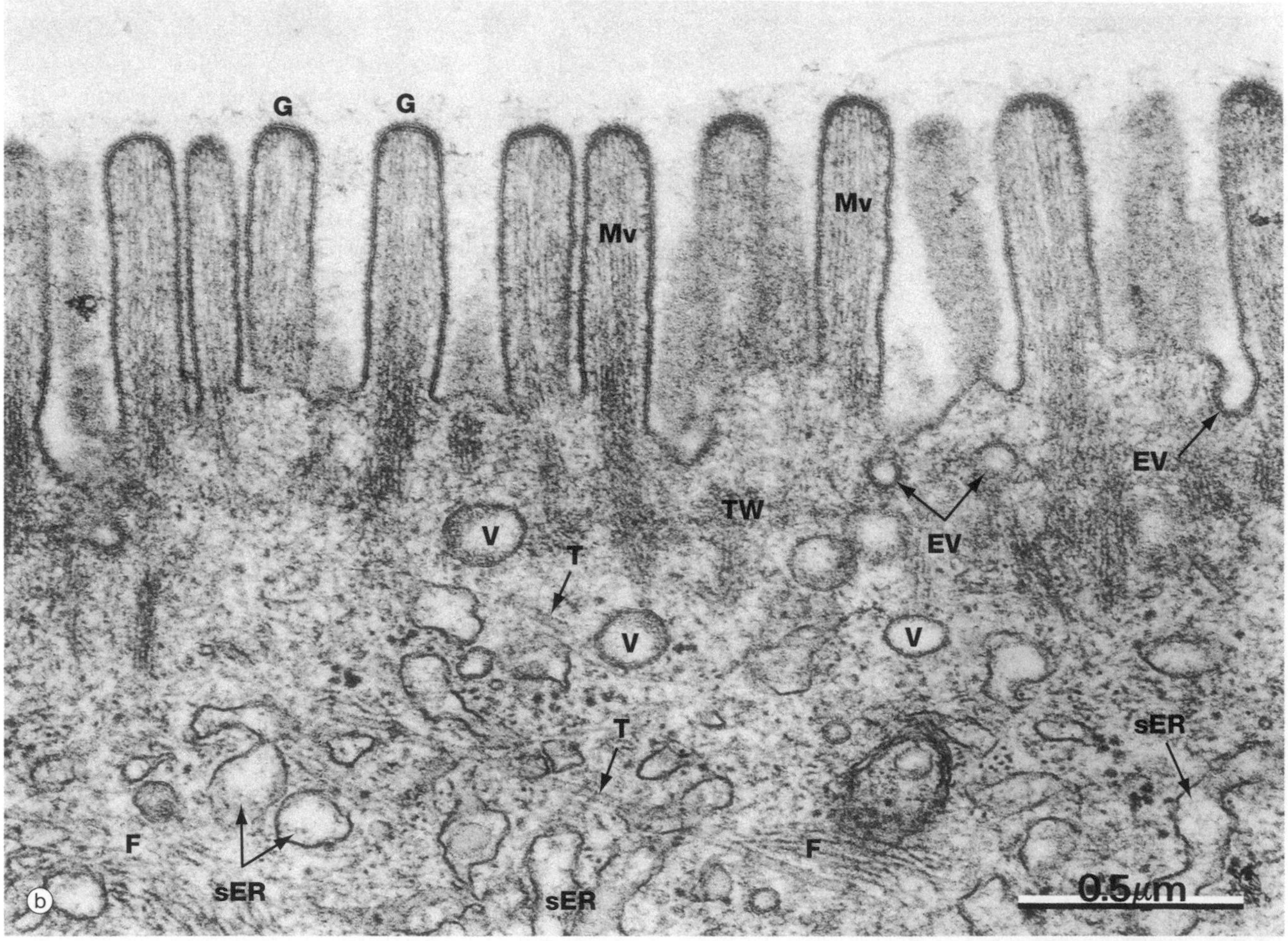

FIG. 14.25 Enterocytes *(caption and illustration (c) opposite)*
(a) EM ×4540 (b) EM ×5600 (c) EM ×22 000

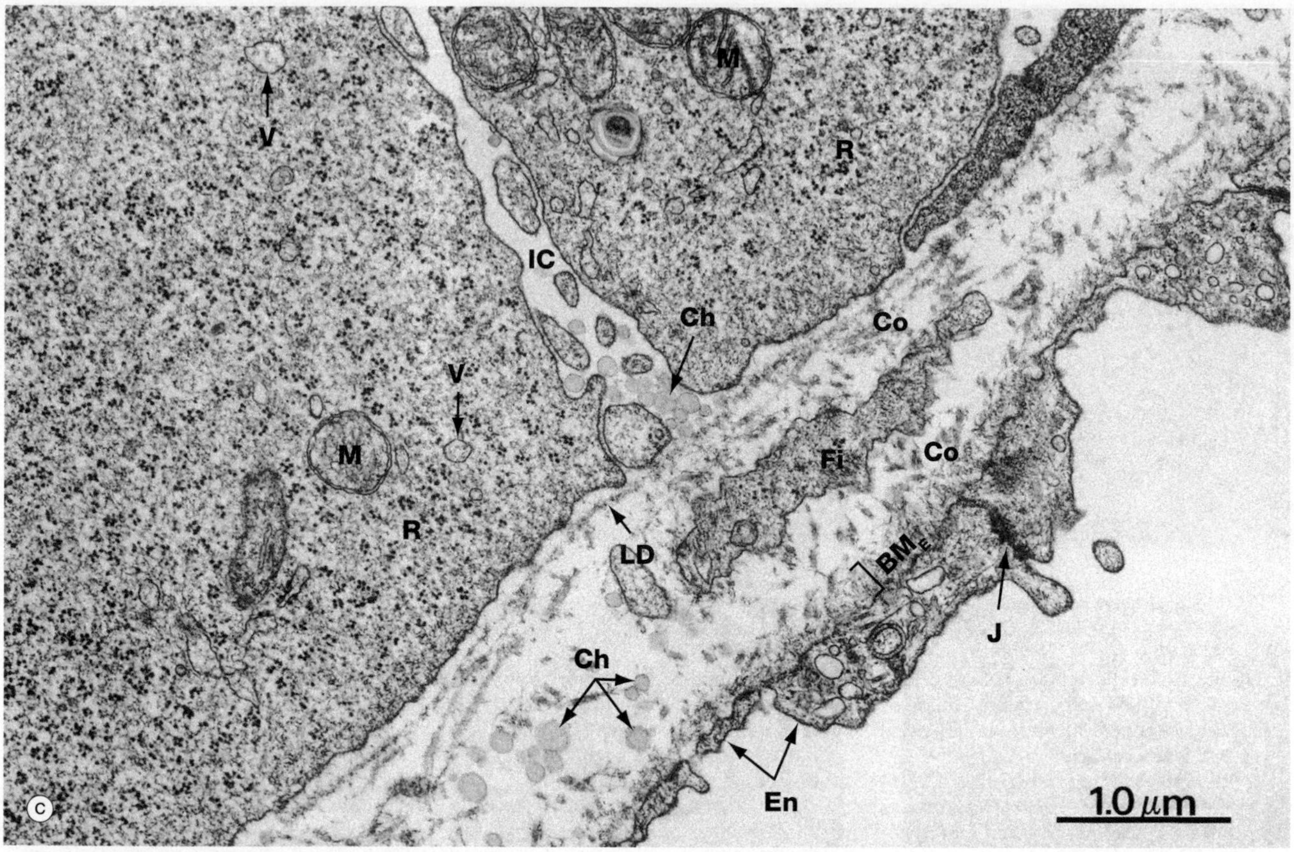

FIG. 14.25 Enterocytes *(illustrations (a) and (b) opposite)*
(a) EM ×4540 (b) EM ×5600 (c) EM ×22 000

These micrographs illustrate the main ultrastructural features of ***enterocytes***, the absorptive cells of the small intestine.

Fig. 14.25a shows the enormous number of ***microvilli* Mv** (up to 3000 per cell), which increase the surface area of the plasma membrane exposed to the lumen by some 30 times. The microvilli are of uniform length (approximately 1 μm) and constitute the ***brush border*** of light microscopy (see Figs 14.22 and 5.14). Most absorption in the small intestine occurs by direct passage of low molecular weight digestion products across the luminal plasma membrane. Mitochondria **M** are particularly abundant within enterocytes, reflecting the high energy demands of such processes. Chylomicrons, assembled in the enterocytes, pass first into the ***intercellular clefts* IC**, then across the basement membrane **BM** into the core of the villus and finally into the ***lacteal***. Lymphocytes **Ly** are commonly found in the intercellular clefts between enterocytes, where they play an important part in the immunological defence of the gastrointestinal tract. Note the close proximity of a blood capillary **C** to the enterocyte basement membrane.

As seen in Fig. 14.25b, the ***glycocalyx* G** of the enterocyte microvilli is unusually prominent. It provides protection against autodigestion and acts as the site for adsorption of pancreatic digestive enzymes. This micrograph also shows the microfilament cytoskeleton of the microvilli **Mv** extending into the superficial cytoplasm. Here, in the terminal web **TW**, it becomes integrated into the cytoskeleton of the body of the cell. Deeper in the cell, microfilaments **F** and microtubules **T** are readily identified. Enterocytes are tightly bound near their luminal surface by junctional complexes (see Fig. 5.9) which prevent direct access of luminal contents into the intercellular spaces, as well as holding the epithelium together.

Endocytotic vesicles* EV** are often seen between the bases of microvilli and ***transport vesicles* V** are common in the superficial cytoplasm. Endocytosis with transfer to the extracellular fluid at the base of the cell (transcytosis***) is an important mechanism of uptake of macromolecules from the gut lumen into the blood. An example of transcytosis is the uptake of maternal antibodies from the milk in breast fed infants. Smooth endoplasmic reticulum **sER** is seen deeper in the cytoplasm.

Fig. 14.25c illustrates the basal aspect of two enterocytes, separated by an intercellular cleft **IC**. Their basement membrane is thin and the lamina densa **LD** appears to be discontinuous. Close beneath the base of the enterocytes is a tiny lymphatic tributary of the central lacteal, its endothelial lining **En** being thin and fenestrated. Note the ***junctional complex* J** binding adjacent endothelial cells and the thin discontinuous endothelial basement membrane $\mathbf{BM_E}$. The delicate supporting tissue between the basement membrane and lymphatic contains fibroblasts **Fi** and fine collagen fibrils **Co**.

The main feature of the basal enterocyte cytoplasm is numerous free ribosomes **R**, scattered mitochondria **M** and membranous vesicles **V** containing lipoprotein droplets en route for exocytosis into the intercellular cleft. The cleft contains numerous small chylomicrons **Ch** that cluster near the lamina densa, as if temporarily held up in their passage towards the lymphatic. In the lamina propria, the chylomicrons are larger, probably due to fusion of smaller ones coursing through from the intercellular cleft. Note that the chylomicrons in the extracellular environment are not membrane-bound but have a fine electron-dense limiting layer of protein.

BM basement membrane $\mathbf{BM_E}$ endothelial basement membrane **C** capillary **Ch** chylomicron **Co** collagen fibrils **En** endothelium **EV** endocytotic vesicles **F** microfilaments **Fi** fibroblast **G** glycocalyx **IC** intercellular cleft **J** junctional complex **LD** lamina densa **Ly** lymphocyte **M** mitochondrion **Mv** microvilli **R** ribosomes **sER** smooth endoplasmic reticulum **T** microtubules **TW** terminal web **V** membranous transport vesicle

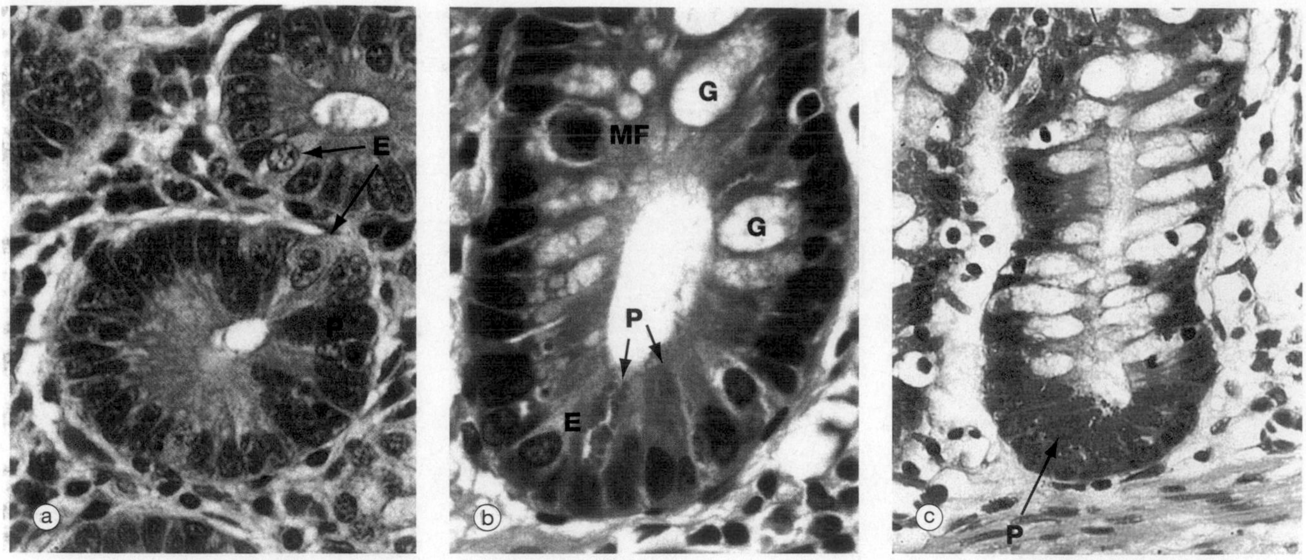

FIG. 14.26 Crypts of Lieberkühn
(a) H&E, TS (HP) (b) H&E, LS (HP) (c) Phloxine–tartrazine, LS (HP)

The majority of cells in the crypt bases are stem cells that divide regularly to replenish the epithelial cells of the villi. Immature goblet cells **G** are readily seen in Fig. 14.26b. A single mitotic figure **MF** is identifiable.

With H&E staining in Fig. 14.26a and b, Paneth cells **P**, which form part of the innate immune system, exhibit intensely eosinophilic apical cytoplasmic granules. These are stained bright scarlet by the phloxine–tartrazine method in Fig. 14.26c. The granules of Paneth cells contain antimicrobial peptides (***defensins***) and protective enzymes such as ***lysozyme*** and ***phospholipase A***. These products, secreted into the small bowel, provide the first line of defence against any pathogens that survive passage through the stomach. The lumen of the small bowel is virtually sterile. Paneth cells are long-lived (weeks) in comparison to the short lifespan (3–5 days) of enterocytes and goblet cells.

Endocrine cells **E** also contain eosinophilic cytoplasmic granules which are found in a subnuclear position, in contrast to the apical granules of Paneth cells. Secretory products of gut endocrine cells include hormones such as ***secretin, somatostatin*** and ***5-HT*** (***serotonin***). In general, each endocrine cell produces only one hormone.

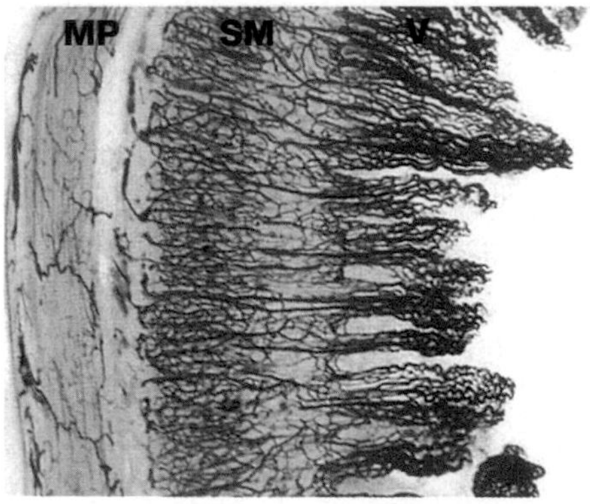

FIG. 14.27 Intestinal villi
Carmine perfused (LP)

Fig. 14.27 of small intestine has been perfused before fixation with a red dye to demonstrate the blood supply of the mucosa. Long loops of branching capillaries originating from a dense capillary network in the submucosa **SM** extend up to the tips of the villi **V**. Note also the capillary network supplying the muscularis propria **MP**. Most of the absorbed food products, with the exception of triglycerides, enter the capillaries and pass via the portal vein to the liver.

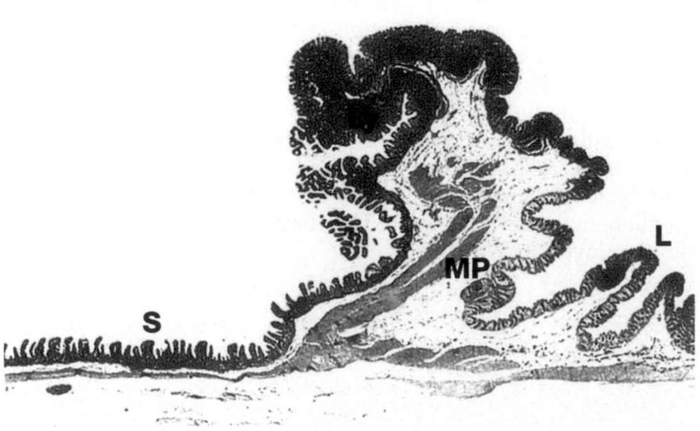

FIG. 14.28 Ileocaecal junction
H&E (LP)

Indigestible food residues from the ileum are propelled by peristalsis into the distended first part of the large intestine, the ***caecum***, through the cone-shaped ***ileocaecal valve*** (Fig. 14.28). There is an abrupt transition in the lining of the valve from the small intestinal villiform pattern **S** to the glandular form in the large intestine **L**. The ileocaecal valve consists of a thickened extension of the muscularis propria **MP** that provides robust support for the mucosa. Lymphoid tissue **Ly** in the form of large ***Peyer's patches*** is found in the mucosa.

CM circular muscle **E** endocrine cell **G** goblet cell **L** large intestine **LM** longitudinal muscle **Ly** lymphoid tissue **MF** mitotic figure **MM** muscularis mucosae **MP** muscularis propria **P** Paneth cell **S** small intestine **SM** submucosa **T** T lymphocyte **V** villus

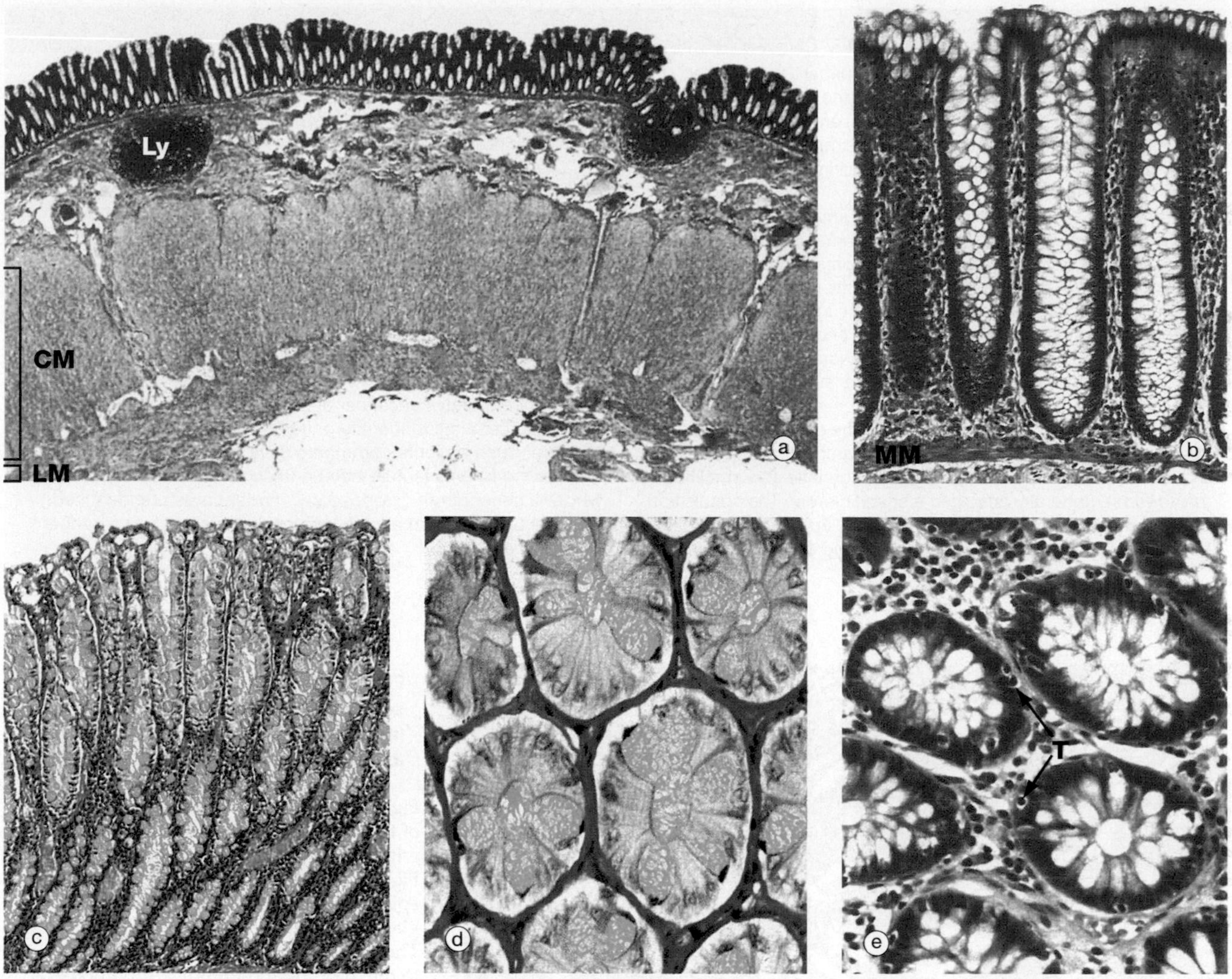

FIG. 14.29 Colon
(a) H&E (LP) (b) H&E (MP) (c) Alcian blue/van Gieson (MP) (d) Alcian blue/van Gieson (HP) (e) H&E (HP)

The principal functions of the large intestine are the recovery of water and salt from faeces and the propulsion of increasingly solid faeces to the rectum prior to defaecation.

As shown in Fig. 14.29a, the muscular wall is consequently thick and capable of powerful peristaltic activity. As in the rest of the gastrointestinal tract, the muscularis propria of the large intestine consists of inner circular **CM** and outer longitudinal layers **LM** but, except in the rectum, the longitudinal layer forms three separate longitudinal bands called ***taeniae coli***.

The mucosa is the same from caecum to rectum. It is folded in the non-distended state but does not exhibit distinct plicae circulares like those of the small intestine. Immediately above the anal valves, the mucosa forms longitudinal folds called the ***columns of Morgagni***. The muscularis mucosae is a prominent feature of the large intestinal mucosa. Rhythmic contractions prevent clogging of the glands and enhance expulsion of mucus.

Consistent with its functions of water absorption and faecal lubrication, the mucosa consists of cells of two types: ***absorptive cells*** and mucus-secreting ***goblet cells***. As seen in Fig. 14.29b, these are arranged in closely packed straight tubular glands or ***crypts***, which extend down to sit on to the muscularis mucosae **MM**. As faeces pass along the large intestine and become progressively dehydrated, the mucus becomes increasingly important in protecting the mucosa from trauma. The Alcian blue method shown in Fig. 14.29c stains goblet cell mucus a greenish-blue colour, while the absorptive cells remain poorly stained. Goblet cells predominate in the base of the glands, whereas the luminal surface is almost entirely lined by columnar absorptive cells.

Fig. 14.29d and e show transverse sections through the upper part of large intestinal glands, highlighting the closely packed arrangement of the glands in the mucosa. The tall columnar absorptive cells have oval basal nuclei. In contrast, goblet cell nuclei are small and condensed. Stem cells at the base of the glands continually replace the epithelium. Intraepithelial T lymphocytes **T** are easily seen in Fig. 14.29e.

Lamina propria fills the space between the glands and contains numerous blood vessels into which water is absorbed. In the lamina propria, lymphatics are very scanty, if present at all. The lamina propria also contains collagen, which is stained red in Fig. 14.29c and d, as well as lymphocytes and plasma cells. These form part of the defence mechanisms against invading pathogens, along with intraepithelial lymphocytes and the ***lymphoid aggregates*** **Ly**, which are smaller than Peyer's patches. These are found in the lamina propria and submucosa, as seen at low power in Fig. 14.29a.

The large intestine is inhabited by a variety of ***commensal bacteria*** that further degrade food residues. Bacterial degradation is an important mechanism for the digestion of cellulose in ruminants but, in humans, most cellulose is excreted. Small quantities of fat-soluble vitamins derived from bacterial activity are absorbed in the large intestine.

Non-malignant disorders of the colon

The colon and rectum are subject to a variety of conditions including infections, inflammatory disorders (discussed later) and vascular disorders. Acute infections often result in diarrhoea and are usually short lived. More chronic infections such as amoebic colitis and those associated with immunocompromise (e.g. cytomegalovirus) are usually diagnosed on biopsy and require special stains for confirmation.

Diverticulosis, in which the mucosa herniates through the bowel wall, can cause an acute abdomen by becoming inflamed with abscess formation or perforation. Vascular compromise of the bowel can occur as a result of herniation, embolus in the blood supply or volvulus (twisting) of the bowel wall.

Carcinoma of the colon and rectum

Malignant tumours arising in glandular epithelium are called adenocarcinomas. Adenocarcinomas of the colon and rectum (commonly referred to as bowel cancers) are common in older patients, particularly in developed countries. This is in contrast to adenocarcinomas of the small intestine, which are comparatively rare.

Intensive research has identified a number of risk factors for the development of colorectal carcinoma, including the prior existence of benign tumours (adenomas) in the bowel, the presence of long-standing ulcerative colitis (a form of chronic inflammatory disease affecting the colon), inherited syndromes such as familial adenomatous polyposis and Gardner syndrome (in which patients have innumerable adenomas in the bowel due to a genetic abnormality) and also factors such as low dietary fibre intake.

The sequence of events involved in the development of some adenocarcinomas is becoming clearer, and it appears to require the accumulation of a number of genetic abnormalities (***mutations***), generally arising in a specific order. The acquisition of these mutations can be detected as the epithelium changes from normal to an adenoma, with increasing degrees of ***dysplasia*** (pre-malignant change in the epithelium with disordered growth and maturation) through to invasive carcinoma. This is known as the ***adenoma–carcinoma sequence***. A typical colorectal adenocarcinoma is shown in Fig. 14.30a.

Our understanding of the processes involved in the development of cancer is critical in trying to prevent its occurrence. For example, simple public health interventions to promote improved dietary fibre intake have the potential to significantly reduce the risk of cancer development. Many developed countries have cancer screening programmes designed to prevent common cancers by detecting pre-cancerous changes and treating them before cancer develops, or to detect cancers in their earliest stages to allow effective curative treatment. Such systems are widely used to reduce the occurrence of cervical cancer and breast cancer. Screening for bowel cancer aims to identify patients with adenomas and early cancers. Such patients commonly have blood in their faeces and testing for this feature can be used to select those patients who will benefit from colonoscopy. If adenomas are identified, removal of these dramatically reduces the risk of future cancer development.

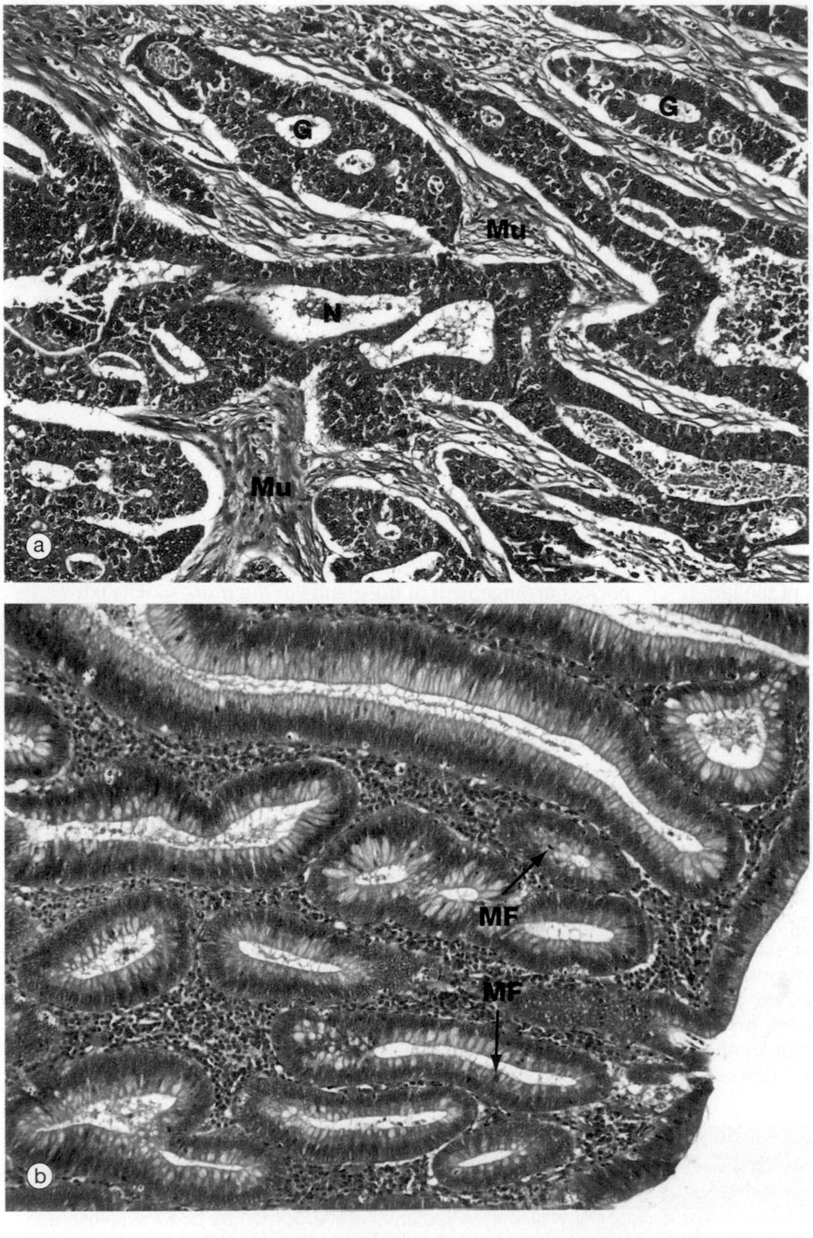

FIG. 14.30 The adenoma–carcinoma sequence
(a) Colonic adenocarcinoma, H&E (MP)
(b) Colonic adenoma, H&E (MP)

Fig. 14.30a shows a typical adenocarcinoma of the colon (see e-Fig. 14.6). Compare this with the normal colonic mucosa seen in Fig. 14.29. In adenocarcinoma, the malignant epithelial cells form disorganised abnormal glands that invade into the adjacent tissues. The depth of invasion and indeed the spread to the draining mesenteric lymph nodes is the basis for ***staging*** the tumour, i.e. giving a prediction of the likely behaviour of the tumour based on the extent of the tumour. Obviously, the further the tumour has spread, the worse the outcome is likely to be. A small superficial adenocarcinoma confined to the colon has a good chance of cure by surgery, whereas a tumour that has spread far and wide (***metastasised***) will have a much worse outlook. In Fig. 14.30a the malignant glands **G** of the tumour have invaded into the muscularis propria. Small bundles of smooth muscle **Mu** can be identified and there are also areas of ***necrosis*** **N** (dead tissue), another feature commonly seen in cancers.

In contrast, Fig. 14.30b shows an adenoma, a benign but pre-cancerous tumour of the colon (see e-Fig. 14.7). These tumours exhibit epithelial dysplasia, showing abnormal disordered growth. When compared against the normal mucosa shown in Fig. 14.29, the epithelial cells are seen to have larger nuclei and there are obvious ***mitotic figures*** **MF**, indicating increased cell proliferation. There are fewer mucus-containing goblet cells, reflecting a lack of normal cellular differentiation. If such pre-malignant changes remain untreated, a significant number of adenomas will progress over time to acquire further genetic abnormalities and invasive adenocarcinoma may develop.

F follicle **G** malignant gland **J** anorectal junction **LP** lamina propria **M** mesoappendix **MF** mitotic figure **Mu** smooth muscle **N** necrosis **RM** rectal mucosa **S** serosa **SM** submucosa **SS** stratified squamous epithelium

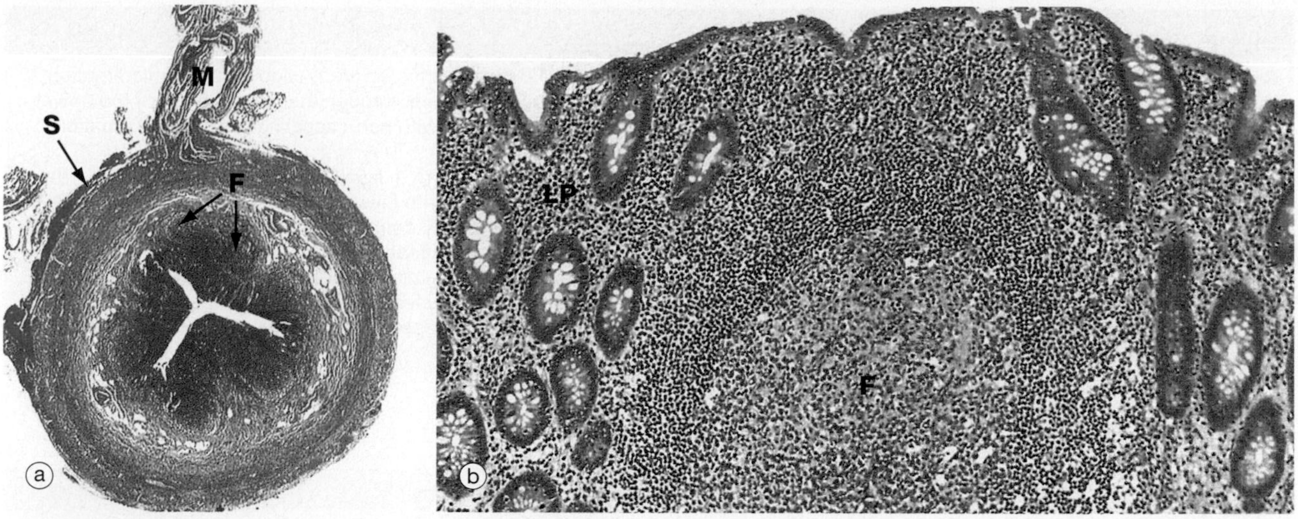

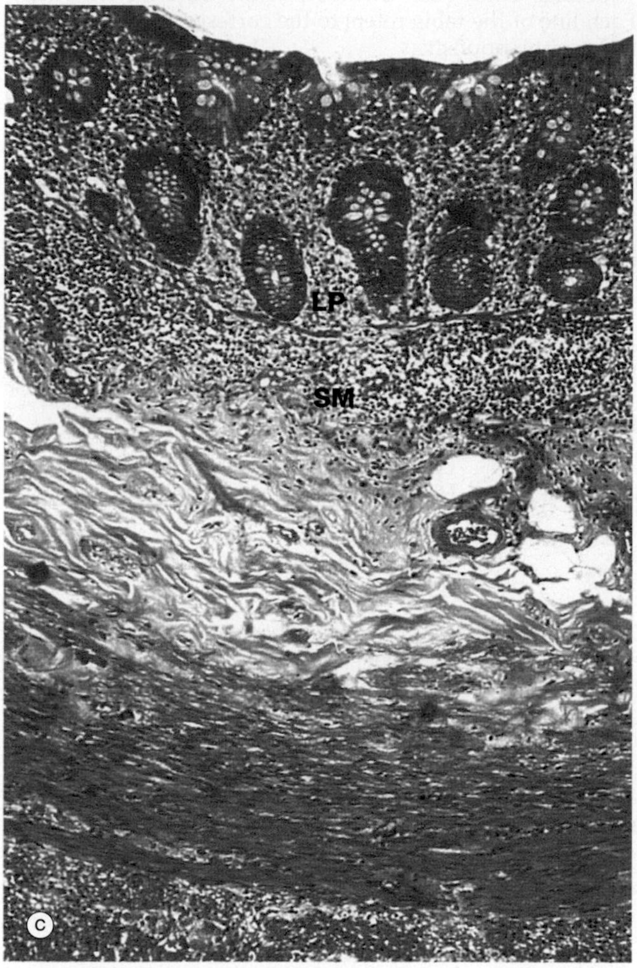

FIG. 14.31 Appendix
(a) H&E (LP) (b) H&E (MP) (c) H&E (MP)

The appendix is a small, blind-ended, tubular sac extending from the caecum just distal to the ileocaecal junction. The general structure of the appendix conforms to that of the rest of the large intestine. In some mammals, the appendix is capacious and is involved in prolonged digestion of cellulose, but in humans its function is unknown.

Fig. 14.31a illustrates the suspensory ***mesentery*** or ***mesoappendix*** **M**, in continuity with the outer serosal layer **S**. The serosa contains extravasated blood due to haemorrhage during surgical removal. The mesenteries of the gastrointestinal tract conduct blood vessels, lymphatics and nerves to and from the gastrointestinal tract.

The most characteristic feature of the appendix, particularly in the young, is the presence of masses of lymphoid tissue in the mucosa and submucosa. As seen in Figs 14.32b and c, the lamina propria **LP** and upper submucosa **SM** are diffusely infiltrated with lymphocytes. Note that the mucosal glands are much less closely packed than in the large intestine. As seen in Figs 14.31a and b, the lymphoid tissue also forms follicles **F**, often containing germinal centres (see Ch. 11). These follicles bulge into the lumen of the appendix and, like the follicles of Peyer's patches in the small intestine, are invested by a simple epithelium of ***M cells*** (see Fig. 11.16), which presumably facilitates sampling of antigen in the lumen.

The most common disorder affecting the appendix is acute appendicitis (inflammation of the appendix) (see e-Fig. 14.8). This typically presents with severe abdominal pain, initially centred in the middle of the abdomen and then later localising to the right iliac fossa. Appendicitis is a fairly common acute surgical emergency. If it is left untreated, the appendix may rupture and discharge infected ***pus*** into the peritoneal cavity, resulting in acute peritonitis.

Primary tumours also occur in the appendix including neuroendocrine tumours (see e-Fig. 14.9), appendiceal mucinous neoplasms and conventional adenocarcinomas.

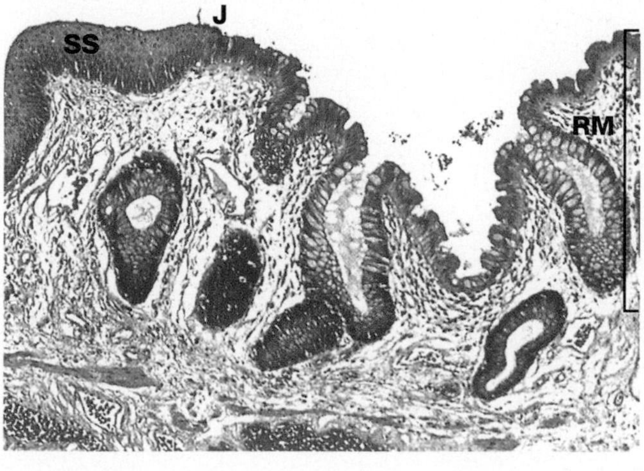

FIG. 14.32 Anorectal junction
H&E (MP)

The rectum is the short, dilated, terminal portion of the large intestine (Fig. 14.32). The rectal mucosa **RM** is the same as the rest of the large bowel except that it has even more numerous goblet cells. At the anorectal junction **J**, it undergoes an abrupt transition to become stratified squamous epithelium **SS** in the ***anal canal***. Branched tubular circumanal glands open at the recto-anal junction into small pits at the distal ends of the ***columns of Morgagni***.

The anal canal forms the last 2 or 3 cm of the gastrointestinal tract and is surrounded by voluntary muscle that forms the ***anal sphincter***. Here, the stratified squamous epithelium undergoes a gradual transition to skin containing sebaceous glands and large apocrine sweat glands (see Ch. 9).

Chronic inflammatory bowel disease (IBD)

Chronic inflammatory bowel disease includes two main conditions: ulcerative colitis (see e-Fig. 14.10) and Crohn's disease (see e-Fig. 14.11). These are relapsing and remitting inflammatory disorders with no known cause. Both conditions cause similar clinical and pathological findings so occasionally it may not be possible to distinguish between the two. Other differential diagnoses (see textbox 'Disorders of the gastrointestinal tract') also need to be considered as many other conditions are mimics of IBD.

Crohn's disease (CD) can affect anywhere in the GI tract though it usually involves the small intestine. CD typically involves the GI tract in a patchy distribution with areas of normal bowel wall between affected areas (skip lesions). Inflammation is usually transmural, i.e. through the full thickness of the bowel wall, and associated with non-caseating granuloma formation (see e-Fig. 14.12).

Ulcerative colitis (UC) usually involves the rectum and can extend proximally to involve the colon. When active, inflammation is usually confined to the mucosa and submucosa. Granulomas are not a feature of UC. As UC is associated with repeated episodes of inflammation, ulceration and epithelial regeneration, this may lead to dysplastic change. This contributes to an increased risk of colorectal cancer in these patients.

REVIEW

Table 14.1 outlines the main structural features of the different components of the gastrointestinal tract for easy reference and revision. Please note that the epithelium of all segments includes stem cells and neuroendocrine cells, which have not been included in the table for simplicity. Each line of the table refers to the correspondingly labelled micrograph opposite.

TABLE 14.1 Review of gastrointestinal tract

Part of the gastrointestinal tract	Type of epithelium	Main cell type of epithelium	Other distinctive features	Figure
Oesophagus	Stratified squamous	Squamous cells	Submucosal glands	14.33a
Body/fundus of stomach	Glandular, straight tubular	Surface mucous cells Neck mucous cells Parietal cells Chief (peptic) cells	Lymphoid cells very sparse No lymphoid aggregates	14.33b
Pylorus and cardia of stomach	Glandular, coiled, branched tubular	Mucous cells May be occasional parietal cells	Lymphoid cells very sparse No lymphoid aggregates	14.33c
Duodenum	Glandular with villi and crypts of Lieberkühn	Enterocytes with microvilli Goblet cells Paneth cells	Brunner's gland Plicae circulares (after distal duodenum)	14.33d
Jejunum and ileum	Glandular with villi and crypts of Lieberkühn	Enterocytes with microvilli Goblet cells Paneth cells	Peyer's patches become more prominent distally Plicae circulares	14.33e
Colon and rectum	Glandular, straight crypts	Goblet cells Absorptive cells	Taeniae coli	14.33f
Appendix	Glandular, straight crypts	Goblet cells Tall columnar cells	Prominent lymphoid tissue	14.33g
Anus	Stratified squamous	Squamous cells	Columns of Morgagni	14.33h

FIG. 14.33 Comparison of histological features throughout the gastrointestinal tract ***(see Table 14.1 opposite)***

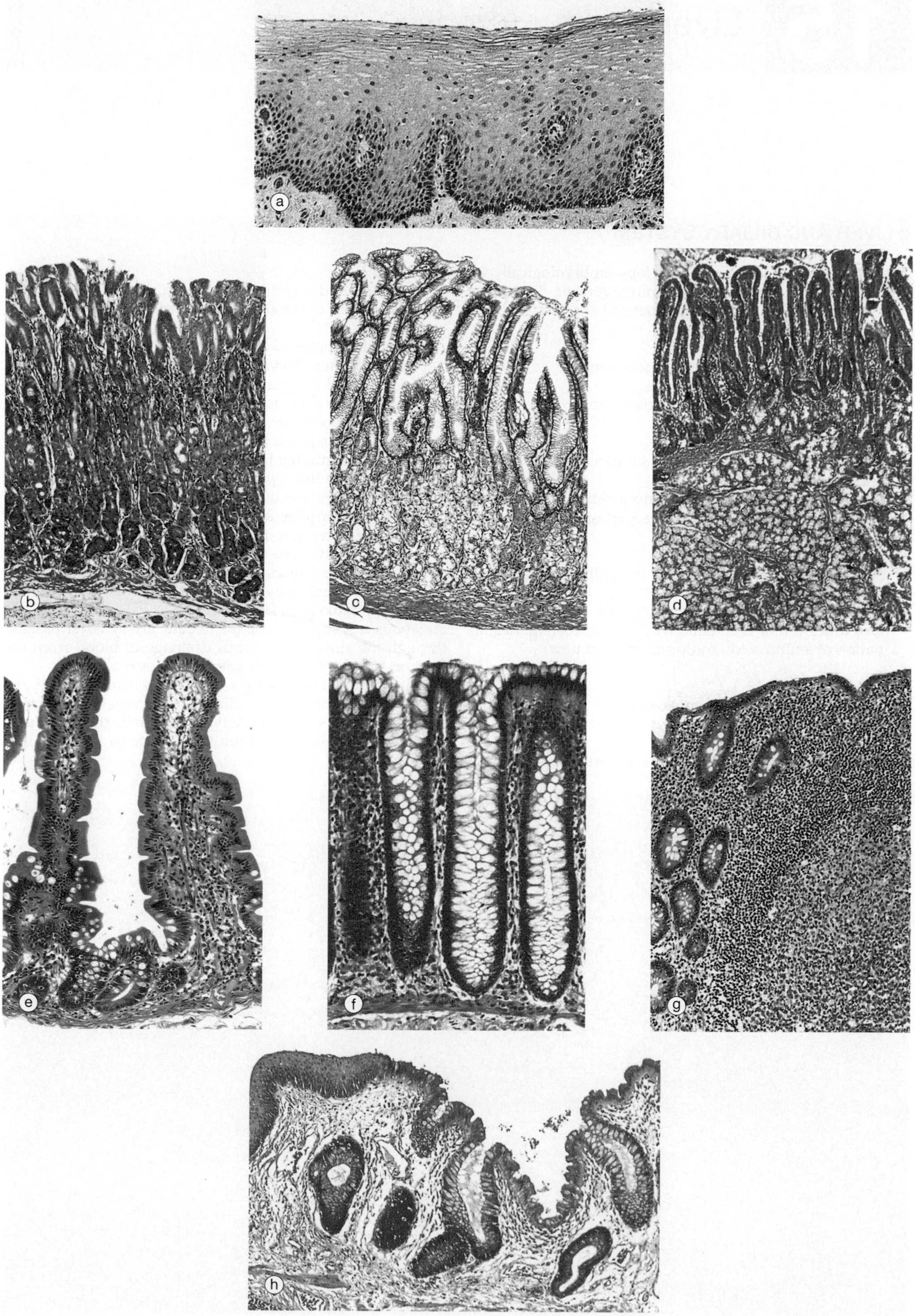

15 Liver and pancreas

LIVER AND BILIARY SYSTEM

The liver, like the pancreas, develops embryologically as a glandular outgrowth of the primitive ***foregut***. The major functions of the liver may be summarised as follows:

Fat metabolism:
- Oxidising triglycerides to produce energy
- Synthesis of plasma lipoproteins
- Synthesis of cholesterol and phospholipid

Carbohydrate metabolism:
- Converting carbohydrates and proteins into fatty acids and triglyceride
- Regulation of blood glucose concentration by glycogenesis, glycogenolysis and gluconeogenesis

Protein metabolism:
- Synthesis of plasma proteins, including albumin and clotting factors
- Synthesis of non-essential amino acids
- Detoxification of metabolic waste products (e.g. deamination of amino acids and production of urea)

Storage:
- Storage of glycogen, vitamins, iron

Intermediary metabolism:
- Detoxification of various drugs and toxins (e.g. alcohol)

Secretion:
- Synthesis and secretion of bile, which contains many of the products of the above processes

The main functional cell in the liver is a type of epithelial cell called the ***hepatocyte***. These cells are arranged as thin plates separated by fine vascular ***sinusoids*** through which blood flows. The close association of liver cells and the circulation allows absorption of nutrients from digestion, as well as secretion of products into the blood.

Blood flow into the liver sinusoids comes from terminal branches of both the ***hepatic portal vein*** and ***hepatic artery***. The liver is therefore unusual in having both arterial and venous blood supplies, as well as separate venous drainage.

With the exception of most lipids, absorbed food products pass directly from the gut to the liver via the hepatic portal vein. This brings blood that is rich in amino acids, simple sugars and other products of digestion but relatively poor in oxygen. The oxygen required to support liver metabolism is supplied via the hepatic artery. After passing through the sinusoids, venous drainage of blood from the liver occurs via the ***hepatic vein*** into the vena cava.

The main blood vessels and ducts run through the liver within a branched collagenous framework termed the ***portal tracts***. These tracts also contain the ***bile ducts*** that transport bile away from the liver to be secreted into the small bowel.

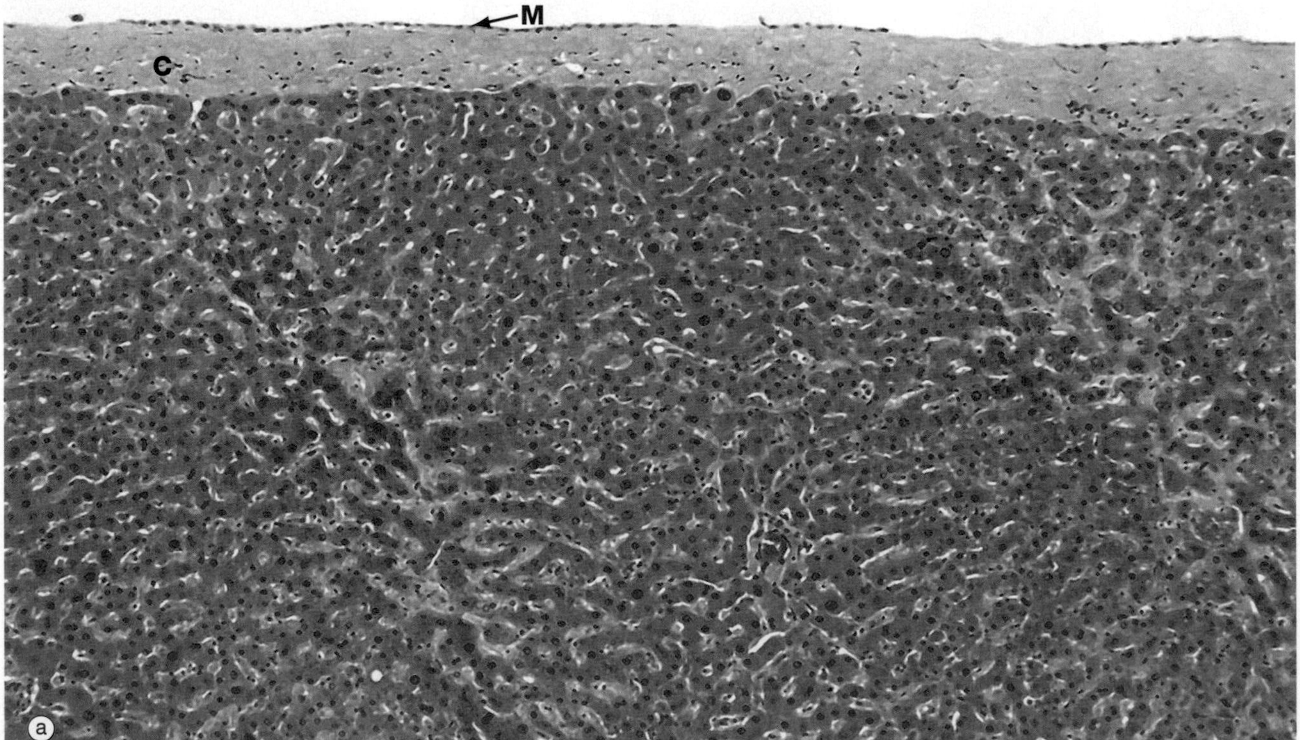

FIG. 15.1 Liver *(caption and illustration (b) opposite)*
(a) Capsule and parenchyma, H&E (MP) (b) Architecture, H&E (LP)

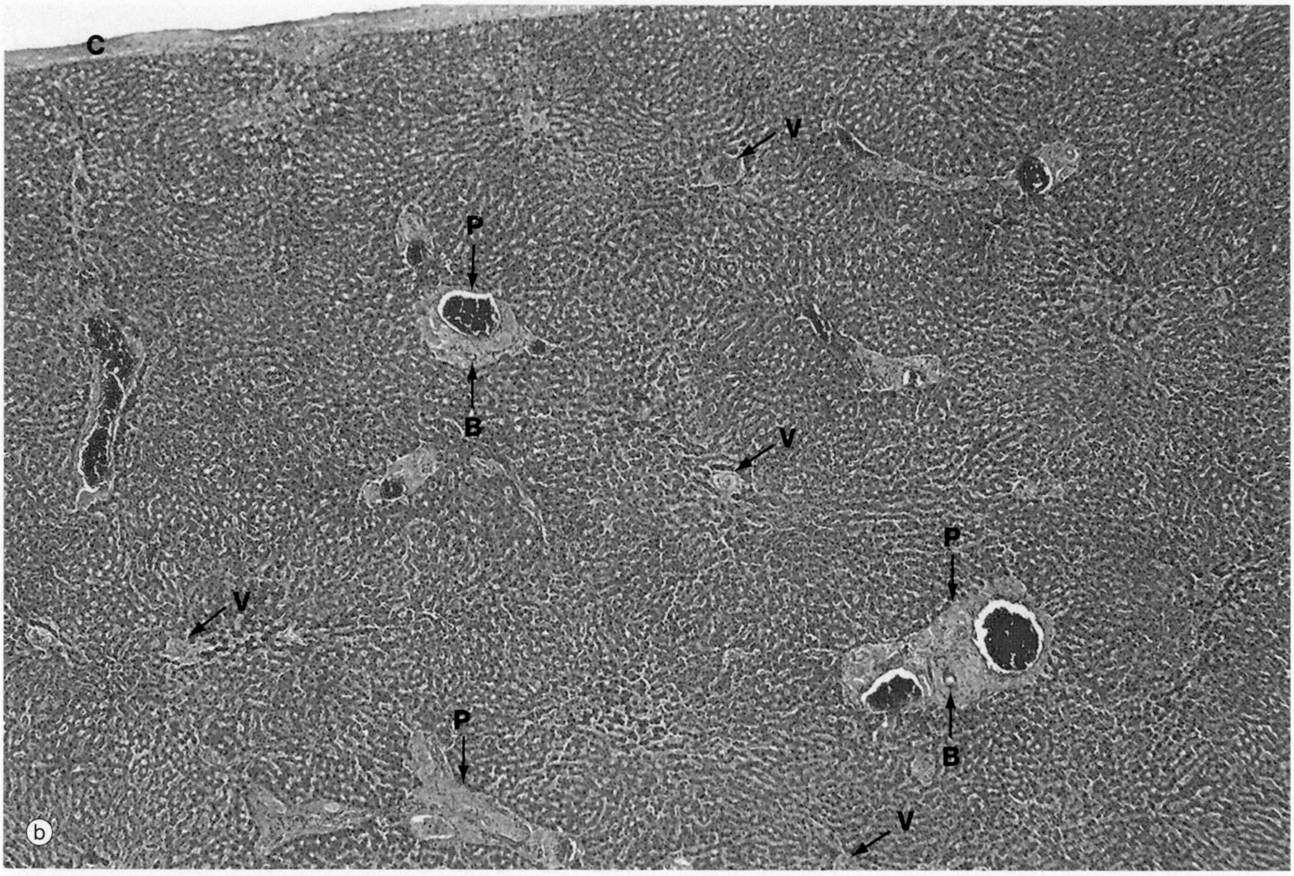

FIG. 15.1 Liver ***(illustration (a) opposite)***
(a) Capsule and parenchyma, H&E (MP) (b) Architecture, H&E (LP)

Fig. 15.1a shows the structure of the liver, which is a solid organ composed of tightly packed pink-staining plates of ***hepatocytes***. The outer surface of the liver is covered by a ***capsule*** composed of collagenous tissue **C** called ***Glisson's capsule,*** covered by a layer of ***mesothelial cells*** **M** from the peritoneum.

The ***sinusoids*** can just be seen as pale-stained spaces between the plates of liver cells. The hepatic sinusoids form a very low-resistance system of vascular channels that allows blood to come into contact with the hepatocytes over a huge surface area.

Fig. 15.1b shows the overall architecture of the liver at a slightly lower magnification. The liver does not contain much in the way of connective tissue. Most of the collagenous connective tissue in the liver is found in the portal tracts **P** which contain the main blood vessels running into the liver. Larger vessels can be seen containing bright red blood, even at this low magnification. The other structures that run in the portal tracts are branches of the ***bile ducts*** **B**.

Less conspicuous than the portal tracts are the ***centrilobular venules*** (***hepatic venules***) **V** that drain the liver. These are tributaries of the hepatic vein and take blood away from the liver.

The very close association of the sinusoidal vasculature of the liver with the hepatocytes is essential for normal function. Certain diseases of the liver cause obliteration of the normal sinusoidal arrangement and this then causes impairment of liver function.

TABLE 15.1 Clinical features of liver disease

The normal liver has very diverse functions (see text). As a result, liver disease can produce a wide range of symptoms and signs affecting multiple body systems, some of which are detailed below.

Sign/symptom	Clinical feature	Mechanism
Jaundice	Yellow colouration of tissues due to bile pigments	Failure of metabolism or excretion of bile
Bleeding	Easy bruising and prolonged clotting time of blood	Failure of hepatic synthesis of clotting factors
Oedema	Swelling of dependent parts secondary to extracellular accumulation of water	Failure of hepatic synthesis of albumin, resulting in reduced plasma oncotic pressure
Ascites	Fluid in peritoneal cavity	Low serum albumin and/or portal hypertension
Gynaecomastia	Enlarged male breasts	Failure to detoxify endogenous oestrogens
Encephalopathy	Altered consciousness, lack of coordination, may lead to coma	Failure to detoxify ammonia and excitatory amino acids derived from protein breakdown
Haematemesis and/or melaena	Vomiting blood and passing blood	Bleeding from oesophageal varices or per rectum owing to portal hypertension

B bile duct **C** liver capsule **M** mesothelial cells **P** portal tract **V** hepatic venule

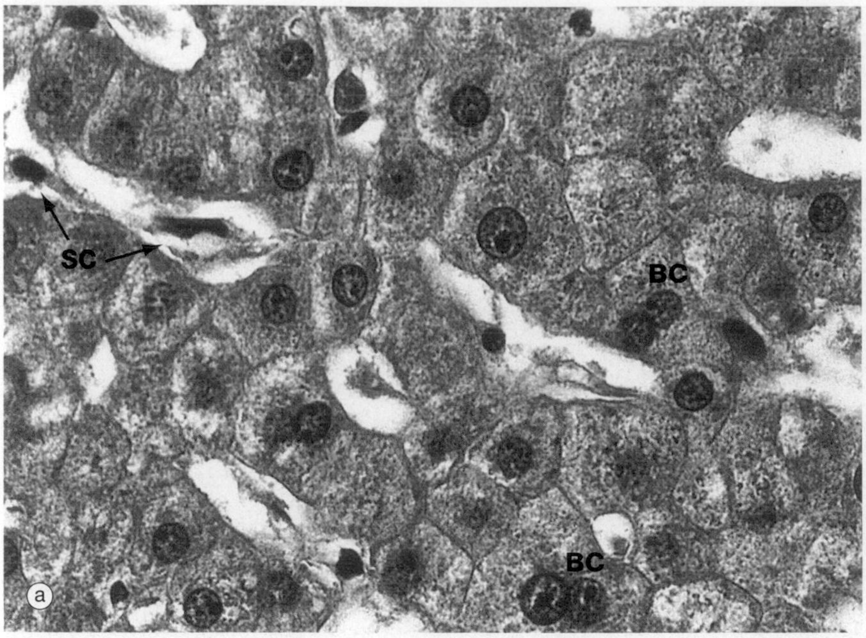

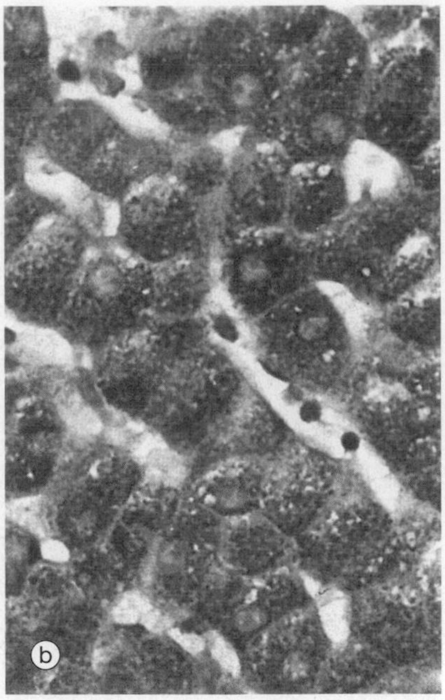

FIG. 15.2 Hepatocytes
(a) H&E (HP) (b) PAS/haematoxylin (HP)

Hepatocytes (Fig. 15.2) are large polyhedral cells with round nuclei, peripherally dispersed chromatin and prominent nucleoli. The nuclei vary greatly in size, reflecting an unusual cellular feature; more than half of the hepatocytes contain twice the normal (diploid) complement of chromosomes within a single nucleus (i.e. they are tetraploid) and some contain four or even eight times this amount (polyploid). Binucleate cells **BC** are also common in normal liver.

The extensive cytoplasm has a variable appearance, depending on the nutritional status of the individual. When well-nourished, hepatocytes store significant quantities of glycogen and process large quantities of lipid. Both of these metabolites are partially removed during routine histological preparation, leaving irregular unstained areas within the cytoplasm. The cytoplasm is otherwise strongly eosinophilic due to numerous mitochondria, with a fine basophilic granularity due to extensive free ribosomes and rough endoplasmic reticulum.

Fine brown granules of the 'wear-and-tear' pigment ***lipofuscin*** (see Fig. 1.26) are present in variable amounts, increasing with age. All of these features are seen in Fig. 15.2a.

The sinusoids are lined by flat endothelial lining cells **SC** which are readily distinguishable from hepatocytes by their flattened condensed nuclei and attenuated poorly stained cytoplasm.

Fig. 15.2b shows glycogen in hepatocytes which, being a polysaccharide, is PAS-positive (i.e. stains magenta). In this preparation, the nuclei are counterstained blue with haematoxylin.

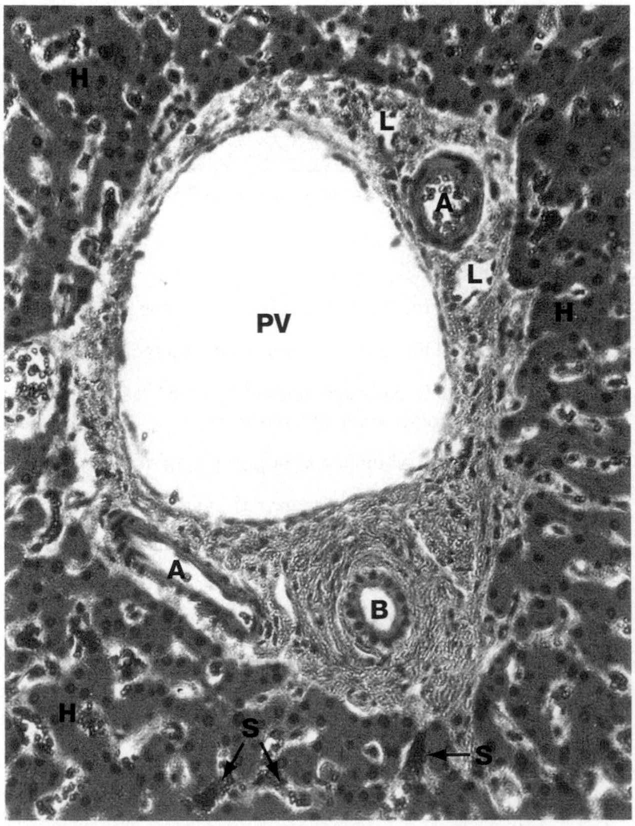

FIG. 15.3 Portal tract
H&E (MP)

Fig. 15.3 shows a typical ***portal tract*** containing three main structures. The largest is a terminal branch of the ***hepatic portal vein*** **PV** (***terminal portal venule***) which has a thin wall lined by endothelial cells. Smaller-diameter thick-walled vessels are terminal branches of the ***hepatic artery*** **A** with the structure of arterioles.

A network of ***bile canaliculi*** is located within each plate of hepatocytes, but these are far too small to be seen at this magnification. These drain into ***bile collecting ducts*** lined by simple cuboidal or columnar epithelium, known as the ***canals of Hering***, which in turn drain into the ***bile ductules*** **B**. The bile ductules are usually located at the periphery of the tract. The bile ductules merge to form larger, more centrally located ***trabecular ducts*** which drain via ***intrahepatic ducts*** into the ***right*** and ***left hepatic ducts***, the ***common hepatic duct*** and then to the duodenum via the ***common bile duct***.

Because these three structures are always found in the portal tracts, the tracts are often referred to as ***portal triads***. ***Lymphatics*** **L** are also present in the portal tracts but, since their walls are delicate and often collapsed, they are less easily identified.

Surrounding the portal tract are anastomosing plates of hepatocytes **H**, between which are the ***hepatic sinusoids*** **S**. These receive blood from both the hepatic portal and hepatic arterial systems. The layer of hepatocytes immediately bordering the portal tract is known as the ***limiting plate***.

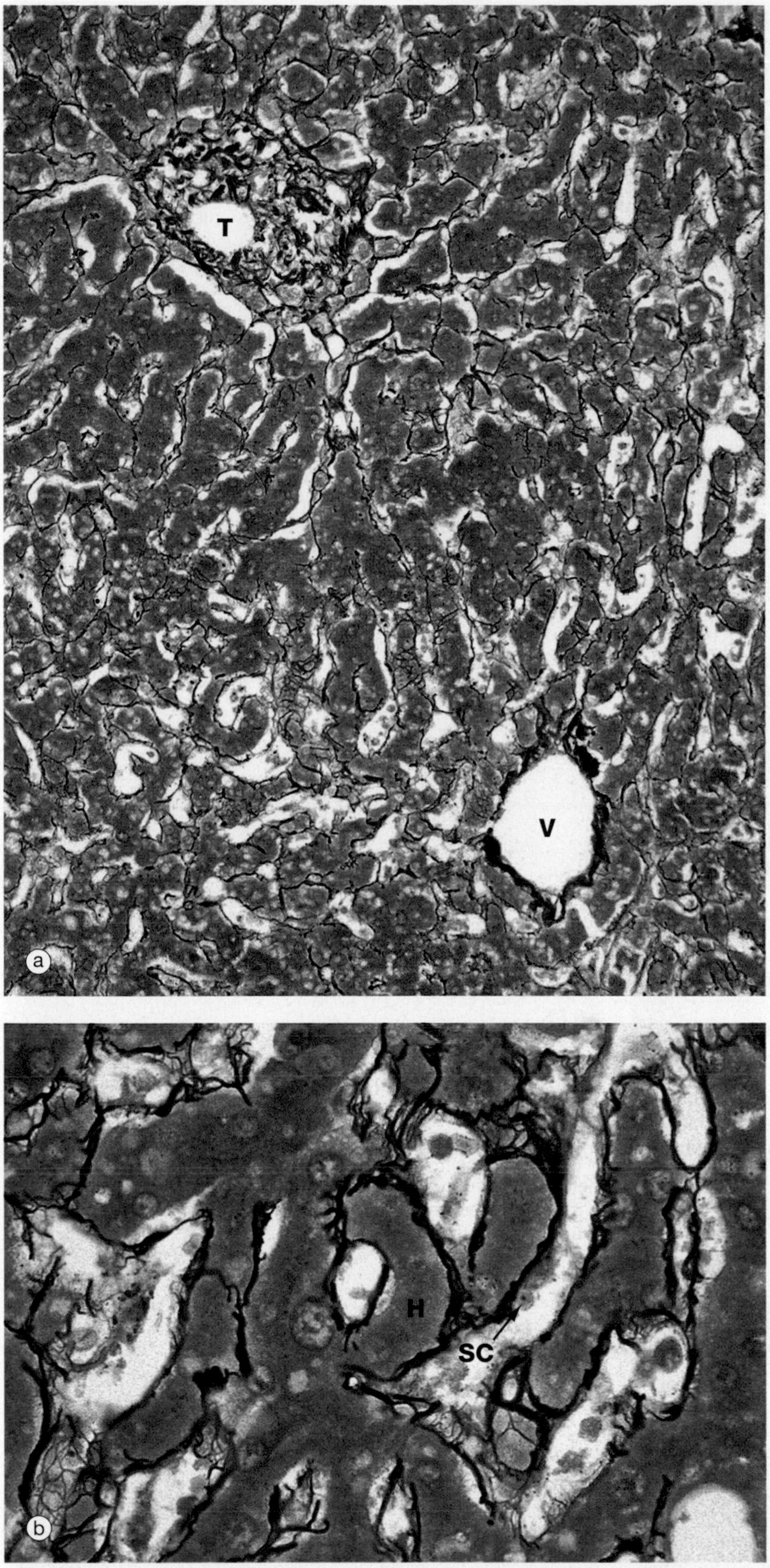

FIG. 15.4 Liver
(a) Reticulin (MP) (b) Reticulin (HP)

The structural integrity of the liver is maintained by a delicate meshwork of extracellular matrix in the form of a fine meshwork of ***reticulin*** fibres (collagen type III). The reticulin meshwork supports both the hepatocytes and the sinusoidal lining cells (endothelial cells). Fig. 15.4a and b have both been stained by a silver method that shows reticulin as a black-stained material.

Fig. 15.4a shows how reticulin is present on both sides of liver cell plates. The sinusoids are also bounded by the same reticulin framework. The reticulin merges with the sparse collagenous supporting tissue of the portal tract **T** and terminal hepatic venule **V**. At the periphery of the liver, the reticulin becomes continuous with Glisson's capsule, which invests the external surface of the liver.

Fig. 15.4b shows more detail of the reticulin scaffolding. Single layers of hepatocytes in the liver cell plates **H** lie immediately upon the reticulin framework. On the other side of the reticulin layer are the hepatic sinusoidal spaces. Some sinusoidal lining cells **SC** can just be seen.

The sinusoids are lined by a discontinuous ***fenestrated endothelium*** which has no basement membrane and is separated from the hepatocytes by a narrow space (the ***space of Disse***) which drains into the lymphatics of the portal tracts.

Liver biopsy examination

Liver disease is a common problem worldwide and its causes are diverse. Some forms of liver disease are readily diagnosed using a combination of clinical features and blood tests. Such investigations may include standard liver function tests, studies to assess for autoimmune disease, serological testing for viral hepatitis, etc.

Direct examination of tissue biopsies from the liver may be necessary in some cases for a range of reasons, such as to determine the underlying diagnosis, assess disease severity or seek evidence of disease progression.

Special staining methods such as the reticulin preparations shown here are very useful in the pathological assessment of liver biopsies, serving to highlight different aspects of the liver structure. Further details on special stains can be found in Appendix 2.

A hepatic artery branch **B** bile ductule **BC** binucleate cell **H** hepatocyte plate **L** lymphatic **PV** terminal portal venule **S** sinusoid **SC** sinusoid lining cell **T** portal tract **V** terminal hepatic venule

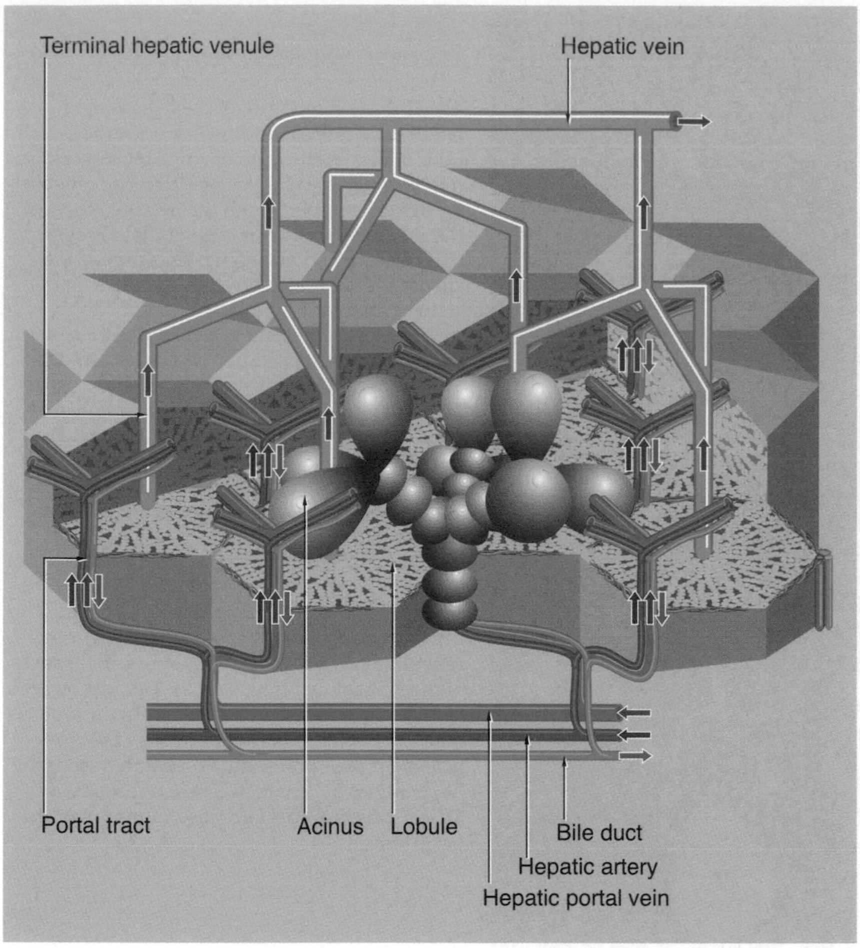

FIG. 15.5 Hepatic vasculature and biliary system

Fig. 15.5 shows the hepatic vascular system and the bile collecting system. The hepatic portal vein and hepatic artery branch repeatedly within the liver. Their terminal branches run within the portal tracts and empty into the sinusoids. Blood from both systems percolates between plates of hepatocytes in the sinusoids, which converge to drain into a terminal hepatic (centrilobular) venule. These drain to intercalated veins and then to the hepatic vein, which drains into the inferior vena cava.

Bile is secreted into a network of minute bile canaliculi situated between the plasma membranes of adjacent hepatocytes. These canaliculi are too small to be represented in this diagram. The canalicular network drains into a system of bile ducts located in the portal tracts. Bile then flows through the extrahepatic biliary tree and is finally discharged into the second part of the duodenum. The hepatic lobule and acinus are explained in Fig. 15.7.

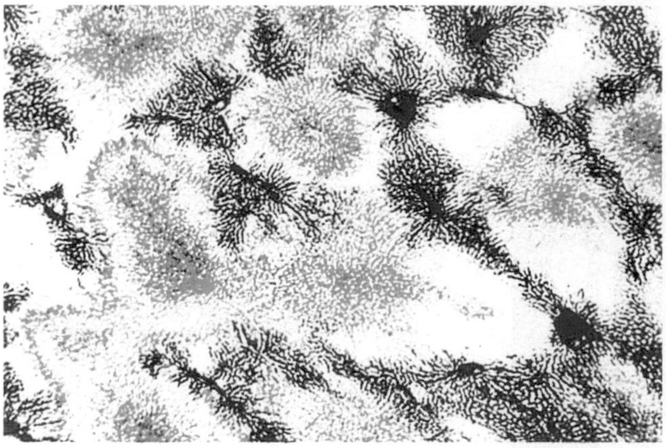

FIG. 15.6 Perfusion method (LP)

This preparation shows one of the techniques used by early histologists in mapping hepatic blood flow. The hepatic portal vein (supplying the liver) has been perfused with a red dye, and the hepatic vein (draining the liver) has been back-perfused with a blue-green dye. Thus it can be seen how liver units can be defined by a number of portal tracts peripherally (stained red), with blood draining to a single terminal hepatic venule (stained blue-green) at the centre.

FIG. 15.7 Liver architecture *(illustrations (a) to (e) opposite)*
(a) Diagram of the liver lobule (b) Pig, H&E (LP) (c) Human, H&E (LP) (d) Diagram of the simple acinus (e) Diagram of acinar agglomerate

The structural unit of the liver can be considered as a conceptually simple ***hepatic lobule***. However, the physiology of the liver is more accurately represented by a unit structure known as the ***hepatic acinus***.

The hepatic lobule (Fig. 15.7a) is roughly hexagonal in shape and is centred on a ***terminal hepatic venule*** (***centrilobular venule***) **V**. The portal tracts **T** are positioned at the angles of the hexagon. The blood from the portal vein and hepatic artery branches flows away from the portal tract to the adjacent central veins. In some species, such as the pig (Fig. 15.7b), the lobule is outlined by bands of fibrous tissue **F**, giving a well-defined structural unit.

In humans (Fig. 15.7c) and most other species, no such clear structural definition exists, although lobules can be roughly outlined as an hexagonal array of portal tracts **T** arranged around a terminal hepatic venule **V**.

The hepatic acinus (Fig. 15.7d) is a more physiologically useful model of liver anatomy, although more difficult to define histologically. The acinus is a roughly berry-shaped unit of liver parenchyma centered on a ***portal tract***. The acinus lies between two or more terminal hepatic venules and blood flows from the portal tracts through the sinusoids to the venules. The acinus is divided into zones 1, 2 and 3 and the hepatocytes in these zones have different metabolic functions.

Zone 1 is closest to the portal tract and receives the most oxygenated blood, while zone 3 is furthest away and receives the least oxygen. Liver cells in zone 3 contain high levels of esterases and low levels of oxidative enzymes. Large branches of the portal vein and hepatic artery supply an agglomerate of acini, each of which is in turn composed of several complex acini which, at the lowest level, are made of simple acini, each supplied by terminal vascular branches. Although the structure looks on paper like a bunch of grapes, it must be remembered that this is a functional grouping and in reality the hepatic parenchyma is uniform and continuous.

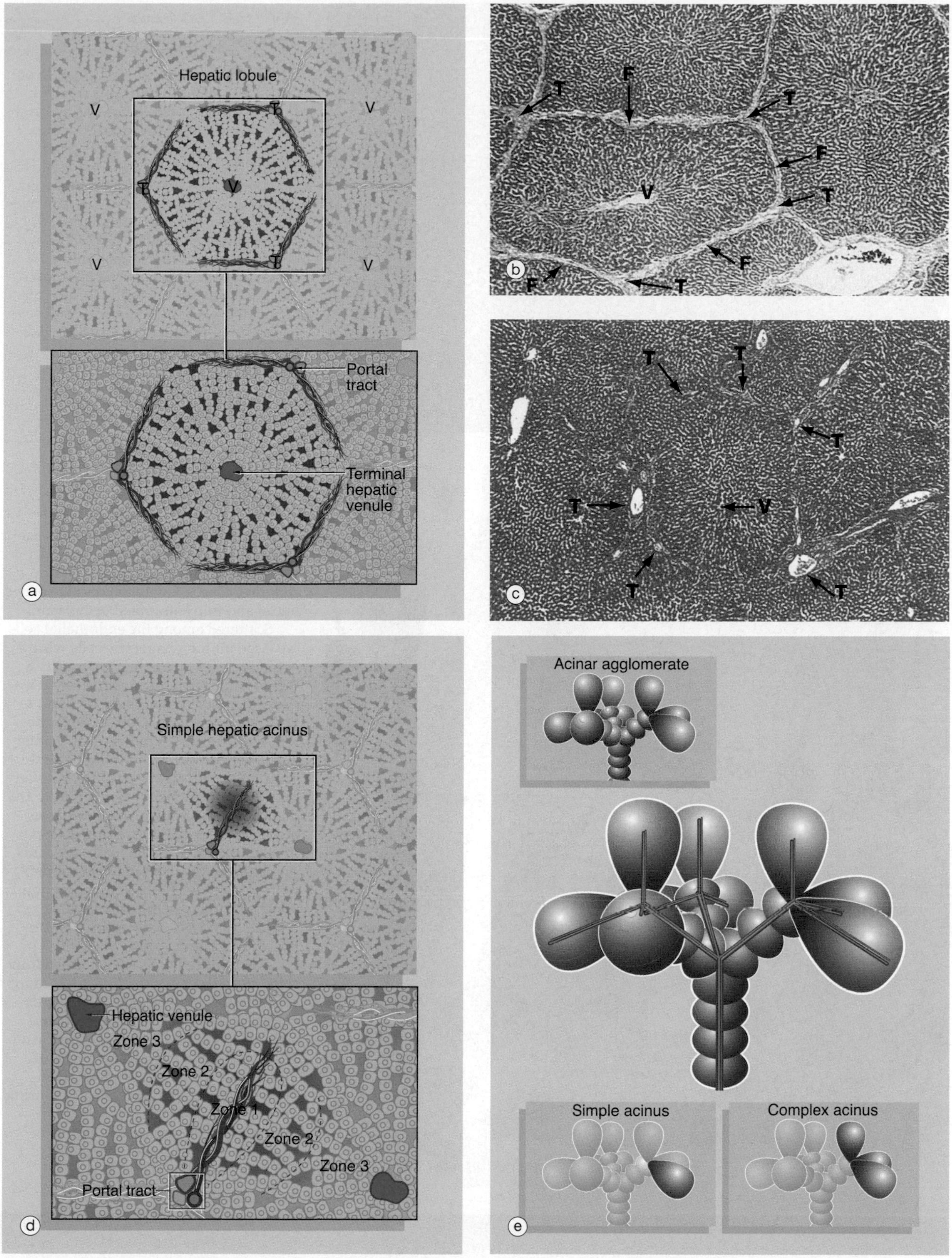

FIG. 15.7 Liver architecture *(caption opposite)*
(a) Diagram of the liver lobule (b) Pig, H&E (LP) (c) Human, H&E (LP) (d) Diagram of the simple acinus (e) Diagram of acinar agglomerate

F fibrous septum **T** portal tract **V** terminal hepatic venule

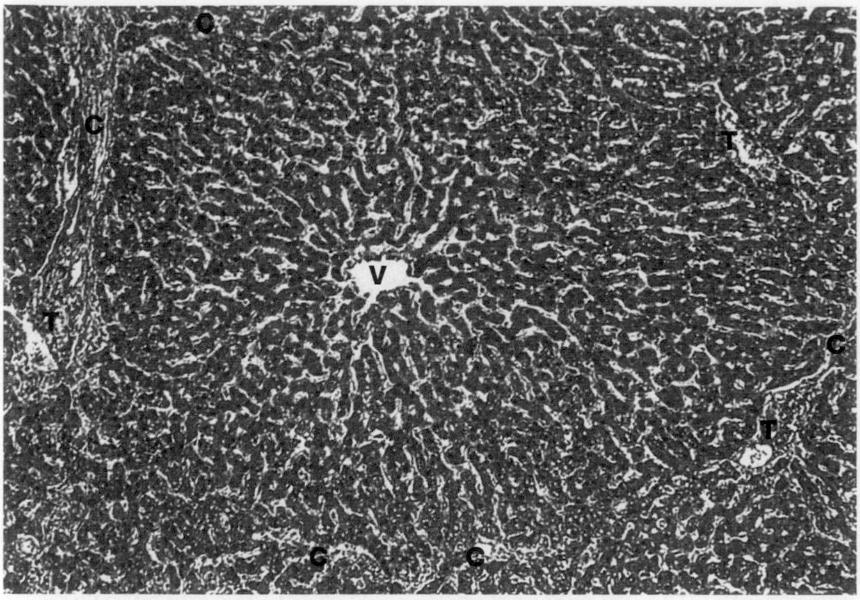

FIG. 15.8 Liver lobule H&E (MP)

Fig. 15.8 illustrates a single human liver lobule and includes parts of a number of hepatic acini, each centred on a portal tract. The irregular hexagonal boundary of the lobule is defined by portal tracts **T** and sparse collagenous tissue **C**. Sinusoids originate at the lobule margin and course between plates of hepatocytes to converge upon the terminal hepatic (centrilobular) venule **V**. The plates of hepatocytes are usually only one cell thick and so each hepatocyte is exposed to blood on at least two sides. The plates of hepatocytes branch and anastomose to form a three-dimensional structure like a sponge.

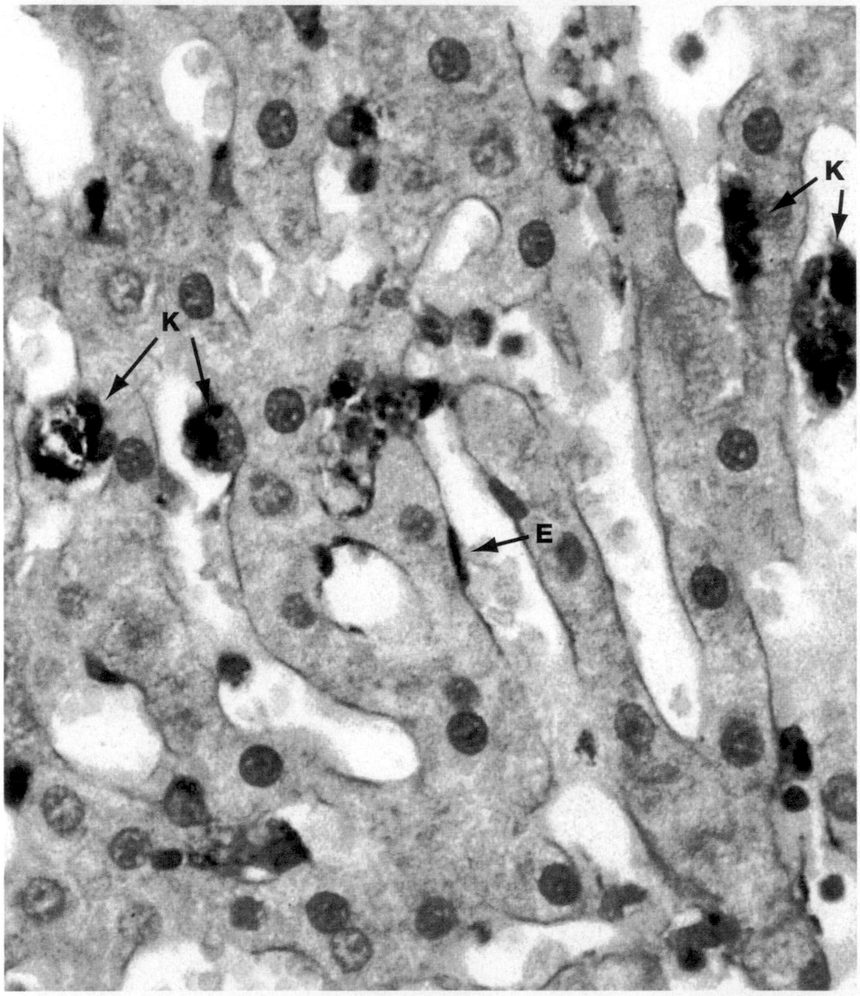

FIG. 15.9 Sinusoid lining cells Perls Prussian blue (HP)

The sinusoid lining cells include at least three cell types (Fig. 15.9). The majority of cells lining the hepatic sinusoids are ***endothelial cells*** **E** with flat darkly stained nuclei and thin fenestrated cytoplasm.

Scattered among the endothelial cells are large plump phagocytic cells with ovoid nuclei. Known as ***Küpffer cells*** **K**, these form part of the monocyte–macrophage defence system (see Chs 3 and 4) and, with the spleen, participate in the removal of spent erythrocytes and other particulate debris from the circulation. The phagocytic capability of the Küpffer cells can be demonstrated when they are 'fed', either artificially or under pathological conditions, with appropriate particulate matter. The animal used for this preparation was injected intravenously with a particulate iron–sugar compound which, with this staining method, is demonstrated as a dark deposit within the sinusoid lining cells.

The third cell type, known as ***stellate cells, Ito cells*** or ***hepatic lipocytes***, cannot be easily distinguished by light microscopy. This cell type has lipid droplets containing vitamin A in their cytoplasm. These cells have the dual functions of vitamin A storage and production of extracellular matrix and collagen. During liver injury, these cells are thought to produce greatly increased amounts of collagen, causing the fibrosis which is a characteristic of hepatic cirrhosis.

Hepatic cirrhosis

In diseases where there is repeated liver cell destruction, the liver responds by cell division to replace dead liver cells (***regeneration***) and by depositing collagenous tissue (***scarring***). The combination of nodules of regenerated liver cells separated by bands of scar tissue is termed ***cirrhosis*** (see e-Fig. 15.1).

In cirrhosis, the liver cells that are separated from a normal sinusoidal blood flow have reduced function (e.g. reduced synthesis of albumin and reduced secretion of bile). The scarring and interruption of the low-resistance sinusoidal system has important consequences. Blood from the portal vein cannot drain from the liver and ***portal hypertension*** develops.

The common causes of cirrhosis are diseases in which there is continued liver cell damage and death. Chronic ethanol abuse is an important cause. Infection with hepatitis viruses B and C often leads to ***chronic hepatitis*** (see e-Fig. 15.2) and a risk of cirrhosis. Certain autoimmune diseases are also recognised to cause chronic hepatitis and cirrhosis in susceptible patients. Rare causes include excessive storage of iron and copper due to genetic metabolic diseases.

B binucleate hepatocyte **C** collagenous tissue **Ca** bile canaliculus **E** endothelial cell **EP** erythroid precursors **K** Küpffer cell **M** megakaryocyte **MP** myeloid precursor **T** portal tract **V** terminal hepatic venule

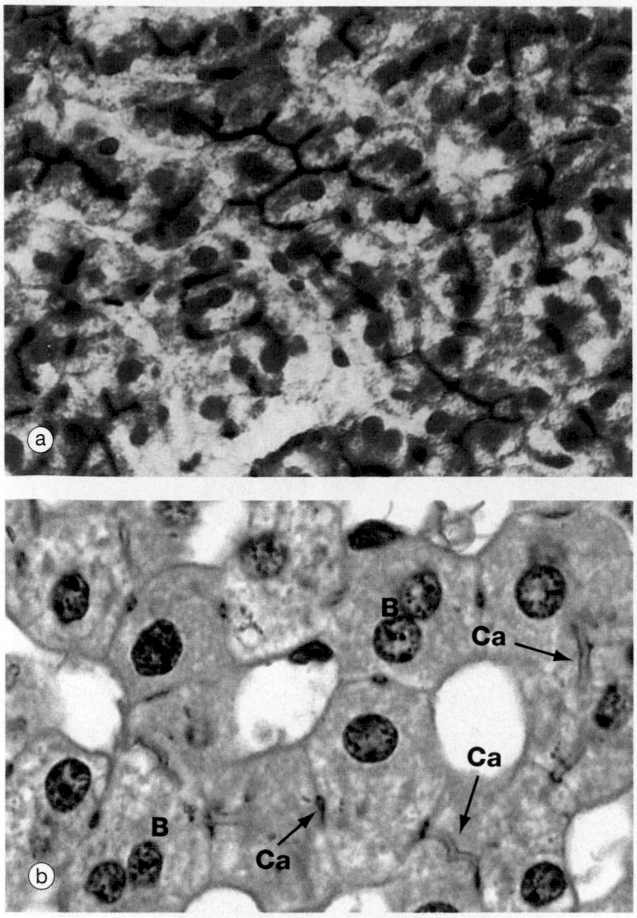

FIG. 15.10 Bile canaliculi
(a) Enzyme histochemical staining for ATPase (HP)
(b) Iron haematoxylin (HP)

Bile is synthesised by all hepatocytes and is secreted into a system of minute ***canaliculi*** which form an anastomosing network within the plates of hepatocytes. The canaliculi have no discrete structure of their own but consist merely of fine channels formed by the plasma membranes of adjacent hepatocytes. The ultrastructural features are shown in Fig. 15.12. Bile canaliculi of adjacent hepatocyte plates merge to form ***canals of Hering*** before draining into the ***bile ductules*** of the portal tracts.

The hepatocyte plasma membranes forming the walls of the canaliculi contain the enzyme ***ATPase***, which suggests that bile secretion is an energy-dependent process. A histochemical method for ATPase has been used in Fig. 15.10a to demonstrate bile canaliculi (stained brown), which are difficult to demonstrate with routine light microscopy methods. Within each hepatocyte plate, the canaliculi form a regular hexagonal network reminiscent of chicken wire, each hexagon enclosing a single hepatocyte.

In Fig. 15.10b, a black stain has been deposited in the walls of the bile canaliculi **Ca**. Note two binucleate hepatocytes **B**. The biliary canalicular membrane also contains ***alkaline phosphatase***. In diseases which cause obstruction of bile flow, this enzyme is released from the hepatocyte canalicular membrane into the blood, where it can be detected. Measurement of the serum alkaline phosphatase level forms part of a typical set of ***liver function*** tests, a common biochemical assay used in routine practice. Elevated blood levels of hepatic alkaline phosphatase are therefore a feature of ***obstructive jaundice*** (see textbox 'Jaundice').

Jaundice

Jaundice is a yellow discolouration of the tissues due to increased levels of bilirubin and associated deposition of bile pigments. It is a common consequence of liver and biliary tract disease but its causes are very diverse. ***Hyperbilirubinaemia*** (raised blood level of bilirubin) can be classified as ***prehepatic, hepatic*** or ***posthepatic***.

Prehepatic jaundice occurs due to increased production of bilirubin, exceeding the liver's capacity to excrete it in its water-soluble conjugated form. The majority of bilirubin comes from metabolism of haemoglobin and so this form of jaundice is usually associated with conditions in which there is excessive red cell breakdown, such as sickle cell anaemia and other haemoglobinopathies. In this type of jaundice, there is predominantly ***unconjugated hyperbilirubinaemia***.

Hepatic jaundice occurs when there is acute or chronic damage to the liver, reducing its ability to metabolise and excrete bilirubin. In this condition, there is usually a mixture of conjugated and unconjugated hyperbilirubinaemia.

Posthepatic jaundice is also known as ***obstructive jaundice*** and reflects some form of mechanical blockage which interrupts the flow of bile into the biliary system. Most commonly, this occurs due to ***gallstones*** (see Fig. 15.13) blocking the common bile duct or due to tumour arising in the head of the pancreas (see Fig. 15.16). In obstructive jaundice, there is predominantly conjugated hyperbilirubinaemia, since there is no intrinsic metabolic problem but, rather, a simple mechanical blockage. Sometimes this type of jaundice is referred to as ***surgical jaundice*** because its treatment often requires surgical input.

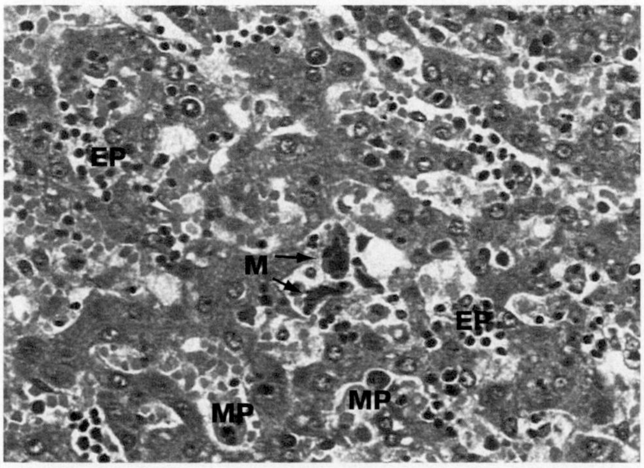

FIG. 15.11 Fetal liver
H&E (MP)

In fetal life, the liver and spleen are important sites of haematopoiesis (see Ch. 3). When haematopoiesis in bone marrow begins, some time after the fourth month of gestation, the importance of the liver and spleen for this function gradually declines. In this micrograph of fetal liver, the hepatocyte plates are two cells thick, a normal finding up to the age of about 7 years. The sinusoids are packed with blood precursors including ***megakaryocytes*** **M** and ***erythroid*** **EP** and ***myeloid*** precursors **MP**.

In adult life, the liver does not normally have haematopoietic tissue. If the capacity of the bone marrow is inadequate for demand, then the fetal function of hepatic haematopoiesis can be re-established. Important causes include fibrosis of bone marrow, replacement of bone marrow by malignancy or some genetic disorders of haemoglobin formation. Haematopoiesis occurs in liver and spleen, both of which may become abnormally enlarged.

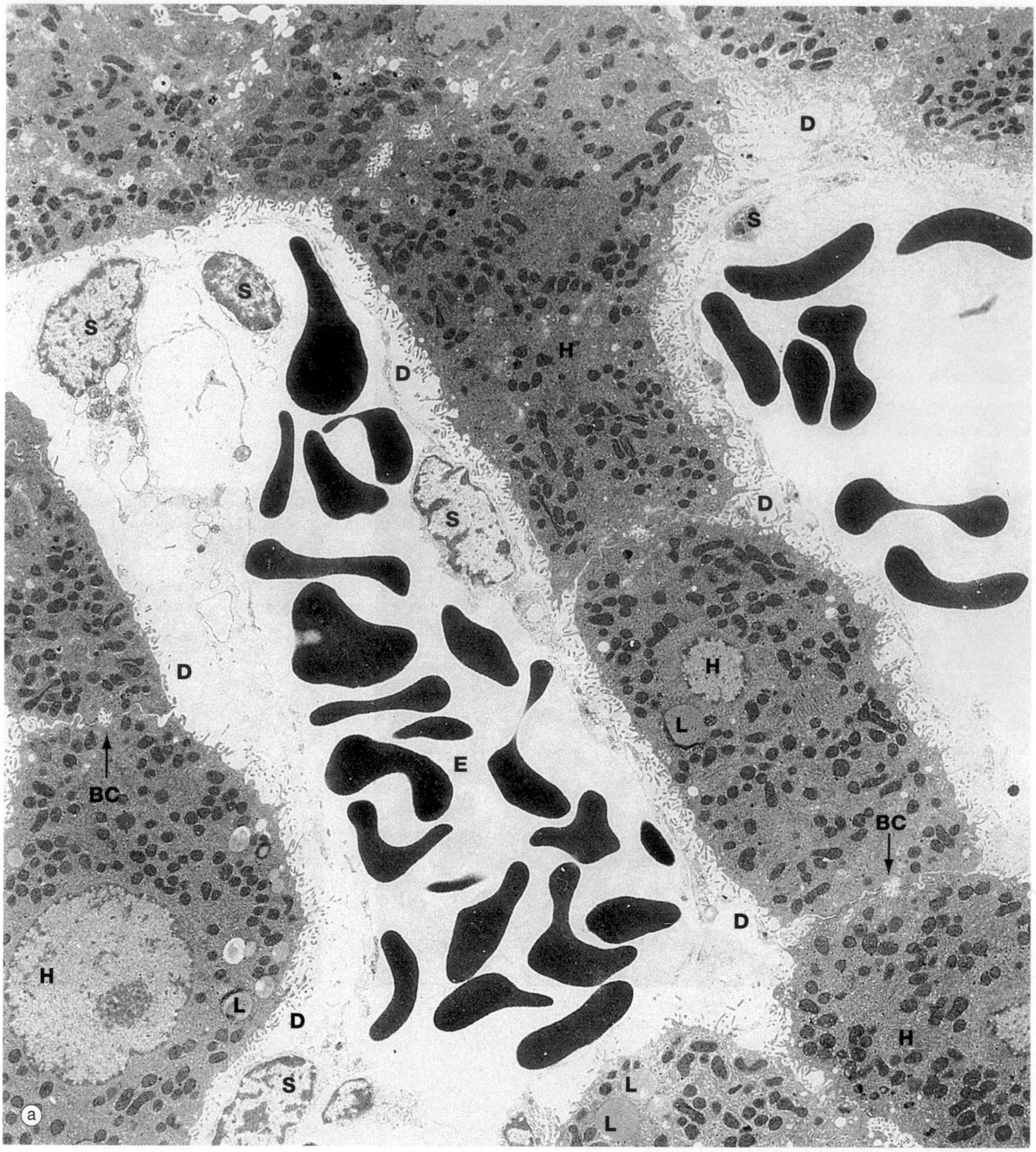

FIG. 15.12 Liver *(illustration (b) opposite)*
(a) EM ×4400 (b) EM ×15 200

Figs 15.12a and b demonstrate the main ultrastructural features of the liver. Hepatocytes **H** are exposed on each side to the sinusoids which are lined by a discontinuous layer of sinusoid lining cells **S**. These are supported by the fine reticulin framework of the liver (see Fig. 15.4), with the ***space of Disse*** **D** between the lining cells and the hepatocyte surface. Via the gaps in the sinusoid lining, the space of Disse is continuous with the sinusoid lumen, thus bathing the hepatocyte surface with plasma. Numerous irregular microvilli **Mv** extend from the hepatocyte surface into the space of Disse, greatly increasing the surface area for metabolic exchange. Between the bases of the microvilli, there are coated pits involved in endocytosis. Erythrocytes **E** can be seen within the sinusoids.

Reflecting their extraordinary range of biosynthetic and degradative activities, the hepatocyte cytoplasm (Fig. 15.12b) is crowded with organelles, particularly rough endoplasmic reticulum **rER**, smooth endoplasmic reticulum **sER**, Golgi stacks, free ribosomes, mitochondria **M**, lysosomes **Ly** and peroxisomes.

Lipid droplets **L** and glycogen rosettes are present in variable numbers depending on nutritional status.

Bile canaliculi **BC** are seen to be formed from the plasma membranes of adjacent hepatocytes, the plasma membranes being tightly bound by junctional complexes **J**. Small microvilli project into the canaliculi. The subjacent cytoplasm contains a network of actin filaments, contraction of which reduces canalicular diameter, thus reducing flow rate.

BC bile canaliculus **D** space of Disse **E** erythrocytes **H** hepatocyte **J** junctional complex **L** lipid droplet **Ly** lysosome **M** mitochondrion **Mv** microvilli **rER** rough endoplasmic reticulum **S** sinusoid lining cells **sER** smooth endoplasmic reticulum

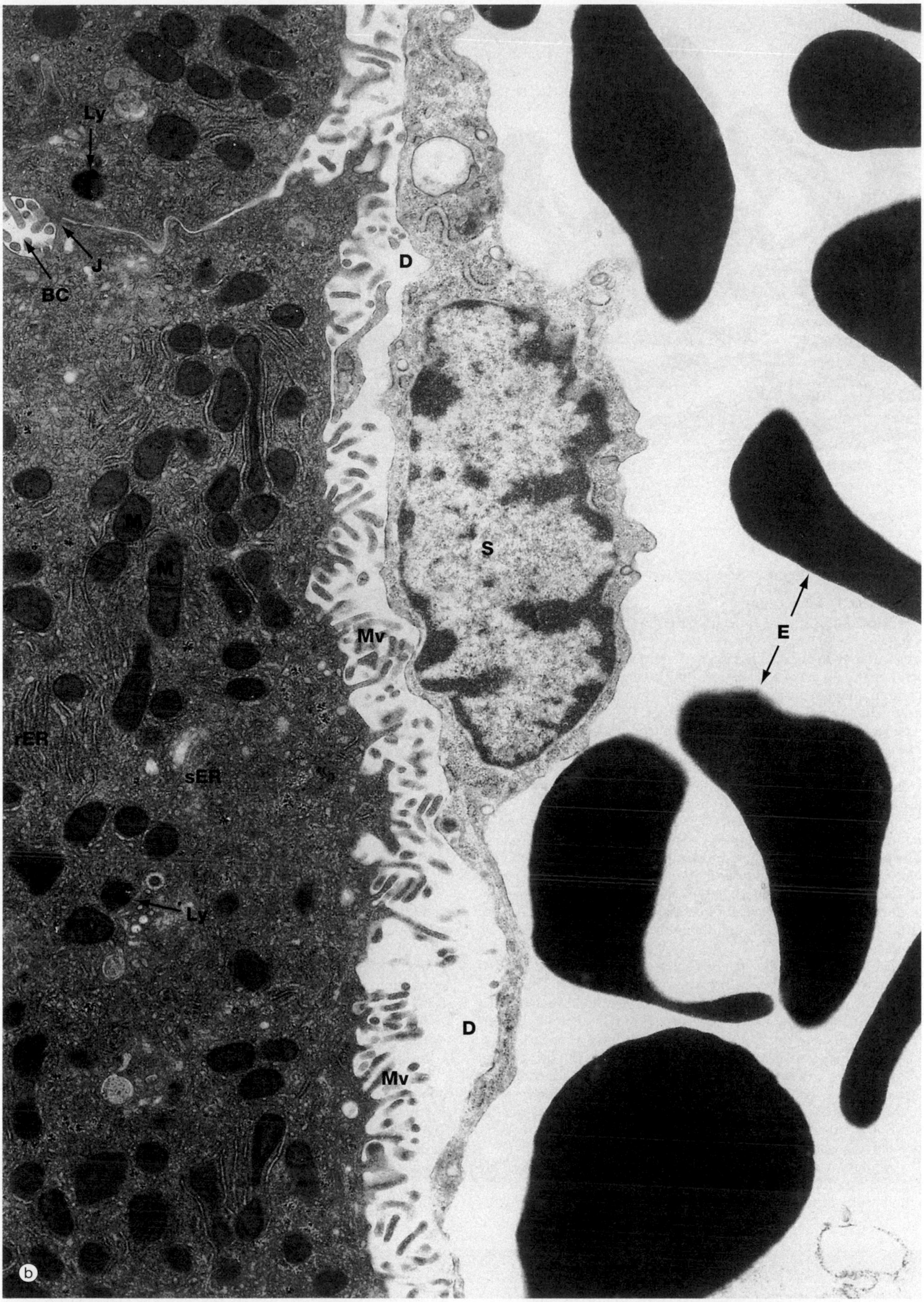

FIG. 15.12 Liver *(caption and illustration (a) opposite)*
(a) EM ×4400 (b) EM ×15 200

Hepatocellular carcinoma (HCC)

Any cause of cirrhosis of the liver predisposes to HCC which is a primary liver carcinoma (see e-Fig. 15.3). Tumours can present as one large tumour nodule or multiple nodules. Histologically, the tumour cells resemble hepatocytes unless very poorly differentiated. Alpha-fetoprotein is often secreted by these tumours and therefore can be used as a tumour marker.

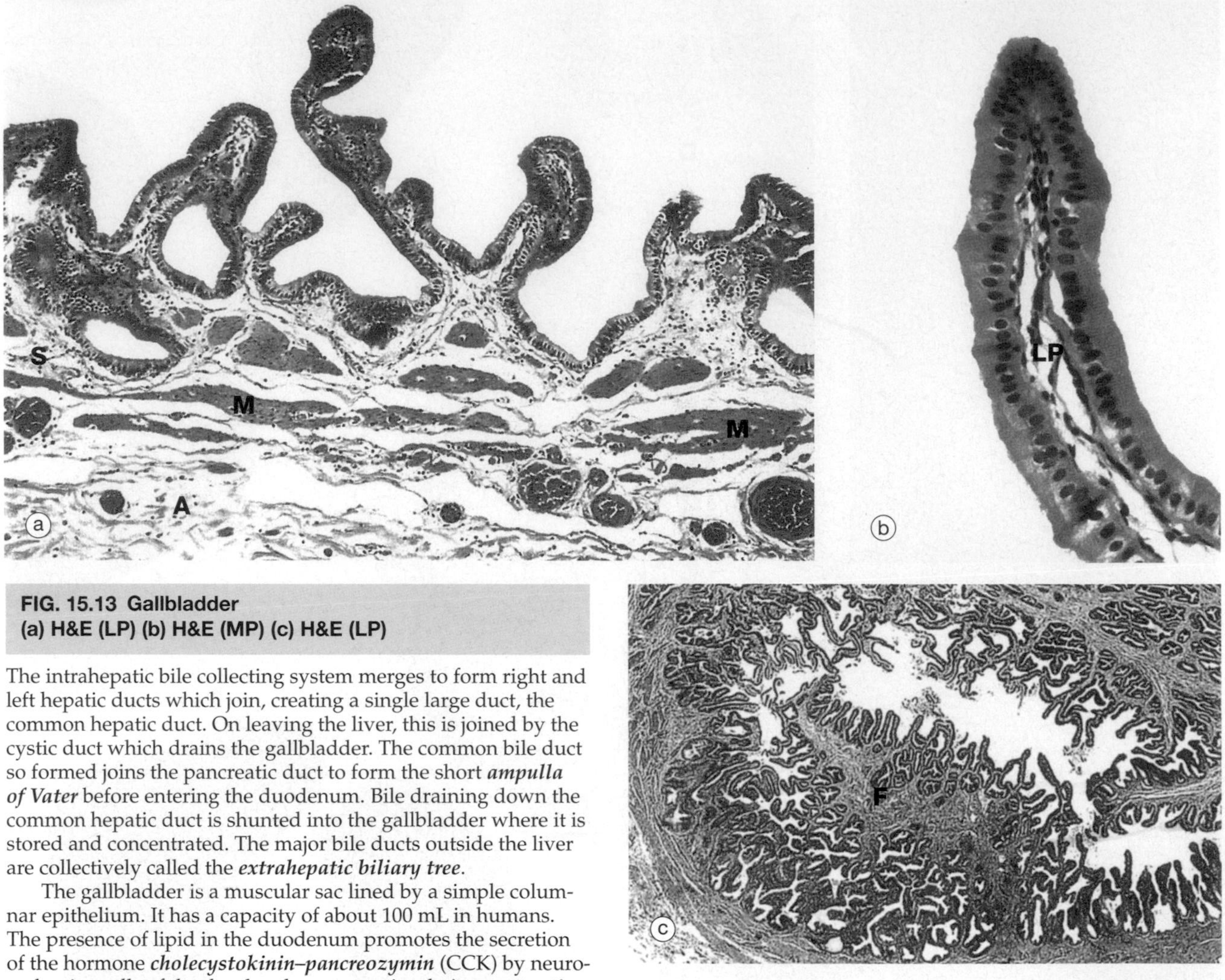

FIG. 15.13 Gallbladder
(a) H&E (LP) (b) H&E (MP) (c) H&E (LP)

The intrahepatic bile collecting system merges to form right and left hepatic ducts which join, creating a single large duct, the common hepatic duct. On leaving the liver, this is joined by the cystic duct which drains the gallbladder. The common bile duct so formed joins the pancreatic duct to form the short ***ampulla of Vater*** before entering the duodenum. Bile draining down the common hepatic duct is shunted into the gallbladder where it is stored and concentrated. The major bile ducts outside the liver are collectively called the ***extrahepatic biliary tree***.

The gallbladder is a muscular sac lined by a simple columnar epithelium. It has a capacity of about 100 mL in humans. The presence of lipid in the duodenum promotes the secretion of the hormone ***cholecystokinin–pancreozymin*** (CCK) by neuroendocrine cells of the duodenal mucosa, stimulating contraction of the gallbladder and forcing bile into the duodenum. Bile is an emulsifying agent, facilitating the hydrolysis of dietary lipids by pancreatic lipases.

Fig. 15.13a shows the wall of a gallbladder in the non-distended state in which the mucosa is thrown up into many folds. The relatively loose submucosa **S** is rich in elastic fibres, blood vessels and lymphatics which drain water reabsorbed from bile during the concentration process. The fibres of the muscular layer **M** are arranged in longitudinal, transverse and oblique orientations but do not form distinct layers. Externally, there is a thick collagenous adventitial (serosal) coat **A**, conveying the larger blood and lymphatic vessels. In the neck of the gallbladder and in the extrahepatic biliary tree, mucous glands are found in the submucosa. Mucus may provide a protective surface film for the biliary tract.

At high magnification in Fig. 15.13b, the simple epithelial lining of the gallbladder is seen to consist of very tall columnar cells with basally located nuclei. Numerous short, irregular microvilli account for the unevenness of the luminal surface. The lining cells concentrate bile 5- to 10-fold by an active process, the resulting water passing into lymphatics in the lamina propria **LP**.

Fig. 15.13c illustrates the wall of the cystic duct, which is formed into a twisted mucosa-covered fold **F** known as the ***spiral valve of Heister***.

The flow of bile and pancreatic juice into the duodenum is controlled by the complex arrangement of smooth muscle known as the ***sphincter of Oddi***. The components of this structure include the ***choledochal sphincter*** at the distal end of the common bile duct, the ***pancreatic sphincter*** at the end of the pancreatic duct, and a meshwork of muscle fibres around the ampulla. This arrangement controls the flow of bile and pancreatic juice into the duodenum and, at the same time, prevents reflux of bile and pancreatic juice into the wrong parts of the duct system. When the choledochal sphincter is closed, bile is directed into the gallbladder where it is concentrated.

Cholelithiasis

Abnormal concentration and precipitation of the constituents of bile may form stones (***calculi*** or ***gallstones***) within the gallbladder or the extrahepatic biliary system. A stone may become impacted in a duct, leading to blockage. Complete blockage of the common bile duct by a stone leads to failure of bile secretion and clinical ***jaundice*** (see textbox 'Jaundice'). If the gallbladder is affected by stones, then it may become inflamed, leading to pain (***chronic cholecystitis*** (see e-Fig. 15.4)). The term ***cholelithiasis*** is used to refer to the presence of stones within the biliary system.

Gallstones are formed from the constituents of bile and so they may be composed of cholesterol, bile pigments or a mixture of these. In broad terms, they occur due to an imbalance in the ratio of these normal bile constituents. This is well illustrated by the frequent occurrence of pigment stones in patients with chronic ***haemolytic anaemias***. Excess breakdown of erythrocytes results in increased excretion of the haem breakdown products bilirubin and biliverdin in bile. These then precipitate to form dark, crystalline gallstones which may cause biliary obstruction.

PANCREAS

The ***pancreas*** is a large gland which, like the liver, develops embryologically as an outgrowth of the primitive foregut. The pancreas has both exocrine and endocrine components. The ***endocrine pancreas*** is described in detail in Ch. 17. The ***exocrine pancreas***, which forms the bulk of the gland, secretes an enzyme-rich alkaline fluid into the duodenum via the pancreatic duct. The high pH of pancreatic secretions is due to a high content of bicarbonate ions and serves to neutralise the acidic chyme as it enters the small intestine from the stomach. The pancreatic enzymes degrade proteins, carbohydrates, lipids and nucleic acids by the process of ***luminal digestion*** (see Fig. 14.18). Like pepsin in the stomach, the pancreatic proteolytic enzymes ***trypsin*** and ***chymotrypsin*** are secreted in an inactive form. ***Enterokinase***, an enzyme secreted by the duodenal mucosa, activates ***protrypsin*** to form ***trypsin***. ***Trypsin*** then activates ***prochymotrypsin*** to form ***chymotrypsin***. This mechanism prevents autodigestion of the pancreas. The other pancreatic enzymes are secreted in the active form.

Pancreatic secretion occurs continuously, the rate being modulated by hormonal and nervous influences. ***Secretin***, a hormone released by neuroendocrine cells scattered in the duodenum, promotes the secretion of copious watery fluid rich in bicarbonate. ***Cholecystokinin–pancreozymin*** (CCK), also derived from duodenal neuroendocrine cells, stimulates the secretion of enzyme-rich pancreatic fluid. ***Gastrin***, secreted by neuroendocrine cells of the gastric pylorus, has a similar action on the pancreas to that of CCK. The pancreas is richly innervated by the autonomic nervous system, which also modulates secretory activity.

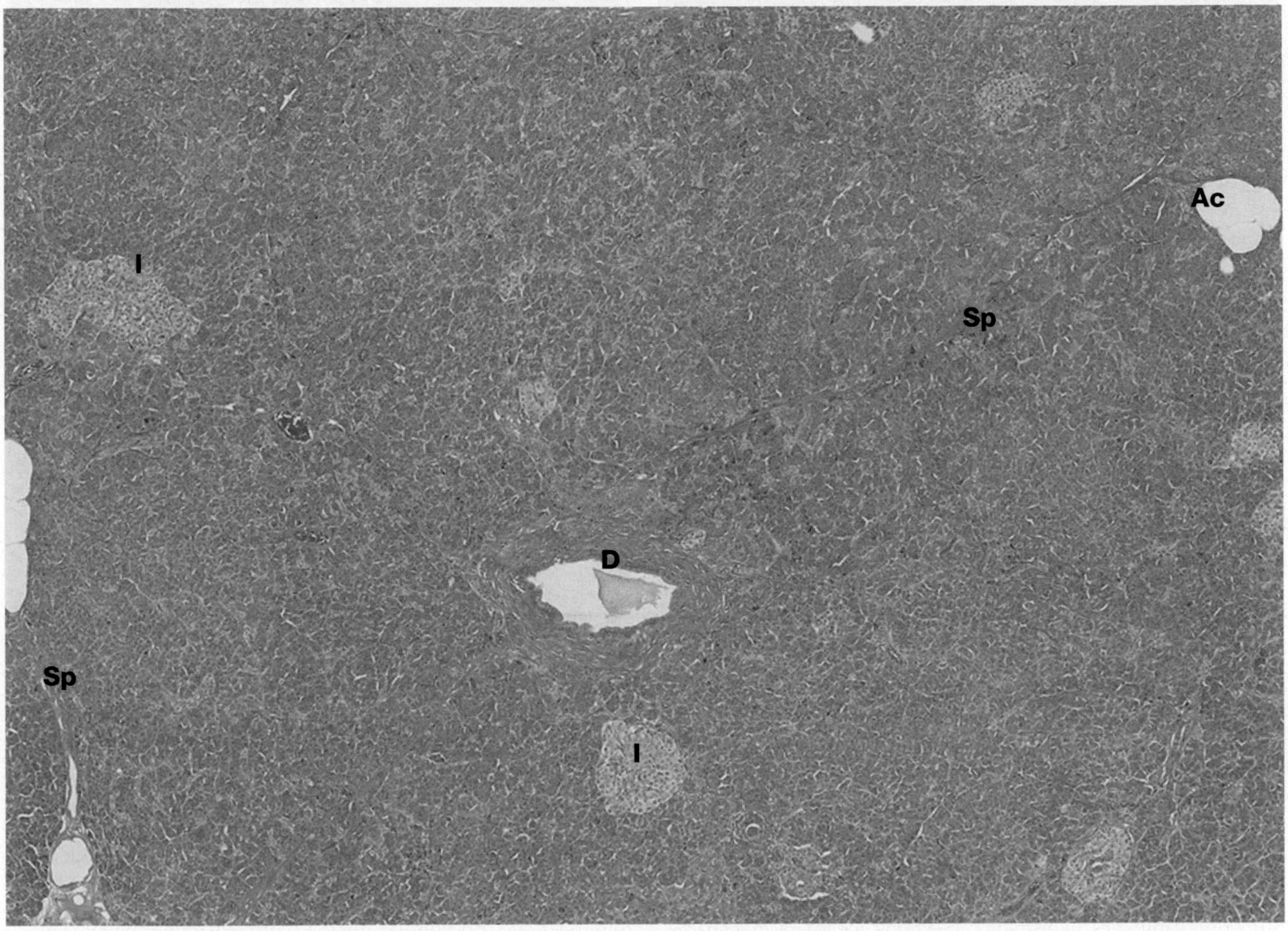

FIG. 15.14 Pancreas
H&E (LP)

The pancreas (Fig. 15.14) is a lobulated gland covered by a thin collagenous capsule which extends as delicate septa **Sp** between the lobules. The exocrine component of the pancreas consists of closely packed secretory ***acini*** which drain into a highly branched duct system. Most of the secretion drains into the main ***pancreatic duct***, which joins the ***common bile duct*** to drain into the duodenum via the ***ampulla of Vater***. In most people, a small accessory pancreatic duct drains into the duodenum more proximally. Interlobular ducts **D** can be seen in this micrograph.

Their surrounding supporting tissue reinforces the septal framework.

The endocrine tissue of the pancreas forms ***islets of Langerhans*** **I** of various sizes scattered throughout the exocrine tissue. Occasional adipocytes **Ac** are scattered throughout the parenchyma. These are scanty in young adults but are seen in increasing numbers in older people, reflecting the natural atrophy of the gland with age.

Acute pancreatitis

Damage to pancreatic acinar cells releases pancreatic enzymes into the local tissues. These powerful enzymes cause death of pancreatic tissue and severe inflammation termed acute pancreatitis (see e-Fig. 15.5). The release of pancreatic lipase causes death of local fat cells (fat necrosis). Pancreatic amylase is released and can be detected at high levels in the blood. This is a severe and life threatening condition.

A adventitia **Ac** adipocyte **D** interlobular duct **F** mucosal fold **I** islet of Langerhans **LP** lamina propria **M** muscle layer **S** submucosa **Sp** septum

Chronic pancreatitis

Chronic pancreatitis (CP) is a chronic condition which results from repeated inflammation in the pancreas and is characterised by loss of secretory cells and fibrous replacement of the pancreas. Alcohol excess and gallstones are the commonest causes of CP.

Recurrent bouts of inflammation result in fibrosis and atrophy of the exocrine glands (acini). This can lead to pain, pancreatic insufficiency and is a risk factor for cancer.

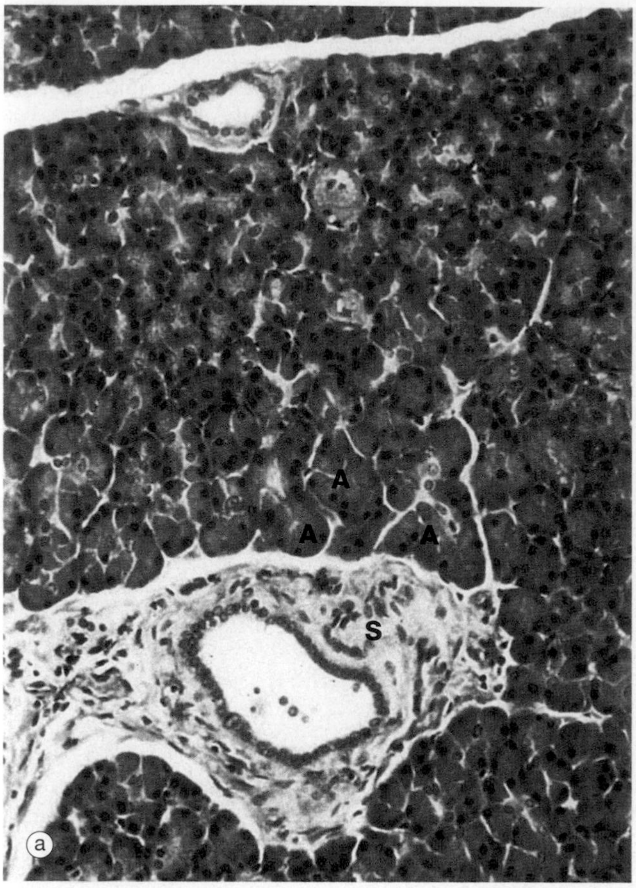

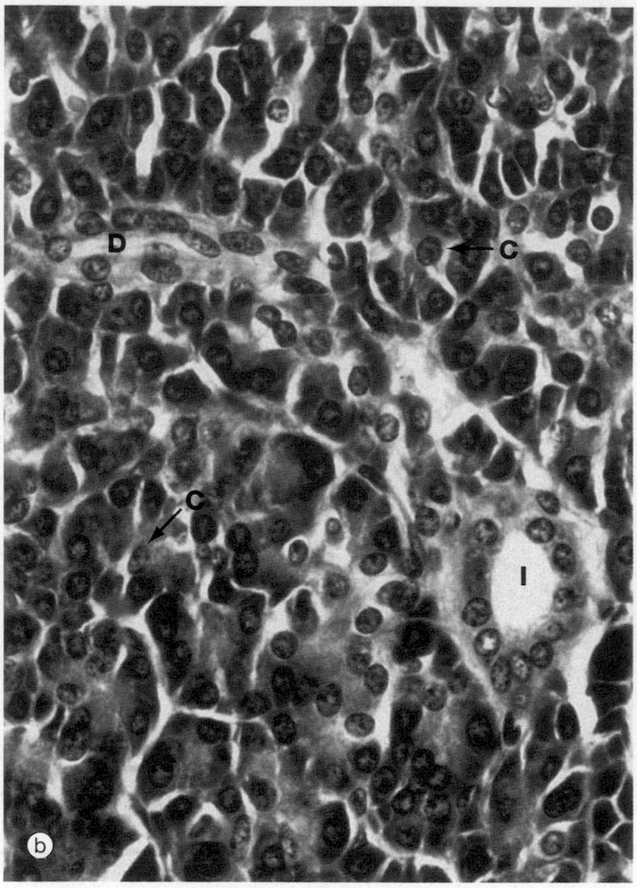

FIG. 15.15 Exocrine pancreas *(illustration (c) opposite)* (a) H&E (MP) (b) H&E (HP) (c) EM ×8500

Details of the pancreatic acini and duct system can be seen in these micrographs. Each ***acinus*** is made up of an irregular cluster of pyramid-shaped secretory cells, the apices of which surround a minute central lumen which represents the end of the duct system. The smallest of the tributaries are known as ***intercalated ducts***. Adjacent acini are separated by inconspicuous supporting tissue containing numerous capillaries. In histological sections, the interacinar spaces tend to appear wider than they do in vivo, due to a fixation artefact.

The intercalated ducts drain into small ***intralobular ducts***, which in turn drain into the ***interlobular ducts*** in the ***septa*** of the gland. The intercalated ducts are lined by simple low cuboidal epithelium, which becomes stratified cuboidal in the larger ducts. With increasing size, the ducts are invested by a progressively thicker layer of dense collagenous supporting tissue. The wall of the main pancreatic duct contains smooth muscle.

Fig. 15.15a shows the general arrangement of the glandular acini **A**. An intralobular duct is seen in upper midfield and a larger interlobular duct in lower midfield, the latter having a much broader sheath of supporting tissue **S**.

At higher magnification in Fig. 15.15b, the cells of each pancreatic acinus have a roughly triangular shape in section, their apices projecting towards a central lumen of a minute duct. The acinar cells are typical protein-secreting cells. The nuclei are basally located and surrounded by basophilic cytoplasm which is crammed with rough endoplasmic reticulum. The apices of the cells are packed with eosinophilic secretory granules containing proenzymes. The centres of the acini frequently contain one or more nuclei of ***centroacinar cells*** **C** with pale nuclei and sparse pale-stained cytoplasm. These represent the terminal lining cells of intercalated ducts. Cells of similar appearance can be seen between the acini and those of intercalated ducts **D** passing to join the larger intralobular ducts **I**. The cells lining the intercalated ducts secrete water and bicarbonate ions into the pancreatic juice.

Fig. 15.15c illustrates part of a pancreatic acinus with its central lumen **L** using electron microscopy. The pyramid-shaped secretory cells have round, basally located nuclei with dispersed chromatin and prominent nucleoli **Nu**, both characteristic features of highly active cells. The basal cytoplasm is packed with lamellar profiles of rough endoplasmic reticulum **rER**, among which elongated mitochondria **M** are scattered. A large Golgi apparatus **G** is located in a supranuclear position and is responsible for packaging enzymes synthesised on the rough endoplasmic reticulum to form ***zymogen granules***. Newly packed secretory or zymogen granules $\mathbf{Z_1}$ are large and much less electron-dense than the smaller mature granules $\mathbf{Z_2}$ which aggregate in the apical cytoplasm. Zymogen granules are released into the acinar lumen by exocytosis. Small irregular microvilli associated with this process are seen projecting into the lumen. Note small capillaries **Ca**, a fibroblast **F** and collagen **Coll** in the fine supporting tissue which surrounds the acinus.

A glandular acinus **C** centroacinar cell **Ca** capillary **Coll** collagen **D** intercalated duct **F** fibroblast **G** Golgi apparatus **I** interlobular duct **L** lumen **M** mitochondrion **Nu** nucleolus **rER** rough endoplasmic reticulum **S** supporting tissue **Z** zymogen granule

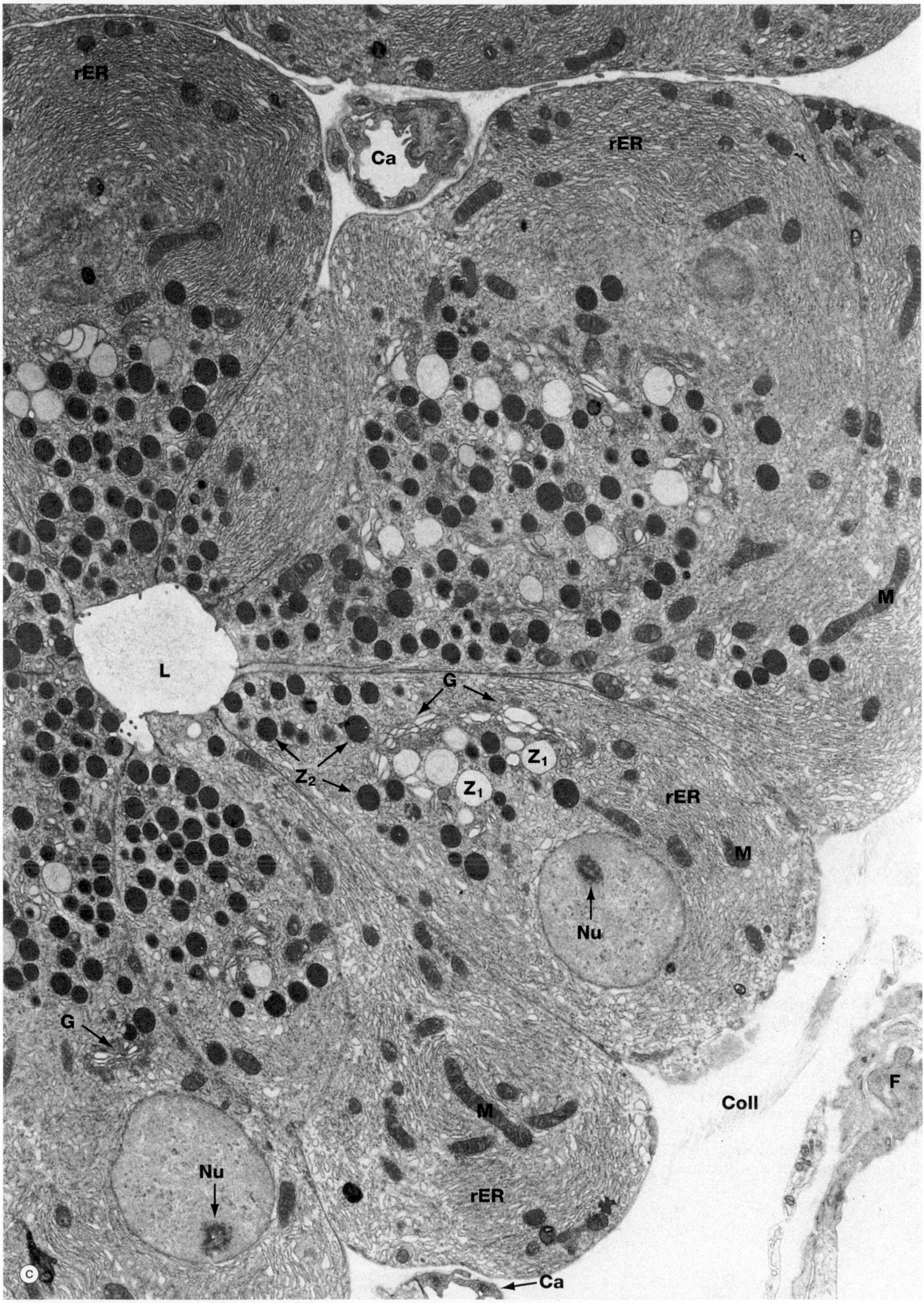

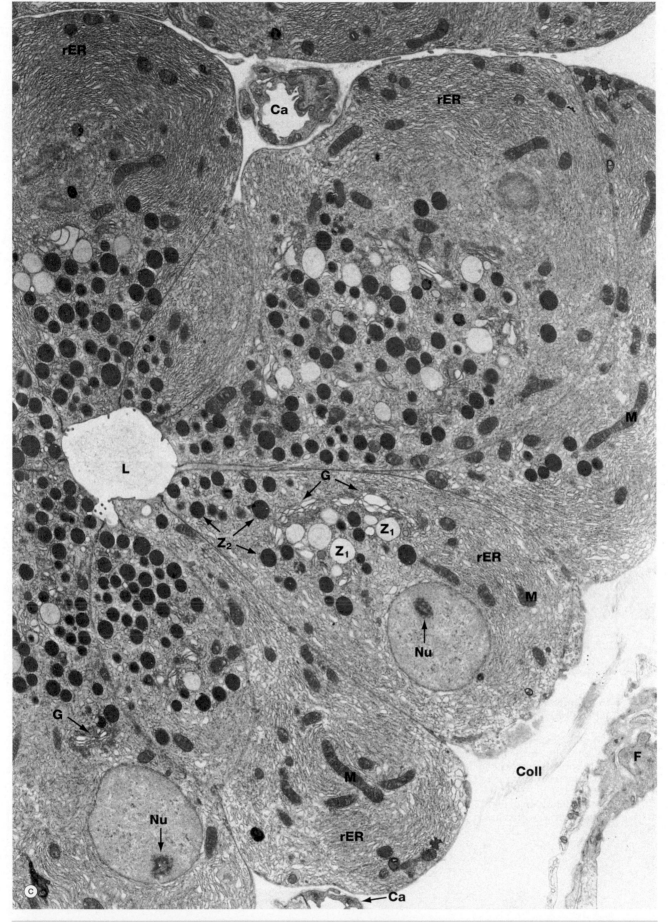

FIG. 15.15 Exocrine pancreas ***(caption and illustrations (a) and (b) opposite)***
(a) H&E (MP) (b) H&E (HP) (c) EM ×8500

Pancreatic tumours

The most common tumour arising in the pancreas is pancreatic ductal adenocarcinoma (PDAC) (see e-Fig. 15.6). These tumours usually arise from the pancreatic ductal epithelium and are of great importance because of their insidious manner of growth, often remaining undetected until a very advanced stage. A typical PDAC is illustrated in Fig. 15.16. Most arise in the head of the gland where they tend to obstruct the common bile duct, thus presenting with painless obstructive jaundice.

This pattern of presentation is the basis of the old clinical adage known as Courvoisier's Law: 'A painless jaundice in the presence of a palpable gallbladder is rarely due to gallstones'. The pathological basis of this rule is that chronic gallstone disease typically causes scarring and fibrosis of the gallbladder wall and, as a result, obstruction of the biliary tree due to gallstones will not result in dilatation of the shrunken, scarred gallbladder. In contrast, occlusion of the biliary tree due to a tumour in the head of pancreas will cause back pressure, and so the (presumably) normal thin-walled gallbladder will become distended with bile such that it can be palpated.

Malignant tumours arising in the body and tail of the pancreas are very difficult to detect and, frequently, these are only identified following autopsy examination in patients with disseminated malignancy of unknown origin.

Other rarer tumours may arise from the endocrine cells of the islets of Langerhans. These lesions belong to the neuroendocrine group of tumours and are usually named according to their secretory products, for example, insulinoma and glucagonoma (see e-Fig. 15.7).

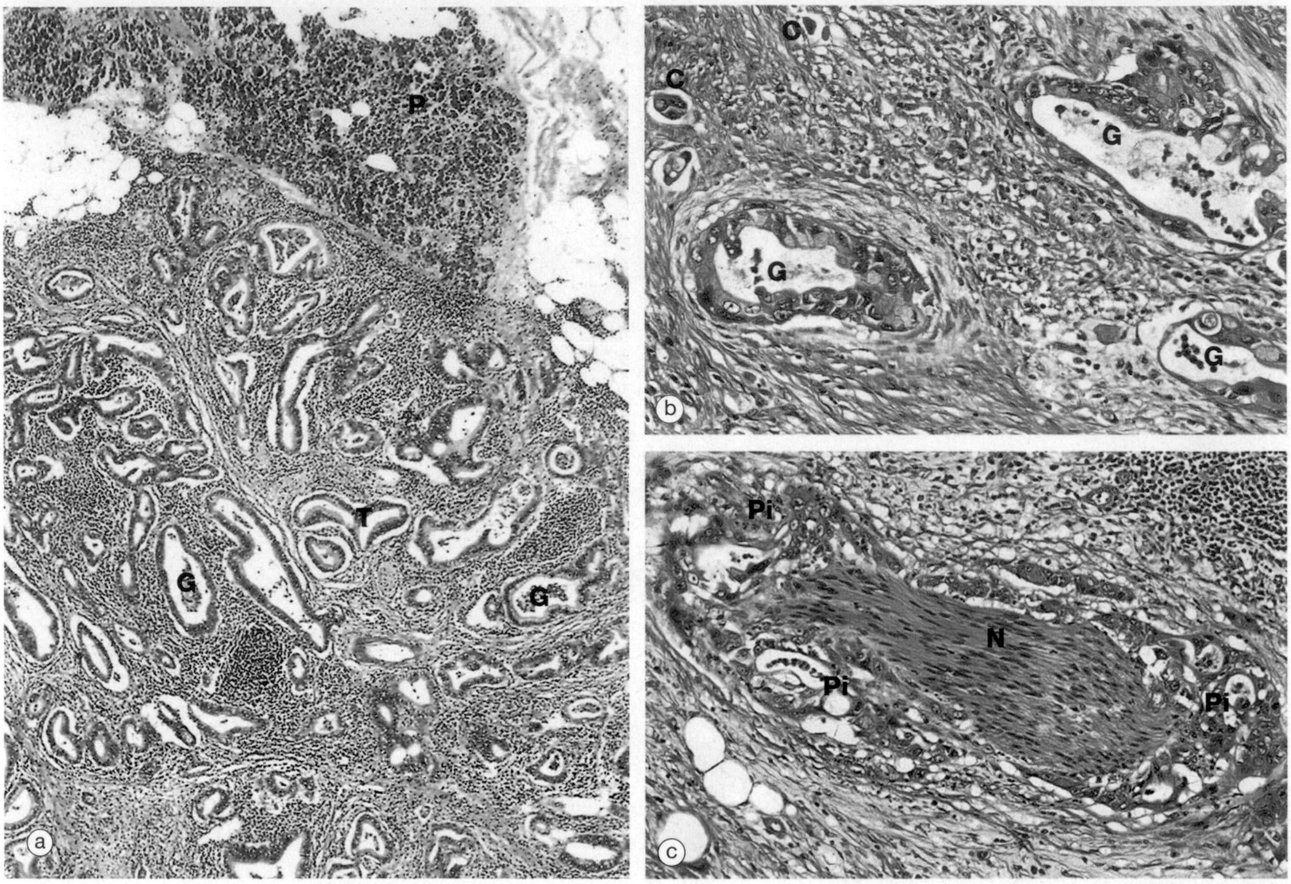

FIG. 15.16 Adenocarcinoma of pancreas
(a) H&E (LP) (b) H&E (HP)

Pancreatic adenocarcinomas usually arise in the head of the gland and present with obstructive jaundice. Fig. 15.16a shows tumour **T**, with normal pancreas **P** in the upper field. Note the characteristic tortuous irregular glands **G** within a dense collagenous stroma.

At higher magnification in Fig. 15.16b, the tumour is seen to have a ductal pattern, with marked variation in the size and shape of neoplastic glands **G** and single infiltrating cells **C**. The cells of these malignant glands have large nuclei with prominent nucleoli. In Fig. 15.16c there is perineural invasion **Pi** of malignant glands, i.e. infiltration around a small peripheral nerve **N**. This is commonly seen in pancreatic ductal cancers and illustrates the aggressive and infiltrative nature of these tumours.

Diagnosis of pancreatic cancer

Pancreatic cancer is usually diagnosed by cytological assessment of cells from a fine needle aspirate of pancreas or bile duct brushings following endoscopic ultrasound assessment (EUS). This is further discussed in Fig. 15.17. The pancreas can also be assessed by other imaging techniques such as CT and MRI scanning in order to stage the tumour and determine if surgery to remove the tumour is possible. Unfortunately, due to the often late stage of presentation, only a small proportion of patients are able to undergo definitive surgical resection. Recent advances in chemotherapy treatments incorporating genomic profiling results may provide more personalised treatment options in the future.

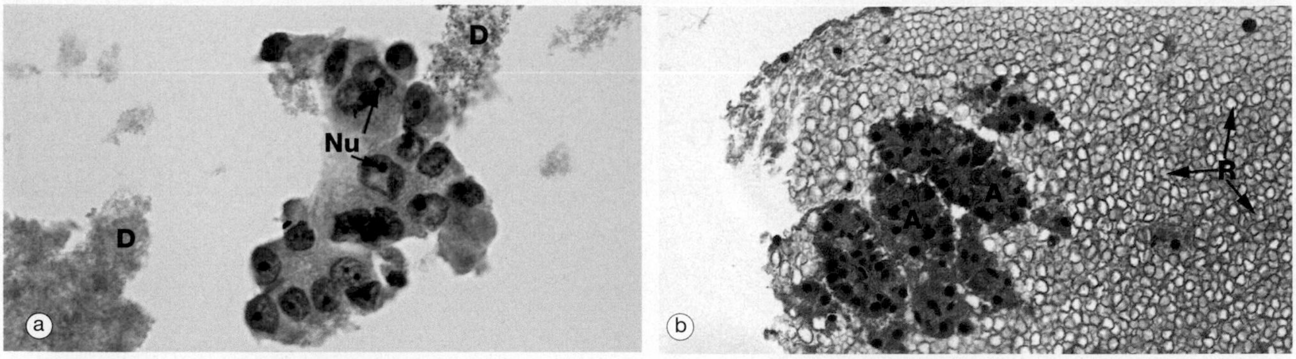

FIG. 15.17 Pancreatic FNA cytology
(a) Malignant adenocarcinoma cells (HP) (b) Cell block normal pancreatic acinar cells H&E (HP)

Fig. 15.17a is from a pancreatic **fine needle aspirate** sample (FNA), showing groups of malignant adenocarcinoma cells with irregular pleomorphic nuclei, prominent nucleoli **Nu** and moderate cytoplasm. There is acellular debris **D** in the background of the sample. Contrast this with the benign pancreatic acinar **A** cells in Fig. 15.17b. In this sample, the FNA fluid has been fixed and processed into a cell block to allow sections to be cut and stained, similar to a standard H&E section (see Appendix 1). The cells form small acinar structures. In the background, the outline of blood constituents can be seen including red blood cells **R**.

REVIEW

TABLE 15.2 Review of liver and pancreas

Structure	Key components and features	Figures
Liver	Solid organ composed of plates of hepatocytes with network of portal tracts	15.1
	Hepatocytes • Large eosinophilic cells with central nuclei and prominent nucleoli • Cells arranged in plates one cell thick with intervening sinusoids • Diverse metabolic functions • Secretion of bile into canaliculi	15.2, 15.10
	Portal tracts • Branches of: – Bile duct – Portal vein – Hepatic artery • Surrounded by limiting plate of hepatocytes	15.3
	Blood supply • Dual vascular supply: – Portal vein (products of digestion but deoxygenated blood) – Hepatic artery (oxygenated blood from systemic circulation) • Drainage via hepatic vein back to systemic circulation	15.5, 15.6
	Architecture • Classical liver lobule is hexagonal with central venule and peripheral portal tracts • Liver acinus more functionally relevant, centred around portal area with zonation of hepatocytes	15.4, 15.7, 15.8
Gallbladder and bile ducts	Bile produced by liver drains via right and left hepatic ducts into common hepatic duct	15.13
	Bile is stored and concentrated in gallbladder, entering via cystic duct	
	Gallbladder consists of simple columnar mucosa with loose submucosa and a rather thin muscular wall	
	Common bile duct is formed by union of cystic duct and common hepatic duct	
	Common bile duct enters second part of duodenum via ampulla of Vater after uniting with pancreatic duct	
Pancreas	Exocrine and endocrine components • Exocrine secretory acini draining into ducts • Endocrine islets of Langerhans produce hormones including insulin (see Ch. 17)	15.14, 15.15
	Exocrine pancreas produces alkaline fluid and digestive enzymes including: • Trypsin • Chymotrypsin • Pancreatic lipase	

A acinar cells **C** single cell infiltration **D** debris **G** malignant glands **N** peripheral nerve **Nu** tumour nucleoli
P normal pancreas **Pi** perineural invasion **R** red blood cells **T** tumour

16 Urinary system

INTRODUCTION

The principal function of the urinary system is the maintenance of water, electrolyte and acid–base ***homeostasis***, which requires that any input into the system is balanced by an equivalent output. The ***kidney*** provides the mechanism by which excess water and electrolytes are eliminated from the body, while the ***ureters***, ***bladder*** and ***urethra*** form the storage and outflow tract. A second major function of the urinary system is the excretion of many toxic metabolic waste products, particularly the nitrogenous molecules urea and creatinine, compounds that can conveniently be excreted dissolved in water. The end product of these processes is ***urine***. Since all body fluids are maintained in dynamic equilibrium with one another by the circulatory system, any adjustment in the composition of the blood results in similar changes in the other fluid compartments of the body. Thus regulation of the osmotic concentration of blood plasma by the kidneys (***osmoregulation***) ensures the osmotic regulation of all other body fluids. The third major function of the kidney is the maintenance of normal blood pressure.

The functional and structural unit of the kidney, the ***nephron***, consists of a ***renal corpuscle*** (including the ***glomerulus***) plus a long, folded ***renal tubule***. The human kidney contains approximately 1 million nephrons that perform the functions of osmoregulation and excretion by the following processes:

- Filtration in the glomerulus of most small molecules from blood plasma to form an ultrafiltrate of plasma.
- Selective reabsorption in the tubule of most of the water and some other molecules from the ultrafiltrate, leaving behind excess and waste materials to be excreted.
- Secretion in the tubule of some excretory products directly from blood into the urine.
- Maintenance of the acid–base balance by selective secretion by the tubule of H^+ ions into the urine.

The kidney also has hormonal and metabolic functions:

- ***Renin***, synthesised in the kidney, is a component of the ***renin–angiotensin–aldosterone*** mechanism that controls blood pressure.
- ***Erythropoietin***, synthesised in the kidney, stimulates the production of erythrocytes in the bone marrow and thus regulates the oxygen-carrying capacity of the blood.
- ***Vitamin D***, which regulates calcium balance, is converted to an active form in the kidney.

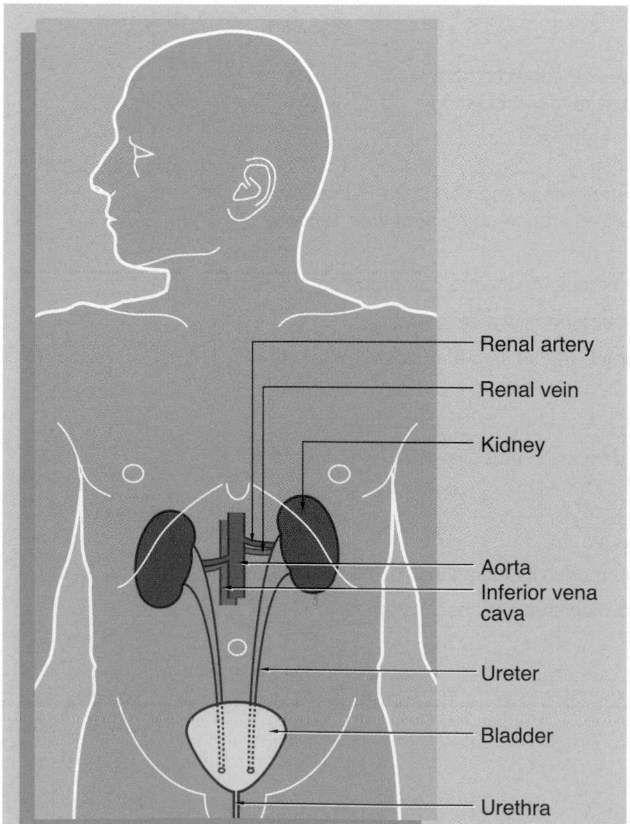

FIG. 16.1 The urinary system

The urinary system comprises two ***kidneys***, two ***ureters***, a ***bladder*** and a ***urethra***. Urine is produced in the kidneys and flows down the ureters to the bladder where it is stored until voided via the urethra. No further modification of the urine takes place after it leaves the kidneys. The kidneys and ureters are found in the retroperitoneum, while the urinary bladder is in the anterior part of the pelvis.

Blood is supplied to each kidney by the ***renal arteries***, which arise from the aorta. One or more ***renal veins*** drains the blood from each kidney to the inferior vena cava. The total blood volume of the body is circulated through the kidneys about 300 times each day.

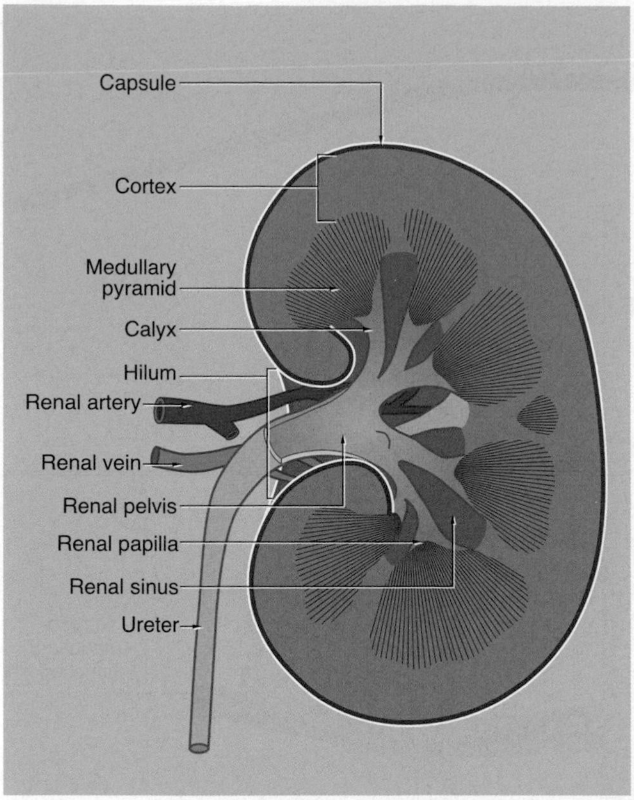

FIG. 16.2 Kidney

The kidney is a bean-shaped organ lying in the upper retroperitoneal area and oriented with the concave surface directed medially. In adults, the kidney measures 10 to 12 cm. The ***hilum*** is the site of entry and exit of the renal blood vessels and the ureter.

The archetypal kidney of lower mammals consists of a single lobe made up of a ***medullary pyramid*** (actually cone-shaped), the base of which is enveloped by the cortex containing the renal corpuscles and the proximal and distal parts of the tubules. Nephrons arise in the cortex, loop down into the medulla and return to the cortex. From here they drain into ***collecting ducts*** that descend again into the medulla to discharge urine from the apex of the medullary pyramid. The apical part of the pyramid (known as the ***renal papilla***) is enveloped by a funnel-shaped ***renal pelvis***, which represents the dilated proximal part of the ureter.

The human kidney is made up of 10 to 18 lobes. In the adult, the cortical components of the lobes are fused so that the cortex forms a continuous smooth outer zone which extends down between the pyramids. The ***renal medulla*** is made up of multiple medullary pyramids, separated by medullary extensions of the cortex. Each renal papilla is surrounded by a branch of the renal pelvis called a ***calyx***; the whole urinary collecting system within the kidney being described as the ***pelvicalyceal system***. The space between the branches of the pelvicalyceal system is filled with fatty supporting tissue and is known as the ***renal sinus***.

The kidney is invested by a tough fibrous capsule which is surrounded by a thick layer of perinephric fat that is in turn encased in a delicate condensation of connective tissue known as ***Gerota's fascia***. The fat around the kidney cushions it against trauma.

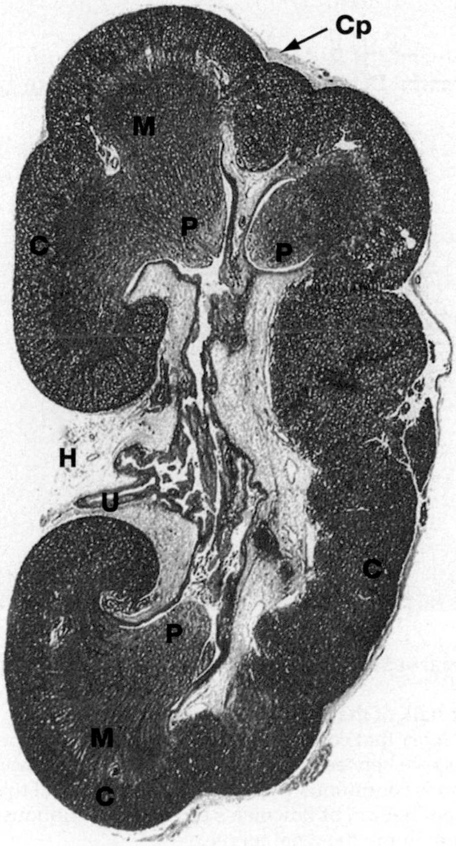

FIG. 16.3 Kidney
H&E (LP)

This micrograph of a kidney from an infant illustrates at low power the features of the kidney described in Fig. 16.2. The kidney of a baby has been chosen as it is small enough to section and photograph in its entirety. Furthermore its convex surface is irregular, reflecting the development of the many lobes making up the organ. In histological section, only a single plane through the pelvicalyceal system can be visualised. This plane of section includes the axes of three lobes, the papilla **P** of each one projecting into the central pelvicalyceal space; this drains into the ureter **U** that leaves the kidney via the hilum **H**.

The darker-stained cortex **C** can be clearly differentiated from the paler-stained medulla **M**. The cortex contains large numbers of tiny spheroidal structures, the developing renal corpuscles (see Fig. 16.8). The medullary pyramids are characterised by the numerous tubules converging towards the tips of the renal papillae. Note the continuity of the cortex throughout the outer zone of the kidney and the cortical extension between the two medullary pyramids at the top of the field. The fibrous ***capsule*** **Cp** of the kidney is continuous at the hilum with fatty supporting tissue, which packs the space (known as the renal sinus) between the hilar structures. The renal artery and vein also pass through the hilum but are not seen in this plane of section.

C cortex **Cp** capsule **H** hilum **M** medulla **P** papilla **U** ureter

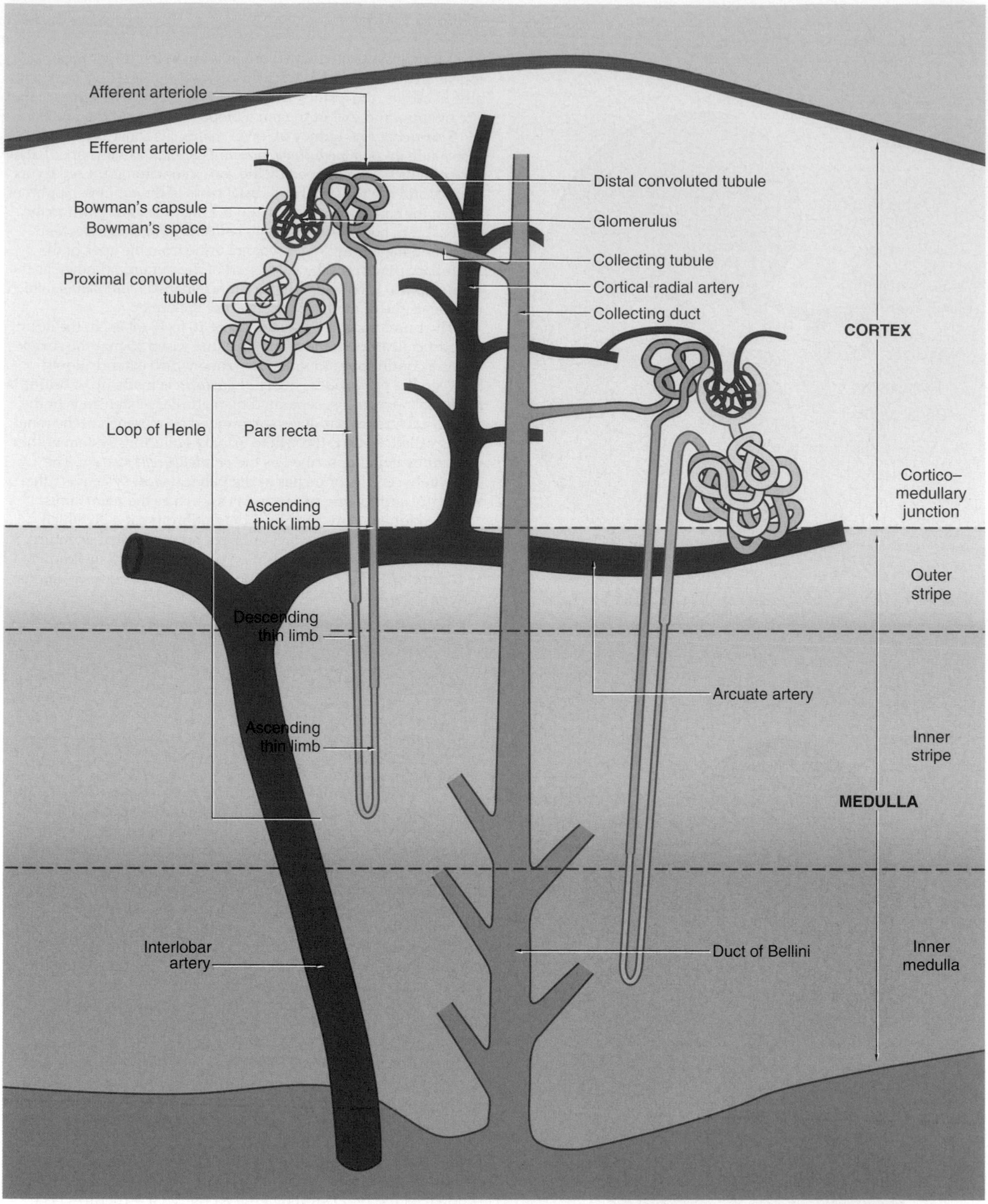

FIG. 16.4 Basic organisation of the nephron, collecting system and renal vasculature ***(caption continues opposite)***

The ***nephron***, the functional unit of the kidney, consists of two major components, the ***renal corpuscle*** and the ***renal tubule***. A normal adult kidney contains between 0.6 and 1.2×10^6 nephrons.

Renal corpuscle

The renal corpuscle is responsible for the filtration of plasma and is a combination of two structures, ***Bowman's capsule*** and the ***glomerulus***.

Bowman's capsule consists of a single layer of flattened cells resting on a basement membrane; it is derived from the distended blind end of the renal tubule. The glomerulus is a globular network of anastomosing capillaries which invaginates Bowman's capsule (see Fig. 16.7). Thus the capillary loops of the glomerulus are invested by the ***visceral layer of Bowman's capsule***, a highly specialised layer of epithelial cells called ***podocytes*** (see Fig. 16.12). The visceral layer is reflected around the vascular stalk of the glomerulus to become continuous with the ***parietal layer*** that constitutes Bowman's capsule proper.

The space between the two layers is known as ***Bowman's space*** and is continuous with the lumen of the renal tubule; the parietal epithelium of Bowman's capsule is continuous with the epithelium lining the renal tubule.

In the renal corpuscle, water and low molecular weight constituents of plasma are filtered from the glomerular capillaries into Bowman's space to form the ***glomerular ultrafiltrate***, which then passes into the renal tubule. Thus the filtration barrier between the capillary lumen and Bowman's space consists of the capillary endothelium, the podocyte layer and their common basement membrane known as the ***glomerular basement membrane*** (see Fig. 16.14); these three components are sometimes called the ***glomerular filtration barrier***.

FIG. 16.4 Basic organisation of the nephron, collecting system and renal vasculature *(illustration opposite)*

The ***afferent arteriole***, which supplies the glomerulus, and the ***efferent arteriole***, which drains it, enter and leave the corpuscle at the ***vascular pole*** that is usually situated opposite the entrance to the renal tubule, the ***urinary pole*** (see Fig. 16.8).

Renal tubule

The renal tubule extends from Bowman's capsule to its junction with a collecting duct. The renal tubule is up to 55 mm long in humans and is lined by a single layer of epithelial cells. The primary function of the renal tubule is the selective reabsorption of water, inorganic ions and other molecules from the glomerular filtrate. In addition, some inorganic ions are secreted directly from blood into the lumen of the tubule. In humans, glomerular filtrate is produced at a steady rate of approximately 120 mL/min; of this, all but about 1 mL is reabsorbed by the renal tubules, giving a normal rate of urine production of around 1 mL/min. The renal tubule has a convoluted shape and has four distinct zones, each of which has a different role in tubular function and a corresponding difference in histological appearance.

1. ***The proximal convoluted tubule*** (***PCT***) is the most convoluted section of the tubule and is responsible for the reabsorption of approximately 65% of the ions and water of the glomerular filtrate. PCTs are confined to the renal cortex and make up the greater part of its bulk.
2. ***The loop of Henle*** includes the distal straight part of the proximal tubule, the ***pars recta***, the ***thin descending*** and ***ascending limbs*** and the ***thick ascending limb***. The difference between these parts is due to differences in the epithelium. The thin segments of the loop of Henle dip down into the medulla where they form a hairpin bend. The length of the loop of Henle varies from short to long, depending on the location of the renal corpuscle of the particular nephron. The corpuscles of short-looped nephrons tend to be located in the superficial and midcortical regions, the loops extending very little beyond the corticomedullary junction. Long-looped nephrons are mainly associated with juxtamedullary corpuscles; a small proportion of long loops almost reach the tips of the renal papillae, but successively greater numbers turn back at higher levels as necessitated by the tapering shape of the medullary pyramids. The limbs of the loop of Henle are closely associated with parallel wide capillary loops, the ***vasa recta*** (not shown in this diagram), which arise from the efferent arterioles of glomeruli located near the corticomedullary junction. The vasa recta descend into the medulla then loop back on themselves to drain into veins at the junction of the medulla and cortex. The main function of the loops of Henle is to generate a high osmotic pressure in the extracellular fluid of the renal medulla; the mechanism by which this is achieved is known as the ***counter-current multiplier system*** (see Fig. 16.26). In some animals, the loop of Henle plays a major role in reabsorption of water from the glomerular filtrate back into the circulation via the vasa recta; however, this function is of lesser importance in the human kidney. The medulla can be divided into different zones according to the components of the loop of Henle that are present: the ***inner medulla*** contains only thin limbs of the loop of Henle, the ***inner stripe*** of the outer medulla contains thick descending limbs as well as thin limbs and the ***outer stripe*** of the outer medulla contains thick ascending limbs as well as thick descending limbs and thin limbs.
3. ***The distal convoluted tubule*** (***DCT***) is a continuation of the thick limb of the loop of Henle after its return to the cortex. Shorter and less convoluted than the PCT, the DCT is responsible for reabsorption of sodium ions, an active process controlled by the adrenocortical hormone ***aldosterone***. Sodium reabsorption is coupled with the secretion of hydrogen or potassium ions into the DCT, the secretion of hydrogen ions resulting in a net loss of acid from the body.
4. ***The collecting tubule*** is the straight terminal portion of the nephron, several collecting tubules converging to form a ***collecting duct***. The collecting ducts descend through the cortex in parallel bundles called ***medullary rays*** (see Fig. 16.5), progressively merging in the medulla to form the large ***ducts of Bellini***, which open at the tips of the renal papillae to discharge urine into the pelvicalyceal system. The collecting tubules and ducts are not normally permeable to water. However, in the presence of ***antidiuretic hormone*** (***ADH***, also known as ***arginine vasopressin*** or ***AVP***) secreted by the posterior pituitary, the collecting tubules and ducts become permeable to water. Thus the high osmotic pressure generated by the counter-current multiplier system into the interstitial tissues of the medulla removes water that is returned to the general circulation via the vasa recta. The loops of Henle and ADH thus provide a mechanism for the production of urine that is hypertonic with respect to plasma.

Renal vasculature

In most cases, each kidney is supplied by a single renal artery which divides in the hilum into two main branches; in some individuals, however, there are two or even more renal arteries that derive directly from the aorta. Each of these gives rise to several ***interlobar arteries*** which ascend between the pyramids to the corticomedullary junction. Here they branch to form the ***arcuate arteries***, which run in an arc-like course parallel to the capsule of the kidney. The arcuate arteries give rise to numerous ***interlobular*** (***cortical radial***) ***arteries*** that radiate towards the capsule, branching to form the afferent arterioles of the glomeruli.

As previously described, the vasa recta form a continuation of the efferent arterioles of juxtamedullary glomeruli and form the microcirculation of the renal medulla. The efferent arterioles of the rest of the cortex divide to form the plexus of capillaries that surround the tubules of the renal cortex. The cortical and medullary capillaries drain via ***cortical radial*** (***interlobular***) ***veins*** to ***arcuate veins*** at the cortico-medullary junction and thence to the ***renal vein***.

Renal failure

Renal failure occurs for a variety of reasons and may be acute or chronic. Irreversible severe renal failure is inevitably fatal unless some form of renal replacement therapy is undertaken. Current options for renal replacement therapy include renal dialysis and renal transplantation. Dialysis may take the form of haemodialysis or, less commonly, peritoneal dialysis. Renal transplantation requires a donor, which can often involve a long wait until a suitable HLA-compatible donor is found. Those individuals lucky enough to have a compatible and willing family member are able to receive a donated kidney from them. This highlights the inbuilt redundancy of the kidneys whereby an individual can survive and be perfectly healthy with only one kidney. Stem cell research may in future provide a third option for renal replacement, the possibility of growing one's own perfectly matched new kidney (or heart or pancreas) from one's own stem cells.

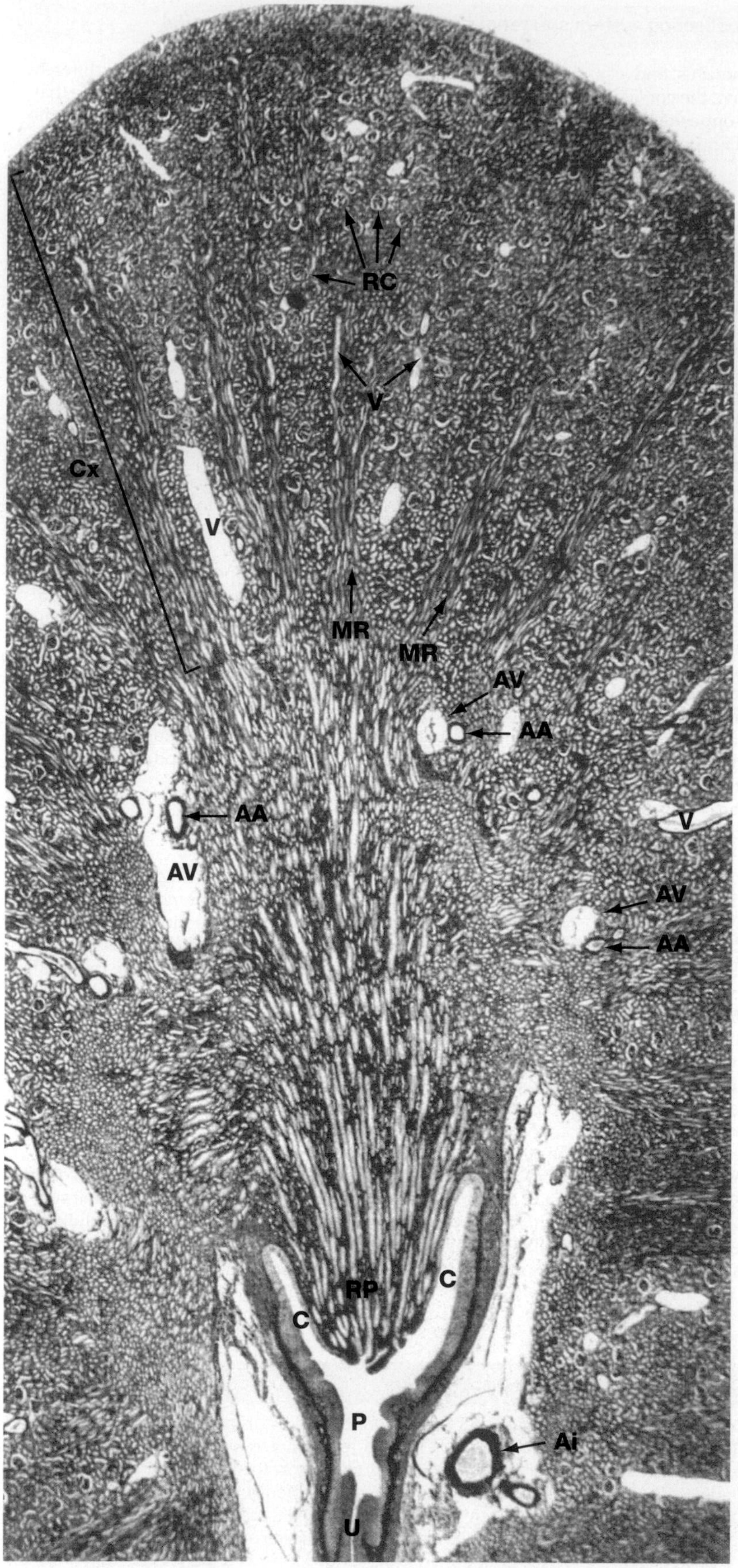

FIG. 16.5 Kidney, monkey
Jones methenamine silver H&E (LP)

The basic geography of the kidney can be seen in this unilobar kidney that has been sectioned through the axis of the medullary pyramid. Note the cup-shaped calyx **C** surrounding the renal papilla **RP**. The calyces fuse to form the pelvis **P** that in turn leads to the ureter **U**.

In the cortex **Cx**, numerous renal corpuscles **RC** (200 μm in diameter) are just visible at this magnification. The corpuscles tend to be arranged in parallel rows at right angles to the capsule, separated by interlobular arteries from which they derive their blood supply. Interlobular arteries are too narrow to be identified at this magnification, but a number of their accompanying thin-walled interlobular veins **V** are easily seen.

Most of the cortical parenchyma surrounding the renal corpuscles consists of proximal and distal convoluted tubules. From the cortex, medullary rays **MR** course towards the medulla; they consist of collecting tubules and ducts draining nephrons located high in the cortex. The collecting ducts merge in the medulla to form the larger ducts of Bellini that converge towards the tip of the renal papilla. Although not visible at this magnification, long loops of Henle dip into the medulla between and parallel with the collecting ducts. The long, straight vasa recta also dip down into the medulla alongside the loops of Henle; these vessels, too small to be seen at this magnification, absorb water from the loops of Henle and collecting ducts.

The corticomedullary junction is marked by several arcuate arteries **AA** and their associated thin-walled arcuate veins **AV**. Note a large interlobar branch of the renal artery **Ai** in the hilar supporting tissue.

AA arcuate artery **Ai** interlobar artery **AV** arcuate vein **C** calyx **Cx** cortex **G** glomerulus **IA** interlobular artery **MR** medullary ray **P** renal pelvis **RC** renal corpuscle **RP** renal papilla **T** tubule **U** ureter **V** interlobular vein

THE RENAL CORTEX

The renal cortex is easily identified even at low magnification by the presence of renal corpuscles, which are absent in the renal medulla. However, the bulk of the cortex is occupied by the proximal and distal convoluted tubules. The arcuate arteries and veins help to demarcate the cortex from the medulla.

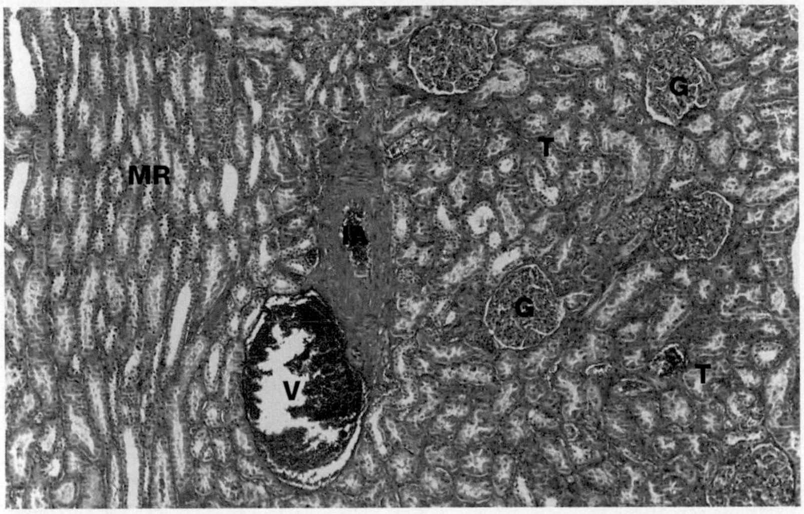

FIG. 16.6 Renal cortex H&E (MP)

At higher magnification, the renal corpuscles are dense rounded structures, the ***glomeruli* G**, surrounded by narrow Bowman's spaces, normally filled with plasma ultrafiltrate and only just visible at this magnification. The tubules **T** fill the bulk of the parenchyma between the corpuscles. The cortex consists mainly of proximal convoluted tubules lined by more eosinophilic epithelial cells, with smaller numbers of distal convoluted tubules and collecting tubules. At the left side of the micrograph, part of a medullary ray **MR** composed of collecting tubules is easily identified. An interlobular artery **IA** and vein **V** are also easily identified.

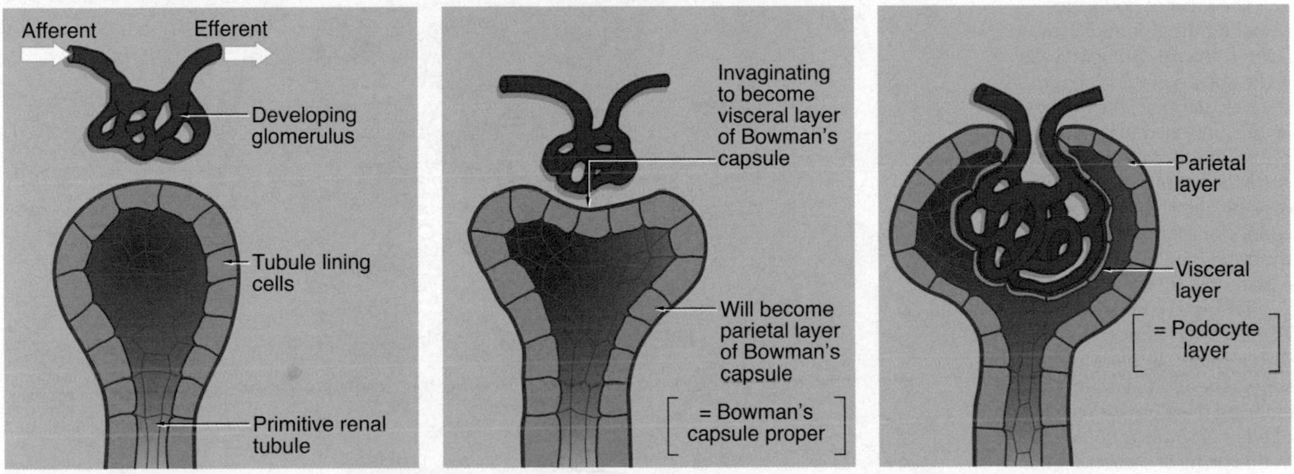

FIG. 16.7 Development of the renal corpuscle

The three-dimensional structure of the renal corpuscle can be clarified by studying its development. The renal tubules develop from the embryological ***metanephros*** as blind-ended tubes consisting of a single layer of cuboidal epithelium. The ends of the tubules dilate and become invaginated by a tiny mass of mesoderm tissue that differentiates to form the glomerulus. The layer of invaginated epithelium flattens and differentiates into podocytes that become closely applied to the outer surfaces of glomerular capillaries (the visceral layer of Bowman's capsule). Most of the intervening tissue disappears so that the basement membranes of glomerular endothelial cells and podocytes effectively fuse, forming the glomerular basement membrane. A small amount of tissue remains to support the capillary loops and differentiates to form the ***mesangium***. Where the mesangium stretches between the capillary loops, its urinary surface is invested by podocyte cytoplasm with underlying basement membrane.

FIG. 16.8 Renal corpuscle
(a) Schematic diagram
(b) PAS (HP)

The main structural features of the renal corpuscle are demonstrated in Fig. 16.8a. The relatively wide-diameter ***afferent arteriole*** enters Bowman's capsule at the vascular pole of the renal corpuscle and then branches to form an anastomosing network of glomerular capillaries, each major branch giving rise to a ***lobule***. The glomerulus is thus suspended in Bowman's space from the vascular pole. The spaces between the capillary loops in each glomerular lobule are filled by ***mesangium*** which contains ***mesangial cells*** (not shown).

The efferent vessel draining the glomerulus is unusual in that it has the structure of an arteriole and is thus called the efferent arteriole (not venule). The efferent arteriole is of smaller diameter than the afferent arteriole, and a pressure gradient is thus maintained that drives the filtration of plasma into Bowman's space.

The layer of podocytes investing the glomerular capillaries (***visceral epithelial cells***) is not shown in this diagram. At the vascular pole, the podocyte layer is reflected to become continuous with the ***parietal epithelial cells*** of Bowman's capsule, which in turn becomes continuous with the first part of the renal tubule, the proximal convoluted tubule.

The renal corpuscle in Fig. 16.8b has been sectioned through the vascular pole and shows the afferent arteriole **A** entering the glomerulus. The efferent arteriole is not seen in this plane of section. At the urinary pole, the start of the proximal convoluted tubule **PCT** is seen. Other proximal convoluted tubules can be seen cut in various planes of section embedded in the renal ***interstitium*** **I**. Glomerular capillaries **C** are cut in transverse, longitudinal and oblique sections. The numerous nuclei in the glomerulus are those of capillary endothelial cells, mesangial cells and podocytes.

The PAS stain picks out the glomerular basement membrane **GBM** and the mesangium **M**, which consists of basement membrane–like material. Mesangial cells are found embedded within the mesangium, but only their nuclei **N** can be discerned at this magnification. The capillary lumina are lined by endothelial cells, again only identifiable by their nuclei **E**.

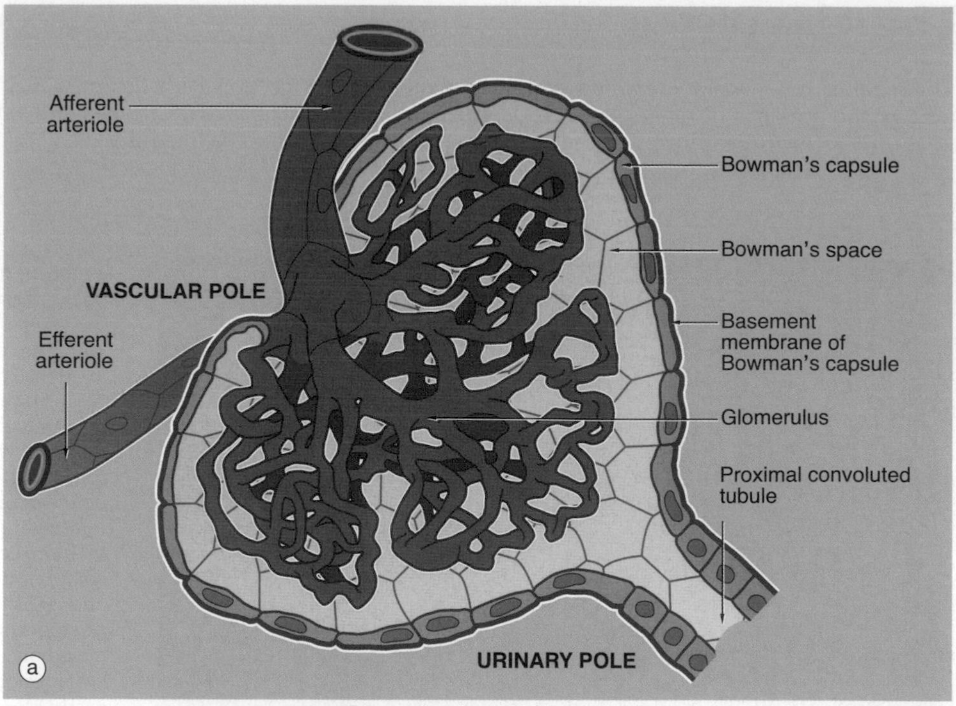

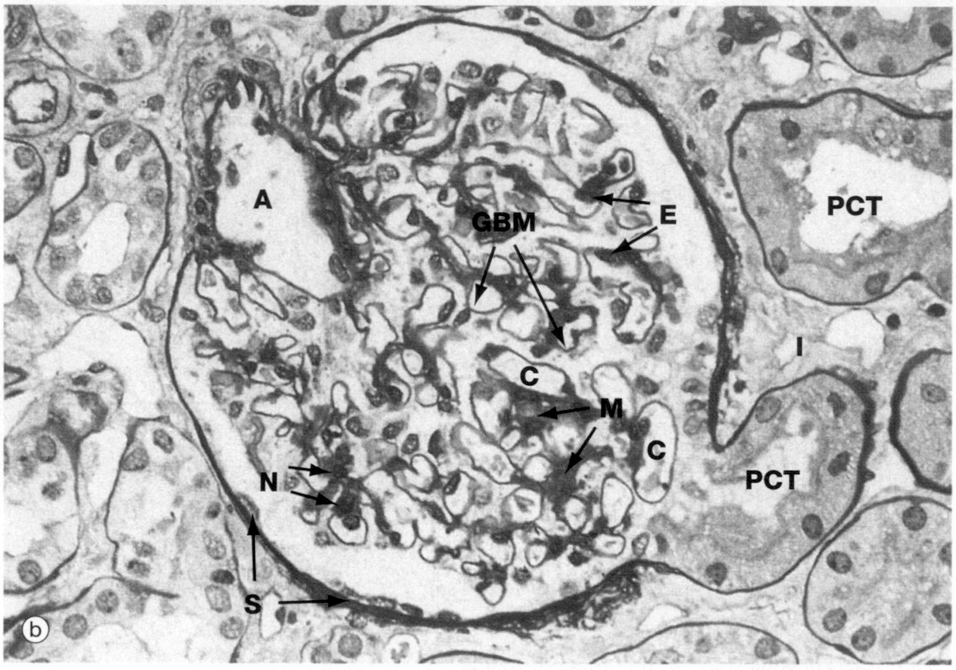

Note the flattened nuclei of the parietal epithelial cells **S** lining Bowman's capsule. This squamous epithelium is continuous with the epithelium of the proximal convoluted tubule and undergoes an abrupt transition to cuboidal form at the urinary pole. The basement membrane of Bowman's capsule is a thick basement membrane which is highlighted by the PAS stain; it is most likely synthesised by the overlying epithelial cells. Bowman's capsule is a permeability barrier preventing escape of the plasma ultrafiltrate into the interstitium. The epithelial cells are connected by tight junctions and also contribute to the permeability barrier.

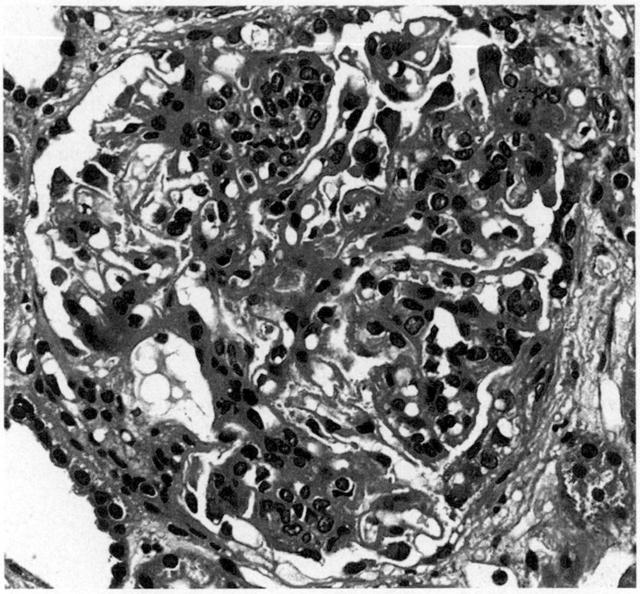

FIG. 16.9 Glomerulonephritis
H&E (HP)

This glomerulus is from a patient with glomerulonephritis (see e-Fig. 16.1). Compare this glomerulus with the normal one in Fig. 16.8. Note how the glomerulus seems full of cells and is virtually solid.

The glomerular capillary loops are partially obstructed by a mixture of activated endothelial cells and mesangial cells. Less obvious with this staining method is the thickening of the glomerular basement membrane. This patient has the autoimmune disease systemic lupus erythematosus (SLE), and the histological changes in the glomerulus result from the deposition of immune complexes and the response of the intrinsic glomerular cells to these immune complexes. The immune complexes consist of antibodies and antigen, such as double-stranded DNA, a normal body component. The clinical symptoms and signs of lupus nephritis include haematuria, proteinuria including nephrotic syndrome, hypertension and, in some cases, eventual chronic renal failure.

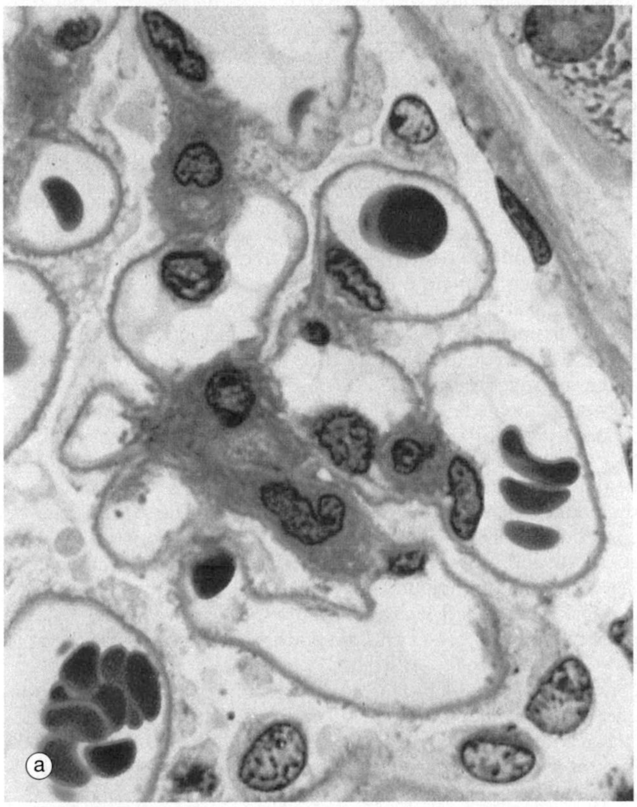

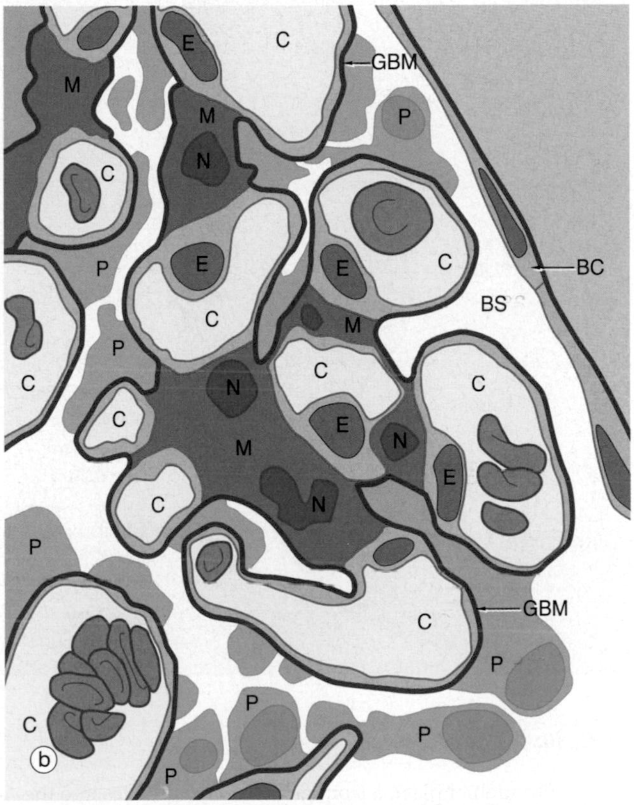

FIG. 16.10 Glomerulus
(a) Thin epoxy resin section, toluidine blue (HP) (b) Schematic diagram

Using resin-embedding techniques it is possible to cut thin sections (approximately 0.5 to 1.0 μm thick) which permit much greater resolution at high magnification.

In this preparation, the glomerular capillaries **C**, some of which contain erythrocytes, are defined by the prominent glomerular basement membranes **GBM**. Occasional capillary endothelial cell nuclei **E** are seen bulging into the capillary lumina. The mesangium **M** consists of material similar to basement membrane and contains mesangial cells, identifiable by their nuclei **N**. Mesangial cells, which have features resembling smooth muscle cells, are contractile and are thus able to modify the diameter of the glomerular capillaries in response to vasoactive substances, some of which they themselves produce. Thus mesangial cells have an important role in the control of capillary flow in the glomerulus. They also secrete the mesangial matrix and have a phagocytic function.

The mesangium is separated from the capillary lumen only by a thin layer of fenestrated endothelial cell cytoplasm, the basement membrane of which merges with the mesangial matrix. Thus particulate matter from blood may pass into the mesangium where it can be phagocytosed and degraded by mesangial cells. The podocytes and their basement membrane invest the outer surface of the mesangium.

Podocytes **P** also invest the capillary loops exposed to Bowman's space **BS**. The podocytes have extensive branching pale-stained cytoplasm and large, round pale-stained nuclei. Note the nuclei of two squamous cells of Bowman's capsule **BC**.

A afferent arteriole **BC** Bowman's capsule **BS** Bowman's space **C** glomerular capillary **E** endothelial cell **GBM** glomerular basement membrane **I** interstitium **M** mesangium **N** mesangial cell nucleus **P** podocyte **PCT** proximal convoluted tubule **S** parietal epithelial cell

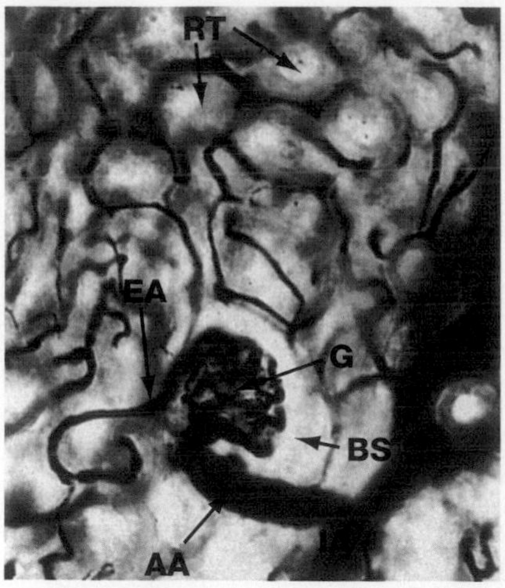

FIG. 16.11 Blood supply of the glomerulus
Carmine–gelatine perfused (MP)

This section is from a kidney that has been perfused with a red dye in order to demonstrate the renal blood supply; the nephrons remain unstained.

An interlobular artery **IA** can be seen branching to form the afferent arteriole **AA** of a glomerulus **G**. The efferent arteriole **EA** leaving the glomerulus is of much smaller diameter than the afferent arteriole, an arrangement which maintains pressure within glomerular capillaries necessary for blood plasma to be filtered into Bowman's space **BS**. Blood pressure within the glomerulus is controlled by variation of the diameter of the afferent and efferent arterioles, a function shared by podocytes and mesangial cells.

In the superficial and midcortex as shown here, efferent arterioles give rise to a network of capillaries, the ***peritubular capillaries***, which surround the renal tubules **RT**; towards the medulla, efferent arterioles give rise to the vasa recta. Molecules reabsorbed from glomerular filtrate are returned to the general circulation via this capillary network which drains into the renal venous system.

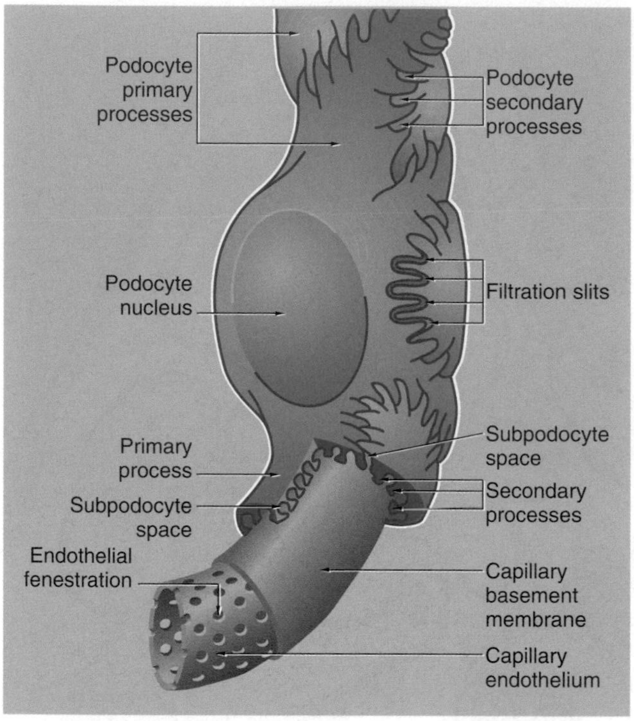

FIG. 16.12 The glomerular filter

During filtration of plasma from glomerular capillaries into the renal tubule, the filtrate passes through at least four layers of the ***glomerular filtration barrier*** (***GFB***): ***capillary endothelium***, ***glomerular basement membrane***, the ***podocyte foot processes with slit diaphragms*** and the ***subpodocyte space***. All four contribute to the filtration process.

The capillary endothelium contains numerous large round fenestrations (60–100 nm in diameter) which occupy 20% to 50% of the endothelial surface area. It was previously thought that the fenestrations do not exhibit diaphragms as in fenestrated capillaries elsewhere in the body (see Fig. 8.16). The endothelial cells, including their fenestrations, are covered on the capillary side by a thick glycocalyx (220–400 nm) composed of glycoproteins, glycosaminoglycans and sialoglycoproteins. This glycocalyx contributes to the filtration barrier.

The glomerular basement membrane (approximately 350 nm in adults) is much thicker than other basement membranes and appears to be produced by both capillary endothelial cells and podocytes. As with basement membranes elsewhere (see Ch. 4), it consists of a feltwork of type IV collagen, structural glycoproteins (fibronectin and laminin) and proteoglycans rich in heparan sulphate, the interstices of this highly cross-linked structure being occupied by water molecules. By electron microscopy, the glomerular basement membrane consists of three layers, a dense central layer, the ***lamina densa*** with a thinner electron-lucent layer on either side of it, the ***lamina rara interna*** under the endothelium and the ***lamina rara externa*** supporting the podocytes. Both laminae rarae are negatively charged.

The podocytes have long cytoplasmic extensions called ***primary processes*** that embrace the capillaries, giving rise to short secondary ***foot processes*** (***pedicels***), which interdigitate with those of other primary processes. The secondary foot processes are directly applied to the lamina rara externa and bound to it by fine filaments. The gaps between adjacent secondary foot processes, known as ***filtration slits***, are of uniform width (40 nm) and are bridged by ***slit diaphragms***. The slit diaphragm is composed of a single layer of the transmembrane protein, ***nephrin***, whose extracellular domains from adjacent foot processes link together rather in the manner of a zip. A glycocalyx rich in negatively charged ***podocalyxin*** covers the urinary surface of the podocytes, including the slit diaphragms. The intracellular component of nephrin is bound to the actin cytoskeleton of the podocyte and it has been suggested that the slit diaphragm is in fact a modified tight junction.

The ***subpodocyte space*** (***SPS***), the space between the podocyte foot processes and the podocyte cell bodies, has been recently shown to be a restricted space that comprises a fourth component of the GFB. The SPS covers approximately 60% of the glomerular capillary surface. Ultrafiltrate in this confined space can only leave it via the ***subpodocyte space exit pore***, which leads into the ***interpodocyte space*** between the podocyte cell bodies and finally into Bowman's space proper. The SPS has higher hydrostatic pressure than Bowman's space, and it is thought that the podocytes, by altering the size of the SPS and the exit pore, are able to regulate filtration though the GBM.

As mentioned above, all layers contribute to the selective filtration barrier. Clinical evidence demonstrates that free haemoglobin (MW 65 000) and smaller molecules pass freely through the glomerular filter, whereas albumin (MW 68 000) and larger molecules are retained. For macromolecules, three factors determine permeability: charge, size and configuration. Negatively charged (anionic) molecules are blocked by the negatively charged endothelial cell coat and laminae rarae of the basement membrane, while the meshwork of the lamina densa of the basement membrane discriminates on the basis of molecular size and configuration. The slit diaphragm restricts the passage of any large molecules, but its main role is in controlling water flow, which is also held back by the colloidal osmotic pressure of retained albumin and other large molecules.

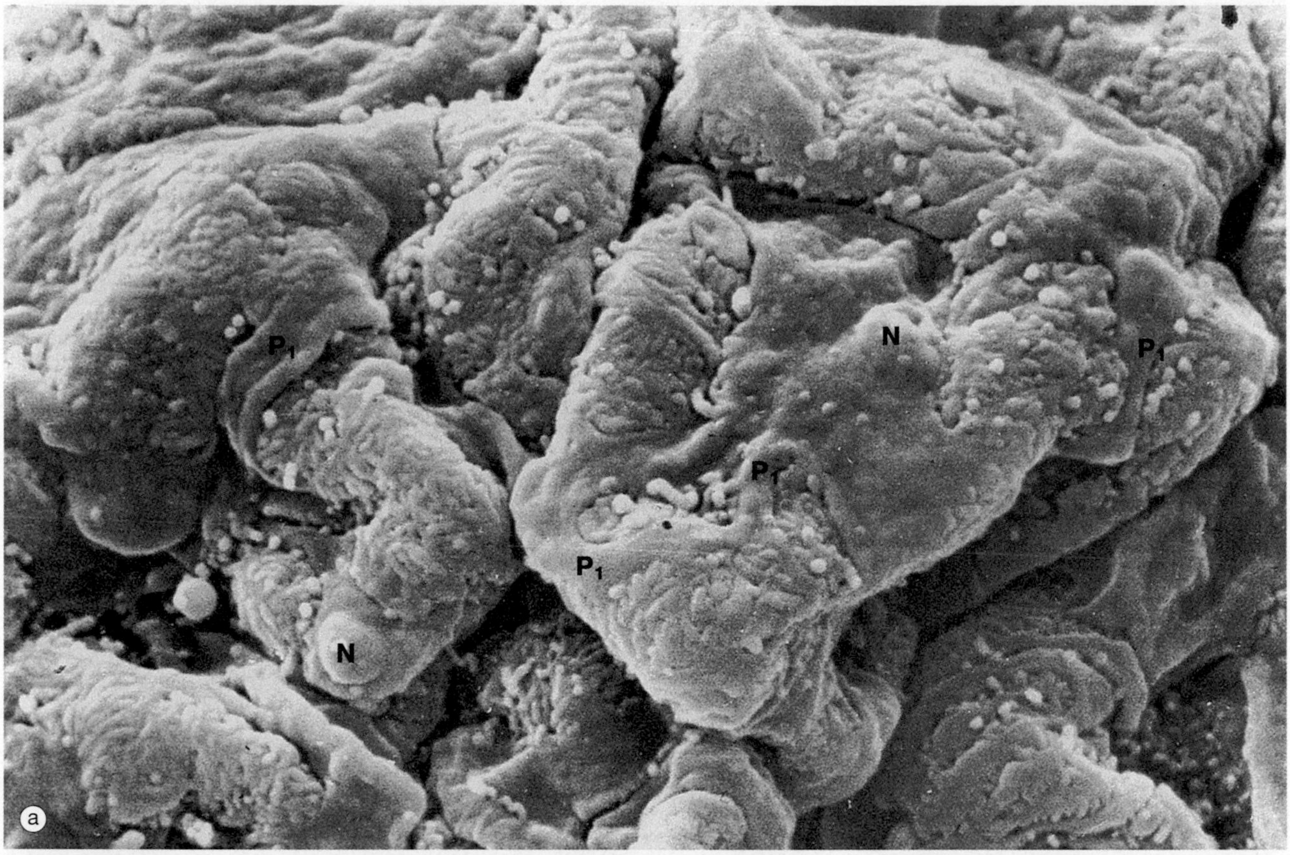

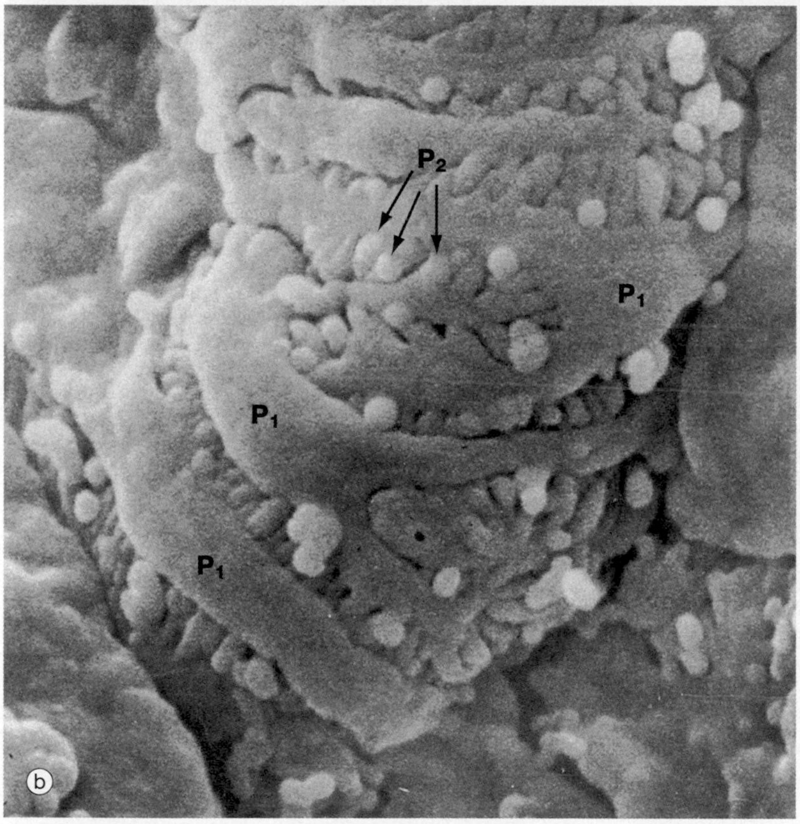

FIG. 16.13 Glomerulus
(a) SEM ×1500 (b) SEM ×6000

Scanning electron microscopy readily demonstrates the three-dimensional relationships of podocytes and their processes that extend like octopus tentacles over the whole surface of the glomerulus.

Fig. 16.13a shows part of a glomerular capillary tuft. The capillaries are enveloped by podocytes which have large flattened cell bodies and bulging nuclei **N**. Each podocyte has several long primary processes $\mathbf{P_1}$ that embrace one or more capillaries. Each primary process has numerous secondary ***foot processes*** (***pedicels***) which rest on the lamina rara externa of the glomerular basement membrane.

At higher magnification in Fig. 16.13b, the secondary foot processes $\mathbf{P_2}$ can be seen as extensions of the large primary processes $\mathbf{P_1}$. The secondary foot processes interdigitate with those of other primary processes, separated by filtration slits of uniform width.

AA afferent arteriole **BS** Bowman's space **EA** efferent arteriole **G** glomerulus **IA** interlobular artery **N** podocyte nucleus $\mathbf{P_1}$ podocyte primary process $\mathbf{P_2}$ podocyte secondary process **RT** renal tubule

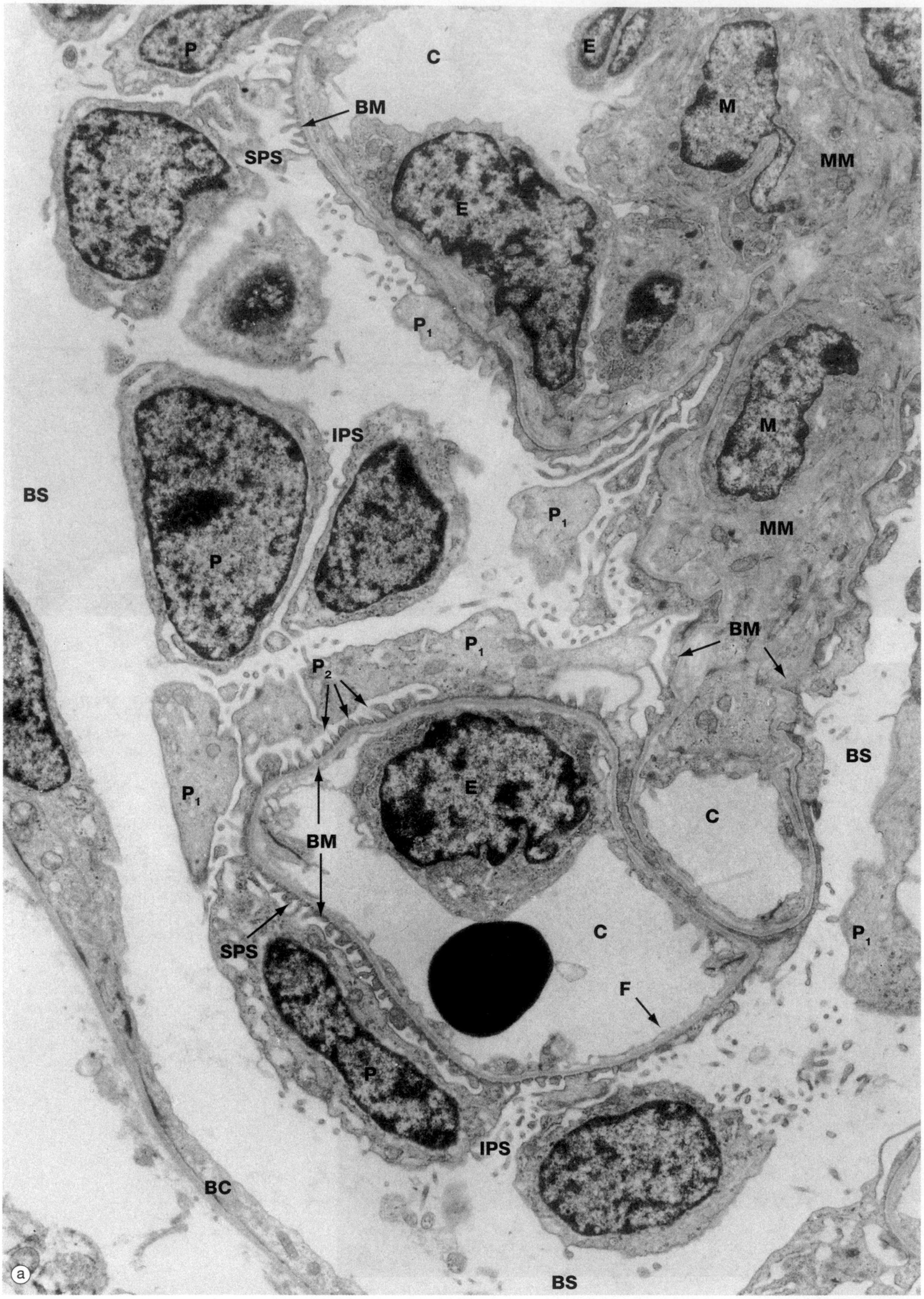

FIG. 16.14 Glomerulus *(caption and illustrations (b) and (c) opposite)*
(a) EM ×4800 (b) EM ×14 000 (c) EM ×30 000

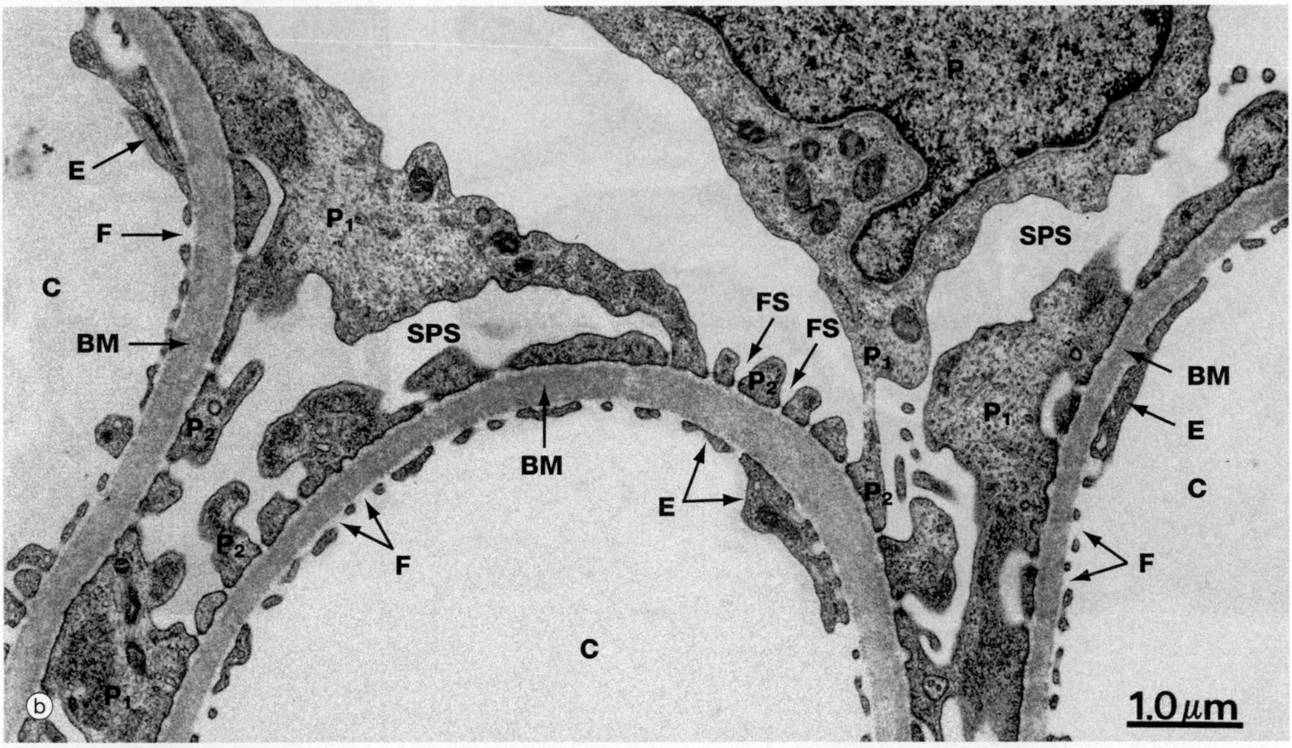

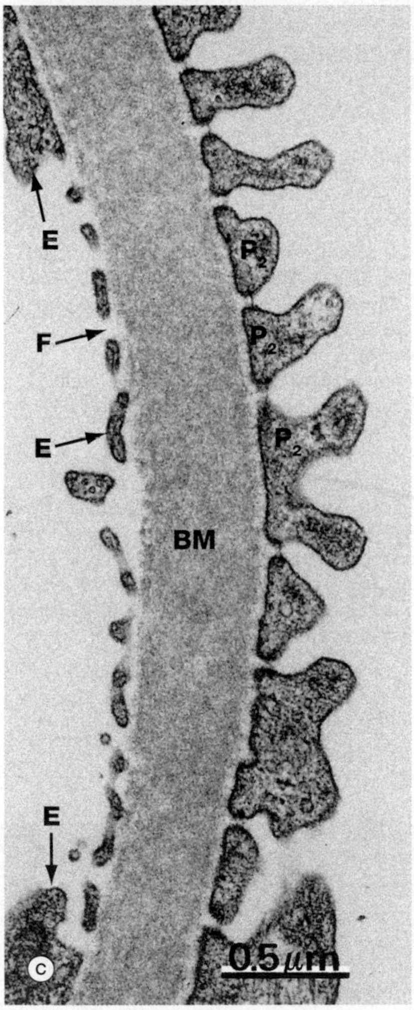

FIG. 16.14 Glomerulus *(illustration (a) opposite)*
(a) EM ×4800 (b) EM ×14 000 (c) EM ×30 000

When examining both light and electron microscope specimens of glomeruli, the podocytes, endothelial cells and mesangium are identified most easily by tracing out the glomerular basement membrane. Fig. 16.14a shows several capillary loops **C** lined by a thin layer of fenestrated endothelial cytoplasm. The endothelial cell nuclei **E** can be seen bulging into the capillary lumina. The capillary endothelial fenestrations **F** are better seen at higher magnification in Fig. 16.14b and c. The nuclei of several podocytes **P** can be seen, their primary processes $\mathbf{P_1}$ giving rise to numerous secondary foot processes $\mathbf{P_2}$ that rest on the glomerular basement membrane **BM**. At right midfield a branched mesangial stalk comprising mesangial cells **M** and mesangial matrix **MM** provides support for the capillary loops. The mesangium is separated from the capillary lumen only by the cytoplasm of the endothelial cells, while the podocytes and their basement membrane continue around the mesangial stalk, separating it from Bowman's space. Part of Bowman's capsule **BC** is seen at the periphery, consisting of a squamous epithelial cell and underlying basement membrane. The subpodocyte space **SPS** and interpodocyte space **IPS** are easily identified, although the subpodocyte space exit pore is not seen. At the periphery of the glomerulus, Bowman's space **BS** is delineated by the podocyte cell bodies on one side and the parietal epithelial cells on the other.

Fig. 16.14b shows three glomerular capillaries **C** lined by attenuated endothelial cytoplasm **E** with wide fenestrations **F**. A podocyte **P** extends several primary processes $\mathbf{P_1}$ onto the capillaries, these in turn giving rise to multiple secondary foot processes $\mathbf{P_2}$ separated by filtration slits **FS**. The subpodocyte space **SPS** can again be identified. The glomerular basement membrane **BM** separates the podocytes and capillary endothelium. The thickness of the basement membrane appears variable, but this is due to the slightly oblique plane of section; the basement membranes are in fact of uniform width.

At even higher magnification in Fig. 16.14c three of the components of the glomerular filter are seen. The fenestrated capillary endothelium **E** is closely applied to the luminal surface of the glomerular basement membrane **BM**; on the opposite side are podocyte secondary foot processes $\mathbf{P_2}$, separated by filtration slits of uniform width and bridged by the slit diaphragms. Part of the subpodocyte space is seen, but the podocyte cell body which delimits the subpodocyte space is not apparent. The wide central lamina densa of the glomerular basement membrane can be seen bordered on each side by a narrow lamina rara. The glycocalyces of the endothelial cells and podocytes are not apparent in these micrographs; special fixation and processing techniques are required to demonstrate them.

BC Bowman's capsule **BM** glomular basement membrane **BS** Bowman's space **C** capillary loop **E** endothelial cell **F** fenestration **FS** filtration slit **IPS** interpodocyte space **M** mesangial cell **MM** mesangial matrix **P** podocyte $\mathbf{P_1}$ podocyte primary process $\mathbf{P_2}$ podocyte secondary foot process **SPS** subpodocyte space

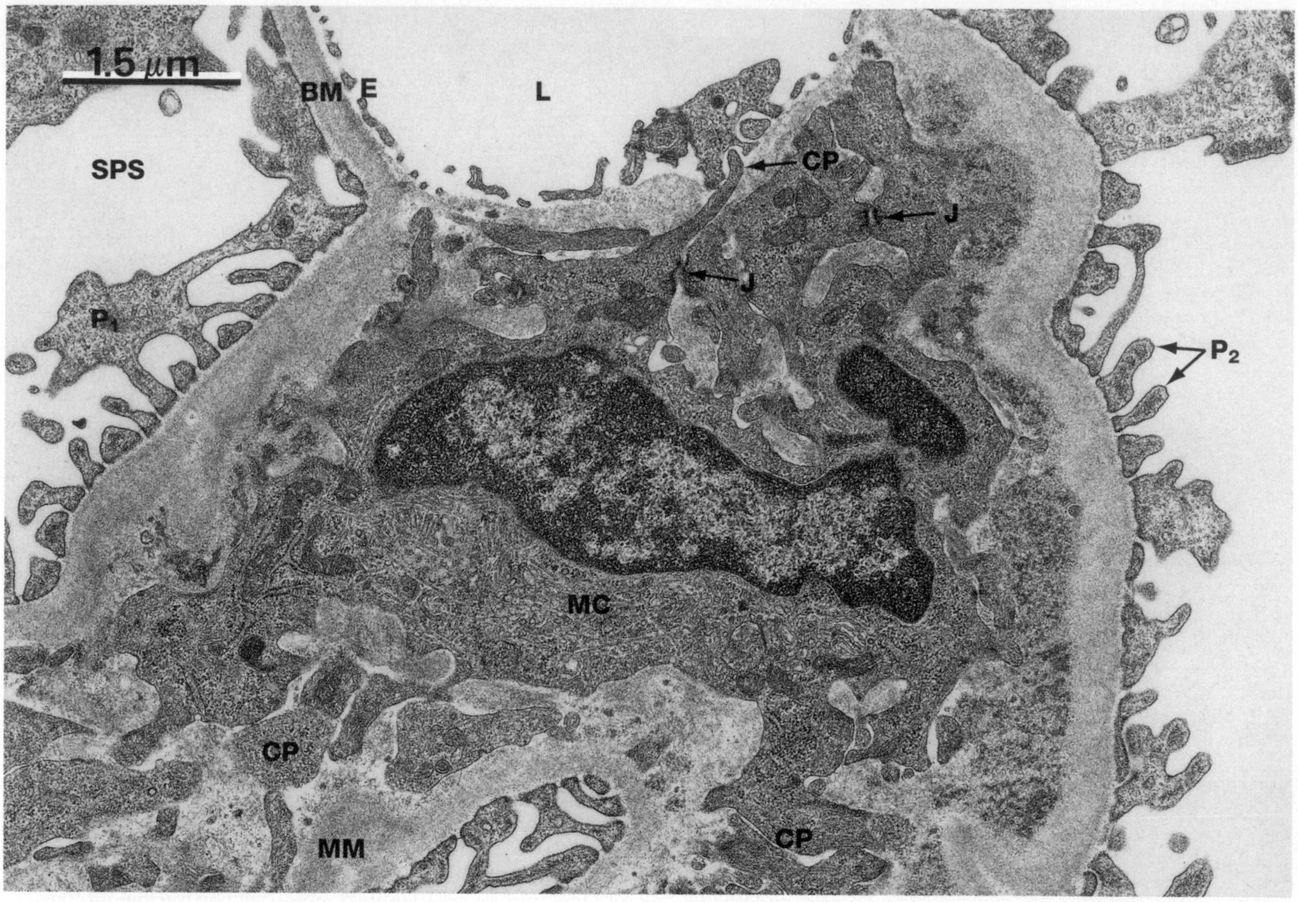

FIG. 16.15 The mesangium, rat
EM ×14 000

Fig. 16.15 shows an area of mesangium along with part of a glomerular capillary lumen **L**. The capillary lumen is lined by the delicate fenestrated endothelium **E**. Podocyte primary processes $\mathbf{P_1}$ and secondary foot processes $\mathbf{P_2}$ are easily seen, as well as subpodocyte space **SPS**. The mesangium is composed of fibrillary basement membrane-like material **MM** within which is embedded a mesangial cell **MC**. Mesangial cells have long cytoplasmic processes **CP** that ramify through the mesangium and form cell junctions with the processes of other mesangial cells. Several of these cell junctions **J** can be seen in this field. Thus the mesangial cells form a network supporting the glomerular capillaries.

One function of mesangial cells is the secretion of mesangial matrix; they also secrete vasoactive factors and cytokines and phagocytose particles such as immune complexes from the blood. The majority of mesangial cells have a well-developed filamentous cytoskeleton rich in actin and are thought to be specialised pericytes, but a small proportion of these cells display phagocytic characteristics such as the expression of surface Fc and C3 receptors. Mesangial cells with this phagocytic phenotype are able to phagocytose and destroy large particles such as immune complexes taken up from the blood.

Fig. 16.15 demonstrates the close relationship between the mesangial and endothelial cells. These are not separated from each other by a basement membrane and in fact lie within the same basement membrane–bound compartment. Conceptually it might be helpful to consider the mesangium as a modified segment of the glomerular capillary wall. Also in this electron micrograph the morphological difference between the glomerular basement membrane **BM** and the mesangial matrix **MM** is apparent; this reflects the differences in chemical composition between the two. The main structural components of mesangial matrix are type IV collagen, laminin, fibronectin and proteoglycans such as decorin and biglycan.

Diabetic renal disease

Diabetic nephropathy is the most common cause of renal failure in affluent countries (see e-Fig. 16.2). The incidence of type 2 diabetes is increasing, an increase that is felt to be largely due to changing lifestyles, with increasing obesity and decreasing exercise, although there is little doubt that genetic factors are also important. Usually one of the earliest signs of diabetic nephropathy is proteinuria, which may eventually progress to the nephrotic syndrome and progressive chronic renal failure. The microscopic features in these cases include thickening of the mesangial basement membrane and an increase in mesangial matrix, often called diabetic glomerulosclerosis. In normal glomeruli, the balance between deposition of new and removal of old mesangial matrix is very tightly controlled. Recent research is beginning to tease out the mechanisms underlying these clinical features, including chemical mediators such as transforming growth factor β (TGF-β) that induce increased deposition of mesangial matrix in response to high glucose concentrations. This mesangial matrix has a different composition to normal matrix, including increased amounts of type I and type III collagen which are not easily removed from the glomerulus. However, other factors, including direct podocyte injury and changes in the slit pore membrane, also contribute to the characteristic proteinuria that precedes frank renal failure.

Diabetics also tend to suffer from vascular disease, hypertension and increased infections in the kidney, and all of these tend to contribute to the development of end-stage renal failure (see e-Fig. 16.3).

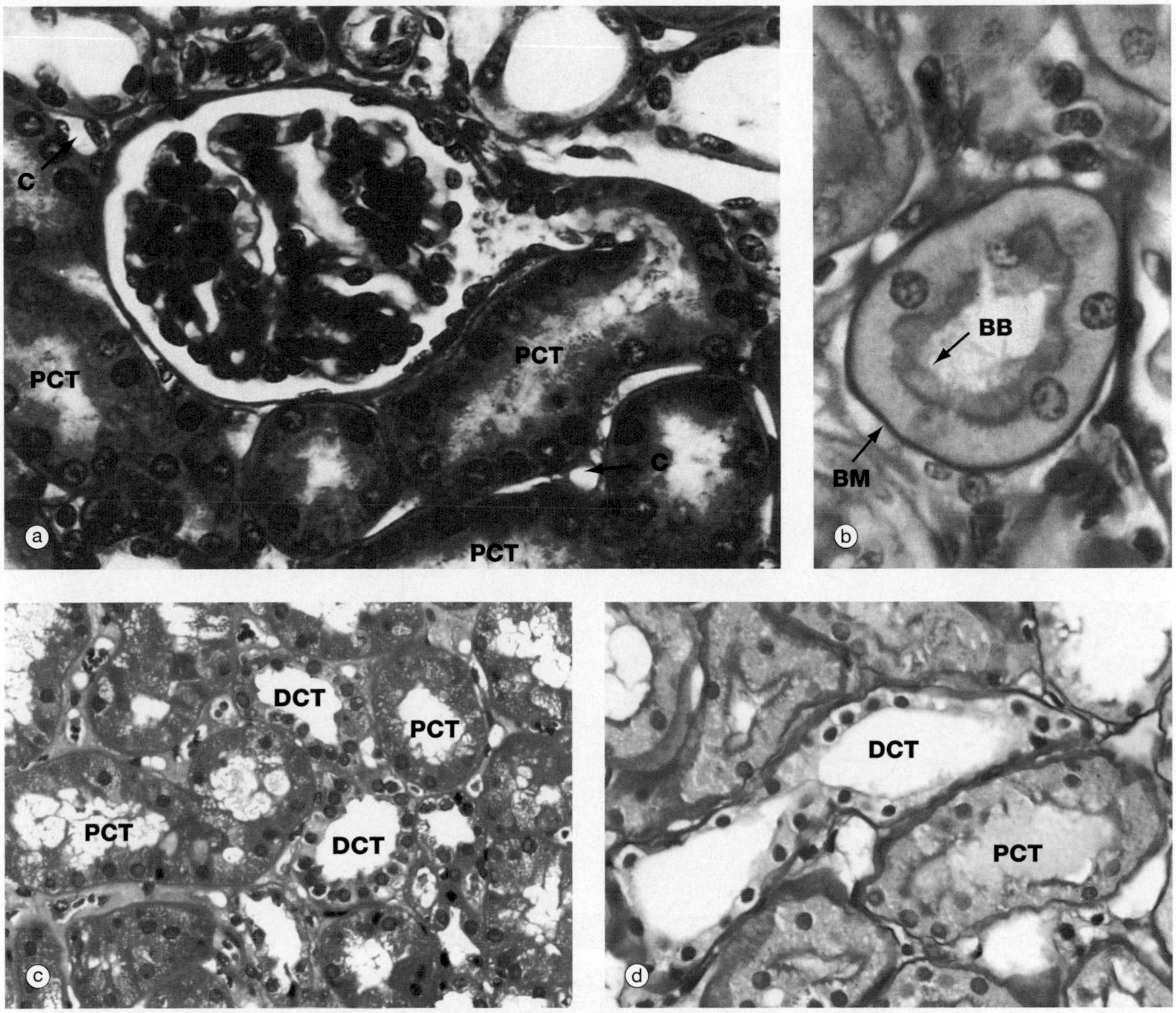

FIG. 16.16 Proximal and distal convoluted tubules
(a) PCT, Azan (HP) (b) PCT, PAS (HP) (c) DCT, H&E (HP) (d) DCT, PAS (HP)

Figs 16.16a–d compare the appearances of the proximal and distal convoluted tubules. The intervening loop of Henle is discussed in Fig. 16.19. The proximal convoluted tubule (PCT) is a coiled tube measuring approximately 14 mm in length and random sections of PCT thus occupy most of the renal cortex. Approximately 65% of the glomerular filtrate is reabsorbed from the PCT, a function reflected in the structure of the epithelial lining.

Fig. 16.16a shows a proximal convoluted tubule **PCT** arising from a renal corpuscle; convolutions of the PCT are also seen in longitudinal, oblique and transverse sections. The simple cuboidal epithelium has a prominent blue-stained brush border of tall microvilli, increasing the surface area of the plasma membrane some 20-fold. The cytoplasm of PCT epithelial cells stains intensely due to a high content of organelles, principally mitochondria. Basement membranes stain blue by this technique, thus highlighting the tubular and glomerular basement membranes and that of Bowman's capsule.

The PAS staining method has been used in Fig. 16.16b to demonstrate the prominent brush border **BB** projecting into the lumen of the PCT. The brush border is PAS-positive, since the surfaces of the microvilli are coated with a prominent glycocalyx (see Fig. 1.2). Like those elsewhere, the basement membrane **BM** supporting the tubular epithelium is strongly PAS-positive. In both micrographs, note that the epithelial cells of the PCT have round nuclei with prominent nucleoli.

A rich network of peritubular capillaries **C** arising from the efferent arteriole of the glomerulus (see Fig. 16.11) surrounds the proximal tubules and returns molecules reabsorbed from the glomerular filtrate back into the general circulation.

The distal tubule is a continuation of the thick ascending limb of the loop of Henle after its return to the cortex and forms the third segment of the renal tubule. Distal tubules are thus found within the cortex among the proximal convoluted tubules. The first part of the distal tubule forms the ***macula densa*** (see Fig. 16.18) while the remainder makes up the distal convoluted tubule (DCT). In the DCT, sodium ions are reabsorbed from the tubular fluid, with one hydrogen or potassium ion being secreted in exchange. This adjustment of acid–base balance is controlled by the hormone ***aldosterone*** secreted by the adrenal cortex (see Fig. 16.18).

As seen in Fig. 16.16c, distal convoluted tubules **DCT** may be differentiated from proximal convoluted tubules **PCT** by the absence of a brush border, a larger more clearly defined lumen, more nuclei per cross-section (since DCT cells are smaller than PCT cells) and paler cytoplasm (due to fewer organelles). In addition, sections of DCT are less numerous than sections of PCT, since the DCT is much shorter than the PCT. In Fig. 16.16d the prominent brush border of the proximal convoluted tubule **PCT** is contrasted with the lack of brush border in the distal convoluted tubule **DCT**.

BB brush border **BM** basement membrane **C** peritubular capillaries **CP** mesangial cell cytoplasmic process
DCT distal convoluted tubule **E** endothelial cell **J** cell junction **L** glomerular capillary lumen **PCT** proximal convoluted tubule
MC mesangial cell **MM** mesangial matrix **P_1** podocyte primary process **P_2** podocyte secondary foot process
SPS subpodocyte space

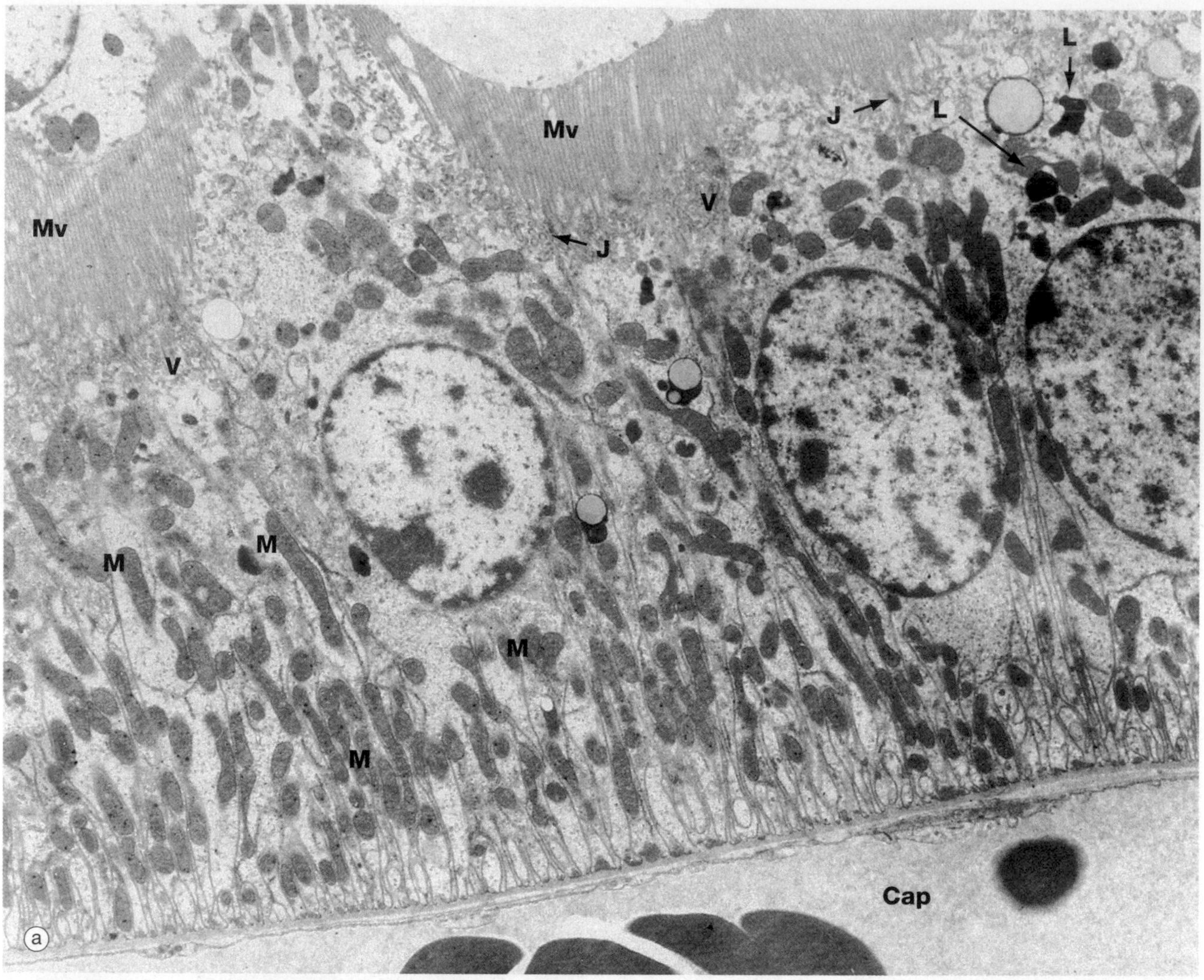

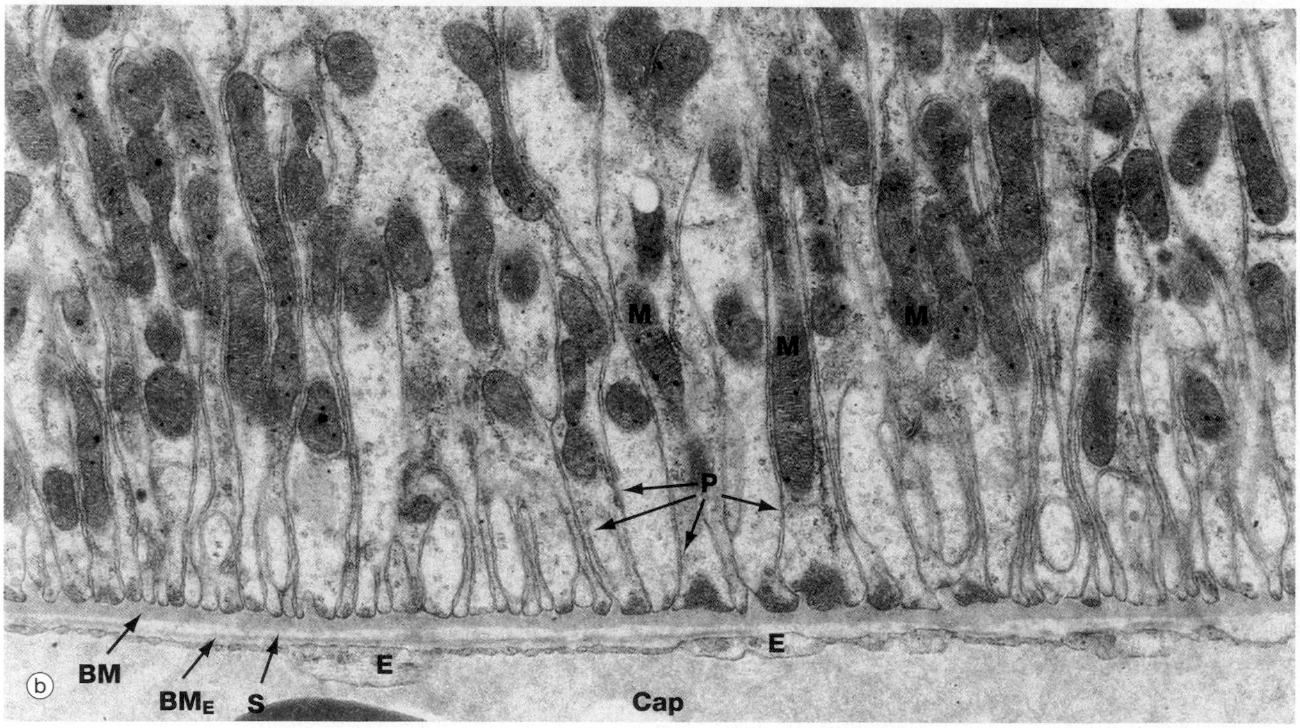

FIG. 16.17 Proximal and distal convoluted tubules *(caption and illustration (c) opposite)*
(a) PCT, EM ×10 000 (b) PCT, EM ×19 000 (c) DCT, EM ×5000

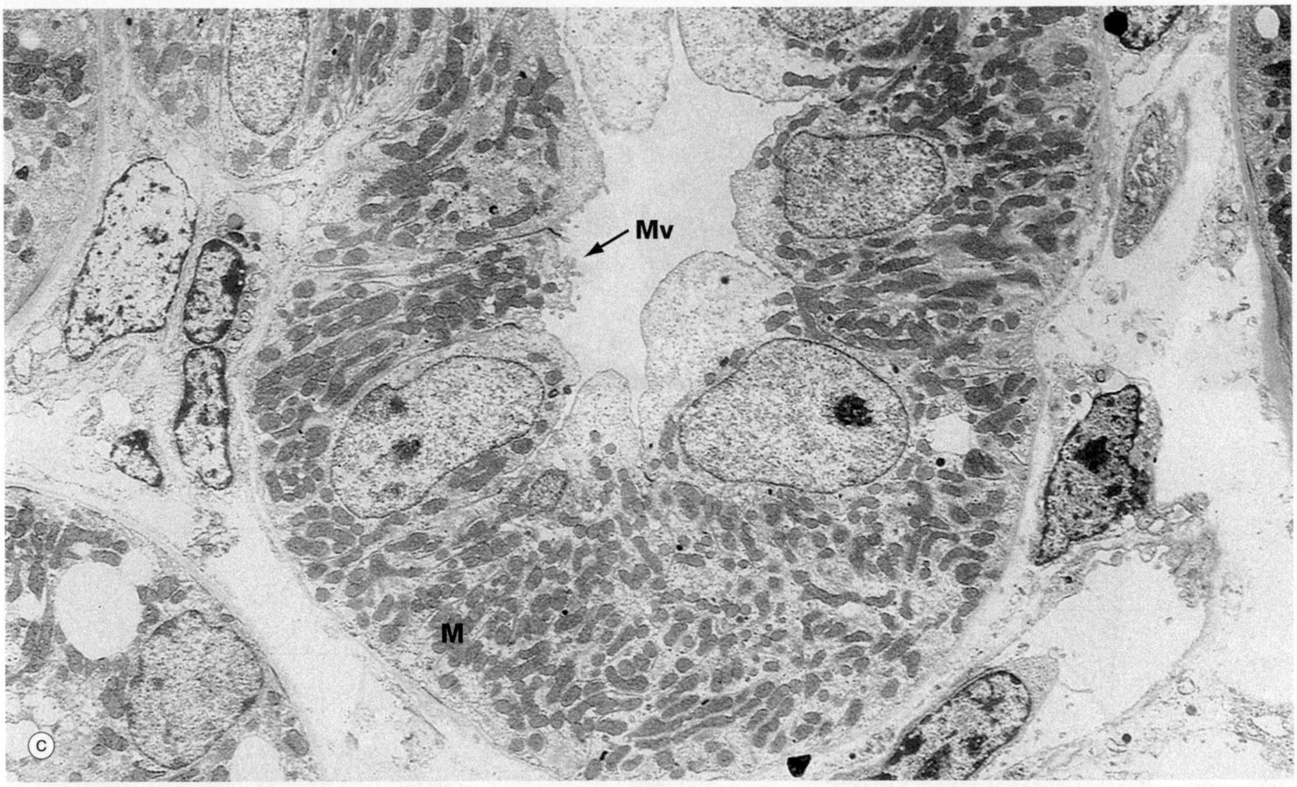

FIG. 16.17 Proximal and distal convoluted tubules *(illustrations (a) and (b) opposite)* (a) PCT, EM ×10 000 (b) PCT, EM ×19 000 (c) DCT, EM ×5000

These electron micrographs compare the ultrastructure of the proximal and distal convoluted tubules. Fig. 16.17a of the proximal tubule reveals profuse tall microvilli **Mv** constituting the brush border seen with light microscopy. The cytoplasm immediately beneath the brush border contains many pinocytotic vesicles **V** (that are just visible at this magnification) and lysosomes **L**, both of which are involved in reabsorption and degradation of small amounts of protein that have leaked through the glomerular filter. Reabsorbed solutes are transported into surrounding peritubular capillaries **Cap**, with attenuated endothelium **E** resting on a very thin basement membrane $\mathbf{BM_E}$; note the narrow intervening supporting tissue layer **S** in Fig. 16.17b.

The epithelial cells of the PCT form multiple lateral processes **P** (Fig. 16.17b) which interdigitate with each other to form a complex ***lateral intercellular space***, with a plasma membrane area equivalent to the luminal plasma membrane. The lateral intercellular space is separated from the lumen of the PCT by a ring of junctional complexes **J** near the luminal surface. The mitochondria **M** in these processes are elongated and arranged at right angles to the basement membrane **BM**. These mitochondria supply ATP for the active transport of Na^+ by the Na^+–K^+ ATPase (sodium pump) located in the basolateral plasma membrane. Thus active transport of Na^+ occurs across the plasma membrane into the lateral intercellular space. This active transport of Na^+ out of the cell is accompanied by facilitated transport into the cells of Na^+, glucose and amino acids by means of transport proteins found in the membrane of the brush border. Almost 100% of the filtered glucose and amino acids is reabsorbed by the PCT.

The distal convoluted tubule (Fig. 16.17c) has many ultrastructural features in common with the proximal convoluted tubule, in particular the lateral cell interdigitations and large numbers of mitochondria **M**. The basolateral plasma membrane contains the Na^+–K^+ ATPase which drives active transport of sodium ions. The most striking difference is that the DCT lacks a brush border, having only a few irregular microvilli **Mv** at the luminal surface. The DCT cells have less cytoplasm than those of the PCT, although the nucleus is of about the same size and consequently occupies much more of the cell. The nuclei of the DCT cells lie close to the luminal surface and tend to bulge into the lumen; the overlying cytoplasm is devoid of mitochondria but contains large numbers of tiny pinocytotic vesicles (not seen at this magnification).

Renal tubular damage

Damage to the renal tubules is a fairly common cause of acute renal failure. ***Acute tubular necrosis*** usually occurs due to a sudden drop in the blood supply to the kidney, for example due to severe dehydration or massive blood loss. The cells of the renal tubules are highly metabolically active and so they are very susceptible to damage when the blood supply is compromised. As noted above, this is particularly so for the cells of the proximal convoluted tubule as they have a very high oxygen requirement.

The tubular epithelial cells will often recover if the underlying cause is treated and the patient is supported effectively during the acute phase of their illness. Often, during the recovery phase, the patient will produce very large volumes of dilute urine (***polyuria***), highlighting the key role of the tubular epithelial cells in reabsorbing water from the glomerular ultrafiltrate (see e-Fig. 16.4). Careful management of fluid balance is critical during recovery.

BM basement membrane $\mathbf{BM_E}$ basement membrane of endothelium **Cap** capillary **E** endothelium **J** junctional complex **L** lysosome **M** mitochondrion **Mv** microvilli **P** cell process **S** supporting tissue **V** pinocytotic vesicle

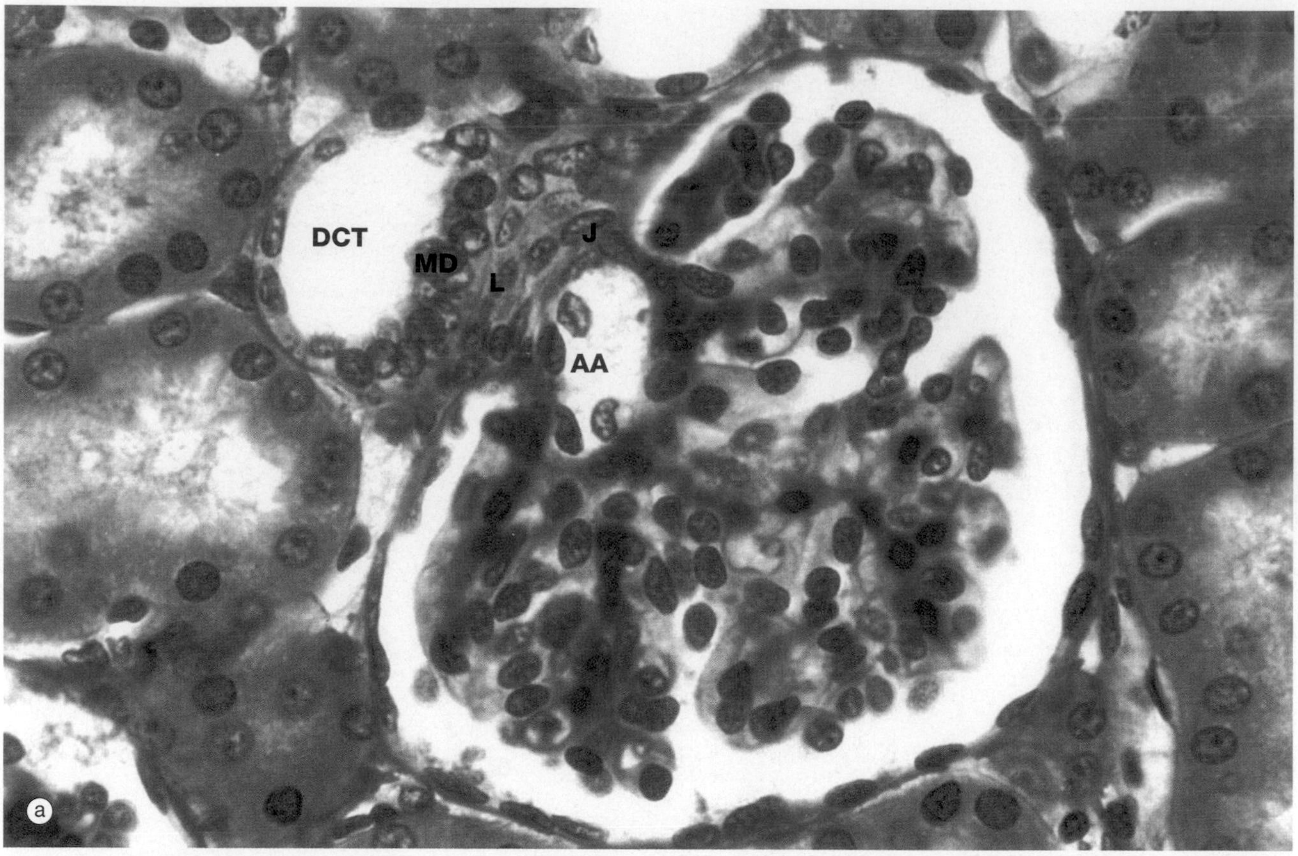

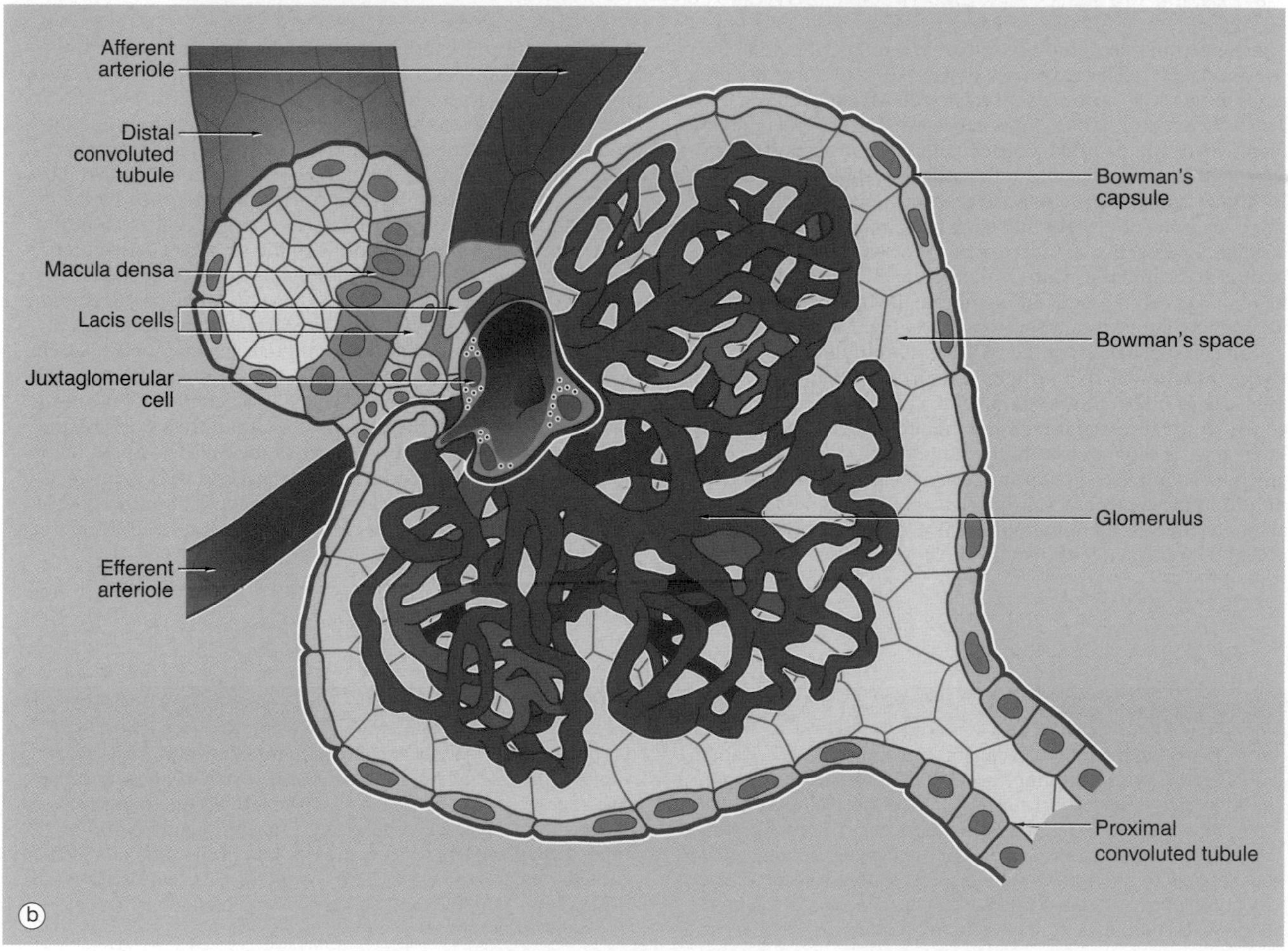

FIG. 16.18 Juxtaglomerular apparatus *(caption and illustration (c) opposite)*
(a) Azan (HP) (b) Diagram (c) Control of blood pressure

AA afferent arteriole **DCT** distal convoluted tubule **J** juxtaglomerular cell **L** lacis cell **MD** macula densa

FIG. 16.18 Juxtaglomerular apparatus *(illustrations (a) and (b) opposite)*
(a) Azan (HP) (b) Diagram (c) Control of blood pressure

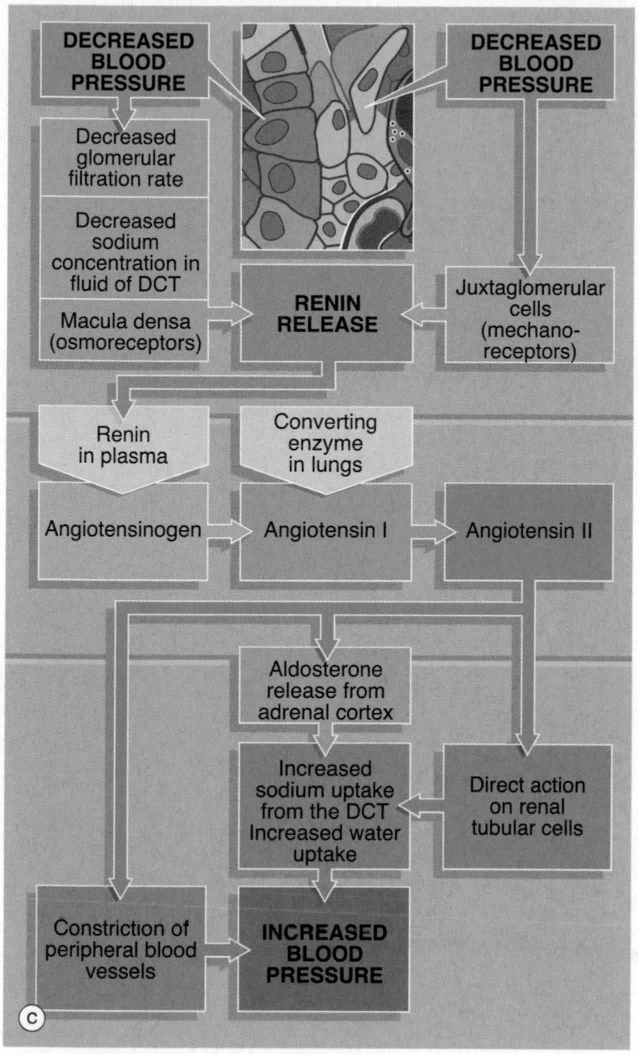

The *juxtaglomerular apparatus* (*JGA*) is a specialisation of the glomerular afferent arteriole **AA** and the distal convoluted tubule **DCT** of the same nephron and is involved in the regulation of systemic blood pressure via the *renin–angiotensin–aldosterone system* (*RAAS*). The juxtaglomerular apparatus is made up of three components: the *macula densa* of the DCT, renin-secreting *juxtaglomerular cells* of the afferent arteriole and *extraglomerular mesangial cells*.

- **Macula densa**. On returning to the cortex from the renal medulla, the ascending thick limb of the loop of Henle becomes the first part of the distal tubule and comes to lie in the angle between the afferent and efferent arterioles at the vascular pole of the glomerulus. The macula densa **MD** is an area of closely packed, specialised DCT epithelial cells where the DCT abuts the vascular pole of the glomerulus.

  Compared with other DCT lining cells, the cells of the macula densa are taller and have larger, more prominent nuclei situated towards the luminal surface. Mitochondria are scattered throughout the cytoplasm and Na^+ pump activity is absent. The basement membrane between the macula and underlying cells is extremely thin. The cells of the macula densa are sensitive to the concentration of sodium ions in the fluid within the DCT; a decrease in systemic blood pressure results in decreased production of glomerular filtrate and hence decreased concentration of sodium ions in the distal tubular fluid.
- **Juxtaglomerular cells**. Juxtaglomerular cells **J** are modified smooth muscle cells of the wall of the afferent arteriole, forming a cluster around it just before it enters the glomerulus. Juxtaglomerular cell cytoplasm contains immature and mature membrane-bound granules of the enzyme *renin*.
- **Extraglomerular mesangial cells**. Also called *Goormaghtigh cells* or *lacis cells* **L**, these cells form a conical mass, the apex of which is continuous with the mesangium of the glomerulus; laterally it is bounded by the afferent and efferent arterioles and its base abuts the macula densa. The lacis cells are flat and elongated, with extensive fine cytoplasmic processes extending from their ends and surrounded by a network ('lacis') of mesangial material. These cells participate in the *tubuloglomerular feedback mechanism* by which changes in Na^+ concentration at the macula densa give rise to signals that directly control glomerular blood flow. The extraglomerular mesangial cells are thought to be responsible for transmission of a signal arising in the macula densa to the intraglomerular mesangial cells, which then contract or relax to make the capillary loops narrower or wider.

Role of the JGA in the control of blood pressure

The juxtaglomerular apparatus is believed to act as both a *baroreceptor* and a *chemoreceptor*, controlling systemic blood pressure by the secretion of renin by the juxtaglomerular cells. The juxtaglomerular cells are suitably placed to monitor systemic blood pressure, with a fall in blood pressure resulting in renin secretion. Reduction in blood pressure results in reduced glomerular filtration and consequently a lower concentration of sodium ions in the DCT.

Acting as chemoreceptors, the cells of the macula densa in some way then promote renin secretion. Renin diffuses into the bloodstream, catalysing the conversion of *angiotensinogen*, an α_2-globulin synthesised by the liver, into the decapeptide *angiotensin I*. In the lungs, *angiotensin converting enzyme* (*ACE*) cleaves two amino acids from angiotensin I to form *angiotensin II*, which is a potent vasoconstrictor.

Angiotensin II raises blood pressure in three ways: constriction of peripheral blood vessels, release of aldosterone from the adrenal cortex and via a direct effect on the renal tubules, where it promotes the reabsorption of sodium ions (and therefore water) from the DCT, thus expanding the plasma volume and increasing blood pressure. As mentioned above, the tubuloglomerular feedback mechanism is also thought to operate at a local level to control glomerular blood flow and therefore indirectly influencing systemic blood pressure.

Hypertension and the kidney

Hypertension is a common condition in middle-aged and elderly persons. Most cases are considered to be idiopathic (which simply means that the mechanism has not yet been elucidated). However, there are certainly genetic factors as well as lifestyle components underlying many, if not most, cases. A much smaller proportion of hypertensive patients, especially younger patients, have hypertension associated with renal disease. Many different types of renal disease may lead to hypertension; a classic example is the acute hypertension seen in patients with post-infectious glomerulonephritis. Many other chronic renal conditions, including diabetic nephropathy, IgA nephropathy and a range of other common conditions lead to secondary hypertension.

Conversely, hypertension can also lead to renal failure. The classic example of this is patients with ***accelerated hypertension*** (see e-Fig. 16.5) who have acute renal failure with classic vascular changes in their renal biopsy at presentation. However, chronic untreated lower-level hypertension also typically leads to chronic renal damage in a pattern sometimes called 'benign nephrosclerosis', a misleading name as it can lead to chronic renal failure which may require renal replacement therapy.

THE RENAL MEDULLA

The renal medulla consists of closely packed tubules of two types: the loop of Henle and the collecting tubules and ducts, as well as the vasa recta. The loop of Henle is a continuation of the proximal convoluted tubule. It dips down into the medulla, where it loops back on itself and returns to the cortex to its own renal corpuscle, becoming the first part of the distal convoluted tubule.

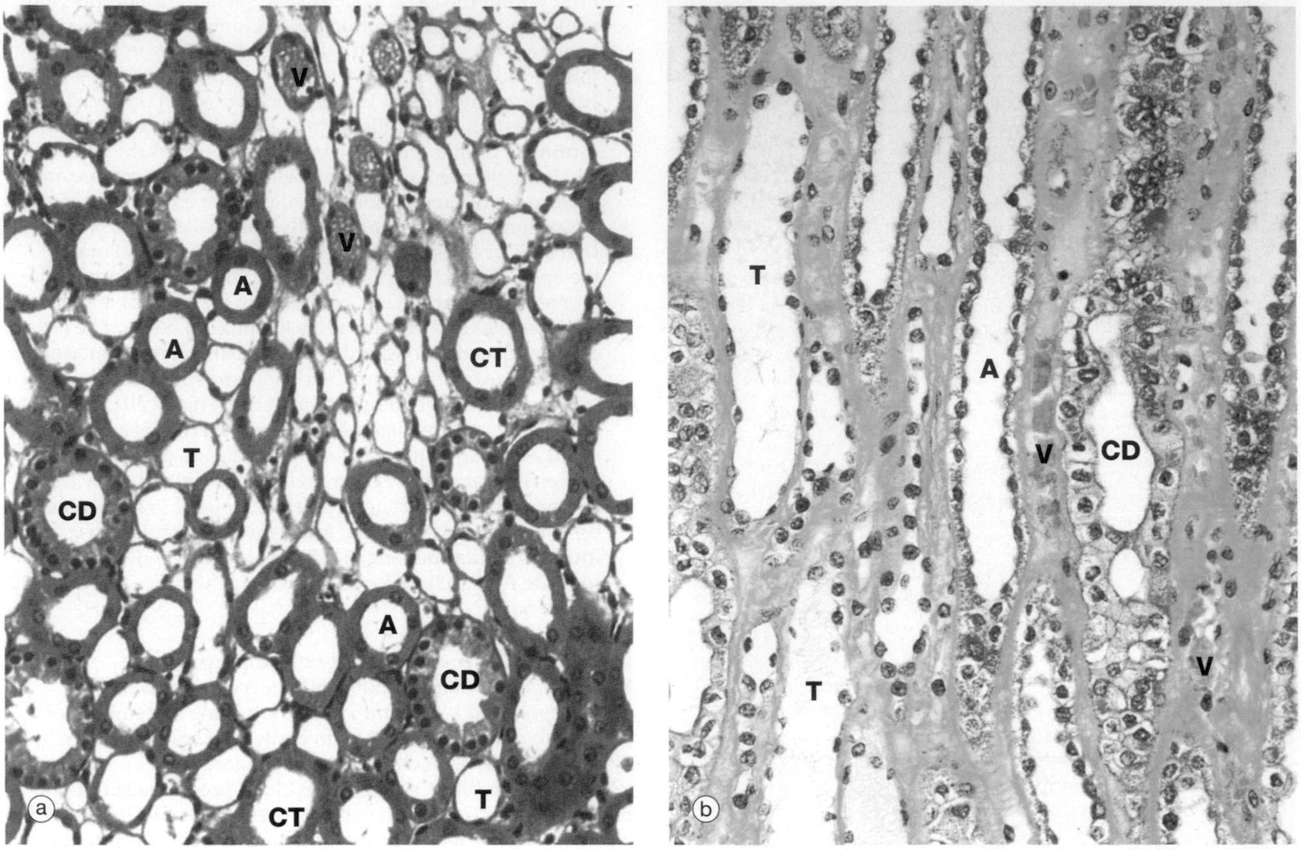

FIG. 16.19 Loop of Henle
(a) H&E, TS (HP) (b) EMSB, LS (HP)

The loop of Henle is made up of four parts:

- ***Thick descending limb (pars recta of the PCT)***
- ***Thin descending limb***
- ***Thin ascending limb***
- ***Thick ascending limb (pars recta of the DCT)***

The thick descending limb is the second, straight part of the proximal tubule that extends down into the outer medulla.

There is an abrupt transition to the thin descending limb, which loops down into the medulla for a variable distance. The thin limbs of juxtamedullary nephrons extend down to the inner medulla before turning back on themselves, while those in the outer cortex only extend a short way into the medulla. After the hairpin bend, the tubule becomes the thin ascending limb for a short distance before abruptly changing into the thick ascending limb. Thus the thin descending limb is longer than the thin ascending limb.

The thin limbs **T** have a simple squamous epithelium and may be differentiated from the vasa recta **V** by the absence of erythrocytes and their regular rounded shape in transverse section (Fig. 16.19a). Erythrocytes, stained orange by this staining method, are easily seen in the vasa recta in Fig. 16.19b. The thick ascending limbs **A** are lined by low cuboidal epithelium and are also round in cross-section. Neither thick nor thin limbs of the loop of Henle have a brush border. Collecting tubules **CT** have a similar epithelial lining to the ascending limbs but are wider and less regular in shape.

The collecting ducts **CD** are easily recognised by their large diameter and pale stained columnar epithelial lining.

The function of the loop of Henle is to produce an increasing osmotic gradient from the cortex to the tip of the renal papilla by the ***counter-current multiplier mechanism*** (see Fig. 16.26). In brief, the parts of the loop of Henle with a thick (cuboidal) epithelium participate in active transport of various ions and molecules out of the lumen and into the interstitium. On the other hand, the thin limbs are lined by a flattened squamous epithelium with little capacity for active transport. The thin descending limb allows free diffusion of H_2O but is fairly impermeable to NaCl, while the thin ascending limb is permeable to NaCl but not to H_2O. The vasa recta take up water from the medullary interstitium and return it to the general circulation.

As the urine flows into the thick ascending limb, active transport of NaCl again occurs, and this correlates with the appearances of the epithelium. Here the cuboidal epithelium exhibits basolateral processes that interdigitate with each other, forming an extensive basolateral intercellular space in a similar manner to the PCT. This active transport process is fuelled by ATP produced by the many mitochondria found in these processes. The thick ascending limb is also impermeable to water. ***Tamm–Horsfall protein*** is a unique glycoprotein produced only by the epithelium of the thick ascending limb. Tamm–Horsfall protein has protective functions, including binding to certain types of *Escherichia coli* to prevent the bacteria adhering to the renal tubular epithelium and prevention of the formation of renal calculi.

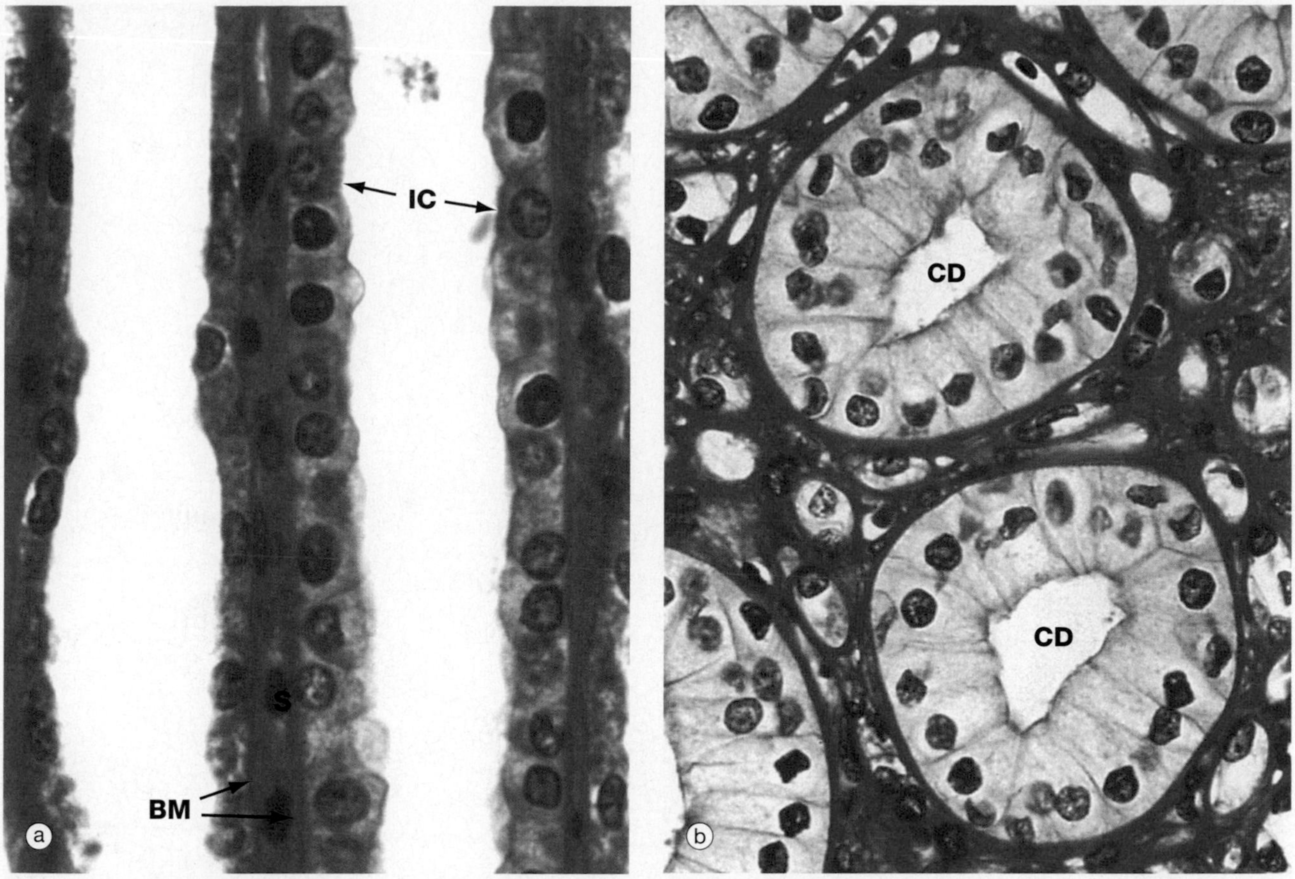

FIG. 16.20 Collecting tubules and ducts
(a) Azan, LS (HP) (b) Azan, TS (HP)

The ***collecting segment*** or ***connecting tubule*** joins the distal convoluted tubule to the collecting duct. Several collecting tubules merge to form each ***collecting duct***. The collecting tubules and ducts descend in the medullary rays (see Fig. 16.5) towards the renal medulla where they progressively merge to form the large ***ducts of Bellini*** which drain urine from the tip of the renal papilla into the pelvicalyceal system.

The collecting tubules and ducts concentrate urine by passive reabsorption of water into the medullary interstitium following the osmotic gradient created by the counter-current multiplier system of the loops of Henle (see Fig. 16.26). The vasa recta return this water to the general circulation. The amount of water reabsorbed is controlled by ***antidiuretic hormone*** (***ADH***, ***vasopressin***) secreted by the posterior pituitary in response to dehydration. ADH acts by increasing the permeability to water of the collecting tubule and ducts, resulting in retention of water by the body and the production of hypertonic urine. Conversely, ADH secretion is inhibited by water overload and an increased volume of hypotonic urine is thus produced. The collecting tubules and ducts are also the final site of H^+, K^+, Na^+ and HCO^- secretion and/or reabsorption to achieve homeostasis; these functions are modified and controlled by the RAAS and local paracrine factors such as kallikrein.

The simple low columnar epithelium of the collecting ducts consists of two cell types, ***principal cells*** and ***intercalated cells***. Principal cells have pale cytoplasm with scanty organelles and short microvilli. These cells have prominent infoldings of the basolateral plasma membrane but no lateral interdigitations. Principal cells actively reabsorb Na^+ and secrete K^+, as well as reabsorbing water. Intercalated cells have darker cytoplasm due to the content of multiple mitochondria, polyribosomes and membrane-bound vesicles. These cells secrete H^+ and reabsorb bicarbonate and are thus important in acid–base homeostasis. The number of intercalated cells varies between different parts of the collecting duct and they are virtually absent in the inner medullary segment.

The collecting tubules are lined by a mixture of DCT cells, collecting tubule cells, principal cells and intercalated cells. Overall, the epithelium is cuboidal and becomes increasingly tall distally until it merges with the columnar epithelium of the collecting duct.

Fig. 16.20a illustrates two collecting tubules in the renal cortex, the tubule on the left being more proximal and the tubule on the right more distal, as shown by the flatter cuboidal lining of the former. The majority of the lining cells are relatively poorly stained. The different cell types cannot be differentiated by light microscopy, except for a small number of dark intercalated cells **IC** with surface microvilli. Note the blue-stained tubular basement membranes **BM** and narrow intervening supporting tissue **S**, mainly occupied by capillaries.

Fig. 16.20b is from the renal medulla and illustrates two collecting ducts **CD** surrounded by loops of Henle and vasa recta that cannot be readily distinguished from one another. In the medullary portion of the collecting ducts, principal cells are predominant and no intercalated cells can be seen in this section.

A thick ascending limb of loop of Henle **BM** tubular basement membrane **CD** collecting duct **CT** collecting tubule
IC intercalated cell **S** supporting tissue **T** thin limb of loop of Henle **V** vasa recta

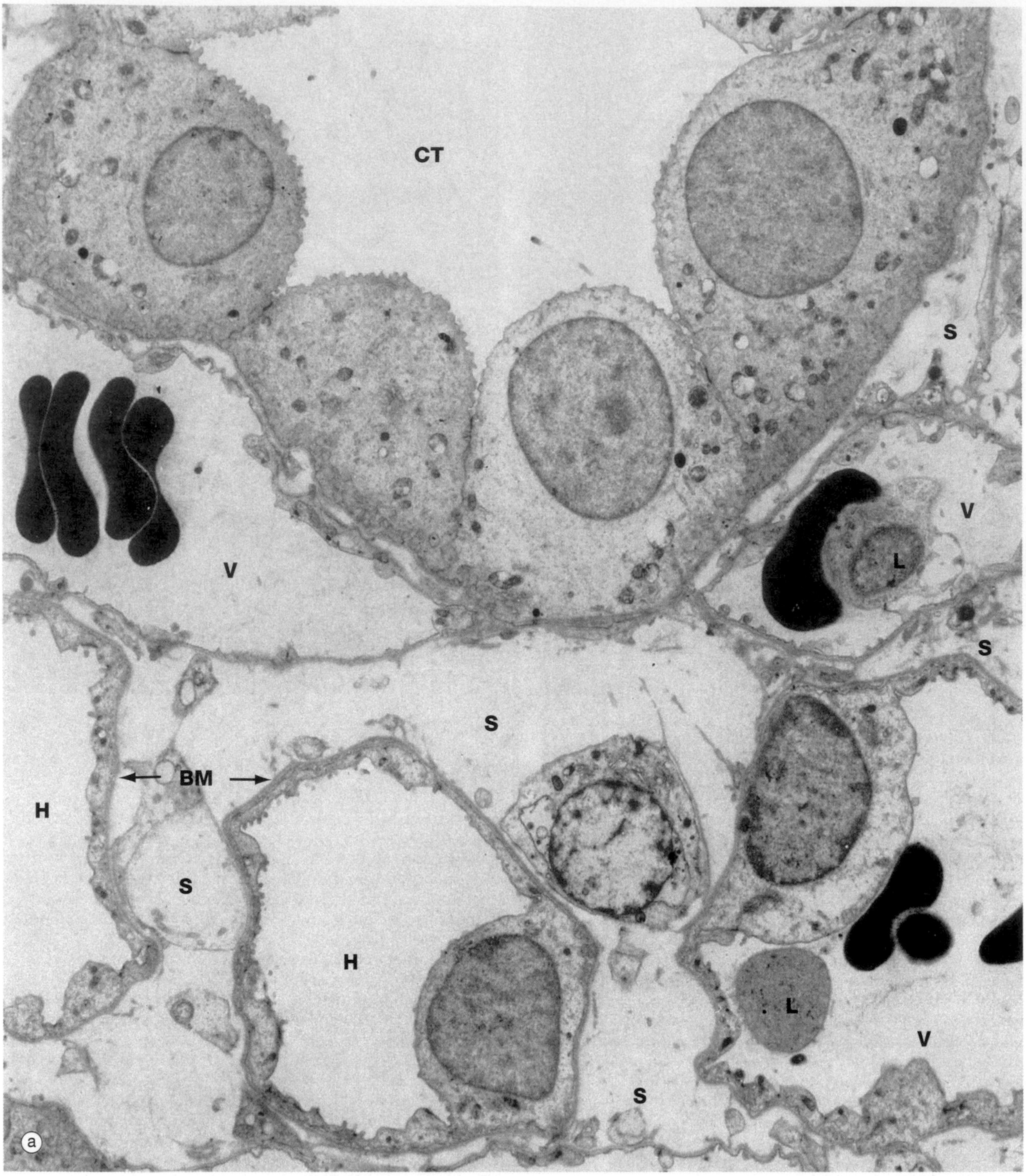

FIG. 16.21 Renal medulla, rat *(illustration (b) opposite)*
(a) EM ×4000 (b) EM ×8000

Fig. 16.21a, a transverse section of the outer medulla, illustrates the ultrastructural features of a collecting tubule **CT**, thin loops of Henle **H** and vasa recta **V**. Lying between the vasa recta and nephrons is the delicate interstitial supporting tissue **S** containing a little collagen along with ***renal interstitial medullary cells*** (***RIMC***).

The collecting tubule in this section is lined mainly by principal cells whose basal mitochondria, associated with infoldings of the plasma membrane, can just be identified at this power and are seen clearly in Fig. 16.21b in the collecting tubule **CT** in the right upper corner. The cells of the thin limbs of loops of Henle are similar to capillary endothelial cells in structure, most of the wall consisting of a thin irregular layer of cytoplasm with a few very short luminal microvilli and the nucleus bulging into the lumen. The epithelium is supported by a thin basement membrane **BM**. The vasa recta can only be readily distinguished from the thin limbs by their content of erythrocytes, occasional leukocytes **L** and precipitated plasma proteins.

The interstitium of the inner medulla in some species, including humans, contains unusual cells called renal interstitial medullary cells. These are illustrated in Fig. 16.21b, a longitudinal section of the medulla, where the cell bodies of two such cells are identifiable by their nuclei **N**. These cells have plentiful lipid droplets **D** within the cytoplasm and long cytoplasmic processes **P** that form a network throughout the loose supporting tissue containing collagen fibrils **C** that fills the intervening space. Interestingly, there are also fragments of redundant basal lamina **BL** in the supporting tissue, implying that these RIMC may change their position over time. These cells are often arranged at right angles to the collecting tubules **CT** and vasa recta **V**. The function of these cells is not yet clear, but they may be involved in the production of prostaglandins and/or hormones that regulate blood pressure.

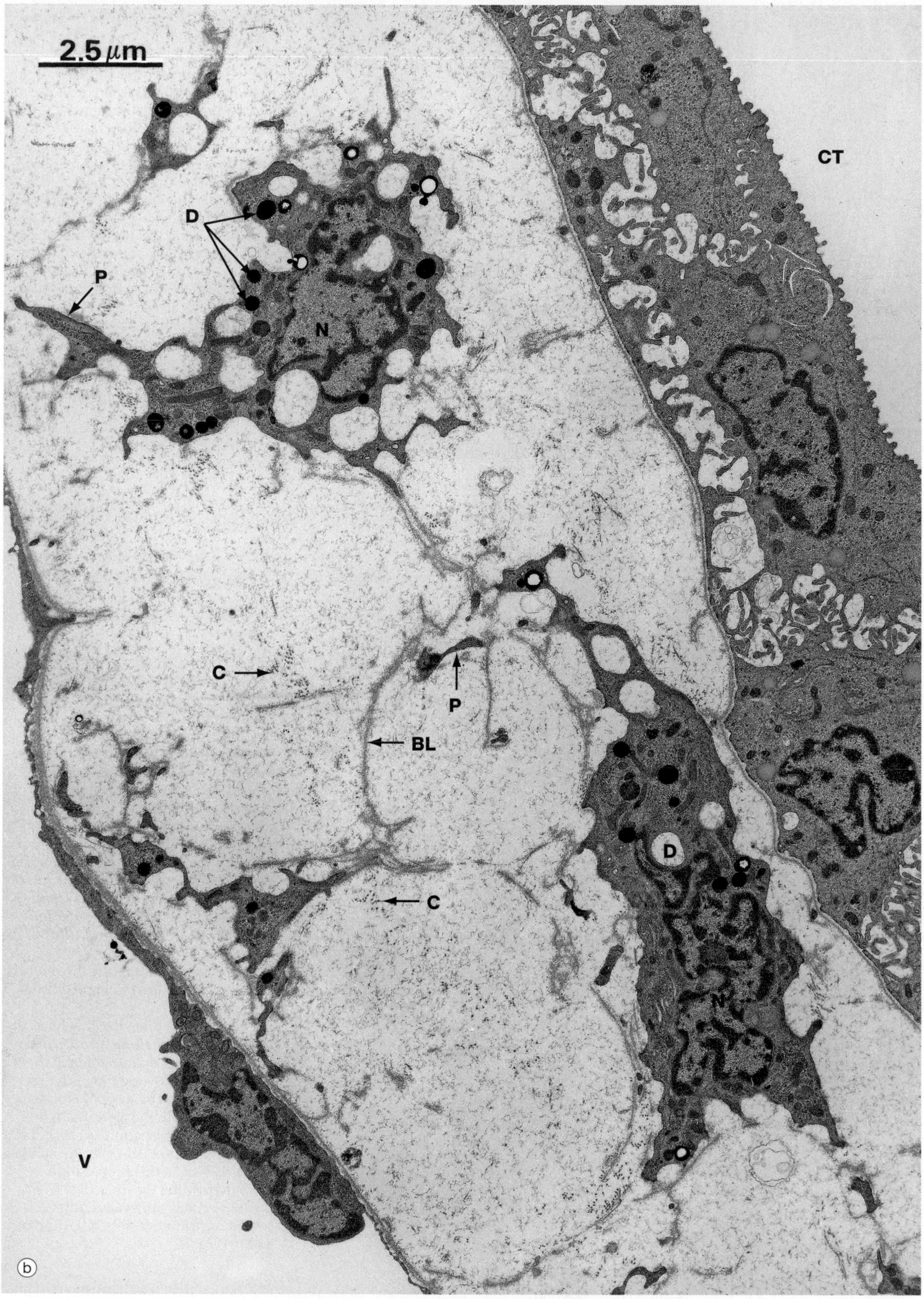

FIG. 16.21 Renal medulla, rat *(caption and illustration (a) opposite)*
(a) EM ×4000 (b) EM ×8000

BL basal lamina **BM** basement membrane **C** collagen fibrils **CT** collecting tubule **D** lipid droplet **H** loop of Henle **L** leukocyte **N** nucleus of interstitial medullary cell **P** cytoplasmic process of interstitial medullary cell **S** supporting tissue **V** vasa recta

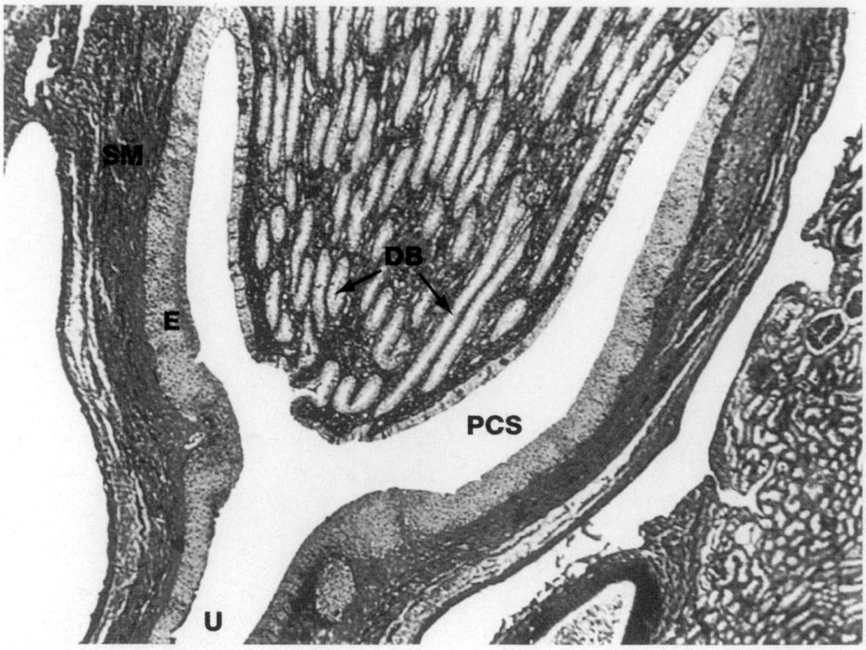

FIG. 16.22 Renal papilla, monkey Azan (LP)

The renal papilla forms the apex of the medullary pyramid, where it projects into the pelvicalyceal system **PCS**. Ducts of Bellini **DB**, the largest of the collecting ducts, converge to drain urine through a number of holes (***cribriform area***) at the tip of the papilla.

Between the ducts are the longest loops of Henle and vasa recta (not visible at this magnification). This papilla is a simple papilla, but at the poles of the human kidney, the papillae are often fused to form complex papillae.

The pelvicalyceal system represents the proximal end of the ureter **U** and, as such, is lined by typical urinary (transitional) epithelium **E**. The wall of the pelvis contains smooth muscle **SM**, continuous with that of the ureter.

THE LOWER URINARY TRACT

The lower urinary tract includes the renal pelvis and calyces, the ureters, the urinary bladder and the urethra. The lower urinary tract is specialised for the storage and excretion of urine at a convenient time; no further modification of the urine is possible after it leaves the renal medulla.

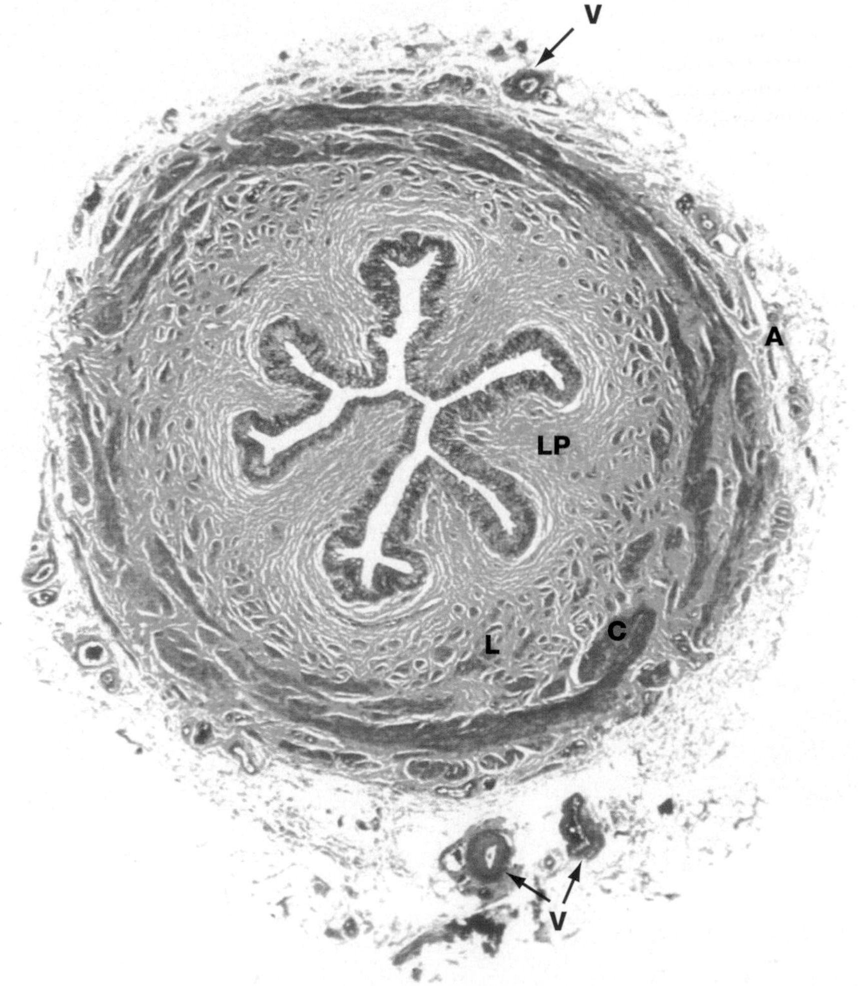

FIG. 16.23 Ureter Masson trichrome (LP)

The ureters are muscular tubes that carry urine from the kidneys to the bladder. Urine is transported from the pelvicalyceal system as a bolus, propelled by peristaltic action of the ureteric wall. The wall of the ureter contains two layers of smooth muscle, arranged as an inner elongated spiral but traditionally known as the ***longitudinal layer*** **L** and an outer tight spiral traditionally described as the ***circular layer*** **C**. Another ***outer longitudinal layer*** is present in the lower third of the ureter.

However, in reality the three layers are often difficult to distinguish from each other.

The lumen of the ureter is lined by ***transitional epithelium*** (***urothelium***) which is thrown up into folds in the relaxed state, allowing the ureter to dilate during the passage of a bolus of urine. Beneath the epithelium is a broad collagenous lamina propria **LP**, the collagen fibres of which are stained greenish-blue in this preparation.

Surrounding the muscular wall is a loose collagenous adventitia **A** containing blood vessels **V**, lymphatics and nerves.

A adventitia **C** circular muscle layer **DB** duct of Bellini **E** transitional epithelium **IL** inner longitudinal muscle layer of bladder **L** longitudinal muscle layer of ureter **LP** lamina propria **OL** outer longitudinal muscle layer of bladder **PCS** pelvicalyceal space **SM** smooth muscle **U** ureter **Um** umbrella cell **V** blood vessel

FIG. 16.24 Bladder
Masson trichrome (LP)

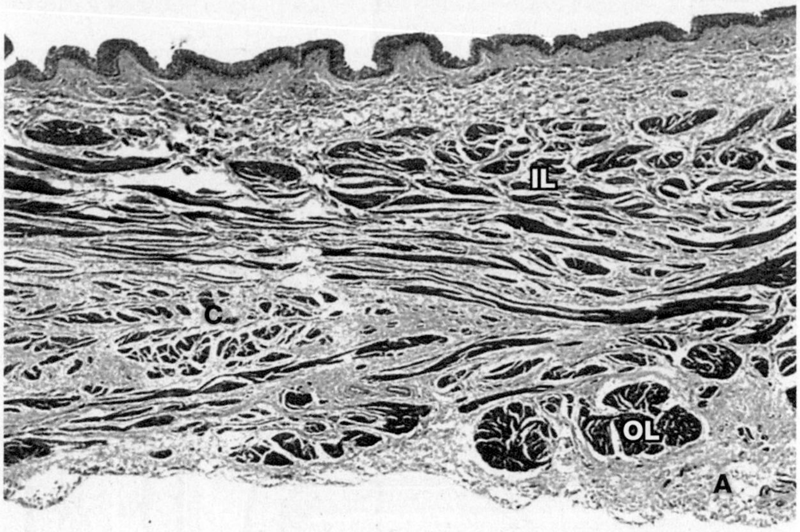

The urinary bladder serves as a urine store in which urine can be held until a convenient time and place for its excretion (***micturition***). The general structure of the bladder wall resembles that of the lower third of the ureters. The wall of the bladder consists of three loosely arranged layers of smooth muscle and elastic fibres that contract during micturition. Note the ***inner longitudinal*** **IL**, ***outer circular*** **C** and ***outermost longitudinal*** **OL** layers of smooth muscle; together the three layers are called the ***detrusor muscle***. As in the ureter, the layers are often difficult to distinguish. The transitional epithelium lining the bladder is thrown into many folds in the relaxed state. A delicate, often incomplete muscularis mucosae (not identifiable at this magnification) separates the lamina propria from the submucosa in some but not all individuals.

The outer adventitial coat **A** contains arteries, veins and lymphatics.

The urethra, the final conducting portion of the urinary tract, is discussed as part of the male reproductive tract in Ch. 18.

FIG. 16.25 Transitional epithelium
H&E (HP)

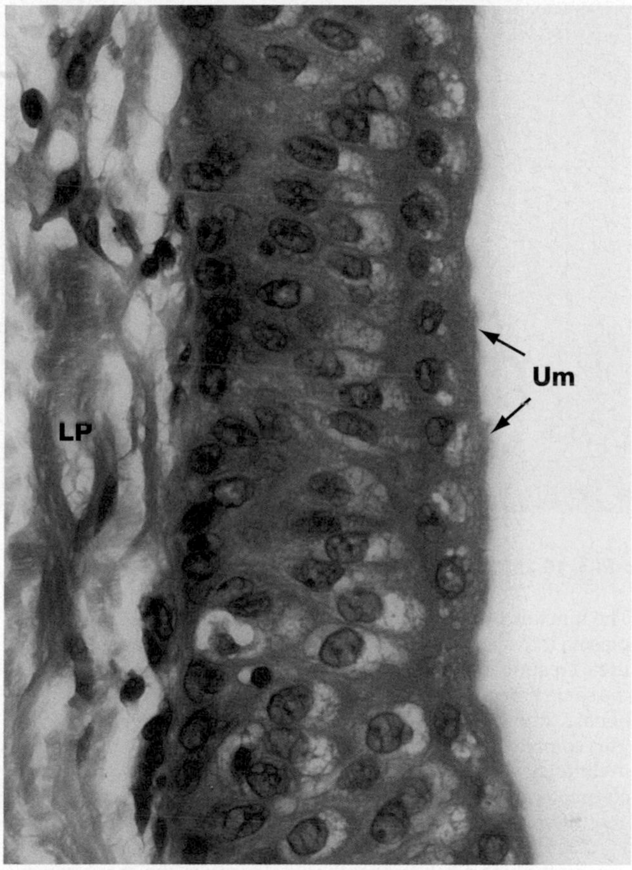

Transitional epithelium, also called ***urothelium***, is found only within the conducting passages of the urinary system, for which it is especially adapted. The epithelium is stratified, comprising three to six layers of cells, the number of layers being greatest when the epithelium is least distended at the time of fixation.

The cells of the basal layer are compact and cuboidal in form, while those of the intermediate layers are more columnar, with their nuclei orientated at right angles to the basement membrane. The surface cells are called ***umbrella*** **Um** or ***dome cells*** and have unique features that allow them to maintain the impermeability of the epithelium to urine, even when at full stretch. This permeability barrier also prevents water from being drawn through the epithelium into hypertonic urine. The umbrella cells are large and ovoid with round nuclei and plentiful eosinophilic cytoplasm; some surface cells are binucleate (not illustrated). The surface outline has a characteristic scalloped appearance and the superficial cytoplasm is fuzzy, indistinct and more intensely stained than the rest of the cytoplasm.

Ultrastructural studies have revealed that much of the surface plasma membrane consists of thickened inflexible ***plaques***, often called ***asymmetrical unit membrane***, interspersed with narrow zones of normal membrane. These normal areas act as 'hinges', allowing sections of the membrane to fold inwards somewhat like a concertina, forming deep clefts and stacks of flattened plasma membrane segments, inappropriately called ***fusiform vesicles***. This structure allows the umbrella cells to expand greatly and quickly when the bladder is distended and the epithelium is at full stretch. Plentiful junctional complexes between the cells maintain the cohesion of adjacent cells. These features of the urothelium allow it to store chemically toxic urine in considerable volumes for quite long periods of time without damage to the tissues.

Urinary epithelium rests on a basement membrane that is often too thin to be resolved by light microscopy. The loose lamina propria **LP** is seen underlying the epithelium.

REVIEW

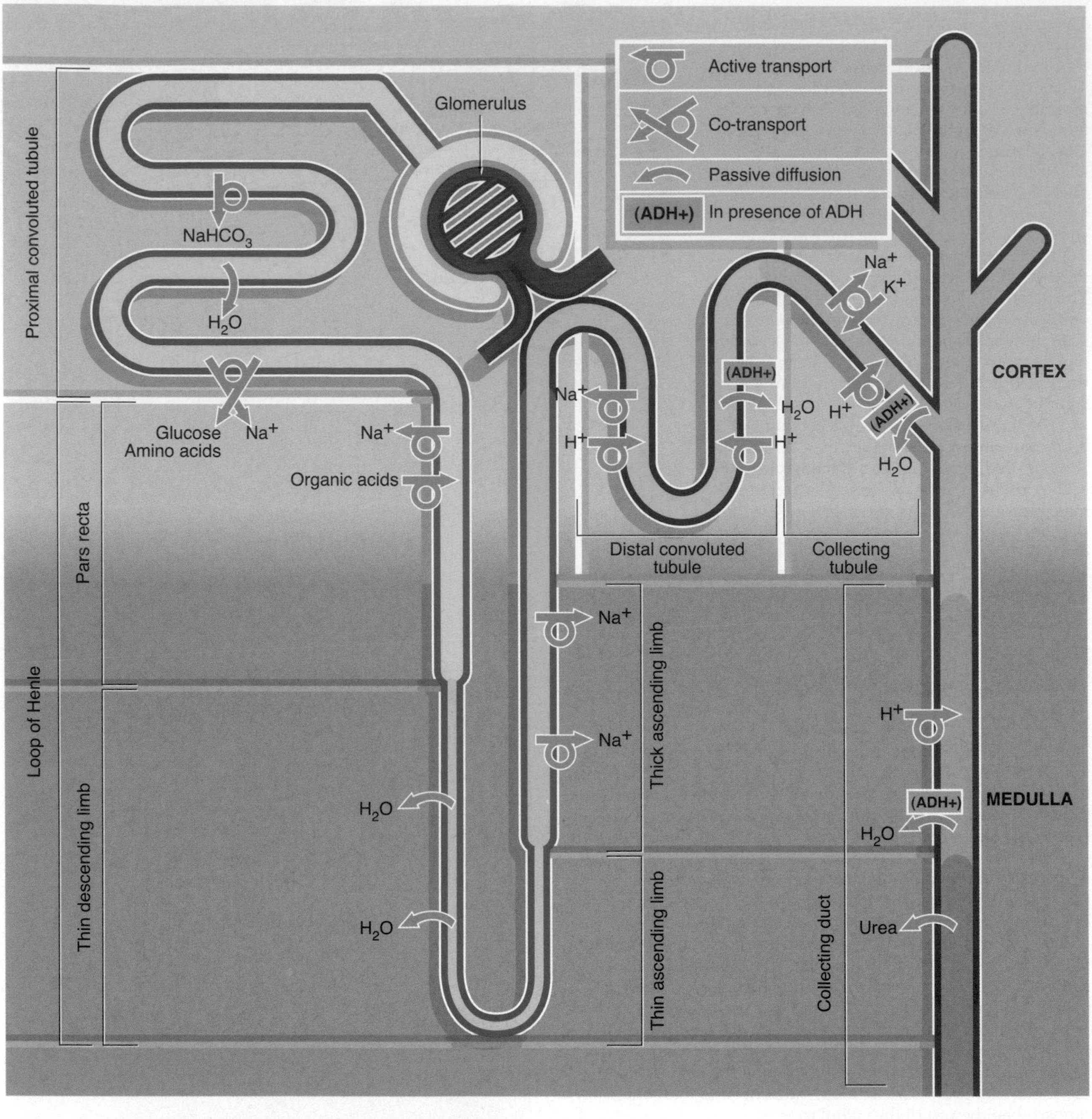

FIG. 16.26 Summary of major activities of different parts of the renal tubule

The function of the renal tubule is to transform an ultrafiltrate of plasma into a concentrated solution of waste products such as urea, creatinine, excess H^+ and K^+ and many other substances. At the same time, the tubule conserves essential water, Na^+, bicarbonate, amino acids, glucose and low molecular weight proteins. This complex procedure is carried out by a variety of mechanisms in different segments of the tubule, including active transport, co-transport, passive diffusion, facilitated diffusion (see Ch. 1) and differential permeability of different parts of the tubule.

The ability of the tubule to produce concentrated urine is dependent on the high osmolarity of the renal medulla, which is created by the unique structure of the loops of Henle and vasa recta dipping down into the medulla. This is known as the ***counter-current multiplier mechanism***. In the presence of ADH, which renders the collecting tubule and duct permeable to water, the high osmolarity of the interstitium of the renal medulla draws water passively out of the tubule and into the medulla where it is carried away by the vasa recta. The counter-current multiplier mechanism is set up by the ability of the thick ascending limb of the loop of Henle to pump large amounts of NaCl into the interstitium against a concentration gradient while remaining impermeable to water. The thin descending limb is permeable to water but not NaCl, and water is reabsorbed into the medulla, resulting in hyperosmolar urine reaching the hairpin bend of the loop. This water, however, is removed by the vasa recta. The hyperosmolarity of the medulla is also partly due to the high concentrations of urea resulting from passive diffusion of urea from the medullary collecting duct into the interstitium along its concentration gradient.

This diagram outlines the major movements of solutes and water into and out of the different parts of the renal tubule. For further detail of these processes the reader is referred to current physiology texts.

REVIEW

TABLE 16.1 Review of the urinary system

Kidney

Part of nephron	Important structural components	Special features	Functional significance	Figures
Glomerulus	Endothelium, glomerular basement membrane and podocytes with foot processes	Glomerular filtration barrier (GFB)	Allow water, ions and small molecules to pass into subpodocyte space while retaining large protein molecules	16.8, 16.10–16.15
Juxta-glomerular apparatus	Macula densa of distal convoluted tubule (DCT)	Specialised cells acting as osmoreceptors of DCT, abutting afferent arteriole (AA)	Sensitive to Na^+ concentration in DCT, indicating reduced BP	16.18
	Juxtaglomerular cells of AA	Modified smooth muscle cells in wall of AA, mechanoreceptors, contain renin	Release renin in response to reduced BP	
	Extraglomerular mesangial cells (lacis cells)	Flattened network of mesangial cells abutting macula densa	Role in tubuloglomerular feedback (changes in Na^+ concentration act to control glomerular flow)	
Proximal convoluted tubule (PCT)	Simple cuboidal epithelium	Microvilli (brush border)	Facilitated diffusion of glucose and amino acids	16.16, 16.17
		Extensive basolateral interdigitations	Na^+ pump	
		Plentiful mitochondria	Energy for active transport	
Pars recta of proximal tubule	Simple cuboidal epithelium	Microvilli (brush border)	Secretion of organic acids	16.19
		No basolateral interdigitations		
Thin descending/ ascending limbs	Simple squamous epithelium	No basolateral interdigitations or microvilli	No active transport	16.19
		Mitochondria scanty	Low energy requirement	
Thick ascending limb	Simple cuboidal epithelium	Microvilli absent	No facilitated diffusion	16.19
		Extensive basolateral interdigitations	Active transport of Na^+	
Distal convoluted tubule (DCT)	Simple cuboidal epithelium	Active transport of Na^+	Extensive basolateral interdigitations	16.16, 16.17
		Mitochondria plentiful	Energy for active transport	
Collecting tubule	Simple cuboidal epithelium	Principal cells	Na^+ reabsorption, ADH-dependent H_2O reabsorption, K^+ secretion	16.19–16.21
		Intercalated cells	Acid–base balance, K^+ reabsorption	
		Collecting tubule cells		
		DCT cells	Active transport of Na^+	
Cortical collecting duct	Simple columnar epithelium	Principal cells	Na^+ reabsorption, ADH-dependent H_2O reabsorption, K^+ secretion	16.20
Medullary collecting duct	Simple columnar epithelium	Mainly principal cells	ADH-dependent water reabsorption	16.22

Lower urinary tract

Component	Muscle structure	Lining epithelium	Function	Figures
Pelvicalyceal system	Smooth muscle, no distinct layer structure	Transitional epithelium (urothelium)	Conveys urine from the tips of the renal papillae into the ureter	16.2, 16.3, 16.5, 16.22, 16.25
Ureter	3 muscle layers: inner spiral (longitudinal) and outer spiral (circular) layers and outermost longitudinal layer in lower third	Transitional epithelium (urothelium)	Carries urine to the bladder	16.1, 16.2, 16.23, 16.25
Bladder	3 muscle layers: inner and outermost longitudinal and middle circular	Transitional epithelium (urothelium)	Stores urine	16.1, 16.24, 16.25

17 Endocrine system

INTRODUCTION

The endocrine system is responsible for the synthesis and secretion of chemical messengers known as ***hormones***. Hormones may be disseminated throughout the body by the bloodstream, where they may act on specific ***target organs*** or affect a wide range of organs and tissues. Other hormones act locally, often arriving at their site of action by way of a specialised microcirculation. In conjunction with the nervous system, hormones coordinate and integrate the functions of all the physiological systems.

As a general rule, endocrine glands are composed of islands of secretory epithelial cells with intervening supporting tissue, rich in blood and lymphatic capillaries. The secretory cells discharge hormone into the interstitial spaces and it is rapidly absorbed into the circulatory system.

Reflecting their active hormone synthesis, cells of the endocrine system have prominent nuclei and abundant mitochondria, endoplasmic reticulum, Golgi bodies and secretory vesicles. The nature of the secretory vesicles varies according to the hormone secreted. There are four main groups of chemicals which can act as hormones:

- Protein and glycoprotein molecules, e.g. insulin, growth hormone, parathyroid hormone (PTH).
- Small peptide molecules, e.g. vasopressin, products of enteroendocrine cells, e.g. glucagon-like peptide 1 (GLP-1).
- Amino acid derivatives, e.g. thyroxine, adrenaline (epinephrine) and noradrenaline (norepinephrine).
- Steroids derived from cholesterol, e.g. adrenal cortical hormones, ovarian and testicular hormones.

Endocrine cells which produce hormones based on amino acids, peptides and proteins often have characteristic membrane-bound secretory vacuoles with electron-dense central cores (***dense core granules***).

The endocrine system can be divided into three parts:

- **The major endocrine organs** in which the sole or major function of the organ is the synthesis, storage and secretion of hormones (e.g. thyroid and adrenal glands)
- **Endocrine components within other solid organs**, for example, the endocrine components of the pancreas, ovary, testis and kidney, in the form of clusters of endocrine cells within other tissues
- **The diffuse endocrine system**, scattered individual hormone cells (or small clumps), usually within an extensive epithelium (e.g. gastrointestinal and respiratory tracts). The major function of these cells is probably ***paracrine*** (i.e. acting on adjacent non-endocrine cells, rather than entering the bloodstream and producing systemic effects).

PITUITARY GLAND

The ***pituitary gland*** (***hypophysis***) is a small bean-shaped gland, about 1 cm diameter, at the base of the brain beneath the third ventricle, sitting in a bony cavity in the base of the skull (the ***sella turcica***). The gland is divided into anterior and posterior parts which have different embryological origins, functions and control mechanisms.

The secretion of all major pituitary hormones is controlled by the hypothalamus, which itself is under the influence of nervous stimuli from higher centres in the brain. Control is mainly by feedback from the levels of circulating hormones produced by pituitary-dependent endocrine tissues.

The pituitary hormones fall into two functional groups:

- Hormones which act directly on non-endocrine tissues: growth hormone (GH), prolactin, antidiuretic hormone (ADH, vasopressin), oxytocin and melanocyte stimulating hormone (MSH).
- Hormones which modulate the secretory activity of other endocrine glands (trophic hormones): thyroid stimulating hormone (TSH), adrenocorticotrophic hormone (ACTH) and the gonadotrophic hormones, follicle stimulating hormone (FSH) and luteinising hormone (LH).

Thus the thyroid gland, adrenal cortex and gonads may be described as ***pituitary-dependent endocrine glands***.

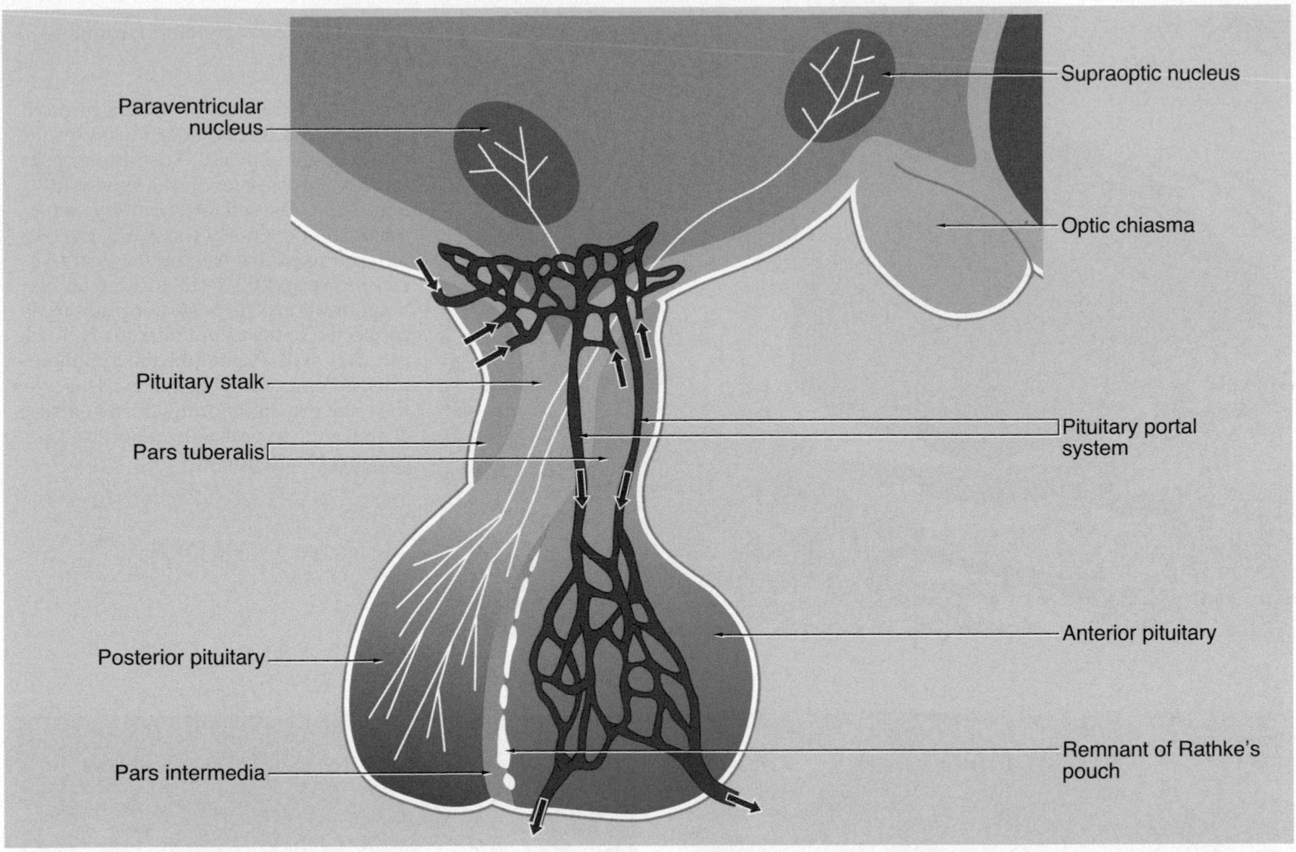

FIG. 17.1 Pituitary gland

The anterior and posterior parts of the pituitary originate from different embryological sources and this is reflected in their structure and function (Fig. 17.1).

The ***posterior pituitary***, also called the ***neurohypophysis*** or ***pars nervosa***, is derived from a downgrowth of nervous tissue from the hypothalamus, to which it remains joined by the ***pituitary stalk***.

The ***anterior pituitary*** arises as an epithelial upgrowth from the roof of the primitive oral cavity known as ***Rathke's pouch***. This specialised glandular epithelium is wrapped around the anterior aspect of the posterior pituitary and is often called the ***adenohypophysis***. The adenohypophysis may contain a cleft or group of cyst-like spaces which represent the vestigial lumen of Rathke's pouch. This vestigial cleft divides the major part of the anterior pituitary from a thin zone of tissue lying against the posterior pituitary known as the ***pars intermedia***. An extension of the adenohypophysis surrounds the neural stalk and is known as the ***pars tuberalis***.

The type and mode of secretion of the posterior pituitary differs greatly from that of the anterior pituitary. The posterior pituitary secretes two hormones, ***antidiuretic hormone*** (***ADH***), also called ***vasopressin*** or ***arginine vasopressin***, and the hormone ***oxytocin***, both of which act directly on non-endocrine tissues.

ADH is synthesised in the neurone cell bodies of the ***supraoptic nucleus***, and oxytocin is synthesised in those of the ***paraventricular nucleus*** of the hypothalamus. Bound to glycoproteins, the hormones pass down the axons of the hypothalamo-pituitary tract through the pituitary stalk to the posterior pituitary where they are stored in the distended terminal parts of the axons. Release of posterior pituitary hormones is controlled directly by nervous impulses passing down the axons from the hypothalamus, a process known as ***neurosecretion***.

Hypothalamic control of anterior pituitary secretion is mediated by specific hypothalamic releasing hormones, such as ***thyroid stimulating hormone releasing hormone*** (***TSHRH***); exceptions to this rule are prolactin secretion, which is under the inhibitory control of ***dopamine***, and secretion of growth hormone, which is controlled by both releasing and inhibitory hormones. These releasing and inhibitory hormones are conducted from the ***median hypothalamic eminence*** to the anterior pituitary by a unique system of ***portal veins*** (***pituitary portal system***).

The pars intermedia synthesises and secretes ***melanocyte-stimulating hormone*** (***MSH***); in humans, the pars intermedia is rudimentary and the physiological importance of MSH and the control of its secretion are poorly understood.

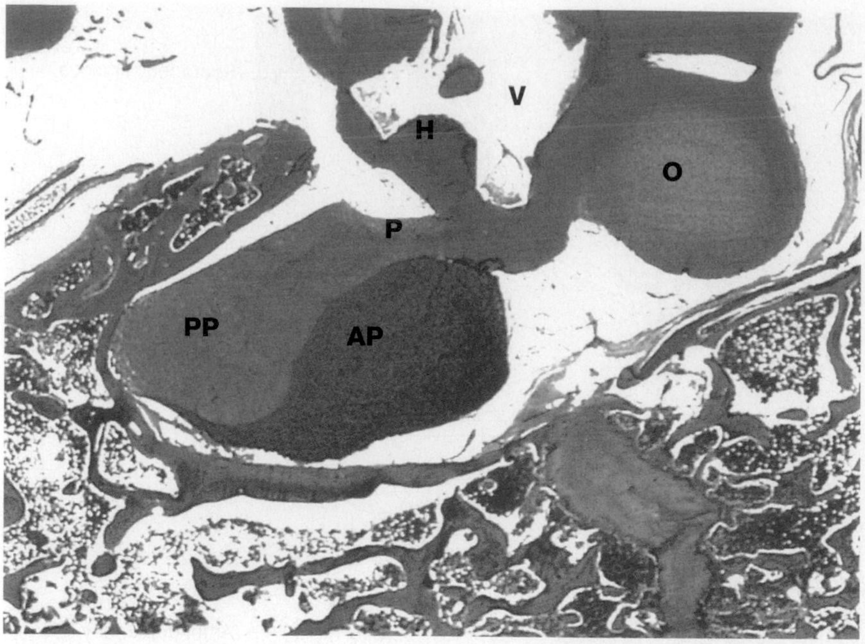

FIG. 17.2 Pituitary gland, monkey H&E (LP)

Fig. 17.2 from a midline section through the brain and cranial floor illustrates the pituitary gland in situ. The pituitary sits in a bony depression in the sphenoid bone called the ***sella turcica***. The two major components of the gland, the ***anterior pituitary*** **AP** and the ***posterior pituitary*** **PP**, are easily seen at this magnification. The posterior pituitary is connected to the hypothalamus **H** by the pituitary stalk **P** and, like the hypothalamus, is composed of nervous tissue. Note the close proximity of the third ventricle **V** above the hypothalamus and the optic chiasma **O** anteriorly.

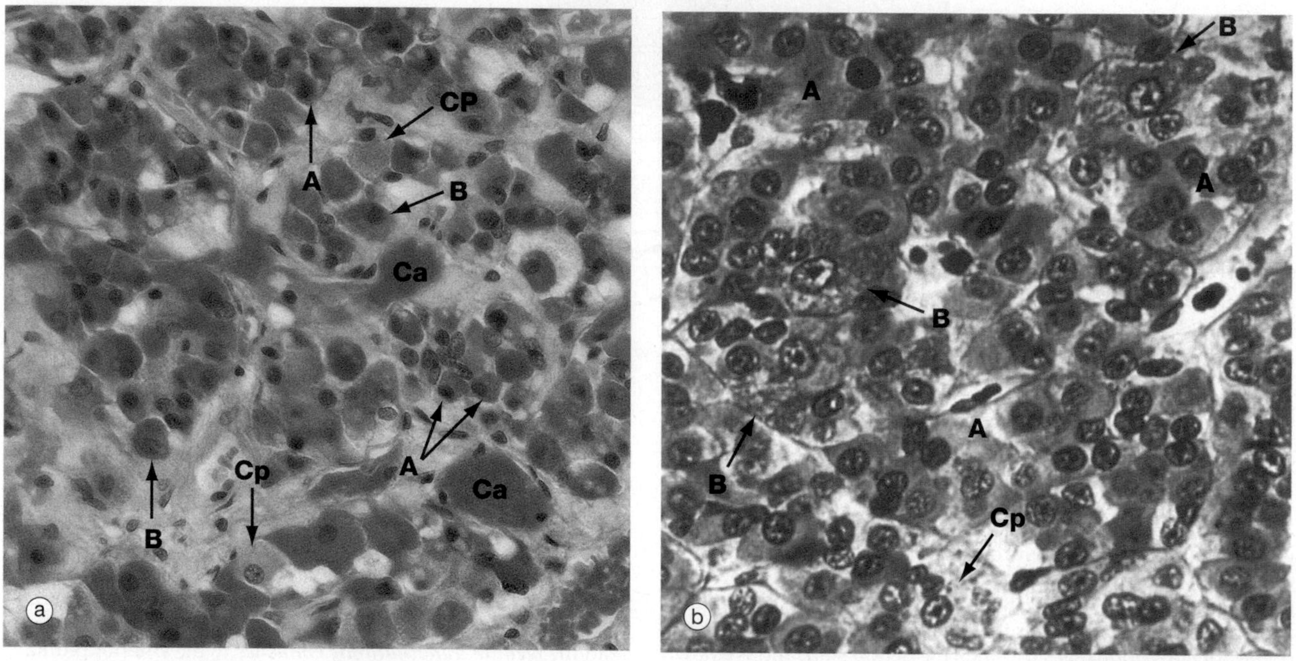

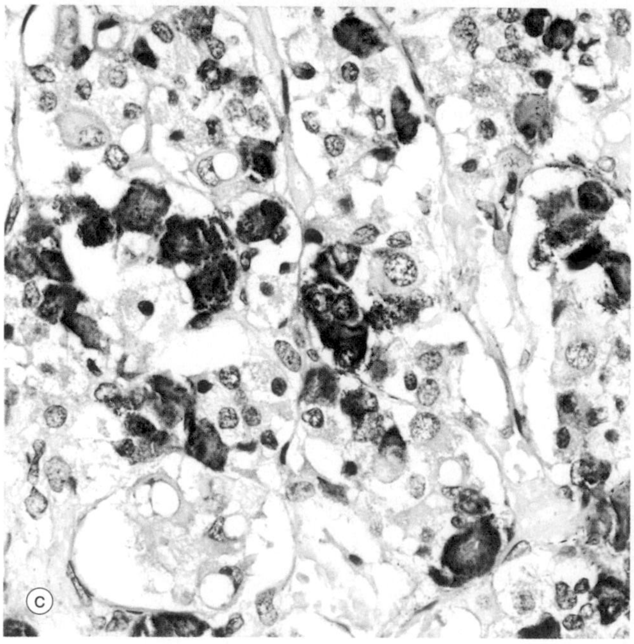

FIG. 17.3 Anterior pituitary *(illustration (d) opposite)* (a) H&E (HP) (b) Azan (HP) (c) Immunohistochemical method for GH (HP) (d) EM ×4270

Fig. 17.3a is an H&E-stained preparation of anterior pituitary and shows two main populations of cells, those with strongly staining cytoplasm (***chromophils***) and those with weakly staining cytoplasm (***chromophobes*** **Cp**). The chromophils can be separated further into basophils **B** and acidophils **A** based on their cytoplasmic staining properties. This is more easily seen in Fig. 17.3b. Note the prominent capillaries **Ca** lying between clumps of secretory cells. The most accurate identification of cell types is given by immunohistochemical methods and electron microscopy. The number of granules in the cytoplasm of these cells may depend on whether they are in a resting phase or actively secreting.

These methods show that chromophobes have very few secretory granules but may produce small amounts of any of the hormones. Chromophobes probably represent cells at the end of a secretory phase, rather than a distinct cell.

Fig. 17.3c shows a section of anterior pituitary stained by the immunohistochemical technique for growth hormone (GH). The brown-stained GH-containing cells can be seen scattered at random among the other cell types.

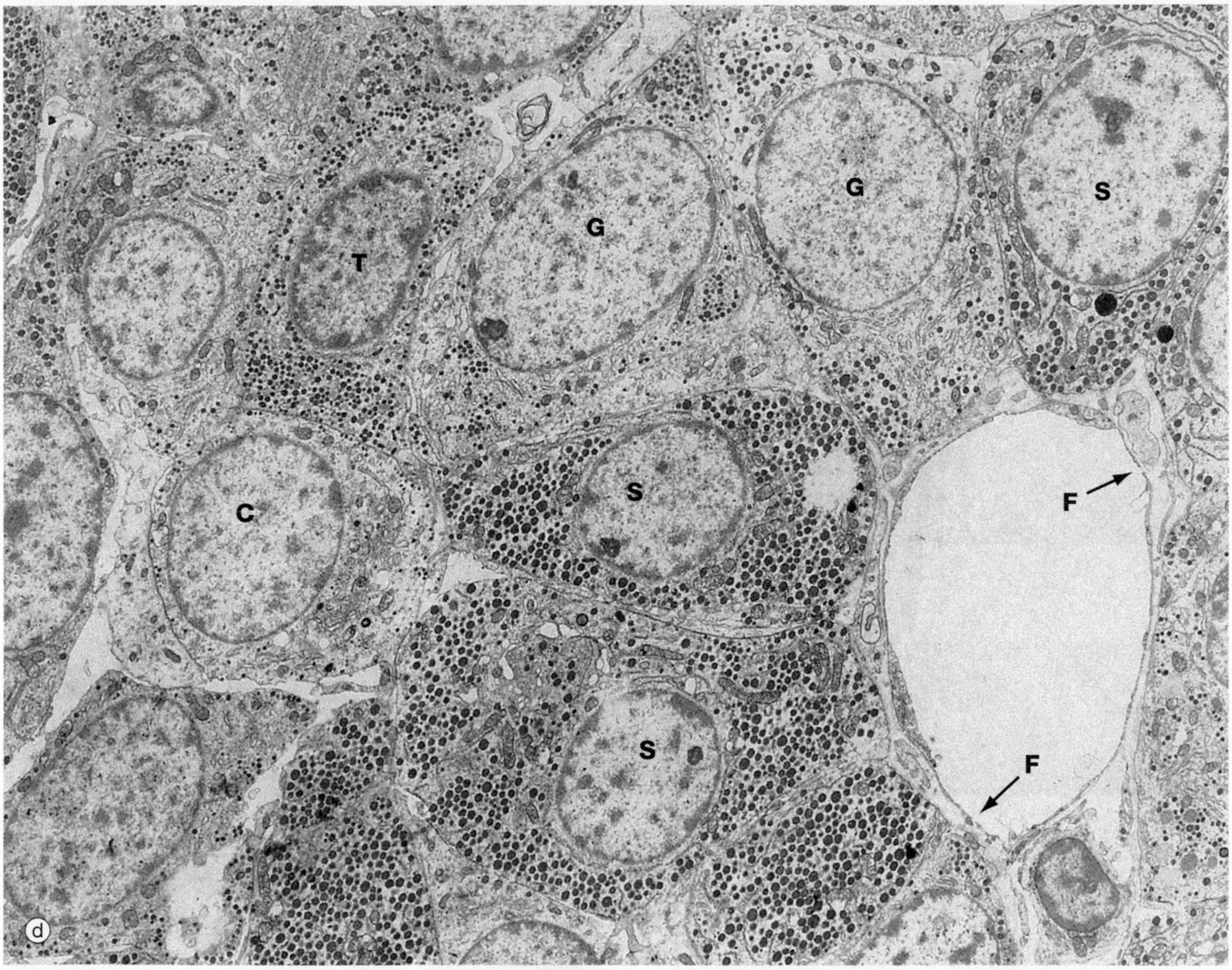

FIG. 17.3 Anterior pituitary *(illustrations (a), (b) and (c) opposite)*
(a) H&E (HP) (b) Azan (HP) (c) Immunohistochemical method for GH (HP) (d) EM ×4270

The different cell types are now named as follows:

- ***Somatotrophs***, the cells responsible for growth hormone secretion, are the most numerous, making up almost 50% of the bulk of the anterior pituitary. These cells predominate in the lateral lobes of the gland and have large numbers of secretory dense granules.
- ***Mammotrophs*** (***lactotrophs***), the prolactin secreting cells, comprise up to 20% of the anterior pituitary, increasing in number during pregnancy; prolactin controls milk production during lactation. They are mainly situated in the posterolateral areas of the gland.
- ***Corticotrophs*** secrete ACTH (***corticotrophin***) and constitute about 20% of the anterior pituitary mass. ACTH is a polypeptide which becomes split from a much larger peptide molecule known as ***pro-opiomelanocortin*** (***POMC***). ***Lipotropins*** (involved in regulation of lipid metabolism), ***endorphins*** (endogenous opioids) and various species of MSH can be derived from the same molecule; this explains the hyperpigmentation associated with excessive ACTH secretion. Corticotrophs are located mainly in the central part of the gland.
- ***Thyrotrophs***, which secrete TSH (***thyrotrophin***), are much less numerous, making up only about 5% of the gland; they are mainly found in the central anterior area of the gland.
- ***Gonadotrophs***, the cells responsible for the secretion of FSH and LH, make up the remaining 5% of the anterior pituitary and are widespread throughout the gland.

In general, one cell produces a single hormone, except for gonadotrophs, which mostly produce both LH and FSH. The different cell types are not evenly distributed throughout the gland, but rather particular cell types tend to congregate in particular zones of the gland.

The secretory granules of each cell type have a characteristic size, shape and electron density by which the different cell types can be recognised with electron microscopy as in Fig. 17.3d. Somatotrophs **S** are packed with secretory granules of moderate size. Thyrotrophs **T** have smaller granules which tend to be more peripherally located. Gonadotrophs **G** are large cells with secretory granules of variable size. Corticotrophs **C** have sparse secretory granules located at the extreme periphery of the cell.

The clumps and cords of cells have a rich capillary network. The endothelial lining of capillaries in endocrine tissue is characteristically fenestrated (see Fig. 8.16), facilitating the passage of hormones into the sinusoids. Note the fenestrations **F** in the sinusoid seen in Fig. 17.3d.

A acidophil **AP** anterior pituitary **B** basophil **C** corticotroph **Ca** capillary **Cp** chromophobe **F** fenestration **G** gonadotroph **H** hypothalamus **O** optic chiasma **P** pituitary stalk **PP** posterior pituitary **S** somatotroph **T** thyrotroph **V** third ventricle

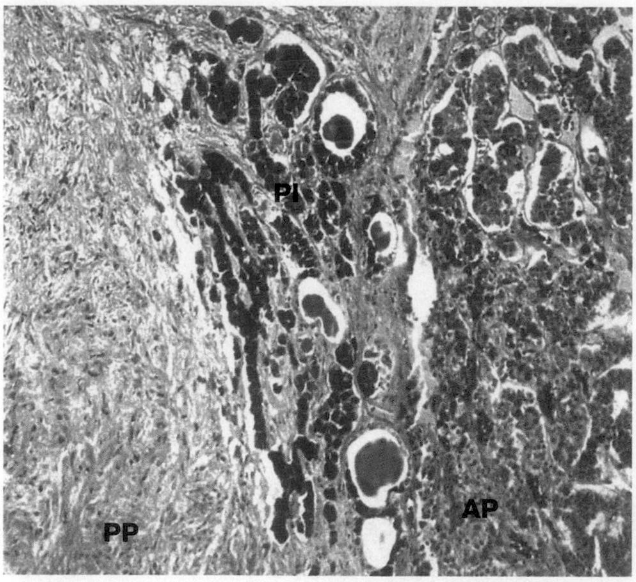

FIG. 17.4 Pituitary, pars intermedia Isamine blue/eosin (MP)

The pars intermedia **PI**, like the anterior pituitary, is derived embryologically from Rathke's pouch (Fig. 17.4). The cells are basophilic (stained blue here), lying in irregular clusters between the anterior **AP** and posterior **PP** pituitary. The pars intermedia also contains small cystic spaces filled with eosinophilic material.

Ultrastructurally, the cells of the pars intermedia contain secretory granules similar to those of corticotrophs. These cells produce α-MSH from pro-opiomelanocortin, usually at low levels.

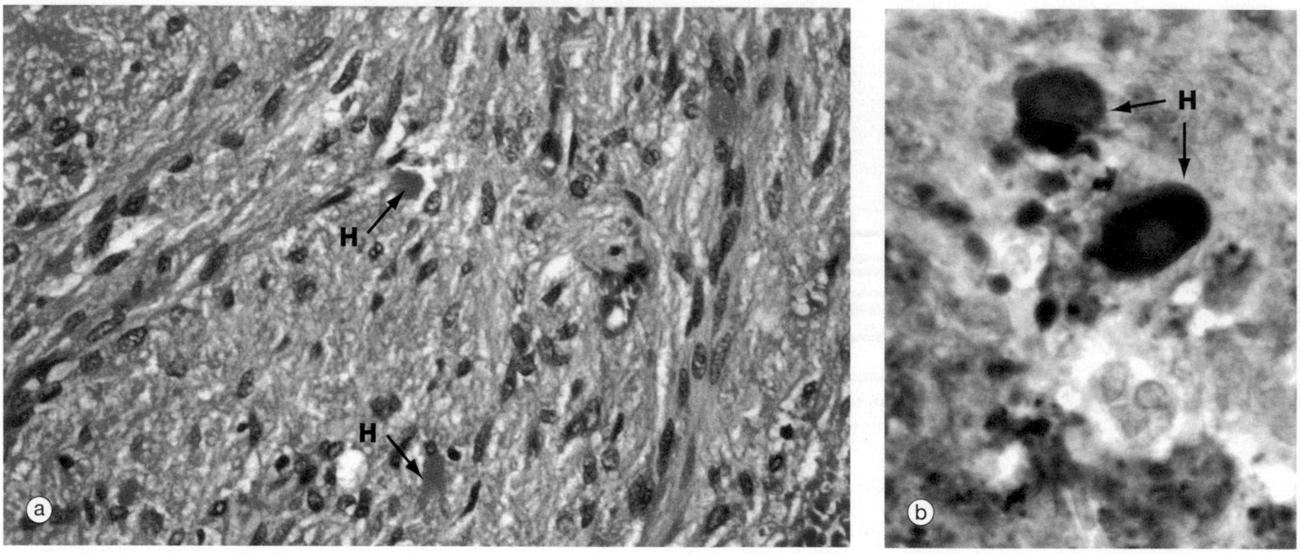

FIG. 17.5 Posterior pituitary (a) H&E (MP) (b) Immunohistochemical method for synaptophysin (HP)

The posterior pituitary is largely composed of the ***non-myelinated axons*** of specialised neurones which have considerable neurosecretory activity. The cell bodies of these neurones are located in the supraoptic and paraventricular nuclei of the hypothalamus and it is here that the posterior pituitary peptide hormones ***oxytocin*** and ***ADH*** are produced. They are passed down the axons in ***neurosecretory granules*** which accumulate in the distended terminations of the axons where they contact capillaries. These distensions are called ***Herring bodies*** **H**. The axons are supported by specialised highly branched glial cells called ***pituicytes***, the cytoplasm of which sometimes contains small amounts of yellowish-brown pigment.

Fig. 17.5a shows the structure of posterior pituitary; the fibrillar structures are the axons of the hypothalamic neurones with distended terminal Herring bodies **H**. The nuclei are those of supporting pituicytes. Fig. 17.5b is an immunohistochemical preparation for neurosecretory granules (synaptophysin). Although granules are scattered in the axons, they are particularly concentrated in the round Herring bodies **H**.

Anterior pituitary disorders

The most common disease of the pituitary is a pituitary adenoma (see e-Fig. 17.1). These tumours are classified as benign because they do not invade adjacent tissues. However, they may have serious or even fatal consequences. They cause their effects by the excessive, continuous production of hormone, uncontrolled by any feedback mechanisms. Thus a tumour of corticotrophs secretes excess ACTH, stimulating the adrenals to produce large quantities of corticosteroid, leading to Cushing's disease. Tumours of somatotrophs produce excess growth hormone (see e-Fig. 17.2), causing gigantism in children or acromegaly in adults. Some pituitary adenomas produce no hormones but grow locally so large that they grow upwards out of the sella turcica to compress and damage the overlying optic chiasma and nerves, leading to visual disturbance and eventual blindness.

The pituitary gland can rarely be destroyed by disease compromising its blood supply, leading to necrosis of the cells and failure of hormone output (panhypopituitarism).

THYROID GLAND

The thyroid gland is a butterfly-shaped endocrine gland lying in the neck in front of the upper part of the trachea. The thyroid gland produces hormones of two types:

- Iodine-containing hormones ***tri-iodothyronine*** (*T_3*), and ***thyroxine*** (***tetra-iodothyronine***, *T_4*); T_4 is converted to T_3 in the general circulation by removal of one iodothyronine unit, although a small amount of T_3 is secreted directly. T_3 is much more potent than T_4 and appears to be the metabolically active form of the hormone. Thyroid hormone regulates the basal metabolic rate and has an important influence on growth and maturation, particularly of nerve tissue. The secretion of these hormones is regulated by TSH secreted by the anterior pituitary.
- The polypeptide hormone ***calcitonin***; this hormone regulates blood calcium levels in conjunction with parathyroid hormone. Calcitonin lowers blood calcium levels by inhibiting the rate of decalcification of bone by osteoclastic resorption and by stimulating osteoblastic activity. Control of calcitonin secretion is dependent only on blood calcium levels and is independent of pituitary and parathyroid hormone levels.

The thyroid gland is unique among the human endocrine glands in that it stores large amounts of hormone in an inactive form within extracellular compartments in the centre of follicles; in contrast, other endocrine glands store only small quantities of hormones in intracellular sites.

The main bulk of the gland develops from an epithelial downgrowth from the fetal tongue, whereas the calcitonin-secreting cells are derived from the ultimobranchial element of the fourth branchial pouch.

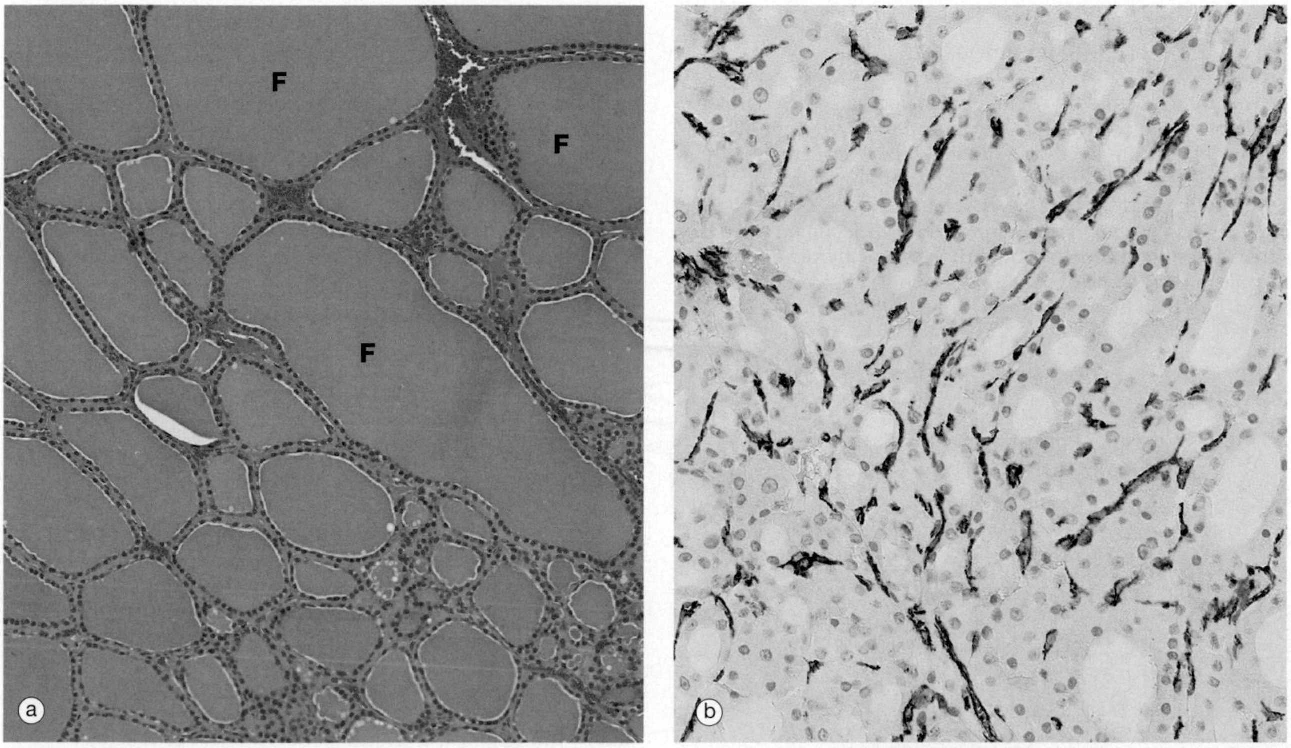

FIG. 17.6 Thyroid gland
(a) H&E (LP) (b) Immunohistochemical method for CD31 (MP)

The functional units of the thyroid gland are the ***thyroid follicles*** **F**, spheroidal structures composed of a single layer of cuboidal epithelial cells, bounded by a basement membrane (see also Fig. 5.27). As seen in this micrograph of a normal thyroid, the follicles are variable in size and contain a homogeneous ***colloid***, which is stained pink in this preparation.

The thyroid gland is enveloped by a fibrous capsule from which fine collagenous septa (not shown in this micrograph) extend into the gland, dividing it into lobules. The septa convey a rich blood supply, together with lymphatics and nerves. Tiny capillaries percolate through the thyroid tissue and surround the follicles and, although these are difficult to see in an H&E preparation, they can be highlighted using an immunohistochemical method for an endothelial marker (CD31), as seen in Fig. 17.6b.

AP anterior pituitary **F** thyroid follicle **H** Herring body **PI** pars intermedia **PP** posterior pituitary

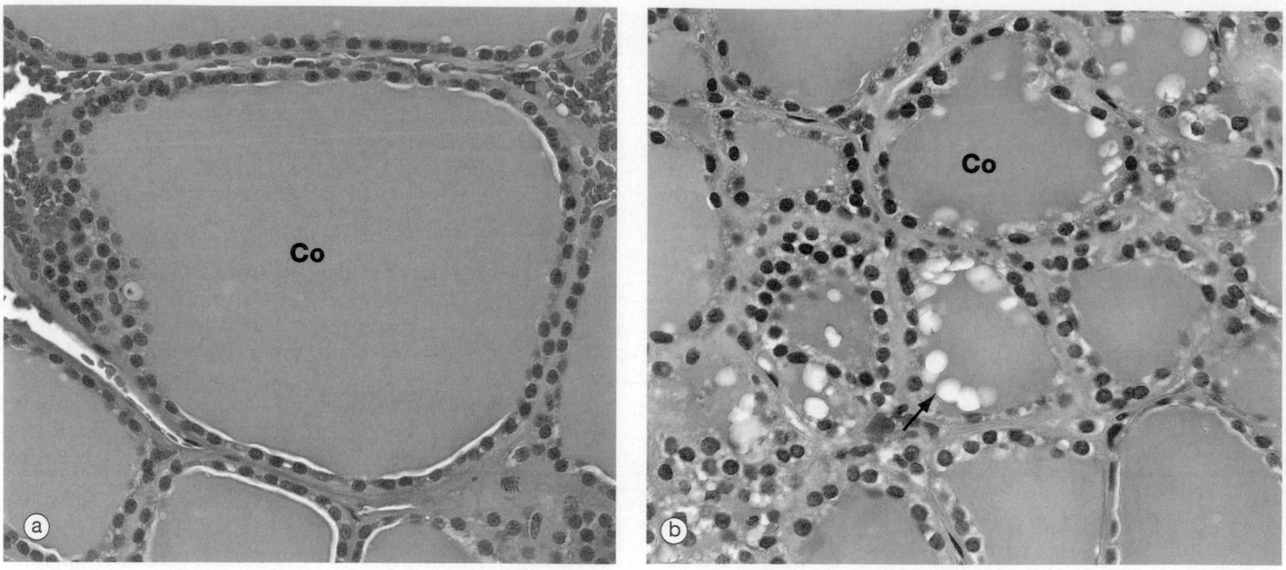

FIG. 17.7 Thyroid follicle
(a) Inactive, H&E (HP) (b) Active, H&E (HP)

Thyroid follicles store thyroglobulin, an iodinated glycoprotein, the storage form of thyroxine (T_4) and tri-iodothyronine (T_3).

The follicles are lined by epithelial cells which are initially responsible for the synthesis of the glycoprotein component of thyroglobulin and for the conversion of iodide to iodine, the iodine linking to the glycoprotein in the follicle lumen. When active thyroid hormone is required, the same thyroid epithelial cells remove some of the stored thyroid colloid and detach T_3 and T_4, which then pass through the cell into an adjacent capillary. When inactive, thyroid epithelial cells are simple flat or cuboidal cells, as in Fig. 17.7a which shows inactive epithelial cells lining follicles filled with stored thyroglobulin (colloid **Co**). Fig. 17.7b, in contrast, shows cells actively synthesising or secreting thyroid hormone; they are tall and columnar. In this follicle, they are extracting stored thyroid colloid **Co** from the lumen and converting it into active thyroid hormones. The 'scalloped' pale edge of the colloid (arrow) indicates where the colloid has been removed from the follicle lumen.

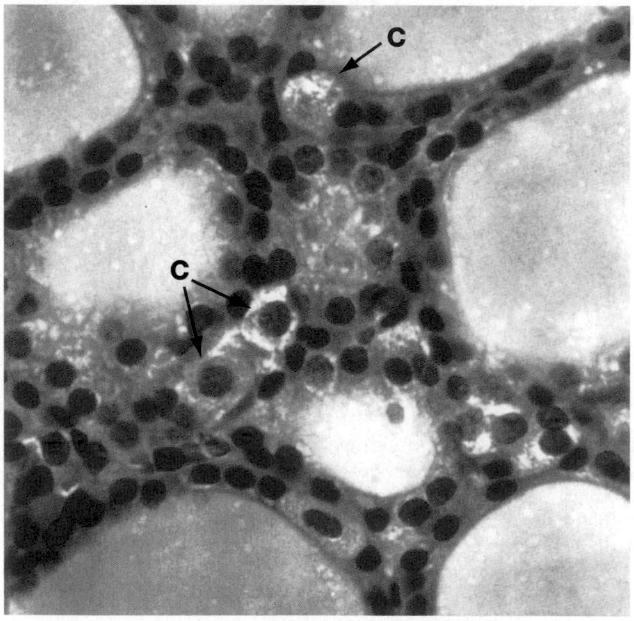

FIG. 17.8 Thyroid C cell
H&E (HP)

A second type of endocrine cell with the ultrastructural characteristics of neuroendocrine cells, the ***C cell*** or ***parafollicular cell*** **C**, is found in the thyroid gland as individual scattered cells in the follicle lining or as small clumps in the interstices between follicles (Fig. 17.8). They are particularly prominent in dogs, where they are identifiable in H&E sections as pale-staining cells with granular cytoplasm. In humans they are much less prominent and can usually only be identified ultrastructurally (see Fig. 17.9) and by immunohistochemical methods. These cells secrete ***calcitonin***, which is a physiological antagonist to parathyroid hormone and therefore lowers blood calcium levels by suppressing the osteoclastic resorption of bone.

Thyrotoxicosis and hypothyroidism

An excess of circulating thyroid hormone causes clinical symptoms due to the systemic effects of thyroid hormone. This is called ***thyrotoxicosis***. Clinical symptoms include palpitations, fatigue, weight loss and anxiety. Blood tests for thyroid stimulating hormone and thyroid hormones (T_3 and T_4) can help to determine the underlying cause of thyroid disease. If TSH is elevated, and T_3 and T_4 are reduced, then a primary cause in the thyroid gland is likely, e.g. Graves disease (see e-Fig. 17.3). If TSH is elevated and T_3/T_4 are elevated, then a secondary cause, e.g. a pituitary adenoma that secretes TSH, could be the cause. A lack of production of thyroid hormone leads to symptoms of thyroid hormone deficiency, termed ***hypothyroidism***. These symptoms include tiredness, weight gain and poor tolerance to cold weather. The most common cause of hypothyroidism is the auto-immune condition Hashimoto's thyroiditis (see e-Fig. 17.4).

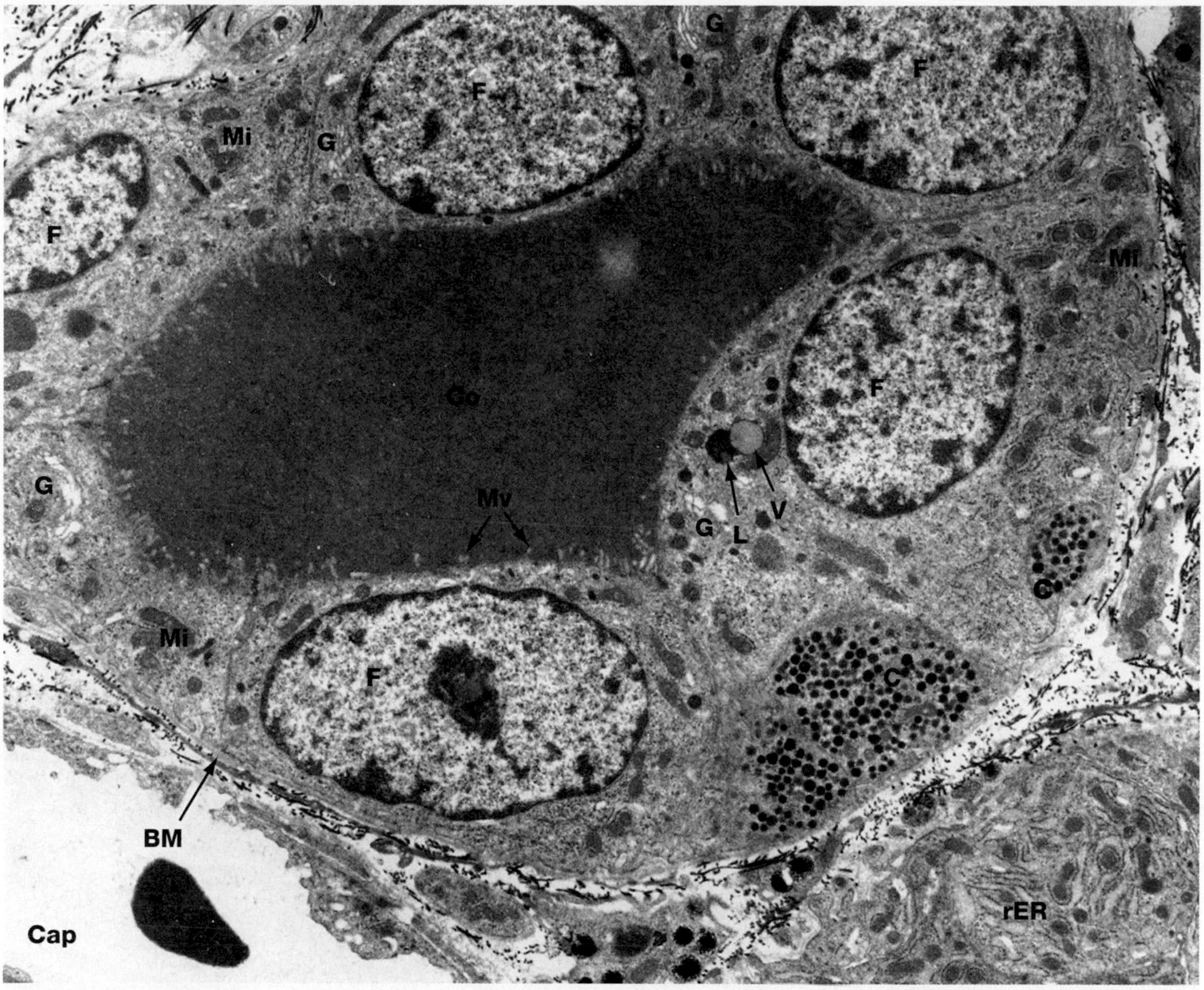

FIG. 17.9 Thyroid follicle, rat
EM ×6800

Fig. 17.9 demonstrates a thyroid follicle composed of cuboidal follicular cells **F** surrounding a lumen containing the homogeneous colloid, thyroglobulin **Co**. A basement membrane **BM** delineates the follicle. Two portions of the cytoplasm of a C cell **C** are seen within the follicular epithelium, typically located on the basement membrane and not exposed to the follicular lumen. The cytoplasm contains numerous electron-dense secretory granules of the hormone calcitonin. A fenestrated capillary **Cap** containing an erythrocyte is closely applied to the follicular basement membrane.

Follicular cells concentrate iodide from the blood by means of an iodide pump in the basal plasma membrane. Within the cell, iodide is oxidised to iodine and transported to the follicular plasma membrane where it is released into the follicular lumen. The glycoprotein thyroglobulin is synthesised in the rough endoplasmic reticulum, glycosylated and packaged by the Golgi apparatus, then released into the follicular lumen by exocytosis. Within the follicular lumen (not within the follicular cells), iodine combines with tyrosine residues of the thyroglobulin to form the hormones tri-iodothyronine (T_3) and tetra-iodothyronine (thyroxine, T_4) which remain bound to the glycoprotein in an inactive form.

Secretion of these hormones involves pinocytosis of the thyroglobulin-hormone complex to form cytoplasmic vacuoles. The vacuoles then fuse with lysosomes of the follicular cell cytoplasm, and hydrolytic enzymes cleave the hormone from the thyroglobulin. The hormones are released in the basal cytoplasm, from which they diffuse into the bloodstream. The synthetic and secretory activity of the thyroid gland is dependent on thyroid stimulating hormone (TSH), secreted by the anterior pituitary.

In this micrograph, rough endoplasmic reticulum **rER** is best demonstrated in the basal aspect of a secretory cell of an adjacent follicle. Mitochondria **Mi** are closely associated with the endoplasmic reticulum and are also scattered throughout the cytoplasm. Golgi complexes **G** are a prominent feature. Small microvilli **Mv**, associated with the exocytosis of thyroglobulin and the endocytosis of the thyroglobulin-hormone complex, protrude into the follicular lumen. In one cell a vacuole **V** of thyroglobulin-hormone is seen about to fuse with a large lysosome **L**. Electron-dense lysosomes are also seen scattered throughout the cytoplasm.

BM basement membrane **C** C cell **Cap** capillary **Co** colloid **F** follicular cell **G** Golgi complex **L** lysosome
Mi mitochondrion **Mv** microvilli **rER** rough endoplasmic reticulum **V** vacuole

PARATHYROID GLAND

The parathyroid glands are small, oval endocrine glands which are closely associated with the thyroid gland. In mammals, there are usually two pairs of glands, one pair situated on the posterior surface of the thyroid gland on each side, although occasional individuals possess five or even six parathyroids. The embryological origins of the parathyroid glands are from the third and fourth branchial (pharyngeal) pouches. The parathyroid glands regulate serum calcium and phosphate levels via ***parathyroid hormone*** (***PTH***).

Parathyroid hormone raises serum calcium levels in three ways:

- Direct action on bone, increasing the rate of osteoclastic resorption and promoting breakdown of the bone matrix
- Direct action on the kidney, increasing the renal tubular reabsorption of calcium ions and inhibiting the reabsorption of phosphate ions from the glomerular filtrate
- Promotion of the absorption of calcium from the small intestine; this effect involves vitamin D.

Secretion of parathyroid hormone is stimulated by a decrease in blood calcium levels. In conjunction with calcitonin secreted by the C cells of the thyroid gland, blood calcium levels are maintained within narrow limits. Parathyroid hormone is the most important regulator of blood calcium levels and is essential to life, whereas calcitonin appears to provide a complementary mechanism for fine adjustment and is not essential to life.

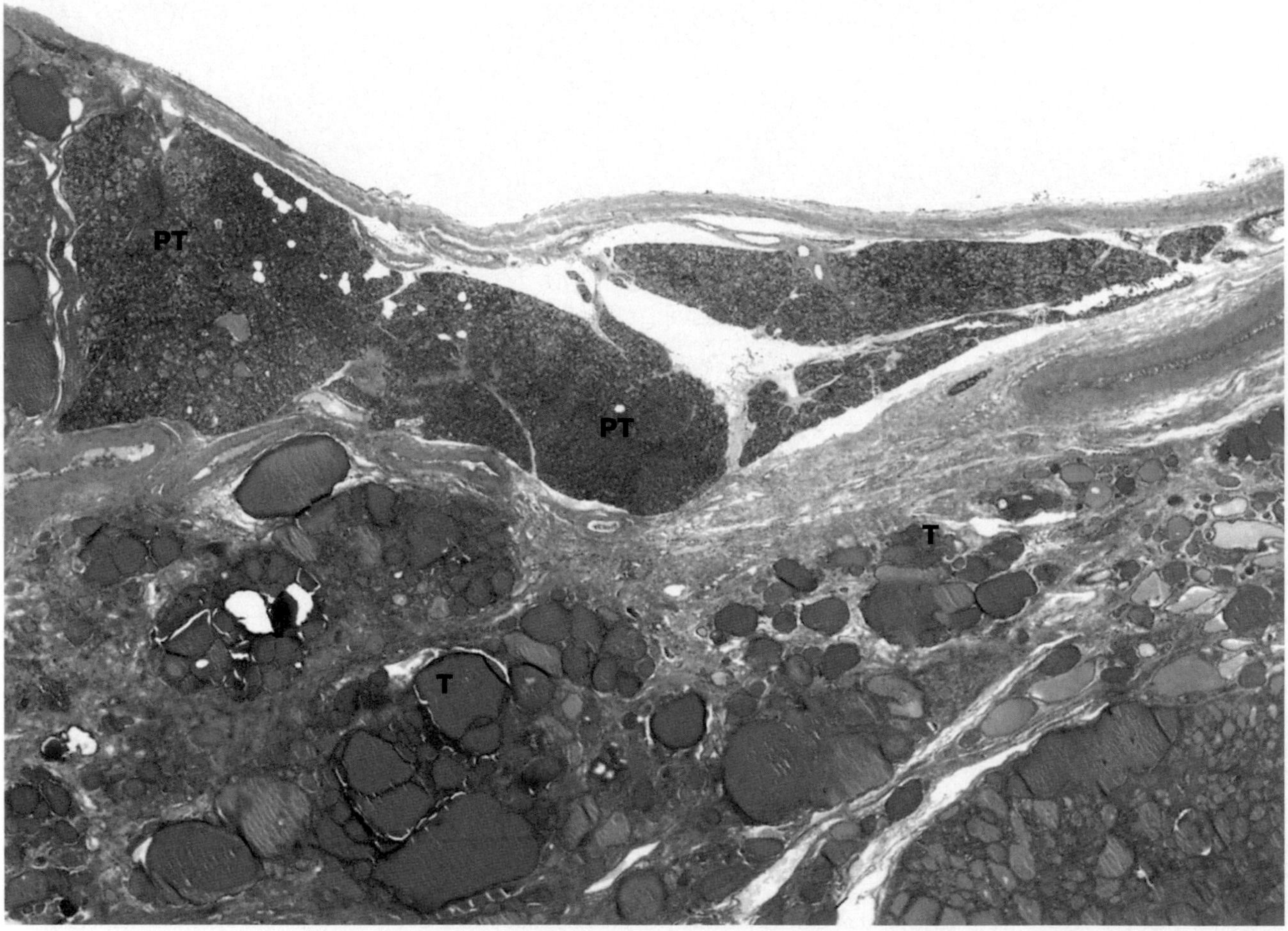

FIG. 17.10 Parathyroid gland
H&E (LP)

Fig. 17.10 shows a parathyroid gland **PT**, embedded under the capsule of a thyroid gland **T**. Some parathyroids are actually found embedded in the thyroid tissue proper.

The thin fibrous capsule of the parathyroid gland gives rise to delicate septa which divide the parenchyma into nodules of secretory cells. They are very prone to shrinkage artefact during histological preparation. The septa carry blood vessels, lymphatics and nerves.

A adipose tissue **C** capillary **G** glandular elements **O** oxyphil cells **P** principal or chief cells **PT** parathyroid gland
T thyroid gland

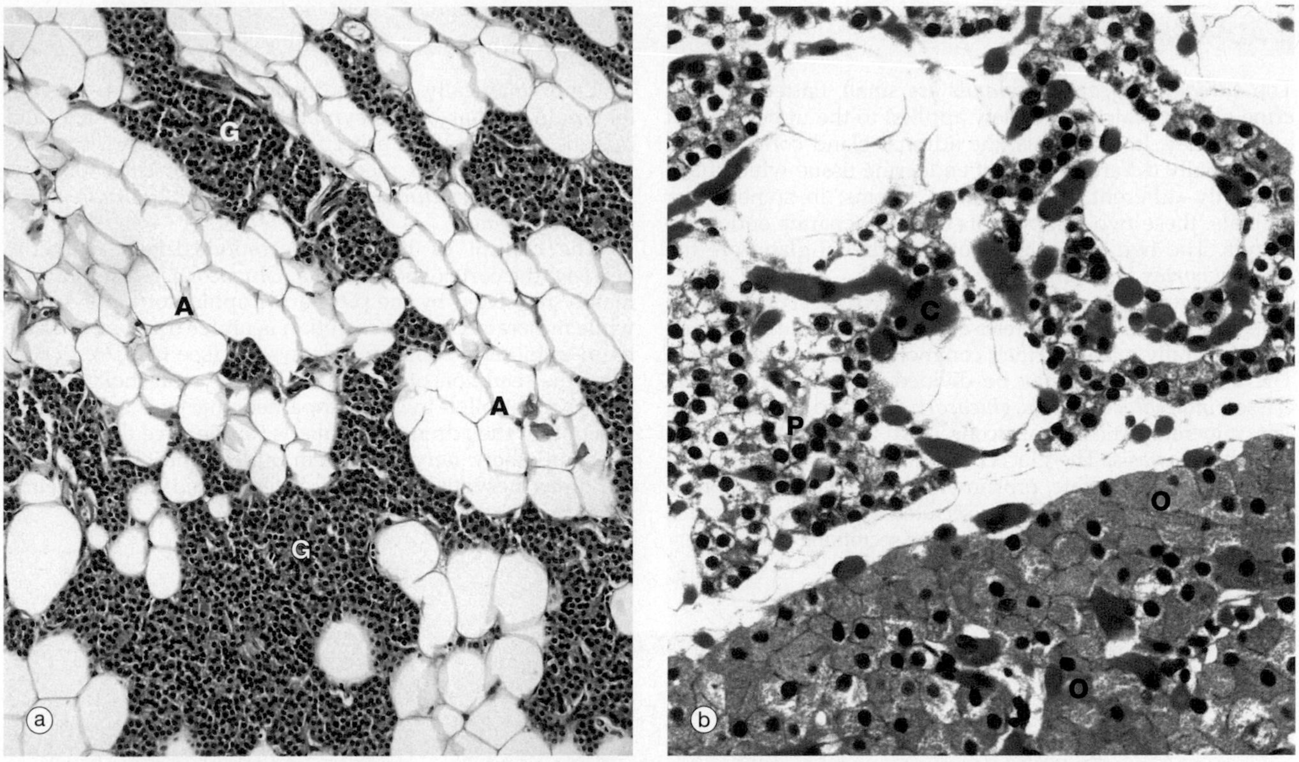

FIG. 17.11 Parathyroid gland
(a) H&E (MP) (b) H&E (HP)

Fig. 17.11a is a medium-power view of normal adult parathyroid, showing the glandular elements **G** intermixed with adipose tissue **A**, which begins to accumulate after puberty and makes up 25% to 40% of the total tissue in normal adults. The glandular cells are of two types: ***chief*** or ***principal cells*** and ***oxyphil cells***. The glandular cells are arranged as clusters, ribbons or glands.

At higher power in Fig. 17.11b, the chief cells **P** are small, with round central nuclei and pale eosinophilic or clear cytoplasm. These are the cells which synthesise and secrete PTH. The staining intensity of the cytoplasm depends on whether the cells are actively secreting PTH, in which case the cytoplasm contains plentiful rough endoplasmic reticulum and stains strongly. On the other hand, resting cells have pale cytoplasm and make up about 80% of the total in normal adults.

Oxyphil cells **O**, which tend to occur in nodules, have copious eosinophilic cytoplasm that ultrastructurally is seen to be packed with mitochondria. These cells do not secrete PTH and increase in number with age.

Note the many delicate capillaries **C** between the nests of endocrine cells.

Disorders of the parathyroid gland

The parathyroid glands may either overwork, producing excessive PTH (***hyperparathyroidism***) or underwork, producing little or no hormone (***hypoparathyroidism***).

The commonest cause of hyperparathyroidism is a benign tumour of one of the parathyroid glands (parathyroid adenoma) (see e-Fig. 17.5) which constantly produces excessive PTH, unresponsive to normal feedback mechanisms related to the blood calcium levels. The excess parathormone stimulates excessive osteoclastic erosion of bone (see Fig. 10.6), with the release of bone calcium into the blood to produce ***hypercalcaemia***. The results include bone pain with X-ray abnormalities and an increased risk of kidney stones. This pattern is called primary hyperparathyroidism. Secondary hyperparathyroidism is a secondary response of all the parathyroid glands to a persistent low serum calcium level in patients with kidney failure who are constantly losing calcium in their urine. The feedback mechanism is triggered and all of the parathyroids become enlarged (***parathyroid hyperplasia***) and secrete excess PTH in an attempt to bring the serum calcium level back to normal.

Tertiary hyperparathyroidism occurs when the hyperplastic glands of secondary hyperparathyroidism cease to respond to serum calcium levels. The glands secrete high levels of PTH autonomously.

Hypoparathyroidism is rare and is usually due to inadvertent surgical removal of all parathyroid glands during total thyroidectomy.

ADRENAL GLAND

The ***adrenal*** (***suprarenal***) ***glands*** are small, flattened endocrine glands which are closely applied to the upper pole of each kidney. In mammals, the adrenal gland contains two functionally different types of endocrine tissue which have distinctly different embryological origins; in some lower animals, these two components exist as separate endocrine glands. The two components of the adrenal gland are the ***adrenal cortex*** and ***adrenal medulla***.

The adrenal cortex has a similar embryological origin to the gonads and, like them, secretes a variety of ***steroid hormones***, all structurally related to their common precursor ***cholesterol***. The adrenal steroids may be divided into three functional classes, ***mineralocorticoids***, ***glucocorticoids*** and ***sex hormones***. The mineralocorticoids are concerned with electrolyte and fluid homeostasis. The glucocorticoids have a wide range of effects on carbohydrate, protein and lipid metabolism. Small quantities of sex hormones are secreted by the adrenal cortex and supplement gonadal sex hormone secretion.

Embryologically, the adrenal medulla has a similar origin to that of the sympathetic nervous system and may be considered as a highly specialised adjunct of this system. The adrenal medulla secretes the catecholamine hormones, ***adrenaline*** (***epinephrine***) and ***noradrenaline*** (***norepinephrine***).

The control of hormone secretion differs markedly between the cortex and medulla. Glucocorticoid secretion is mainly regulated by the pituitary trophic hormone ACTH, while mineralocorticoid secretion is under the control of the renin–angiotensin–aldosterone system (see Ch. 16). In contrast, the secretion of adrenal medullary catecholamines is directly controlled by the sympathetic nervous system. The function of the adrenal medulla is to reinforce the action of the sympathetic nervous system under conditions of stress, the direct nervous control of adrenal medullary secretion permitting a rapid response.

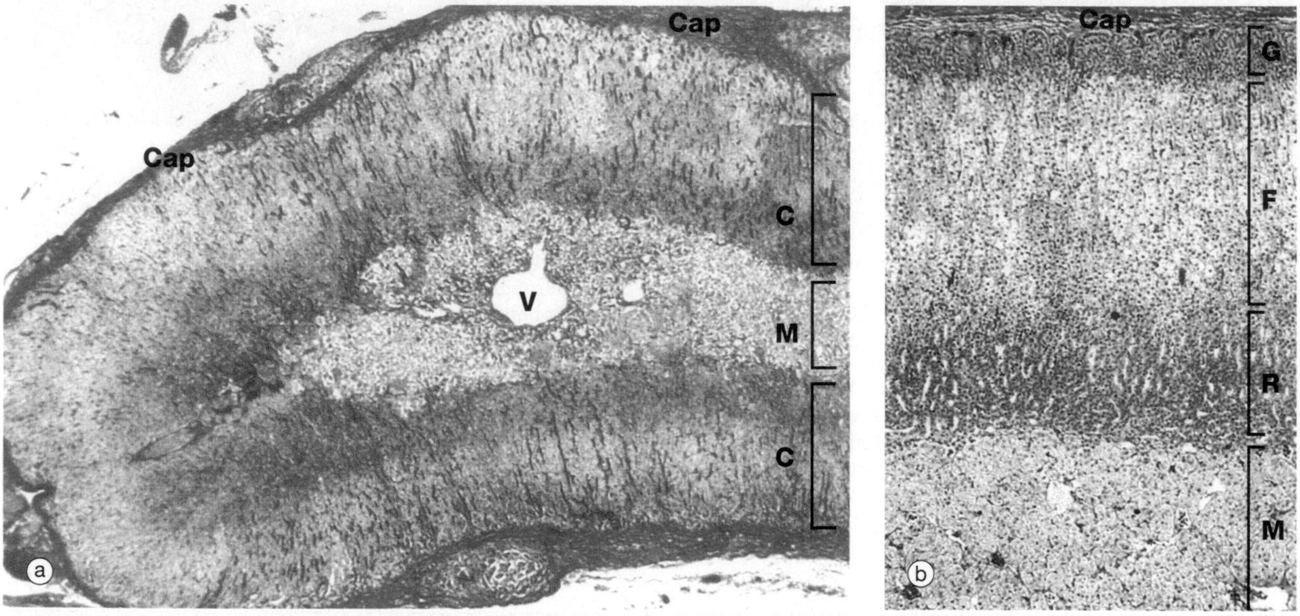

FIG. 17.12 Adrenal gland
(a) Azan (LP) (b) Azan (MP)

At low magnification in Fig. 17.12a, the adrenal gland is seen to be divided into an outer cortex **C** and a pale-stained inner medulla **M**. A dense fibrous tissue capsule **Cap**, stained blue in this preparation, invests the gland and provides external support for a delicate collagenous framework supporting the secretory cells. A prominent vein **V** is characteristically located in the centre of the medulla.

At higher magnification in Fig. 17.12b, the adrenal cortex can be seen to consist of three histological zones which are named according to the arrangement of the secretory cells: ***zona glomerulosa***, ***zona fasciculata*** and ***zona reticularis***.

The zona glomerulosa **G**, lying beneath the capsule, contains secretory cells arranged in rounded clusters. The intermediate zona fasciculata **F** consists of parallel cords of secretory cells disposed at right angles to the capsule. The zona reticularis **R**, which lies adjacent to the medulla **M**, consists of small closely packed cells arranged in irregular cords. Often the borders of the zones are less regular and less easily recognised than in this specimen.

Familial cancer syndromes and adrenal tumours

Around 10% of adrenal tumours are associated with familial cancer syndromes. Phaeochromocytoma (see e-Fig. 17.6) is a tumour of the adrenal medulla (see Fig. 17.4). A diagnosis of phaeochromocytoma necessitates investigations for familial cancer syndromes. An example is succinic dehydrogenase B deficiency (SDH-B deficiency) (see e-Fig. 17.7). Adrenal cortical carcinomas are malignant tumours of the adrenal cortex. These tumours can be seen in association with Li Fraumeni syndrome (caused by a mutation in TP53, a tumour suppressor gene) and Beckwith–Weidemann syndrome (caused by a mutation in chromosome 11p15).

C cortex **Cap** capsule **F** zona fasciculata **G** zona glomerulosa **M** medulla **R** zona reticularis **T** trabecula **V** vein

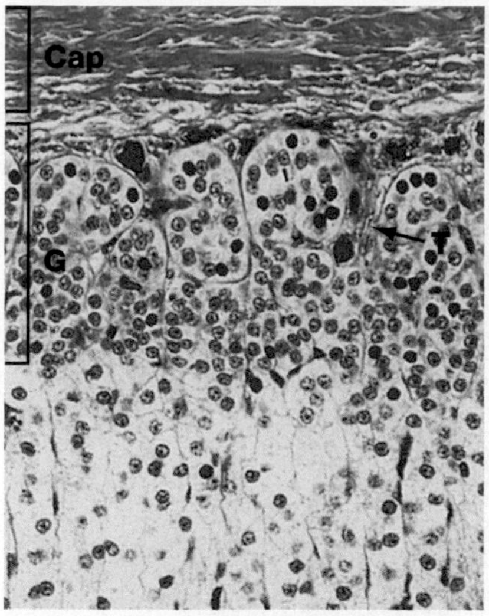

FIG. 17.13 Adrenal cortex, zona glomerulosa
Azan (MP)

Fig. 17.13 shows the outer zone of the adrenal cortex. The zona glomerulosa **G** is composed of cells arranged in irregular ovoid clusters separated by delicate fibrous trabeculae **T**, which are continuous with the fibrocollagenous capsule **Cap**; both the trabeculae and inner capsule contain prominent capillaries. The cells have round nuclei and less cytoplasm than the cells in the adjacent zona fasciculata. The cytoplasm contains plentiful smooth endoplasmic reticulum and numerous mitochondria, but with only scanty lipid droplets.

This zone secretes the mineralocorticoid hormones, principally ***aldosterone***, the secretion of which is controlled by the renin–angiotensin system (see Ch. 16), which in turn is controlled by the macula densa of the distal renal tubule. Aldosterone acts directly on the renal tubules to increase sodium and therefore water retention. This increases extracellular fluid volume and therefore increases arterial blood pressure.

Aldosterone secretion is independent of ACTH control.

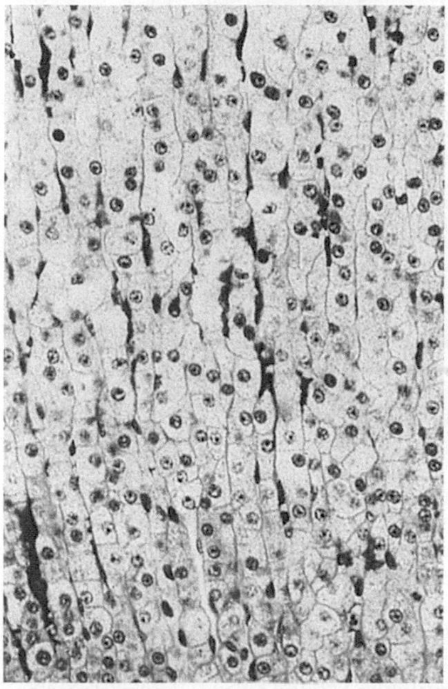

FIG. 17.14 Adrenal cortex, zona fasciculata
Azan (MP)

The zona fasciculata is the middle and broadest of the three cortical zones (Fig. 17.14). It consists of narrow columns and cords of cells, often only one cell thick, separated by fine strands of collagen and wide-bore capillaries. The cell cytoplasm is abundant and pale staining due to the large number of lipid droplets present; mitochondria and smooth endoplasmic reticulum are also abundant. The zona fasciculata secretes glucocorticoid hormones, mainly ***cortisol***, which have many metabolic effects, one of which is to raise blood glucose levels and increase cellular synthesis of glycogen. They also increase the rate of protein breakdown and the rate of liberation of lipid from tissue stores.

Cortisol secretion is controlled by the hypothalamus via the anterior pituitary trophic hormone ACTH. By this means, many stimuli, such as stress, promote glucocorticoid secretion.

The zona fasciculata is also the site of secretion of small amounts of androgenic sex hormones.

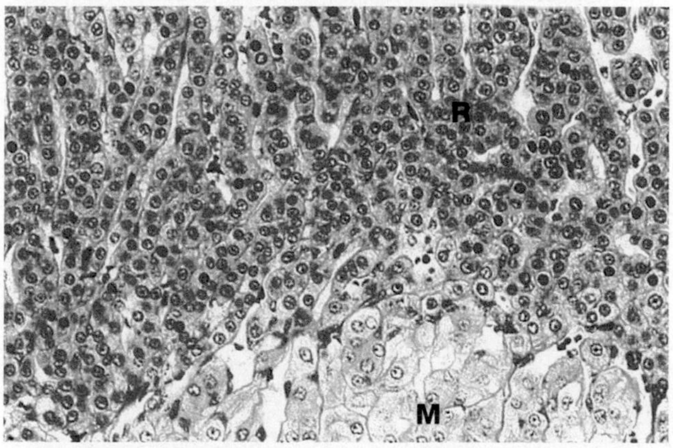

FIG. 17.15 Adrenal cortex, zona reticularis
Azan (LP)

The zona reticularis **R** is the thin, innermost layer of the adrenal cortex and lies next to the adrenal medulla **M** (Fig. 17.15). It consists of an irregular network of branching cords and clusters of glandular cells, separated by numerous wide-diameter capillaries. The zona reticularis cells are much smaller than those of the adjacent zona fasciculata, with less cytoplasm. The cytoplasm is darker staining because it contains considerably fewer lipid droplets. Brown lipofuscin pigment (see Fig. 1.26) is sometimes seen in the cells of this layer. The zona reticularis secretes small quantities of androgens and glucocorticoids.

Disorders of the adrenal cortex

Destruction of both adrenals (e.g. by autoimmune adrenalitis or, in former years, by tuberculosis) leads to failure of secretion of all adrenal cortical hormones (***hypoadrenalism***), leading to the clinical syndrome called Addison's disease (weakness, tiredness, skin pigmentation, postural hypotension, hypovolaemia and low blood sodium). More common is ***hyperadrenalism*** where there is excess secretion of one or more of the cortical hormones, mainly glucocorticoids (producing Cushing's syndrome) or mineralocorticoids (producing Conn's syndrome). The excess hormone may be produced by a benign tumour (adrenal cortical adenoma, see e-Fig. 17.8) or a malignant tumour (adrenal cortical carcinoma) or by diffuse hyperplasia of the adrenal cortex (see e-Fig. 17.9). In adrenal cortical carcinoma, the excessive output may affect all three types of cortical hormone, including androgens, and hirsutism or virilisation are sometimes present.

Ectopic ACTH syndrome occurs when some types of tumour elsewhere in the body (e.g. neuroendocrine carcinomas in the lung) secrete excessive amounts of an ACTH-like substance which stimulates the zona fasciculata to produce excess glucocorticoids.

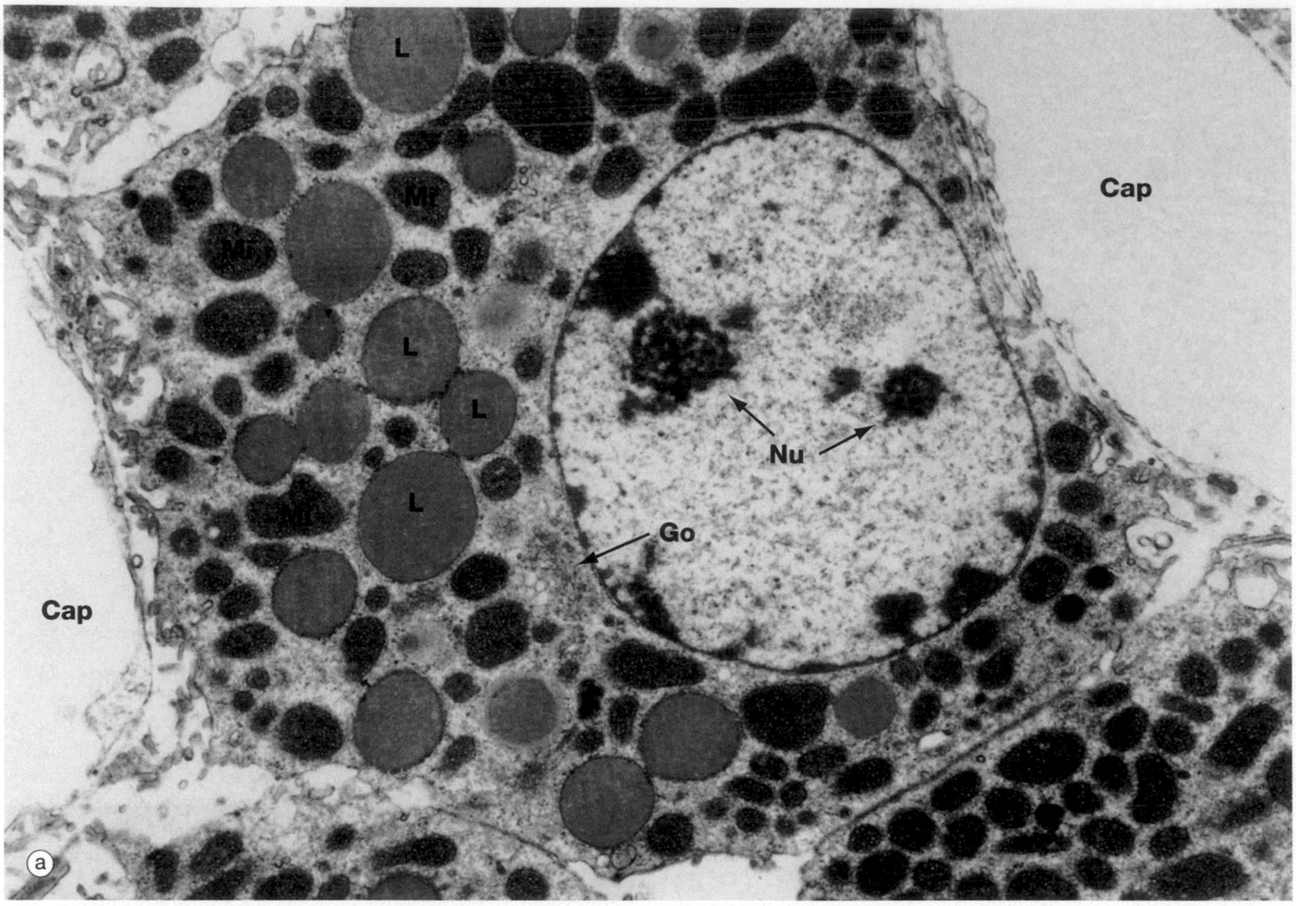

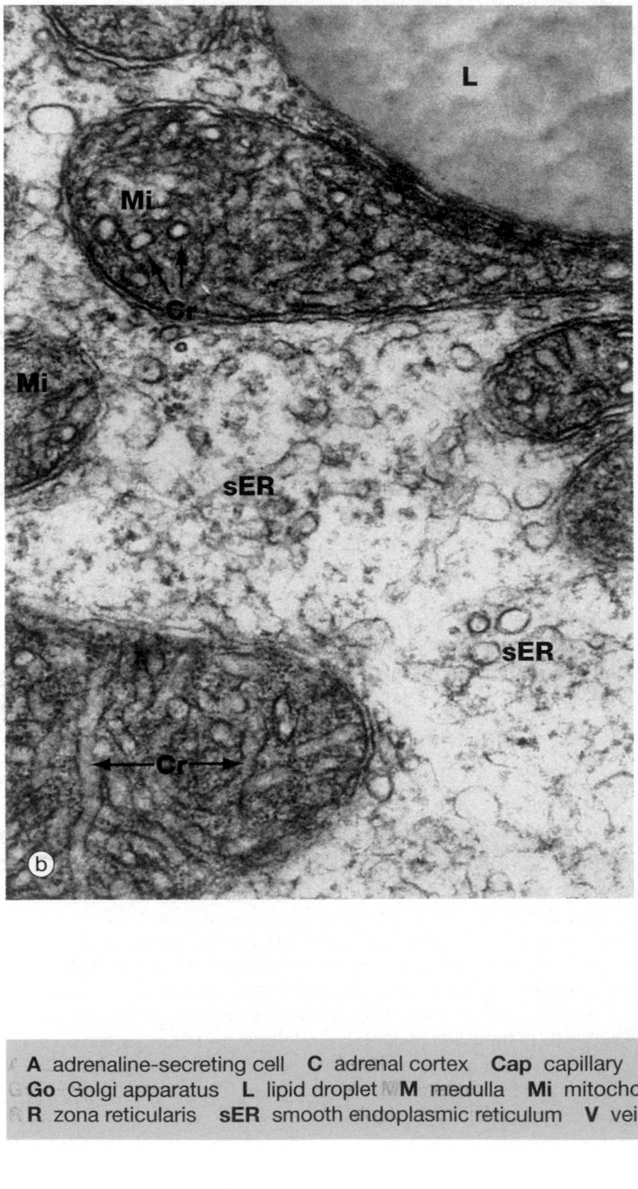

FIG. 17.16 Steroid-secreting cell
(a) EM ×8500 (b) EM ×110 500

Fig. 17.16a and b illustrate the typical ultrastructural features of steroid-secreting cells, which are seen not only in the cells of the adrenal cortex but also in the steroid-secreting cells of the ovaries and testes (see Chs 18 and 19). At low magnification in Fig. 17.16a, a secretory cell is seen, intimately associated with fenestrated capillaries **Cap**. Note the short microvillous projections of the secretory cell plasma membrane subjacent to the capillary endothelium. The rounded secretory cell nucleus is characterised by one or more prominent nucleoli **Nu**.

The abundant cytoplasm contains many large lipid droplets **L** containing stored cholesterol esters. A small Golgi apparatus **Go** is seen close to the nucleus. Numerous variably shaped mitochondria **Mi** crowd the cytoplasm. As seen in Fig. 17.16b at high magnification, the mitochondria have unusual tubular cristae **Cr**. The cytoplasm contains a prolific system of smooth endoplasmic reticulum **sER**.

Synthesis of steroid hormones begins with the liberation of cholesterol esters from lipid droplets. The cholesterol molecule is modified to form a wide range of steroid hormones by enzyme systems found in the smooth endoplasmic reticulum and in the mitochondria.

A adrenaline-secreting cell **C** adrenal cortex **Cap** capillary **Cr** cristae **F** zona fasciculata **G** zona glomerulosa **Go** Golgi apparatus **L** lipid droplet **M** medulla **Mi** mitochondrion **Na** noradrenaline-secreting cell **Nu** nucleolus **R** zona reticularis **sER** smooth endoplasmic reticulum **V** vein

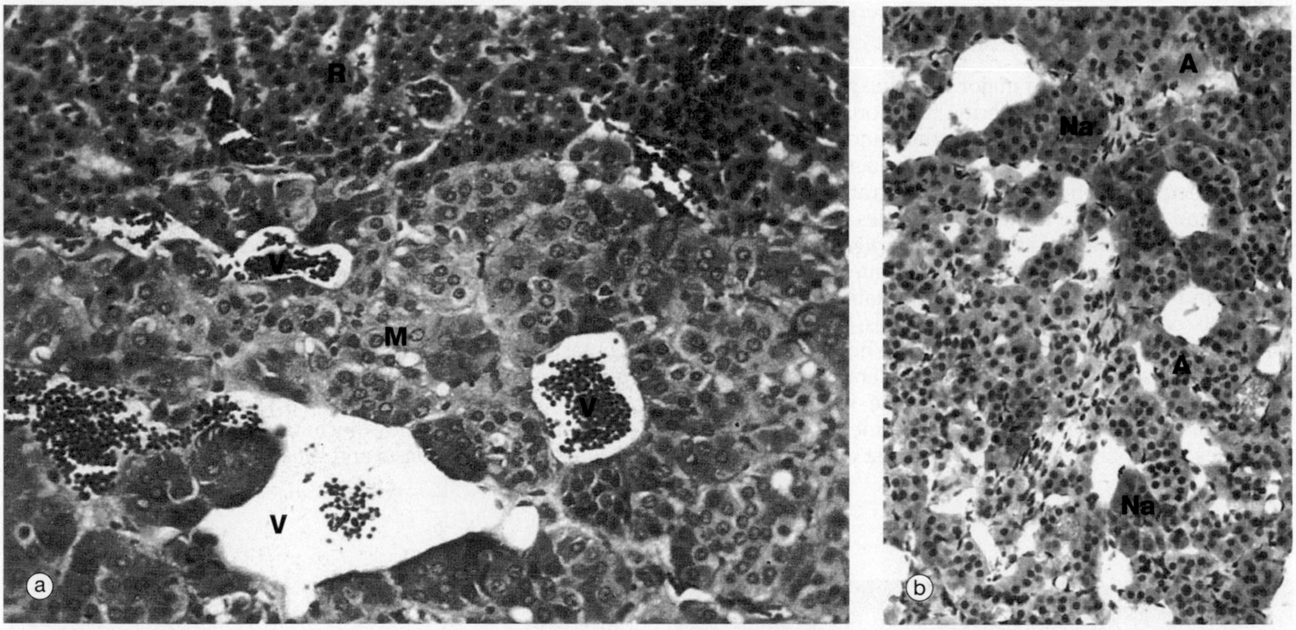

FIG. 17.17 Adrenal medulla
(a) H&E (MP) (b) Chrome salt fixation, H&E (MP)

The adrenal medulla secretes the amines ***adrenaline*** (***epinephrine***) and ***noradrenaline*** (***norepinephrine***) under the control of the sympathetic nervous system. When stained with the standard H&E method the adrenal medulla **M**, as shown in Fig. 17.17a, is composed of clusters of cells with granular, faintly basophilic cytoplasm, with numerous capillaries in their fine supporting stroma. Venous channels **V** draining blood from the sinusoids of the cortex pass through the medulla towards the central medullary vein. This photomicrograph also shows part of the zona reticularis **R** of the cortex.

When fixed in chrome salts as in Fig. 17.17b, the stored catecholamine granules of adrenal medullary cells are oxidised to a brown colour; consequently the name ***chromaffin cells*** was often applied to the secretory cells of the adrenal medulla. Some adrenal medullary cells synthesise noradrenaline; however, the majority synthesise adrenaline by the addition of a further N-methyl group to noradrenaline. Those cells containing noradrenaline **Na** exhibit a much more strongly positive chromaffin reaction than adrenaline-secreting cells **A**. Ultrastructurally, the cytoplasm of the medullary cells contains ***dense core granules*** similar to those illustrated in Fig. 17.23. The granules in adrenaline-secreting cells have a narrow clear halo surrounding the dense core, while those containing noradrenaline have a much wider clear halo around the dense core.

Secretion of catecholamines by the adrenal medulla is controlled by preganglionic neurones of the sympathetic nervous system; thus, the secretory cells of the adrenal medulla are functionally equivalent to the postganglionic neurones of the sympathetic nervous system. Acute physical and psychological stresses initiate release of adrenal medullary hormones. The released catecholamines act on adrenergic receptors throughout the body, particularly in the heart and blood vessels, bronchioles, visceral muscle and skeletal muscle, producing physiological effects very familiar to those who have ever taken a viva voce examination.

Adrenaline also has potent metabolic effects, such as the promotion of glycogenolysis in liver and skeletal muscle, thus releasing a readily available energy source during stress situations.

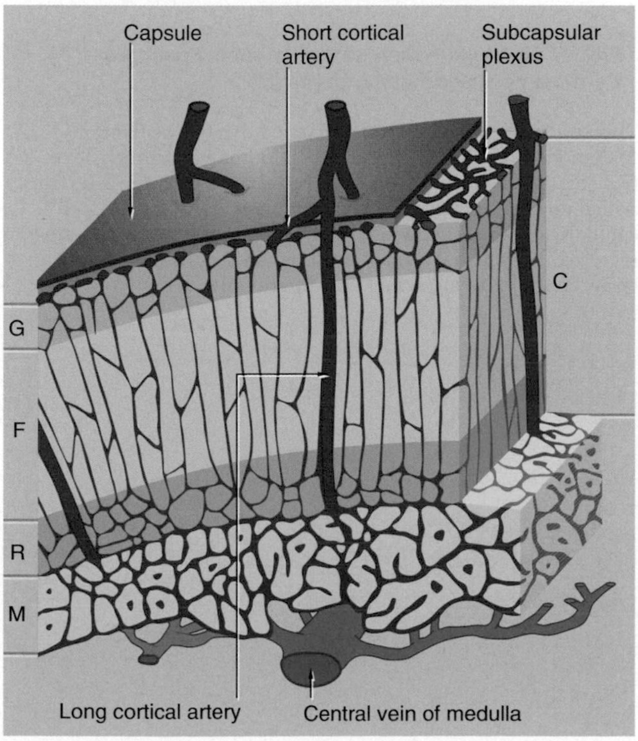

FIG. 17.18 Blood supply of the adrenal

The adrenal gland (Fig. 17.18) is supplied by the ***superior***, ***middle*** and ***inferior suprarenal arteries***, which form a plexus just under the capsule of the gland.

The vascular system of the cortex **C** consists of an anastomosing network of capillary sinusoids supplied by branches of the subcapsular plexus, known as ***short cortical arteries***. The sinusoids descend between the cords of secretory cells in the zona fasciculata **F** into a deep plexus in the zona reticularis **R** before draining into small venules which converge upon the central vein of the medulla **M**. The central medullary veins contain longitudinal bundles of smooth muscle between which the cortical venules enter; contraction of this smooth muscle is thought to hold back cortical blood and thus regulate flow.

The medulla is supplied by ***long cortical arteries*** which descend from the subcapsular plexus through the cortex into the medulla where they ramify into a rich network of dilated capillaries surrounding the medullary secretory cells. The medullary capillaries also drain into the central vein of the medulla. Thus the secretory cells of the medulla are exposed to fresh arterial blood as well as blood rich in adrenocorticosteroids, which are believed to have an important influence on the synthesis of adrenaline by the medulla.

ENDOCRINE PANCREAS

The *pancreas* is not only a major exocrine gland (see Ch. 15) but also has important endocrine functions.

The embryonic epithelium of the pancreatic ducts consists of both potential exocrine and endocrine cells. During development, the endocrine cells migrate from the duct system and aggregate around capillaries to form isolated clusters of cells known as ***islets of Langerhans***, scattered throughout the exocrine glandular tissue. The islets vary in size and are most numerous in the tail of the pancreas. The islets contain a variety of cell types, each responsible for secretion of one type of polypeptide hormone.

The main secretory products of the endocrine pancreas are ***insulin*** and ***glucagon***, polypeptide hormones which play an important role in carbohydrate metabolism. Insulin promotes the uptake of glucose by most cells, particularly those of the liver, skeletal muscle and adipose tissue, thus lowering plasma glucose concentration. In general, glucagon has metabolic effects that oppose the actions of insulin. Apart from their role in carbohydrate metabolism, these hormones have a wide variety of other effects on energy metabolism, growth and development.

At least five other types of endocrine cells are present in the islets or else scattered singly or in small groups between the exocrine acini and along the ducts. Their secretory products include ***somatostatin*** (which has a wide variety of effects on gastrointestinal function and may also inhibit insulin and glucagon secretion), and ***pancreatic polypeptide (PP)***. Another cell type, the ***enterochromaffin (EC)*** cell, appears to secrete several different peptides including ***motilin, 5-hydroxytryptamine (5-HT, serotonin)*** and ***substance P***.

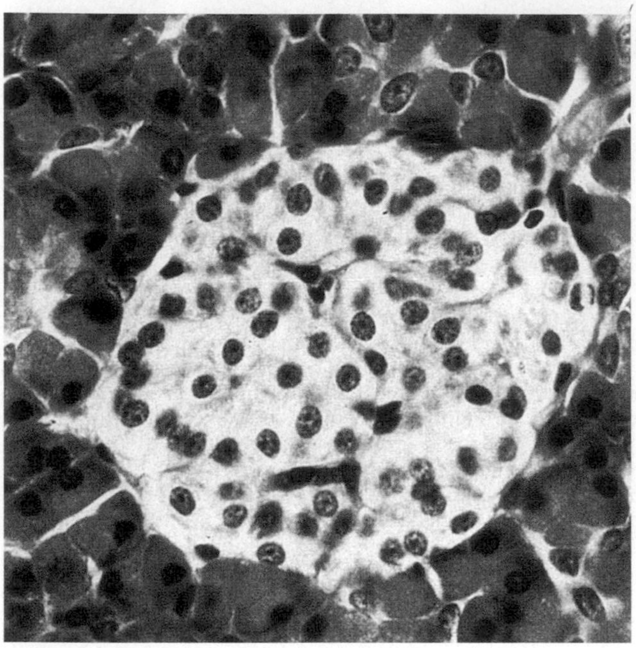

FIG. 17.19 Islet of Langerhans
H&E (HP)

The islets of Langerhans (Fig. 17.19) are composed of groups of up to 3000 secretory cells supported by a fine collagenous network containing numerous fenestrated capillaries. A delicate capsule surrounds each islet. The endocrine cells are small with a pale-stained granular cytoplasm: in contrast, the large cells of the surrounding exocrine pancreatic acini stain strongly.

The endocrine pancreas contains secretory cells of several types; however, in H&E stained preparations the cell types are indistinguishable from one another and special staining methods are required to differentiate between them.

Glucagon-, insulin-, somatostatin-, pancreatic polypeptide-, and ghrelin-secreting cells have been designated as ***alpha, beta, delta, gamma and epsilon*** cells, respectively. However, with the advent of immunohistochemical methods for identification of secretory products, it is most appropriate to identify cells by their products.

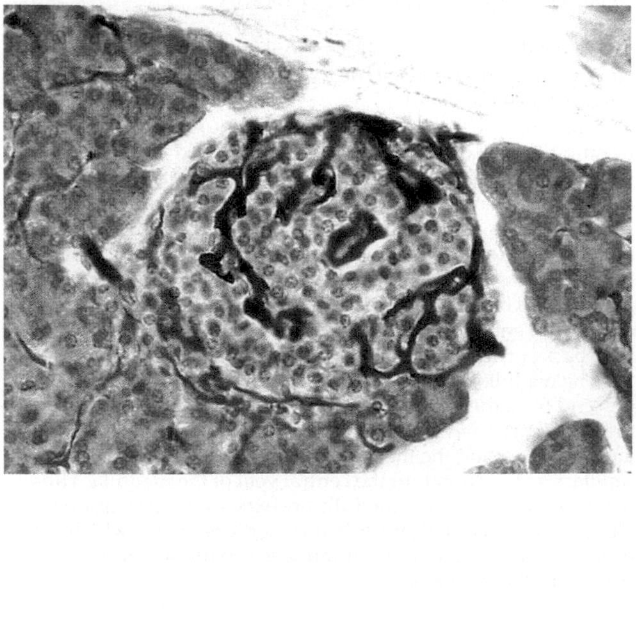

FIG. 17.20 Blood supply of the endocrine pancreas
Carmine perfused/haematoxylin (MP)

This specimen was perfused with a red dye before fixation to demonstrate the rich blood supply of the pancreatic islets (Fig. 17.20). Each islet is supplied by as many as three arterioles, which ramify into a highly branched network of fenestrated capillaries, into which the hormones produced in the islet are secreted. The islet is drained by about six venules, passing between the exocrine acini to the interlobular veins.

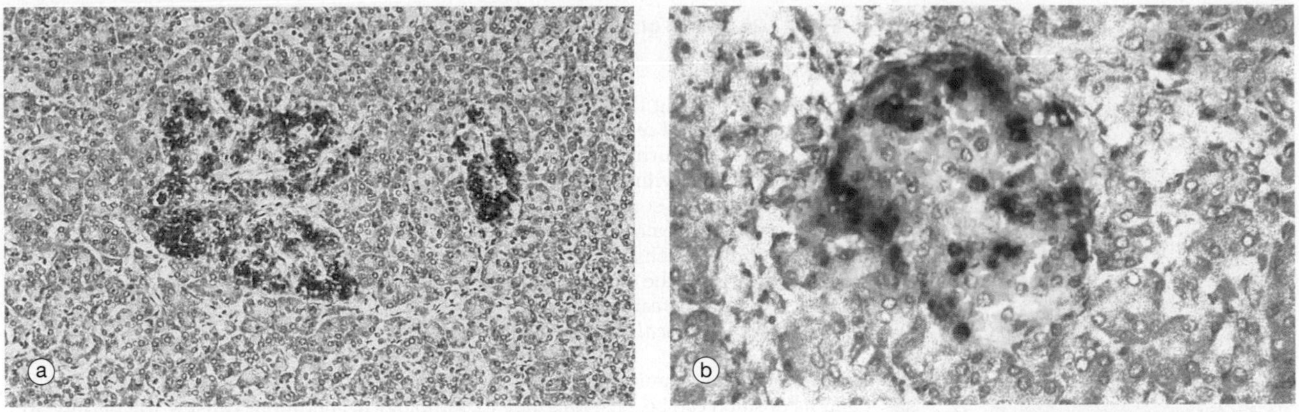

FIG. 17.21 Islet of Langerhans
(a) Immunohistochemical stain for insulin (MP) (b) Immunohistochemical stain for glucagon (HP)

In the past, empirical staining methods were used to demonstrate the different cell types in the islets of Langerhans. These have now been superseded by the immunohistochemical techniques which are able to detect specific intercellular products, in this case insulin and glucagon. The insulin-producing beta cells, which constitute over 60% of the cells in the islet, are stained brown in Fig. 17.21a. Beta cells are distributed throughout the islet, while in contrast, glucagon-producing alpha cells (about 25% of the total) are arranged around the periphery, as in Fig. 17.21b. Other hormone-producing cells are unstained in these micrographs. The close proximity of these cells facilitates their interaction for control of blood glucose levels and other metabolic functions.

Insulin, a small protein, is synthesised in the rough endoplasmic reticulum as ***preproinsulin*** which is then cleaved to form ***proinsulin***. Proinsulin is cleaved again, this time in the Golgi apparatus, to form insulin, which is then packaged with a small amount of uncleaved proinsulin into membrane-bound secretory granules which remain in the cytoplasm until insulin secretion is triggered.

Disorders of the endocrine pancreas

The islets of Langerhans contain endocrine cells which produce a range of hormones, but the most important disease is that associated with the production and function of insulin.

Diabetes mellitus

Diabetes mellitus is a common and important disease of insulin metabolism, resulting in hyperglycemia. There are two main types:

- Type 1 diabetes usually begins in childhood or adolescence and is the result of loss of endocrine cells in the pancreatic islets, including those which secrete insulin. The islet cell destruction is thought to be due to an abnormal autoimmune response, possibly triggered by a viral infection, and results in insulin deficiency. This has widespread metabolic effects on carbohydrate, protein and fat metabolism, leading to complex metabolic and structural effects.
- Type 2 diabetes is the result of the resistance of target cells to the effect of insulin, rather than a failure of insulin production by the pancreatic islets. It is becoming more common due to the increasing incidence of obesity.

Tumours of the islets of Langerhans

Rarely, tumours of the islets of Langerhans may produce disease as a result of excessive secretion of one of the islet hormones, for example, an insulin-secreting tumour produces ***hyperinsulinism*** with ***hypoglycaemic*** symptoms.

PINEAL GLAND

The ***pineal gland*** is a small, roughly spherical gland 6 to 10 mm in diameter which lies in the midline of the brain, just below the posterior end of the corpus callosum. It represents an evagination of the posterior part of the roof of the third ventricle. It is connected to the brain by a short stalk containing nerve fibres, some of which communicate with the hippocampus. The pineal gland synthesises the hormone ***melatonin*** which acts as an endocrine transducer, inducing rhythmical changes in the endocrine activity of the hypothalamus, pituitary, ovaries and testes in response to changes in light received by the retina. Melatonin production by the pineal is induced by darkness and inhibited by light, probably via sympathetic nerves transmitting messages from the eye through the suprachiasmatic nucleus, central sympathetic pathways and the superior cervical ganglion.

Effects of melatonin in man include an influence on the onset of puberty and body biorhythms. In other animals, it plays a role in the timing of seasonal reproductive cycles and, in reptiles and other lower vertebrates, is responsible for changing skin colour through its action on melanophores, pigmented cells analogous to melanocytes in mammals. Melatonin is also synthesised in many peripheral tissues, where it appears to have paracrine effects. In recent years, melatonin has been used as a treatment for sleep disturbance (e.g. jet lag) and melatonin analogues are also used to treat depression.

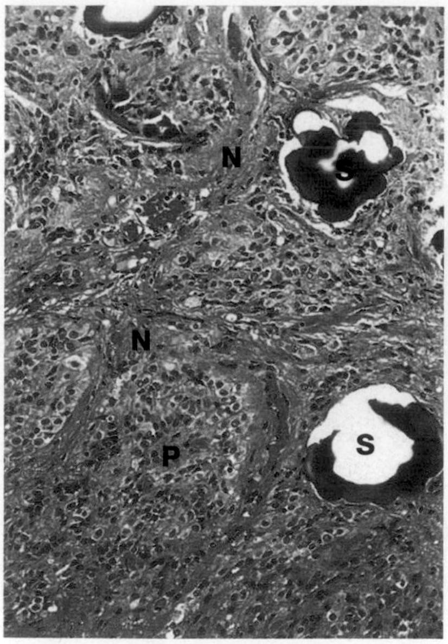

FIG. 17.22 Pineal gland
H&E (MP)

The pineal gland (Fig 17.22) consists of two main cell types: ***pinealocytes*** (***pineal chief cells***) and ***neuroglial cells***. Pinealocytes **P** are highly modified neurones, arranged in clusters and cords surrounded by a rich network of fenestrated capillaries. Pinealocytes have round nuclei with prominent nucleoli and granular cytoplasm and many highly branched processes, some of which terminate near or upon blood vessels. The cytoplasmic granules of pinealocytes contain melatonin and its precursor, 5-HT.

The neuroglial cells **N**, which are similar to the astrocytes of the rest of the CNS, are dispersed between the clusters of pinealocytes and in association with capillaries.

A characteristic feature of the ageing pineal is the presence of basophilic extracellular bodies called ***pineal sand*** **S**, consisting of concentric layers of calcium and magnesium

phosphate in an organic matrix. The calcified pineal can be seen on X-rays of the skull and its position can be a useful guide to pathological conditions causing the midline to be displaced to one side.

DIFFUSE NEUROENDOCRINE SYSTEM

This is the name given to a scattered system of neuroendocrine cells which secrete hormones and active peptides. Neuroendocrine cells possess characteristic membrane-bound neurosecretory vesicles, usually spherical, with an electron-dense central core (***dense core vesicles***). Although neuroendocrine-type cells form part of other endocrine organs (e.g. adrenal medulla) and some non-endocrine organs (e.g. islets of Langerhans in the pancreas, juxtaglomerular apparatus in the kidney), they are particularly important in the diffuse neuroendocrine systems in the gastrointestinal and respiratory tracts.

Gastrointestinal neuroendocrine cells are found scattered in the mucosa of the gastrointestinal tract and in the pancreatic and biliary ducts. These cells secrete more than 20 different peptide and amine hormones, including gastrin, secretin, CCK, 5-HT, enteroglucagon, somatostatin, substance P, vasoactive intestinal peptide (VIP), bombesin, gastric inhibitory polypeptide (GIP), motilin and pancreatic polypeptide (PP). These hormones constitute a system of interacting mediators which collectively regulate and coordinate most aspects of gastrointestinal activity, in concert with the autonomic nervous system.

While some of these substances are true ***endocrine hormones***, acting at a distance from their site of origin, others are locally acting mediators known as ***paracrine hormones***. A third mechanism of action (***neurocrine***) is by neurotransmitter activity and indeed some of these substances also act as neurotransmitters within the central nervous system (gastrin, VIP, CCK and many others).

The lower respiratory tract contains scattered peptide- and amine-secreting endocrine cells, analogous to those in the gastrointestinal tract, which are probably involved in local and autonomically mediated regulation of respiratory tract function, particularly in early childhood. The endocrine cells are scattered individually in the epithelium or in clumps (see Fig. 12.11) protruding into the airway and have a variety of secretory products including 5-HT, calcitonin, bombesin and leu-enkephalin.

Tumours of the diffuse neuroendocrine system

The cells of the diffuse neuroendocrine system may occasionally give rise to tumours. The most frequent, and most important, is a highly malignant tumour of neuroendocrine cells of the bronchial tree, called small cell carcinoma (see e-Fig. 17.10). This tumour grows very rapidly and infiltrates and destroys nearby tissues, but also spreads to distant sites such as bones, liver, and brain (***metastases***). Some of these tumours retain some capacity to synthesise and secrete hormones or hormone-precursor molecules and, rarely, excessive secretion of these can cause fatal metabolic disorders. Small cell carcinoma of the lung often secretes an ACTH-like substance which stimulates excessive and uncontrolled secretion of hormones from the adrenal cortex.

A tumour of the neuroendocrine cells (see e-Fig. 17.11) in the alimentary tract is called a neuroendocrine tumour (NET). These are most common in the small intestine and appendix and grow slowly. They secrete 5-HT which usually has no systemic effect because it passes from the tumour in the gut via the hepatic portal vein to the liver where it is broken down into inactive products. Although these tumours are slow-growing, they are potentially malignant and can spread to secondary sites away from the gut. In this case, 5-HT can enter the systemic blood circulation and produce metabolic effects; this is called carcinoid syndrome (see e-Fig 17.12).

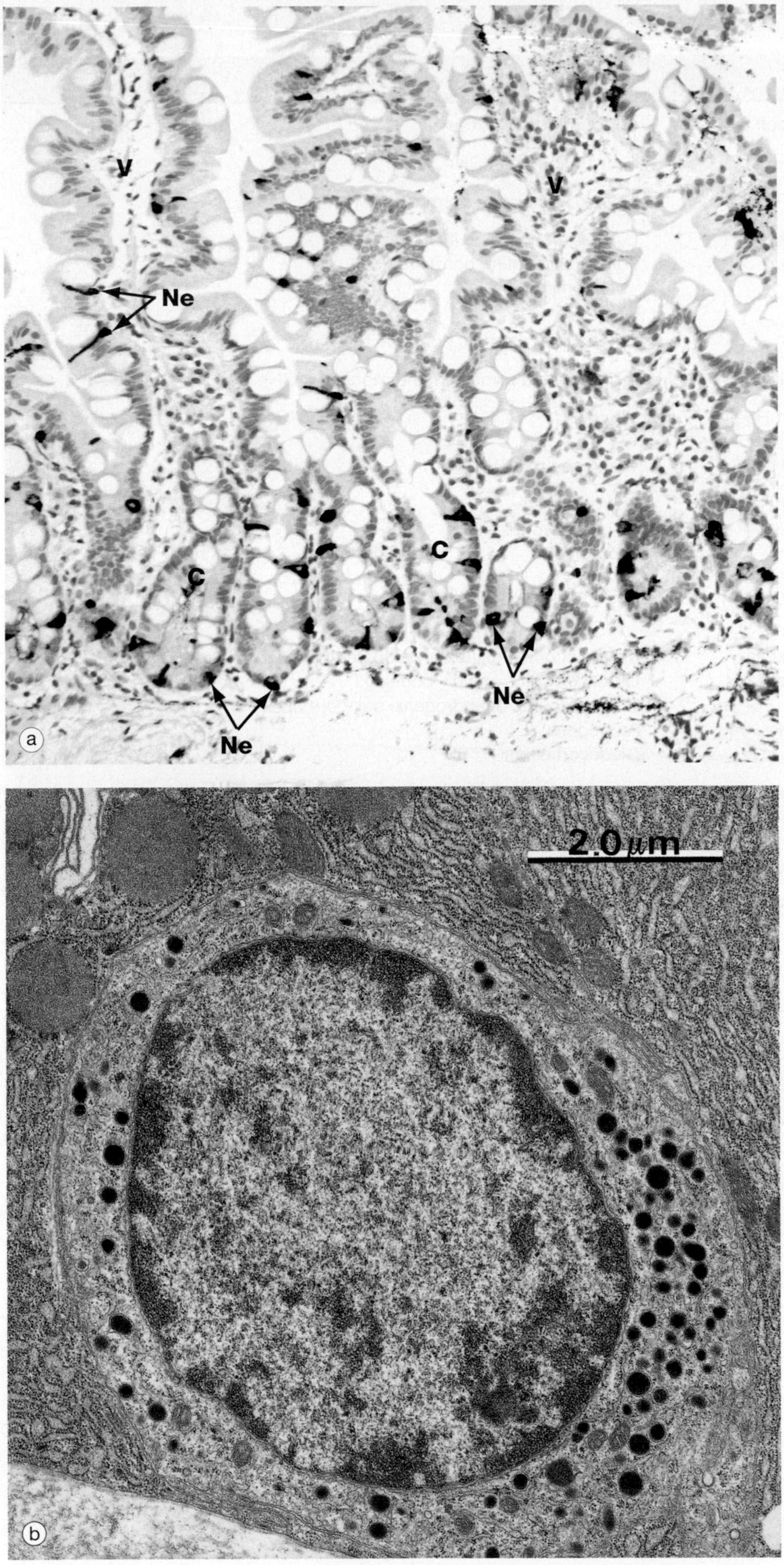

FIG. 17.23 Gastrointestinal neuro-endocrine cells
(a) Immunohistochemical stain for chromogranin A (MP) (b) EM ×12 500

Neuroendocrine cells are very difficult to identify on H&E stained sections, but immunohistochemistry and electron microscopy make the task easy. Fig. 17.23a shows duodenal mucosa with the crypts **C** as well as the lower segments of the villi **V** stained by an immunohistochemical method for chromogranin A. Chromogranin A is a component of all neurosecretory granules and so merely identifies the cells as neuroendocrine cells, without giving any clue as to their secretory product. The neuroendocrine cells **Ne** (dark brown) are pyramidal-shaped, with a broad base sitting on the basement membrane of the epithelium and a narrower part approaching the lumen of the gland. In so-called open-type mucosal neuroendocrine cells, the narrow end of the cell is in contact with the lumen and its contents. Note that the neuroendocrine cells are concentrated in the crypts, but occasional cells are also seen within the villous epithelium.

Fig. 17.23b shows a somatostatin-secreting neuroendocrine cell in the gastric mucosa. The cytoplasm contains large numbers of electron-dense neurosecretory vacuoles (dense core granules); they are mainly spherical, of various sizes, and are particularly concentrated towards the base of the cell.

C duodenal crypt **V** duodenal villus **N** neuroglial cells **Ne** neuroendocrine cell **P** pinealocytes **S** pineal sand

REVIEW

TABLE 17.1 Review of endocrine system

Specialised tissue type	Specialised cell type	Functional attributes	Figure
Anterior pituitary	Somatotrophs	Growth hormone (GH)	17.3, 17.4
	Thyrotrophs	Thyroid stimulating hormone (TSH)	
	Gonadotrophs	Luteinising hormone (LH) Follicle stimulating hormone (FSH)	
	Lactotrophs	Prolactin	
	Corticotrophs	Adrenocorticotrophic hormone (ACTH)	
Pars intermedia	Corticotroph-like cells	α-Melanocyte stimulating hormone (α-MSH)	17.4
Posterior pituitary	Neurones with Herring bodies Pituicyte (glial cells)	Oxytocin Vasopressin (ADH)	17.5
Thyroid	Follicular epithelial cells C-cells	Thyroxine (T_4) Tri-iodothyronine (T_3) Calcitonin	17.6–17.9
Parathyroid	Chief cells Oxyphil cells	Parathyroid hormone (PTH)	17.10, 17.11
Adrenal cortex	Zona glomerulosa Zona fasciculata Zona reticularis	Mineralocorticoids (mainly aldosterone) Glucocorticoids (mainly cortisol) Small amounts of androgenic sex hormones Androgens Glucocorticoids	17.13 17.14 17.15
Adrenal medulla	Chromaffin cells	Adrenaline (epinephrine) Noradrenaline (norepinephrine)	17.17
Islets of Langerhans (pancreas)	Alpha cells Beta cells Gamma cells PP cells	Glucagon Insulin Somatostatin Pancreatic polypeptide	17.19–17.21
Pineal	Pinealocytes	Melatonin	17.22
Diffuse neuroendocrine system (gastrointestinal and respiratory tracts)	Neuroendocrine cells	Many different products including gastrin, secretin, CCK, 5-HT, enteroglucagon, somatostatin, substance P, vasoactive intestinal polypeptide (VIP), bombesin, gastric inhibitory polypeptide (GIP), motilin, PP, leu-enkephalin, calcitonin	17.23

18 Male reproductive system

INTRODUCTION

The male reproductive system is responsible for the production of ***spermatozoa*** and their delivery into the female reproductive tract and may be divided into four major functional components:

- The ***testes*** or male gonads, paired organs lying in the ***scrotal sac***, are responsible for production of the male gametes, ***spermatozoa***, and secretion of male sex hormones, principally ***testosterone***.
- A system of ducts consisting of ***ductuli efferentes, epididymis, ductus (vas) deferens*** and ***ejaculatory duct*** collects, stores and carries spermatozoa from each testis. The ejaculatory ducts converge on the urethra, from which spermatozoa are expelled into the female reproductive tract during copulation.
- Two exocrine glands, the paired ***seminal vesicles*** and the single ***prostate gland***, secrete a nutritive and lubricating fluid medium called ***seminal fluid*** in which spermatozoa are conveyed to the female reproductive tract. ***Semen***, the fluid expelled during ejaculation, consists of seminal fluid and spermatozoa, plus some desquamated duct-lining cells.
- The ***penis*** is the organ of copulation. A pair of small accessory glands, the ***bulbourethral glands of Cowper***, secrete a fluid which lubricates the urethra for the passage of semen during ejaculation.

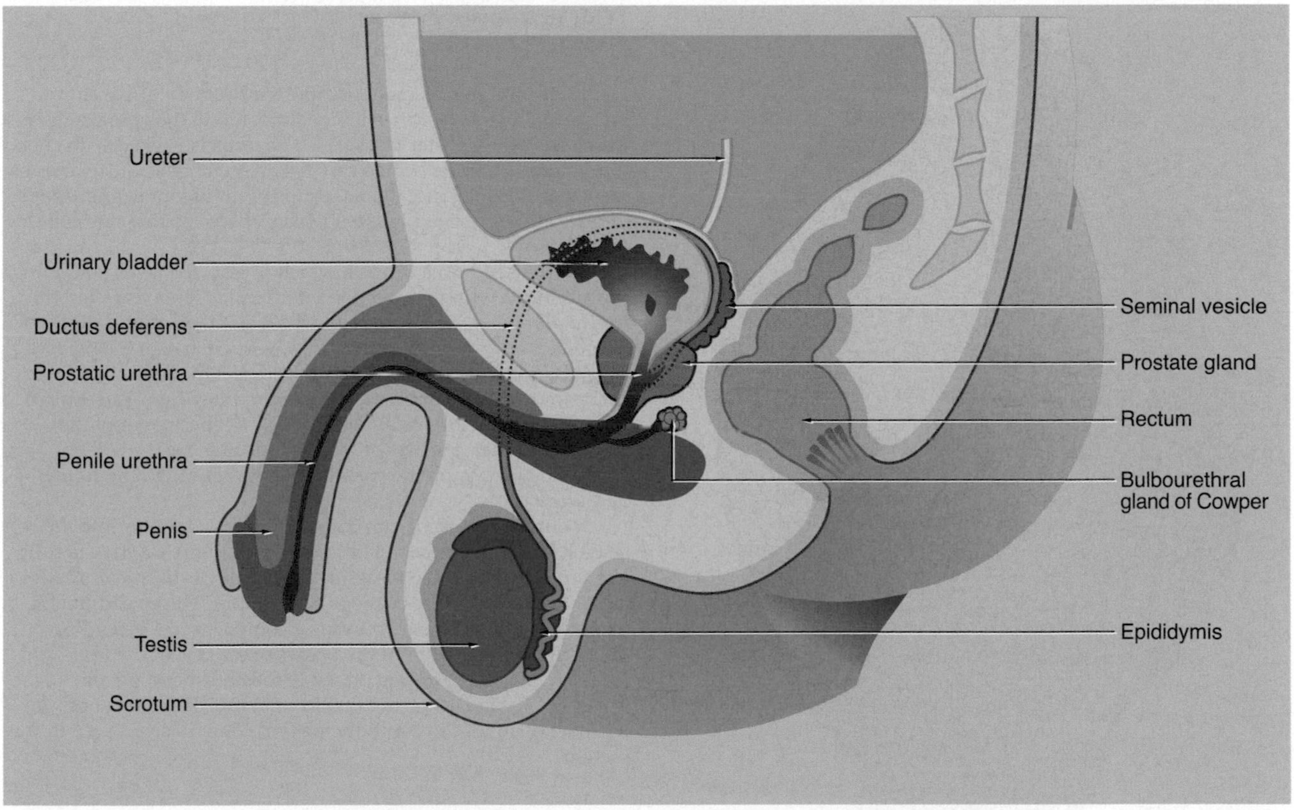

FIG. 18.1 Male reproductive system

Embryology of the male genital tract

Many of the structures of the male genital tract are derived from the paired ***Wolffian*** or ***mesonephric ducts***. These give rise to the right and left epididymis, vas deferens, ejaculatory duct and seminal vesicle. The prostate gland develops from the urogenital sinus whilst the testes have a separate origin, developing from mesoderm high in the posterior abdominal wall and later descending into the scrotum via the processus vaginalis. Testicular descent begins after the third month of pregnancy and is generally complete by term. Failure of this process may cause ***cryptorchidism***. Uncorrected, this can be associated with later subfertility. If the processus vaginalis fails to close and regress after testicular descent, this can predispose to the development of a ***hydrocoele*** (a collection of fluid around the testis) or an ***indirect inguinal hernia***, where abdominal contents can pass along the inguinal canal to the scrotum.

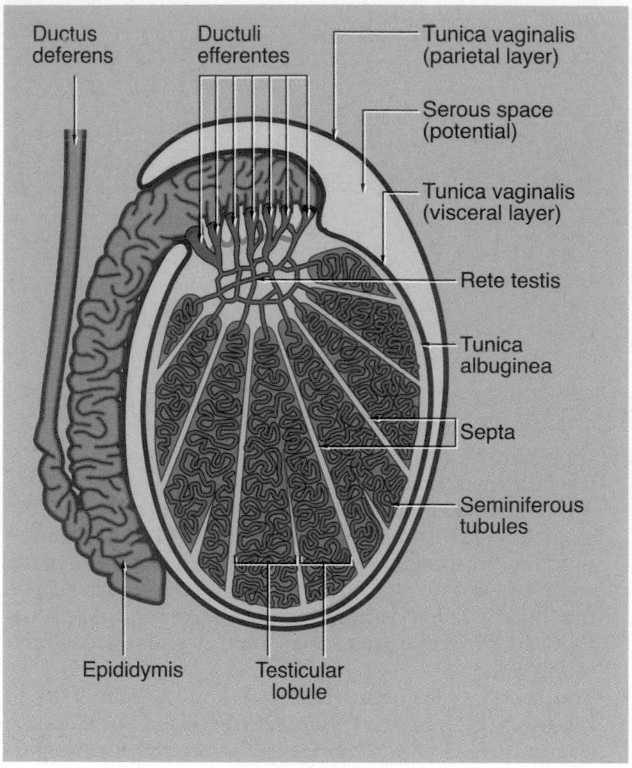

FIG. 18.2 Testis

During embryological development, each testis with the first part of its duct system, blood vessels, lymphatics and nerves descends from the posterior wall of the peritoneal cavity to the scrotum. During migration, the testis carries with it an investing layer of peritoneum so that in the scrotum the testis is almost completely surrounded by a double layer of mesothelium, enclosing a potential space. This double lining is called the ***tunica vaginalis*** and, like the pleura, consists of ***visceral*** and ***parietal layers***, separated by a thin layer of serous fluid. The fluid is secreted by the mesothelial cells and acts as a lubricant, allowing the testis to move freely in the scrotal sac. The visceral layer of the tunica vaginalis rests on the capsule of the testis, the ***tunica albuginea***, which gives rise to numerous incomplete collagenous septa. These divide the testis into about 250 ***testicular lobules***. Within each lobule, there are one to four highly convoluted tubes, the ***seminiferous tubules***, in which spermatozoa are produced. The seminiferous tubules converge upon a plexus of channels, the ***rete testis***. From the rete testis, 15 to 20 small ducts called the ***ductuli efferentes*** carry spermatozoa to the extremely tortuous first part of the ***ductus deferens***, which is known as the ***epididymis***.

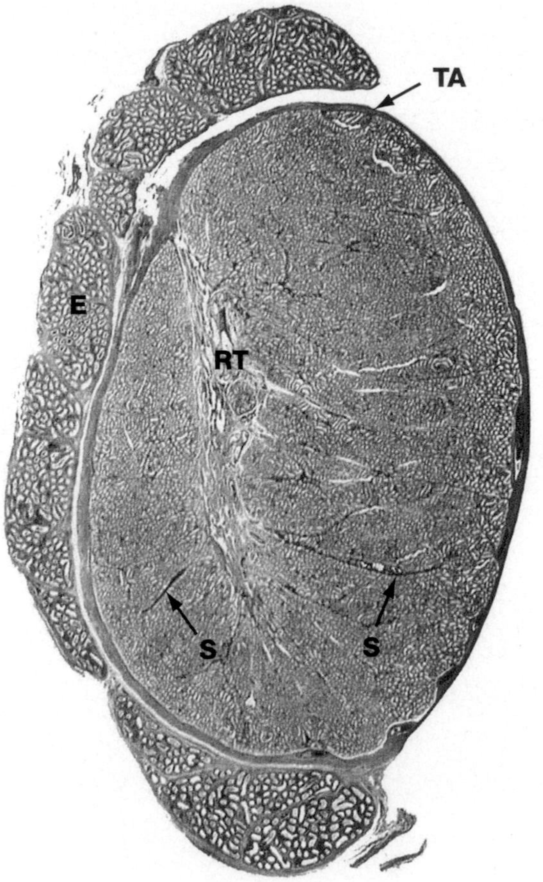

FIG. 18.3 Testis, monkey
H&E (LP)

Fig. 18.3 illustrates the macroscopic features of a testis; cut in the sagittal plane, it shows the relationship to the epididymis **E**, which lies on its posterior aspect. The testis is packed with coiled seminiferous tubules which can just be seen in various planes of section at this magnification. Groups of up to four seminiferous tubules are segregated into testicular lobules by fine interlobular septa **S**.

The dense fibrous capsule which invests the testis, and which is continuous with many of the interlobular septa, is called the ***tunica albuginea*** **TA**. It contains fibroblasts and abundant myofibroblasts and smooth muscle cells, particularly in the posterior aspect close to the rete testis, which subject the seminiferous tissue to rhythmic contractions. Scattered Leydig cells are also found within the tunica albuginea. The deepest layer of the tunica albuginea consists of loose connective tissue containing blood and lymphatic vessels, sometimes called the ***tunica vasculosa***.

Spermatozoa pass from the seminiferous tubules into the rete testis **RT**, which is connected to the epididymis via the ductuli efferentes at the upper posterior pole of the testis; the ductuli are not included in the plane of this section. The epididymis is a tightly coiled tube which forms a compact mass extending down the whole length of the posterior surface of the testis and is the major site of storage of newly formed spermatozoa. At the lower pole of the testis, the epididymal tube becomes continuous with the relatively straight ductus (vas) deferens, not seen in this section.

The testes

Most of the structures of the male reproductive system arise from the Wolffian (mesonephric) duct system as described above (see textbox, 'Embryology of the male genital tract'), however the testes arise from the ***genital ridge***, a thickening in the mesothelium high on the posterior wall of the peritoneal cavity. The organs later descend to their adult position in the scrotum. As a result, the blood supply and lymphatic drainage of the testes is derived from the upper abdomen, with the paired testicular arteries arising from the abdominal aorta, just distal to the origin of the renal arteries. This embryological fact is important in understanding why testicular (and also ovarian) tumours typically spread to para-aortic lymph nodes, rather than to local lymph nodes in the pelvic or inguinal area.

GAMETOGENESIS

In all somatic cells, cell division (***mitosis***) results in the formation of two daughter cells, each one genetically identical to the mother cell. Somatic cells contain a full complement of chromosomes (the ***diploid number***) which function as homologous pairs (see Ch. 2). The process of sexual reproduction involves the fusion of specialised male and female cells called ***gametes*** to form a ***zygote***, which has the diploid number of chromosomes. Each gamete contains only half the diploid number of chromosomes, one representative of each pair; this half complement of chromosomes is known as the ***haploid number***.

The production of haploid cells involves a unique form of cell division called ***meiosis***, which occurs only in the germ cells of the gonads during the formation of gametes; meiotic cell division is thus also called ***gametogenesis***. Meiosis involves two cell division cycles, of which only the first is preceded by duplication of chromosomes (see Ch. 2). Thus, meiotic cell division of a single diploid germ cell gives rise to four haploid gametes. In the male, each of the four gametes undergoes morphological development into a mature ***spermatozoon***. In contrast, in the female, unequal distribution of the cytoplasm during meiosis results in one gamete gaining almost all the cytoplasm from the mother cell, while the other three acquire almost no cytoplasm; the large gamete matures to form an ***ovum*** and the other three, called ***polar bodies***, degenerate.

The primitive germ cells of the male, the ***spermatogonia***, are present only in small numbers in the male gonads before sexual maturity. After puberty, spermatogonia multiply continuously by mitosis to provide a supply of cells which then undergo meiosis to form male gametes. In contrast, the germ cells of the female, called ***oogonia***, multiply by mitosis only during early fetal development, thereby producing a fixed complement of cells with the potential to undergo gametogenesis. Gametogenesis in the female is discussed more fully in Ch. 19. The production of male gametes is called ***spermatogenesis*** and the subsequent development of the male gamete into a motile spermatozoon is called ***spermiogenesis***, the whole process taking approximately 70 days; both these processes occur within the testes, although final maturation of spermatozoa occurs in the epididymis.

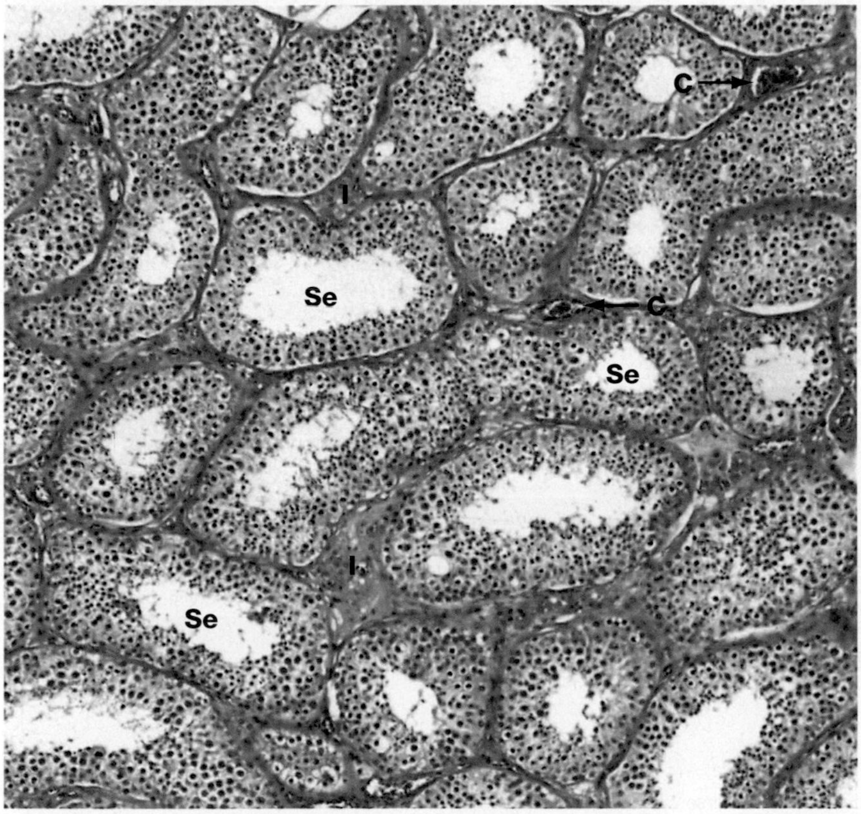

FIG. 18.4 Seminiferous tubules H&E (MP)

This micrograph illustrates seminiferous tubules cut in various planes of section. The seminiferous tubules are highly convoluted and are lined by:

- Germ cells in various stages of spermatogenesis and spermiogenesis, which are collectively referred to as the ***spermatogenic series***
- Non–germ cells, called ***Sertoli cells***, which support and nourish the developing spermatozoa are also found within the seminiferous tubules.
- In the interstitial spaces between the tubules, endocrine cells called ***Leydig cells*** are found either singly or in groups in the supporting tissue.

In this micrograph of normal testis at medium power, note the seminiferous tubules **Se** cut in various planes of section, giving round and ovoid profiles. Between the seminiferous tubules the interstitium **I** contains Leydig cells (which cannot be discerned at this magnification) and small capillaries **C**. Larger arteries and veins are found in the fibrous septa that divide the organ into lobules.

Testicular pathology

Common disorders affecting the testis include infective and inflammatory processes (causing ***orchitis***), ***torsion*** (twisting of the organ which blocks off the blood supply, see e-Fig. 18.1) and a variety of tumours. These can arise in any of the normal components of the testis but the majority are derived from the multipotent cells of the seminiferous tubules and these are called ***germ cell tumours*** (see e-Table. 18.1). This is a very diverse group of tumours but, in broad terms, most of these are malignant tumours and they may be divided very broadly into ***seminoma*** (resembling the normal cells in the seminiferous tubules, see e-Fig. 18.2) and ***non seminomatous germ cell tumours*** (resembling a variety of embryonal or extra-embryonal structures). Combinations of these types are common (see e-Fig. 18.3). This division reflects important differences in tumour management and prognosis.

C capillary **E** epididymis **I** interstitium **RT** rete testis **S** interlobular septum **Se** seminiferous tubule **TA** tunica albuginea

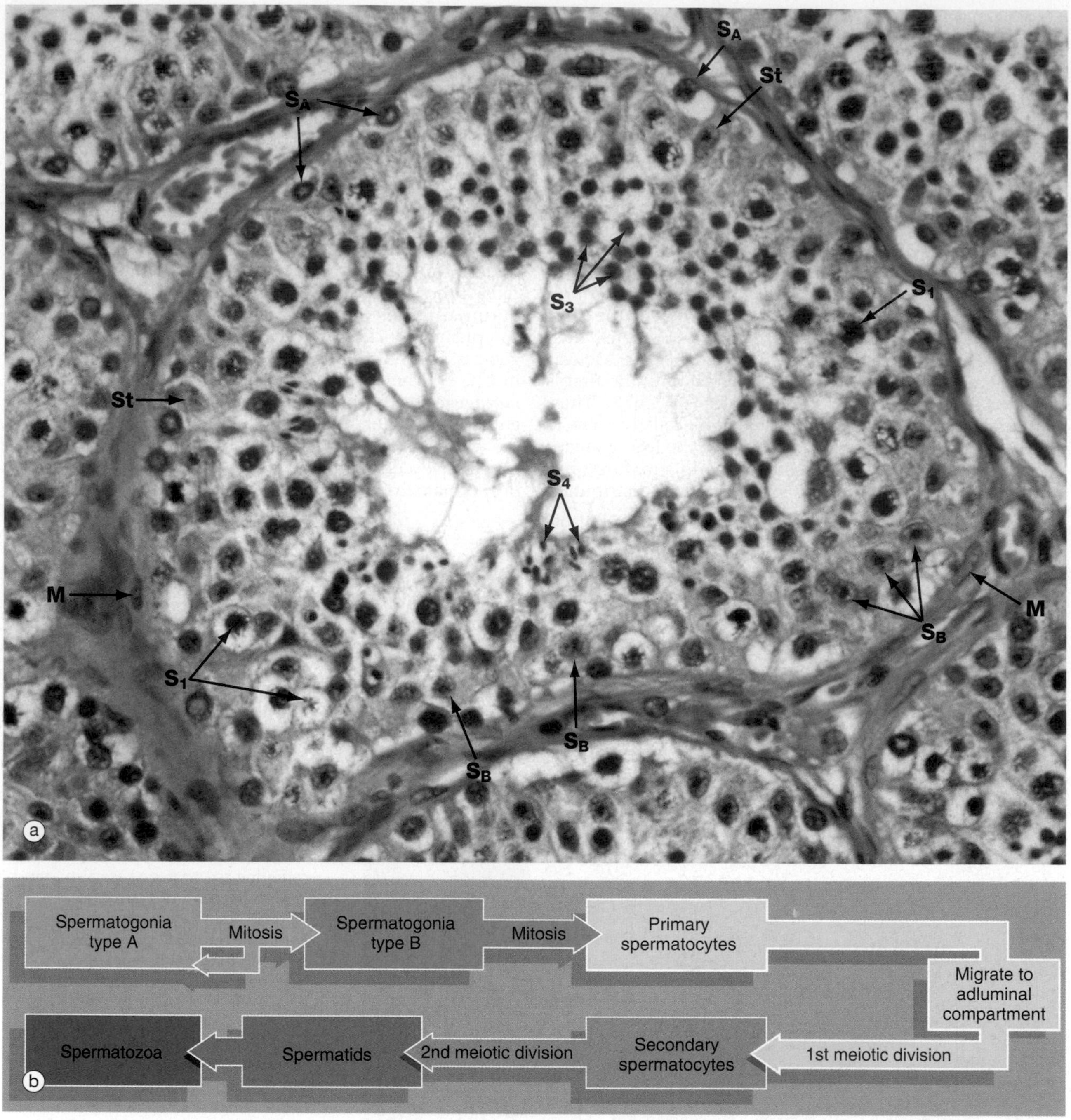

FIG. 18.5 Seminiferous tubule
(a) H&E (HP) (b) Diagram

Fig. 18.5a illustrates an adult seminiferous tubule cut in transverse section. The processes of ***spermatogenesis*** and ***spermiogenesis*** are synchronised, with waves of activity occurring sequentially along the length of each tubule. Thus in a single cross-section of a tubule, not all development phases will be represented (Fig. 18.5b).

The undifferentiated diploid germ cells, found in the basal compartment of the seminiferous tubule, are called ***type A spermatogonia***. These go through several cycles of mitosis to produce further type A spermatogonia, which maintain the germ cell pool, and ***type B spermatogonia***, which are committed to production of spermatozoa. Spermatogonia type A $\mathbf{S_A}$ are characterised by a large round or oval nucleus with condensed chromatin; peripheral nucleoli and a nuclear vacuole may be prominent. Spermatogonia type B $\mathbf{S_B}$ have dispersed chromatin, central nucleoli, and no nuclear vacuole. Both types of spermatogonia have sparse poorly stained cytoplasm.

Type B spermatogonia undergo further mitotic divisions to produce ***primary spermatocytes***. These migrate to the adluminal compartment of the seminiferous tubule before commencing the first meiotic division. Primary spermatocytes $\mathbf{S_1}$ are readily recognised by their copious cytoplasm and large nuclei containing coarse clumps or thin threads of chromatin; dividing cells may be seen. In humans, the first meiotic division cycle takes approximately 3 weeks to complete, after which time the daughter cells become known as ***secondary spermatocytes***. The smaller secondary spermatocytes rapidly undergo the second meiotic division and are therefore seldom seen.

The gametes thus produced, called ***spermatids*** $\mathbf{S_3}$, then proceed through the long maturation process known as spermiogenesis to become recognisable as spermatozoa. During this process, the nuclei of the spermatids assume the small pointed form of spermatozoa $\mathbf{S_4}$ (Fig. 18.7). Examination of different sections of the tubules of a normal testis shows about half the spermatogenic cells to be in the late spermatid stage.

During the developmental process, the cells of the spermatogenic series are supported by ***Sertoli cells*** **St**, whose nuclei are usually found towards the basement membrane of the seminiferous tubule. The Sertoli cell nucleus is typically triangular or ovoid in shape with a prominent nucleolus and dispersed chromatin.

The basal layer of germinal cells is supported by a basement membrane which is surrounded by a lamina propria containing several layers of spindle-shaped myofibroblasts **M** and fibroblasts.

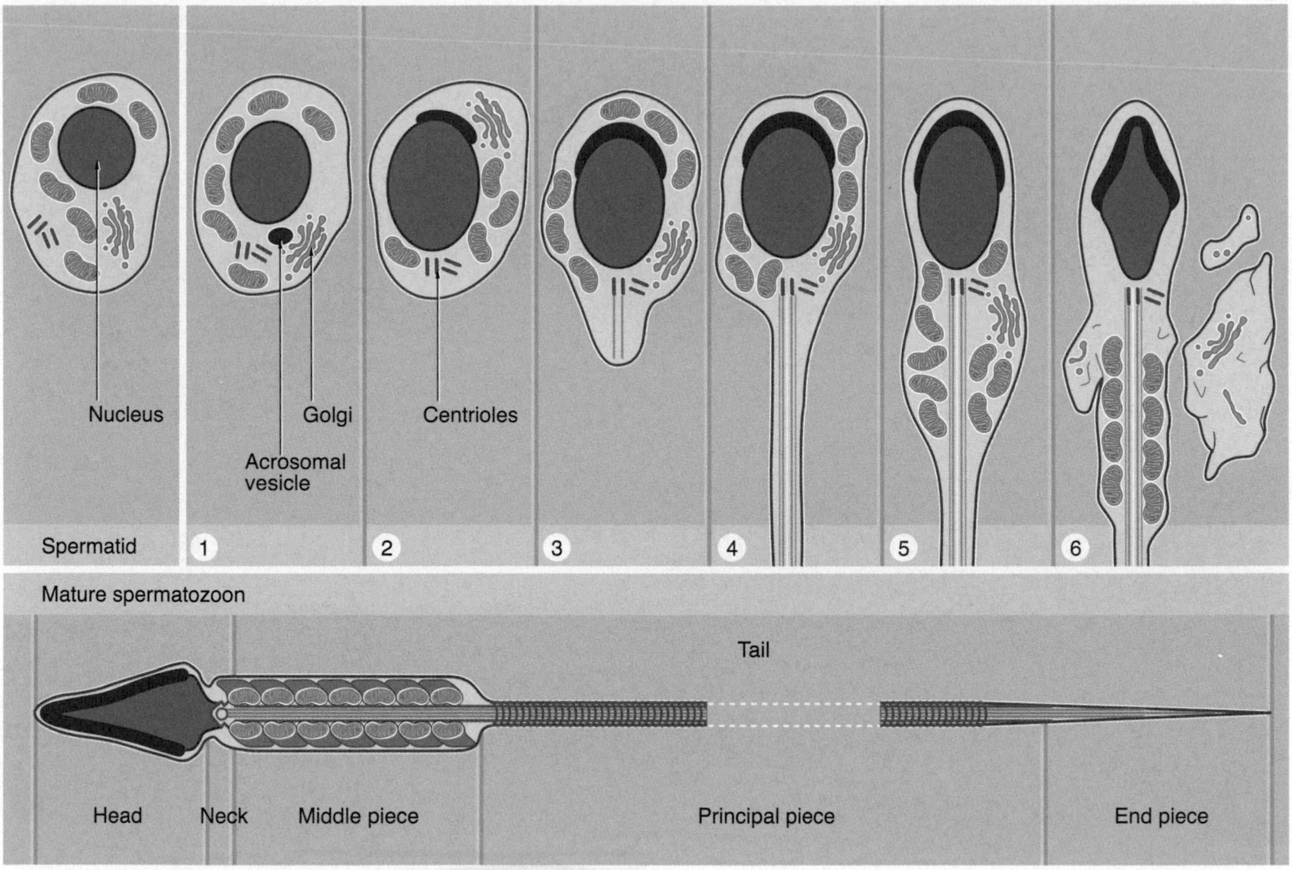

FIG. 18.6 Spermiogenesis

Spermiogenesis is the process by which spermatids, the gametes produced by meiotic division, are transformed into motile mature spermatozoa. This involves the following major stages:

1. The Golgi apparatus elaborates a large membrane-bound vesicle, the ***acrosomal vesicle***, which accumulates carbohydrates and hydrolytic enzymes.
2. The acrosomal vesicle becomes applied to one pole of the progressively elongating nucleus to form a structure known as the ***acrosomal head cap***.
3. Meanwhile, both centrioles migrate to the end of the cell opposite to the acrosomal head cap; the centriole aligned parallel to the long axis of the nucleus elongates to form a flagellum which has a basic structure similar to that of the cilium (see Fig. 5.13).
4. As the flagellum elongates, nine ***coarse fibrils***, which may contain contractile proteins, become arranged longitudinally around the core of the flagellum. Further rib-like fibrils then become disposed circumferentially around the whole flagellum.
5. The cytoplasm migrates to surround the first part of the flagellum. The remainder of the flagellum appears to project from the cell but in fact remains surrounded by plasma membrane. This migration of cytoplasm thus concentrates mitochondria in the flagellar region.
6. As the flagellum elongates, excess cytoplasm is phagocytosed by the enveloping Sertoli cell prior to release of the spermatid into the lumen, a process called ***spermiation***.

The mitochondria become arranged in a helical manner around the fibrils which surround the first part of the flagellum.

The structure of fully formed spermatozoa varies in detail from species to species but conforms to the basic structure seen in this diagram of a human spermatozoon.

Throughout the entire developmental process from spermatogonia to spermatozoa, hundreds of spermatids remain connected to one another by narrow cytoplasmic bridges which only break down upon release of spermatozoa into the lumen of the seminiferous tubule. This explains the synchronous development of spermatozoa at any one part of the tubule.

Sertoli cells are important in the regulation of spermatogenesis and spermiogenesis. Sertoli cells form tight junctions with each other as well as with the developing germ cells. It is well established that high concentrations of androgen hormones, secreted by Leydig cells of the testicular interstitium (Fig. 18.10), are essential for production and maturation of spermatogenic cells. Sertoli cells secrete an androgen-binding protein which transports testosterone and dihydrotestosterone to the lumen of the seminiferous tubule. These hormones are also necessary for function of the epithelium of the rete testis and epididymis; production of this binding protein is believed to be dependent on the pituitary gonadotrophin follicle stimulating hormone (FSH).

M myofibroblast **S_A** type A spermatogonium **S_B** type B spermatogonium **S_1** primary spermatocyte **S_3** spermatid **S_4** spermatozoon **St** Sertoli cell

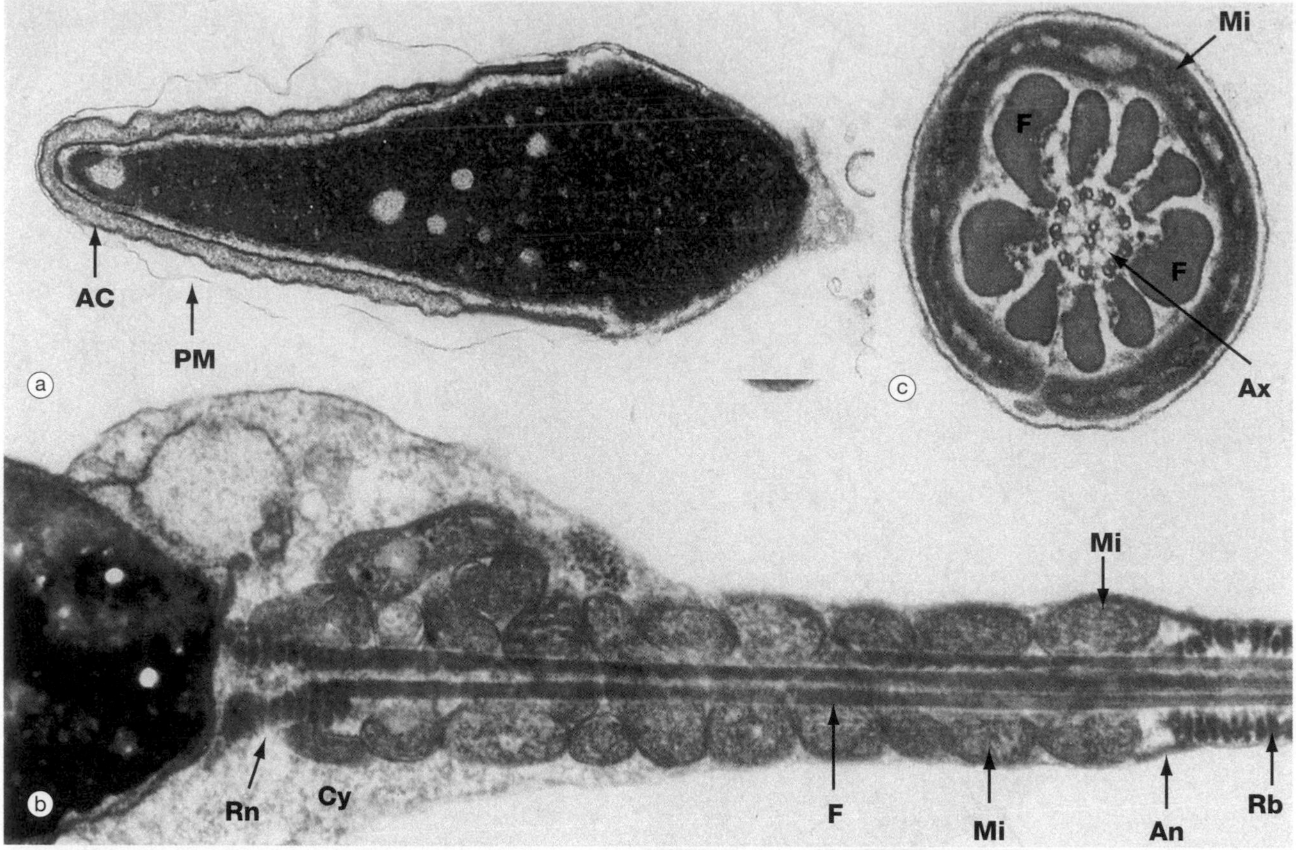

FIG. 18.7 Spermatozoa
(a) Head, LS, EM ×14 000 (b) Neck (middle piece and principal piece), LS, EM ×17 000 (c) Middle piece, TS, EM ×48 000

The ultrastructural features of human spermatozoa are shown in these micrographs. The spermatozoon is an extremely elongated cell (about 65 μm long) consisting of three main components: the ***head***, ***neck*** and ***tail***. The tail is subdivided into three segments: the ***middle piece***, ***principal piece*** and ***end piece*** (see Fig. 18.6).

The head is the most variable structure between different mammalian species. In humans the head is about 7 μm long and has a flattened pear shape. As seen in Fig. 18.7a, the nucleus, which occupies most of the head, is composed of very condensed chromatin; in humans, this contains a variable number of areas of dispersed chromatin called ***nuclear vacuoles***. Surrounding the anterior two-thirds of the nucleus is the acrosomal cap **AC**, a flattened membrane-bound vesicle containing a range of glycoproteins and a variety of hydrolytic enzymes, principally hyaluronidase; the enzymes disaggregate the cells of the corona radiata and dissolve the zona pellucida during fertilisation (see Ch. 19). Note the plasma membrane **PM**, which has become partially separated during preparation.

The neck is a very short segment connecting the head with the tail. It contains vestiges of the centrioles, one of which gives rise to the axoneme **Ax** of the flagellum, which is seen in Fig. 18.7c. The axoneme has the standard 'nine plus two' arrangement of microtubule doublets seen in cilia (see Fig. 5.13). The axoneme of the neck is surrounded by several condensed fibrous rings **Rn** seen in Fig. 18.7b. In human spermatozoa, a significant amount of cytoplasm **Cy** often remains in the neck region.

The middle piece, the first part of the tail, is about the same length as the head and consists of the flagellar axoneme surrounded by nine coarse (outer dense) fibres **F** arranged longitudinally. External to this core, elongated mitochondria **Mi** are arranged in a tightly packed helix providing the energy required for flagellar movement. A fibrous thickening beneath the plasma membrane, called the ***annulus*** **An**, prevents the mitochondria from slipping into the principal piece. The principal piece, which constitutes most of the tail length, consists of a central core comprising the axoneme and the nine coarse fibres continuing from the middle piece. Surrounding this core are numerous fibrous ribs **Rb** arranged in a circular manner and seen in Fig. 18.7b. Two of the longitudinal fibrils of the core are fused with the surrounding ribs so as to form dorsal and ventral columns extending throughout the length of the principal piece (not illustrated). This arrangement divides the principal piece longitudinally into two functional compartments, one containing three coarse fibrils and the other containing four. Little is known of the mechanism of flagellar motion, but this asymmetry may account for the more powerful stroke of the tail in one direction, the so-called power stroke; this can easily be observed in fresh live preparations of spermatozoa viewed with the light microscope. The end piece, not shown in these micrographs, is merely a short, tapering portion of the tail containing the axoneme only.

AC acrosomal cap **An** annulus **AV** acrosomal vesicle **Ax** axoneme **BM** basement membrane **C** chromatin body **Cy** cytoplasm **F** outer dense fibres **G** Golgi apparatus **M** myofibroblast **Mi** mitochondrion **Nu** nucleolus **PM** plasma membrane **Rb** fibrous ribs **Rn** fibrous rings **S** spermatogonium **St** Sertoli cell S_1 primary spermatocyte S_3 spermatid S_4 spermatozoon

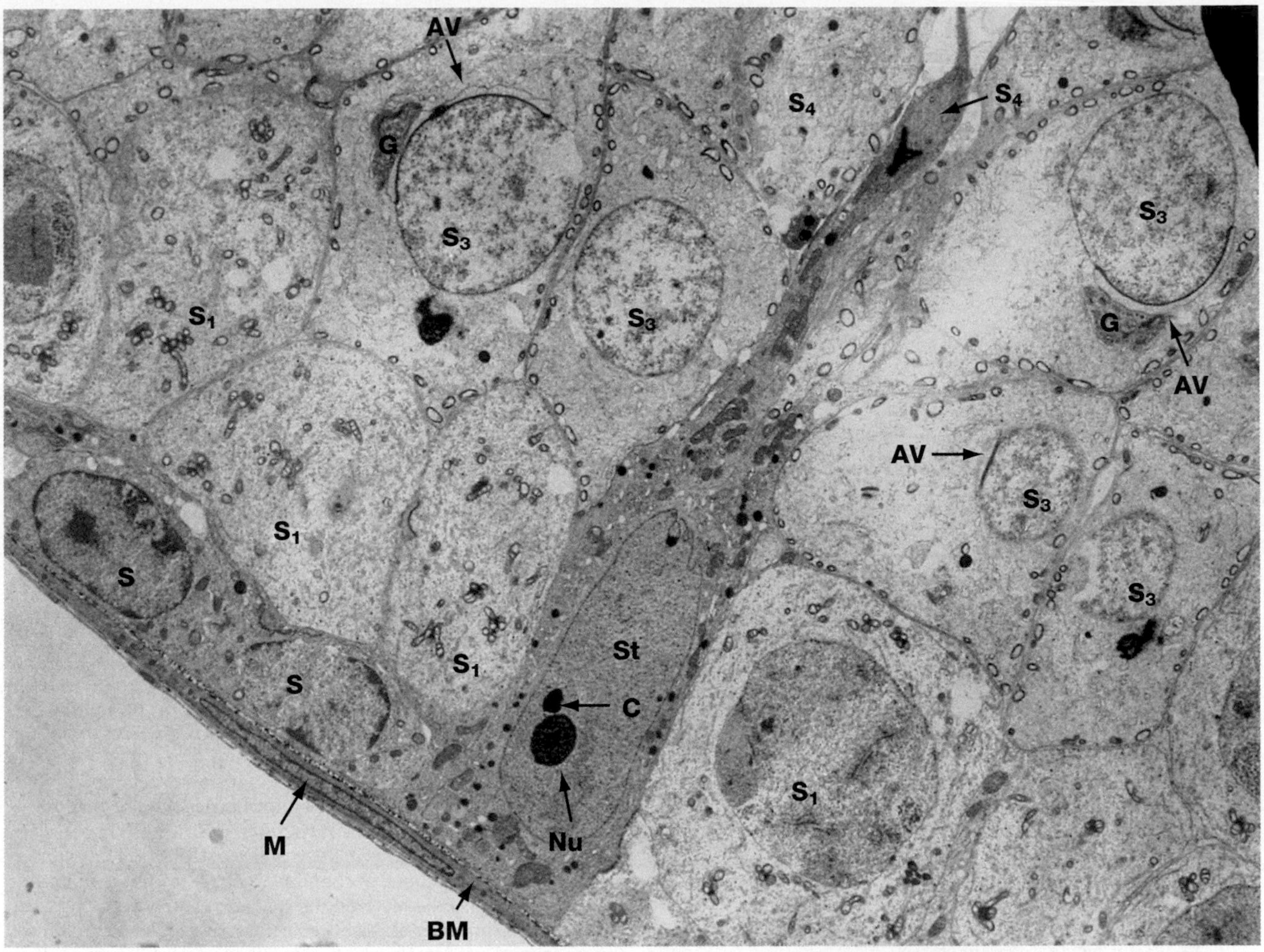

FIG. 18.8 Sertoli cell
EM ×3400

The intimate relationship of a Sertoli cell **St** to cells of the spermatogenic series is demonstrated in this electron micrograph.

The Sertoli cell rests on the basement membrane **BM** of the seminiferous tubule and its cytoplasm extends to the lumen of the tubule. Sertoli cells have an extensive cytoplasm which ramifies throughout the whole germinal epithelium, enclosing all the cells of the spermatogenic series. The cytoplasmic outline of the Sertoli cell is thus highly irregular and constantly changing to permit the progressive movement of developing spermatozoa towards the luminal surface. The oval nucleus of the Sertoli cell is characteristically orientated at right angles to the basement membrane and often exhibits a deep indentation. A prominent nucleolus **Nu** is a constant feature and dense chromatin bodies **C** are often associated with the nucleolus. The cytoplasm contains a moderate number of mitochondria, lipid droplets and a small amount of rough endoplasmic reticulum. Plentiful smooth endoplasmic reticulum is also present, as well as lamellar protein arrays known as ***Charcot–Bottcher crystals*** (not shown in this cell).

Sertoli cells are bound to one another by junctional complexes containing extensive tight junctions (see Ch. 5). The junctional complex is located towards the basal layer of the spermatogenic epithelium so as to divide the tubule into ***basal*** and ***adluminal compartments***. The latter contains the spermatids, which are thus isolated by a ***blood–testis barrier***.

The Sertoli cells mediate all metabolic exchange with the systemic compartment. The function of this barrier is to prevent exposure of gametes, which are antigenically different from somatic cells, to the immune system, thus preventing an autoimmune response. Sertoli cells have multiple functions including:

- Secretion of factors which regulate spermatogenesis and spermiogenesis
- Secretion of factors which regulate the function of Leydig cells and peritubular cells
- Secretion of ***inhibin*** which regulates hormone production
- Secretion of tubular fluid
- Phagocytosis of discarded spermatid cytoplasm

A variety of cells of the spermatogenic series are seen in this micrograph. Spermatogonia **S** rest upon the basement membrane **BM**, beneath which there is a myofibroblast **M**. Above the germ cell layer, primary spermatocytes $\mathbf{S_1}$ are seen; secondary spermatocytes are short-lived and therefore rarely seen. Spermatids $\mathbf{S_3}$ in different phases of spermiogenesis are seen in upper layers; these cells have developing acrosomal vesicles **AV** elaborated by a large Golgi apparatus **G** (see Fig. 18.6). At the luminal surface, the Sertoli cell partly envelops the head of an almost fully formed spermatozoon $\mathbf{S_4}$.

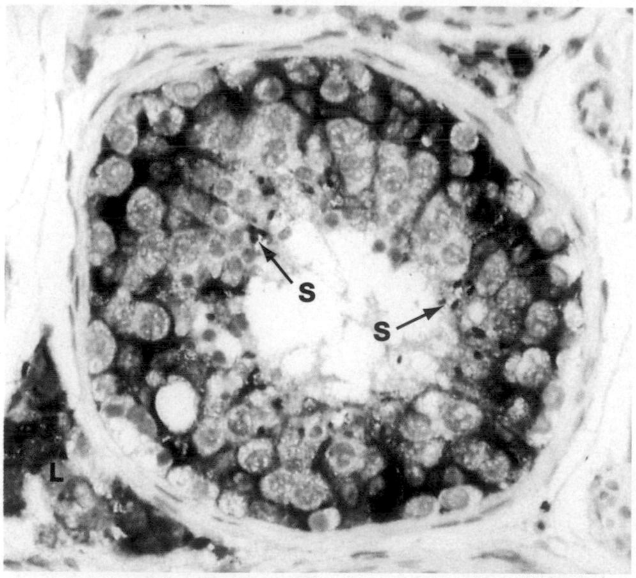

FIG. 18.9 Sertoli cells (HP)
Immunohistochemical method for inhibin

Sertoli cells can be difficult to identify in standard H&E-stained sections. However, Fig. 18.9 demonstrates the extensive cytoplasm of the Sertoli cells as they ramify around the cells of the spermatogenic series. The immunohistochemical stain uses an antibody directed against ***inhibin***, a product of ***Sertoli*** and ***Leydig*** cells, and so the cytoplasm of both of these cell types is strongly stained brown; note the cluster of Leydig cells **L** in the interstitium. The nuclei are not stained. Note the maturing spermatozoa **S** towards the lumen of the seminiferous tubules.

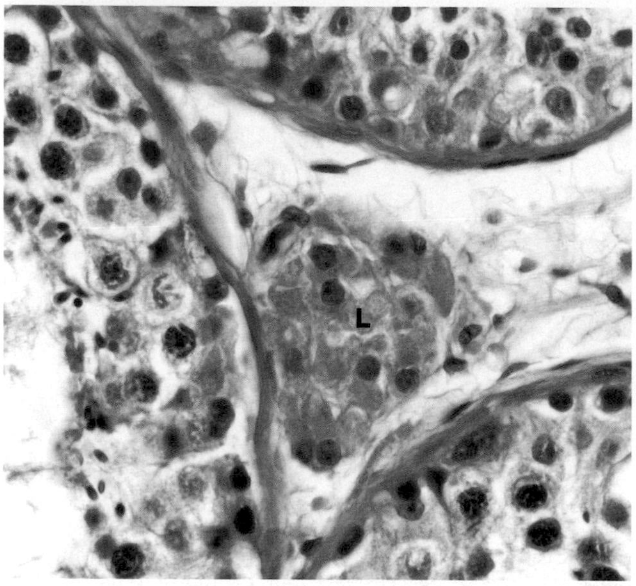

FIG. 18.10 Interstitial (Leydig) cells of the testis
H&E (HP)

Leydig cells **L**, the principal cell type found in the interstitial supporting tissue between the seminiferous tubules, synthesise and secrete the male sex hormones and other non-steroid substances. They occur singly or in clumps and are embedded in the rich plexus of blood and lymph capillaries which surrounds the seminiferous tubules. The nucleus is round with dispersed chromatin and one or two nucleoli at the periphery. The extensive eosinophilic cytoplasm contains variable numbers of lipid vacuoles and, seen by electron microscopy, closely resembles the steroid-secreting cells of the adrenal cortex (see Fig. 17.16). In humans (and wild bush rats) but no other species, Leydig cells also contain elongated cytoplasmic ***crystals of Reinke*** which are large enough to be seen with light microscopy when suitably stained; these crystals are found only in adults but their function is unknown.

Testosterone is the main hormone secreted by Leydig cells. Testosterone is not only responsible for the development of male secondary sexual characteristics at puberty but is also essential for the continued function of the seminiferous epithelium. The secretory activity of Leydig cells is controlled by the pituitary gonadotrophic hormone ***luteinising hormone***, sometimes called ***interstitial cell stimulating hormone (ICSH)*** in the male.

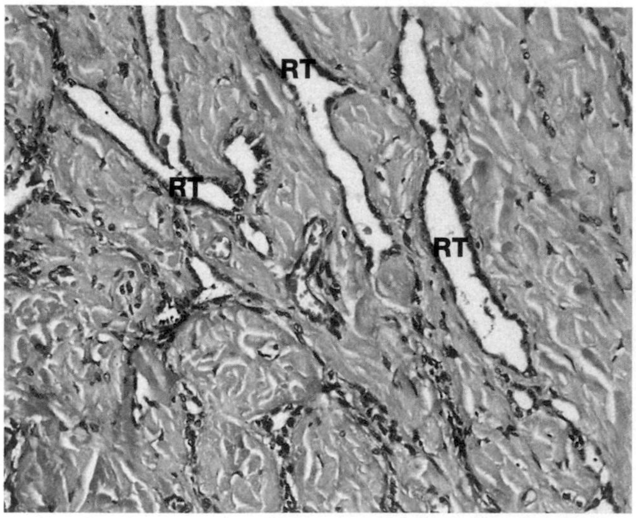

FIG. 18.11 Rete testis
H&E (LP)

The seminiferous tubules converge upon the ***mediastinum testis***, which consists of a plexiform arrangement of channels, the ***rete testis*** **RT**, surrounded by highly vascular collagenous supporting tissue containing myoid cells. The rete testis (Fig. 18.11) is lined by a single layer of low cuboidal epithelial cells with surface microvilli and a single cilium.

Myoid cell contraction helps to mix the spermatozoa and move them towards the epididymis. The lining epithelium reabsorbs protein and potassium from the seminal fluid. Ciliary activity is presumed to aid the progress of spermatozoa, which do not become motile until after maturation is completed in the epididymis.

A appendix testis **B** basal cell **DE** ductulus efferens **L** Leydig cells **RT** rete testis **S** spermatozoa **SM** smooth muscle **ST** seminiferous tubule

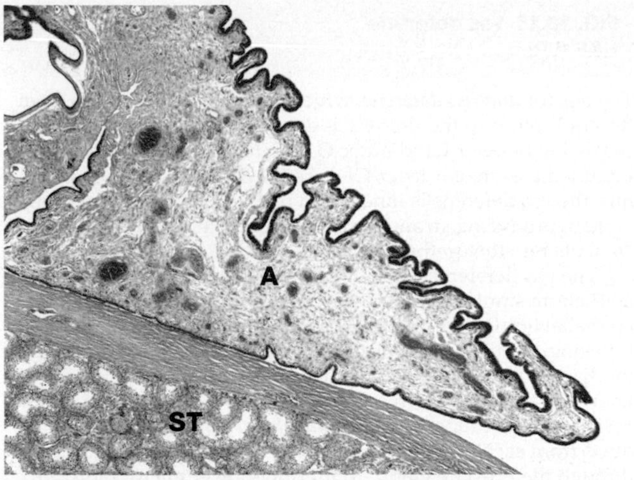

FIG. 18.12 Appendix testis
H&E (LP)

The ***appendix testis (hydatid of Morgagni)*** is a tiny tag of tissue protruding from the antero-superior aspect of the testis. It is important because it may undergo torsion leading to loss of blood supply and necrosis (infarction), an extremely painful process. The appendix testis is a remnant of the Müllerian duct and is present in approximately 80% of men.

The appendix testis **A** has a fibrovascular core and a cuboidal to columnar surface epithelium which may be ciliated (not visible at this magnification). Note the seminiferous tubules **ST** in the adjacent testis.

Other appendages in this area are the less common appendix epididymis, the vas aberrans (organ of Haller) and the paradidymis (organ of Giraldes).

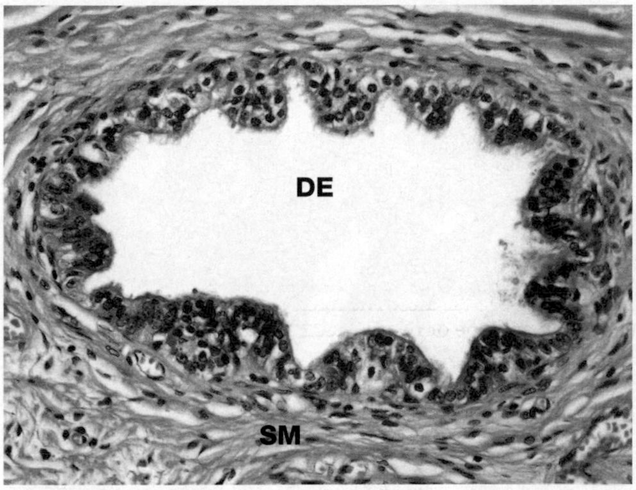

FIG. 18.13 Ductulus efferens
H&E (MP)

The rete testis drains into the head of the epididymis via some 15 to 20 convoluted ducts, the ***ductuli efferentes*** **DE**. The ductuli are lined by a single layer of epithelial cells, some of which are tall columnar and ciliated and others which are short and non-ciliated; both cell types often contain a brown pigment of unknown composition. Ciliary action in the ductuli propels the still non-motile spermatozoa towards the epididymis. The non-ciliated cells reabsorb some of the fluid produced by the testis. Basal cells, which do not reach the lumen, are also present and probably act as stem cells. A thin band of circularly arranged smooth muscle **SM** surrounds each ductulus and aids propulsion of the spermatozoa towards the epididymis.

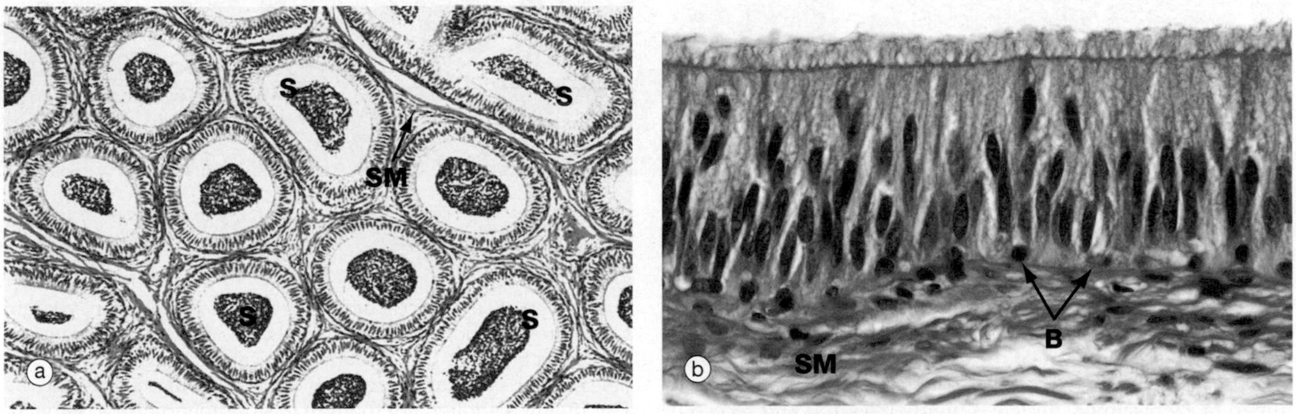

FIG. 18.14 Epididymis
(a) H&E (LP) (b) H&E (HP)

The ***epididymis*** is a long, extremely convoluted duct extending down the posterior aspect of the testis to the lower pole where it becomes the ***ductus (vas) deferens***. The epididymis consists of a ***head*** at the upper pole of the testis, a ***body*** lying along the posterior margin and a ***tail*** at the lower pole of the testis. The major function of the epididymis is the accumulation, storage and maturation of spermatozoa **S**; in the epididymis, the spermatozoa develop motility.

The epididymis is a tube of smooth muscle lined by a pseudostratified epithelium. From the proximal to the distal end of the epididymis, the muscular wall increases from a single circular layer **SM** to three layers organised in the same manner as in the ductus deferens (Fig. 18.15). Proximally, the smooth muscle exhibits slow, rhythmic contractility which gently moves spermatozoa towards the ductus deferens.

Distally, the smooth muscle is richly innervated by the sympathetic nervous system, which produces intense contractions of the lower part of the epididymis during ejaculation.

The epithelial lining of the epididymis exhibits a gradual transition from a tall pseudostratified columnar form in the head, as seen in Fig. 18.14b, to a shorter pseudostratified form at the tail. The principal cells of the epididymal epithelium bear tufts of very long microvilli, inappropriately called ***stereocilia*** (see Fig. 5.15), which are thought to be involved in absorption of an excess of fluid accompanying the spermatozoa from the testis. The ultrastructure of the cells strongly suggests an additional secretory function but the nature of epididymal secretory products, if any, remains unknown. Basal cells **B** are prominent at the base of the epithelium.

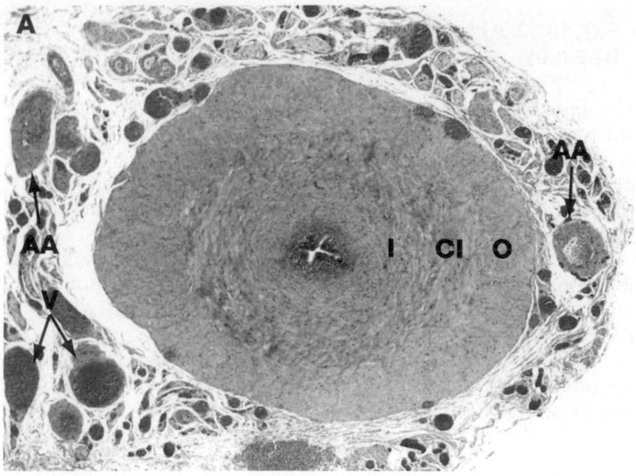

FIG. 18.15 Vas deferens
H&E (LP)

The ***vas*** (or ***ductus***) ***deferens***, which conducts spermatozoa from the epididymis to the urethra, is a thick-walled muscular tube consisting of inner **I** and outer **O** longitudinal layers and a thick intermediate circular layer **CI**. Like the distal part of the epididymis, the vas deferens is innervated by the sympathetic nervous system, producing strong peristaltic contractions to expel its contents into the urethra during ejaculation.

The vas deferens is lined by a pseudostratified columnar epithelium similar to that of the epididymis (see Fig. 18.14); the epithelial lining and its supporting lamina propria are thrown into longitudinal folds, permitting expansion of the duct during ejaculation. The dilated distal portion of each vas deferens, known as the ***ampulla***, receives a short duct draining the seminal vesicle, thus forming the short ***ejaculatory duct***; the ejaculatory ducts from each side converge to join the urethra as it passes through the prostate gland. In this low-power micrograph, the adipose tissue **A**, arteries **AA** and veins **V** that accompany the vas are easily seen; together these structures comprise the ***spermatic cord***.

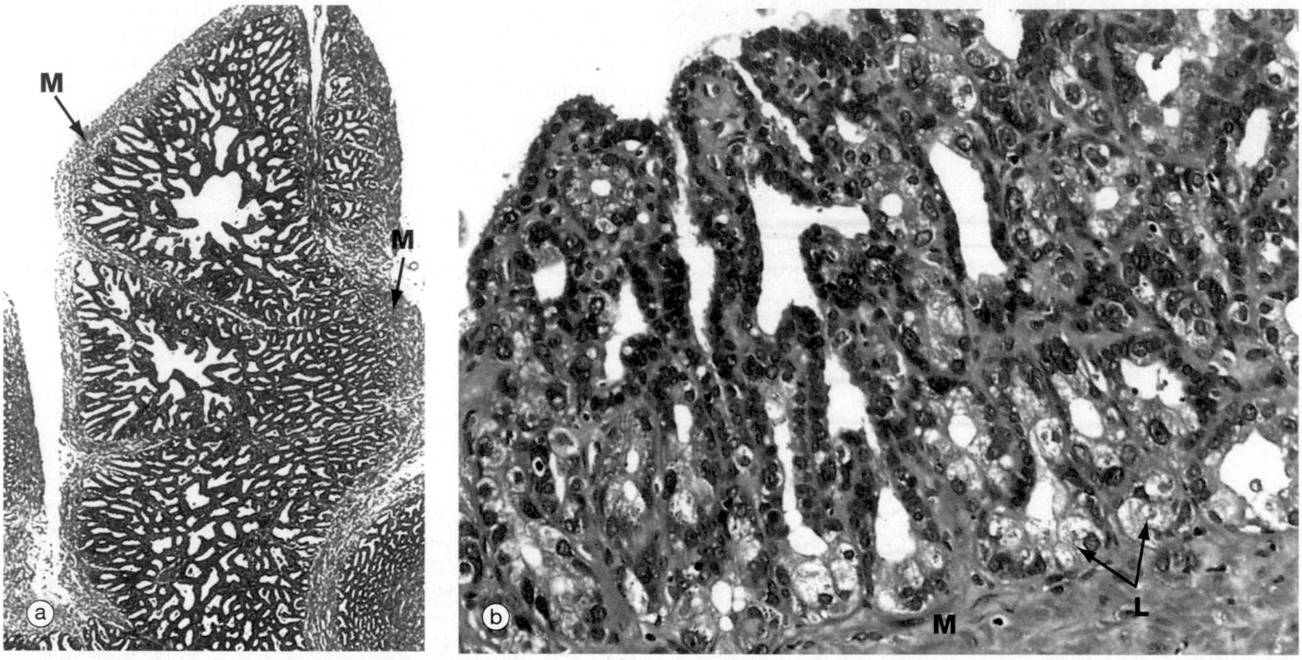

FIG. 18.16 Seminal vesicle
(a) H&E (LP) (b) H&E (HP)

Each seminal vesicle is a complex glandular diverticulum of the associated ductus deferens. Between them, the seminal vesicles secrete 50%–70% of the total volume of seminal fluid, most of the rest being secreted by the prostate gland. The lumen of each seminal vesicle is highly irregular and recessed, giving a honeycomb appearance at low magnification (Fig. 18.16a).

The epithelial lining is usually of a pseudostratified tall columnar type and consists of secretory cells with lipid droplets in the cytoplasm, giving it a foamy appearance. The seminal vesicles produce a yellowish viscid alkaline fluid containing a wide range of substances, including fructose, fibrinogen, vitamin C and prostaglandins. The epithelial cells often contain brown lipofuscin granules **L** and characteristically have rather variable nuclear shape and size. Both of these features are seen in Fig. 18.16b. Although not thought to store spermatozoa, seminal vesicles are often seen to contain spermatozoa which have probably entered by reflux from the ampulla. The prominent muscular wall **M** is arranged into inner circular and outer longitudinal layers and is supplied by the sympathetic nervous system; during ejaculation, muscle contraction forces secretions from the seminal vesicles into the urethra via the ampullae.

A adipose tissue **AA** artery **C** verumontanum **Cap** capsule **CI** intermediate circular muscle layer **CZ** central zone **ED** ejaculatory duct **I** inner longitudinal muscle layer **L** lipofuscin granules **M** muscular wall **O** outer longitudinal muscle layer **PZ** peripheral zone **St** fibrous stroma **Sp** fibrous septum **TZ** transitional zone **U** urethra **V** vein

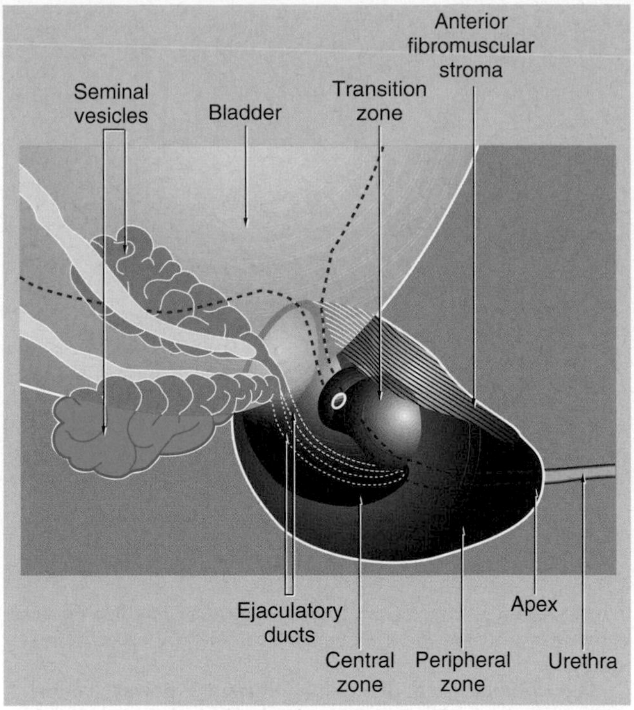

FIG. 18.17 Prostate gland

The prostate gland, which in young adults is about the size of a walnut, surrounds the bladder neck and the first part of the urethra, known as the ***prostatic urethra***. The urethra courses through the prostate to become the ***membranous urethra*** at the apex of the prostate. In the substance of the gland, the urethra merges with the ***ejaculatory ducts*** and at this point angles anteriorly.

The prostate consists of branched tubulo-acinar glands, embedded in a fibromuscular stroma. There is a partial capsule enclosing the posterior and lateral aspects of the prostate but the anterior and apical surfaces are bounded by the ***anterior fibromuscular stroma***, a part of the gland consisting, as the name implies, only of collagenous stroma and muscle fibres.

In the past, the prostate was described as consisting of a number of ill-defined lobes. However, this terminology has been replaced by the concept of prostate zones and the gland is now described as consisting of four zones of unequal size:

- The ***transition zone*** surrounds the proximal prostatic urethra and comprises about 5% of the glandular tissue.
- The ***central zone*** (20%) surrounds the ejaculatory ducts.
- The ***peripheral zone*** makes up the bulk of the gland (approximately 70%).
- The ***anterior fibromuscular stroma*** contains no glandular tissue and lies anteriorly.

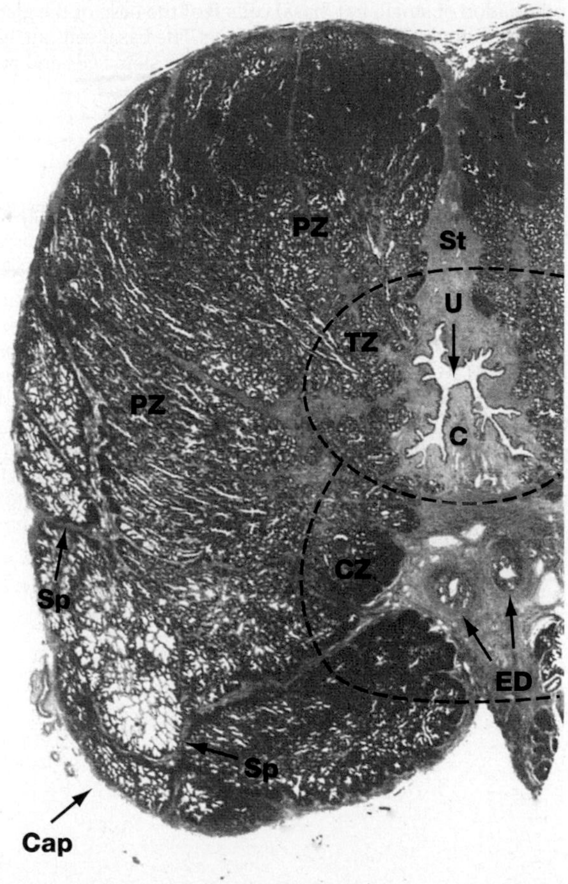

FIG. 18.18 Prostate gland, dog H&E (LP)

This low-power view of the prostate of a dog shows the general architectural features of the gland. The ***urethra*** **U** lies centrally, surrounded by a fibrous stroma **St**. The ejaculatory ducts **ED** also lie in this central stroma as they course towards their junction with the prostatic urethra. The zones of the prostate are not clearly demarcated from each other anatomically. Partial fibrous septa **Sp** separate the gland into lobules. The transition zone **TZ** surrounds the first part of the prostatic urethra. The central zone **CZ** lies posterior to the transition zone and encircles the ejaculatory ducts **ED**. The peripheral zone **PZ** makes up the main bulk of the gland. The ducts of the peripheral zone glands empty into the posterolateral recesses of the urethra on either side of the ***verumontanum (urethral crest)*** **C**.

The different zones of the prostate are important because they tend to be the sites of different disease processes. Most cases of carcinoma of the prostate arise in the peripheral zone (see e-Fig. 18.5), while the transition zone harbours almost all cases of benign nodular hyperplasia (see below).

At this power the anterior fibromuscular stroma appears continuous with the capsule **Cap** and its content of muscle fibres cannot be discerned.

Common prostatic disease

The most common disease of the prostate is called benign prostatic hyperplasia and occurs in men over 50 (see e-Fig. 18.4). The prostatic glands around the urethra (transition zone, see Fig. 18.17) become greatly increased in size and number and the gland lumina become distended by secretions and corpora amylacea. At the same time, the stromal smooth muscle fibres become greatly enlarged. This increase in bulk enlarges the prostate gland as a whole, and compresses the urethra, leading to interference with bladder emptying.

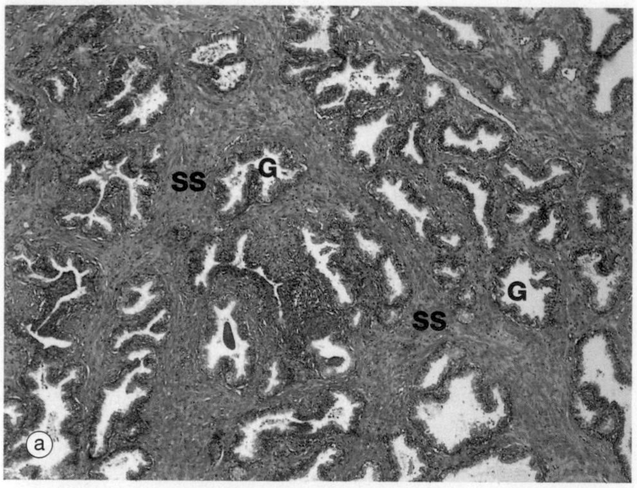

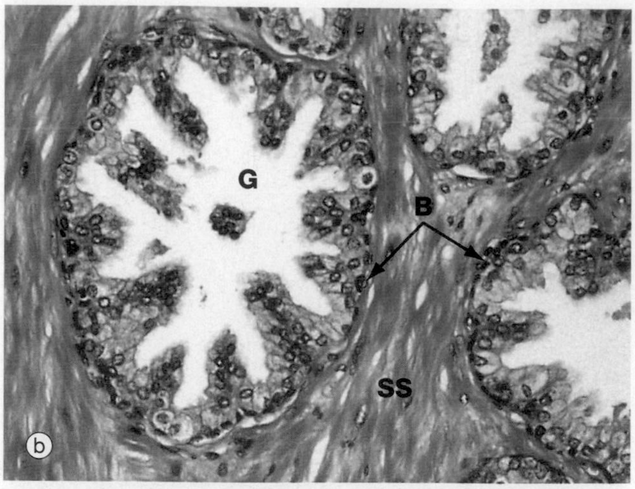

FIG. 18.19 Prostate gland
(a) H&E (LP) (b) H&E (HP)

The prostate gland is composed of glands and stroma (Fig. 18.19a). The supporting stroma **SS** is a mixture of collagenous fibrous tissue and smooth muscle fibres, which are best seen at higher magnification in Fig. 18.19b. The glands **G** show a convoluted pattern with the epithelium thrown up into folds, sometimes into almost a papillary pattern.

The secretory product of the prostate, which makes up about 30%–50% the seminal fluid volume, is a thin liquid rich in citric acid and proteolytic enzymes, including fibrinolysins, which liquefies the coagulated semen after it has been deposited in the vagina. Inspissated secretions may accumulate in some glands to form spherical concretions (***corpora amylacea***) which increase in number with age and may become calcified (not seen in this example).

Fig. 18.19b, taken at higher magnification, shows the detail of the epithelium of the prostate glands. The main epithelial cell type is the tall columnar secretory cell with prominent round basal nuclei and pale-staining cytoplasm. There is also a scanty population of small, flat, basal cells **B** at the base of the gland in contact with the basement membrane. The basal cells are easily seen in this micrograph. These cells act as stem cells and may become quite prominent in prostatic hyperplasia.

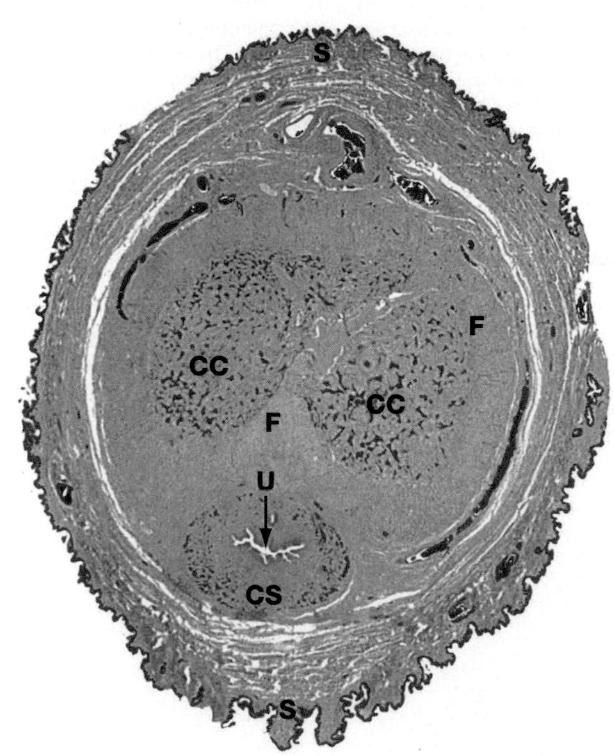

FIG. 18.20 Penis
H&E (LP)

This transverse section of the human penis shows the arrangement of the erectile tissues, which exist in the form of three columns. The two dorsal columns are called the ***corpora cavernosa*** **CC** and the single ventral column is the ***corpus spongiosum*** **CS** through which runs the ***penile urethra*** **U**. At its distal end, the corpus spongiosum expands to form the ***glans penis***. The erectile corpora are enclosed within and separated by a fibrocollagenous capsule **F**. The erectile centre of the penis is enclosed in a sheath of skin **S** to which it is connected by a loose subcutis containing prominent blood vessels.

B basal cell **CC** corpus cavernosum **CS** corpus spongiosum **F** fibrocollagenous capsule **G** gland **HA** helicine artery **P** para-urethral gland **S** skin **Si** vascular sinus **SS** supporting stroma **U** urethra

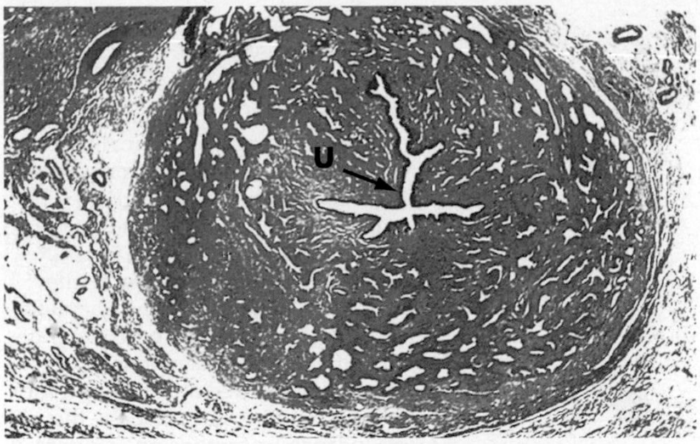

FIG. 18.21 Corpus spongiosum H&E (LP)

The corpus spongiosum is composed of erectile tissue, large irregular interconnected vascular channels with fibrocollagenous stroma between; the stroma contains some smooth muscle fibres. Running through the centre of the corpus spongiosum is the penile urethra **U**. Small paraurethral mucus glands open into the urethra.

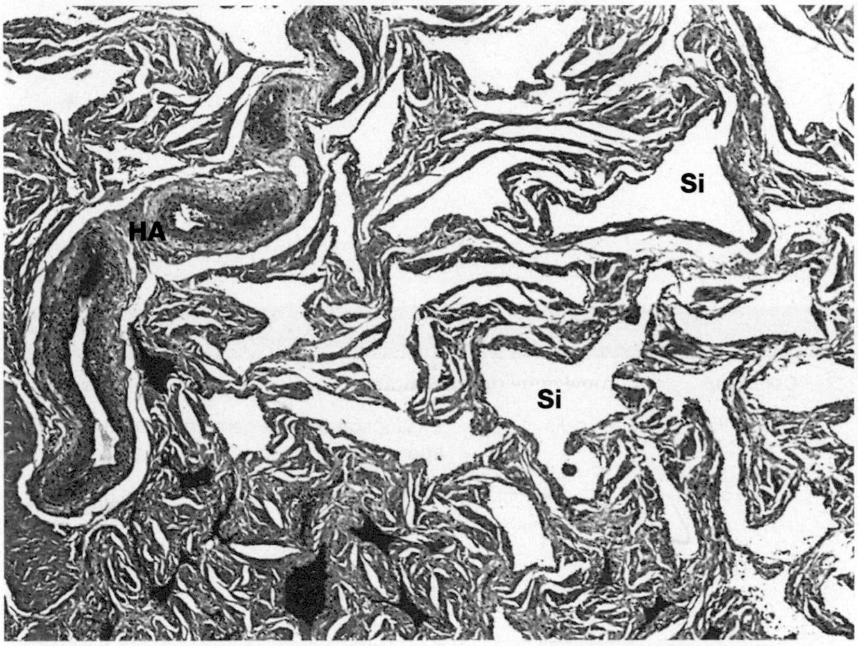

FIG. 18.22 Penile erectile tissue H&E (LP)

The vascular sinuses **Si** of the cavernous bodies of the penis are supplied by numerous anastomosing thick-walled arteries and arterioles called ***helicine arteries*** **HA**, since they follow a spiral course in the flaccid state. Blood drains from the sinuses via veins which lie immediately beneath the dense fibroelastic tissue investing the cavernous bodies. During erection, dilatation of the helicine arteries, mediated by the parasympathetic nervous system, results in engorgement of the vascular sinuses, which enlarge, compressing and restricting venous outflow. The process is enhanced by relaxation of smooth muscle cells in the trabeculae of the cavernous bodies.

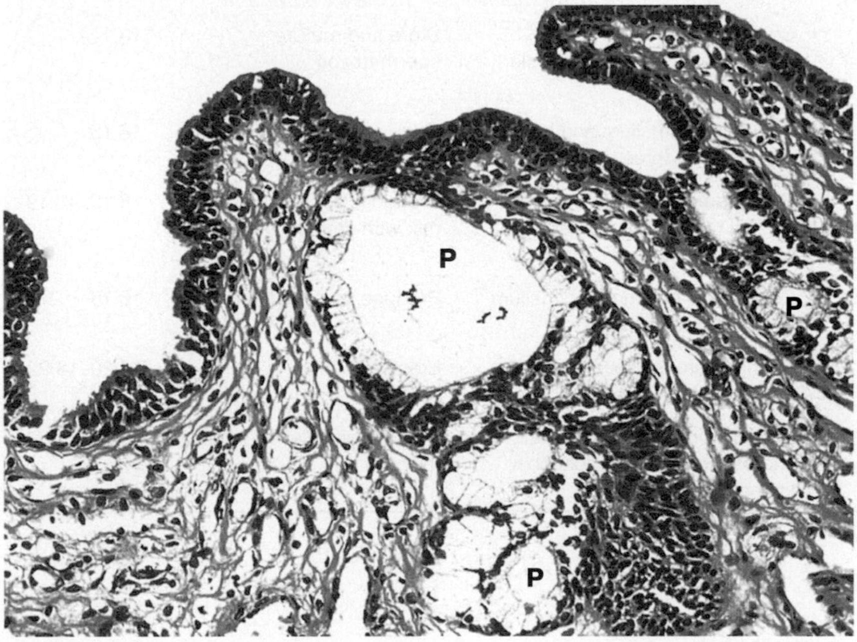

FIG. 18.23 Penile urethra H&E (HP)

Apart from the prostatic urethra, which is lined by transitional epithelium, the male urethra is lined by stratified or pseudostratified columnar epithelium, although small areas of stratified squamous epithelium may also be found in human adult males. The external opening (***urethral meatus***) is lined by stratified squamous epithelium which becomes continuous with the epithelium of the glans.

The urethra is lubricated by mucous secretions from the para-urethral glands **P** and the ***bulbo-urethral glands of Cowper*** (see Fig. 18.1), which have a similar but more discrete organisation.

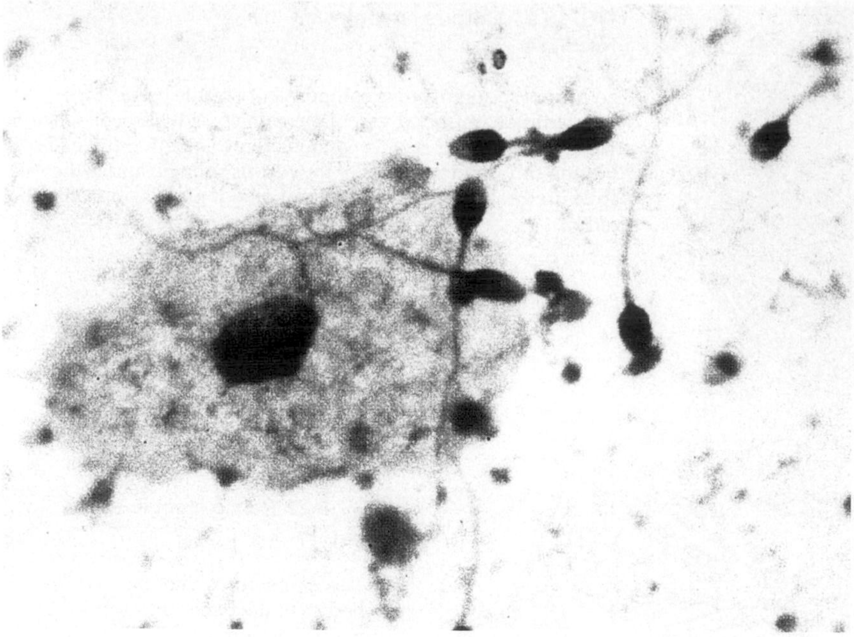

FIG. 18.24 Semen
H&E (HP)

Semen, the product of ejaculation, consists of spermatozoa and seminal fluid, which is derived principally from the seminal vesicles and prostate gland. The volume of each human ejaculate is about 3.5 mL, containing from 50 to 150 × 10^6 spermatozoa per mL. In normal fertile human males, up to 25% of the ejaculated spermatozoa are abnormal or degenerate forms. By the time of ejaculation, spermatozoa have matured and acquired the property of motility; nevertheless, they remain incapable of fertilising an ovum until after undergoing a process called ***capacitation*** within the female genital tract.

REVIEW

TABLE 18.1 Review of the male genital tract

Organ	Main components	Cell types	Functions	Figures
Testis	Seminiferous tubules	Spermatogenic series cells	Production of male gametes, spermatozoa	18.3–18.5, 18.7
		Sertoli cells	Support cells for spermatogenesis	18.5, 18.8, 18.9
	Interstitium	Leydig cells	Synthesis of androgenic hormones, principally testosterone	18.9, 18.10
	Rete testis	Cuboidal epithelium with cilia and smooth muscle coat	Convey spermatozoa to ductuli efferentes and thence to epididymis	18.11
Epididymis	Head, body, tail	Columnar epithelium with stereocilia and smooth muscle coat	Store and mature spermatozoa	18.14
Vas deferens		Columnar epithelium and smooth muscle coat, three layers	Carry sperm to urethra during ejaculation	18.15
Prostate	Central, transition and peripheral zones and anterior fibromuscular stroma	Epithelium with two cell layers, luminal tall columnar layer and basal cell layer	Produces secretions that mix with seminal fluid	18.18, 18.19
Seminal vesicle		Cuboidal to columnar epithelium with muscular wall	Produce seminal fluid	18.16
Penis	Corpus spongiosum and corpora cavernosa	Spongy fibrous tissue containing anastomosing vascular sinuses	Erectile tissue	18.20–18.22
	Urethra	Lined by urothelium proximally and pseudostratified columnar epithelium distally	Duct for ejaculation (and micturition)	18.23

19 Female reproductive system

INTRODUCTION

The female reproductive system has six major functions:

- Production of female gametes, the *ova*, by the process of *oogenesis*
- Reception of male gametes, the *spermatozoa*
- Provision of a suitable environment for the *fertilisation* of ova by spermatozoa
- Provision of an environment for the development of the fetus
- Expulsion of the developed fetus to the external environment
- Nutrition of the newborn

These functions are all integrated by an elegant system of hormonal and nervous mechanisms. The female reproductive system may be divided into three structural units on the basis of function:

- The **ovaries**, which are the site of oogenesis, are paired organs lying on either side of the uterus adjacent to the lateral wall of the pelvis. In sexually mature mammals, ova are released by the process of ovulation in a cyclical manner, either seasonally or at regular intervals throughout the year. This cycle is suspended during pregnancy. The ovaries are also endocrine organs, producing the hormones *oestrogen* and *progesterone*. Both ovulation and ovarian hormone production are controlled by the cyclical release from the anterior pituitary of the gonadotrophic hormones *luteinising hormone* (LH) and *follicle stimulating hormone* (FSH). Oestrogen and progesterone in turn regulate LH and FSH production by feedback mechanisms. Thus, ovulation is coordinated with preparation of the uterus to receive the fertilised ovum.
- The **genital tract** extends from near the ovaries to an opening at the external surface and provides an environment for reception of male gametes, fertilisation of ova, development of the fetus and expulsion of the fetus at birth. The genital tract begins with a pair of *Fallopian tubes*, also called *oviducts* or *uterine tubes*, which conduct ova from the ovaries to the uterus where fetal development occurs. Fertilisation of ova by spermatozoa occurs within the Fallopian tubes. The *uterus* is a muscular organ, the mucosal lining of which undergoes cyclical proliferation under the influence of ovarian hormones. This provides a suitable environment for implantation of the fertilised ovum and subsequent development of the *placenta*. This is the means by which the developing fetus is nourished throughout gestation. At birth (*parturition*), strong contractions of the muscular uterine wall expel the fetus through the lower part of the uterus, the *uterine cervix*, into the birth canal or *vagina*. The vagina is an expansile muscular tube specialised for the reception of the penis during coitus and for the passage of the fetus to the external environment. At the external opening of the vagina there are thick folds of skin, the *labia* which, along with the *clitoris*, constitute the *vulva*.
- The **breasts** are highly modified apocrine sweat glands which, in the female, develop at puberty and regress at menopause. During pregnancy, the secretory components expand greatly in size and number in preparation for milk production (*lactation*).

In the non-pregnant state, the female reproductive system undergoes continuous cyclical changes from puberty to menopause. When ovulation is not followed by the implantation of a fertilised ovum, the thickened mucosal lining, the *endometrium*, degenerates and a new ovulation cycle commences. In humans, the thickened endometrium is shed in a period of bleeding known as *menstruation*. The first day of bleeding marks the beginning of a new cycle of endometrial proliferation which is known as the *menstrual cycle*. In humans, the standard menstrual cycle is of 28 days duration, but there is considerable variation among normal individuals. Ovulation usually occurs at the midpoint of the cycle.

In other mammals, the proliferated uterine mucosa is absorbed rather than shed, and the female is receptive to the male only during the period of ovulation, which is known as *oestrus* (or heat). The remaining part of the cycle is called the *dioestrus*, and the whole cycle is known as the *oestrus cycle*.

The general anatomy of the female genital tract is illustrated in Figs. 19.1 and 19.2.

Embryology of the female genital tract

Most of the structures of the female genital tract are derived from the paired ***Müllerian*** or ***paramesonephric ducts***. These give rise to the right and left Fallopian tubes and fuse centrally to form the structures of the uterus, cervix and vagina.

Occasionally, congenital anomalies can occur because of failure of this process of embryological fusion. This can result in a persistent short septum dividing the fundus of the uterus resulting in a ***bicornuate*** or ***septate uterus***. In more extreme cases, reduplication of the uterus (***didelphys***), cervix and vagina may occur.

The structures of the male genital tract are derived from the ***Wolffian*** or ***mesonephric duct*** system; in the female, these structures normally regress during fetal life. Small embryological remnants of the Wolffian ducts may persist into adulthood and can be noted in sites such as the paratubal tissue (or mesosalpinx) and in the lateral walls of the cervix. An awareness of these embryological remnants is important for diagnostic pathologists, as the unexpected finding of small epithelial-lined tubules in unusual sites may lead to misdiagnosis of malignancy.

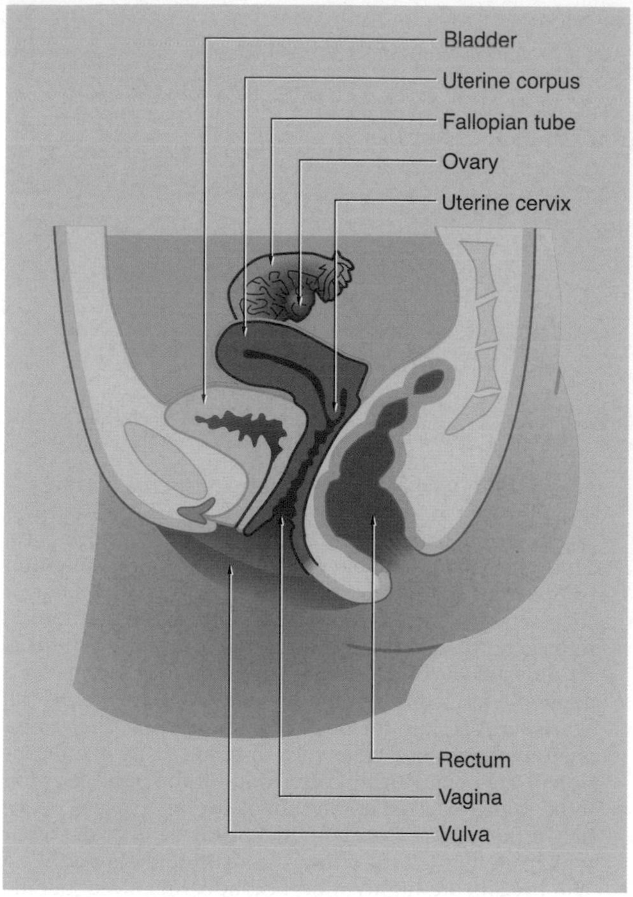

FIG. 19.1 Female reproductive system, sagittal view

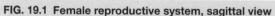

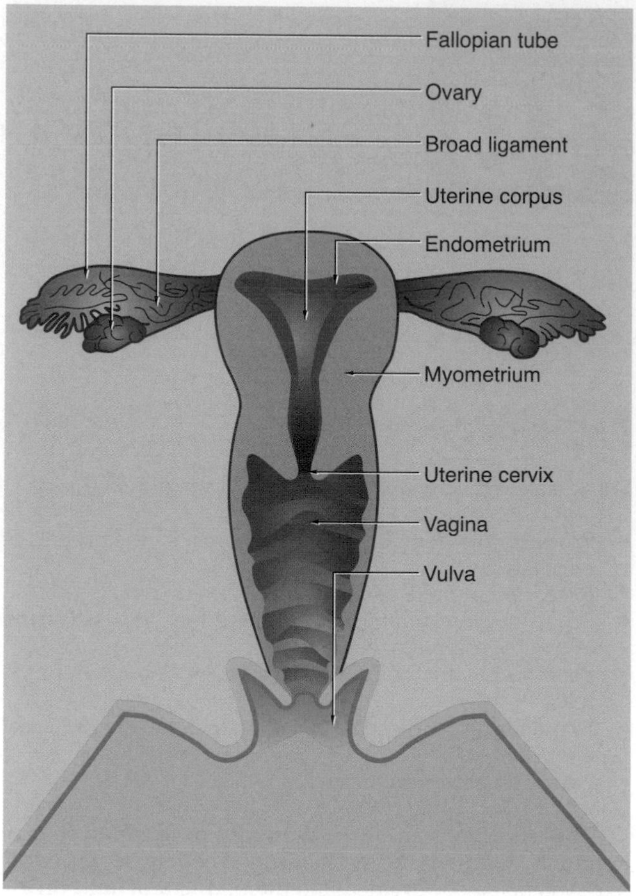

FIG. 19.2 Female reproductive system, coronal view

The ovaries

Whilst most of the structures of the female reproductive system arise from the Müllerian duct system as described above (see textbox), the ovaries arise from the ***genital ridge***, a thickening in the mesothelium high on the posterior wall of the peritoneal cavity. The ovaries later descend to their adult position in the pelvis. As a result, the blood supply and lymphatic drainage of the ovaries is derived from the upper abdomen, with the paired ovarian arteries arising from the abdominal aorta, just proximal to the origin of the renal arteries. This rather unexpected fact is important in understanding why ovarian (and, indeed, testicular) tumours typically spread to para-aortic lymph nodes, rather than to local lymph nodes in the pelvic or inguinal area.

FIG. 19.3 Ovary *(illustrations (a) and (b) opposite)*
(a) Monkey, Azan (LP) (b) Human, H&E (LP)

The ovaries of all mammals have a similar basic structure. There are, however, considerable variations in accordance with species differences in the ovarian cycle and the stage in the cycle at which the ovary is examined. Figs 19.3a and b compare the ovarian appearance of the monkey with that of the human.

The ovaries, which are some 3 to 5 cm long in humans, have a flattened ovoid shape. The body of the ovary consists of spindle-shaped cells, fine collagen fibres and ground substance that together constitute the ***ovarian stroma***. The stromal cells resemble fibroblasts, but some contain lipid droplets. Bundles of smooth muscle cells are also scattered throughout the stroma. In the peripheral zone of the stroma, known as the ***cortex***, there are numerous ***follicles*** that contain female gametes in various stages of development. In addition, there may also be post-ovulatory follicles of various kinds, namely ***corpora lutea*** (responsible for oestrogen and progesterone production, see Fig. 19.8), degenerate and former corpora lutea (***corpora albicantia***, see Fig. 19.11) and degenerate (***atretic***) follicles (see Fig. 19.10).

The superficial cortex is more fibrous than the deep cortex and is often called the ***tunica albuginea***. However, unlike the testis, this is not an anatomically distinct capsule. On the surface of the ovary is an epithelial covering, misleadingly called ***germinal epithelium***, which is a continuation of the peritoneum.

In the monkey ovary, numerous ***follicles*** **F** are seen in various sizes and states of development. In contrast, developing follicles are difficult to see in the human ovary (see Fig. 10.3b) at this magnification. An active corpus luteum **CL** and several degenerating corpora lutea **D** and corpora albicantia **A** dominate this human ovary.

The central zone of the ovarian stroma, the ***medulla*** **M**, is highly vascular and contains ***hilus cells***, which are morphologically very similar to Leydig cells of the testis. The ovarian artery (a branch of the aorta) and ovarian branches of the uterine artery form anastomoses in the mesovarium and the broad ligament **L**. From this arterial plexus, approximately 10 coiled arteries, the ***helicine arteries*** **H** enter the hilum of the ovary, best seen in Fig. 19.3a. Smaller branches form a plexus at the corticomedullary junction, giving rise to straight cortical arterioles that radiate into the cortex. Here, they branch and anastomose to form vascular arcades, giving rise to a rich network of capillaries around the follicles. Venous drainage follows the course of the arterial system, the medullary veins being large and tortuous. Lymphatics arise in the perifollicular stroma, draining to larger vessels which coil around the medullary veins. Innervation of the ovary is by sympathetic fibres that not only supply blood vessels but also terminate on smooth muscle cells in the stroma around the follicles, possibly playing some part in follicular maturation and ovulation. In Fig. 19.3b, the nearby Fallopian tube **FT** is included in the plane of section.

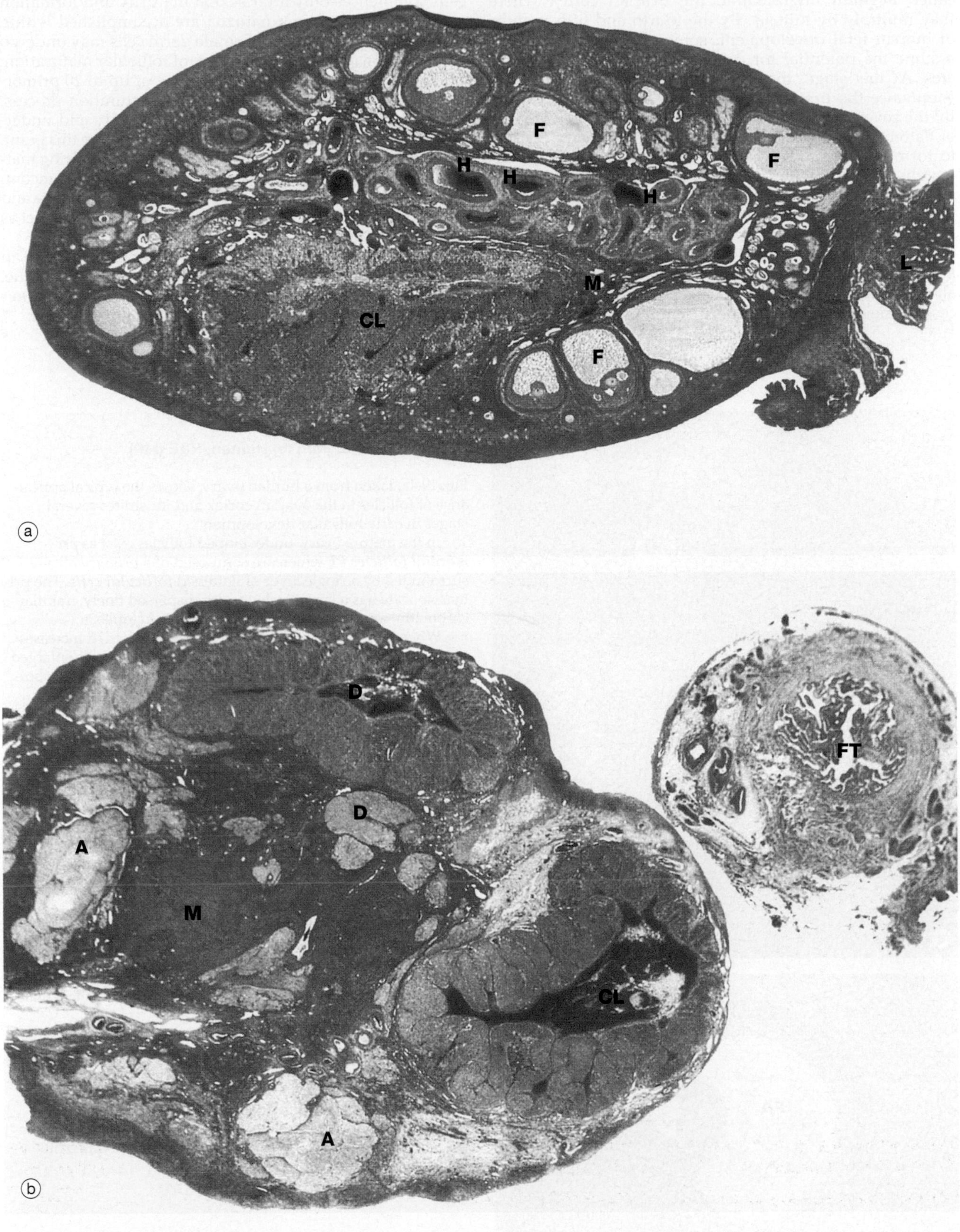

FIG. 19.3 Ovary *(caption opposite)*
(a) Monkey, Azan (LP) (b) Human, H&E (LP)

A corpus albicans **CL** corpus luteum **D** degenerating corpus luteum **F** follicle **FT** Fallopian tube **H** helicine artery
L broad ligament **M** medulla

FOLLICULAR DEVELOPMENT

During early fetal development, primordial germ cells called ***oogonia*** migrate into the ovarian cortex where they multiply by mitosis. By the fourth and fifth months of human fetal development, some oogonia enlarge and assume the potential for development into mature gametes. At this stage, they are called ***primary oocytes*** and commence the first stage of ***meiotic division*** (see Ch. 2). By the seventh month of fetal development, a single layer of flattened ***follicular cells*** surrounds the primary oocytes to form ***primordial follicles***, of which there are approximately 500 000 in the human ovary at birth. This encapsulation arrests the first meiotic division and no further development of primordial follicles then occurs until after the female reaches sexual maturity (***puberty***). The process of meiotic division is only completed during follicular maturation, leading up to ovulation and fertilisation. Thus, all the female germ cells are present at birth, but the process of meiotic division is only completed some 15 to 50 years later! In contrast, in males, meiotic division of germ cells commences only after sexual maturity and formation and maturation of spermatozoa are accomplished within about 70 days (see Ch. 18). Female germ cells may undergo degeneration (***atresia***) at any stage of follicular maturation.

During each ovarian cycle, a cohort of up to 20 primordial follicles is activated to begin the maturation process. Usually, only one follicle reaches full maturity and undergoes ovulation while the remainder regress before this point. The reason for this apparent wastage is unclear. During maturation, however, the follicles have an endocrine function which may be far beyond the capacity of a single follicle and so the primary purpose of the other follicles may be to act as an endocrine gland.

Follicular maturation involves changes in the oocyte, in the follicular cells and in the surrounding stromal tissue. Follicular maturation is stimulated by ***FSH*** (***follicle stimulating hormone***) secreted by the anterior pituitary gland.

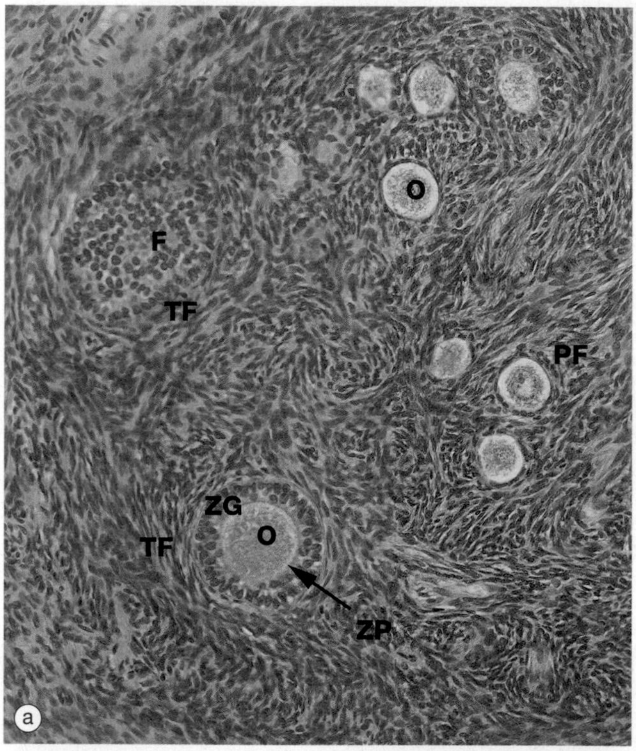

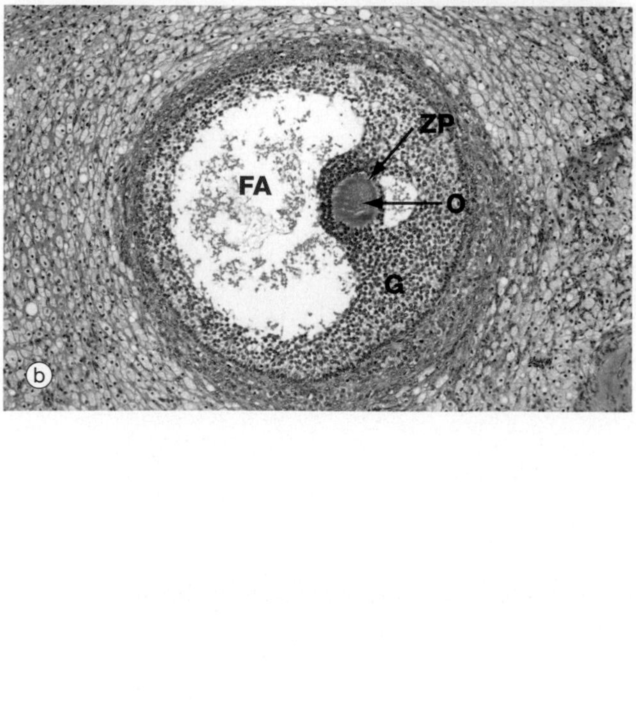

FIG. 19.4 Ovarian cortex
(a) Human, H&E (MP) (b) Human, H&E (MP)

Fig. 19.4a, taken from a human ovary, shows the typical appearance of follicles in the ovarian cortex and illustrates several stages in early follicular development.

In the mature ovary, undeveloped follicles exist as ***primordial follicles*** **PF** which are composed of a ***primary oocyte*** surrounded by a single layer of flattened ***follicular cells***. The primary oocyte has a large nucleus with dispersed finely granular chromatin, a prominent nucleolus and little cytoplasm.

When a primordial follicle has been stimulated, it increases in size to form a ***primary follicle***. Its oocyte **O** becomes enlarged and the follicular cells **F** multiply by mitosis and become cuboidal in shape. They are now known as ***granulosa cells***. A thick homogeneous layer of glycoprotein and acid proteoglycans, the ***zona pellucida*** **ZP**, develops between the oocyte and the follicular cells. Both cell types probably contribute to its formation.

With further follicular development, as seen in the larger follicles on the left, the surrounding stromal cells begin to form an organised layer around the follicle called the ***theca folliculi*** **TF**, separated from the granulosa cells by a basement membrane. Theca cells are derived from the fibroblast-like cells of the ovarian stroma. The primary follicle continues to enlarge and the granulosa cells continue to proliferate, forming a layer several cells thick called the ***zona granulosa*** **ZG**.

The surface of the ovary has a fibrous ***tunica albuginea*** and a single layer of low cuboidal mesothelial cells. This layer is continuous with the mesothelial lining of the peritoneal cavity and was formerly known as the ***germinal epithelium***, based upon the mistaken belief that these cells were the origin of the female germ cells.

Fig. 19.4b illustrates a section of human ovary, showing the next stage in follicular maturation. Fluid-filled spaces develop between the granulosa cells **G**, and these begin to coalesce to form the ***follicular antrum*** **FA**. This is now known as a ***secondary follicle***. The zona pellucida **ZP** is well seen in this micrograph, but the nucleus of the oocyte **O** does not lie in this plane of section. Details of the secondary follicle are illustrated at higher magnification in Fig. 19.5.

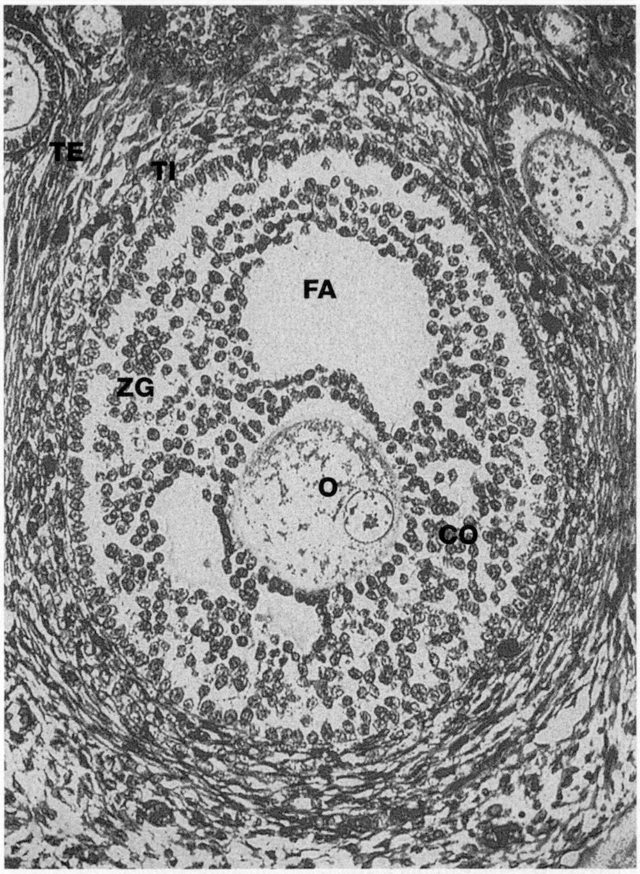

FIG. 19.5 Secondary follicle
Azan (MP)

Primary follicles continue to develop to form ***secondary follicles*** and acquire the features seen in Fig. 19.5. By now they are usually situated deeper in the ovarian cortex.

The ***zona granulosa*** **ZG** continues to proliferate, and small fluid-filled spaces appear within it. These fuse to form the ***follicular antrum*** **FA**, in which follicular fluid accumulates. At this stage, the oocyte **O** has almost reached its full size and becomes situated eccentrically in a thickened area of the granulosa called the ***cumulus oophorus*** **CO**.

At the periphery of the follicle, the ***theca folliculi*** has developed two layers, the ***theca interna*** **TI**, comprising several layers of rounded cells, and the less well-defined ***theca externa*** **TE**, consisting of spindle-shaped cells that merge with the surrounding stroma.

The cells of the theca interna have the features of typical steroid-secreting cells (see Fig. 17.16) and produce oestrogen precursors (e.g. androstenedione), oestrogen and, in the preovulatory stage, progesterone. In the ovary, these steroid-secreting cells are often described as ***luteinised***. Follicular hormones promote proliferation of the endometrium in readiness for the implantation of a fertilised ovum.

The theca externa is composed of flattened stromal cells and has no endocrine function. The granulosa cells also produce hormones from the stage of antral formation onwards.

Oestrogen is produced from precursors secreted by the theca interna, as well as small amounts of intrafollicular FSH and, at ovulation, the FSH inhibitor ***inhibin F***.

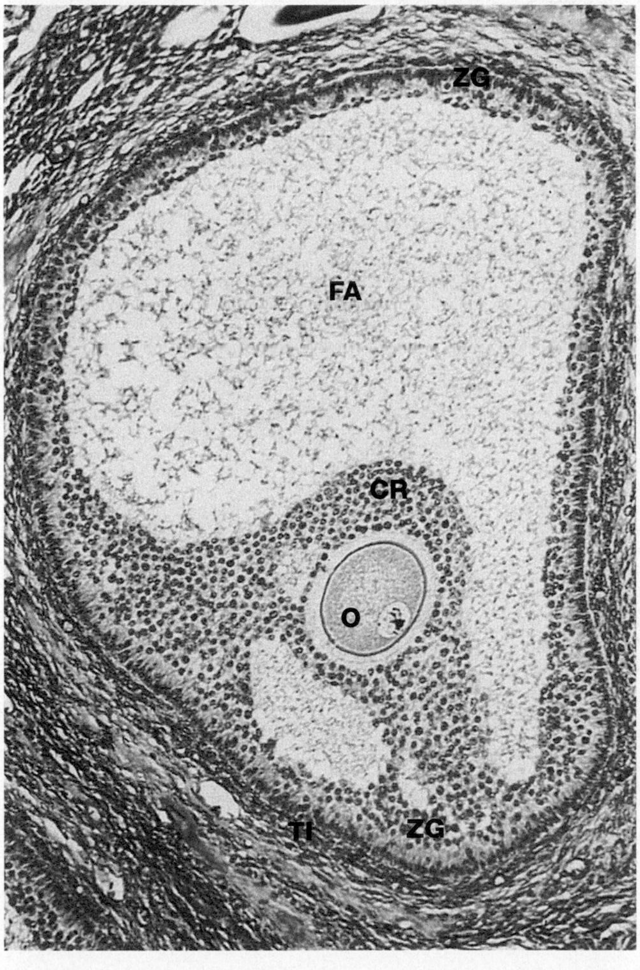

FIG. 19.6 Graafian follicle
Azan (LP)

Approaching maturity, further growth of the oocyte ceases and the first meiotic division is completed just before ovulation (Fig. 19.6). At this stage, the oocyte becomes known as the ***secondary oocyte*** and commences the second meiotic division. The first polar body (see Ch. 2), containing very little cytoplasm, remains inconspicuously within the zona pellucida. The follicular antrum **FA** enlarges markedly and the zona granulosa **ZG** now forms a layer of even thickness around the periphery of the follicle. The cumulus oophorus diminishes, leaving the oocyte **O** surrounded by a layer several cells thick, the ***corona radiata*** **CR**, which remains attached to the zona granulosa by thin bridges of cells. Before ovulation, these bridges break down and the oocyte, surrounded by the corona radiata, floats free inside the follicle.

Note the surrounding theca interna **TI**, consisting of plump luteinised cells. By this stage, the follicle has reached between 1.5 and 2.5 cm in diameter and bulges under the ovarian surface. The overlying surface epithelial cells are flattened and atrophic and the thin intervening stroma becomes degenerate and avascular.

At ***ovulation***, the mature follicle ruptures and the ovum, made up of the secondary oocyte, zona pellucida and corona radiata, is expelled into the peritoneal cavity near the entrance to the Fallopian tube. The second meiotic division of the oocyte is not completed until after penetration of the ovum by a spermatozoon.

CO cumulus oophorus **CR** corona radiata **F** follicular cells **FA** follicular antrum **G** granulosa cells **O** oocyte
PF primordial follicle **TE** theca externa **TF** theca folliculi **TI** theca interna **ZG** zona granulosa **ZP** zona pellucida

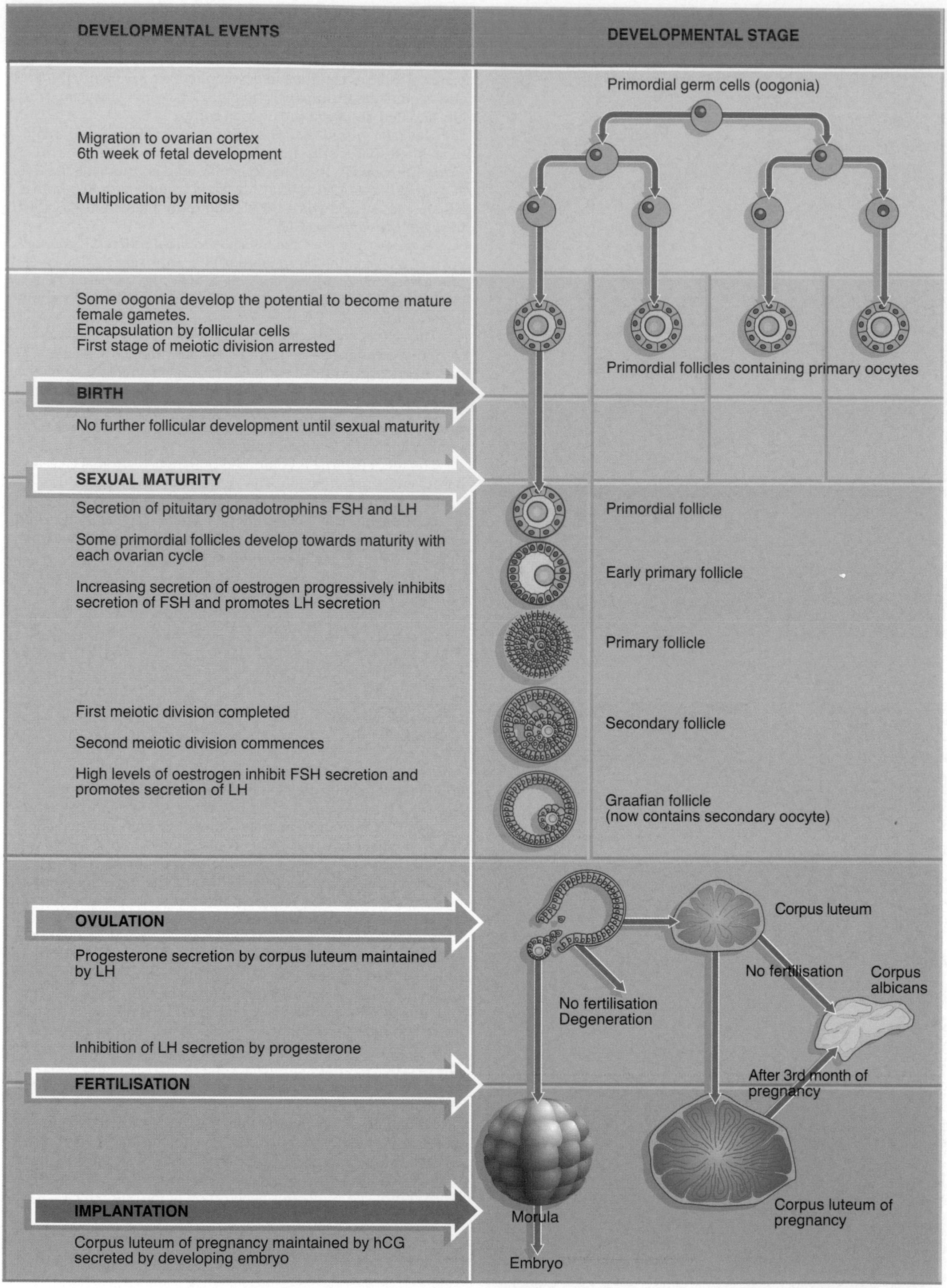
DEVELOPMENTAL EVENTS
DEVELOPMENTAL STAGE
Primordial germ cells (oogonia)
Migration to ovarian cortex
6th week of fetal development
Multiplication by mitosis
Some oogonia develop the potential to become mature female gametes.
Encapsulation by follicular cells
First stage of meiotic division arrested
Primordial follicles containing primary oocytes
BIRTH
No further follicular development until sexual maturity
SEXUAL MATURITY
Secretion of pituitary gonadotrophins FSH and LH
Some primordial follicles develop towards maturity with each ovarian cycle
Increasing secretion of oestrogen progressively inhibits secretion of FSH and promotes LH secretion
Primordial follicle
Early primary follicle
Primary follicle
First meiotic division completed
Second meiotic division commences
High levels of oestrogen inhibit FSH secretion and promotes secretion of LH
Secondary follicle
Graafian follicle
(now contains secondary oocyte)
OVULATION
Progesterone secretion by corpus luteum maintained by LH
Corpus luteum
No fertilisation
Corpus albicans
No fertilisation
Degeneration
Inhibition of LH secretion by progesterone
FERTILISATION
After 3rd month of pregnancy
IMPLANTATION
Corpus luteum of pregnancy maintained by hCG secreted by developing embryo
Morula
Embryo
Corpus luteum of pregnancy

FIG. 19.7 Follicular development

B blood clot **G** granulosa lutein cells **S** septum **Sh** vascular sheath of theca cells **T** theca lutein cells
TE theca externa cells **TI** theca interna cells **V** blood vessel

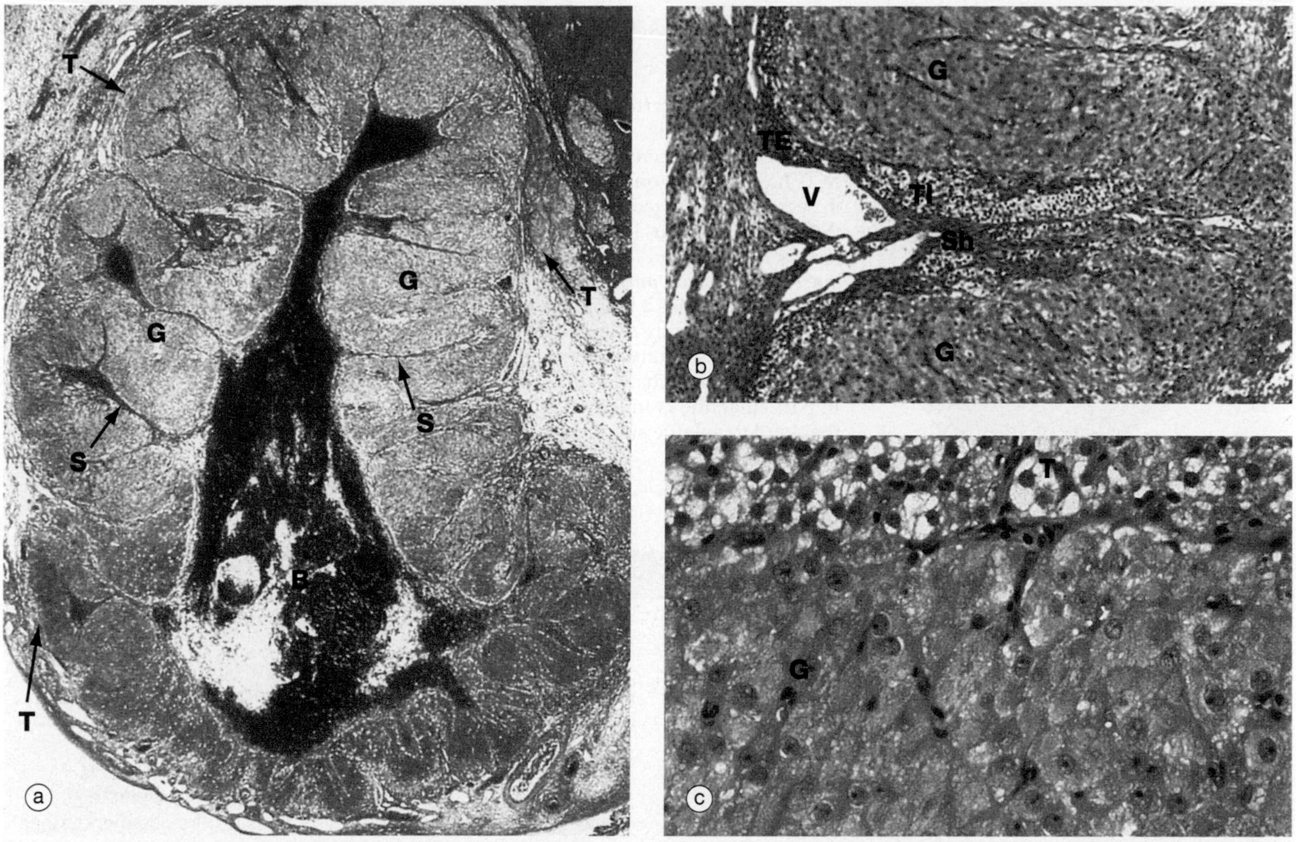

FIG. 19.8 Corpus luteum of menstruation
(a) H&E (LP) (b) H&E (MP) (c) H&E (HP)

Following ovulation, the ruptured follicle collapses and fills with a blood clot to form the ***corpus luteum of menstruation***, which has a brief career as an endocrine organ.

The corpus luteum of menstruation is about the same size as the antecedent ovulatory follicle (i.e. 1.5 to 2.5 cm). Under the influence of luteinising hormone (LH) secreted by the anterior pituitary, granulosa cells increase greatly in size and begin secretion of progesterone. The granulosa cells acquire the characteristics of steroid-secreting cells and are now called ***granulosa lutein cells***. Progesterone promotes the changes in the endometrium that make it ready for implantation of the embryo should fertilisation occur (see Figs 19.15 to 19.19). Thus the cycles of production of oocytes and the preparation of the endometrium (the menstrual cycle) are coordinated by the same set of hormones.

The cells of the theca interna also increase somewhat in size and acquire similar cytoplasmic features to the luteinised granulosa cells. Although interrupted by ovulation, these cells (as well as the granulosa cells) continue to secrete oestrogens which are necessary to maintain the thickened uterine mucosa. These cells become known as ***theca lutein cells***.

The basement membrane between the zona granulosa and the theca interna breaks down and these layers are invaded by capillaries and larger vessels from the theca externa to form a rich vascular network, characteristic of endocrine glands.

Progesterone production by the corpus luteum is dependent on LH from the anterior pituitary, but rising progesterone levels inhibit LH production. Without the continuing stimulus of LH, the corpus luteum cannot be maintained and, 12 to 14 days after ovulation, it regresses, ultimately forming a functionless ***corpus albicans*** (see Fig. 19.11). Once the corpus luteum regresses, secretion of both oestrogen and progesterone ceases. Without these hormones, the endometrial lining of the uterus collapses, resulting in the onset of ***menstruation***.

Fig. 19.8a shows a corpus luteum of menstruation. In the centre, the remnant of the post-ovulatory blood clot **B** is seen, surrounded by a broad zone of granulosa lutein cells **G**, penetrated by septa **S** containing the larger blood vessels.

Peripherally, a thin zone of theca lutein cells **T** can be seen. Externally, the corpus luteum is bounded by a zone of condensed stromal tissue, representing the theca externa of the antecedent Graafian follicle.

Fig. 19.8b shows the margin of a corpus luteum at intermediate magnification. Most of the field is occupied by granulosa lutein cells **G**, large polygonal cells with abundant pale eosinophilic (pink-stained) cytoplasm and round nuclei. The cytoplasm contains plentiful smooth endoplasmic reticulum, abundant mitochondria, lipid droplets and some lipofuscin, giving the corpus luteum a yellow colour macroscopically.

At the periphery, there are theca cells which also extend in a finger-like extension, forming a sheath **Sh** around blood vessels **V**. The theca externa cells **TE** have darker-stained cytoplasm while the luteinised theca interna cells **TI** have pale cytoplasm due to their content of lipid droplets.

At high magnification in Fig. 19.8c, granulosa lutein cells **G** may be compared with theca lutein cells **T**. The eosinophilic cytoplasm of the granulosa lutein cells contains numerous small lipid droplets which give rise to the vacuolated appearance seen in this preparation. Their larger spherical nuclei contain one or two prominent nucleoli. Theca lutein cells are smaller, with a more densely staining cytoplasm but with larger lipid vacuoles. Their ovoid nucleus has a single large nucleolus. The ultrastructure of the endocrine cells of the corpus luteum is characteristic of all steroid secretory cells (see Fig. 17.16).

As previously described, the granulosa lutein cells secrete progesterone (and a small amount of oestrogen) and the theca lutein cells secrete oestrogen precursors which are converted to oestrogen by the granulosa cells.

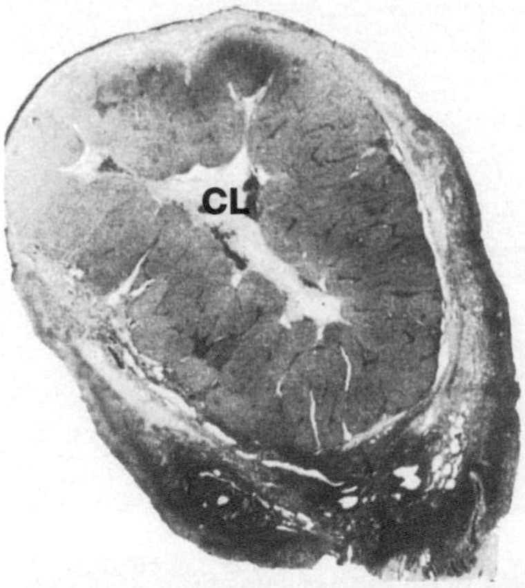

FIG. 19.9 Corpus luteum of pregnancy
H&E (LP)

Implantation of a fertilised ovum in the uterine wall interrupts the integrated ovarian and menstrual cycles. After implantation, a hormone called ***human chorionic gonadotrophin*** (***hCG***) is secreted into the maternal circulation by the developing placenta; hCG has an analogous function to LH and maintains the function of the ***corpus luteum*** in secreting oestrogen and progesterone until about the 9th week of pregnancy. After this time, the corpus luteum of pregnancy slowly regresses to form a functionless ***corpus albicans*** and the placenta takes over the major role of oestrogen and progesterone secretion until ***parturition***.

Fig. 19.9 shows a human ovary during the first trimester of pregnancy. The corpus luteum **CL** is greatly enlarged and by now occupies most of the ovary. The organisation of the corpus luteum of pregnancy is similar to that of menstruation, but there are some histological changes that are almost specific for the corpus luteum of pregnancy. In particular, the granulosa lutein cells contain hyaline, eosinophilic inclusion bodies that tend to enlarge and then calcify as the pregnancy progresses.

Ovarian cysts

Ovarian cysts are common and can be broadly divided into neoplastic and non-neoplastic cysts. Non-neoplastic cysts include follicular cysts, due to enlargement of normal follicles, and corpus luteum cysts, which result from a similar expansion of a normal corpus luteum (see e-Fig. 19.1).

There are many different types of neoplastic cysts. Most are derived from epithelial cells and are classed as benign (cystadenoma), borderline or malignant. There are many subtypes of epithelial cyst such as serous and mucinous (see e-Fig. 19.2). High grade serous carcinoma, the commonest malignant tumour found in the ovary, is now thought to arise from pre-cancerous (dysplastic) lesions at the end of the fallopian tube (see e-Fig. 19.3). A fairly common type of ovarian cyst in young women is the dermoid cyst or mature cystic teratoma, which is usually benign (see e-Fig. 19.4).

Another common type of cyst is the endometriotic cyst or endometrioma, where abnormal deposits of endometrial glands and stroma are found in the ovary and, indeed, in many other sites in the body (see e-Fig. 19.5).

Endometriosis is often associated with infertility, as is polycystic ovarian syndrome, a condition where multiple follicular cysts are associated with obesity, hirsuitism and other metabolic abnormalities such as impaired glucose tolerance.

The type of cyst, along with other pathological factors influences the treatment (surgical and/or oncological). Diagnosis often requires biopsy, oophorectomy (removal of the ovary) or cystectomy (removal of the cyst).

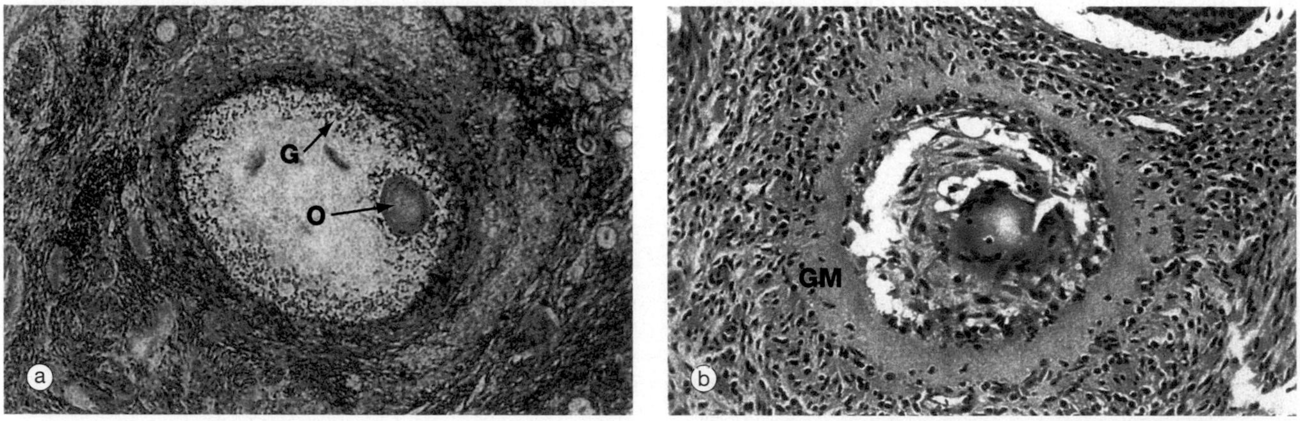

FIG. 19.10 Atretic follicles
(a) H&E (LP) (b) H&E (MP)

The process of ***follicular atresia*** (degeneration) may occur at any stage in the development of the ovum. By the sixth month of development, the fetal ovary contains several million primordial follicles yet, by the time of birth, only about half a million remain. Atresia continues until puberty and thereafter through the reproductive years. In addition, with each ovarian cycle approximately 20 follicles begin to mature, usually all but one becoming atretic at some stage before complete maturity.

The histological appearance of atretic follicles varies enormously, depending on the stage of development reached and the progress of atresia. The atretic follicle seen in Fig. 19.10a is a secondary follicle in early atresia. The oocyte **O** has degenerated and the granulosa cells **G** have begun to disaggregate.

Advanced atresia, as seen in Fig. 19.10b, is characterised by gross thickening of the basement membrane between the granulosa cells and the theca interna, forming the so-called ***glassy membrane*** **GM**. Atretic follicles are ultimately replaced completely by collagenous tissue known as the ***corpus fibrosum***. Most corpora fibrosa eventually disappear completely. In the postmenopausal woman, primordial follicles are absent, and the cortex consists of stroma and corpora albicantes only, with no developing follicles. The postmenopausal ovary is smaller than that in premenopausal women.

C corpus albicans **CL** corpus luteum **G** granulosa cells **GM** glassy membrane **M** macrophages **O** oocyte **P** primordial follicle **S** stroma

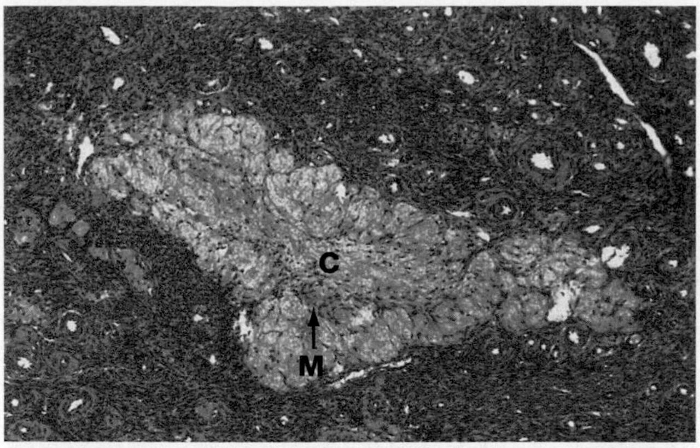

FIG. 19.11 Corpus albicans
H&E (LP)

The ***corpus albicans*** **C** is the inactive fibrous tissue mass that forms following the involution of a corpus luteum (Fig. 19.11). The secretory cells of the degenerate corpus luteum undergo autolysis and are phagocytosed by macrophages **M**, a few of which, containing cytoplasmic haemosiderin pigment, can be seen here. The vascular supporting tissue regresses to form a relatively acellular collagenous scar containing a few fibroblasts. In the human ovary, corpora albicantes are a dominant feature, increasing in number with age and often appearing to occupy almost the whole ovarian stroma. Most regress completely leaving no trace, otherwise the postmenopausal ovary would contain approximately 500 corpora albicantia.

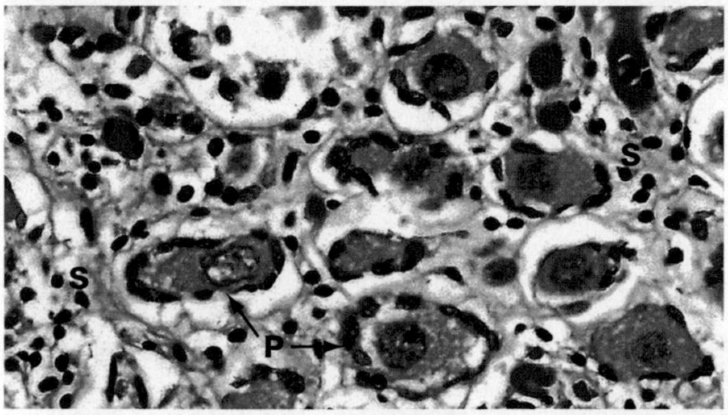

FIG. 19.12 Fetal ovary
H&E (HP)

In this micrograph of ovary (Fig. 19.12) from a term fetus, the ovarian cortex is seen to be packed with ***primordial follicles*** **P**. The surrounding stroma **S** is much more delicate than in an adult woman. These ova are arrested in the first meiotic division and remain so until the onset of puberty signals the waves of maturation of follicles that occur with each cycle in the reproductive years.

THE GENITAL TRACT

The genital tract consists of the ***Fallopian tubes***, the ***uterus*** and the ***vagina***, all of which have the same basic structure, consisting of a wall of smooth muscle with an inner mucosal lining and an outer layer of loose supporting tissue.

The mucosal and muscular components vary greatly according to their location and functional requirements. The whole tract undergoes cyclical changes under the influence of ovarian hormones which are released during the ovarian cycle. The cyclical changes which occur in the genital tract facilitate the entry of ova into the Fallopian tube, the passage of spermatozoa through the uterine cervix and into the Fallopian tube, the passage of the fertilised ovum into the uterus and the implantation and development of the fertilised ovum in the mucosal lining (***endometrium***) of the uterus.

Implantation of a fertilised ovum results in secretion of hormones that inhibit the ovarian cycle and produce changes in the genital tract necessary for fetal development and parturition.

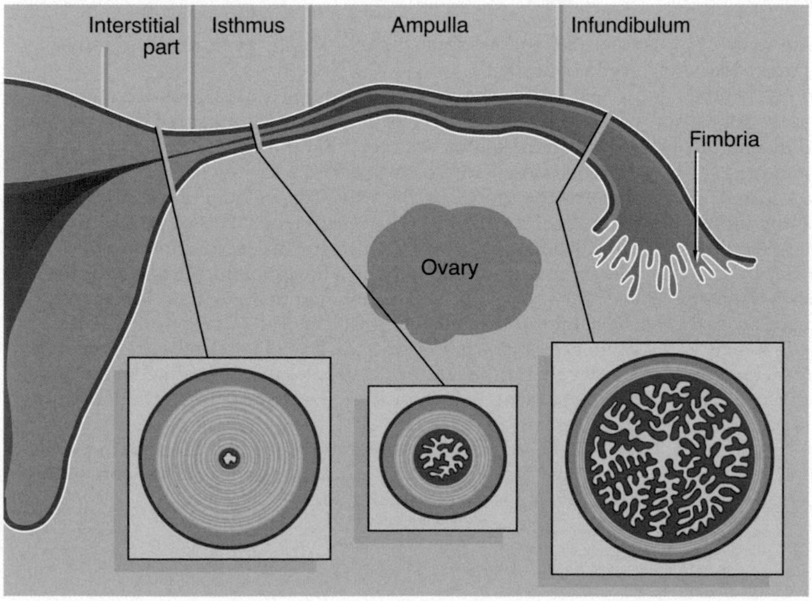

FIG. 19.13 Fallopian tubes

The ***Fallopian tubes*** (also called ***uterine tubes*** or ***oviducts***) carry ova from the surface of the ovaries to the uterine cavity and are also the site of fertilisation by spermatozoa. The Fallopian tube is shaped like an elongated funnel and is divided anatomically into four parts as shown in the diagram.

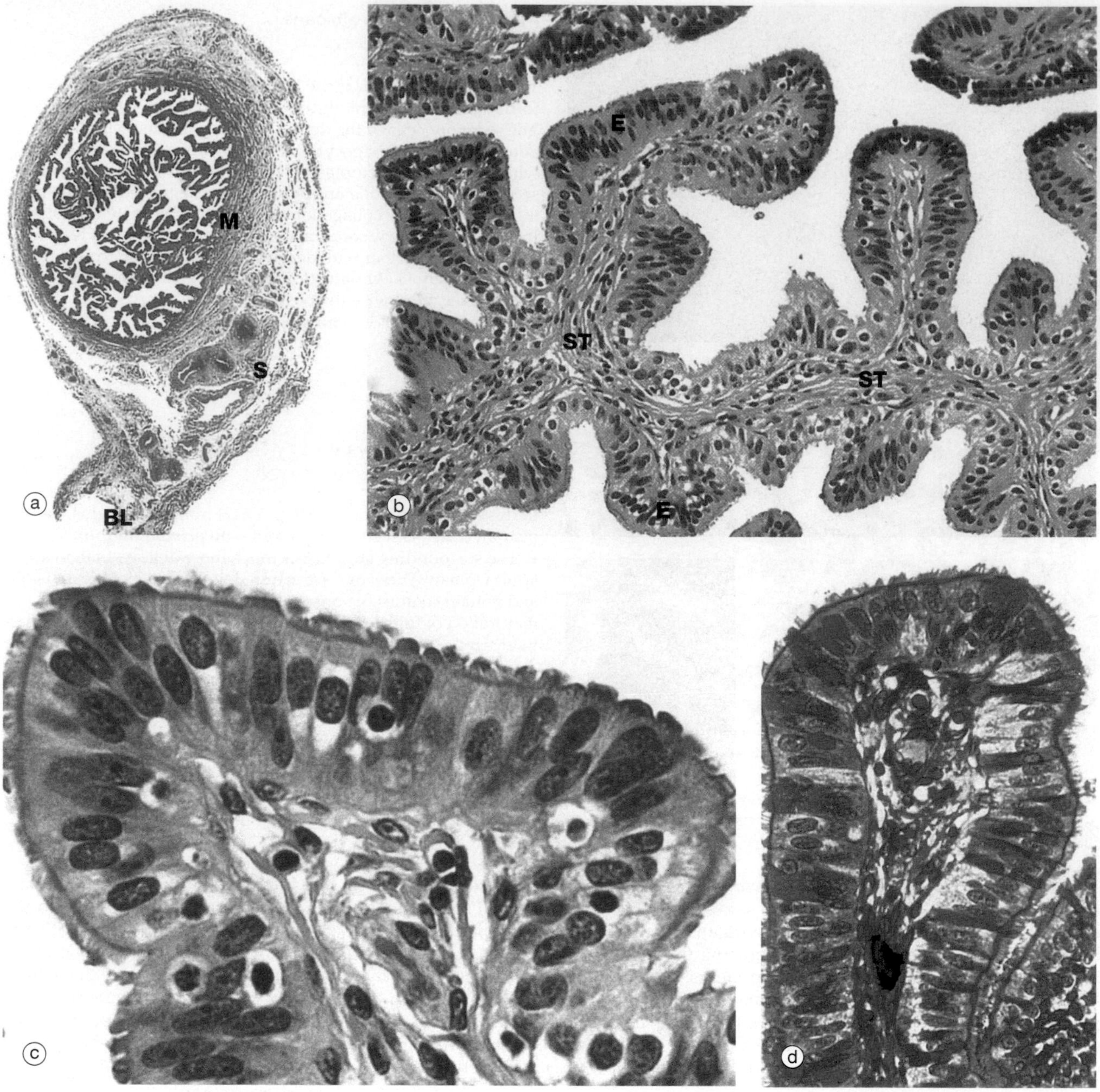

FIG. 19.14 Fallopian tube
(a) H&E (LP) (b) H&E (MP) (c) H&E (HP) (d) Azan (HP)

At the time of ovulation, the ***infundibulum*** moves so as to overlie the site of rupture of the Graafian follicle. Finger-like projections called ***fimbriae*** extending from the end of the tube envelop the ovulation site and direct the ovum into the tube. Movement of the ovum along the tube is mediated by gentle peristaltic action of the longitudinal and circular smooth muscle layers of the oviduct wall. This is aided by a current of fluid, propelled by the action of the ciliated epithelium lining the tube. The mucosal lining of the Fallopian tube is thrown into a labyrinth of branching longitudinal folds, a feature that is most prominent in the ***ampulla*** (Fig. 19.14a), which is the usual site of fertilisation. Note also in Fig. 19.14a, the muscular wall **M** and the vascular supporting tissue of the serosa **S**, which is continuous with the broad ligament **BL**. The serosal layer and broad ligament have a surface lining of mesothelium. The muscular wall has two layers, an ***inner circular*** and an ***outer longitudinal***, not discernible at this magnification.

Fig. 19.14b focuses on one of the mucosal folds of the ampulla. These have a branching core of vascular supporting tissue **ST** and are invested by a single layer of tall columnar epithelial cells **E**.

Fig. 19.14c shows the tip of a mucosal fold at high magnification. The columnar cells of the epithelium are of three types: ciliated, non-ciliated secretory and ***intercalated cells***.

The non-ciliated cells produce a secretion that is propelled towards the uterus by the wave-like beating of the cilia of the ciliated cells, carrying with it the ovum. This secretion probably also has a role in the nutrition and protection of the ovum. The intercalated cells may be a morphological variant of the secretory cells. The ratio of ciliated to non-ciliated cells and the height of the cells undergo cyclical variations under the influence of ovarian hormones. The ciliated cells are generally shorter than the secretory cells, making the epithelial surface somewhat irregular in outline. Scattered intraepithelial lymphocytes are also present.

Fig. 19.14d employs a method that stains the secretory cells blue. Note that the collagen of the supporting tissue core of the mucosal fold is also stained blue.

Pathology of the Fallopian tube

The Fallopian tube can be damaged by a variety of pathological processes and such tubal injury may then lead to a range of other problems including subfertility and even tubal ectopic pregnancy, where the fertilised ovum implants in the wall of the Fallopian tube, rather than passing along to enter the uterine cavity.

Common causes of tubal injury include pelvic inflammatory disease (where tubal inflammation and scarring occurs due to infection with organisms such as *Chlamydia* or *Gonococcus*) and endometriosis, a disorder in which small deposits of endometrium are found outside the uterine cavity.

Endometriosis often affects the Fallopian tubes and, again, this results in scarring and peritoneal adhesions which can block the Fallopian tubes, leading to reduced fertility. As well as preventing the normal passage of the ovum to the uterus, such tubal blockage can result in cystic dilatation of the tube, forming a hydrosalpinx. If such a fluid collection becomes infected and consists of pus, it is called a pyosalpinx.

THE HUMAN MENSTRUAL CYCLE

The uterus is a flattened pear-shaped organ approximately 7 cm long in the non-pregnant state. Its mucosal lining, the ***endometrium***, provides the environment for fetal development. The thick smooth muscle wall, the ***myometrium***, expands greatly during pregnancy and provides protection for the fetus and a mechanism for the expulsion of the fetus at ***parturition***.

The endometrium is variable in thickness, measuring between 1 and 5 mm at different stages of the menstrual cycle. The myometrium makes up the bulk of the uterus, measuring up to about 20 mm in a woman of reproductive age (see Fig. 19.2).

In women of child-bearing age, the endometrial lining of the uterine cavity consists of a pseudostratified columnar ciliated epithelium forming numerous simple tubular glands, supported by the cellular ***endometrial stroma***. Under the influence of oestrogen and progesterone secreted during the ovarian cycle, the endometrium undergoes regular cyclical changes so as to offer a suitable environment for implantation of a fertilised ovum. These changes are summarised in Fig. 19.15. For successful implantation, the fertilised ovum requires an easily penetrable, highly vascular tissue and an abundant supply of glycogen for nutrition until vascular connections are established with the maternal circulation.

The cycle of changes in the endometrium proceeds through three distinct phases: ***menstruation***, ***proliferation*** and ***secretion***. These changes involve both the epithelium and supporting stroma.

- The **menstrual phase**. The first day of menstruation is, by convention, taken as the first day of the cycle, simply because it is easily identified. This is the phase of endometrial shedding that only occurs if there is failure of fertilisation and/or implantation of the ovum. Progesterone production by the corpus luteum is inhibited by negative feedback on the anterior pituitary, thus suppressing LH release and leading to involution of the corpus luteum. In the absence of progesterone, the endometrium cannot be maintained. Reactivation of FSH secretion initiates a new cycle of follicular development and oestrogen secretion. This, in turn, initiates a new cycle of proliferation of the endometrium from the endometrial remnants of the previous cycle.
- The **proliferative phase**. The endometrial stroma proliferates, becoming thicker and richly vascularised. The simple tubular glands elongate to form numerous long, coiled glands that begin secretion coincident with ovulation. The proliferative phase is initiated and sustained until ovulation by the increasing production of oestrogens from developing ovarian follicles.
- The **secretory phase**. Release of progesterone from the corpus luteum after ovulation promotes production of a copious, thick, glycogen-rich secretion by the endometrial glands.

A typical menstrual cycle is 28 days in length, although there is wide variation among normal women. Menstruation lasts on average 5 days. The proliferative phase continues until about the 14th day when ovulation occurs and the secretory phase begins. The secretory phase culminates at the onset of menstruation on about the 28th day.

The endometrium is divided into three histologically and functionally distinct layers. The deepest or basal layer, the ***stratum basalis***, adjacent to the myometrium, undergoes little change during the menstrual cycle and is not shed during menstruation. The broad intermediate layer is characterised by a stroma with a spongy appearance and is called the ***stratum spongiosum***. The thinner superficial layer, which has a compact stromal appearance, is known as the ***stratum compactum***. The compact and spongy layers exhibit dramatic changes throughout the cycle and both are shed during menstruation. These layers are jointly referred to as the ***stratum functionalis***.

The arrangement of the arterial supply of the endometrium has important influences on the menstrual cycle. Branches of the uterine arteries pass through the myometrium and immediately divide into two different types of arteries, ***straight arteries*** and ***spiral arteries***. Straight arteries are short and pass a small distance into the endometrium, then bifurcate to form a plexus supplying the stratum basalis. Spiral arteries are long, coiled and thick-walled and pass to the surface of the endometrium, giving off numerous branches which give rise to a capillary plexus around the glands and in the stratum compactum. Unlike the straight arteries, the spiral arteries are responsive to the hormonal changes of the menstrual cycle. The withdrawal of progesterone secretion at the end of the cycle causes the spiral arteries to constrict and this precipitates an ischaemic phase that immediately precedes menstruation.

BL broad ligament **E** epithelial cells **M** muscular wall **S** serosa **ST** supporting tissue

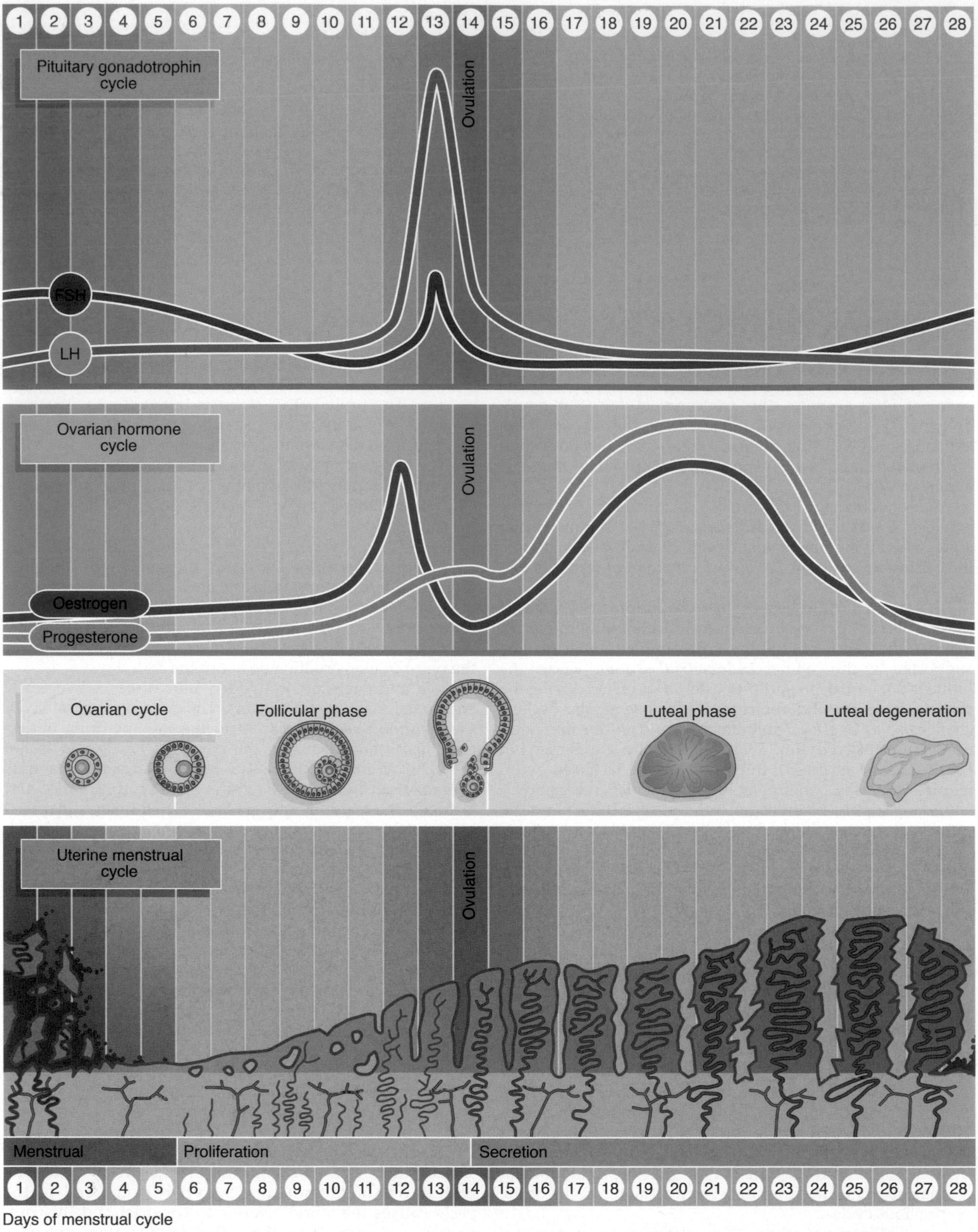

FIG. 19.15 The hormonal integration of the ovarian and menstrual cycles

The menstrual cycle

The illustration above shows the changes which occur during a typical 28-day-long menstrual cycle, but there is significant variation in the length of the menstrual cycle in normal women, often ranging from 21 days up to 40 days or sometimes more. In such cases, there is variation in the duration of both the follicular and the luteal phases of the menstrual cycle, but the luteal phase seems to be of more fixed duration and typically lasts around 14 days, with more of the difference in cycle length being attributable to variation in the duration of the follicular part of the cycle.

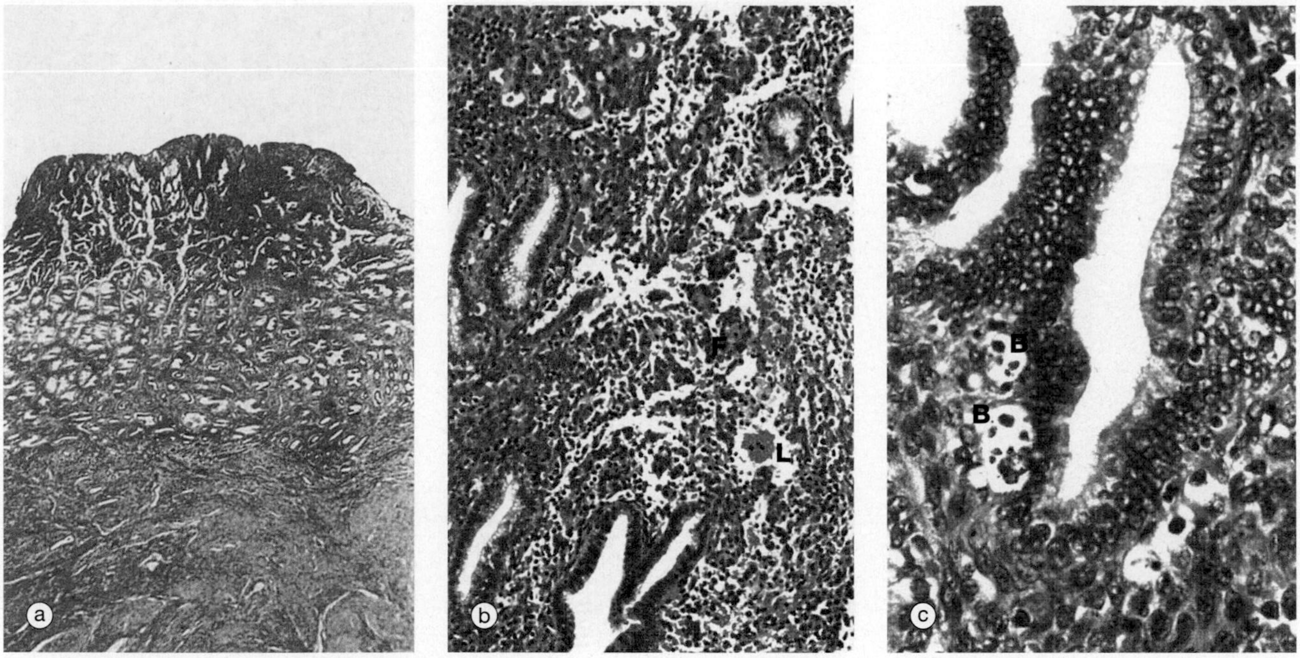

FIG. 19.16 Endometrium, the onset of menstruation
(a) H&E (LP) (b) H&E (MP) (c) H&E (HP)

In the absence of implantation of a fertilised ovum, degeneration of the corpus luteum results in cessation of oestrogen and progesterone secretion. In turn, this initiates spasmodic constriction in the spiral arterioles of the endometrial ***stratum functionalis*** **F**. The resulting ischaemia is initially manifest by degeneration of the superficial layers of the endometrium and leakage of blood **L** into the stroma. This is illustrated in Fig. 19.16a and b. Stromal cells disaggregate and the endometrial glands collapse. These features are indicative of early necrosis of glands and stroma. At high magnification in Fig. 19.16c nuclear debris of endometrial cells (***apoptotic bodies***) **B** can be seen at the onset of menstruation. These cells have died by ***apoptosis*** (see Ch. 2).

Further ischaemia leads to degeneration of the whole stratum functionalis, which is progressively shed as ***menses***. Menses is thus composed of blood, necrotic epithelium and stroma. Normally, menstrual blood does not clot due to the local release of inhibitory (anticoagulant) factors and its expulsion is enhanced by uterine contractions. By day 3 to 4 of menstruation, most of the stratum functionalis has been shed and proliferation of the basal layer of the endometrium has begun again.

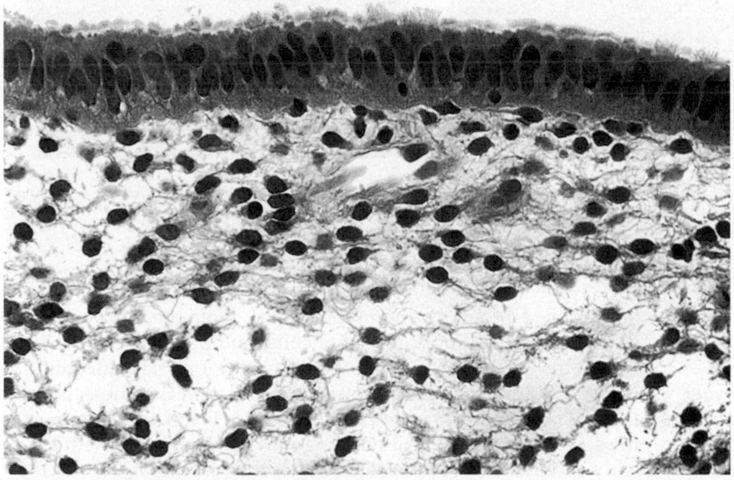

FIG. 19.17 Endometrial surface
H&E (HP)

Fig. 19.17 illustrates the surface epithelium of the endometrium, which is tall and columnar in form. Some of the cells bear cilia, the remainder having surface microvilli. Stromal cells have plump, spindle-shaped nuclei and scanty cytoplasm.

This specimen was obtained during the secretory phase of the menstrual cycle at a time when the stroma is quite oedematous. This can be seen in the clear spaces between the spindle-shaped stromal cells.

Endometrial cancer

Endometrial cancer is the commonest type of gynaecological cancer in women (see e-Fig. 19.6). Risk factors include increasing age, hyperoestrogenic states including certain medications such as oestrogen therapies, high BMI and genetic syndromes. Hormonal overstimulation of the uterus can result in overgrowth (hyperplasia) of the endometrium, which may be associated with invasive cancer. There are many different types of EC, the commonest of which is endometrioid adenocarcinoma, a gland-forming malignant tumour which resembles normal endometrial glands.

B apoptotic bodies **F** stratum functionalis **L** leakage of blood

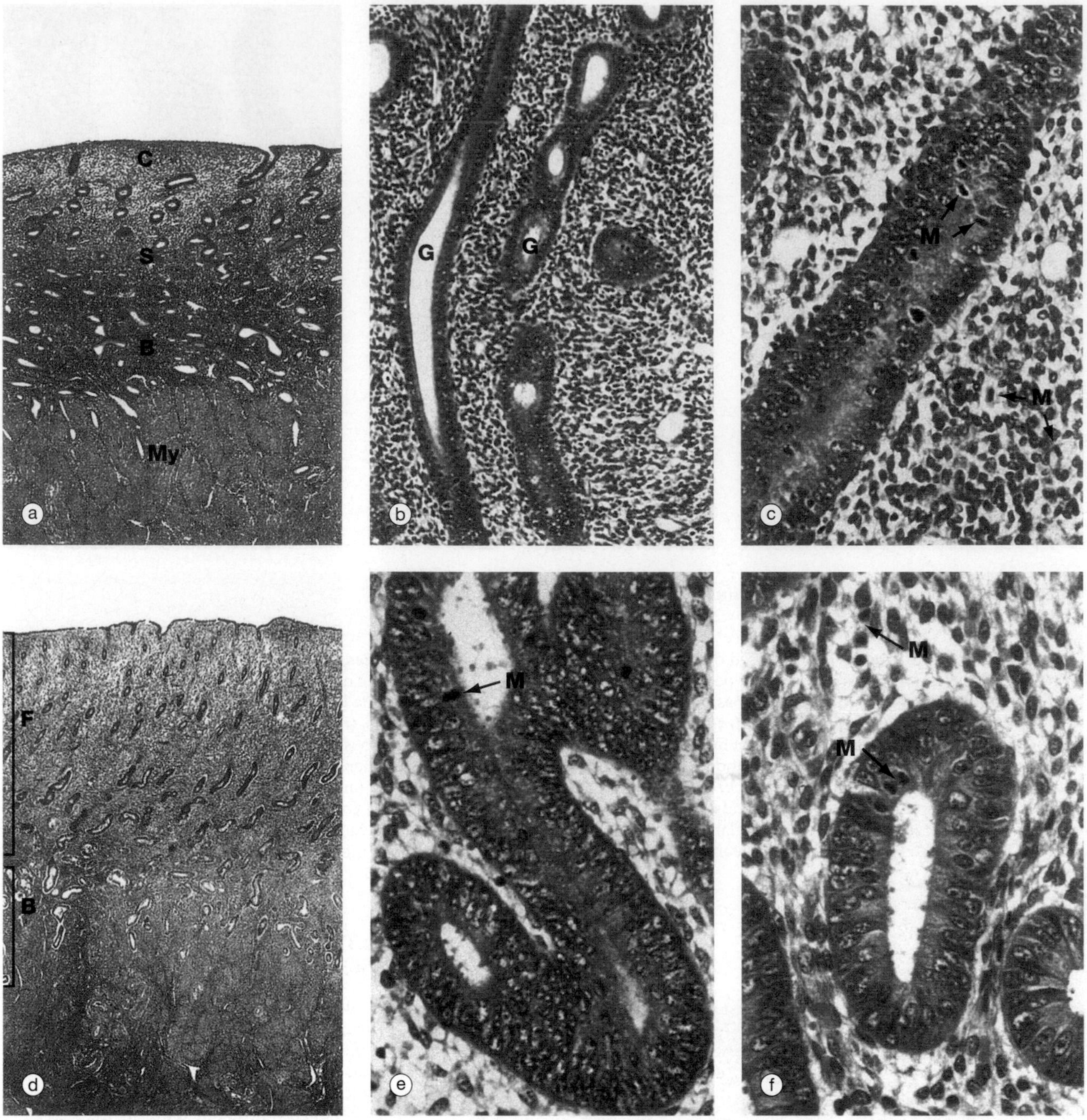

FIG. 19.18 Proliferative endometrium
(a) Early phase, H&E (LP) (b) Early phase, H&E (MP) (c) Early phase, H&E (HP) (d) Late phase, H&E (LP) (e) Late phase, H&E (HP) (f) Late phase, H&E (HP)

Fig. 19.18a illustrates early ***proliferative endometrium*** at low magnification. The bottom of the field includes part of the muscular wall, the ***myometrium*** **My**. The relatively thin endometrium consists of the ***stratum basalis*** **B**, ***stratum spongiosum*** **S** and ***stratum compactum*** **C**. The glands at this stage are fairly sparse and straight.

As the glands, stroma and vessels proliferate, the endometrium gradually becomes thicker. By day 5 to 6 of the cycle, the surface epithelium has regenerated. During the proliferative phase, the epithelial cells acquire microvilli and cilia as well as the cytoplasmic organelles required for the secretory phase.

At higher magnification in Fig. 19.18b, the straight tubular form of the endometrial glands **G** can be seen. At very high magnification in Fig. 19.18c, the proliferating glandular epithelium is seen to consist of columnar cells with basally located nuclei exhibiting prominent nucleoli. Mitotic figures **M** can be seen, both in the epithelium and in the stroma. Note the highly cellular stroma which is almost devoid of collagen fibres.

By the late proliferative stage, shown at low magnification in Fig. 19.18d, the endometrium has doubled in thickness. Note that in contrast to the ***stratum functionalis*** **F**, the appearance of the stratum basalis **B** is little changed when compared with the early proliferative phase. With further magnification, Fig. 19.18e shows that the tubular glands are now becoming coiled and more closely packed. At very high magnification in Fig. 19.18f, mitotic figures **M** are more prevalent in both the glandular epithelium and the supporting stroma. The stroma is also somewhat oedematous at this stage. During the proliferative phase, there is a continuum of change that makes the precise dating of the cycle inaccurate in histological specimens. Lymphocytes and occasional lymphoid aggregates are a normal feature of late proliferative phase endometrium, but plasma cells are abnormal, indicating chronic infection (***endometritis***).

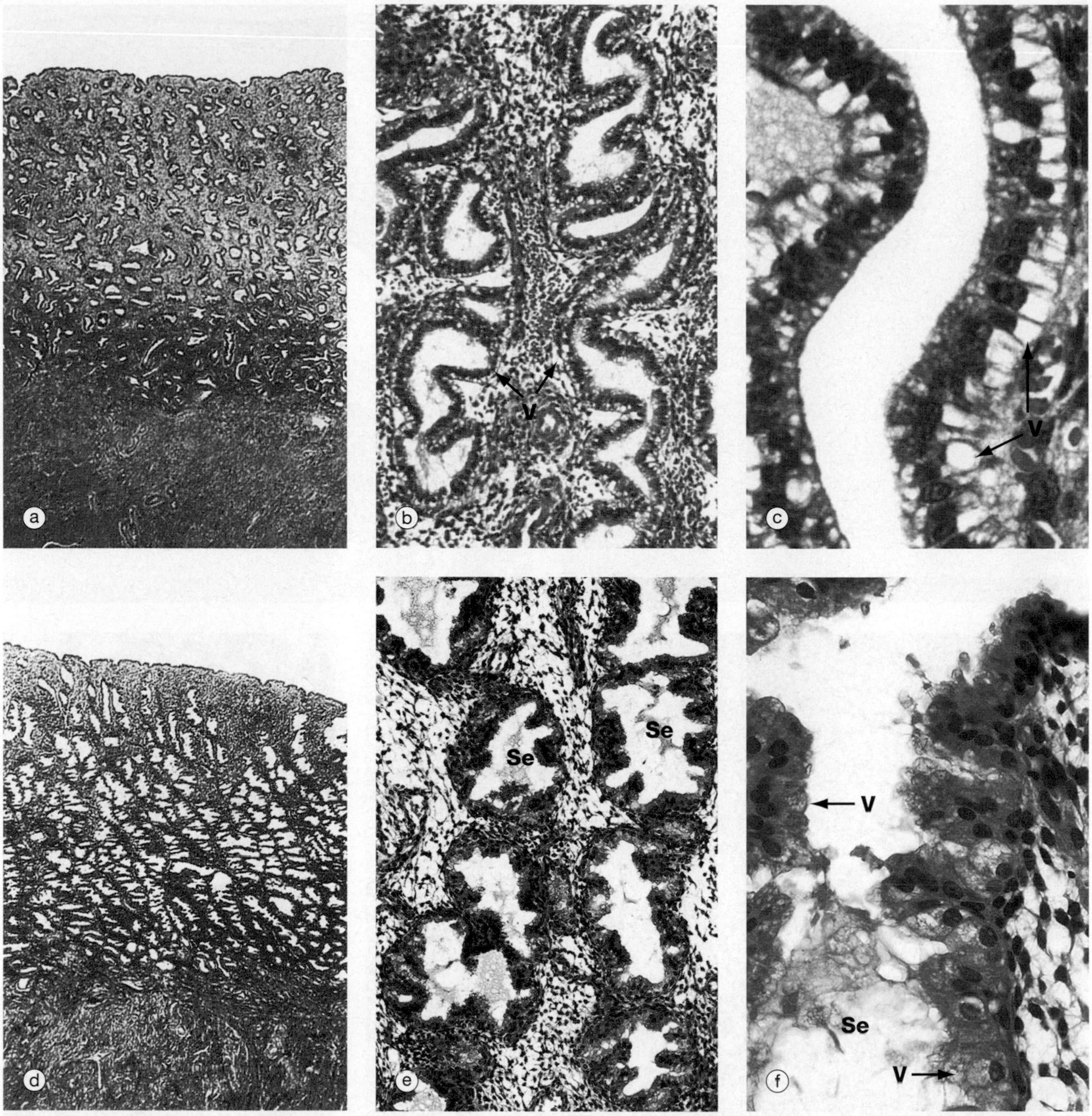

FIG. 19.19 Secretory endometrium
(a) Early phase, H&E (LP) (b) Early phase, H&E (MP) (c) Early phase, H&E (HP) (d) Late phase, H&E (LP) (e) Late phase, H&E (MP) (f) Late phase, H&E (HP)

Ovulation marks the onset of the secretory phase, although endometrial cell division continues for several days. At low magnification in Fig. 19.19a, the coiled appearance of the glands is now more pronounced and the endometrium approaches its maximum thickness.

Under the influence of progesterone, the glandular epithelium is stimulated to synthesise glycogen. Initially, the glycogen accumulates to form vacuoles **V** in the basal aspect of the cells, thus displacing the nuclei towards the centre of the now tall columnar cells. This ***basal vacuolation*** of the cells appears on day 16 and is the characteristic feature of early secretory endometrium as seen at intermediate and high magnification in Fig. 19.19b and c, respectively. Glycogen is an important source of nutrition for the fertilised ovum.

The late secretory phase is characterised by a saw-tooth appearance of the glands, containing copious thick glycogen- and glycoprotein-rich secretions **Se**. This is illustrated at low and intermediate magnification in Fig. 19.19d and e, respectively.

At very high magnification in Fig. 19.19f, the cytoplasmic vacuoles **V** can now be seen on the luminal aspect of the cell, and the nucleus has returned to its basal position. These vacuoles contain glycogen and glycoproteins that are secreted **Se** into the glandular lumen by apocrine-type secretion. Mitotic figures are absent. The stroma is by now at its most vascular and interstitial fluid begins to accumulate between the stromal cells. ***Endometrial stromal granulocytes***, which are probably large granular lymphocytes, are found in the stroma at this stage. These changes in secretory phase endometrium make more precise dating possible on histological specimens than in the proliferative phase. Such examinations may be helpful in the investigation of infertility.

B stratum basalis **C** stratum compactum **F** stratum functionalis **G** endometrial gland **M** mitotic figure **My** myometrium **S** stratum spongiosum **Se** secretions **V** vacuoles

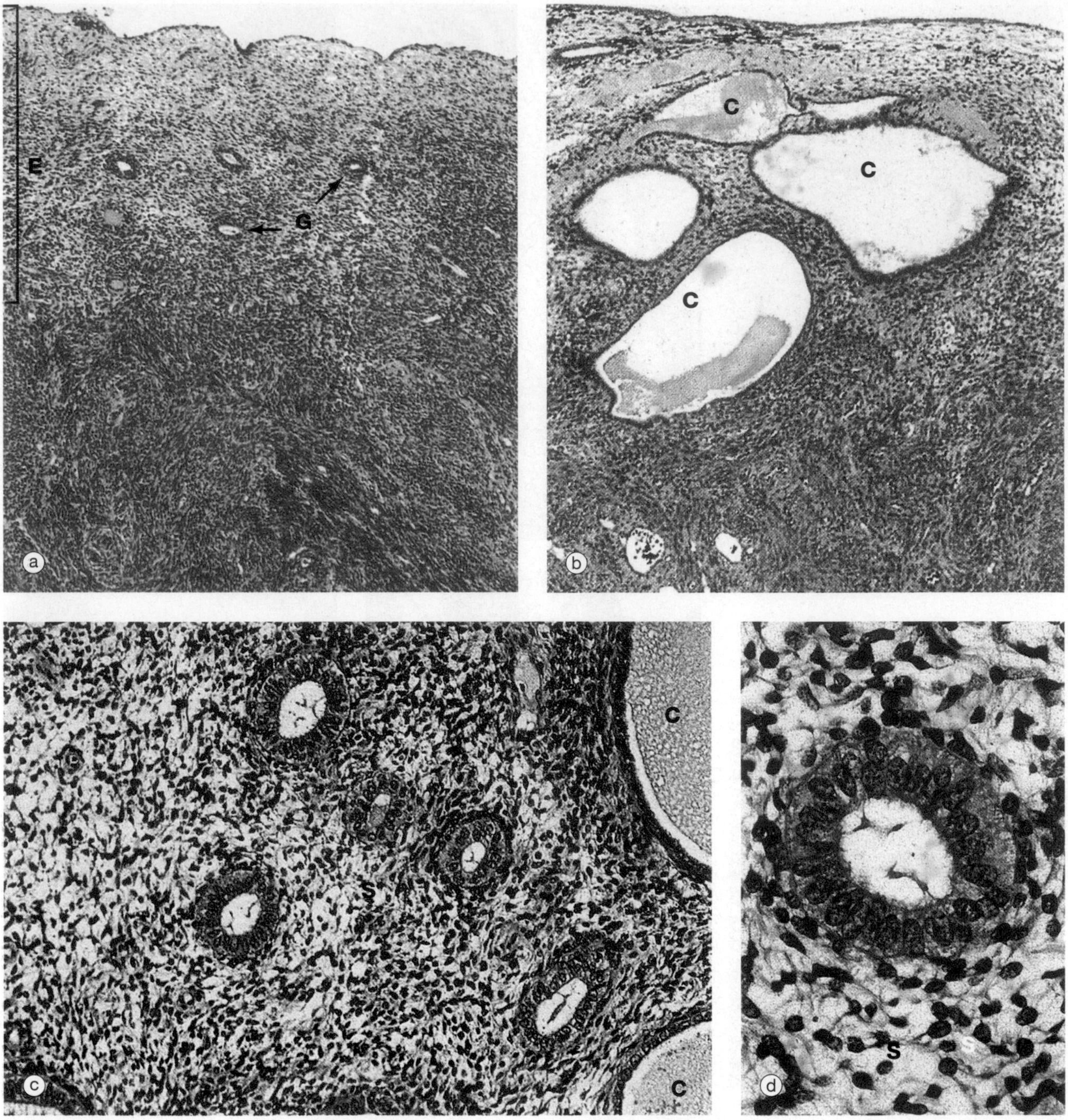

FIG. 19.20 Post-menopausal endometrium
(a) H&E (LP) (b) H&E (LP) (c) H&E (MP) (d) H&E (HP)

After the menopause, the cyclical production of oestrogen and progesterone from the ovaries ceases and the whole genital tract undergoes ***atrophy***. As seen in Fig. 19.20a, the endometrium **E** is thin, consisting only of the stratum basalis, and the glands **G** are sparse and inactive.

In some women, the glands become dilated to form cystic spaces **C** as shown in Fig. 19.20b. The reason for this is unknown, but this appearance is so common as to be considered a normal variant.

At higher magnifications in Fig. 19.20c and d, the glandular epithelial cells are cuboidal or low columnar with no mitotic figures or secretory activity. The epithelium which lines cystically dilated glands **C**, as shown in Fig. 19.20c, is often flattened. The stroma **S** is much less cellular and contains more collagen fibres than during the reproductive years and no mitotic activity is seen. The myometrium also becomes atrophic after the menopause and the uterus shrinks to about half its former size.

Hormonal effects on the endometrium

A variety of drug treatments have effects on the endometrium. Commonly used agents include the oral contraceptive pill (OCP) and post-menopausal hormone replacement therapy (HRT). These treatments may use a combination of oestrogenic and progestogenic agents to mimic the changes of a normal menstrual cycle or sometimes use progestogenic agents alone.

Other drugs used in treatment of malignant disease have hormonal effects, including the anti-oestrogenic drugs which are used in patients with hormone-sensitive breast cancer. These agents may have unpredictable effects on the endometrium.

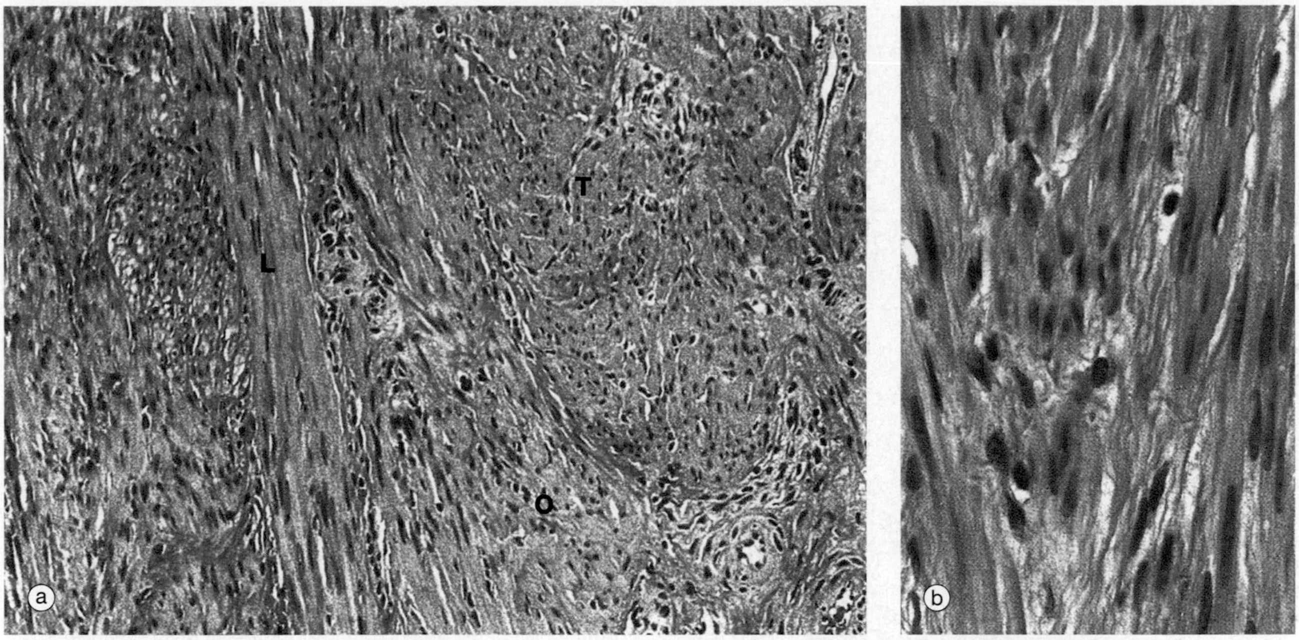

FIG. 19.21 Myometrium
(a) H&E (MP) (b) H&E (HP)

The main bulk of the uterus consists of smooth muscle, the ***myometrium***, which is composed of interlacing bundles of long slender fibres arranged in ill-defined layers. This is readily seen in Fig. 19.21a, which contains bundles of fibres in transverse **T**, longitudinal **L** and oblique sections **O**. Within the muscle, there is a rich network of arteries and veins which are supported by collagenous supporting tissue. Fig. 19.21b shows detail of the smooth muscle cells at high magnification, highlighting the closeness with which the muscle fibres are packed.

During pregnancy, in response to increased levels of oestrogens, the myometrium increases greatly in size, mainly by increasing cell size (***hypertrophy***), although some increase in cell numbers (***hyperplasia***) due to cell division may also occur.

At parturition, strong contractions of the myometrium are reinforced by the action of the hormone ***oxytocin***, secreted by the posterior pituitary. These contractions expel the fetus from the uterus and also constrict the blood supply to the placenta, thus precipitating its detachment from the uterine wall.

Smooth muscle tumours

The uterine leiomyoma, colloquially known as a fibroid, is a very common benign tumour of women of reproductive age. They tend to increase in size and number with age and cause a range of symptoms, including abnormal bleeding, a feeling of pain or dragging in the lower abdomen, urinary frequency if they compress the bladder, and infertility. A typical leiomyoma is illustrated in Fig. 19.22. Uterine fibroids are often multiple.

In contrast, leiomyosarcomas, the malignant counterpart of the benign fibroid, are much rarer, are typically solitary and occur in older women. These tumours are characterised by features such as an infiltrative margin, marked cytological atypia, necrosis and increased mitotic activity.

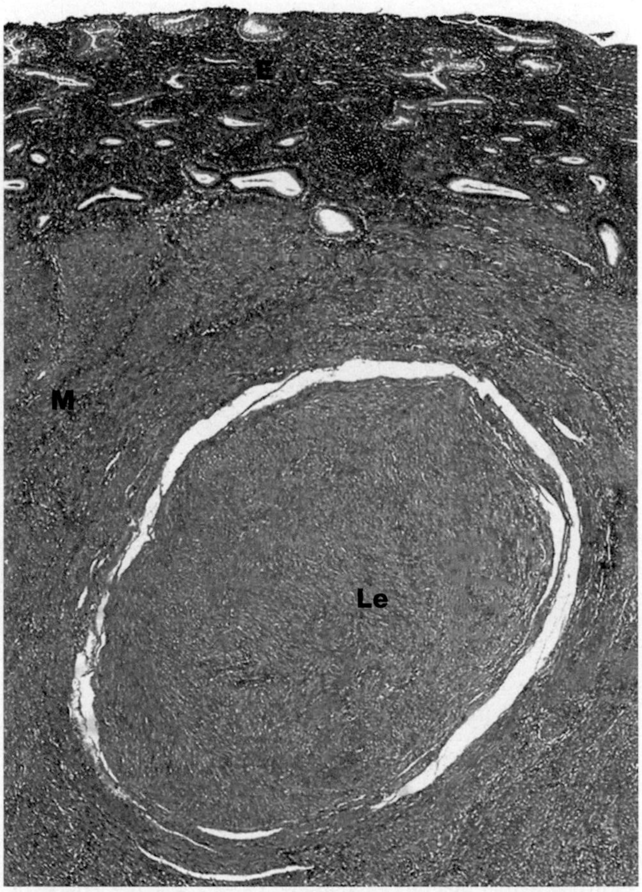

FIG. 19.22 Uterine leiomyoma
H&E (LP)

The leiomyoma (known as a 'fibroid') **Le** consists of bland smooth muscle fibres which are very like their normal counterparts in appearance (Fig. 19.22). The smooth muscle fibres form whorls and are embedded in a fibrous stroma. The resulting nodule has a very well-circumscribed margin and there is a pseudocapsule of compressed smooth muscle separating it from the normal myometrium **M**. The endometrium **E** is seen at the top of this micrograph. Although this example is a small leiomyoma, they may reach considerable size, and examples 15 cm in diameter or larger are not uncommon.

Leiomyomas may be described as submucosal, intramural or subserosal, based upon their position within the myometrium. Submucosal leiomyomas occur just beneath the endometrium and may greatly enlarge and distort the endometrial cavity, resulting in very heavy menses (menorrhagia).

C cystic gland **E** endometrium **G** gland **L** longitudinal smooth muscle bundle **Le** leiomyoma **M** myometrium
O oblique smooth muscle bundle **S** stroma **T** transverse smooth muscle bundle

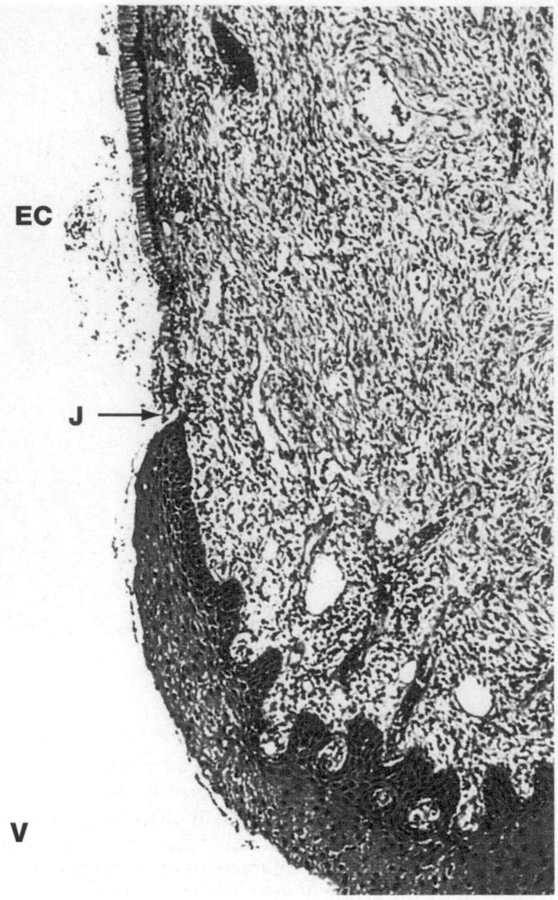

**FIG. 19.23 Uterine cervix
H&E (LP)**

The ***uterine cervix*** protrudes into the upper vagina and contains the ***endocervical canal***, linking the uterine cavity with the vagina. The function of the cervix is to admit spermatozoa to the genital tract at the time when fertilisation is possible, i.e. around the time of ovulation. At other times, including pregnancy, its function is to protect the uterus and upper tract from bacterial invasion. In addition, the cervix must be capable of great dilatation to permit the passage of the fetus during parturition.

As seen in Fig. 19.23, the endocervical canal **EC** is lined by a single layer of tall columnar mucus-secreting epithelial cells. Where the cervix is exposed to the more hostile environment of the vagina **V**, the ***ectocervix***, it is lined by thick stratified squamous epithelium as in the vagina and the vulva. The cells of the ectocervix often have clear cytoplasm due to their high glycogen content (not apparent in this specimen).

The junction **J** between the ecto- and endocervical epithelium is quite abrupt and is normally located at the external os, the point at which the endocervical canal opens into the vagina.

The main bulk of the cervix is composed of tough collagenous tissue containing a little smooth muscle. At the squamocolumnar junction, the cervical stroma is often infiltrated with leukocytes, forming part of the defence against ingress of microorganisms.

The columnar epithelium of the endocervix can undergo metaplasia to squamous epithelium. This 'transformation zone' is sensitive to human papillomavirus (HPV) infection, persistent high risk types of which are associated with squamous intraepithelial lesions (cervical intraepithelial neoplasia; CIN) and invasive cervical cancer (see e-Figs 19.7 and 19.8).

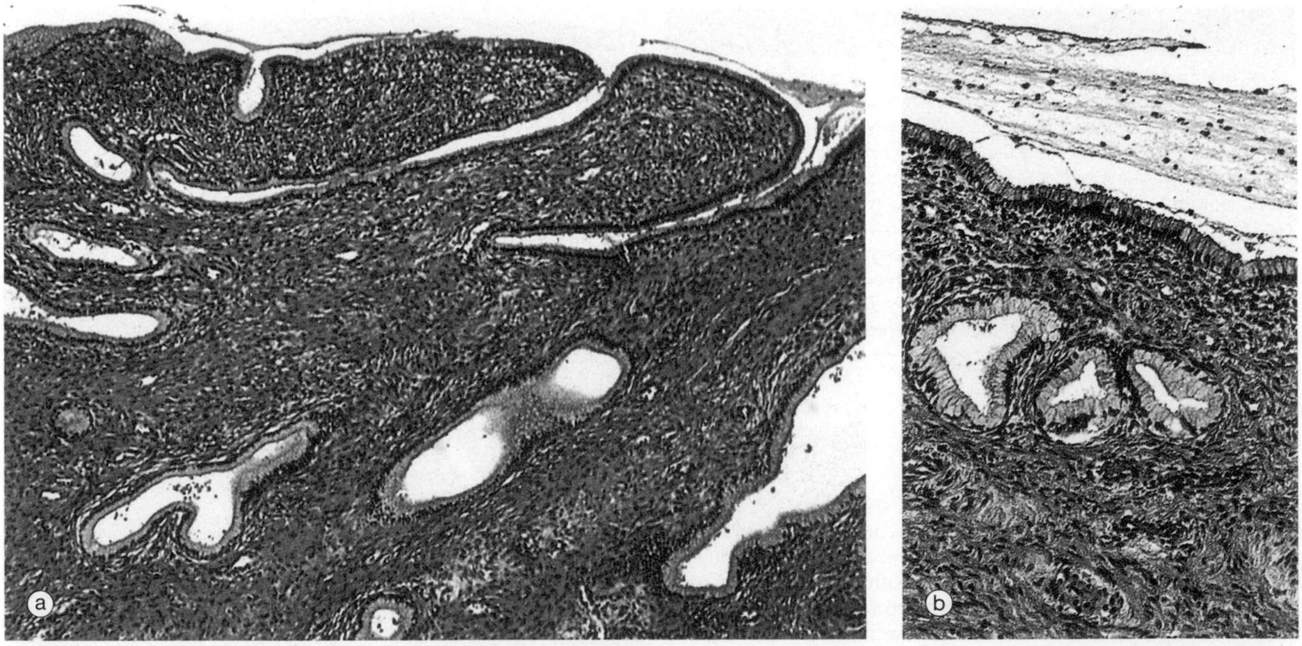

**FIG. 19.24 Endocervix
(a) H&E (LP) (b) H&E (MP)**

As seen in Fig. 19.24a, the mucus-secreting epithelial lining of the endocervical canal is thrown into deep furrows and tunnels, giving the appearance in two dimensions of branched tubular glands, hence the rather inaccurate term ***endocervical glands***. The columnar mucus-secreting cells lining the 'glands' are shown at higher magnification in Fig. 19.24b. Note the leukocytic infiltrate in the superficial stroma and the presence of leukocytes in the endocervical mucus on the surface. Some inflammation is considered to be normal at this site.

During the menstrual cycle, the endocervical epithelium undergoes cyclical changes in secretory activity. In the proliferative phase, rising levels of oestrogen promote secretion of thin, watery mucus which permits the passage of spermatozoa into the uterus around the time of ovulation.

Tunnel clusters are lobular groups of dilated endocervical glands found in the wall of the cervix (see e-Fig. 19.9) that are of no clinical significance.

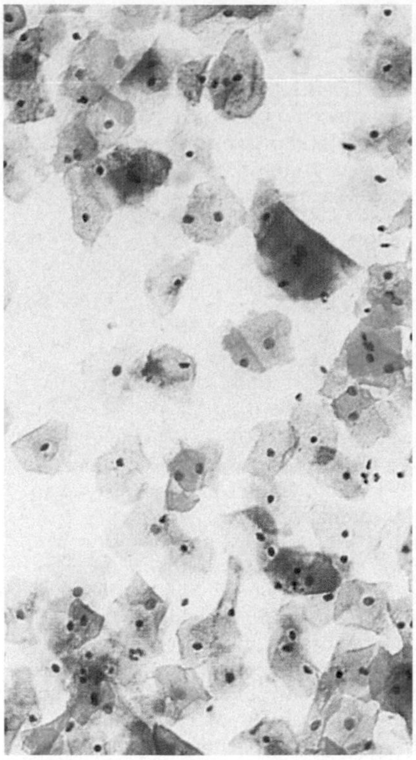

FIG. 19.25 Cervical cytology Papanicolou (HP)

The cervical stroma is influenced by ovarian hormones, particularly oestrogens, which soften the tissues by reducing collagenous cross-linkages and increasing uptake of water by the ground substance. At its most extreme, this provides the means by which the cervix stretches, thins and dilates in late pregnancy and during parturition. To a much lesser extent, similar changes occur during the normal menstrual cycle. One effect of this is that the volume of the cervical stroma varies during each cycle, causing eversion of the columnar epithelium near the squamocolumnar junction and exposing it to the vaginal environment. This ***ectropion*** is known colloquially as '***cervical erosion***'. This induces the growth of stratified squamous epithelium (***squamous metaplasia***) over the exposed area, considered a normal variant in women of reproductive age. The importance of this ***transformation zone*** is that it may undergo malignant change, causing cancer of the cervix.

This area can be studied by scraping cells from the surface using various types of spatula or brush, smearing them on a glass slide and staining them by the ***Papanicolaou method*** (the cervical smear or 'Pap test'). This technique is known as ***exfoliative cytology*** and is demonstrated here from a normal healthy cervix (Fig. 19.25 and e-Fig. 19.10). The surface cells of the stratified squamous epithelium have small, contracted nuclei and are stained pink due to the cytoplasmic keratin. Deeper cells have plump nuclei of normal appearance, and the cytoplasm is stained blue/green. An adequate Pap smear should also contain some endocervical cells (demonstrating that the transformation zone has been sampled), as well as cervical mucin and inflammatory cells.

A more recent development of the cervical smear suspends the exfoliated cells in a special alcohol-based fixative medium and then layers them evenly onto a glass slide, a technique known as ***liquid-based cytology***. This gives superior visibility of the cells and improves the ability of the cytologist to see abnormal cells. Various computerised technologies are also becoming available to screen the slides and detect abnormal cells. Furthermore, cervical screening programmes, such as that available in the UK, are now utilising molecular tests to detect high risk human papillomavirus (HR-HPV) types in smear samples. If HR-HPV is detected, samples then go on to have cytological assessment of the cells in the sample.

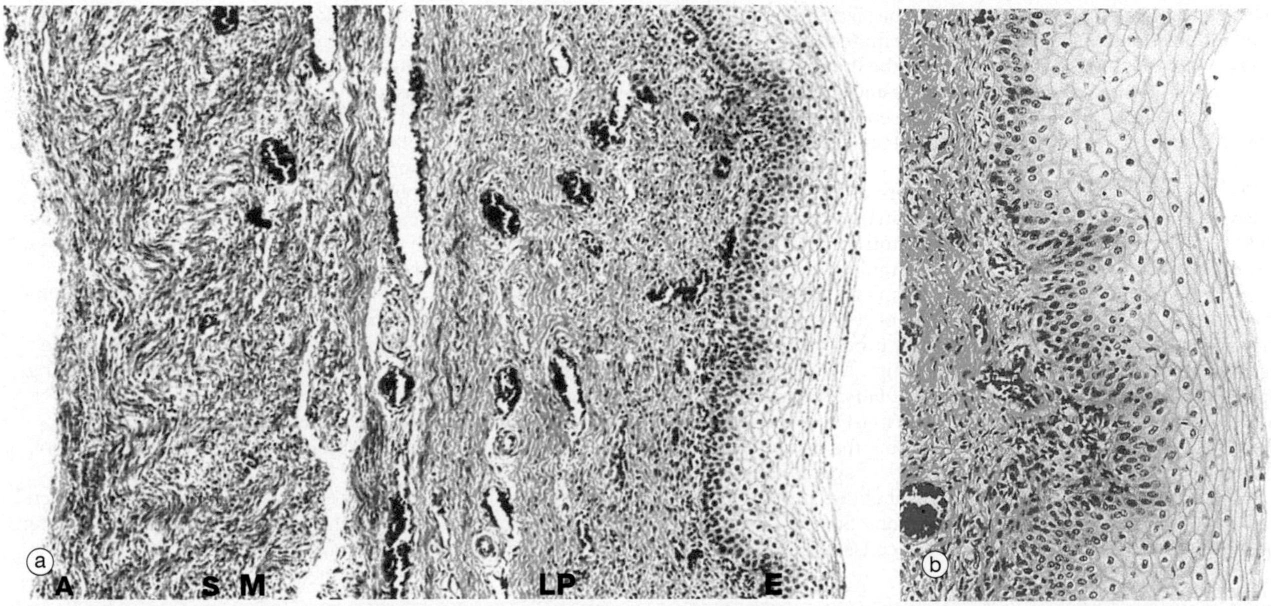

FIG. 19.26 Vagina
(a) Masson trichrome (LP) (b) Masson trichrome (MP)

The wall of the ***vagina***, Fig. 19.26a, consists of a mucosal layer lined by stratified squamous epithelium **E**, a layer of smooth muscle **SM** and an outer adventitial layer **A**. In the relaxed state, the vaginal wall collapses to obliterate the lumen, and the vaginal epithelium is thrown up into folds. The fibrous lamina propria **LP** contains many elastin fibres, has a rich plexus of small veins and is devoid of glands.

The vagina is lubricated by cervical mucus, a fluid transudate from the rich vascular network of the lamina propria, and mucus secreted by glands of the labia minora. The smooth muscle bundles of the muscular layer are arranged in ill-defined ***inner circular*** and ***outer longitudinal*** layers. The adventitial layer of the vagina merges with the adventitial layers of the bladder anteriorly and rectum posteriorly.

The combination of a muscular layer and a highly elastic lamina propria and outer adventitia permits the gross distension that occurs during parturition. Conversely, after coitus, involuntary contraction of the smooth muscle layer ensures that a pool of semen remains in the cervical region.

Fig. 19.26b illustrates the stratified squamous epithelium that lines the vagina. During the menstrual cycle, this epithelium undergoes cyclical changes in glycogen levels. Throughout the cycle, the superficial cells produce glycogen that is anaerobically metabolised by vaginal commensal bacteria to form lactic acid which inhibits the growth of pathogenic microorganisms.

A adventitia **E** stratified squamous epithelium **EC** endocervical canal **J** squamocolumnar junction **LP** lamina propria **SM** smooth muscle **V** vagina

THE PLACENTA

The placenta is formed from elements of the membranes that surround the developing fetus, as well as the uterine endometrium, and provides the means for physiological exchange between the fetal and maternal circulations. The structure of the placenta varies greatly from one species to another and the following discussion is thus necessarily confined to the human placenta. At various stages during fetal development, the placenta performs a remarkable range of functions until the fetal organs become functional. These include gaseous exchange, excretion, maintenance of homeostasis, hormone secretion, haematopoiesis and hepatic metabolic functions.

FIG. 19.27 Fertilisation and implantation *(illustrations below and opposite)*

Within about 24 to 48 hours after ovulation, fertilisation of an ovum by a spermatozoon occurs in the ampulla of the Fallopian tube, with the formation of a ***zygote***. The zona pellucida remains intact (see Fig. 19.4). Within 24 hours, the zygote undergoes its first mitotic cell division, the process continuing until there are some 12 to 16 cells called ***blastomeres***, each with a small portion of the original cytoplasm. The mass, now called a ***morula*** (for its resemblance to a mulberry), remains enclosed by the zona pellucida, through which it is nourished by diffusion of oxygen and low molecular weight metabolites from Fallopian tube secretions.

The morula reaches the uterus 2 to 3 days after fertilisation and begins to absorb uterine fluid, forming a central cavity. The ***blastocyst***, as it is now known, consists of a peripheral layer of blastomeres forming the ***trophoblast***, with a mass of cells at one aspect, the ***polar trophoblast***, bulging into the central lumen and known as the ***inner cell mass***. The trophoblast (along with a maternal contribution) eventually gives rise to the placenta while the inner cell mass develops into the embryo. By this time, the blastocyst has grown to about twice the size of the original ovum and the zona pellucida has become quite thin.

When the blastocyst has been within the uterine cavity for 2 to 3 days, the zona pellucida disappears and ***implantation*** occurs. The polar trophoblast invades the endometrium so that, by the 10th day after conception, the blastocyst is completely buried.

The trophoblast gives rise to two layers, an inner ***cytotrophoblast*** layer of mononuclear cells and an outer ***syncytiotrophoblast*** layer, formed by fusion of cytotrophoblast cells to form a continuous multinucleate syncytium in which there is no internal cytoplasmic demarcation by plasma membranes. The cytotrophoblast remains as a single layer of cells, whereas the syncytiotrophoblast becomes increasingly broad and develops finger-like projections into the endometrium. A third type of trophoblast known as ***intermediate trophoblast*** has histological features intermediate between cytotrophoblast and syncytiotrophoblast and has a major role in invading the endometrium. Within a short time, a sponge-like network of spaces called ***lacunae*** develops within the syncytiotrophoblast, initially filled with tissue fluid and uterine secretions. Soon afterwards, invasion by the intermediate trophoblast causes disintegration of endometrial capillaries with leakage of maternal blood into the lacunae. Progressively, the trophoblast envelops maternal capillaries, expanding the lacunar network and establishing an arterial supply and venous drainage system.

By now, the syncytiotrophoblast also secretes a variety of hormones including ***human chorionic gonadotrophin*** (***hCG***), ***human chorionic somatotrophin*** (previously ***human placental lactogen***, ***hPL***), oestrogen and progesterone, which are necessary to sustain the endometrial tissues. In the meantime, the blastocyst cavity becomes filled with ***extraembryonic mesoderm*** (mesenchyme), which completely surrounds the early embryo, developing from the inner cell mass. The embryo by now comprises plates of embryonic ***endoderm*** and ***ectoderm*** on either side of which lie the ***yolk sac*** and ***amniotic cavities***, enclosed by extraembryonic endoderm and extraembryonic ectoderm, respectively. Subsequently, a cavity forms within the extraembryonic mesoderm; this ***extraembryonic coelom*** eventually surrounds the developing embryo, which remains attached to the trophoblast by a connecting stalk of extraembryonic mesoderm. The trophoblast, along with the mesodermal layer remaining beneath it, now constitutes the ***chorion***.

Meanwhile the ***trabeculae*** of syncytiotrophoblast and intermediate trophoblast between the lacunae are invaded by columns of cytotrophoblastic cells called ***primary chorionic villi***. These grow out to the periphery and spread out over the interface between the trophoblast and endometrium, forming the ***cytotrophoblast shell***. Extraembryonic mesoderm now invades the primary villi, which thus develop a mesenchymal core, becoming known as ***secondary chorionic villi***.

By about 2 weeks after implantation (i.e. about 24 days after fertilisation), primitive blood vessels begin to develop in the chorionic mesoderm simultaneously with development of the primitive embryonic circulatory system, the embryo now being too large to rely on mere diffusion for its growth and metabolic requirements. When the mesenchymal cores of the villi become vascularised, they become known as ***tertiary villi*** (not illustrated).

The form of the placenta is essentially established by the end of the fourth month, after which the placenta grows in diameter, complementing growth in the size of the uterus.

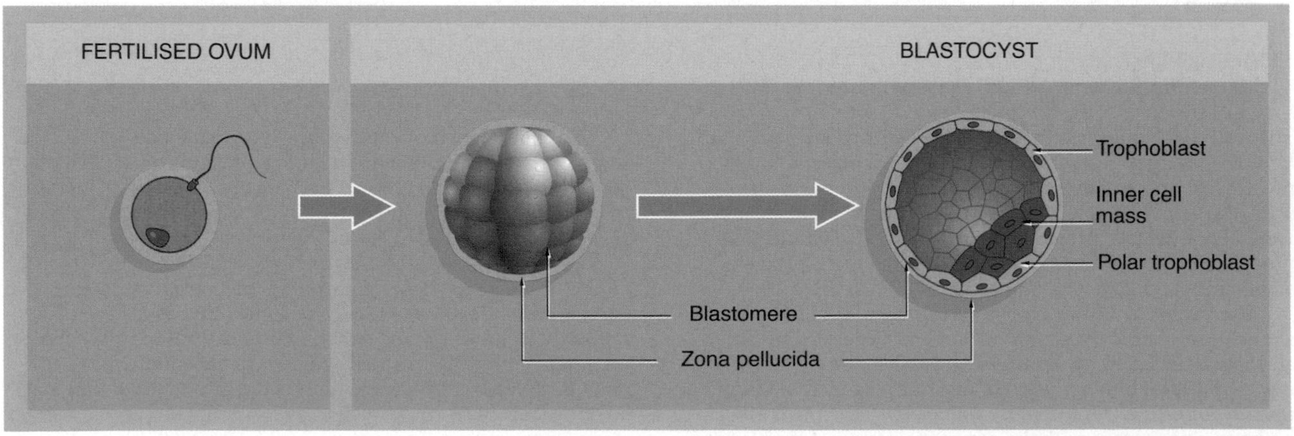

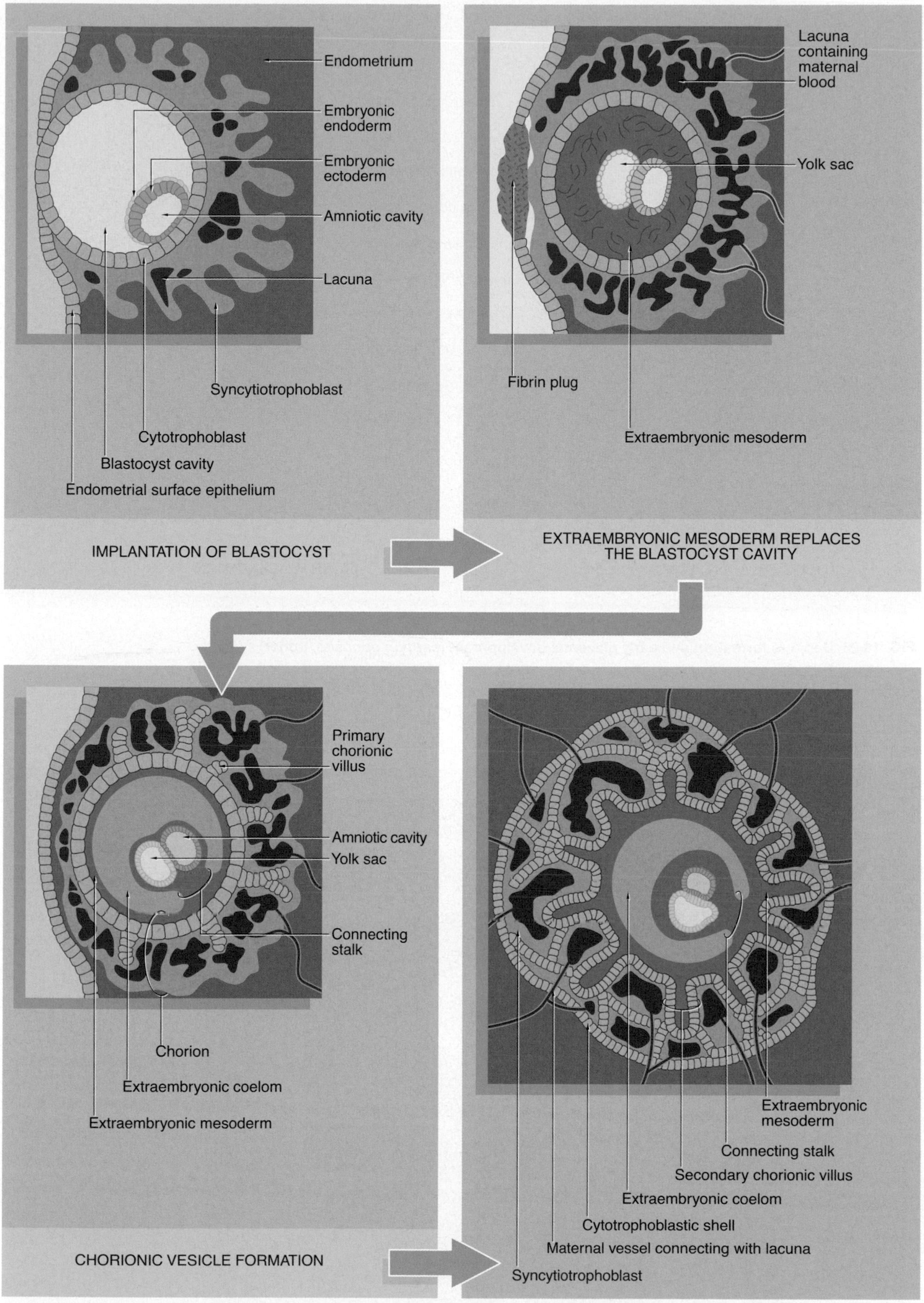
Endometrium
Embryonic endoderm
Embryonic ectoderm
Amniotic cavity
Lacuna
Syncytiotrophoblast
Cytotrophoblast
Blastocyst cavity
Endometrial surface epithelium
IMPLANTATION OF BLASTOCYST
Lacuna containing maternal blood
Yolk sac
Fibrin plug
Extraembryonic mesoderm
EXTRAEMBRYONIC MESODERM REPLACES THE BLASTOCYST CAVITY
Primary chorionic villus
Amniotic cavity
Yolk sac
Connecting stalk
Chorion
Extraembryonic coelom
Extraembryonic mesoderm
CHORIONIC VESICLE FORMATION
Extraembryonic mesoderm
Connecting stalk
Secondary chorionic villus
Extraembryonic coelom
Cytotrophoblastic shell
Maternal vessel connecting with lacuna
Syncytiotrophoblast

FIG. 19.27 Fertilisation and implantation ***(caption opposite)***

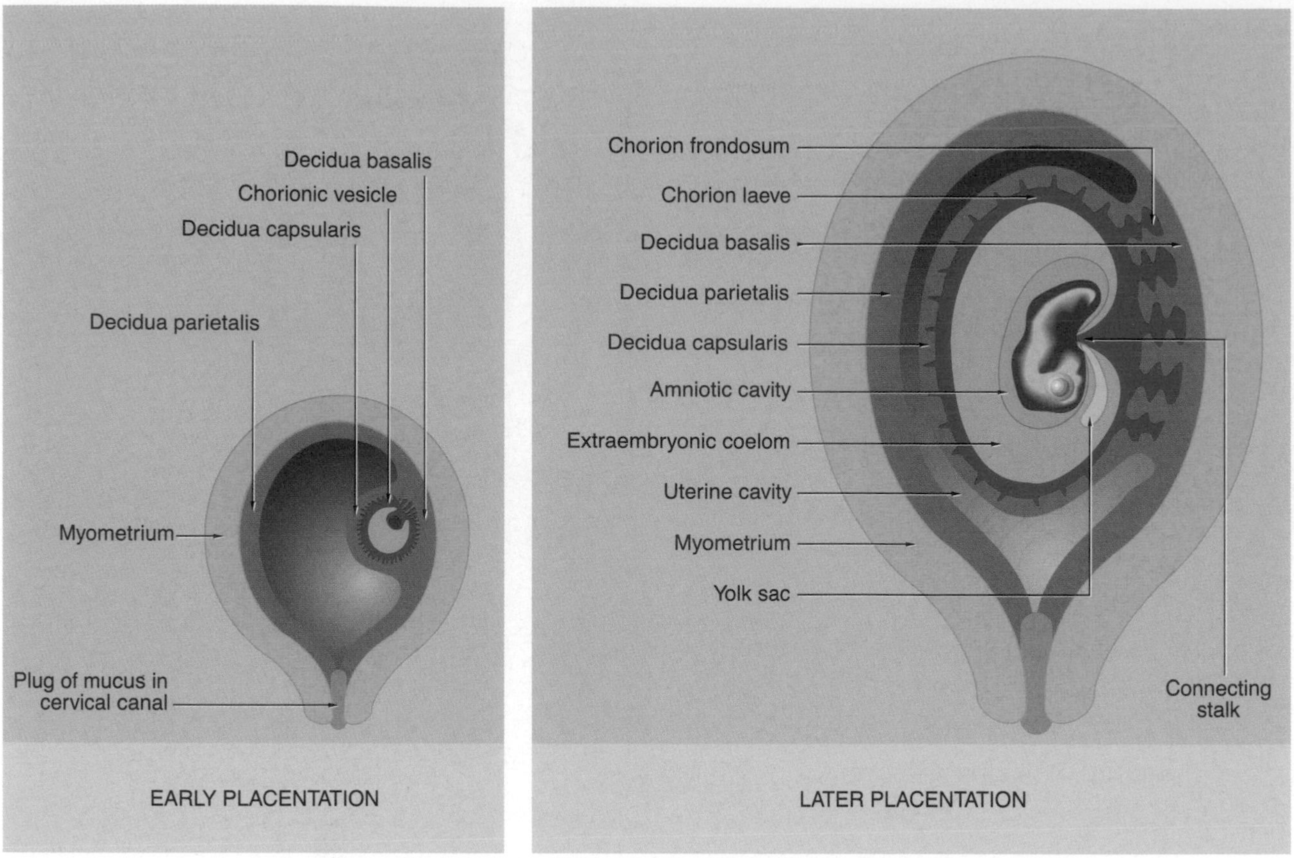

FIG. 19.28 Decidua formation and early placental development ***(caption opposite, upper)***

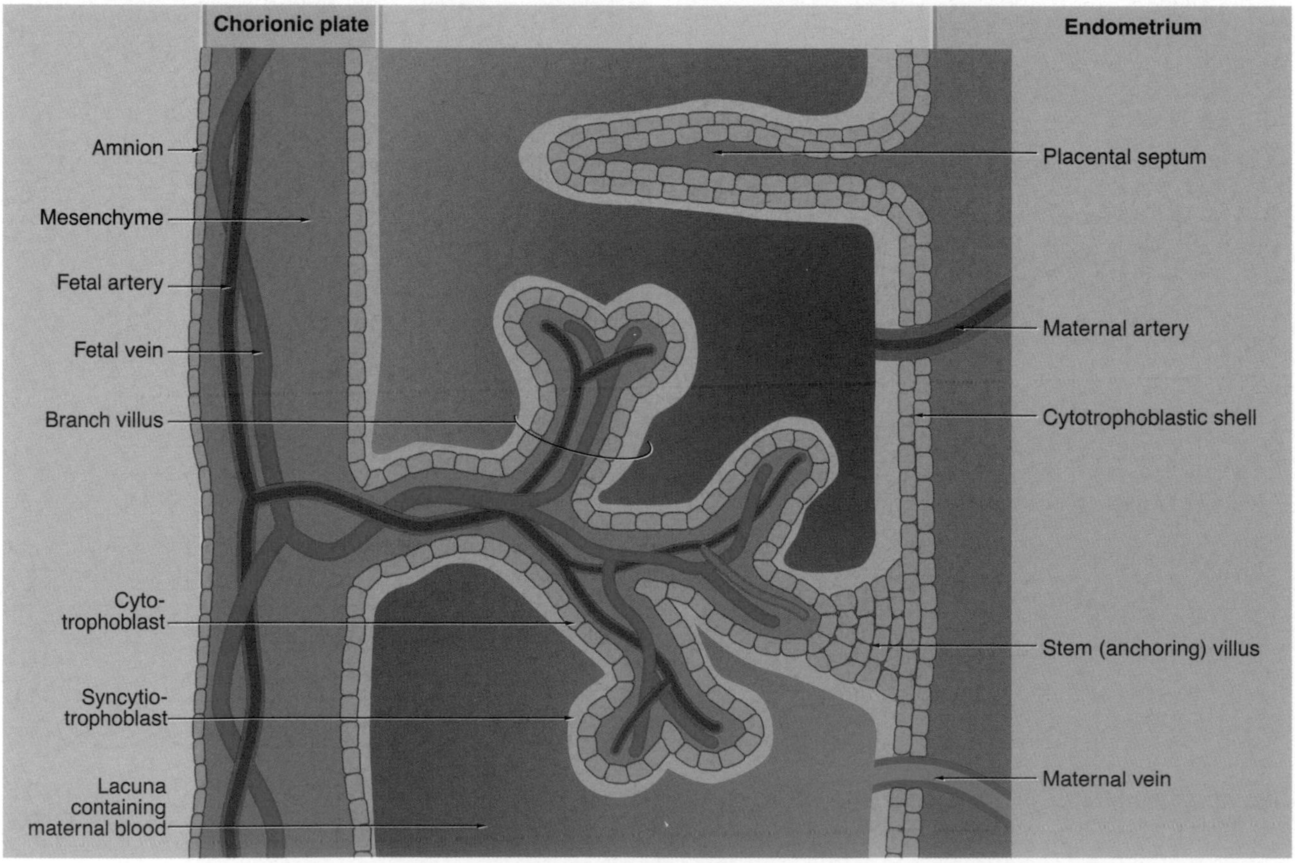

FIG. 19.29 Structure of placental villi ***(caption opposite, lower)***

FIG. 19.28 Decidua formation and early placental development ***(illustration opposite, upper)***

During the process of implantation (Fig. 19.28), secretion by the syncytiotrophoblast of hCG (which is functionally analogous to luteinising hormone) interrupts the ovarian cycle. This results in growth and proliferation of stromal cells of the endometrial stratum functionalis at the implantation site into large polyhedral ***decidual cells***, a change that has already begun in the late secretory phase. The decidua beneath the developing embryo is known as the ***decidua basalis*** and, with the trophoblast, will form the future placenta. The decidua overlying the embryo is known as the ***decidua capsularis***, and the decidual lining of the rest of the uterus is called the ***decidua parietalis***. Ultimately, expansion of the embryo and its enveloping fluid-filled membrane system results in fusion of the capsular and parietal layers of the decidua, with complete obliteration of the uterine cavity.

During the first 2 months of embryological development, the chorion grows fairly uniformly around the whole periphery of the vesicle. From the third month, the chorion in contact with the decidua basalis develops extensive frond-like villous outgrowths into the decidua, becoming known as the ***chorion frondosum***, while the superficial chorion in contact with the decidua capsularis atrophies to become the smooth ***chorion laeve***. Progressively, the chorion frondosum and decidua basalis develop into the flattened ***placenta*** and the vessels connecting the chorion to the embryonic circulation become the ***umbilical cord***.

FIG. 19.29 Structure of placental villi ***(illustration opposite, lower)***

From the time maternal blood appears within the trophoblastic lacunae, the trabeculae between the lacunae become increasingly robust, with ***stem villi*** forming anchorage points with the cytotrophoblastic shell (Fig. 19.29). Side branches grow out into the lacunae, progressively forming a complex villous structure. Each villus has a mesenchymal core containing capillaries served by afferent and efferent fetal blood vessels. Between the villous capillaries and the maternal blood, there is a continuous layer of syncytiotrophoblast supported by a layer of proliferating cytotrophoblast cells. From the fourth month onwards, the cytotrophoblast layer becomes atrophic. As more and more branches are added to the villous tree, the villi become smaller and smaller, and the tissue barrier between fetal capillaries and maternal blood is greatly diminished.

As the placenta develops, the decidua basalis regresses so that all that remains are a number of anastomosing septa of maternal supporting tissue projecting into the cytotrophoblastic shell. When the placenta is shed immediately after childbirth, its maternal surface is seen to be divided into about 20 irregular segments called ***cotyledons*** that are demarcated from each other by the positions of the former maternal (placental) septa.

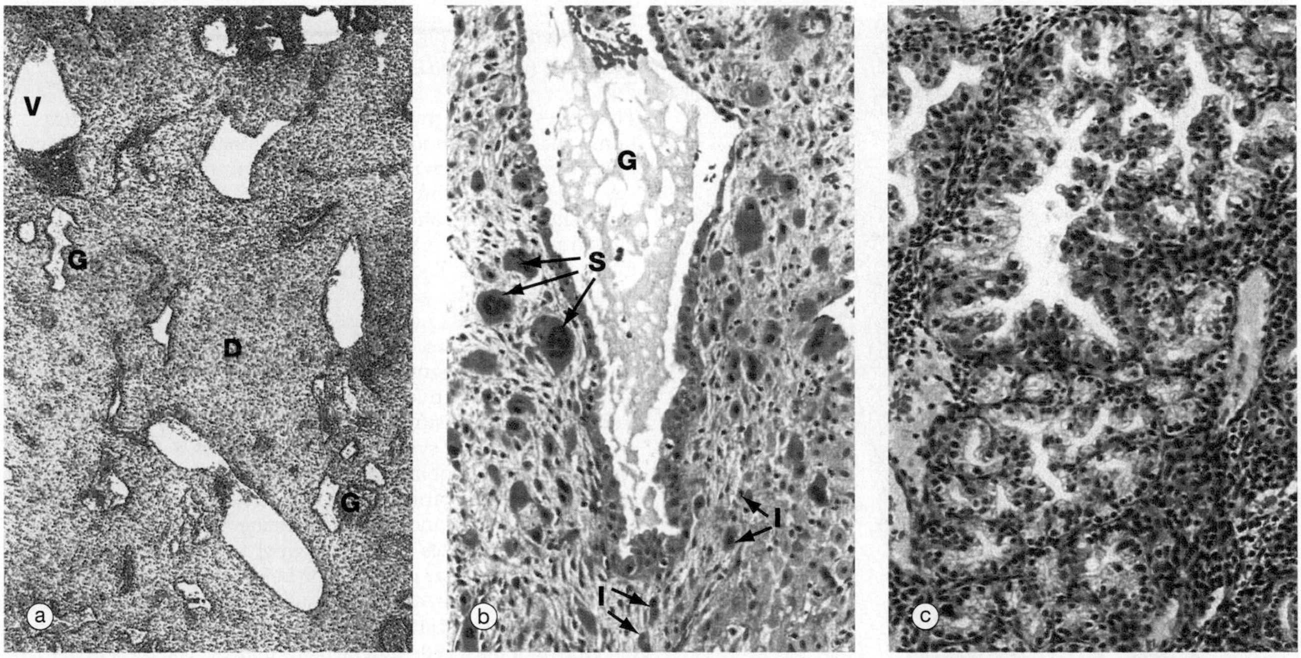

FIG. 19.30 Decidua
(a) H&E (LP) (b) H&E (MP) (c) H&E (HP)

Fig. 19.30a illustrates ***decidual change*** **D** in the endometrial stroma. The decidual cells proliferate and enlarge greatly, their cytoplasm staining pink (eosinophilia) due to the presence of numerous mitochondria and intermediate filaments. Dilated blood vessels **V** and endometrial glands **G** are apparent.

At higher power in Fig. 19.30b, multinucleated syncytiotrophoblast cells **S** can be seen infiltrating the decidua. Intermediate trophoblast cells **I** are actually present in greater numbers than syncytiotrophoblast cells but are less easily identified. In the centre of the field, there is a dilated gland **G**.

Fig. 19.30c shows the deeper part of the endometrium in pregnancy. Here, the decidual reaction is inconspicuous, but the secretory nature of the glands is greatly exaggerated. It is thus often called ***hypersecretory endometrium***. Note the prominent infolding of the glandular epithelium and the vacuolation of the epithelial cell cytoplasm.

D decidua **G** endometrial gland **I** intermediate trophoblast **S** syncytiotrophoblast cell **V** blood vessel

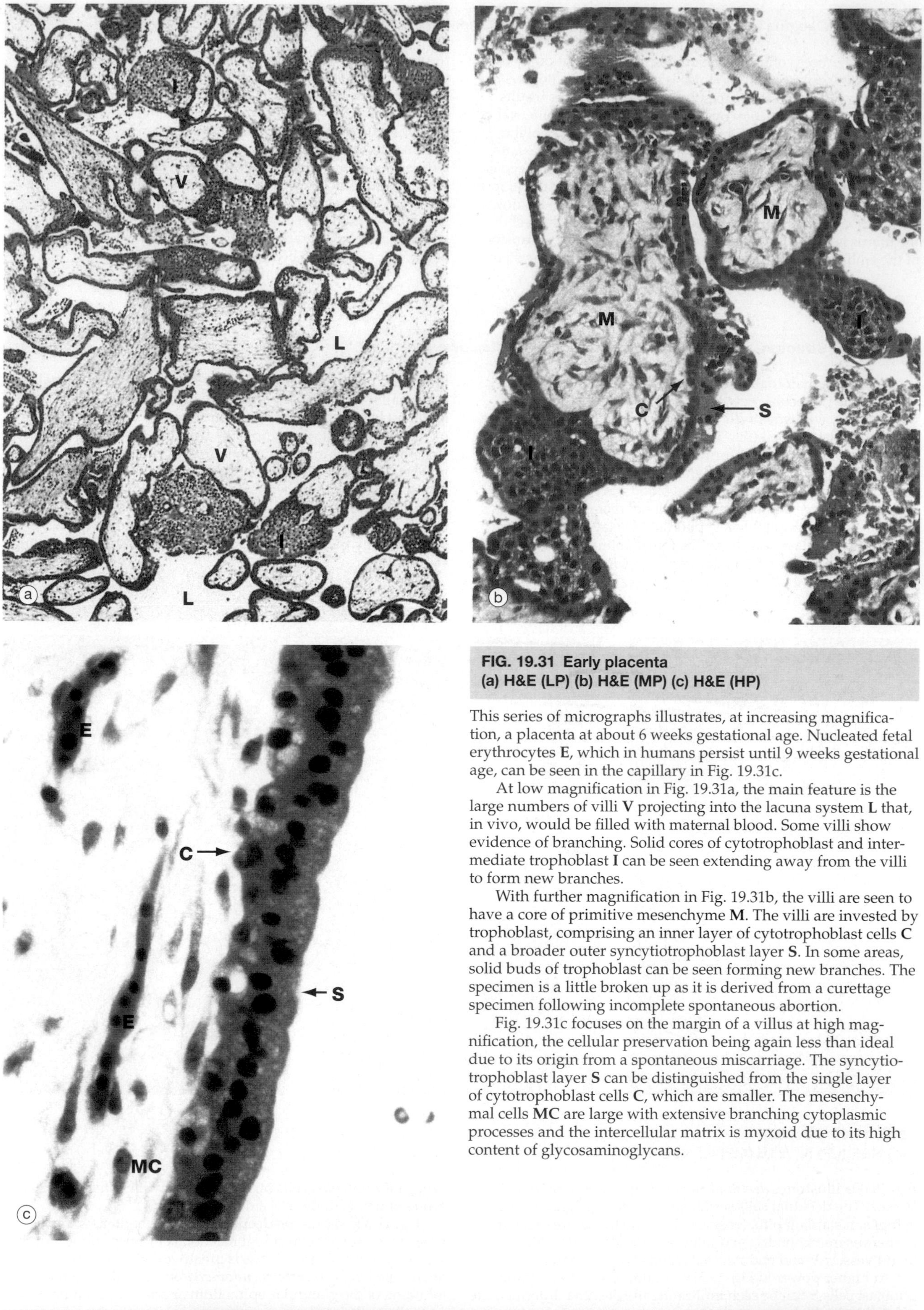

FIG. 19.31 Early placenta
(a) H&E (LP) (b) H&E (MP) (c) H&E (HP)

This series of micrographs illustrates, at increasing magnification, a placenta at about 6 weeks gestational age. Nucleated fetal erythrocytes **E**, which in humans persist until 9 weeks gestational age, can be seen in the capillary in Fig. 19.31c.

At low magnification in Fig. 19.31a, the main feature is the large numbers of villi **V** projecting into the lacuna system **L** that, in vivo, would be filled with maternal blood. Some villi show evidence of branching. Solid cores of cytotrophoblast and intermediate trophoblast **I** can be seen extending away from the villi to form new branches.

With further magnification in Fig. 19.31b, the villi are seen to have a core of primitive mesenchyme **M**. The villi are invested by trophoblast, comprising an inner layer of cytotrophoblast cells **C** and a broader outer syncytiotrophoblast layer **S**. In some areas, solid buds of trophoblast can be seen forming new branches. The specimen is a little broken up as it is derived from a curettage specimen following incomplete spontaneous abortion.

Fig. 19.31c focuses on the margin of a villus at high magnification, the cellular preservation being again less than ideal due to its origin from a spontaneous miscarriage. The syncytiotrophoblast layer **S** can be distinguished from the single layer of cytotrophoblast cells **C**, which are smaller. The mesenchymal cells **MC** are large with extensive branching cytoplasmic processes and the intercellular matrix is myxoid due to its high content of glycosaminoglycans.

Abnormalities of the placenta

The normal placenta invades into the uterine wall in order to establish circulation with a supply of oxygen and nutrients for the developing fetus. In some cases, the placenta becomes abnormally adherent and invades too deeply into the uterus, preventing the normal process of separation which occurs after parturition. This can lead to serious maternal blood loss. The least severe form of this is known as placenta accreta, where the placenta does not invade significantly into the myometrium. Placenta increta describes deeper attachment which extends further into the myometrium. In its most severe form, placenta percreta, the placenta may penetrate through to the serosal surface of the uterus and can even attach to other pelvic organs.

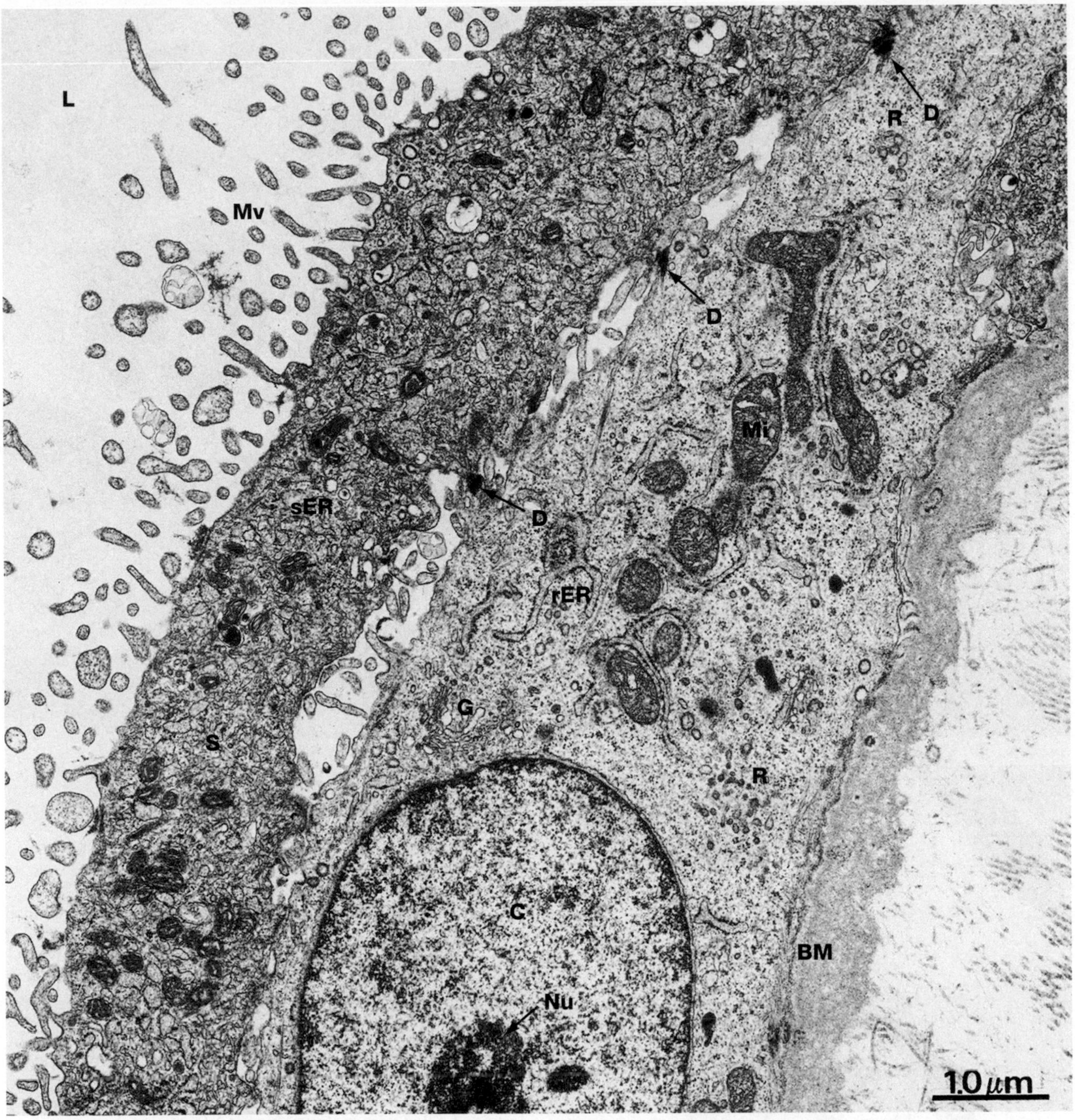

FIG. 19.32 Trophoblast
EM ×16 000

Fig. 19.32 shows the general ultrastructural features of the trophoblastic components. These show considerable variation from one region to another and from early to late stages of placental development.

The syncytiotrophoblast **S** typically presents large numbers of irregular microvilli **Mv** to the lacunae **L**, greatly enhancing the surface area for physiological exchange. The plasma membranes of the microvilli incorporate a wide variety of enzymes and receptors involved in membrane transfer processes, as well as receptors for many hormones and growth factors. Microfilaments extend into the microvilli from a cytoskeletal network concentrated immediately below the free surface. Some areas of the syncytiotrophoblast contain rough endoplasmic reticulum while, in other areas, as shown here, smooth endoplasmic reticulum **sER** predominates, presumably involved in steroid hormone synthesis.

The cytotrophoblast layer **C** has ultrastructural features of relatively undifferentiated stem cells, exhibiting profiles of rough endoplasmic reticulum **rER**, a well-defined Golgi apparatus **G**, relatively few mitochondria **Mi** and numerous polyribosomes **R**. The nucleus is typically large with dispersed chromatin and nucleoli **Nu**. The cytotrophoblast is usually tightly bound to the overlying syncytiotrophoblast by desmosomes **D**, but in some areas, as in this specimen, spaces can be seen between the cell layers. The reason for this is unclear. Separating the cytotrophoblast from the underlying collagenous stroma is a relatively thick basement membrane **BM**.

BM basement membrane **C** cytotrophoblast **D** desmosome **E** nucleated erythrocytes **G** Golgi apparatus **I** intermediate trophoblast **L** lacuna **M** mesenchyme **MC** mesenchymal cell **Mi** mitochondrion **Mv** microvilli **Nu** nucleolus **R** polyribosomes **rER** rough endoplasmic reticulum **S** syncytiotrophoblast **sER** smooth endoplasmic reticulum **V** villus

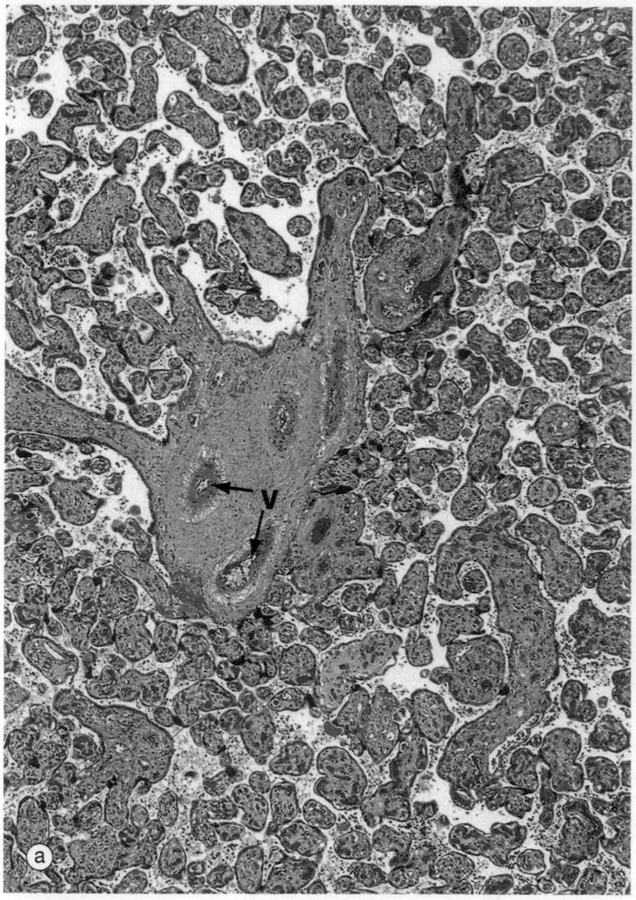

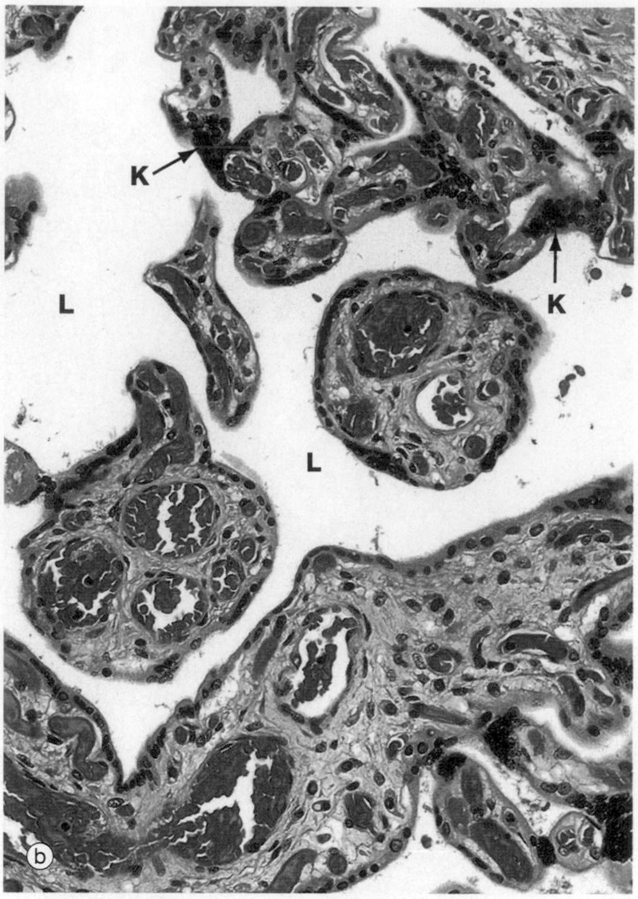

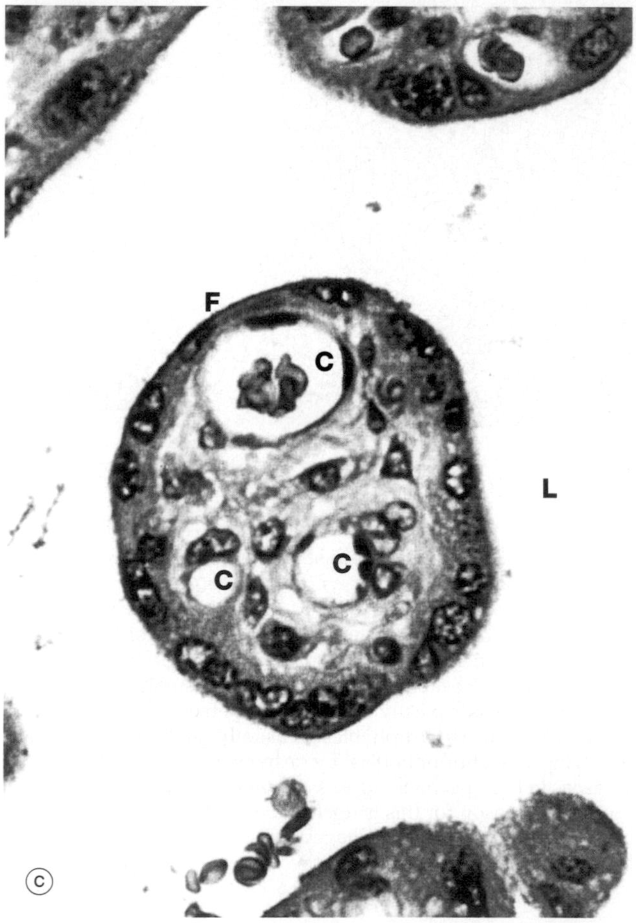

FIG. 19.33 Term placenta
(a) H&E (LP) (b) H&E (MP) (c) H&E (HP)

These micrographs illustrate placenta from a full-term fetus.

At low magnification in Fig. 19.33a, huge numbers of villi can be seen, cut in various planes of section and varying in diameter from large mainstem villi to very small terminal branch villi. Compared with early placenta shown in Fig. 19.31, the villous pattern is much more highly developed and the average villous diameter is much smaller, reflecting the extensive branching growth of the villi as the placenta enlarges. Note the large blood vessels **V** in the largest villi.

Fig. 19.33b demonstrates the branching nature of the villi at higher magnification. Compare the marked vascularity of the villous cores with that of the much earlier placenta in Fig. 19.31 and the greatly increased villous surface area exposed to the lacunae **L** filled with maternal blood. A feature of the term placenta is the ***syncytial knot*** **K**, where syncytiotrophoblast nuclei are aggregated together in clusters, leaving zones of thin cytoplasm devoid of nuclei between.

Fig. 19.33c focuses on a small branch villus and highlights the proximity of blood in fetal capillaries **C** to maternal blood in the surrounding lacuna **L**. The trophoblast is reduced to a thin layer of syncytiotrophoblast only and the capillaries tend to be located in the periphery of the core. The diffusion barrier between maternal and fetal circulations comprises five layers: trophoblast, trophoblast basement membrane, villous core supporting tissue, capillary endothelial basement membrane and endothelium. In many cases, fetal capillaries are so close to the trophoblast that their basement membranes fuse **F**, reducing the diffusion barrier to only three layers.

A umbilical artery **Am** amniotic membrane **BM** basement membrane **C** capillary **Ch** chorionic membrane
D outer collagenous layer **E** epithelial cells **F** fused basement membranes **I** inner collagenous layer of chorionic membrane
In intermediate zone **K** syncytial knot **L** lacuna **M** mesenchymal layer **MC** mesenchymal cell **T** trophoblast
V blood vessel **Ve** umbilical vein **W** Wharton's jelly

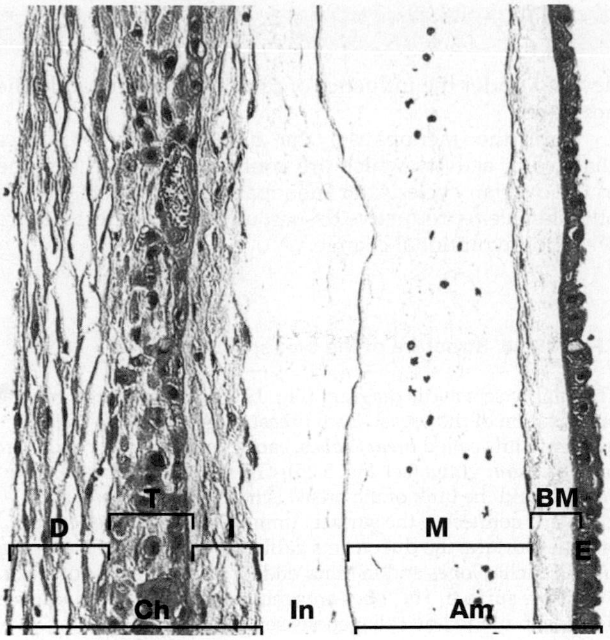

FIG. 19.34 Fetal membranes
H&E (MP)

During early development, the embryo is surrounded by the *extraembryonic coelom* (see Fig. 19.28), but later this is obliterated as the amniotic cavity expands to surround the fetus. The outer mesenchymal layer of the amnion then comes to lie in contact with (and often fuses with) the inner mesenchymal layer of the chorion, forming the *chorioamnion* or *fetal membranes*. The two layers are often difficult to separate from one another at birth.

As shown in Fig. 19.34, the *amniotic membrane* **Am** comprises a single layer of epithelial cells **E** derived from extraembryonic ectoderm, resting on a thick basement membrane **BM**. Beneath this, there is a delicate avascular mesenchymal layer **M** which is a remnant of the extraembryonic mesoderm. The *chorionic membrane* **Ch** consists of three layers. A vascular collagenous inner layer **I** is also derived from extraembryonic mesoderm. The intermediate zone **In**, seen here separating it from the amnion, represents the remnant of the extraembryonic coelom and varies greatly in thickness. The trophoblast **T** of the chorion laeve is represented by the middle layer of eosinophilic epithelial cells, whilst the outermost vascular collagenous layer **D** is of maternal origin, representing the decidua capsularis (see Fig. 19.28).

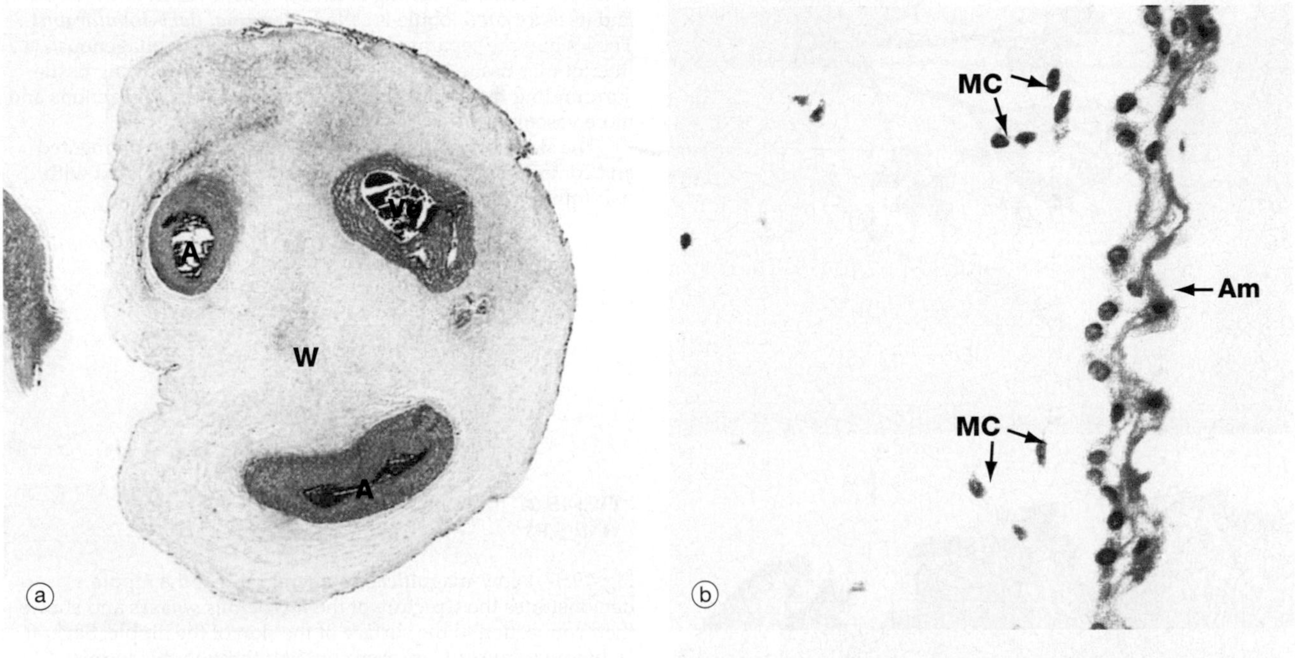

FIG. 19.35 Umbilical cord
(a) H&E (LP) (b) H&E (HP)

The development of the umbilical cord begins with the formation of the extraembryonic coelom which almost surrounds the early embryo and which remains attached to the chorion by the connecting stalk of mesenchyme (see Fig. 19.28). With further embryonic development, the site of attachment of the connecting stalk becomes located ventrally, just caudal to the point where the *vitello-intestinal duct* connects the yolk sac to the mid-gut. As the embryo grows, the amniotic sac expands greatly, filling the extraembryonic coelom and compressing the vitello-intestinal duct and yolk sac remnant (surrounded by a sleeve of extraembryonic coelom) up against the connecting stalk. These structures ultimately fuse to form the *umbilical cord*, which now is surrounded by the amnion and amniotic cavity.

By the middle of the fifth month, the remnants of the vitello-intestinal duct, yolk sac and sheath of extraembryonic coelom atrophy and disappear. As seen in Fig. 19.35a, all that remains are two *umbilical arteries* **A** and a single *umbilical vein* **Ve**, embedded in mesenchyme consisting mainly of ground substance and known as *Wharton's jelly* **W**. Mesenchymal cells **MC** and surface amnion **Am** are shown at high magnification in Fig. 19.35b. The umbilical arteries convey deoxygenated fetal blood to the placenta while the umbilical vein conveys oxygenated blood back to the fetus.

THE BREAST

The breasts (***mammary glands***) are highly modified apocrine sweat glands (see Fig. 9.14) which develop embryologically along two lines, the ***milk lines***, extending from the axillae to the groin. In humans, only one gland develops on each side of the thorax, although accessory breast tissue may be found anywhere along the milk lines.

The breasts of both sexes follow a similar course of development until puberty, after which the female breasts develop under the influence of pituitary, ovarian and other hormones.

Until the menopause, the breasts undergo cyclical changes in activity which are controlled by the hormones of the ovarian cycle. After menopause, the breasts, like the other female reproductive tissues, undergo progressive atrophy and involutional change.

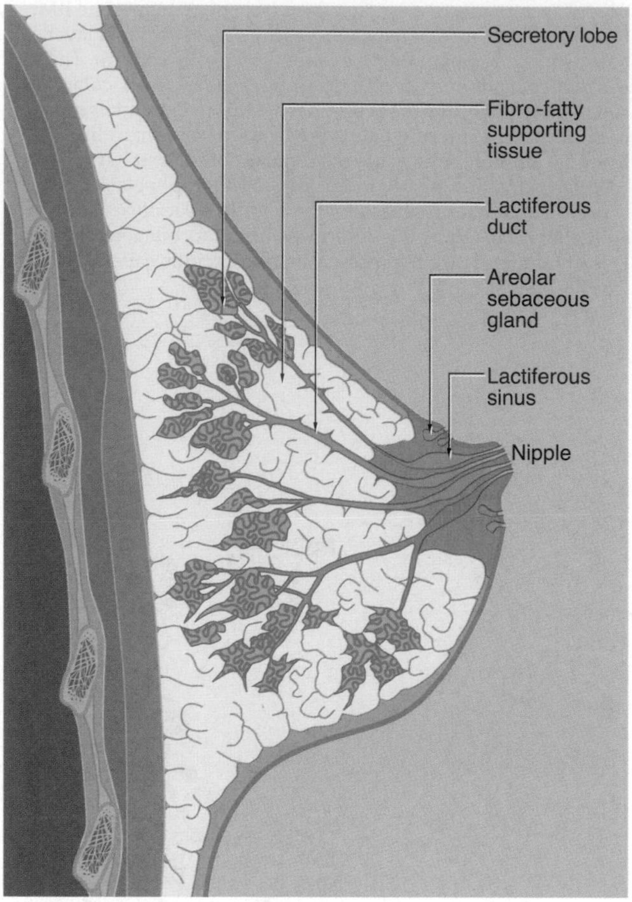

FIG. 19.36 Structure of the breast

This highly schematic diagram (Fig. 19.36) illustrates the general organisation of the breast. Each breast consists of 15 to 25 independent units called ***breast lobes***, each consisting of a ***compound tubulo-acinar gland*** (see Fig. 5.25). The size of the lobes is quite variable and the bulk of the breast is made up of a few large lobes that connect to the surface. Immediately before opening onto the surface, the duct forms a dilatation called the ***lactiferous sinus***. Smaller lobes end in blind ending ducts that do not reach the nipple surface. The lobes are embedded in a mass of adipose tissue, subdivided by collagenous septa.

The ***nipple*** contains bands of smooth muscle, orientated in parallel to the lactiferous ducts and circularly near the base. Contraction of this muscle causes erection of the nipple.

Within each lobe of the breast, the main duct branches repeatedly to form a number of ***terminal ducts***, each of which leads to a ***lobule*** consisting of multiple ***acini***. Each terminal duct and its associated lobule is called a ***terminal duct–lobular unit***. The lobules are separated by moderately dense collagenous interlobular tissue, whereas the intralobular supporting tissue surrounding the ducts within each lobule is less collagenous and more vascular.

The skin surrounding the nipple, the ***areola***, is pigmented and contains sebaceous glands which are not associated with hair follicles.

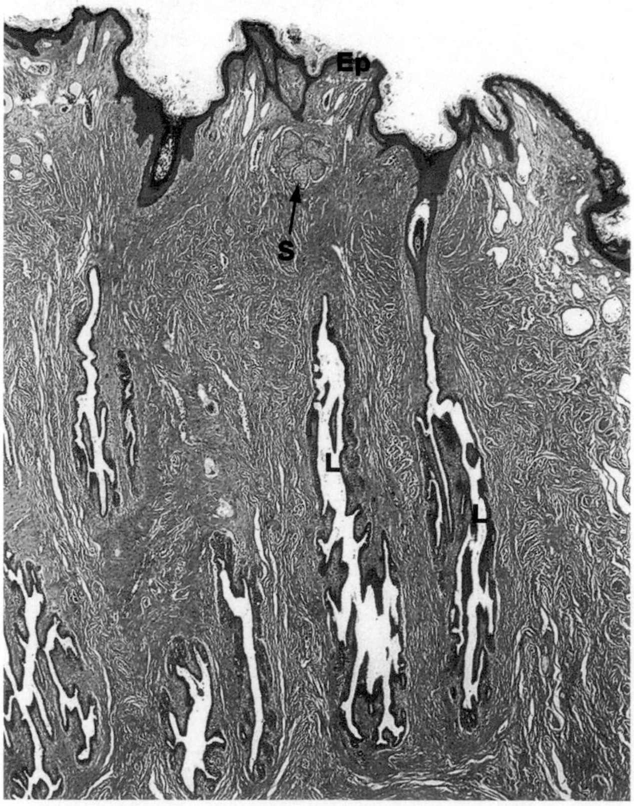

FIG. 19.37 The nipple
H&E (LP)

Fig. 19.37, a low-magnification micrograph of the nipple, demonstrates the structure of the ***lactiferous sinuses*** and shows their connection to the surface of the skin of the nipple. Several lactiferous sinuses **L** are seen coursing through the dermis towards the skin surface. Only the lactiferous sinus on the right can be seen connecting to the surface in this micrograph, but this is probably due to a slightly oblique plane of section, rather than indicating blind-ending sinuses.

The undulating surface of the epidermis **Ep** is seen, and a single sebaceous gland **S** is also identifiable. The epithelium of the lactiferous sinuses is similar to that of the ducts in the rest of the breast until close to the surface, where the epithelium becomes stratified squamous in type.

Paget's disease of breast

Invasive breast cancer or carcinoma in situ (see Fig. 19.42) may spread through ducts and along the lactiferous sinus from the underlying breast lobe and may even spread into the surface epidermis, where it is known as Paget's disease of the breast (see e-Fig. 19.11).

Clinically, this disease typically presents as a patch of red, scaly, seemingly inflamed skin around the nipple, closely mimicking eczema, a common inflammatory skin disease. In this setting, it is important to examine carefully for any underlying breast lump. Skin biopsy may be performed to allow definitive diagnosis.

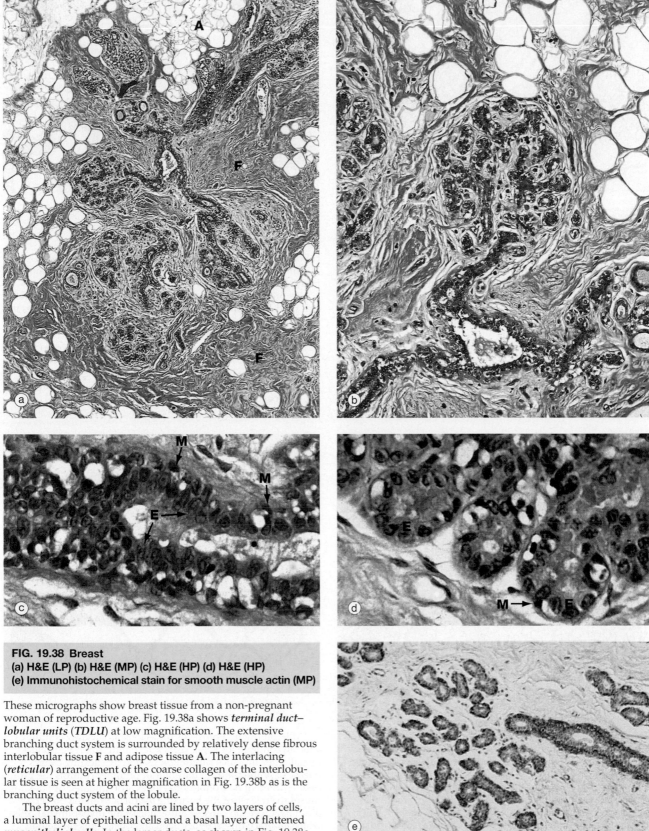

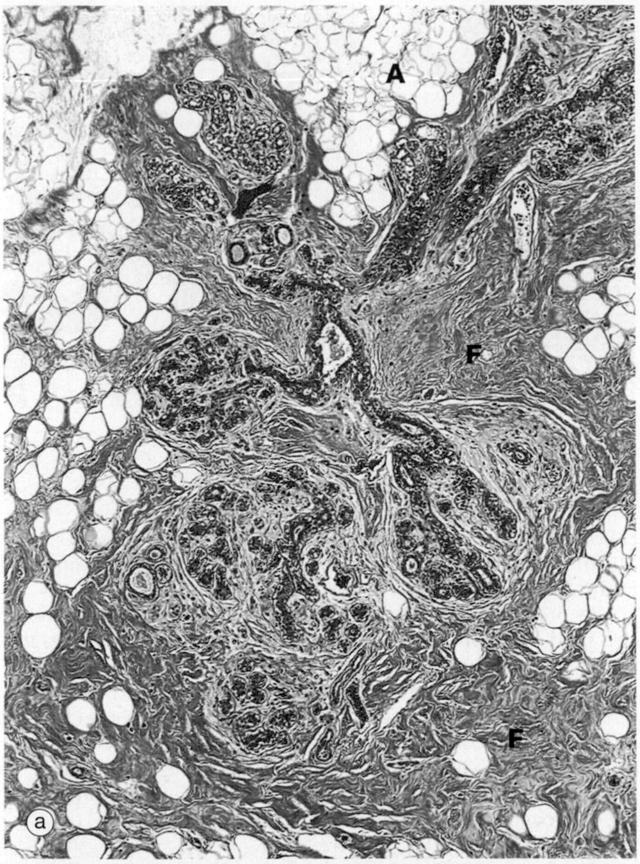

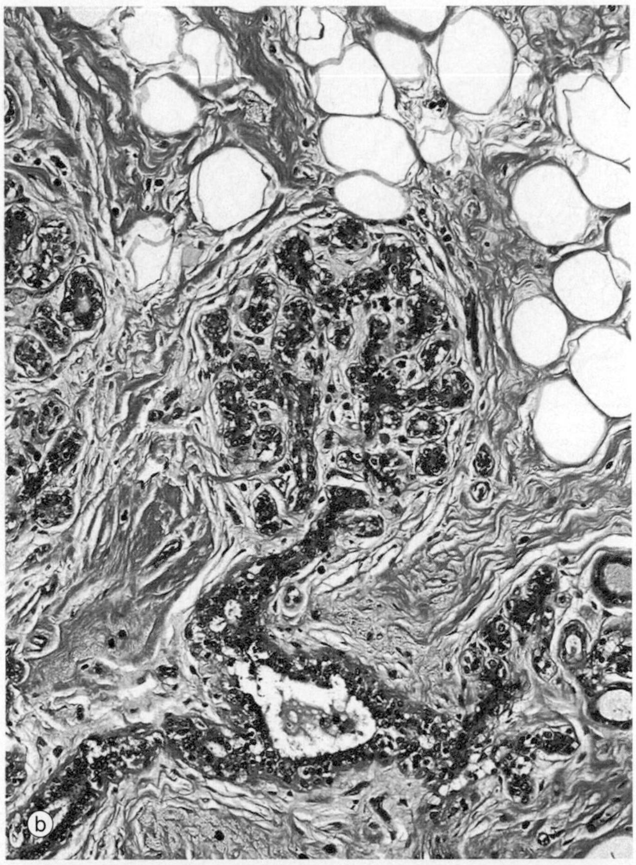

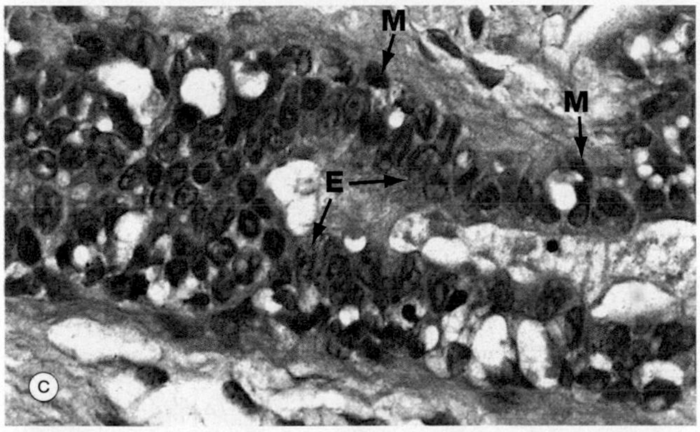

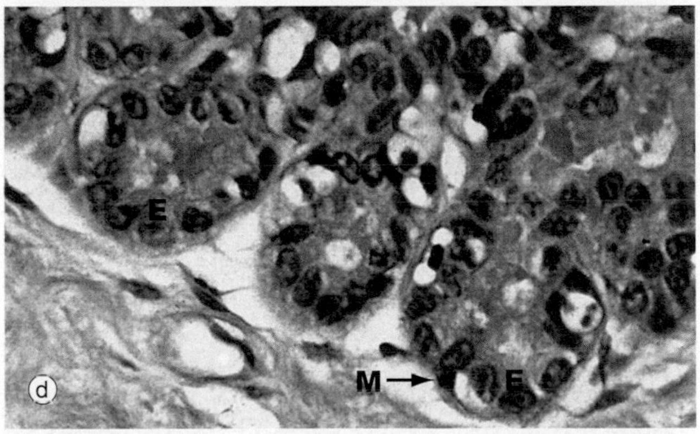

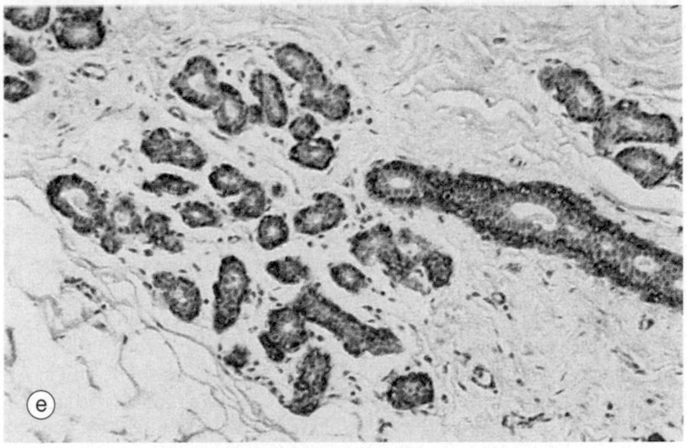

FIG. 19.38 Breast
(a) H&E (LP) (b) H&E (MP) (c) H&E (HP) (d) H&E (HP)
(e) Immunohistochemical stain for smooth muscle actin (MP)

These micrographs show breast tissue from a non-pregnant woman of reproductive age. Fig. 19.38a shows ***terminal duct–lobular units*** (***TDLU***) at low magnification. The extensive branching duct system is surrounded by relatively dense fibrous interlobular tissue **F** and adipose tissue **A**. The interlacing (***reticular***) arrangement of the coarse collagen of the interlobular tissue is seen at higher magnification in Fig. 19.38b as is the branching duct system of the lobule.

The breast ducts and acini are lined by two layers of cells, a luminal layer of epithelial cells and a basal layer of flattened ***myoepithelial cells***. In the larger ducts, as shown in Fig. 19.38c, the luminal epithelial cells **E** are tall columnar in type, whereas in the smaller ducts and acini shown in Fig. 19.38d, the epithelial cells are cuboidal. A discontinuous layer of stellate myoepithelial cells **M** with pale cytoplasm surrounds the ductal lining cells. In Fig. 19.38e, which uses an immunohistochemical technique to stain the myoepithelial cells for actin, the extent and number of the myoepithelial cells (stained brown) are apparent.

During the reproductive years, the duct epithelium undergoes mild cyclical changes under the influence of ovarian hormones. Early in the cycle, the duct lumina are not clearly evident but, later in the cycle, they become more prominent and may contain an eosinophilic secretion.

A adipose tissue **E** epithelial cell **Ep** epidermis **F** fibrous interlobular tissue **L** lactiferous sinus **M** myoepithelial cell **S** sebaceous gland

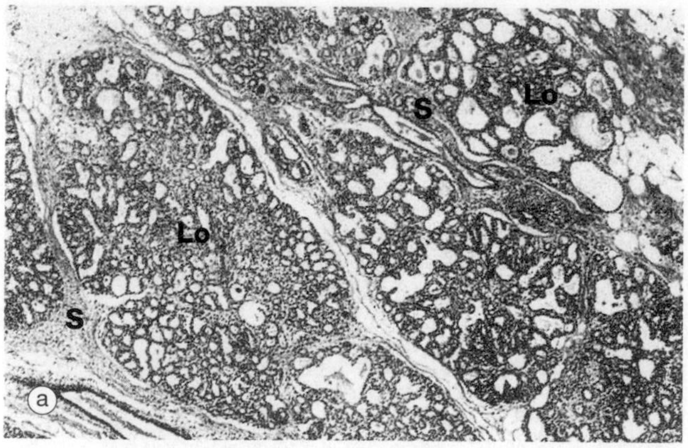

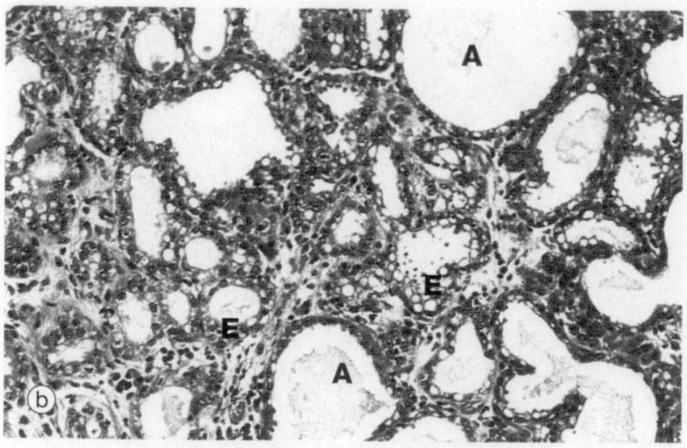

FIG. 19.39 Breast during pregnancy
(a) H&E (LP) (b) H&E (MP)

Under the influence of oestrogens and progesterone produced by the corpus luteum and later by the placenta, the terminal duct epithelium proliferates to form greatly increased numbers of secretory acini. Breast proliferation is also dependent on ***prolactin, human chorionic somatomammotropin*** (a prolactin-like hormone produced by the placenta), ***thyroxine*** and ***corticosteroids***.

At low magnification in Fig. 19.39a, the breast lobules **Lo** are seen to have enlarged greatly at the expense of the intralobular tissue and interlobar adipose tissue, although septa **S** of interlobular tissue still remain. At higher magnification in Fig. 19.39b the acini **A** are dilated. The lining epithelial cells **E** vary from cuboidal to low columnar and contain cytoplasmic vacuoles. The intralobular stroma is much less prominent and contains an infiltrate of lymphocytes, eosinophils and plasma cells.

As pregnancy progresses, the acini begin to secrete a protein-rich fluid called ***colostrum***, the accumulation of which dilates the acinar and duct lumina as seen in Fig. 19.39b. Colostrum is the form of breast secretion available during the first few days after birth. It contains a laxative substance and maternal antibodies. Unlike milk, colostrum contains little lipid. Breast secretion is controlled by the hormone prolactin. During pregnancy, prolactin secretion progressively increases, but high levels of circulating oestrogens and progesterone suppress its activity.

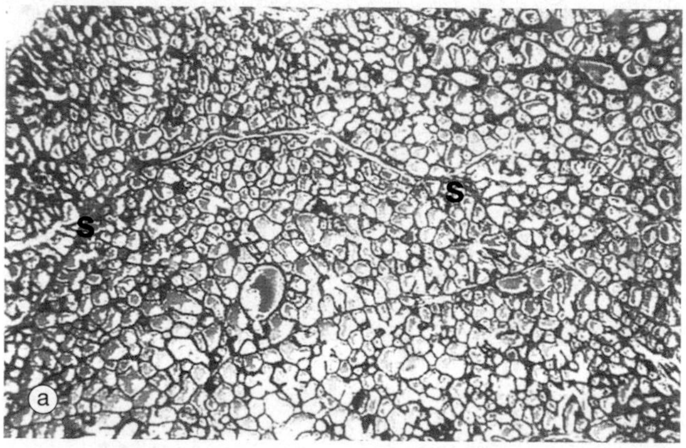

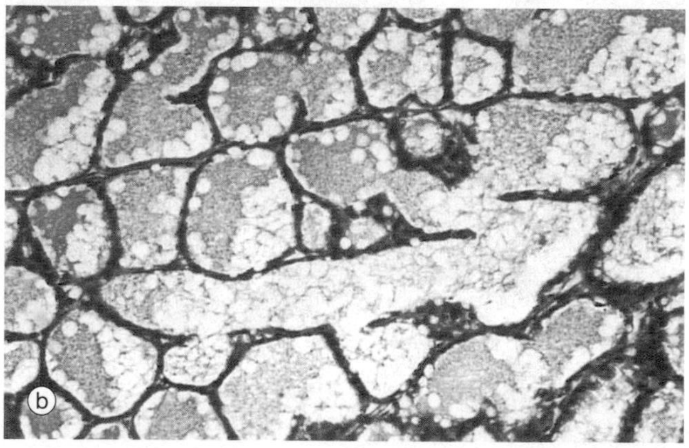

FIG. 19.40 Lactating breast
(a) H&E (LP) (b) H&E (MP)

After parturition, the levels of circulating progesterone and oestrogens, which inhibit milk secretion, fall precipitously. ***Prolactin*** stimulates milk production in conjunction with several other hormones.

As seen in Fig. 19.40a, the lactating breast is composed almost entirely of acini distended with milk, the interlobular tissue now being reduced to thin septa **S** between the lobules. At higher magnification in Fig. 19.40b, the acini are filled with an eosinophilic material containing clear vacuoles caused by lipid droplets which have dissolved out during tissue preparation. The epithelial cells are flattened and the acini distended by secretions. However, in different areas, the epithelium may be thicker and the acinar lumina smaller.

Milk production proceeds for as long as suckling continues and can continue for some years after childbirth. A neurohormonal reflex in which nipple stimulation by suckling causes release of ***prolactin*** from the anterior pituitary controls the process. A different neurohormonal reflex, also initiated by suckling, causes the release of the hormone ***oxytocin*** from the posterior pituitary. Oxytocin causes contraction of the myoepithelial cells which embrace the secretory acini and ducts, thus propelling milk into the lactiferous sinuses (***milk 'let-down'***). Withdrawal of the suckling stimulus, and hence the release of pituitary hormones at weaning, results in regression of the lactating breast and resumption of the normal ovarian cycle.

A acinus **BM** basement membrane **E** epithelial cells **G** Golgi apparatus **L** lipid droplet L_1 large lipid droplet L_2 very large lipid droplet **Lo** lobule **M** myoepithelial cell **N** nucleus **rER** rough endoplasmic reticulum **S** septum **V** secretory vacuole

Other effects of lactation

The hormonal changes which occur during lactation may interrupt resumption of the normal menstrual cycle following pregnancy and childbirth. As a result, a substantial proportion of women have ***lactational amenorrhoea*** whilst breast feeding. High levels of prolactin act to suppress production of LH and so can effectively inhibit ovulation.

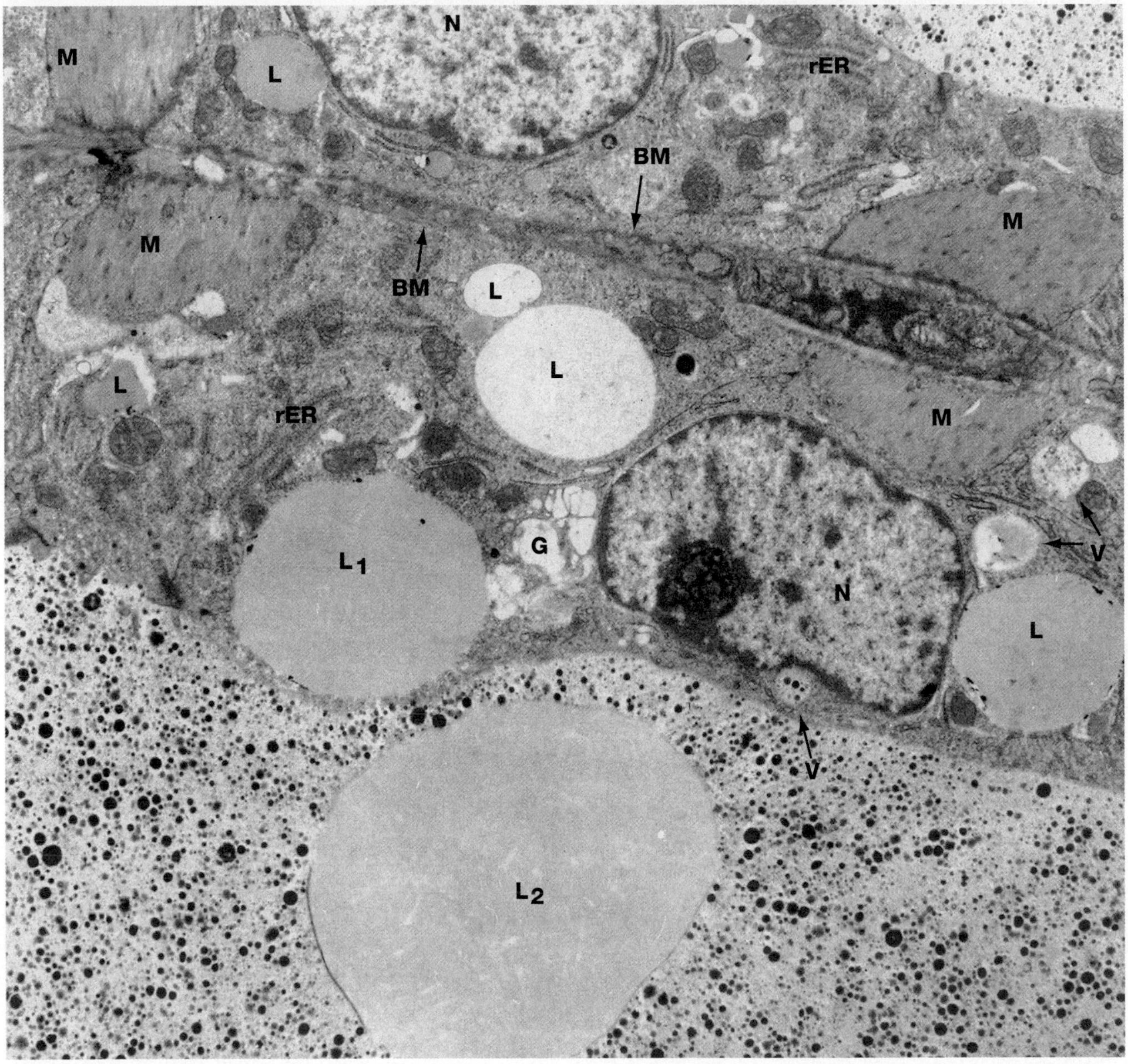

FIG. 19.41 Lactating breast
EM ×9000

Fig. 19.41 shows two secretory cells of adjacent acini in a lactating breast. Their nuclei **N** are large, with prominent nucleoli. Each acinus is bounded by a basement membrane **BM**, the basement membranes in this example being separated by only a shred of intralobular supporting tissue. Between each basement membrane and the secretory cells are the cytoplasmic processes of myoepithelial cells **M**, contraction of which expels milk from the gland.

The composition of milk varies somewhat during lactation and even during each suckling episode, but its main constituents are as follows: water (88%), ions (particularly sodium, potassium, chloride, calcium and phosphate), protein (1.5%, mainly lactalbumin and casein), carbohydrate (7%, mainly lactose), lipids (3.5%, mainly triglycerides), vitamins and antibodies (mainly IgA).

Secretion of different components of the milk occurs by different mechanisms. Water and some ions diffuse freely through the apical cell membrane. Proteins are synthesised on the rough endoplasmic reticulum **rER**, packaged in the Golgi apparatus **G** and secreted in vacuoles **V** by exocytosis. Protein in the milk is represented by small electron-dense granules. The Golgi apparatus is extensive and the protein-containing secretory vacuoles also contain a considerable amount of other less electron-dense material, including lactose and calcium.

The cytoplasm of the secretory cells contains lipid droplets **L** of various sizes which are not bounded by membrane. These contain triglycerides, although whether this is derived directly from blood or synthesised in the secretory cells is uncertain.

The lipid is discharged by ***apocrine secretion***, which involves the lipid droplet, surrounding cytoplasm and plasma membrane being cast off into the lumen. A large lipid droplet $\mathbf{L_1}$ with thin overlying rim of cytoplasm can be seen in the lower acinus, just prior to secretion. An even larger droplet $\mathbf{L_2}$ surrounded by a remnant of cytoplasm and plasma membrane is seen in the lumen close by.

IgA, taken up by ***receptor-mediated endocytosis*** at the base of the cell from the bloodstream, is transported across the cell in small membranous vesicles and released by exocytosis into the milk, a process known as ***transcytosis***.

Breast carcinoma

Carcinoma of the breast is one of the commonest malignant tumours of women, leading to many premature deaths and great morbidity. In many countries, breast cancer screening programmes are in operation in the hope that early detection of cancer or even precancerous lesions will cure the disease.

Many successful breast screening programmes and rapid one stop clinics exist worldwide to identify patients with breast cancer at an early stage. Lesions identified at mammography are biopsied, and the pathologist determines whether the lesion is a cancer or one of many benign breast lesions that may cause a lump or a mammographic abnormality. A typical breast carcinoma is illustrated in Fig. 19.42.

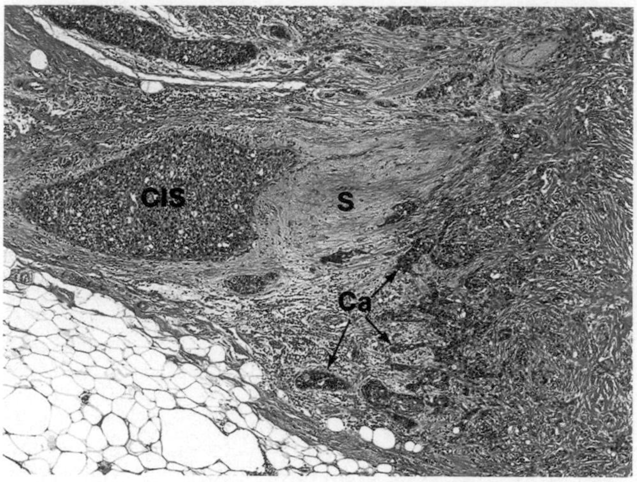

FIG. 19.42 Breast cancer
H&E (MP)

Fig. 19.42 shows a medium-power view of an area of breast carcinoma in a middle-aged woman. The cancer is of the commonest type, known as ductal carcinoma, NOS (not otherwise specified) (see e-Fig. 19.12). Note how clusters of malignant epithelial cells **Ca** invade into the normal breast stroma **S**, destroying it.

In the left side of the field, there is a single expanded duct which appears to be filled and expanded by similar malignant cells. This is an area of ductal carcinoma in situ **CIS**.

Breast carcinoma in situ often calcifies, allowing the disease to be identified on mammograms. Obviously, the earlier the cancer is identified, the better the chance of a complete cure.

Breast cancer is typically treated by a combination of surgery, hormonal therapy, chemotherapy and radiotherapy, depending upon the type and extent of the tumour. Predictive tests are often performed on the biopsy or resection specimen such as detection of oestrogen and progesterone receptors in the tumour which allows more tailored therapy.

REVIEW

TABLE 19.1 Review of the female reproductive system

Part of the female genital tract	Key features	Figure
Ovary	Primordial and developing follicles embedded in ovarian stroma Surface covering of epithelium (mesothelium) Corpora lutea and corpora albicantia	19.43a
Fallopian tube	Muscular wall Folded mucosa Ciliated columnar epithelium	19.43b
Uterus	Muscular wall – the myometrium Lining endometrium consisting of glands and stroma, varies with the menstrual cycle	19.43c
Endocervix	Bulk consists of a dense fibromuscular stroma Surface has deep clefts lined by simple columnar mucus-secreting epithelium	19.43d
Ectocervix	Stroma same as for endocervix Stratified squamous non-keratinising surface epithelium	19.43e
Vagina	Fibromuscular wall Stratified squamous non-keratinising surface epithelium	19.43f
Vulva	Stratified squamous epithelium/modified skin (see Ch. 9)	
Placenta	Chorionic villi with cores of mesenchyme and double surface layer of trophoblast	19.43g
Breast	Stroma consists of adipose tissue with fibrous septa Branching tubulo-acinar glands Glandular epithelium consists of luminal epithelial cells and underlying myoepithelial cells	19.43h

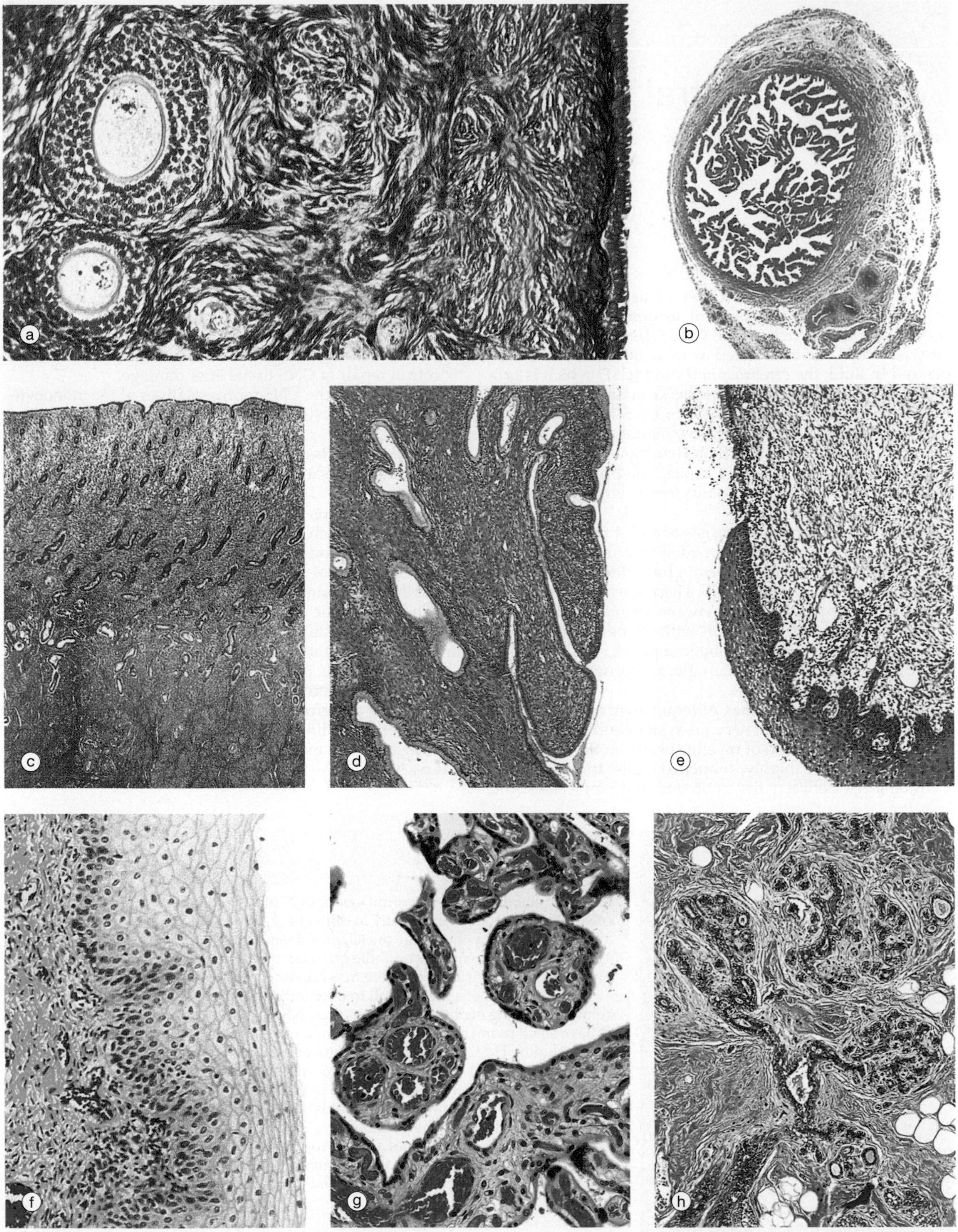

FIG. 19.43 The main components of the female reproductive system ***(see Table 19.1 opposite)***
(a) Azan (MP) (b) H&E (LP) (c) H&E (LP) (d) H&E (MP) (e) H&E (MP) (f) Masson trichrome (MP) (g) H&E (LP) (h) H&E (LP)

Ca invasive carcinoma **CIS** carcinoma in situ **S** fibrous breast stroma

20 Central nervous system

The central nervous system (CNS) consists of the brain and spinal cord and is composed of ***neurones***, neuronal processes, supporting cells of the CNS (***glial cells***) and blood vessels. The CNS is invested with meninges and is suspended in fluid, the ***cerebrospinal fluid (CSF)*** which is produced by specialised choroid plexus structures.

Macroscopically, all parts of the CNS are made up of ***grey matter*** and ***white matter***. Grey matter contains most of the neurone cell bodies and their dendritic processes while the white matter contains the axons. The lipid-rich myelin sheaths around the axons accounts for the white appearance of the white matter.

Central nervous tissue consists of a vast number of neurones and their processes embedded in a mass of support cells, collectively known as ***neuroglia***, which form almost half of the total mass of the CNS. These are highly branched cells that occupy the spaces between neurones; they have intimate functional relationships with the neurones, providing both mechanical and metabolic support.

Four principal types of neuroglia are recognised:

- ***Oligodendrocytes*** are the CNS equivalent of the Schwann cells of the peripheral nervous system and are responsible for the formation of myelin sheaths in the CNS.
- ***Astrocytes*** are highly branched cells that pack the interstices between the neurones, their processes and oligodendrocytes. They provide mechanical support as well as mediating the exchange of metabolites between neurones and the vascular system. They also form part of the blood–brain barrier. Astrocytes play an important role in repair of CNS tissue after damage.
- ***Microglia*** are the CNS representatives of the monocyte–macrophage system and have defence and immunological functions.
- ***Ependymal cells*** make up a specialised epithelium which lines the ventricles and spinal canal.

Central nervous tissue proper lacks collagenous supporting tissue which is confined to the immediate surrounds of penetrating blood vessels and to the meninges that invest the outer surface of the brain. The CNS also contains little extracellular material.

While the basic organisation of grey and white matter remains consistent throughout the brain, in detail they form complex arrangements of the basic components to give a rich microscopic anatomy (histology) which is highly related to the macroscopic anatomy and function. In this chapter after description of the specialised supporting cells and tissues, including CSF production (choroid plexus), we will illustrate the microanatomy of some major structures in the CNS.

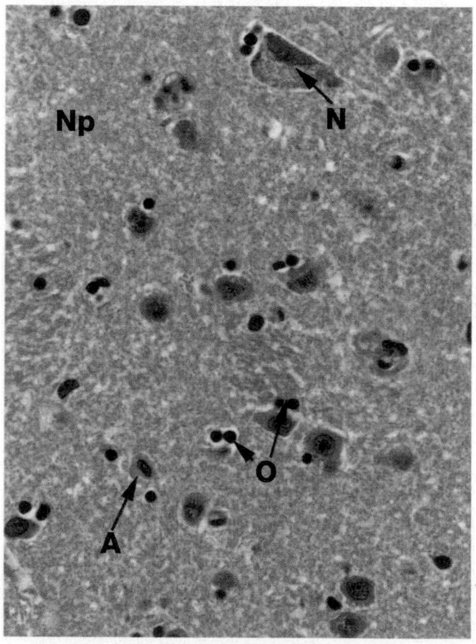

FIG. 20.1 Grey matter
H&E (HP)

Common staining methods permit ***neurones*** **N** to be readily distinguished from glial cells. While neurones vary greatly in different regions of the brain, they are usually recognisable by their large nuclei, prominent nucleoli and dispersed chromatin. There is usually extensive basophilic granular cytoplasm, and parts of one or more processes may be visible, often due to processing artefact.

Types of neuroglia are difficult to differentiate from each other with certainty by common staining methods. In the mature CNS, as in this specimen, ***oligodendrocytes*** **O** have small round condensed nuclei; their cytoplasm is unstained by routine methods, including H&E. In grey matter, oligodendrocytes are not only scattered between the nerve cell bodies along with the astrocytes but also tend to be aggregated around the neurone cell bodies. Other glial cells in the image, marked **A**, are probably ***astrocytes***. Microglia (not shown here) are cells with short processes that are essentially inactive macrophages in the CNS.

The nuclei of both neurones and neuroglia are surrounded by a dense network of branching cytoplasmic cell processes, ***axons*** and ***dendrites***. This is seen as a fibrillar eosinophilic material on H&E and is called ***neuropil*** **Np**. Only some of the fibres are myelinated axons.

Responses of the CNS to injury

Neurones are vulnerable to any significant changes in their environment such as hypoxia following a cardiac arrest. As a result, there is red cell change characterised by cell body swelling, chromatolysis (loss of Nissl substance) and nuclear pyknosis (see e-Fig. 20.1).

Dead neurones are phagocytosed by monocytes and, following this, the astrocytes proliferate to form an astrocytic scar. This whole process is known as ***gliosis*** and is unique to the CNS, due to the absence of fibroblasts that generate granulation tissue and scar tissue at other sites of the body.

A astrocyte **C** astrocyte cytoplasmic extension **IF** intermediate filament bundle **M** myelinated axon **N** neurone **Np** neuropil **O** oligodendrocyte

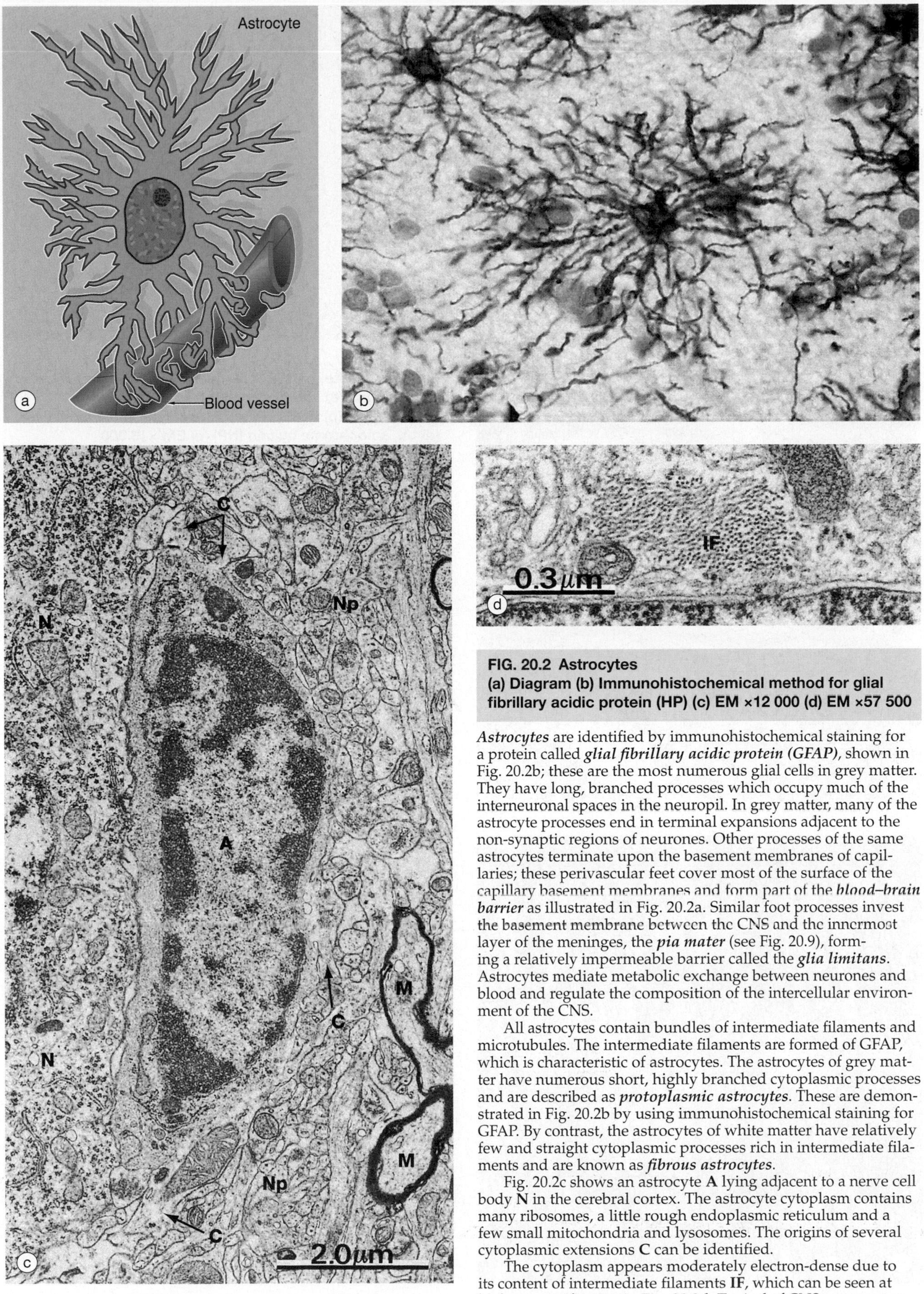

FIG. 20.2 Astrocytes
(a) Diagram (b) Immunohistochemical method for glial fibrillary acidic protein (HP) (c) EM ×12 000 (d) EM ×57 500

Astrocytes are identified by immunohistochemical staining for a protein called ***glial fibrillary acidic protein (GFAP)***, shown in Fig. 20.2b; these are the most numerous glial cells in grey matter. They have long, branched processes which occupy much of the interneuronal spaces in the neuropil. In grey matter, many of the astrocyte processes end in terminal expansions adjacent to the non-synaptic regions of neurones. Other processes of the same astrocytes terminate upon the basement membranes of capillaries; these perivascular feet cover most of the surface of the capillary basement membranes and form part of the ***blood–brain barrier*** as illustrated in Fig. 20.2a. Similar foot processes invest the basement membrane between the CNS and the innermost layer of the meninges, the ***pia mater*** (see Fig. 20.9), forming a relatively impermeable barrier called the ***glia limitans***. Astrocytes mediate metabolic exchange between neurones and blood and regulate the composition of the intercellular environment of the CNS.

All astrocytes contain bundles of intermediate filaments and microtubules. The intermediate filaments are formed of GFAP, which is characteristic of astrocytes. The astrocytes of grey matter have numerous short, highly branched cytoplasmic processes and are described as ***protoplasmic astrocytes***. These are demonstrated in Fig. 20.2b by using immunohistochemical staining for GFAP. By contrast, the astrocytes of white matter have relatively few and straight cytoplasmic processes rich in intermediate filaments and are known as ***fibrous astrocytes***.

Fig. 20.2c shows an astrocyte **A** lying adjacent to a nerve cell body **N** in the cerebral cortex. The astrocyte cytoplasm contains many ribosomes, a little rough endoplasmic reticulum and a few small mitochondria and lysosomes. The origins of several cytoplasmic extensions **C** can be identified.

The cytoplasm appears moderately electron-dense due to its content of intermediate filaments **IF**, which can be seen at higher magnification in Fig. 20.2d. Typical of CNS grey matter, the adjacent neuropil **Np** contains numerous neuronal and glial processes in various planes of section; some myelinated axons **M** are included in the field.

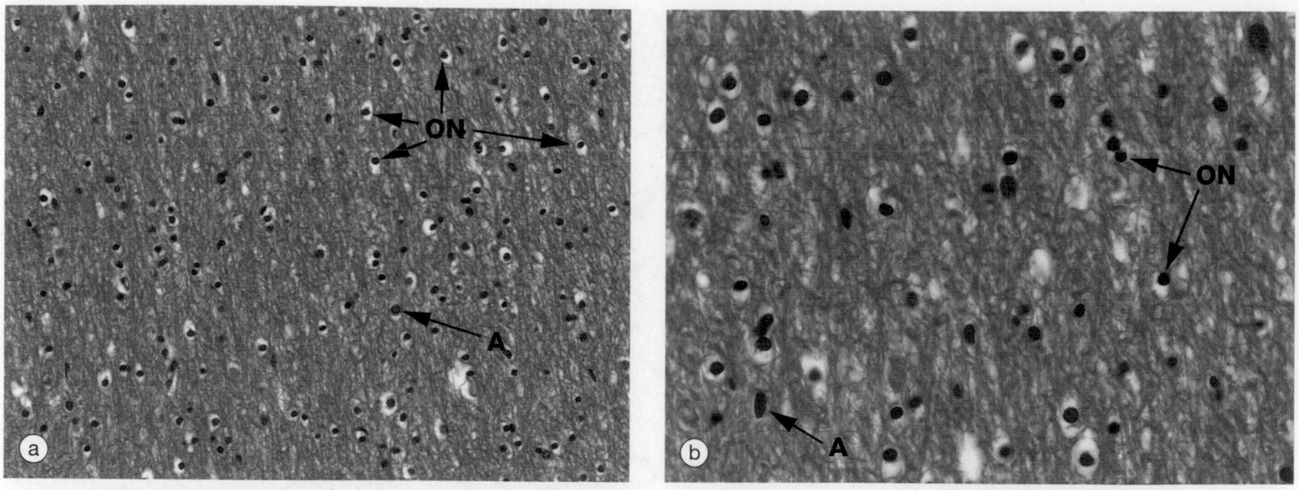

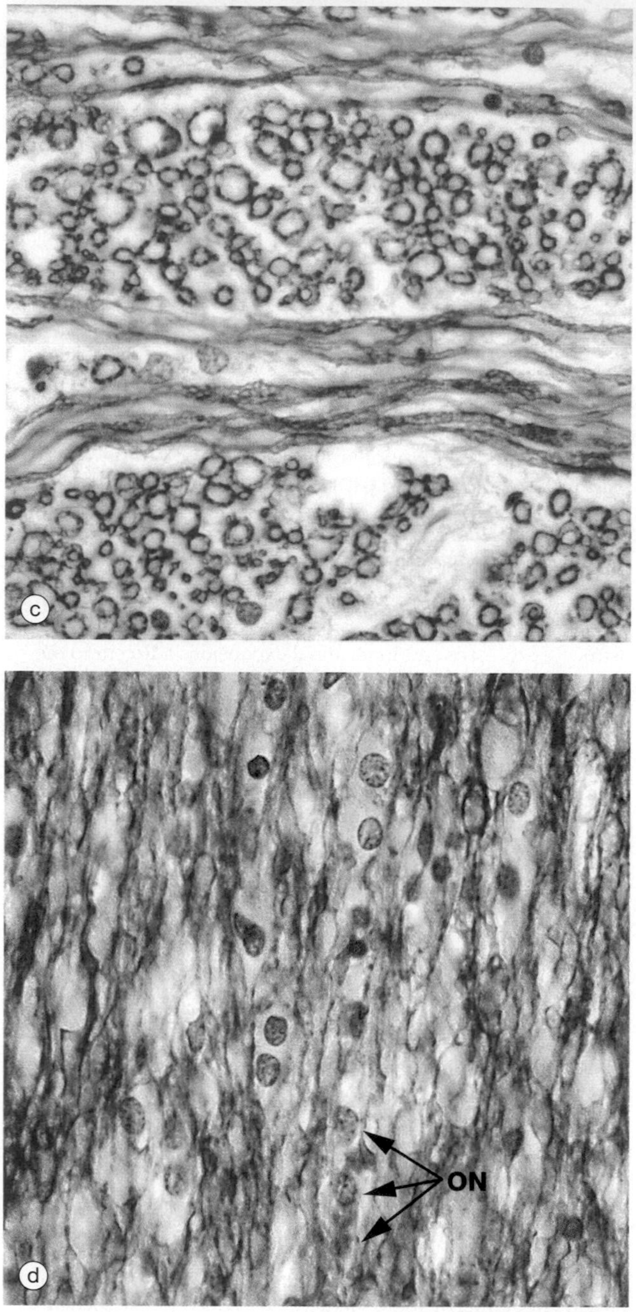

FIG. 20.3 White matter CNS myelin and oligodendrocytes *(illustrations (e) and (f) opposite)*
(a) H&E (MP) (b) H&E (HP) (c) TS, solochrome cyanin (HP) (d) LS, solochrome cyanin (HP) (e) EM ×13 000 (f) Schematic diagram

White matter consists of nerve fibres (***axons***), often myelinated by ***oligodendrocytes***, organised in ***tracts***, with supporting astrocytes, microglia and vessels. Oligodendrocytes were so named because original heavy metal impregnation methods showed that they only had a small number of short, branched processes (Greek: *oligos* = few, *dendron* = tree). It is now known that oligodendrocytes are responsible for myelination of axons and the processes originally described are the short pedicles that connect the cell body to the myelin sheaths.

A single oligodendrocyte can contribute to the myelination of up to 50 axons from the same or different fibre tracts, as illustrated in Fig. 20.3f. Conversely, any one axon will require the services of numerous different oligodendrocytes because of the limited length of the myelin segments (***internodes***) produced by each oligodendrocyte. The mechanism of myelin sheath formation is very similar to that of Schwann cells in peripheral nerve (see Fig. 7.6). Oligodendrocytes are the predominant type of neuroglia in white matter, as well as being abundant in grey matter.

Figs 20.3a and b show CNS white matter, with the oligodendrocyte nuclei **ON** often having an artefactual perinuclear halo and a few larger astrocyte nuclei **A**. Fig. 20.3c shows a myelin stain, with the transverse ring-shaped profiles of blue-stained myelin each surrounding an axon, unstained and not visible in this preparation. Fig. 20.3d demonstrates longitudinal fibres using the same stain. Oligodendrocyte nuclei **ON** can be seen as rounded red-stained profiles.

Oligodendrocytes aggregate closely around nerve cell bodies in the grey matter, where they are thought to have a support function analogous to that of the satellite cells which surround nerve cell bodies in peripheral ganglia (see Fig. 7.20).

Fig. 20.3e shows an oligodendrocyte **O** lying adjacent to a nerve cell body **N**, with a neuronal dendrite **D** at the upper right. The oligodendrocyte contains prominent rough endoplasmic reticulum, ribosomes and Golgi apparatus **G**. The commencement of a cytoplasmic process **C** is seen. The remainder of the image shows the complexity of the neuropil **Np**, comprising glial and neuronal processes including myelinated axons **M**.

Myelin sheath formation begins in the CNS of the human embryo at about 4 months gestation, with the formation of most sheaths at least commenced by about the age of 1 year.

From this time, successive layers continue to be laid down, with final myelin sheath thickness being achieved by the time of physical maturity.

A astrocyte nucleus **C** cytoplasmic process of oligodendrocyte **D** neuronal dendrite **G** Golgi apparatus **M** myelinated axon **N** nerve cell body **Np** neuropil **O** oligodendrocyte **ON** oligodendrocyte nucleus

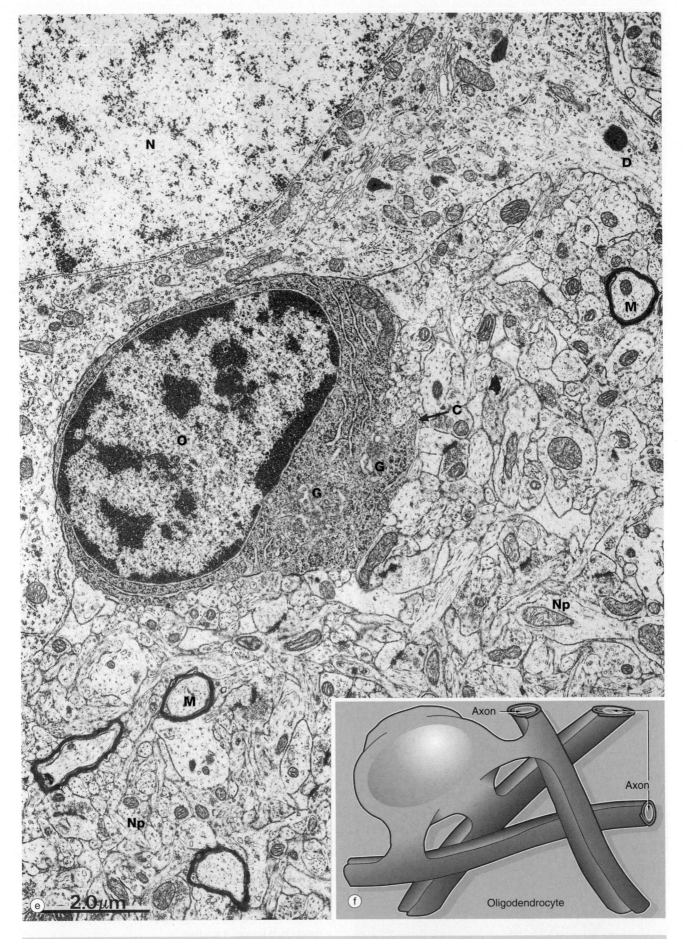

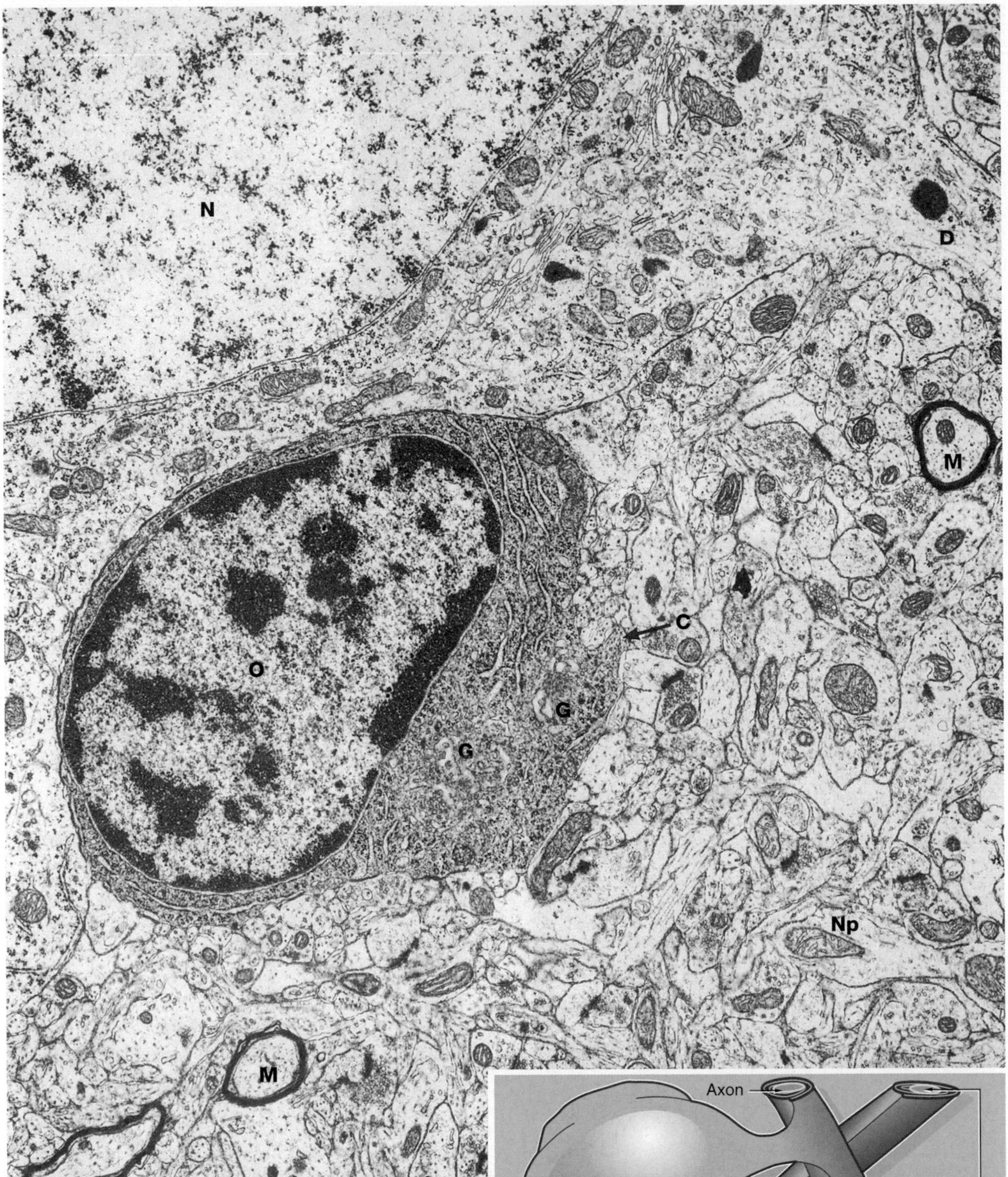

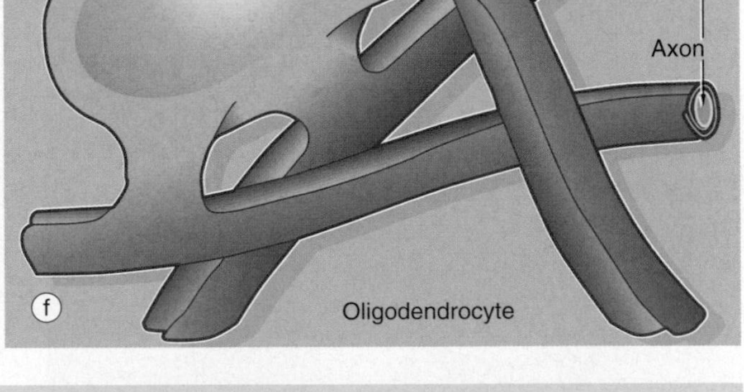

FIG. 20.3 White matter CNS myelin and oligodendrocytes *(caption and illustrations (a) to (d) opposite)*
(a) H&E (MP) (b) H&E (HP) (c) TS, solochrome cyanin (HP) (d) LS, solochrome cyanin (HP) (e) EM ×13 000
(f) Schematic diagram

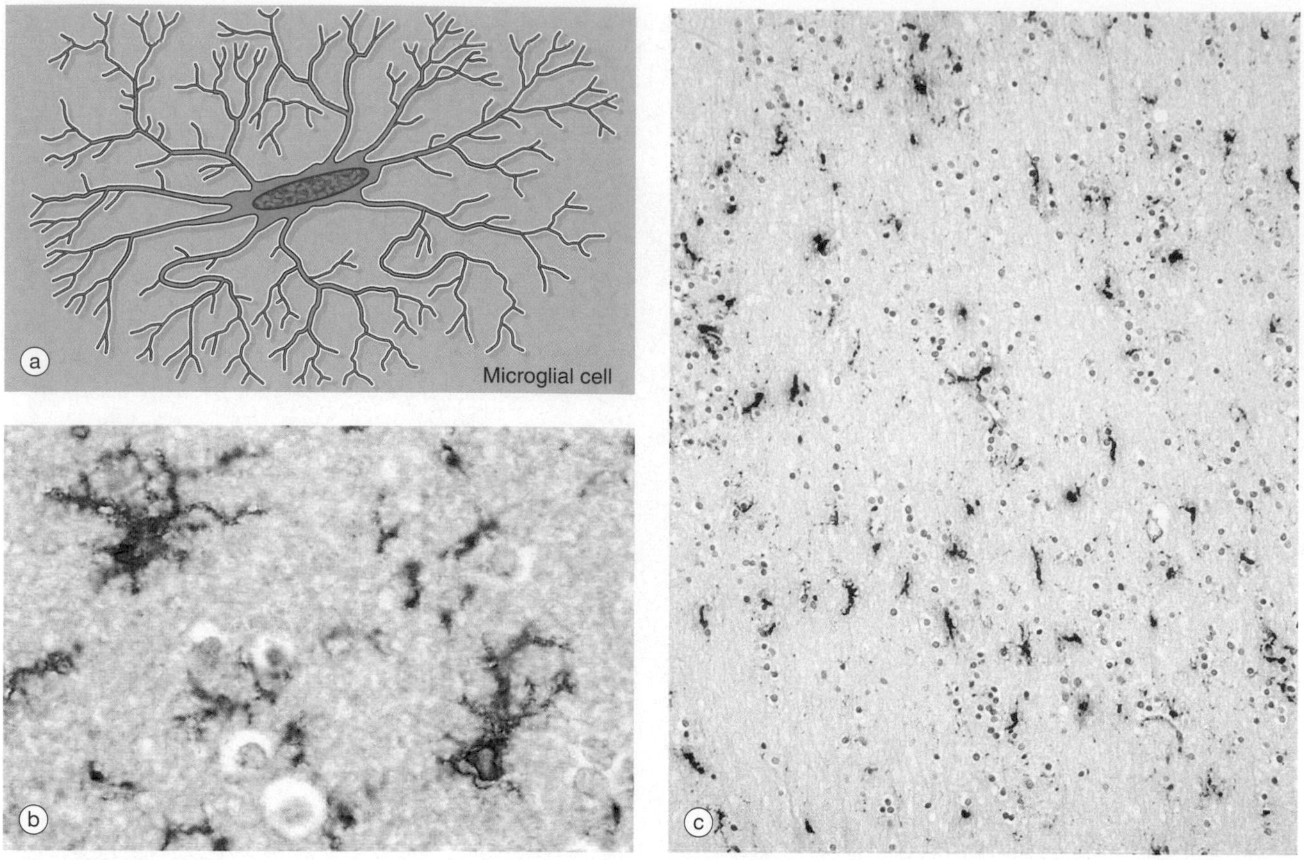

FIG. 20.4 Microglia
(a) Diagram (b) Ricinus communis agglutinin (HP) (c) Immunohistochemical method for CD68 (MP)

Microglia are small cells derived from cells of mesenchymal origin which invade the CNS at a late stage of fetal development. As shown in Fig. 20.4d, microglia have elongated nuclei and relatively little cytoplasm, which forms fine highly branched processes. In consequence, they are difficult to identify in conventional preparations for light microscopy.

Immunohistochemical staining provides the best way to see microglia. Fig. 20.4b shows the ramified profile of microglia cells, identified by staining using ricinus communis agglutinin which binds to sugars on the membrane of this cell type. Fig. 20.4c highlights the distribution of this cell type in white matter from the cerebral hemisphere. The rounded nuclei in the background are mainly oligodendrocytes.

In response to tissue damage, microglia transform into large amoeboid phagocytic cells and are thus the CNS representatives of the macrophage–monocyte defence system (see Fig. 4.19). CD68 stains cells of macrophage lineage, including microglial cells. Other macrophages, distinct from microglia, are present in the space surrounding the CNS capillaries but are separated from the CNS compartment proper by the perivascular feet of astrocytes.

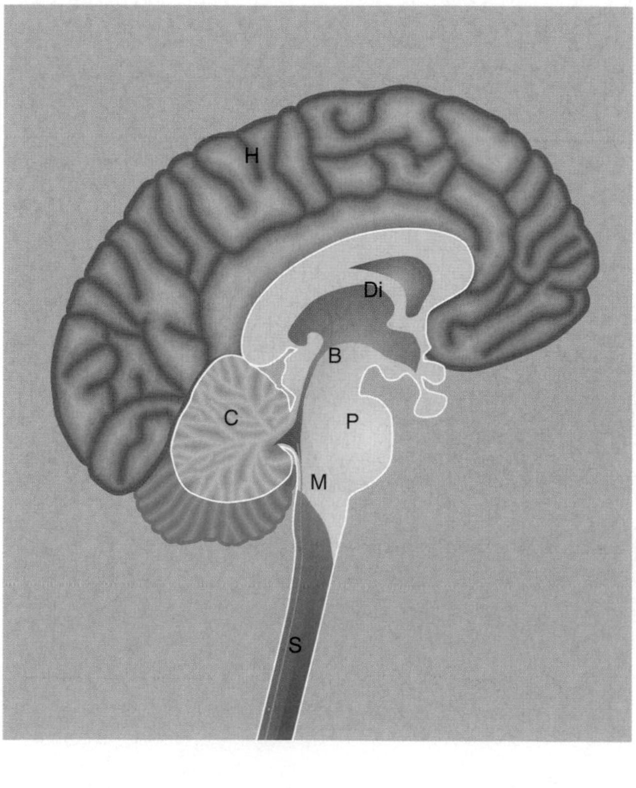

FIG. 20.5 Main anatomical divisions in the CNS

Fig. 20.5 shows the brain and spinal cord viewed in a sagittal section. The main part of the brain consists of the paired ***cerebral hemispheres*** **H** which are invested by the cerebral cortex. Deep within the brain are large grey matter structures which form the ***diencephalon*** **Di**. Included in this region are the ***basal ganglia*** and ***thalamus***. The cerebral hemispheres are connected to structures below by the ***midbrain*** **B**. In this region, there are important nuclei including the ***substantia nigra***. The ***pons*** **P** connects to the medulla **M** as well as to the ***cerebellum*** **C**. The pons, medulla and midbrain are often collectively termed the ***brainstem***. The ***spinal cord*** **S** extends from the lower end of the medulla.

Specific terms are used to describe arrangements of cells and their connections:

- The grey matter over the surface of the brain is termed the ***cortex***.
- A discrete arrangement of neurones, often with a specific function, is termed a ***nucleus***.
- An arrangement of neuronal cells running along the spinal cord is termed a ***column***.
- A defined bundle of axons running in white matter is termed a ***tract*** or a ***fascicle***.
- The crests of folds are termed ***gyri*** (singular: gyrus) while the clefts between folds are termed ***sulci*** (singular: sulcus). In the cerebellum these folds are termed ***folia***.

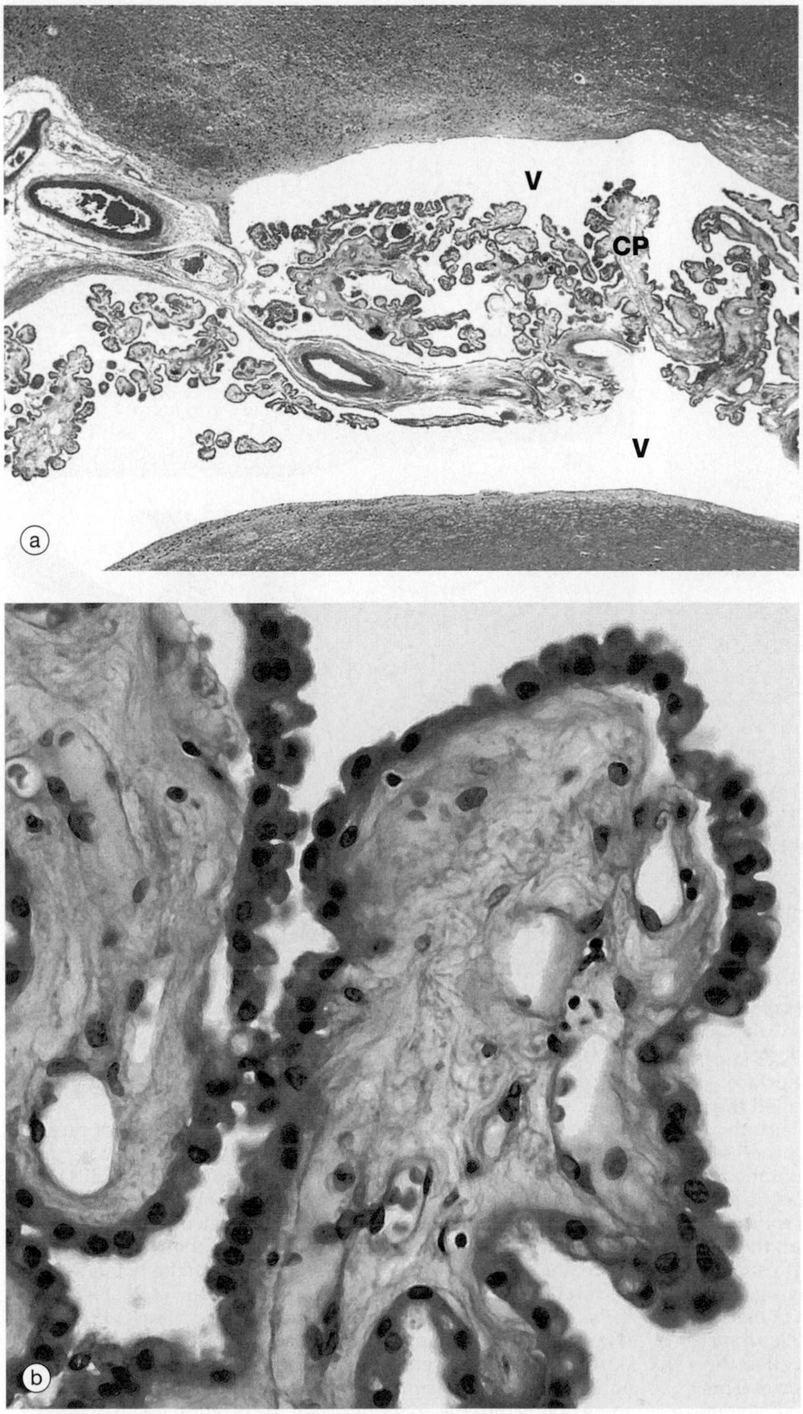

FIG. 20.6 Choroid plexus
(a) H&E (LP) (b) H&E (HP)

The choroid plexus is a vascular structure arising from the wall of each of the four ventricles of the brain and responsible for the production of ***cerebrospinal fluid (CSF)***. CSF drains from the interconnected ventricular cavities via three channels connecting the fourth ventricle with the subarachnoid space which surrounds the CNS. CSF is produced at a constant rate and is reabsorbed from the subarachnoid space into the superior sagittal venous sinus, via finger-like projections called ***arachnoid villi***. Thus the CNS is suspended in a constantly circulating fluid medium which acts as a support and shock absorber.

Each choroid plexus consists of a branching system of blood vessels which run in fronds composed of collagenous tissue and covered by a cuboidal or columnar epithelium. The choroid plexus is therefore a villous structure. Fig. 20.6a shows the choroid plexus **CP** within a ventricle of the brain **V**.

Fig. 20.6b shows detail of one of the choroid plexus processes. The capillaries and vessels of the choroid plexus are large, thin-walled and sometimes fenestrated lying in a fibrous core. The epithelial cells rest on a basal lamina. At the ultrastructural level, long bulbous microvilli project from the luminal surfaces of the choroid plexus epithelial cells and their cytoplasm contains numerous mitochondria, features which suggest that the elaboration of CSF is an active process.

The mode of CSF secretion involves active secretion of sodium ions by choroid epithelial cells into the CSF, followed by passive movement of water from the local vessels.

Continuous tight junctions (***zonula occludens***) between epithelial cells contribute to a ***blood–CSF barrier***, preventing ingress of almost all other molecules.

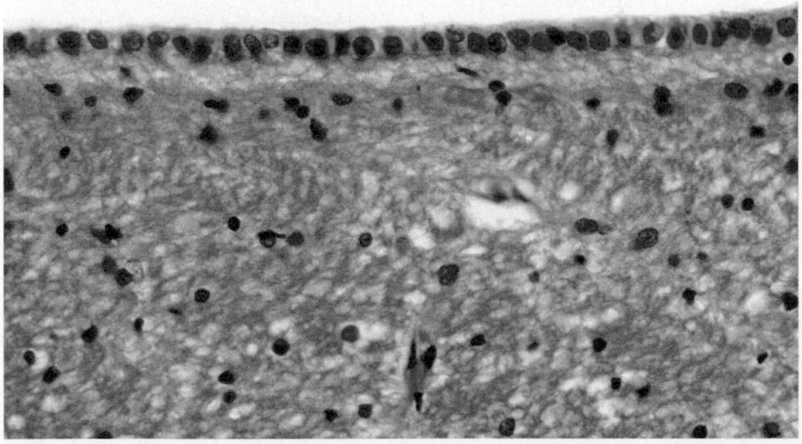

FIG. 20.7 Ependyma
H&E (HP)

Ependymal cells (Fig. 20.7) form the lining of the ventricles and spinal canal. Cuboidal or low columnar in shape, the cells are tightly bound together at their luminal surfaces by the usual epithelial junctional complexes. Unlike epithelia, however, ependymal cells do not rest on a basement membrane but, rather, the bases of the cells taper and then branch into fine processes which ramify within the underlying layer of processes derived from astrocytes. At the luminal surface, there are a variable number of cilia. Microvilli are also present and probably have absorptive and secretory functions. The ependymal layer tends to become incomplete with increasing age.

B midbrain **C** cerebellum **CP** choroid plexus **Di** diencephalon **H** hemisphere **M** medulla **P** pons **S** spinal cord **V** ventricle

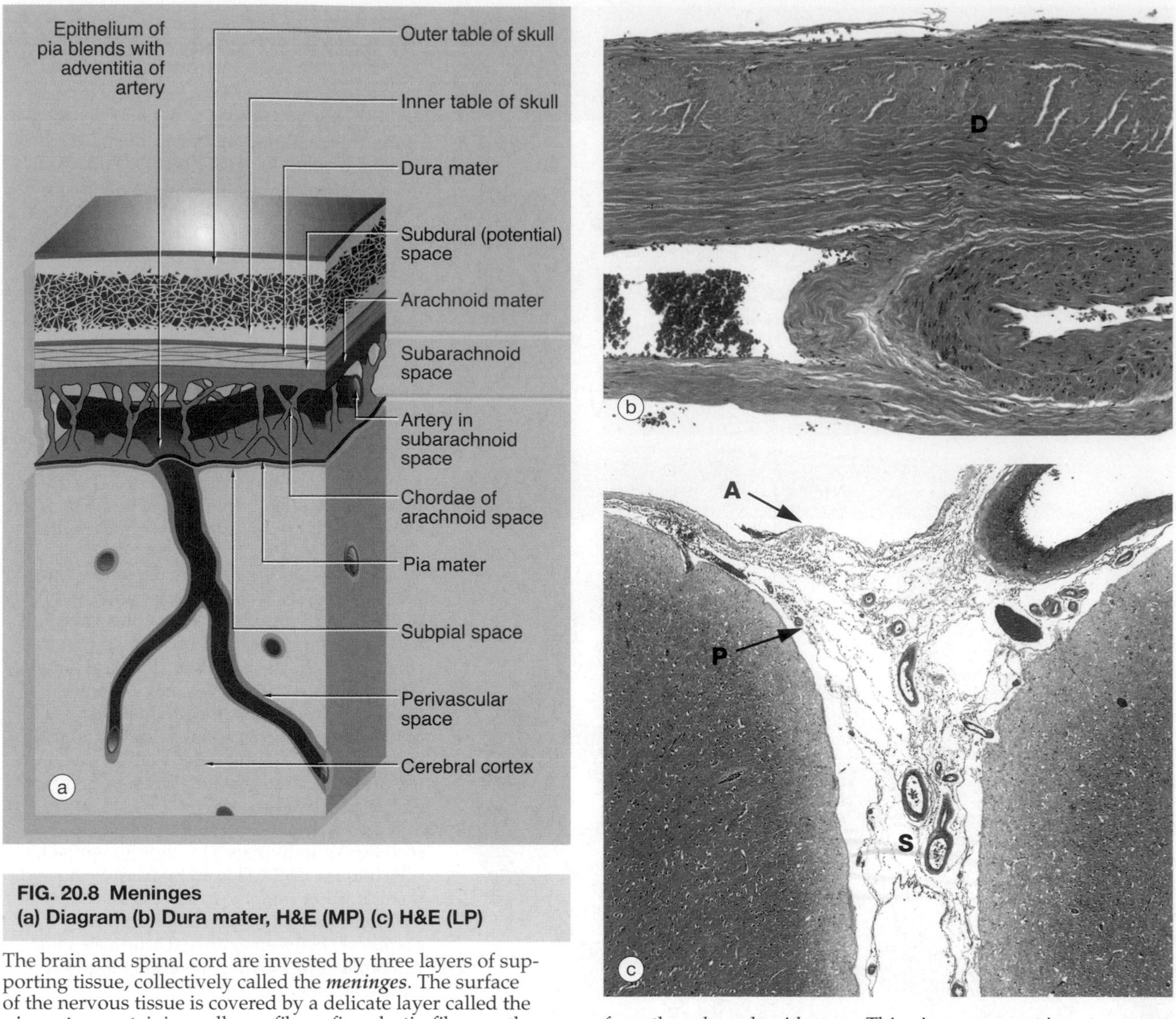

FIG. 20.8 Meninges
(a) Diagram (b) Dura mater, H&E (MP) (c) H&E (LP)

The brain and spinal cord are invested by three layers of supporting tissue, collectively called the ***meninges***. The surface of the nervous tissue is covered by a delicate layer called the ***pia mater***, containing collagen fibres, fine elastin fibres and occasional fibroblasts, separated from the astrocytic processes of underlying CNS parenchyma by a basement membrane. The basement membrane is completely invested by astrocytic processes, the two layers forming the impermeable ***glia limitans***.

Overlying the pia mater is a thicker fibrous layer, the ***arachnoid mater***, which derives its name from the presence of cobweb-like strands which connect it to the underlying pia; since the pia and arachnoid are continuous, they may be considered as a unit, the ***pia–arachnoid***, also called the ***leptomeninges***. The space between the pia and arachnoid is called the ***subarachnoid space*** and, in places, forms large cisterns. This subarachnoid space is connected with the ventricular system by three ***foramina*** in the ***fourth ventricle*** (in the ***brainstem***), and CSF circulates continuously from the ventricles into the subarachnoid space.

The subarachnoid space is lined by flattened arachnoidal cells. The outer surface of the arachnoid mater is also lined by flat cells. As shown in Fig. 20.8a, arteries and veins passing to and from the CNS pass in the subarachnoid space loosely attached to the pia mater and invested by subarachnoid meningothelium. As the larger vessels extend into the nervous tissue, they are surrounded by a delicate sleeve of pia mater. Between the penetrating vessels and the pia there is a ***perivascular space***. In humans, the pia blends with the adventitia of the vessel as it penetrates the brain, thus separating the perivascular space from the subarachnoid space. This pia component is not present around the capillaries of the CNS.

External to the arachnoid mater is a dense fibroelastic layer called the ***dura mater*** **D**, Fig. 20.8b, which is lined on its internal surface by flat cells. The dura is closely applied to but not connected with the arachnoid layer and there is the potential for a space, the ***subdural space***, to develop between the two layers. In the cranium, the dura mater merges with the periosteum of the skull but also extends into the brain space as several folds. A large fold, the ***falx***, extends along the midline from top of the skull into the space between the cerebral hemispheres while a horizontal fold, the ***tentorium***, is attached to the posterior skull and extends into the space between the cerebral hemispheres and cerebellum. These folds help support the brain and contain venous sinuses, forming part of the brain's venous return system.

Around the spinal cord, dura is suspended from the periosteum of the spinal canal by ***denticulate ligaments***, the intervening ***epidural space*** being filled with loose fibrofatty tissue and a venous plexus.

The pia and arachnoid layers of the brain meninges are illustrated in Fig. 20.8c. Pia mater **P** is attached to the surface of the brain and continues into the suclus **S** and around the penetrating vessels. The arachnoid mater **A** appears to be a completely separate layer and bridges the sulcus. Meningeal vessels lie in the subarachnoid space.

Meningitis

In bacterial meningitis, infective organisms invade the CSF, inducing a neutrophillic inflammatory response. The majority of cases are due to haematogenous spread though some may arise due to local spread from the head/neck (e.g. infected air sinuses) or following surgery. Bacterial meningitis is a serious and potentially life-threatening infection, in contrast to viral infections which are rarely fatal and induce a lymphocytic response in the CSF.

A arachnoid mater **D** dura mater **F** fibrous strand **P** pia mater **PVS** perivascular space **S** sulcus **SS** subarachnoid space **V** vessel

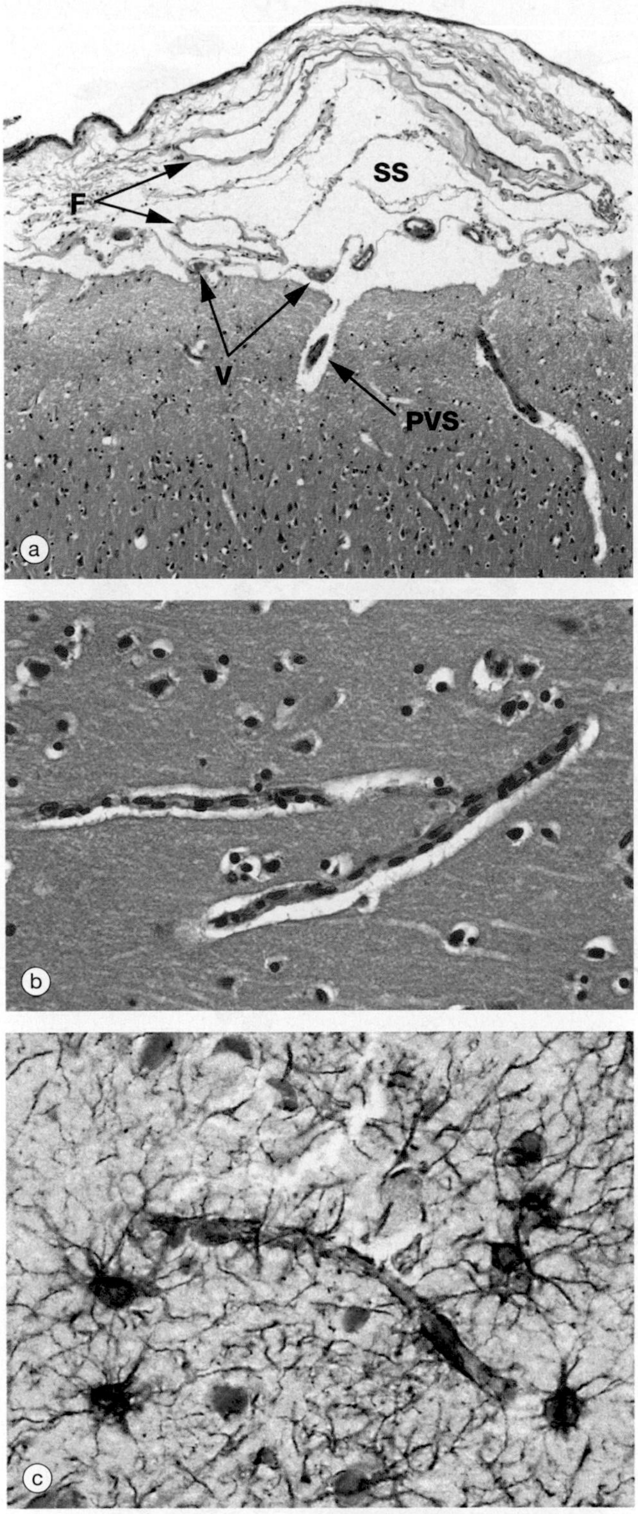

FIG. 20.9 Meninges
(a) H&E (MP) (b) H&E (HP) (c) Immunohistochemical method for GFAP (HP)

The pia and arachnoid layers of the brain meninges are illustrated in Fig. 20.9a. In this micrograph, delicate fibrous strands **F** can be discerned traversing the subarachnoid space **SS** to connect the pia and arachnoid layers. Small vessels **V** can be seen in the subarachnoid space. A penetrating vessel is also seen, surrounded by a perivascular space **PVS**. The perivascular space is extremely narrow, although it often appears artefactually wider as in this micrograph. The CNS contains no lymphatics and interstitial fluid is thought to drain outwards from the brain substance to join the subarachnoid CSF via the perivascular spaces, contributing as much as 20% of its volume.

As seen in Fig. 20.9b by light microscopy, the capillaries of the CNS are similar to those elsewhere in the body, with flattened endothelial cells resting on a basement membrane; however, unlike elsewhere, these endothelial cells are not fenestrated and are bound together by continuous tight intercellular junctions (***zonula occludens***). Externally, the basement membranes are covered by the perivascular foot processes of astrocytes, shown in Fig. 20.9c, where brown-stained processes form a continuous layer.

Perfusion studies show that the CNS capillaries are impermeable to certain plasma constituents, especially larger molecules, forming a ***blood–brain barrier***. The capillary endothelium plays the central role, since the junctions between endothelial cells are sealed; the endothelial cells exhibit little or no pinocytosis. Luminal surface membranes contain various enzymes which destroy neurotoxic metabolites and neuroactive humoral substances.

Maintenance of barrier-type endothelium appears to be under the control of astrocyte foot processes. The blood–brain barrier provides neurones with a relatively constant biochemical and metabolic environment, protection against endogenous and exogenous toxins and infective agents and insulates the neurones from circulating neurotransmitters and other humoral agents. The capillaries of the choroid plexus, the pituitary and pineal glands and the vomiting centre of the hypothalamus are, however, devoid of this barrier to allow for their specialised functions.

The specialised function of the blood brain barrier protects the brain from a variety of infective and toxic agents as discussed above. However this selective function can also create problems when considering drug delivery to the CNS as these macromolecules can be blocked from entering. As such, some drugs need to be delivered directly into the cerebrospinal fluid (intrathecal) in order to reach the target cells in the CNS.

Intracranial haemorrhage

Damage to delicate vessels in the brain (e.g. rupture due to a weakness of the vessel wall) allows blood to escape (haemorrhage), which can result in raised intracranial pressure, stroke (see e-Fig. 20.2) and can ultimately be fatal. Some types of haemorrhage are described below:

- ***Intracerebral haemorrhage*** is most often due to hypertension which weakens the vessel walls. Haemorrhage typically occurs around the basal ganglia.
- The subdural space is the potential space between the dura and the arachnoid. Veins traverse this tissue plane. In the elderly and in patients with impaired blood clotting, minor trauma can tear veins, causing bleeding into this space (***subdural haemorrhage***).
- The dura is firmly attached to the inner surface of the skull. If there is bleeding associated with skull fracture, typically due to injury of the middle meningeal artery, blood can accumulate in this tissue plane between bone and dura, producing an ***extradural haemorrhage***.

FIG. 20.10 Spinal cord transverse sections Luxol fast blue, H&E photomontage, (LP) (a) Cervical (b) Thoracic (c) Lumbar (d) Sacral

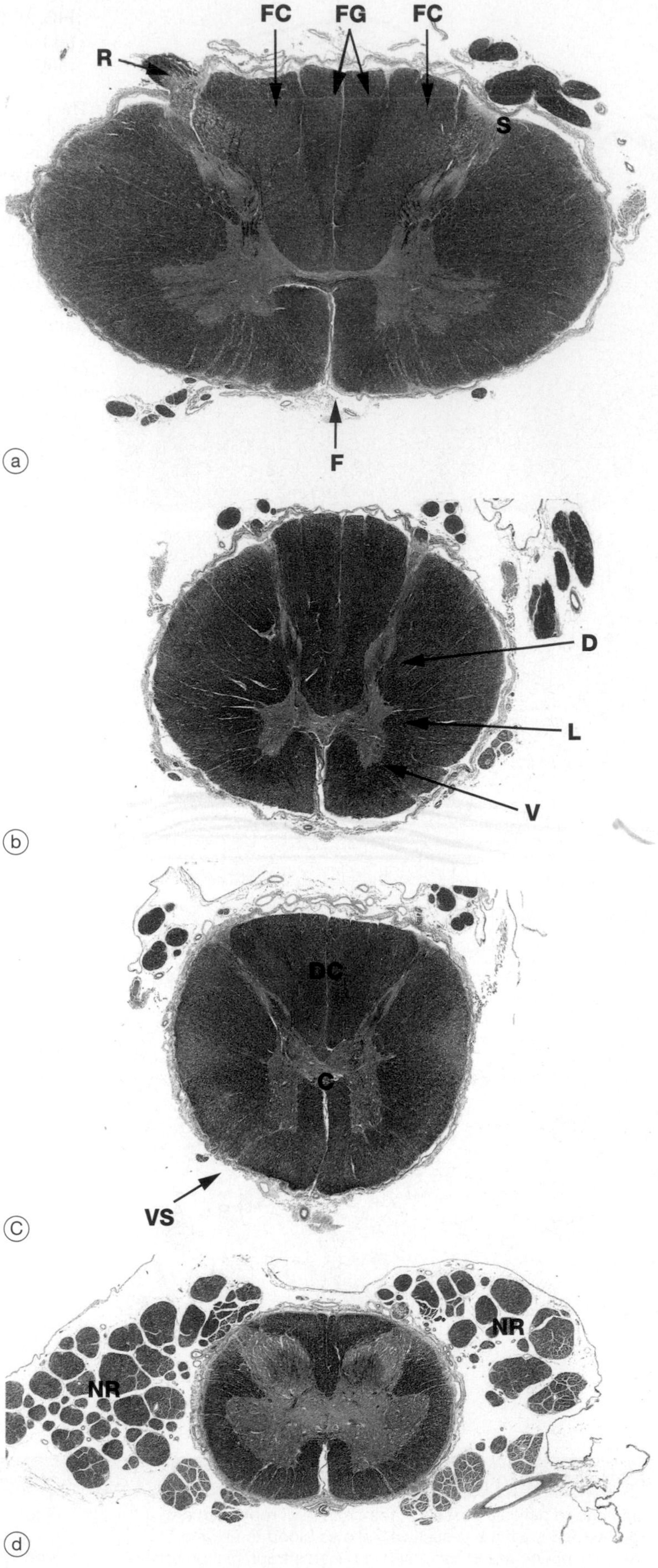

The structure of the spinal cord is similar throughout its length, with four regions demonstrated in this series of micrographs. In transverse sections, the central mass of grey matter has the shape of a butterfly, the ***ventral horns*** **V** being prominent and containing the cell bodies of the large alpha lower motor neurones (Fig. 20.10b). The ***dorsal horns*** **D** contain the cell bodies of small second-order sensory neurones. These relay upwards sensory information on pain and temperature and participate in spinal reflexes. Small ***lateral horns*** **L** are found in the thoracic and upper lumbar regions and contain cell bodies of sympathetic nervous system efferent neurones. The volume of grey matter is more extensive in the cervical and lumbar regions and the cord is larger, corresponding to innervation of the limbs.

The ***central canal*** lies in the ***central commissure*** **C** of grey matter; it is lined by ependymal cells and contains CSF. The white matter consists of ascending tracts of sensory fibres and descending motor tracts; passing up the spinal cord towards the brain, more and more fibres enter and leave the cord so that the volume of white matter increases progressively from the sacral to cervical regions.

The spinal cord has a deep ***ventral (anterior) median fissure*** **F** but, dorsally, there is only a shallow dorsal midline sulcus. On each side, a dorsolateral sulcus **S** marks the line of entry of the dorsal nerve roots **R**, part of which can be seen in Fig. 20.10a. The white matter between the dorsal horns represents the ascending ***dorsal columns*** **DC** (Fig. 20.10c) which convey fibres for senses of vibration, proprioception and fine touch to the medulla where they synapse with second-order sensory neurones in the ***gracile*** and ***cuneate nuclei***. In the cervical region, each dorsal column is subdivided into two fascicles: the medial ***fasciculus gracilis*** **FG**, conveying fibres from the lower limbs, and the lateral ***fasciculus cuneatus*** **FC**, conveying fibres from the upper limbs.

Ventrolateral sulci **VS** may be discernible, marking the line of exit of the ventral nerve roots. The ventrolateral white matter contains most notably the ***lateral spinothalamic tract*** (pain and temperature), the ***ventral spinothalamic tract*** (light touch), the ***spinocerebellar tracts*** and the ***corticospinal tract*** (motor).

The spinal cord is invested by meninges, with the dura mater being loosely connected to the periosteum of the vertebral canal by ***denticulate ligaments***; the residual epidural space is filled by adipose tissue and a venous plexus. During development, the vertebral column lengthens more than the enclosed spinal cord, and the segmental levels of the lower part of the cord therefore lie above the corresponding intervertebral foramina. Below the cervical region, the ***nerve roots*** **NR** pursue an increasingly oblique course in the subarachnoid space before passing through the intervertebral foramina and are thus found adjacent to the cord, particularly in the lumbar and sacral regions (Fig. 20.10d).

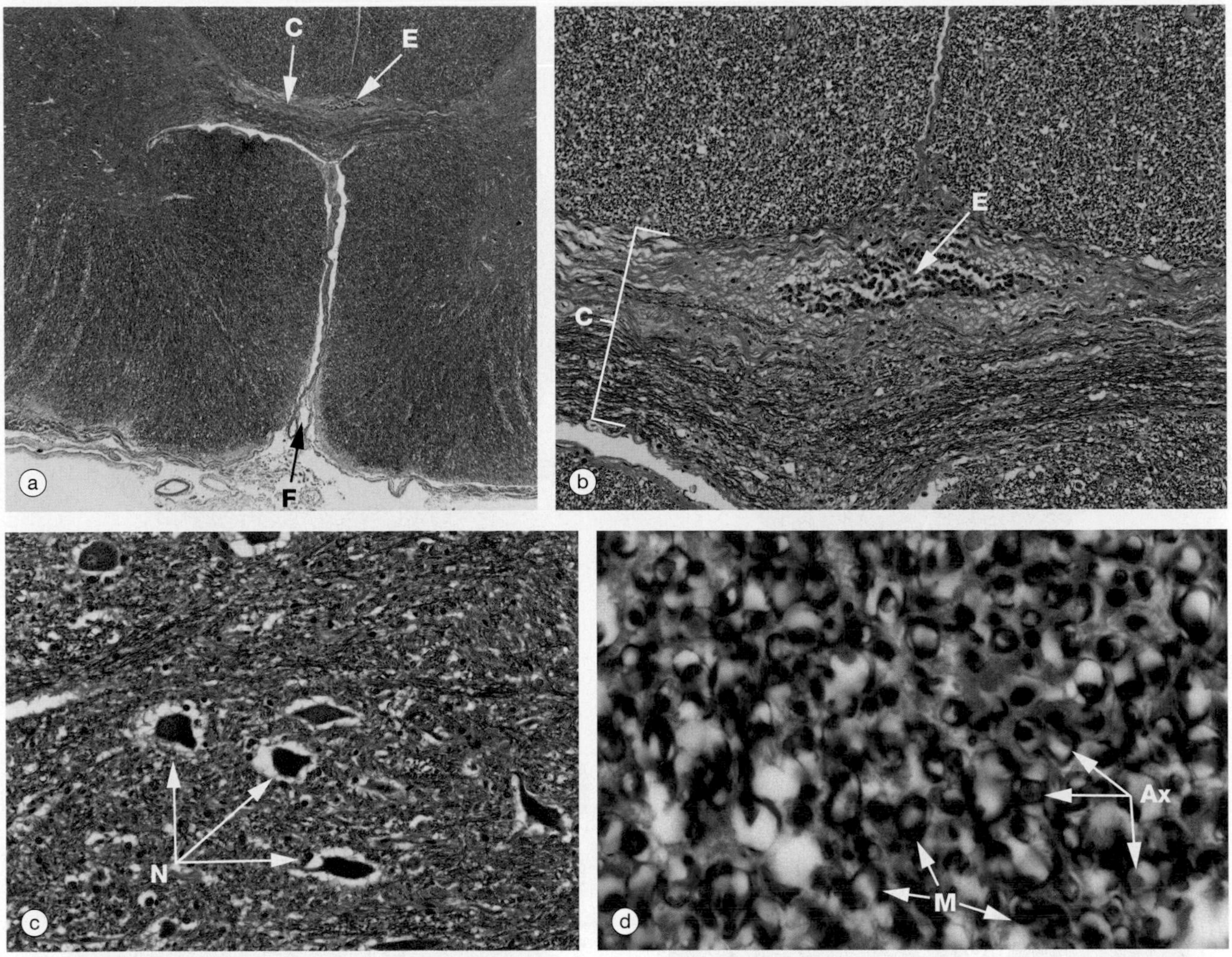

FIG. 20.11 Spinal cord and central canal
Luxol fast blue, H&E (a) Ventral spinal cord (MP) (b) Commissure and spinal canal (HP) (c) Grey matter anterior horn (HP) (d) White matter (HP)

Luxol fast blue stains the myelinated sheaths of nerve fibres a dark blue while the H&E stain colours the cytoplasm of cells and their processes red. Fig. 20.11a illustrates the ***ventral median fissure*** **F** and the anterior spinal vessels which are the cord's main blood supply. Both Figs 20.11a and b illustrate the ***central commissure*** **C** where both grey matter (pink-staining cells and their processes) and blue-staining myelinated nerve fibres cross the midline. The ***spinal canal*** **E** with its ependymal cell lining is identified in both images but can only be seen clearly in Fig. 20.11b. Fig. 20.11c illustrates part of the grey matter, the anterior horn with large neurones with their purple-staining cytoplasmic Nissl substance. Parts of their dendritic processes or axons are visible as a result of shrinkage artefact. These cells are the ***alpha motor neurones*** **N** (lower motor neurones) responsible for voluntary skeletal muscle control and thus voluntary movement. They are situated in a background of small cells, cell processes and nerve fibres.

Fig. 20.11d is a high-power view of the cord white matter, formed of massed nerve fibres with ***axons*** **Ax** and their surrounding ***myelin sheaths*** **M**. Large numbers of small myelinated axons and unmyelinated axons are also present but are not visible at this power and in this kind of section.

Poliomyelitis

Polio viruses, in some infected patients, cause destruction of the alpha motor neurones in the anterior horn of the spinal cord, resulting in permanent paralysis. This is a flaccid paralysis also known as ***lower motor neurone (LMN) paralysis***, where the muscles innervated by the neurones become weak or paralysed, lose tone, cease to resist forced movements and become floppy.

Without their neural stimulation, these muscles then permanently atrophy. Immunisation against poliomyelitis has taken this virus group to the edge of extinction (native type 2 polio has not existed outside laboratories for years). However, other viruses do rarely produce spinal cord inflammation and paralysis.

Ax axon **C** central commissure **D** dorsal horn **DC** dorsal columns **E** ependyma/spinal canal **F** median fissure **FC** fasciculus cuneatus **FG** fasciculus gracilis **L** lateral horn **M** myelin **N** neurone cell body **NR** nerve root **R** dorsal nerve root **S** dorsolateral sulcus **V** ventral horn **VS** ventrolateral sulcus

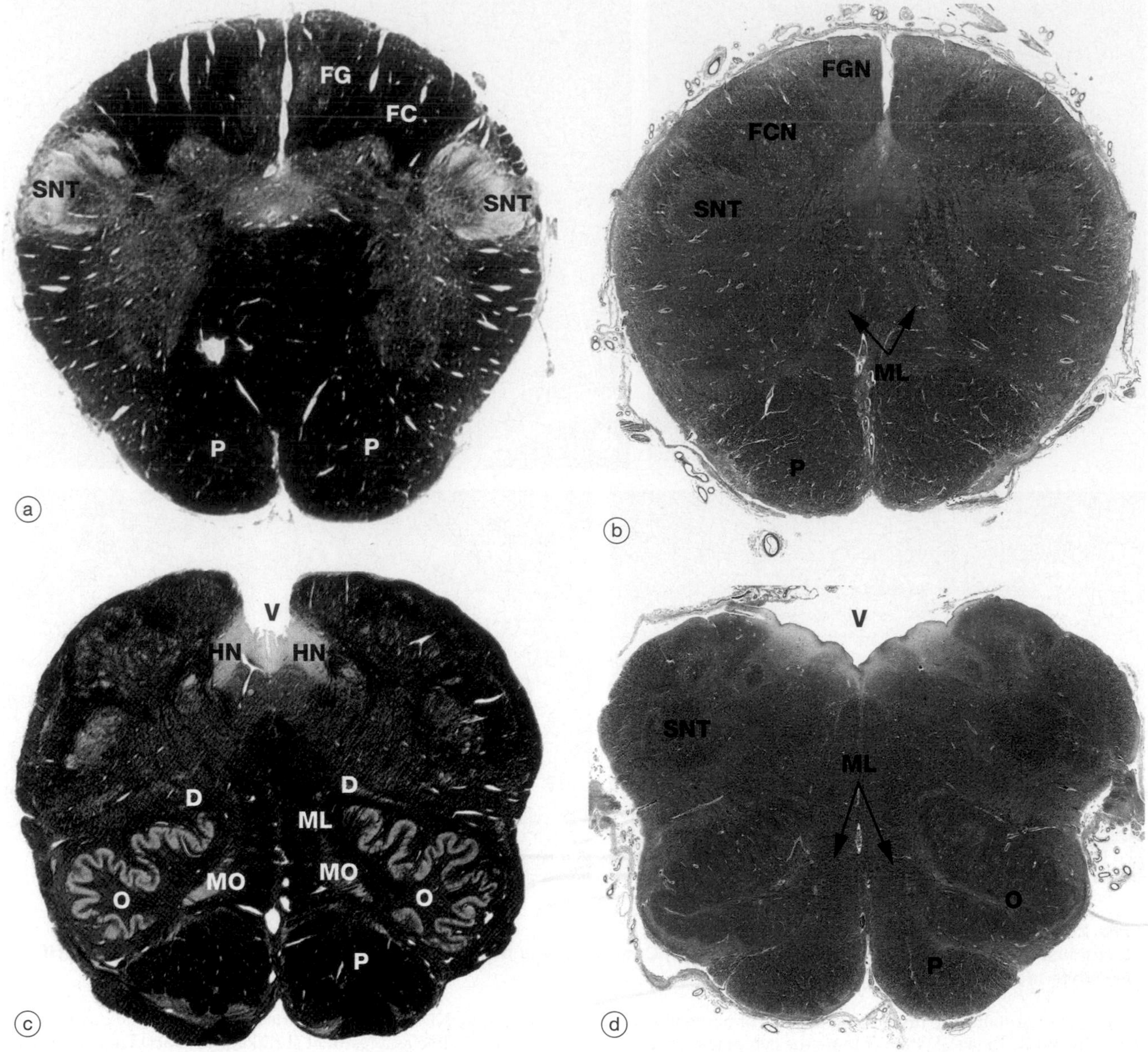

FIG. 20.12 Medulla oblongata
(a) Weigart-Pal (LP) (b) H&E (LP) (c) Weigart-Pal (LP) (d) H&E (LP); (b) and (d) are digitally enhanced photomontages

The medulla oblongata is the most caudal part of the brainstem and connects to spinal cord. Figs 20.12a to 20.12d are in order from ***caudal*** (towards tail) to ***rostral*** (towards head). The Weigart-Pal used in Figs 20.12a and c is a myelin stain which leaves the grey matter relatively unstained.

The prominent ventral ***pyramids*** **P** on each side of the medulla are the corticospinal tracts which transmit voluntary motor signals from the motor cortex to alpha motor neurones in the anterior horns of the spinal cord. About 85% of fibres cross to the opposite side in the ***decussation of the pyramids*** located in the medulla (remember, the left brain cortex supplies the right side of the body).

All of the ascending (sensory) pathways in the spinal cord pass through the medulla, although their arrangement differs from the spinal cord. The easiest traced are the dorsal white matter columns of the spinal cord which convey ascending proprioceptive, vibration and discriminatory touch fibres. These axons relay with neurones in the similarly situated ***gracile*** **FGN** and ***cuneate*** **FCN** nuclei located in the dorsum of medulla, Fig. 20.12b, at the rostral end of the ***gracile*** **FG** and ***cuneate*** **FC** ***fasciculi*** of the dorsal columns, seen in Fig. 20.12a. The axonal fibres of the tract (after the relay) then pass upwards to the thalamus via the ***medial lemniscus*** **ML** which lies medially (see Fig. 20.12d).

The medulla contains numerous other ascending and descending tracts and also includes various tracts and nuclei of the eighth to the twelfth cranial nerves. The medulla also contains a spinal nucleus which is part of the trigeminal nerve (cranial nerve V) and associated tract; this ***spinal nucleus of the trigeminal tract*** **SNT** is recognisable dorsolaterally throughout the medulla, with its tract of white matter lying superficially. The ***hypoglossal nucleus*** **HN** can also be identified in Fig. 20.12c.

In the most caudal medulla, Fig. 20.12a, grey matter can be seen still roughly resembling the butterfly shape seen in sections of the spinal cord. The ventral grey matter horns contain cell bodies of lower motor neurones running in the spinal accessory and first cervical nerves.

A prominent feature of the upper medulla is the ***inferior olivary nucleus*** **O**, named for a gross anatomical resemblance to an olive. It has a convoluted appearance in transverse section and is associated with several smaller ***accessory nuclei***, including the dorsal accessory olivary nucleus **D** and the medial accessory olivary nucleus **MO**. The neurones of this inferior olivary complex relay central and spinal afferent stimuli to the cerebellar cortex. Dorsally, the spinal canal opens into the ***fourth ventricle*** **V**.

Dorsal

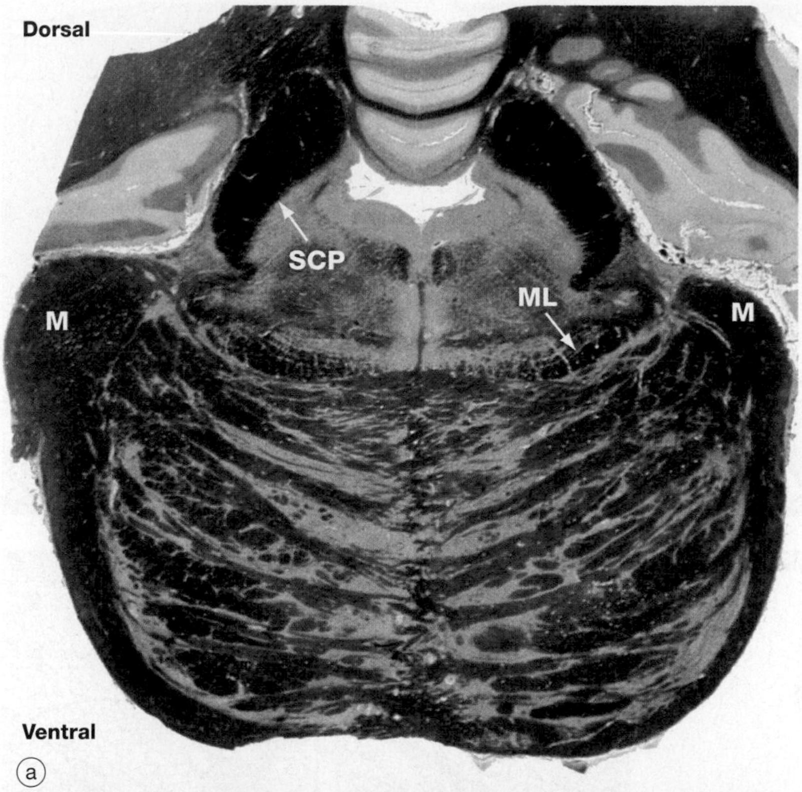

Ventral

(a)

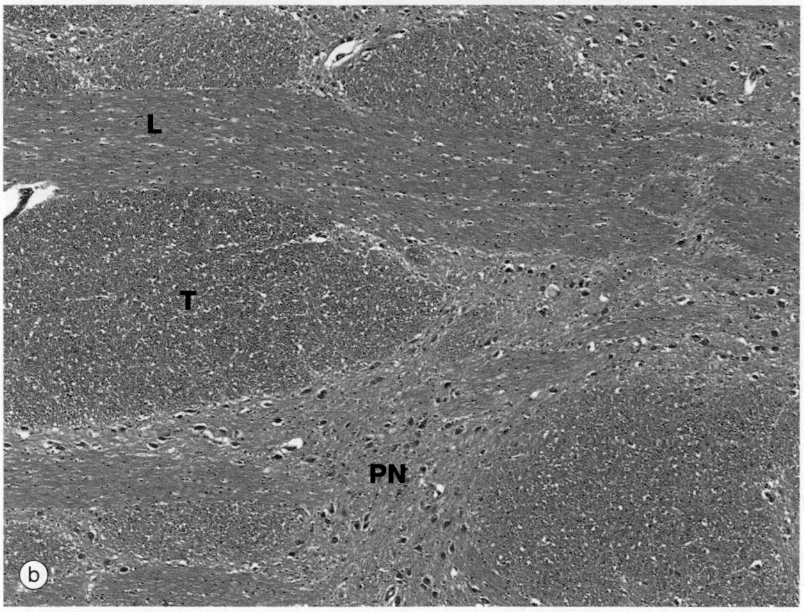

FIG. 20.13 Pons
(a) Mid-pons, Weigart-Pal (LP)
(b) Basal pons, H&E (MP)

The pons is the middle portion of the brainstem, lying between the midbrain rostrally and medulla caudally. In transverse section, it comprises two parts, a bulky ventral region (***basal pons***) and a smaller dorsal (***tegmental***) region. The basal pons consists of crisscrossed bundles of longitudinal and transverse fibres between which lie collections of neurone cell bodies known as ***pontine nuclei***.

The longitudinal fibres of the basal pons consist of descending fibres of two main types. There are axons of the corticospinal tract which transmit voluntary motor signals from the motor cortex to the alpha motor neurones of the ventral horns of the spinal cord. On traversing the pons, these axons converge to form the pyramids of the medulla.

A second group of descending fibres originate in various areas of the cortex and synapse in the pontine nuclei, from which fibres then pass in the transverse bundles, crossing the midline to enter the cerebellum via the ***middle peduncles*** **M**.

The dorsal tegmentum contains the ascending spinothalamic (sensory) tracts and the nuclei of the fifth, sixth and seventh cranial nerves. On each side, the ***medial lemniscus*** **ML** is readily identifiable; this represents the upward continuation of proprioceptive, vibration and fine touch pathways of the spinal dorsal columns, relayed via the gracile and cuneate nuclei of the medulla.

The ***cerebellum*** is located on the dorsum of the brainstem at the pons and is connected via the ***cerebellar peduncles***, which are subdivided into superior, middle, and inferior peduncles reflecting the three main fibre tracts. Part of the ***middle peduncle*** **M** is present in sections through the mid-pontine level, as in Fig. 20.13a, while the ***superior cerebellar peduncles*** **SCP** are very prominent. The main bulk of the superior cerebellar peduncles is made up of fibres from the central nuclei of the cerebellum passing upwards to the thalamus and then to the motor cortex.

Fig. 20.13b is a higher-power view of the basal pons and shows in transverse section **T** the rostral–caudal fibre bundles, including the cortical spinal motor tracts. In longitudinal section **L** are fibres crossing between the cerebellar hemispheres. There is also the interspersed grey matter with its neurones representing the pontine motor nuclei **PN**.

Raised intracranial pressure

The skull is a rigid box containing blood, brain and CSF with a constant volume as stated in the Monro–Kellie hypothesis. The volume of all components of the brain is constant such that an increase in contents (e.g. haemorrhage or tumour) must be compensated by a reduction in one of the other components in the skull (usually blood or CSF). This compensatory mechanism is protective to a point, maintaining intracranial pressure (ICP) within normal ranges; after which the equilibrium is overwhelmed and ICP rises to dangerous levels. A large increase in ICP can cause brain 'shift' of large compartments of the brain and intracranial herniation of important structures, which can be fatal.

D dorsal accessory olivary nucleus **FC** fasciculus cuneatus **FCN** nucleus of fasciculus cuneatus **FG** fasciculus gracilis **FGN** nucleus of fasciculus gracilis **HN** hypoglossal nucleus **L** longitudinal fibre bundles **M** middle cerebellar peduncle **ML** medial lemniscus **MO** medial accessory olivary nucleus **O** inferior olivary nucleus **P** pyramid **PN** pontine nuclei **SCP** superior cerebellar peduncle **SNT** spinal nucleus and tract of trigeminal nerve **T** transverse fibre bundles **V** fourth ventricle

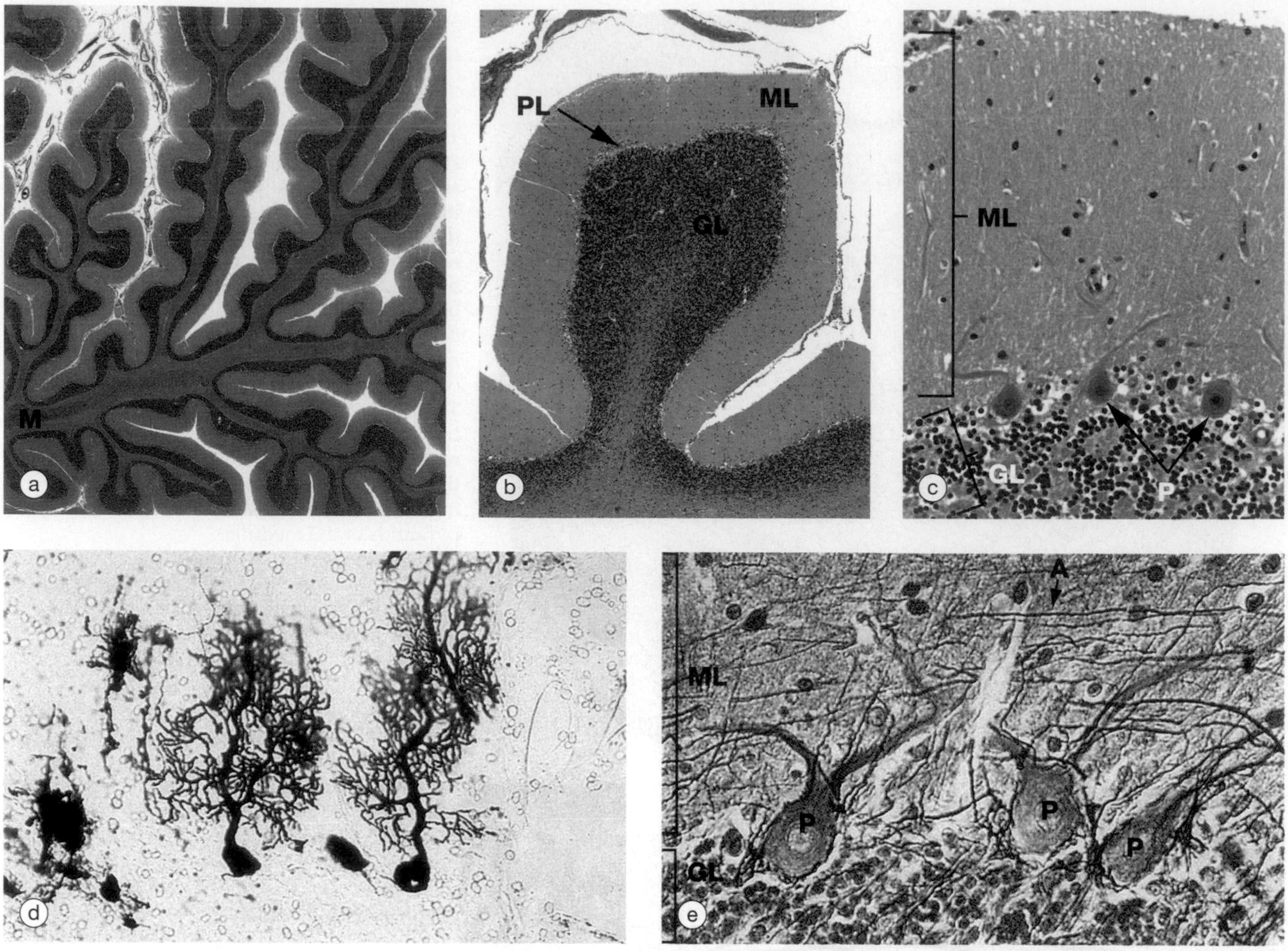

FIG. 20.14 Cerebellum
(a) H&E (LP) photomontage (b) H&E (LP) (c) H&E (MP) (d) Golgi–Cox (MP) (e) Bielschowsky/neutral red (HP)

The cerebellum coordinates muscular activity and maintains posture and equilibrium. It consists of a cortex of grey matter with a central core of white matter containing four pairs of nuclei. Afferent and efferent fibres pass to and from the brainstem via inferior, middle and superior cerebellar peduncles, linking medulla, pons and midbrain, respectively.

As seen in Fig. 20.14a, the cerebellar cortex forms a series of deeply convoluted folds or folia supported by a branching ***central white matter*** **M** (sometimes called the medulla of the cerebellum, but not to be confused with the nearby medulla oblongata). At higher magnification in Fig. 20.14b, the cortex is seen to consist of three layers. The outer ***molecular layer*** **ML** contains relatively few neurones and large numbers of unmyelinated fibres. The inner ***granular cell layer*** **GL** is extremely cellular. Between the two is a single layer of huge neurones called ***Purkinje cells*** **PL**. Purkinje cells **P** are seen at higher magnification in Fig. 20.14c; they have very large cell bodies, a relatively fine axon extending down through the granular cell layer **GL** and an extensively branching dendritic system which arborises in the molecular layer **ML**. The extraordinary dendritic system of Purkinje cells is best demonstrated by heavy metal methods as in Fig. 20.14d.

The deep granular cell layer of the cortex contains numerous small neurones, the non-myelinated axons of which pass outwards to the molecular layer where they bifurcate to run parallel to the surface to synapse with the dendrites of Purkinje cells. Fig. 20.14e demonstrates these granular cell axons in the molecular layer. The axons **A** are stained black with silver and their cell bodies in the granular cell layer **GL** are counter-stained with neutral red. In addition to the Purkinje **P** and granular cells already described, there are three other types of small neurones in the cerebellar cortex: ***stellate cells*** and ***basket cells*** scattered in the molecular layer **ML** and ***Golgi cells*** scattered in the superficial part of the granular cell layer. Note black-stained fibrils of basket cell axons surrounding the Purkinje cell bodies **P** in Fig. 20.14e.

Afferent fibres enter the cerebellum from the brainstem and then pass via the central white matter to make complex connections with granular cells; these, in turn, connect with Purkinje dendrites via basket cells and other neurones of the cerebellar cortex. The efferent fibres from the cerebellar cortex are the Purkinje cell axons which traverse the granular cell layer to synapse in the central nuclei of the cerebellum.

Cerebellar ataxia

Diseases that damage the cerebellar cortex lead to the development of cerebellar ataxia, in which there is poor coordination of voluntary movement and loss of balance.

Causes include tumours, trauma, familial neurodegenerative disease, alcohol and hypoxic damage.

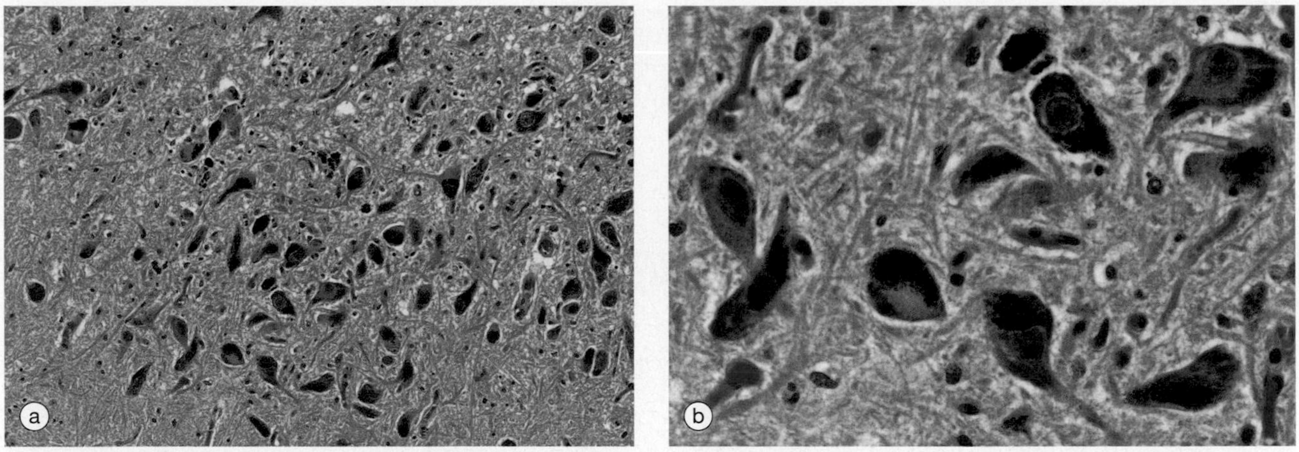

FIG. 20.15 Substantia nigra
(a) H&E (LP) (b) H&E (HP)

The ***substantia nigra*** is a large mass of grey matter extending throughout the midbrain; on each side it divides the cerebral peduncles into dorsal and ventral parts and, in sections of the midbrain as in Fig. 20.15a, it is easily recognised by neurones containing dark pigment from which its name derives. The substantia nigra has extensive connections with the cortex, spinal cord, corpus striatum and reticular formation and appears to play an important part in the fine control of motor function.

The neurones of the substantia nigra are multipolar in form, and, in adults, the cytoplasm contains numerous granules of ***neuromelanin pigment*** as seen in Fig. 20.15b. The pigmented neurones of the substantia nigra contain dopamine, which appears to act as a neurotransmitter causing inhibitory effects, particularly on neurones in the corpus striatum (one of the basal ganglia of the diencephalon).

Neuromelanin is contained in membrane-bound granules. Very little neuromelanin is present at birth, with the amount increasing during childhood and thereafter rising with increasing age. The origin of neuromelanin is still debated, with proposals that it is enzymatically generated or is merely an oxidation byproduct of dopamine synthesis. Functionally, it may sequester metals such as iron, as well as toxic organic compounds.

Parkinson's disease

Parkinson's disease (see e-Fig. 20.3) is a common neurodegenerative disease, usually seen in later life. It is clinically characterised by tremor, muscular rigidity and slowness of movement. Neuropathology shows degeneration and death of neurones in the substantia nigra. This leads to a marked reduction in dopamine levels in the brain that in turn leads to the movement disorder.

Macroscopic examination of the brain of a patient who has died with Parkinson's disease shows abnormal pallor of the substantia nigra, correlating with loss of the pigmented (neuromelanin)-containing nigral neurones. Histologically these neurones contain Lewy body inclusions made up of alpha-synuclein protein.

Symptoms can be alleviated by the drug L-dopa, a dopamine precursor.

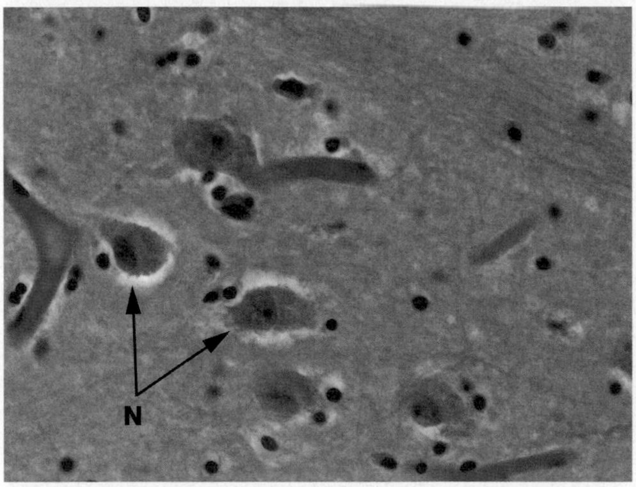

FIG. 20.16 Thalamus
H&E (HP)

The ***thalami*** are large masses of grey matter lying on each side of the third ventricle and comprising the main bulk of the ***diencephalon***, the central core of the cerebrum. Other large basal ganglia include the ***corpus striatum*** and ***caudate nucleus***. Functionally, the thalamus is subdivided into a large number of nuclei, including reticular and motor nuclei as well as specific sensory nuclei containing the cell bodies of neurones with axons projecting to the cerebral cortex. The thalamus constitutes an extremely complex relay and integration centre for information from almost all parts of the CNS. Fig. 20.16 shows the histological appearance of a typical basal nucleus, consisting of a loose aggregation of neurone cell bodies **N** in a background of neuropil. As an age-related change, these neurones have accumulated light brown ***lipofuscin pigment*** consisting of indigestible lipid byproducts.

A axon **GL** granular cell layer **M** medulla (central white matter) of cerebellum **ML** molecular layer **N** neurone cell bodies **P** Purkinje cell **PL** Purkinje cell layer

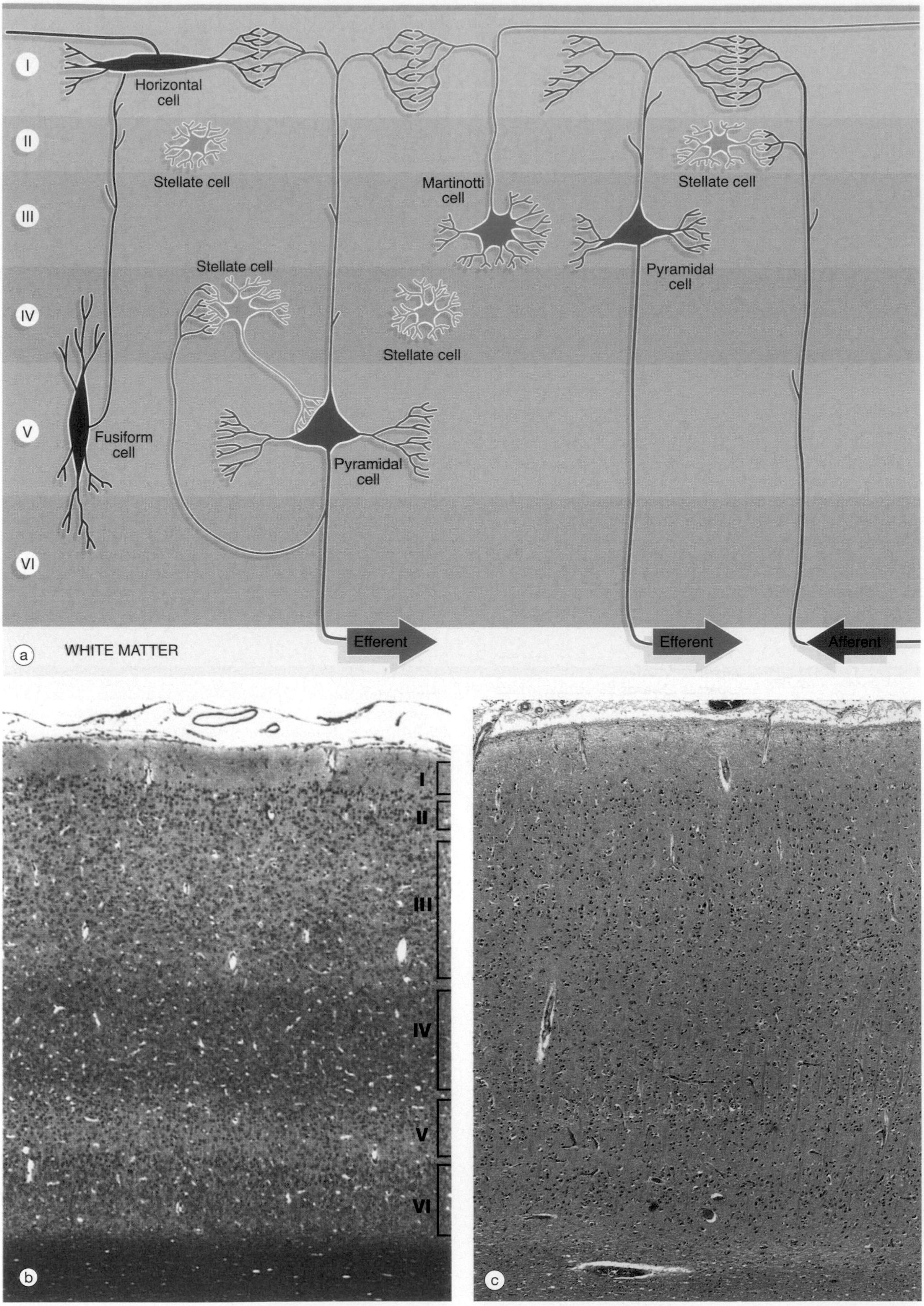

FIG. 20.17 Cerebral cortex *(caption opposite)*
(a) Neuronc cell types diagram (b) Methylene blue (MP) (c) H&E (MP)

FIG. 20.17 Cerebral cortex *(illustrations opposite)*
(a) Neurone cell types diagram (b) Methylene blue (MP) (c) H&E (MP)

The cerebral hemispheres consist of a folded cortex of grey matter overlying white matter which conveys fibres between different parts of the cortex and to and from other parts of the CNS.

Histologically, the neurones of the cerebral cortex can be divided into five different morphological types which are arranged in several layers. The biologically oldest part of the cortex is concerned with ***olfaction*** (smell) and the neurones are arranged into three layers. In mammals, most of the cortex is called ***neocortex*** and consists of six layers. In humans, this constitutes about 90%; the three-layered pattern persists only in the olfactory cortex and in the cortical part of the limbic system in the temporal lobe.

The synaptic interconnections within the cortex are complex, with any one neurone synapsing with several hundred others. However, there are several basic principles of cortical organisation and function:

- Functional units are disposed vertically, corresponding to the general orientation of axons and major dendrites.
- ***Afferent fibres*** (incoming axons) generally synapse high in the cortex with the dendrites of ***efferent neurones*** whose cell bodies sit in deeper layers of the cortex.
- Efferent (outgoing) pathways, typically axons from pyramidal cells, tend to give off branches which pass back into more superficial layers and communicate with their own dendrites via interneuronal connections with other cell types.

The five characteristic types of cortical neurone are shown diagrammatically in Fig. 20.17a, the pyramidal and stellate cells being by far the most common types:

- ***Pyramidal cells*** have pyramid-shaped cell bodies with the apex directed towards the cortical surface. From the apex, a thick branching dendrite passes towards the surface where it has an array of fine dendritic branches. An axon arises from the base of the cell and passes into the white matter though, in the case of small superficial cells, the axon may synapse in the deep layers of the cortex. Short dendrites also arise from the edges of the base and ramify laterally. The size of pyramidal cells varies, with the smallest tending to sit superficially. The huge upper motor neurones of the motor cortex, known as ***Betz cells***, are the largest pyramidal cells in the cortex.
- ***Stellate (granule) cells*** are small neurones with a short vertical axon and several short branching dendrites, giving the cell body the shape of a star, although other shapes have been described. With routine histological methods, the cells look like small granules, giving rise to their alternative name.
- ***Cells of Martinotti*** are small polygonal cells with a few short dendrites; the axon extends towards the surface and bifurcates to run horizontally, usually in the most superficial layer.
- ***Fusiform cells*** are spindle-shaped cells oriented at right angles to the surface of the cerebral cortex. The axon arises from the side of the cell body and passes superficially. Dendrites extend from each end of the cell body, branching into deeper and more superficial layers.
- ***Horizontal cells of Cajal*** are small and spindle-shaped but oriented parallel to the surface. They are the least common cell type and are only found in the most superficial layer, where their axons pass laterally to synapse with the dendrites of pyramidal cells.

In addition to neurones, the cortex contains supporting neuroglial cells (***astrocytes***), ***oligodendroglia*** and ***microglia***.

The neocortex is arranged into six layers, with the layers differing in neurone morphology, size and population density. They merge with one another, rather than being sharply demarcated. They also vary in thickness and detail from one region of the brain to another. Fig. 20.17b and c illustrate the typical layered appearance of the cerebral cortex and its layers:

I. **Plexiform (molecular) layer**. The superficial layer contains dendrites and axons of cortical neurones making synapses with one another; nuclei are sparse and are those of neuroglia and horizontal cells of Cajal.
II. **Outer granular layer**. This contains a dense population of small pyramidal cells and stellate cells, admixed with various axons and dendritic connections from deeper layers.
III. **Pyramidal cell layer**. Pyramidal cells of moderate size predominate in this broad layer, the cells increasing in size deeper in the layer. Martinotti cells are also present.
IV. **Inner granular layer**. This layer consists mainly of densely packed stellate cells.
V. **Ganglionic layer**. Large pyramidal cells and smaller numbers of stellate cells and cells of Martinotti make up this layer, its name originating from the huge pyramidal (ganglion) Betz cells of the motor cortex.
VI. **Multiform cell layer**. This is named for the wide variety of differing morphological forms found in this layer. It contains numerous small pyramidal cells and cells of Martinotti as well as stellate cells, especially superficially, and fusiform cells in the deeper part.

Dementia

Medical conditions with progressive generalised deterioration in brain function, especially higher cortical functions, are called ***dementia***. These are characterised by progressive degeneration of neurones, hence the term ***neurodegenerative disease***. There are many different forms of dementia with varying genetic components, some of which are described below:

- Alzheimer's disease (AD) is the commonest form of dementia, particularly in the older population. Patients present with progressive memory and cognitive impairment. The disease is characterised histologically by accumulations of the abnormal protein amyloid which form plaques in the cerebral cortex and Tau neurofibrillary tangles (see e-Fig. 20.4).
- Dementia with Lewy bodies (see e-Fig. 20.5) is similar to AD though patients also show fluctuating cognition and parkinsonism. Lewy bodies are seen histologically, similar to Parkinson's disease though in a different distribution.
- Vascular dementia is associated with underlying intracerebral vascular disease and classically presents with stepwise deterioration in cognitive function.
- Creutzfeldt–Jacob disease (CJD) (see e-Fig. 20.6) causes rapid onset of dementia often over weeks or months. In the variant form, an infective agent known as a prion protein has been identified as a causative agent.

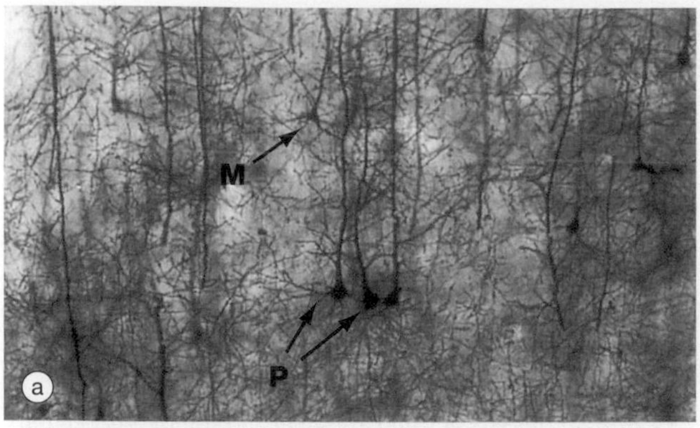

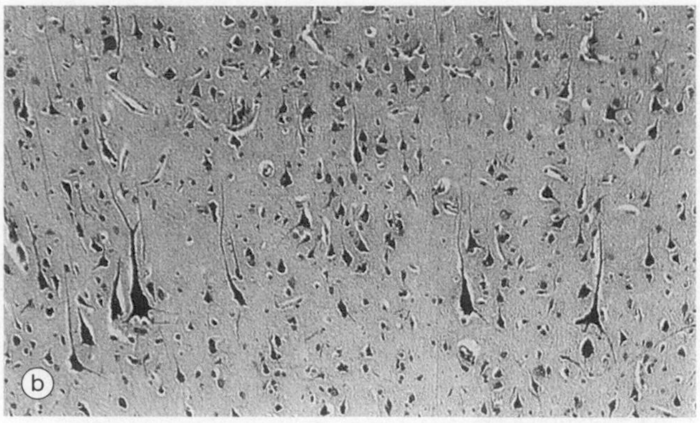

FIG. 20.18 Cortex
(a) Golgi method (MP) (b) Nissl method (MP)

Fig. 20.18a shows a part of layer V; a thick section is employed, stained with a heavy metal impregnation technique which demonstrates considerable morphological detail. Several pyramidal cells **P** are easily identifiable, with their principal dendrites rising towards the cortical surface. Their axons are not seen as they are not in the plane of the section. A cell of Martinotti **M** is identified by its polygonal shape.

Fig. 20.18b also shows layer V but, in this case, the section is thinner and stained by a routine histological method. At this magnification, there is little morphological detail; nevertheless, most of the cells are identifiable as pyramidal cells, increasing in size in the deeper part and including several very large cells.

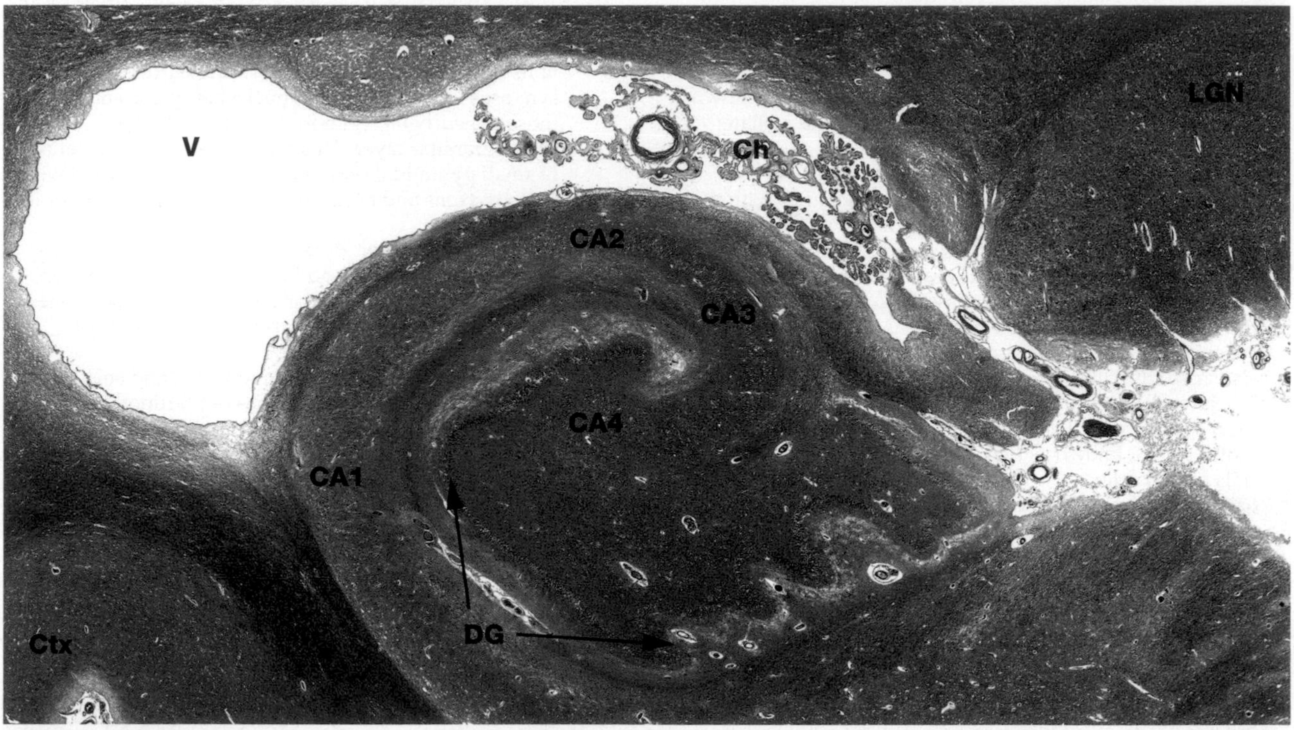

FIG. 20.19 Ammon's horn
Luxol fast blue, H&E (LP)

Ammon's horn, more formally the ***cornus ammonis*** **CA**, is a recognisable structure in the hippocampus in the inferomedial part of the temporal lobe. Ammon's horn is named in reference to the coiled horns of sheep (Fig. 20.19). Its main neurone layer has been traditionally divided into four areas **CA1–CA4**. The irregular folded segment is the end of the ***dentate gyrus*** **DG**, also part of the ***hippocampus***. Above is the anterior part of the temporal horn of the ***lateral ventricle*** **V**, with CSF-producing ***choroid plexus*** **Ch**. Part of the cortex **Ctx** is visible in the lower left of the image. The ***lateral geniculate nucleus*** **LGN** is a relay for visual information from the retina to the visual cortex in the occipital lobe. It has a layered architecture. The hippocampus is an important brain structure involved in long-term memory.

Epilepsy and Ammon's horn

CA1 is particularly susceptible to hypoxia/ischaemia with subsequent loss of neurones and scarring (gliosis), while CA2 is very resistant. This 'hippocampal sclerosis' is a recognised pathological finding in patients with temporal lobe epilepsy. Typically there is segmental sclerosis of segment CA1 and CA4 with gliosis.

CA1-CA4 numbered zones of the cornus ammonis **Ch** choroid plexus **Ctx** cortex **DG** dentate gyrus **LGN** lateral geniculate nucleus **M** cell of Martinotti **P** pyramidal cell **V** lateral ventricle

REVIEW

TABLE 20.1 Review of the central nervous system

Main structures	Sub-structures	Detail and function	Figure
Dura mater		Dense fibrous outer layer of central nervous system (CNS); merges with periosteum of skull	20.8
Leptomeninges	Pia–arachnoid	Outer brain covering; lined by arachnoidal cells; contains cerebrospinal fluid (CSF)	20.9
Choroid plexus		Specialised ventricular structure; produces CSF	20.6
Ependyma		Epithelial-like cells with cilia which line ventricles and spinal canal	20.7
Spinal cord	White matter columns	Numerous nerve fibres, afferent and efferent	20.10
	Anterior horns	Grey matter containing alpha motor neurones	20.11
	Spinal canal	Small; lined by ependymal cells; extends from fourth ventricle	20.10, 20.11
	Commissure	Cross-over of nerve fibres in cord near spinal canal	20.10
Brainstem	Medulla	Afferent and efferent nerve fibres; relays some signals in nuclei but also processes some (olives) and contains cranial nerve nuclei	20.12
	Pons	Afferent and efferent nerve fibres with extensive fibres to cerebellum; pontine nuclei	20.13
Cerebellum		Highly branched folia; three cell layers (molecular, Purkinje and granular); involved in balance and fine motor skills	20.14
Upper brainstem	Substantia nigra	Neuromelanin containing neurones	20.15
Diencephalon	Thalamus and other basal ganglia	Numerous multifunction relay and processing grey matter nuclei	20.16
Cortex	Neocortex	Sensory and motor functions, visual cortex, auditory cortex, language, thought and other higher mental functions	20.17
	Grey matter	Contains neuronal cell bodies along with other microglial cells and neuropil	20.1
	White matter	Nerve fibres (axons) with supporting astrocytes, microglial cells and vessels	20.3
	Ammon's horn	Structure in hippocampus related to long-term memory	20.19

21 Special sense organs

INTRODUCTION

The organs of special sense are sophisticated sensory structures in which the specific neural receptors are incorporated in a non-neural structure which enhances and refines the reception of incoming stimuli. The *eye* and the ***audiovestibular apparatus*** of the ear are the main special sense organs, but the ***gustatory*** (taste) and ***olfactory*** (smell) receptors are usually also included in this category.

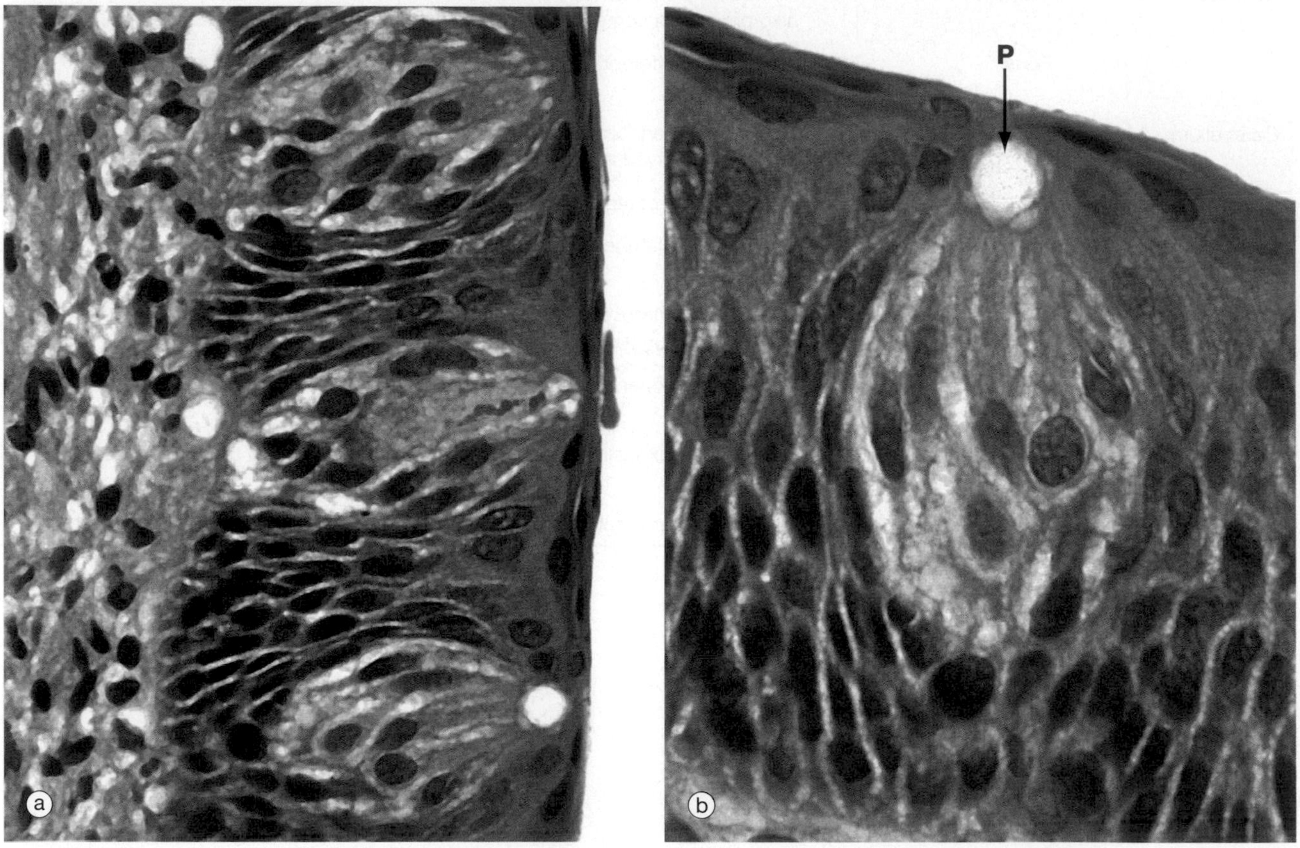

FIG. 21.1 Taste buds
(a) H&E (MP) (b) H&E (HP)

Taste buds, the chemoreceptors for the sense of taste (***gustation***), are in humans mainly located in the epithelium of the ***circumvallate papillae*** of the tongue (see Fig. 13.12), although they are also found scattered in other parts of the tongue, palate, pharynx and epiglottis. In the circumvallate papillae, taste buds face into the deep troughs surrounding the papillae. Serous glands called the ***glands of von Ebner*** secrete a serous fluid into the troughs to act as a solvent for taste-provoking substances. The human tongue has approximately 3000 taste buds.

The taste bud (Figs 21.1a and b) is a barrel-shaped organ, occupying the full thickness of the epithelium and opening at the surface via the taste pore **P**. Each taste bud contains about 50 long, spindle-shaped cells which extend from the basement membrane to the taste pore. Classically, two types of cell are described in the taste bud: light ***gustatory cells*** and dark ***supporting*** or ***sustentacular cells***. A third cell type, the ***basal cell***, is now generally recognised and may constitute the precursor of one or both of the other cell types. Both gustatory and sustentacular cells have long microvilli extending into the taste pore, which contains a glycoprotein substance, thought to be secreted by the sustentacular cells.

Ultrastructural studies have shown that non-myelinated nerve fibres are associated with both cell types, but there appears to be a more intimate synapse-like relationship between the nerve fibres and the gustatory cells. Although the gustatory cells are thought to be the taste receptors, the sustentacular cells may also serve some receptor function. Like the oral epithelium, all the cells of the taste bud, which represent highly specialised epithelial cells, are renewed continuously, although the gustatory and sustentacular cells are replaced at different rates.

Four taste modalities are recognised: ***sweet, bitter, acid*** and ***salt***. Each modality tends to be principally perceived in a specific region of the tongue; however, no structural differences have been demonstrated between taste buds from different areas. The sensations of taste and smell are closely associated, and loss of olfactory sense is accompanied by diminished gustatory perception.

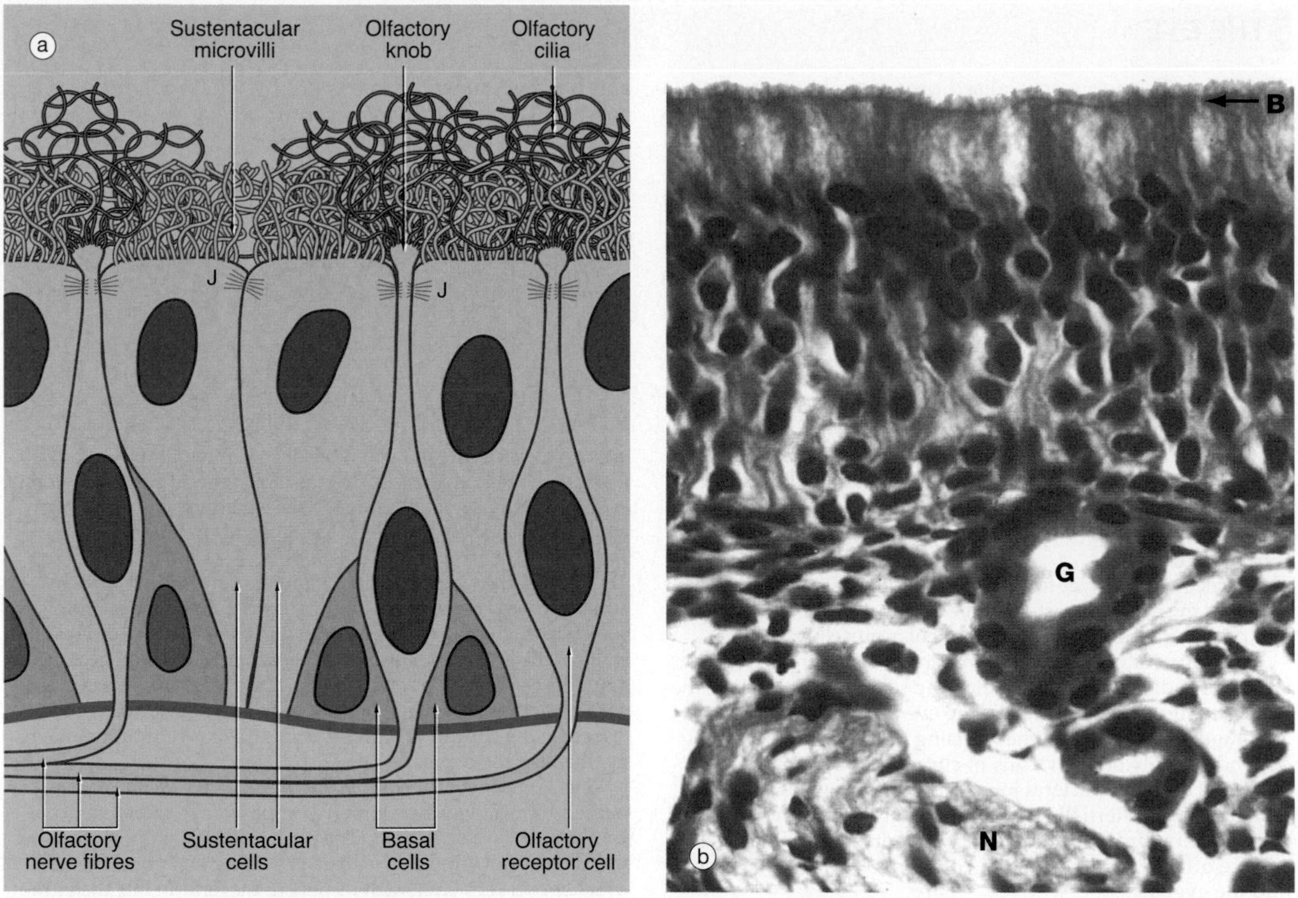

FIG. 21.2 Olfactory receptors
(a) Schematic diagram (b) H&E (HP)

The receptors for the sense of smell are located in a modified form of respiratory epithelium called ***olfactory epithelium*** in the nasal cavity; although extensive in some mammals such as the dog, the olfactory epithelium is restricted to a small area in the roof of the nasal cavity in humans. The olfactory epithelium (Fig. 21.2a) is very tall pseudostratified columnar in form and contains cells of three types: ***olfactory receptor cells, sustentacular*** (supporting epithelial) ***cells*** and ***basal epithelial cells***.

The olfactory receptor cells are true bipolar neurones (see Fig. 7.2), the cell bodies of which are located in the middle stratum of the olfactory epithelium. A single dendritic process extends from the cell body to the free surface where it terminates as a small swelling, the ***olfactory knob***, which gives rise to about a dozen extremely long modified cilia. These cilia, or olfactory hairs, contain the usual 9 plus 2 arrangement of microtubules in their proximal portion but become thinner distally where they contain variable numbers of single microtubules in different species. The cilia are non-motile and lie flattened against the epithelial surface in the surface mucous layer. The cilia are the sites of interaction between odoriferous substances and the receptor cells. At the basal aspect, each receptor cell gives rise to a single fine non-myelinated axon which penetrates the basement membrane to join the axons of other receptor cells. The bundles of axons pass via about 20 small holes on each side of the ***cribriform plate*** of the ethmoid bone to reach the olfactory bulbs of the forebrain where they synapse with second-order sensory neurones.

The supporting or sustentacular cells are elongated with their tapered bases resting on the basement membrane. Many long microvilli extend from their luminal surfaces to form a tangled mat with the cilia of the receptor cells. At the luminal surface, the plasma membranes of the sustentacular and receptor cells are bound together by typical junctional complexes **J**. The functions of the sustentacular cells are poorly understood, but they probably provide mechanical and physiological support for the receptor cells. The basal cells are small conical cells which appear to be stem cells for both olfactory and sustentacular cells.

In histological section, it is difficult to distinguish individual cell types within the olfactory epithelium; however, the nuclei of sustentacular cells occupy the uppermost stratum, those of the receptor cells the middle stratum and those of the basal cells lie close to the basement membrane. Note the terminal bar **B** at the luminal surface, representing junctional complexes; note also the fuzzy surface contour representing the tangled meshwork of microvilli and cilia on the surface.

The olfactory epithelium (Fig. 21.2b) is supported by loose vascular tissue containing bundles of afferent nerve fibres **N** and numerous serous glands called ***Bowman's glands*** **G** which produce the watery surface secretions in which odoriferous substances are dissolved.

Anosmia

Anosmia is the clinical term used to describe loss of smell. The most common cause of loss smell is post-viral anosmia. Other causes include blockage of the nasal passages by nasal polyps and, rarely, due to deficiencies in ciliary function e.g. primary ciliary dyskinesia. Recently, anosmia has been shown to be one of the earliest symptoms of COVID-19. The SARS CoV-2 virus is known to infect cells via the ACE2 receptor protein. This is expressed on the sustentacular cells of the olfactory region. Therefore, in most cases, SARS CoV-2 infection is unlikely to lead to permanent anosmia as the olfactory neurones are not affected.

B terminal bar **G** Bowman's gland **J** junctional complex **N** afferent nerve fibres **P** taste pore

THE EYE

The eye is the highly specialised organ of photoreception, a process which involves the conversion of light energy into nerve action potentials. The photoreceptors are modified dendrites of two types of nerve cells, ***rod cells*** and ***cone cells***. The rods are integrated into a system which is receptive to light of differing intensity; this is perceived in a form analogous to a black and white photographic image. The cones are of three functional types, receptive to the colours blue, green and red, and constitute a system by which coloured images are seen. The rod and cone receptors and a system of integrating neurones are located in the inner layer of the eye, the ***retina***. The remaining structures of the eye serve to support the retina or to focus images of the visual world upon the retina.

In addition, several accessory structures, namely the ***eyelids***, ***lacrimal gland*** and ***conjunctiva***, protect the eye from external damage.

FIG. 21.3 The eye *(illustration opposite)*

The eye is made up of three basic layers: the outer ***corneo-scleral layer***, the intermediate ***uveal layer*** (***uveal tract***) and the inner ***retinal layer***.

Corneo-scleral layer

The corneo-scleral layer forms a tough fibroelastic capsule which supports the eye. The posterior five-sixths, the ***sclera***, is opaque and provides insertion for the extraocular muscles.

The anterior one-sixth, the ***cornea***, is transparent and has a smaller radius of curvature than the sclera. The cornea is the principal refracting medium of the eye and roughly focuses an image onto the retina; the focusing power of the cornea depends mainly on the radius of curvature of its external surface. The corneo-scleral junction is known as the ***limbus*** and is marked internally and externally by a shallow depression. Running from the junction of the cornea and limbus, the surface of the eye is covered by ***conjunctiva*** which is reflected into the eyelids.

Uveal layer

The middle layer, the uvea or uveal tract, is a highly vascular layer which is made up of three components: the ***choroid***, the ***ciliary body*** and the ***iris***. The choroid lies between the sclera and retina in the posterior five-sixths of the eye. It provides support for the retina and is heavily pigmented, thus absorbing light which has passed through the retina. Anteriorly, the choroid merges with the ciliary body, which is a circumferential thickening of the uvea lying beneath the limbus.

The ciliary body surrounds the coronal equator of the lens and is attached to it by the ***suspensory ligament*** or ***zonule***. The lens is a biconvex transparent structure, the shape of which can be varied to provide fine focus of the corneal image upon the retina. The ciliary body contains smooth muscle, the tone of which controls the shape of the lens via the suspensory ligament. The lens, suspensory ligament and ciliary body divide the eye into a large compartment containing a thick gel called the ***vitreous body*** and a compartment part in front containing a watery fluid called the ***aqueous humor***.

The iris, the third component of the uvea, forms a diaphragm extending in front of the lens from the ciliary body, so as to incompletely divide the anterior compartment into two chambers; these are known by the terms ***anterior*** and ***posterior chamber***. The highly pigmented iris acts as an adjustable diaphragm which regulates the amount of light reaching the retina. The aperture of the iris is called the ***pupil***.

The anterior and posterior chambers contain the aqueous humor, which is secreted into the posterior chamber by the ciliary body and circulated through the pupil to drain into a canal at the angle of the anterior chamber, the ***canal of Schlemm***. The aqueous humor is a source of nutrients for the non-vascular lens and cornea and acts as an optical medium which is non-refractive with respect to the cornea. The pressure of aqueous humor maintains the shape of the cornea.

The large posterior compartment of the eye contains a specialised connective tissue largely composed of a transparent gel known as the vitreous body. The vitreous body supports the lens and retina from within, as well as providing an optical medium which is non-refractive with respect to the lens. In life, the vitreous body contains a canal which extends from the exit of the optic nerve to the posterior surface of the lens; this ***hyaloid canal*** represents the course of the hyaloid artery which supplies the vitreous body during embryological development. The vitreous body and hyaloid canal are rarely preserved in histological preparations.

Retinal layer

The photosensitive retina forms the inner lining of most of the posterior compartment of the eye and terminates along a scalloped line, the ***ora serrata***, behind the ciliary body. Anterior to the ora serrata, the retinal layer continues as a non-photosensitive epithelial layer which lines the ciliary body and the posterior surface of the iris.

The visual axis of the eye passes through a depression in the retina called the ***fovea*** which is surrounded by a yellow-pigmented zone, the ***macula lutea***. The fovea is the area of greatest visual acuity.

Afferent nerve fibres from the retina converge to form the ***optic nerve*** which leaves the eye through a part of the sclera known as the ***lamina cribrosa***. The retina overlying the lamina cribrosa, the ***optic papilla*** (***optic disc***), is devoid of photoreceptors and thus represents a blind spot.

Loss of visual acuity

Loss of visual acuity, leading to blurring of vision, is common and can have several causes.

Certain disorders of the eye cause problems with accommodation such that light is not brought into a correct focus on the retina. For example, ageing is associated with difficulty focusing on objects that are close (presbyopia), due to loss of elasticity of the lens.

In other disorders, the normal transparent structures of the eye become opaque and visual acuity is reduced. Diseases of the cornea that cause scarring lead to abnormal opacification and light scattering, reducing visual acuity. Diseases that cause abnormal opacification of the lens (cataracts) lead to loss of visual acuity and, when severe, blindness.

The retina may be the seat of several diseases which cause problems with visual acuity. The retina may become detached from the uvea (retinal detachment), leading to loss of light perception in the affected part. Any condition that causes loss of the specialised photoreceptors from the retina causes loss of visual acuity. Common conditions affecting the retina include macular degeneration, in which there is loss of specialised retinal cells, and diabetes mellitus, in which pathology affecting small blood vessels causes retinal damage and cell death.

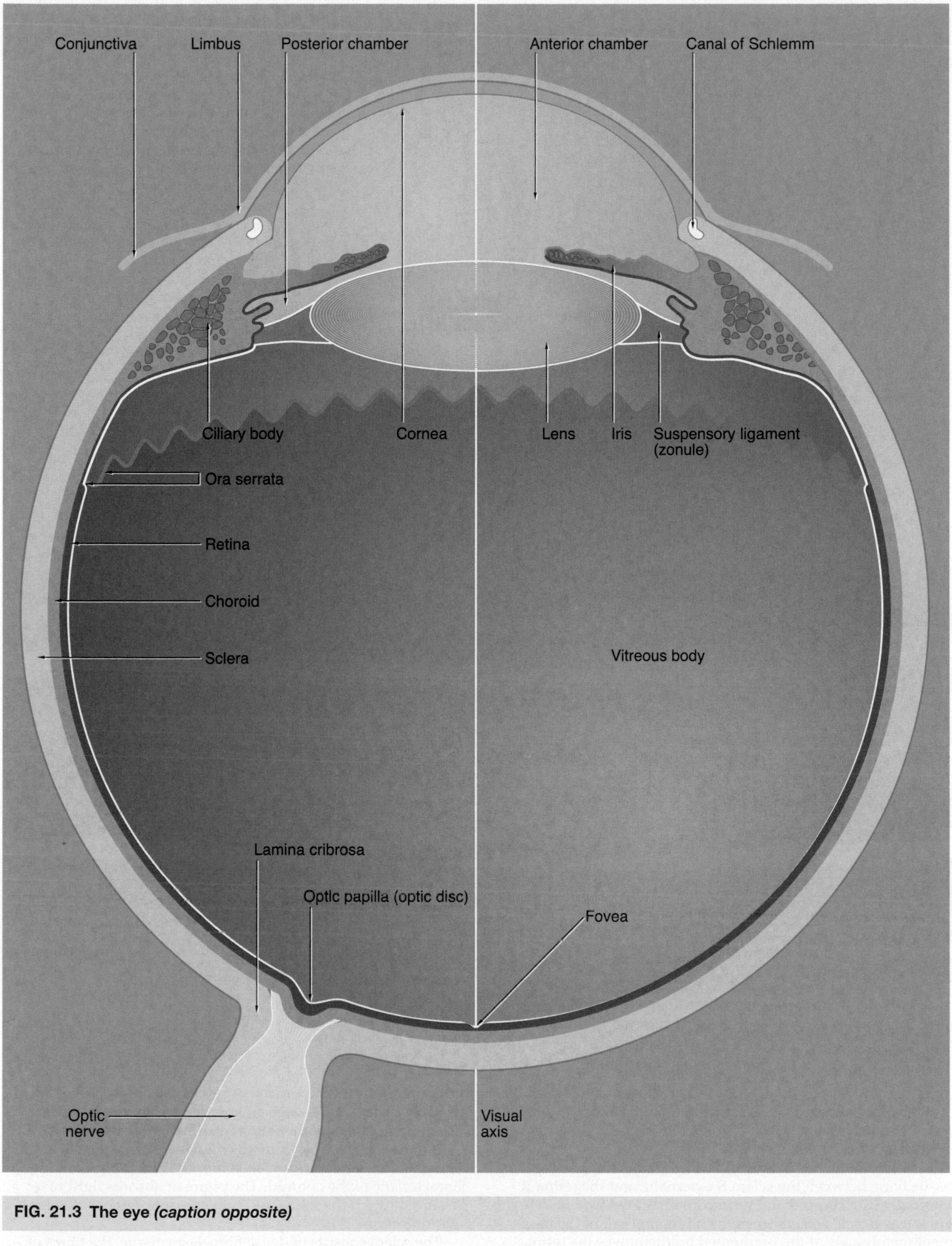

FIG. 21.3 The eye *(caption opposite)*

Inflammatory diseases of the eye

The different compartments of the eye can be the focus of specific inflammatory diseases.

- Conjunctivitis refers to inflammation of the conjunctival surface of the eye, also involving the lining of the eyelids.
- Uveitis describes inflammation of the uveal tract, including the uvea and ciliary body. Uveitis is often caused by autoimmune disease. When uveal inflammation is limited to the iris it is termed iritis.
- Inflammation of the sclera is termed scleritis.
- Certain diseases cause inflammation of the retina known as retinitis.
- Blepharitis refers to inflammation of the eyelids leading to red, itchy and painful eyelids.

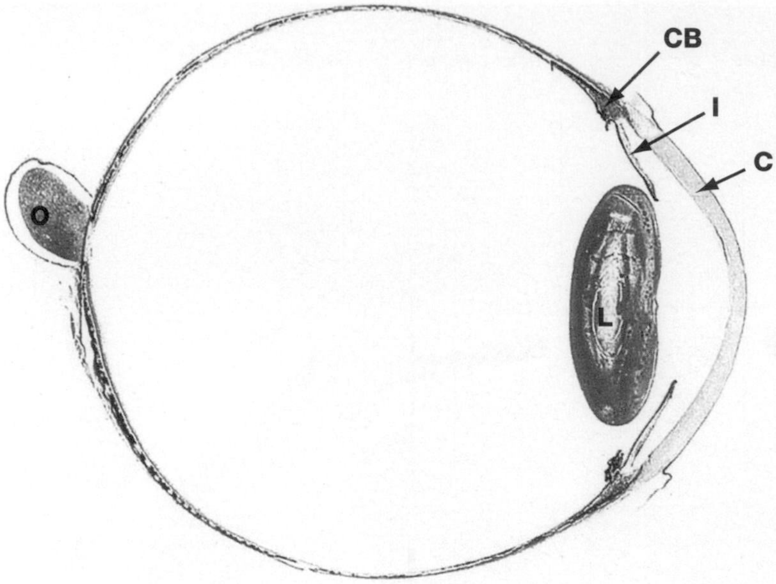

FIG. 21.4 Eye, monkey
H&E (LP)

This horizontal section (Fig. 21.4) shows the relative sizes of the components of the eye. At this magnification, the three layers making up the wall of the globe are not readily distinguishable although, in the wall of the posterior compartment, the middle layer (choroid) is recognisable by its high content of pigment.

The other uveal structures, the ciliary body **CB** and iris **I**, are readily visible. The lens **L** has been artefactually distorted during preparation, and the suspensory ligament by which it is attached to the ciliary body is not preserved. Note the relative thickness of the cornea **C**.

The optic nerve **O** is seen to penetrate the sclera medial to the visual axis; the fovea is not present in this plane of section.

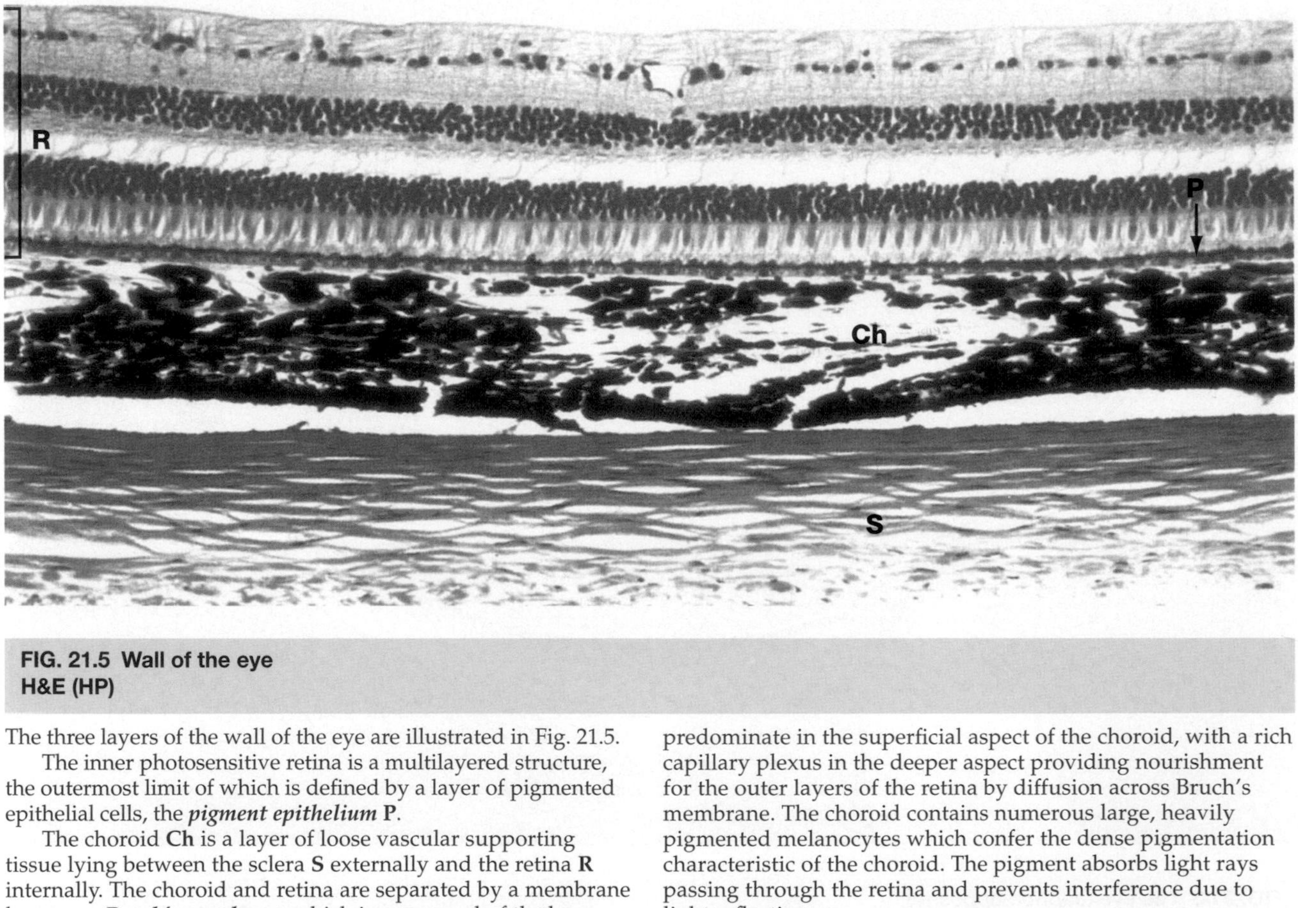

FIG. 21.5 Wall of the eye
H&E (HP)

The three layers of the wall of the eye are illustrated in Fig. 21.5.

The inner photosensitive retina is a multilayered structure, the outermost limit of which is defined by a layer of pigmented epithelial cells, the ***pigment epithelium*** **P**.

The choroid **Ch** is a layer of loose vascular supporting tissue lying between the sclera **S** externally and the retina **R** internally. The choroid and retina are separated by a membrane known as ***Bruch's membrane*** which is composed of the basement membranes of the pigmented epithelium of the retina and the endothelium of the choroid capillaries plus intervening layers of collagen and elastin fibres. The blood supply of the uveal layer of the eye is provided by branches of the ophthalmic artery, which penetrates through the sclera. Larger vessels predominate in the superficial aspect of the choroid, with a rich capillary plexus in the deeper aspect providing nourishment for the outer layers of the retina by diffusion across Bruch's membrane. The choroid contains numerous large, heavily pigmented melanocytes which confer the dense pigmentation characteristic of the choroid. The pigment absorbs light rays passing through the retina and prevents interference due to light reflection.

The sclera consists of dense fibroelastic tissue, the fibres of which are arranged in bundles parallel to the surface. This layer contains little ground substance and few fibroblasts. The sclera varies in thickness, being thickest posteriorly and thinnest at the coronal equator of the globe.

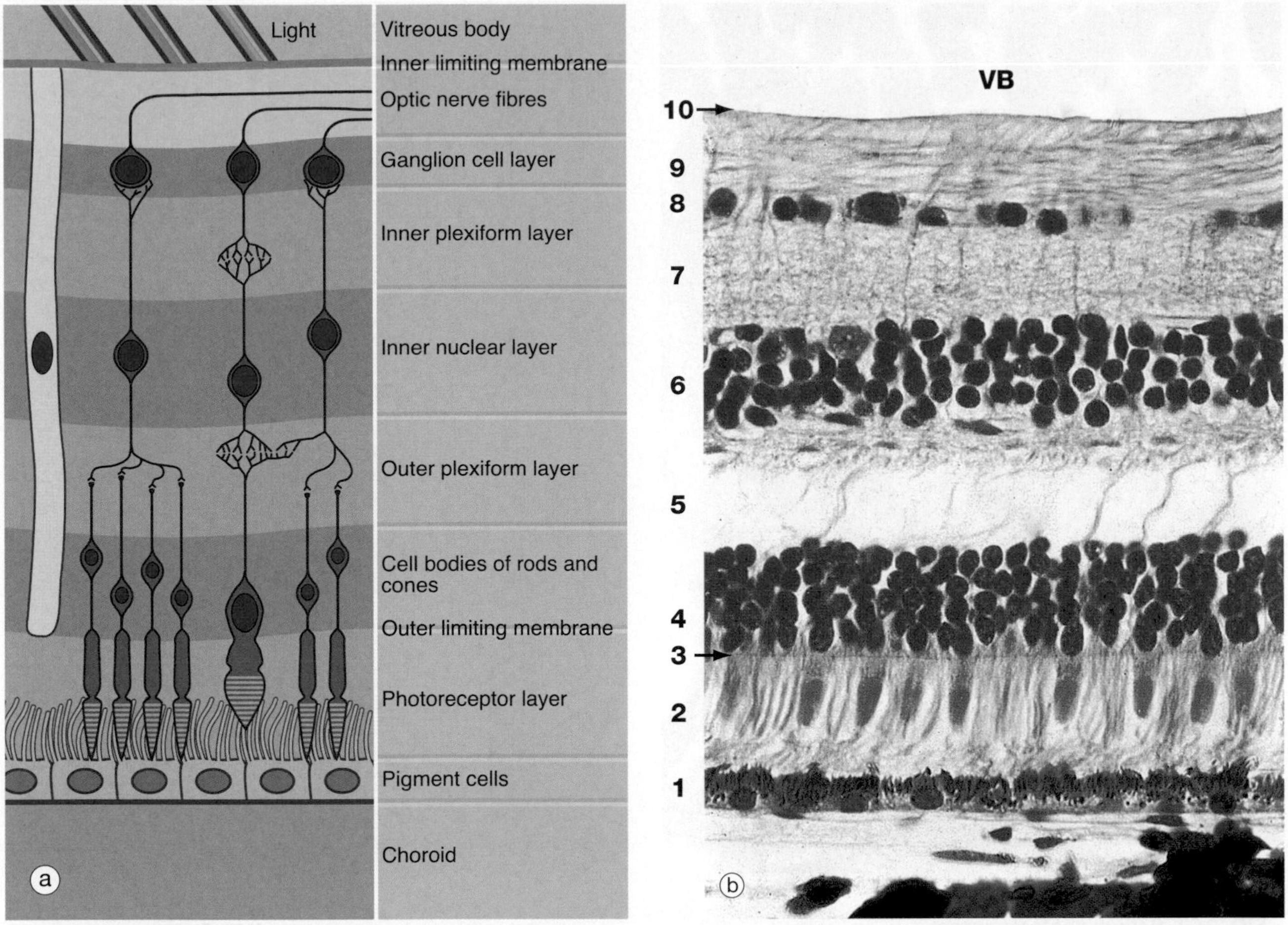

FIG. 21.6 Retina
(a) Schematic diagram (b) H&E (HP)

The retina is made up of three cell types: ***neurones, pigmented epithelial cells*** and ***neurone support cells***. The neurones are divided into three functional groups: photoreceptor cells (rod cells and cone cells), the cells of afferent fibres passing in the optic nerve and a group of neurones interposed between the first two types which integrate sensory input from the photoreceptors before transmission to the cerebral cortex. The integrating neurones are further subdivided into three types: ***bipolar cells, horizontal cells*** and ***amacrine cells***.

Histologically, the retina is traditionally divided into 10 distinct histological layers, as shown in Fig. 21.6b; the distribution of the different cell types being illustrated in a highly schematic manner in Fig. 21.6a.

The outermost layer (1) consists of the ***pigmented epithelial cells*** forming a single layer resting on Bruch's membrane, which separates them from the choroid. The next layer is the ***photoreceptor layer***, made up of the rod and cone processes (2) with a thin eosinophilic structure known as the ***outer limiting membrane*** (3) separating them from a layer of densely packed nuclei described as the ***outer nuclear layer*** (4). The outer nuclear layer contains the cell bodies of the rod and cone photoreceptors. The almost featureless layer next to this is known as the ***outer plexiform layer*** (5) and contains synaptic connections between the short axons of the photoreceptor cells and integrating neurones, the cell bodies of which lie in the ***inner nuclear layer*** (6). In the ***inner plexiform layer*** (7), the integrating neurones make synaptic connections with dendrites of neurones whose axons form the optic tract. The cell bodies of the optic tract neurones (***retinal ganglion cells***) comprise the ***ganglion cell layer*** (8). Internal to this is the layer of afferent fibres (9) passing towards the optic disc to form the optic nerve. Finally, the ***inner limiting membrane*** (10) demarcates the innermost aspect of the retina from the vitreous body **VB**. Note in the diagram that only bipolar cells are represented in the integrating cell layer; this layer also contains the cell bodies of the horizontal and amacrine cells as illustrated in Fig. 21.8.

Note that light impinging on the retina passes through many layers before reaching the photoreceptor cells.

Towards the left of the diagram there is an extremely elongated support cell extending between inner and outer limiting membranes; it has its nucleus in the same layer as the integrating neurones, the inner nuclear layer. These cells, known as ***Müller cells***, are analogous to the neuroglia of the central nervous system and have long cytoplasmic processes which embrace and sometimes even encircle the retinal neurones, filling all the intervening spaces. Müller cells provide structural support and may also mediate the transfer of essential metabolites such as glucose to the retinal neurones.

The outer limiting membrane is not a true membrane but merely represents the line of intercellular junctions between Müller cells and the photoreceptor cells (shown diagrammatically in Fig. 21.7). In contrast, the inner limiting membrane represents the basement membrane of the Müller cells resting on the vitreous body.

C cornea **CB** ciliary body **Ch** choroid **I** iris **L** lens **O** optic nerve **P** pigment epithelium **R** retina **S** sclera **VB** vitreous body

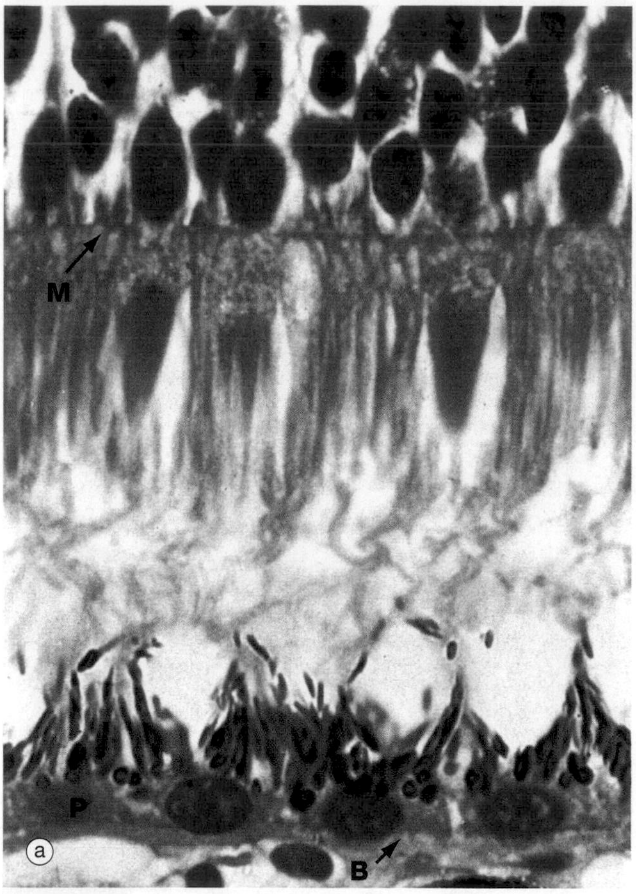

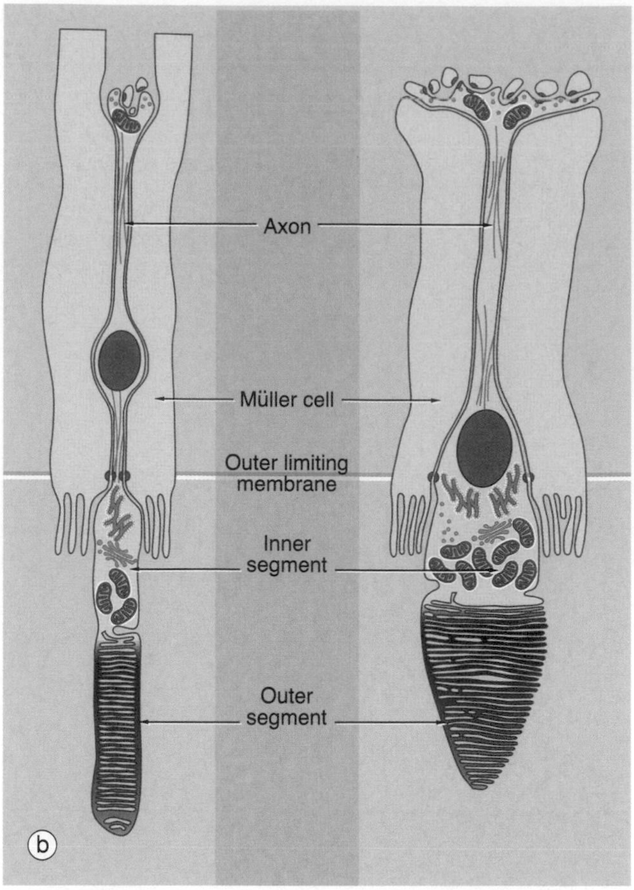

FIG. 21.7 Retinal photoreceptors
(a) H&E (HP) (b) Schematic diagram

The rod and cone photoreceptor layer of the retina is shown at very high magnification in Fig. 21.7a, the cell bodies of the rod and cone cells lying internal to the outer limiting membrane **M**. Peripherally, the rods and cones mingle with long microvilli extending from the pigmented epithelial cells **P**.

As shown in diagram Fig. 21.7b, the rod photoreceptors are long slender bipolar cells, the single dendrite of each cell extending beyond the outer limiting membrane as the rod proper. The rod proper consists of ***inner*** and ***outer segments*** connected by a thin eccentric strand of cytoplasm containing nine microtubule doublets, similar to those of a cilium but without the inner pair of microtubules. The inner segment contains a prominent Golgi apparatus and many mitochondria. The outer segment has a regular cylindrical shape and contains a stack of flattened membranous discs which incorporate the pigment ***rhodopsin*** (visual purple). The membranous discs are continuously shed from the end of each rod and phagocytosed by the pigmented epithelial cells. The discs are continuously replaced from the inner part of the outer segment. In essence, the transduction process involves the interaction of light with rhodopsin molecules which promotes a conformational change in the rhodopsin molecule, thus initiating an action potential. The action potential then passes inwards along the dendrite and axon to the layer of integrating neurones.

Cones are similar in basic structure to the rods, but they differ in several details. The outer segment of the cone is a long conical structure, about two-thirds the length of a rod, and contains a similar number of even more flattened membranous discs. Unlike the situation in the rods, however, the disc membrane is continuous with the plasma membrane so that, on one side, the spaces between the discs are continuous with the extracellular environment. The discs are not shed, although the tips of the cones are invested by processes of pigmented epithelial cells. The cones contain visual pigments similar to rhodopsin, receptive to blue, green and red light, and the mechanism of transduction is probably similar. The bodies of the cone cells are generally continuous with the inner segment of the cone proper, without an intervening dendritic process, and the nuclei of cone cells thus form a row immediately deep to the outer limiting membrane.

As seen in Fig. 21.7a, the pigmented epithelial cells are cuboidal in shape with the nuclei located basally towards ***Bruch's membrane*** **B**. Apically, the cells are crammed with melanin granules, numerous mitochondria and lipofuscin, a residual product of phagocytosis (see Fig. 1.26). The pigmented cell microvilli, which are 5 to 7 μm long, extend between the photoreceptors and, with electron microscopy, are seen to contain membranous lamellae similar to those in the rod outer segments; these appear to disintegrate as they pass deeper into the pigmented cells. In addition to phagocytosis, the pigmented epithelial cells provide structural and metabolic support for the rods and cones and also absorb light, thus preventing back reflection.

Retinal detachment

The specialised photoreceptor cells are normally closely attached to the retinal pigment epithelium so that the pigment epithelium can maintain a vital support function. This junction can be the site of separation of the retinal layers in the condition of ***retinal detachment***. Symptoms include loss of vision corresponding to the detached part of the retina described as 'like a dark curtain' in the visual field. If the retina can be surgically re-attached then vision can be restored.

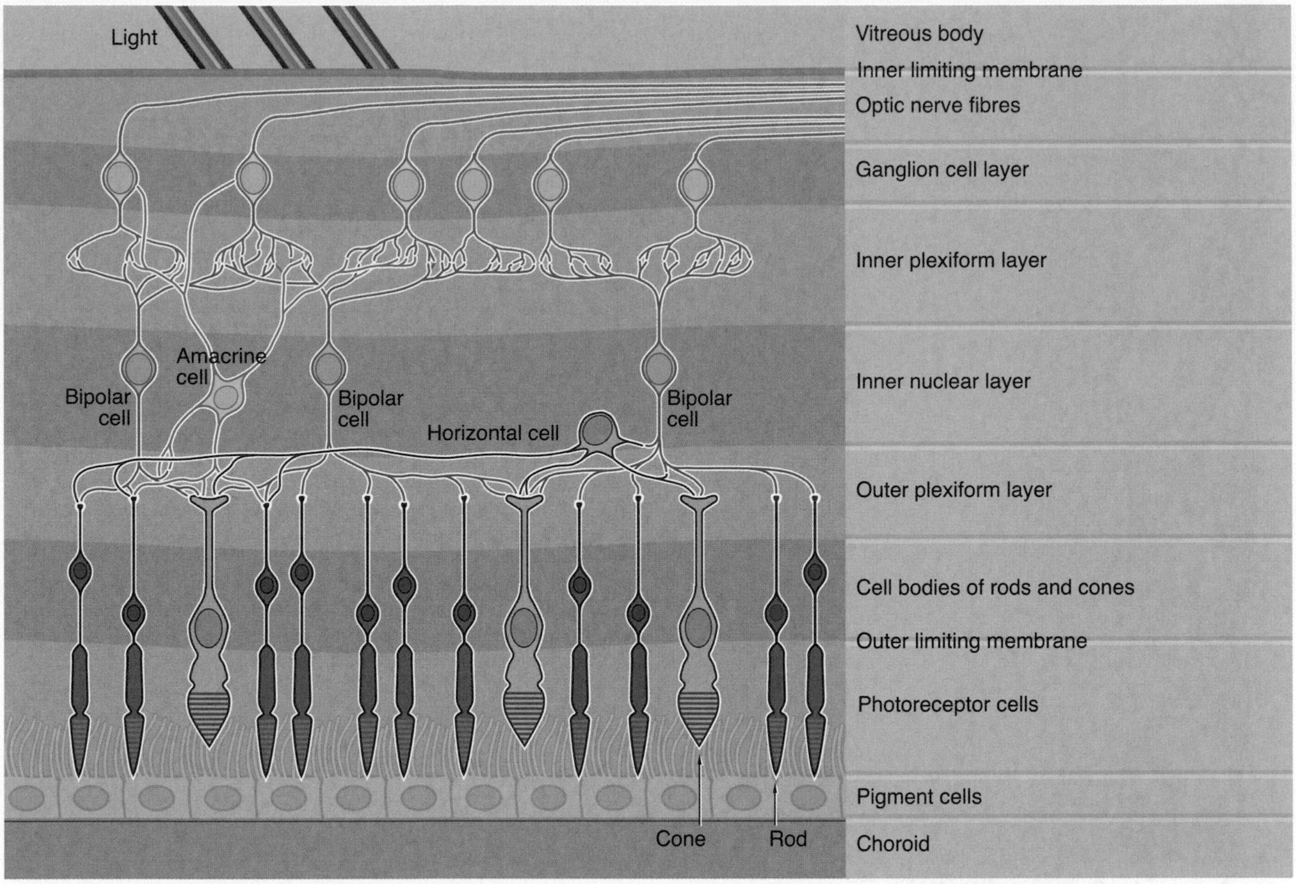

FIG. 21.8 Neuronal interconnections in the retina

Fig. 21.8 demonstrates the basic pattern of neuronal interconnections between the photoreceptor cells and the afferent neurones of the optic tract. The interneurones consist of three basic cell types, ***bipolar cells, horizontal cells*** and ***amacrine cells***, their cell bodies all being located in the inner nuclear layer (along with those of the supporting Müller cells).

Bipolar cells, the most numerous of the integrating neurones, in general make direct connections between one or more photoreceptors and one or more optic tract neurones, as well as with horizontal and amacrine cells. Horizontal cells have several short processes and one long process, the terminal branches of each making lateral connections between adjacent and more distant rods and cones in the outer plexiform layer. Horizontal cells also synapse with the dendrites of bipolar cells. The amacrine cells have numerous dendrites which make connections with bipolar and optic tract neurones in the inner plexiform layer, as well as making occasional feedback connections with photoreceptors in the outer plexiform layer.

As seen in Fig. 21.7b, the axons of the rod photoreceptors terminate in spherical processes into which are invaginated their small number of synaptic connections. In contrast, the cone photoreceptors have a flattened pedicle which accommodates hundreds of intercellular contacts.

In all, there are more than 100 million rods and 6 million cones. The cones are particularly dense in the macula and the immediately surrounding area and, in the fovea itself, the photoreceptors are almost exclusively cones. The density of both rods and cones diminishes towards the retinal periphery. The foveal cones have an almost one-to-one relationship with optic tract neurones, giving maximal visual discrimination.

There are only about 1 million optic tract neurones and, the more peripheral the photoreceptors, the greater the number of photoreceptors synapsing with each optic tract neurone. This is consistent with the main function of the more peripheral receptors (predominantly rods), which is for determination of light and dark, rather than fine two-point discrimination.

Retinal degenerations

The retina is affected by several diseases classed as retinal degenerations. These lead to loss of specialised photoreceptor cells and progressive loss of visual acuity, often causing total blindness.

Macular degeneration is a condition which is mainly seen in people over the age of 60. It is one of the commonest causes of loss of visual acuity in the elderly. Abnormal masses of lipid-rich material accumulate in the choroid (drusen), leading to failure of support for photoreceptor cells. The macula is the retinal region serving fine-detailed colour vision in the centre of the visual field (Fig. 21.9). Loss of receptor cells in this area leads to severe visual impairment, but peripheral vision served by rods is preserved.

Retinitis pigmentosa is the name given to a family of inherited degenerative diseases of the retina. There are several genetic forms of disease which all cause death of specialised retinal elements. In the commonest forms, there is preferential degeneration of rod cells, leading to gradual loss of peripheral vision, sometimes described as 'tunnel vision' as the macula, composed of cones, is affected last.

B Bruch's membrane **M** outer limiting membrane **P** pigment epithelial cell

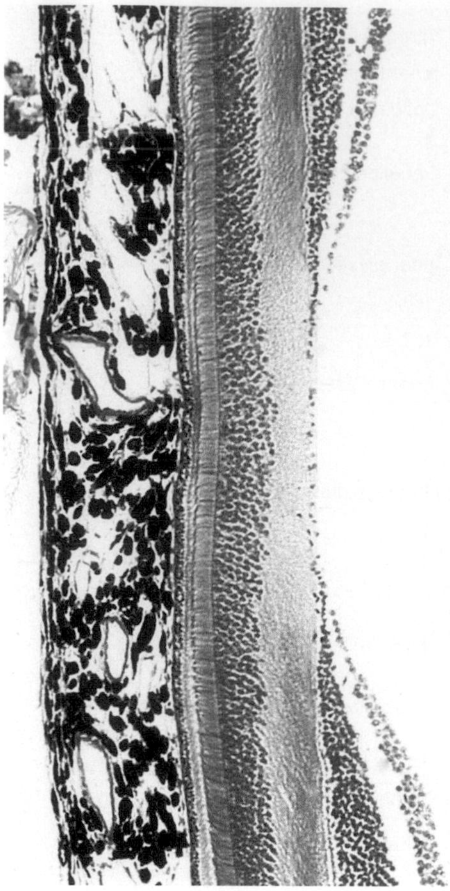

FIG. 21.9 Fovea
Masson trichrome (HP)

The fovea (Fig. 21.9) is a conical depression in the retina, corresponding to the point where the visual axis of the cornea and lens meets the retina and lying about 4 mm lateral and slightly inferior to the exit of the optic nerve fibres at the optic disc. Consequently, the fovea is the area subject to the least refractory distortion. To complement this, the foveal retina is modified to obtain the maximum photoreceptor sensitivity and is thus the area of the retina with the greatest visual discrimination; however, its function is poor in conditions of low light intensity.

Surrounding the fovea is an ovoid yellow area about 1 mm wide called the ***macula lutea***.

As seen in this micrograph, at the fovea the inner layers of the retina are flattened laterally so as to present the least barrier to light reaching the photoreceptors. Retinal blood vessels are absent at the fovea, as can be readily seen with the ophthalmoscope, and the brownish colour of the choroidal melanin shows through the much attenuated retina. At the fovea, the photoreceptors are almost exclusively cones which are elongated and closely packed (approximately 100 000 cones are contained in the fovea). Neuronal interconnections in the bipolar cell layer provide for a one-to-one ratio of these cones to optic nerve fibres, which means that each foveal photoreceptor is individually represented at the visual cortex.

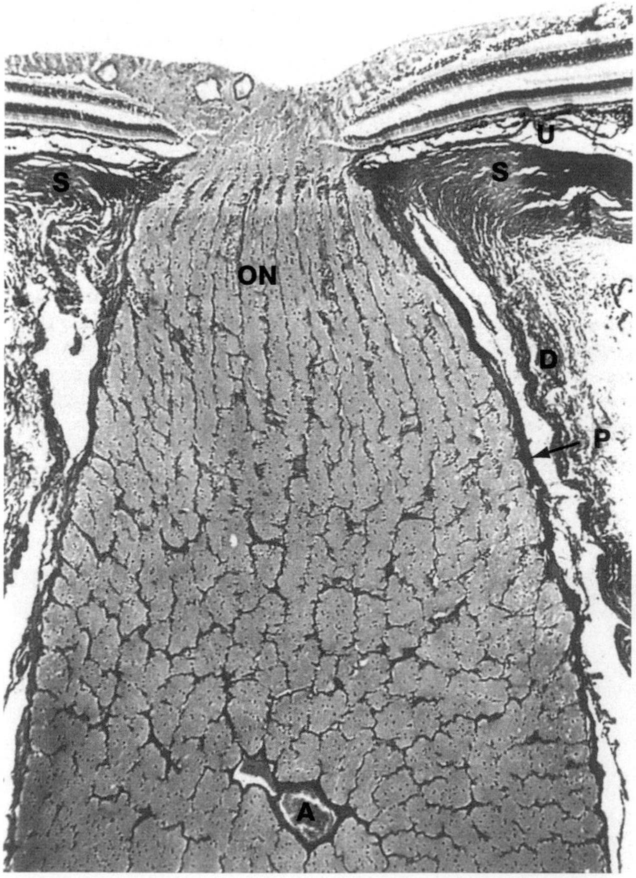

FIG. 21.10 Optic nerve
H&E (LP)

The afferent fibres from the retina converge at a point medial to the fovea, the ***optic papilla*** or ***optic disc***, fibres from the lateral quadrants sweeping above and below the macula to avoid the fovea. The fibres then penetrate the sclera **S** through the ***lamina cribrosa*** to form the optic nerve **ON** (Fig. 21.10). Note the thickness of the optic tract layer overlying the disc and the absence of photoreceptor cells from the optic papilla, which is thus a blind spot on the retina.

In their course across the retina, the afferent fibres are not myelinated as this would obstruct light passing to the photoreceptors. Myelination commences at the optic disc, which imparts the white colour seen with the ophthalmoscope.

The optic nerve and retina develop embryologically as an outgrowth of the primitive forebrain and thus the optic nerve is invested by meninges. The ***dura mater*** **D** becomes continuous with its developmental equivalent, the sclera, while the ***pia–arachnoid*** **P** continues into the eye as the uveal tract **U**.

The main blood supply of the retina is provided by the ***central artery of the retina*** **A**, a branch of the ophthalmic artery. This divides at the optic disc into four branches supplying the quadrants of the retina. These vessels course within the optic nerve fibre layer, breaking up into a rich capillary network which drains back into a venous system, closely following the course of the arterial supply. The vessels are confined to the optic nerve fibre layer and more superficial layers are dependent on diffusion, the most peripheral retinal layers being supplied likewise from the choroid.

A central artery of the retina **C** ciliary process **CB** ciliary body **CS** canal of Schlemm **D** dura mater **E** epithelium **I** iris **ICA** iridocorneal angle **L** lens **M** smooth muscle **ON** optic nerve **P** pia-arachnoid **PC** posterior chamber **S** sclera **SL** suspensory ligament **U** uvea

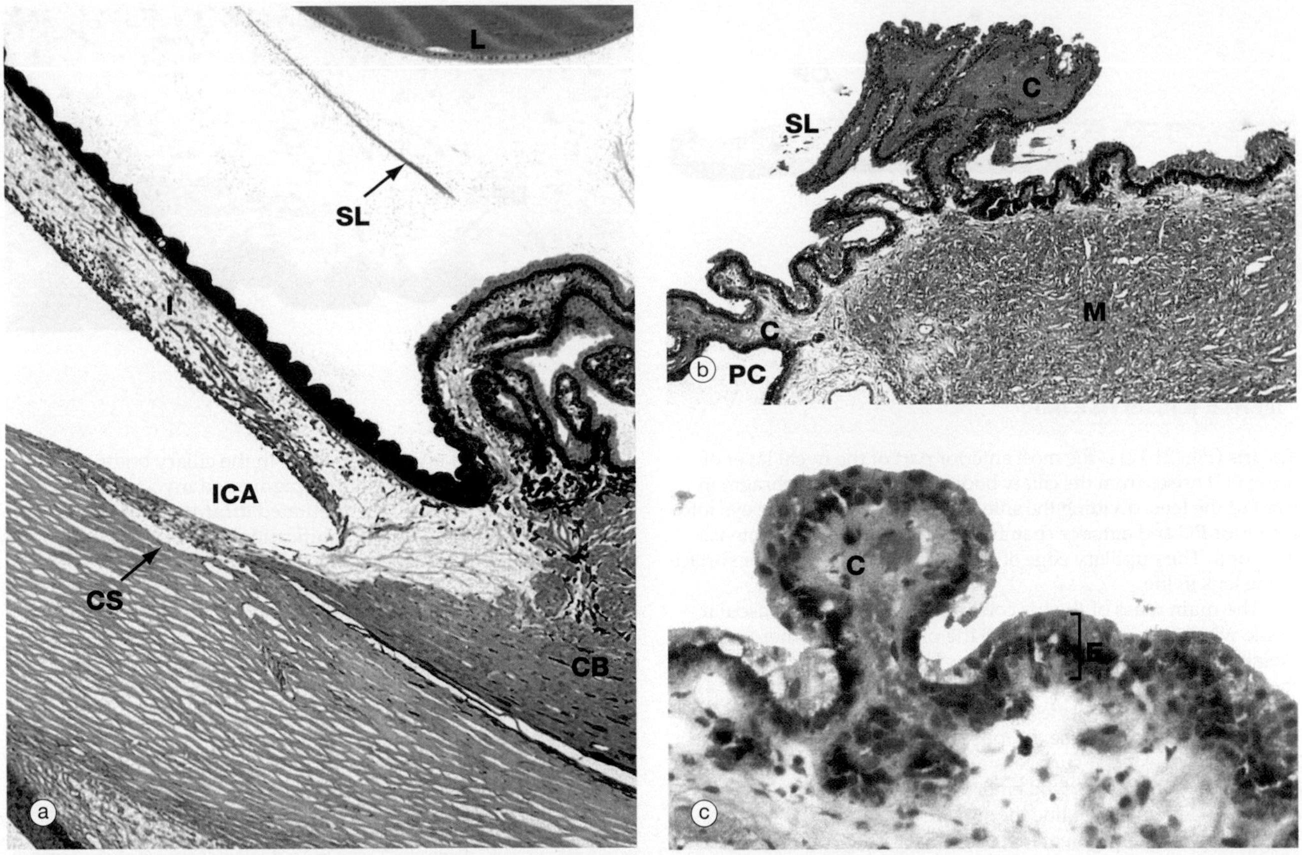

FIG. 21.11 Ciliary body
(a) H&E (LP) (b) H&E (LP) (c) H&E (MP)

The ciliary body is a circumferential structure which bulges into the eye between the ora serrata and the limbus (see Fig. 21.3). As seen in Fig. 21.11a, the ciliary body **CB** represents the forward continuation of the choroid layer of the uveal tract of the posterior five-sixths of the wall of the eye and, like it, is highly vascular and contains a considerable amount of dark-staining melanin pigment. Anteriorly, it is continuous with the third component of the uveal tract, the iris **I**, passing in front of the lens **L**.

As seen in Fig. 21.11c, the ciliary body is lined with a double layer of cuboidal epithelium **E**. The deep layer is highly pigmented and represents a forward continuation of the pigmented epithelial layer of the retina, while the surface layer, which is not pigmented, is a non-photosensitive forward extension of the receptor layer of the retina.

The ciliary body is attached to the coronal equator of the lens by the ***suspensory ligaments*** **SL** which consist of extremely fine strands composed of the protein ***fibrillin*** (Fig. 21.11b). Tension in the suspensory ligament tends to flatten the lens which, in the relaxed state, assumes a more globular shape. The bulk of the ciliary body consists of smooth muscle **M** arranged in such a manner that, when it contracts, tension upon the suspensory ligament is reduced, thus permitting the lens to assume a more convex shape. This mechanism permits fine focusing of images already roughly focused upon the retina by the cornea. The ciliary muscle is innervated by parasympathetic nerve fibres.

From that part of the ciliary body exposed to the angle of the ***posterior chamber*** **PC**, there project a number of branching epithelial folds called ***ciliary processes*** **C** with a supporting tissue core rich in fenestrated capillaries. The ciliary processes are responsible for the continuous production of ***aqueous humor***, which then circulates into the ***anterior chamber*** via the pupil. Aqueous humor is continuously reabsorbed into the ***canal of Schlemm*** **CS** seen at the base of the irido-corneal angle of the anterior chamber **ICA** in Fig. 21.11a.

Aqueous humor is a clear watery fluid, somewhat similar in composition to cerebrospinal fluid and hypotonic with respect to plasma. The production of aqueous humor is an active process, mediated by the two epithelial layers lining the ciliary processes. Balanced rates of secretion and reabsorption of aqueous humor result in the maintenance of a constant intraocular pressure of about 15 mmHg which stabilises the lens and cornea. The flow of aqueous humor also provides for a continuous exchange of metabolites with the cells of the avascular cornea and lens.

Glaucoma

If the drainage of aqueous humor is obstructed and the ciliary body continues to secrete, this may lead to a sustained increase in the intraocular pressure called ***glaucoma***. If untreated this causes damage to the neural retina and can cause blindness.

- Some forms of glaucoma are inherited and are associated with abnormal filtration of aqueous humor at the canal of Schlemm.
- Any disease which causes inflammation or scarring of the iridocorneal angle can lead to glaucoma by blocking the canal of Schlemm.
- Proliferation of blood vessels in the iris root, usually as a response to poor blood supply to the retina, as may happen in patients with diabetes, may block aqueous drainage.

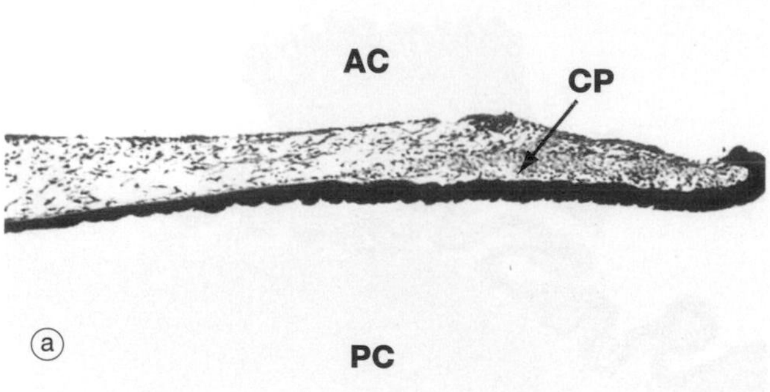

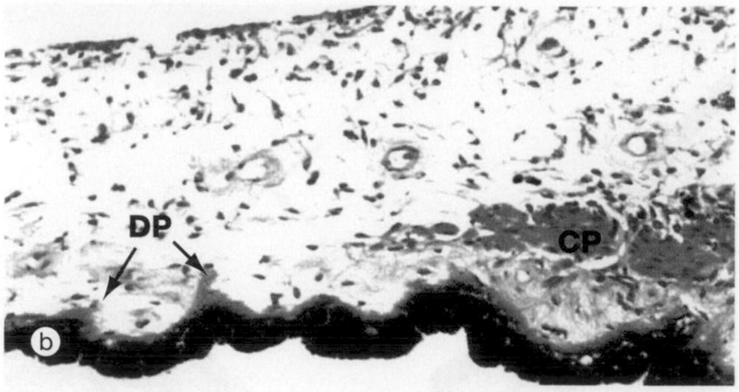

FIG. 21.12 Iris
(a) H&E (LP) (b) H&E (MP)

The iris (Fig. 21.12) is the most anterior part of the uveal layer of the eye. It arises from the ciliary body and forms a diaphragm in front of the lens, dividing the anterior compartment of the eye into posterior **PC** and anterior chambers **AC** which communicate via the pupil. The pupillary edge of the iris rests on the anterior surface of the lens in life.

The main mass of the iris consists of loose, highly vascular tissue which is pigmented due to the presence of numerous melanocytes scattered in the stroma. The anterior surface of the iris is irregular and consists of a discontinuous layer of fibroblasts and melanocytes; in the fetus, the surface is lined by endothelial cells but these disappear during early childhood. In contrast, the posterior surface is relatively smooth and is lined by epithelium which is derived embryologically as a continuation of the two layers which line the surface of the ciliary body. The surface layer, non-pigmented in the ciliary body, becomes heavily pigmented in the iris such that the individual cells are completely obscured. The deep layer, pigmented in the ciliary body, is transformed in the iris into lightly pigmented myoepithelial cells which constitute the radially orientated ***dilator pupillae muscle*** **DP** of the iris. Even at high magnification (Fig. 21.12b), these myoepithelial cells are difficult to distinguish.

The constrictor muscle of the pupil (***constrictor pupillae***) **CP** consists of a band of circumferentially oriented smooth muscle fibres situated in the stroma near to the free edge of the iris. Like the smooth muscle of the ciliary body, the constrictor pupillae is innervated by the parasympathetic nervous system, whereas the myoepithelial cells of the dilator pupillae are innervated by the sympathetic nervous system.

The colour of the iris depends on the amount of pigment in the stroma, the amount of pigment in the posterior epithelial layer being relatively constant between individuals. Blue eyes contain little pigment, whereas brown eyes have plentiful stromal pigment.

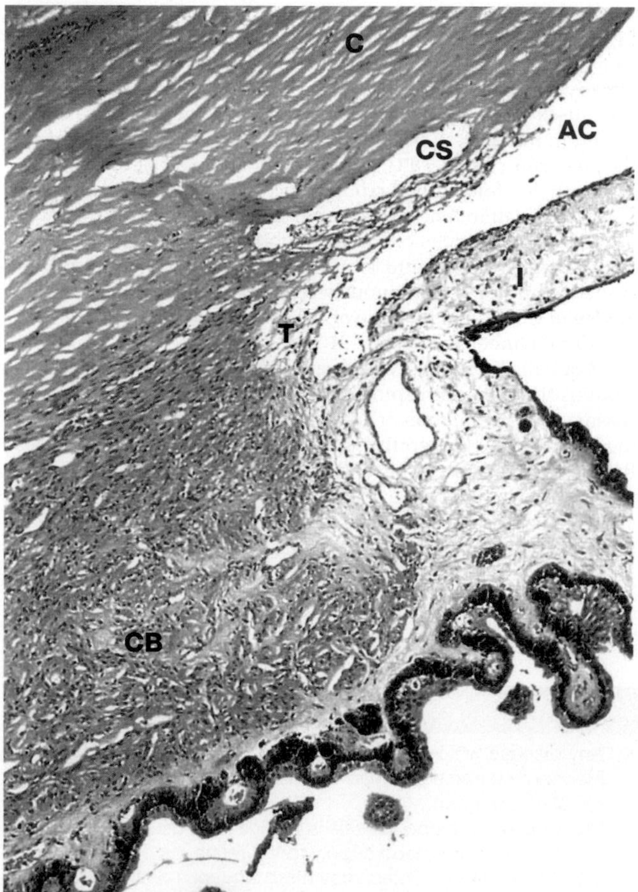

FIG. 21.13 Canal of Schlemm
H&E (MP)

The ***canal of Schlemm*** **CS** (Fig. 21.13) is a circumferential canal lined by endothelium which is situated in the inner aspect of the corneal margin **C**, immediately adjacent to the angle of the anterior chamber **AC**. At the angle of the anterior chamber, there is a meshwork of fine collagenous ***trabeculae*** **T** lined by endothelium; aqueous humor percolates through the spaces between the trabeculae before reaching the canal of Schlemm. There is no direct communication between the trabecular spaces and the canal of Schlemm and thus reabsorption of aqueous humor involves passage across two layers of endothelium and intervening supporting tissue. The canal of Schlemm drains via minute channels through the sclera into the episcleral venous system, a pressure gradient being maintained to prevent reflux of blood. Note the close relationship between the root of the iris **I** and the canal of Schlemm. The smooth muscle of the ciliary body **CB** is easily seen in this micrograph.

A lens epithelium **AC** anterior chamber **C** cornea **CA** lens capsule **CB** ciliary body **CP** constrictor pupillae **CPR** ciliary process **CS** canal of Schlemm **DP** dilator pupillae **E** lens equator **I** iris **J** junction between anterior and posterior lens cells **N** nuclei of peripheral lens fibres **PC** posterior chamber **R** retina **T** trabeculae

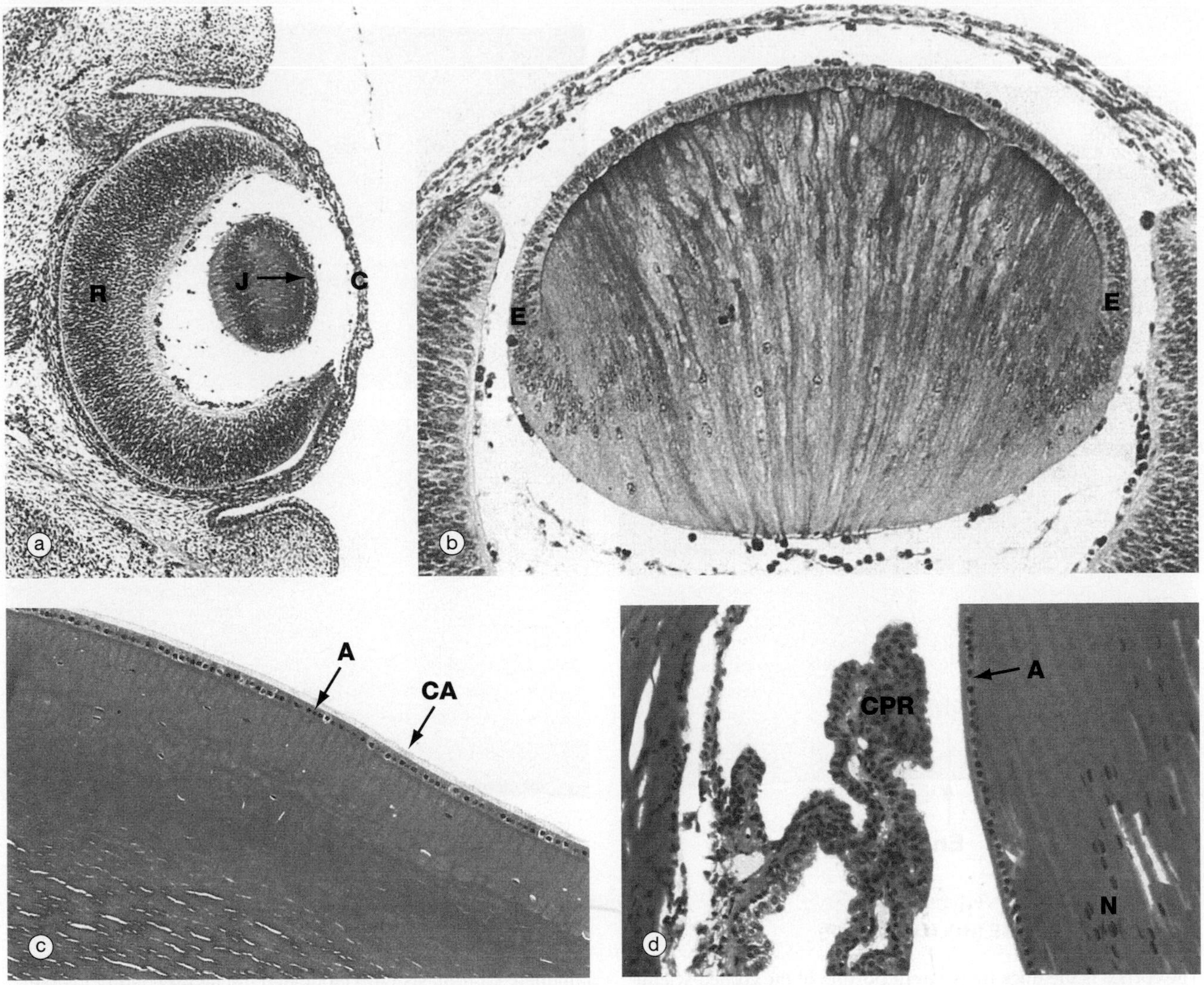

FIG. 21.14 The lens and its development
(a) H&E (MP) (b) H&E (HP) (c) H&E (MP) (d) H&E (MP)

The *lens* is an elastic biconvex structure which, although transparent and apparently amorphous, is almost entirely composed of living cells. The *lens cells* are highly modified epithelial cells, derived embryologically from ectoderm which forms a depression, the *lens pit*, overlying the embryonic *optic vesicle*.

With further development, the lens pit becomes deeper, its margins fusing to form the lens vesicle which becomes detached from the surface and sinks deeper to become enveloped by the growing optic vesicle; at this stage, the lens vesicle merely consists of a single layer of epithelial cells.

The posterior cells of the lens vesicle now become greatly elongated anteroposteriorly, filling the central cavity of the vesicle. This stage of development is shown in Fig. 21.14a, showing the junction **J** between posterior and anterior cells of the former lens vesicle. Note the developing *cornea* **C** and *retina* **R**. The lens cells in the central anteroposterior axis then undergo maturation as seen in Fig. 21.14b losing their nuclei to become known as *lens fibres*. Proliferation of the cells at the lens equator **E** adds further fibres to the central mass, the growth process continuing at a slow rate even into old age.

When fully developed, the lens substance consists of 2000 to 3000 anucleate fibres, each stretching between anterior and posterior poles of the lens. The fibres have the shape of extremely elongated six-sided prisms, the more peripheral fibres curving to follow the anteroposterior surface contour of the lens. The lens fibres are packed with proteins called *crystallins* and the cell membranes of adjacent fibres are fused, leaving little intervening extracellular substance.

The whole lens is enveloped by a thick epithelial basement membrane forming the *lens capsule*, which is connected via the suspensory ligament to the ciliary body. The anterior lens surface is covered by a single layer of cuboidal cells which retain their nuclei, this layer merging with the residual proliferative cells at the equatorial margin of the lens. This cell layer lies deep to the capsule and is absent posteriorly.

Fig. 21.14c shows part of the mature lens, including the *anterior cuboidal epithelium* **A** and lens capsule **CA**. The lens substance is particularly prone to artefactual distortion during histological preparation. Fig. 21.14d shows the equatorial region of the lens and nearby ciliary processes **CPR**. Note the anterior epithelial layer **A** and nuclei **N** in the more recently formed peripheral fibres.

Cataracts

The normal lens is translucent and elastic. If there is damage to the lens fibres or if the normally translucent crystallin proteins aggregate, the lens becomes opaque and light is either diffused or blocked. The lens opacity is called a ***cataract***.

Cataracts can occur due to ageing, trauma to the lens, inflammatory diseases within the eye or in response to some metabolic diseases.

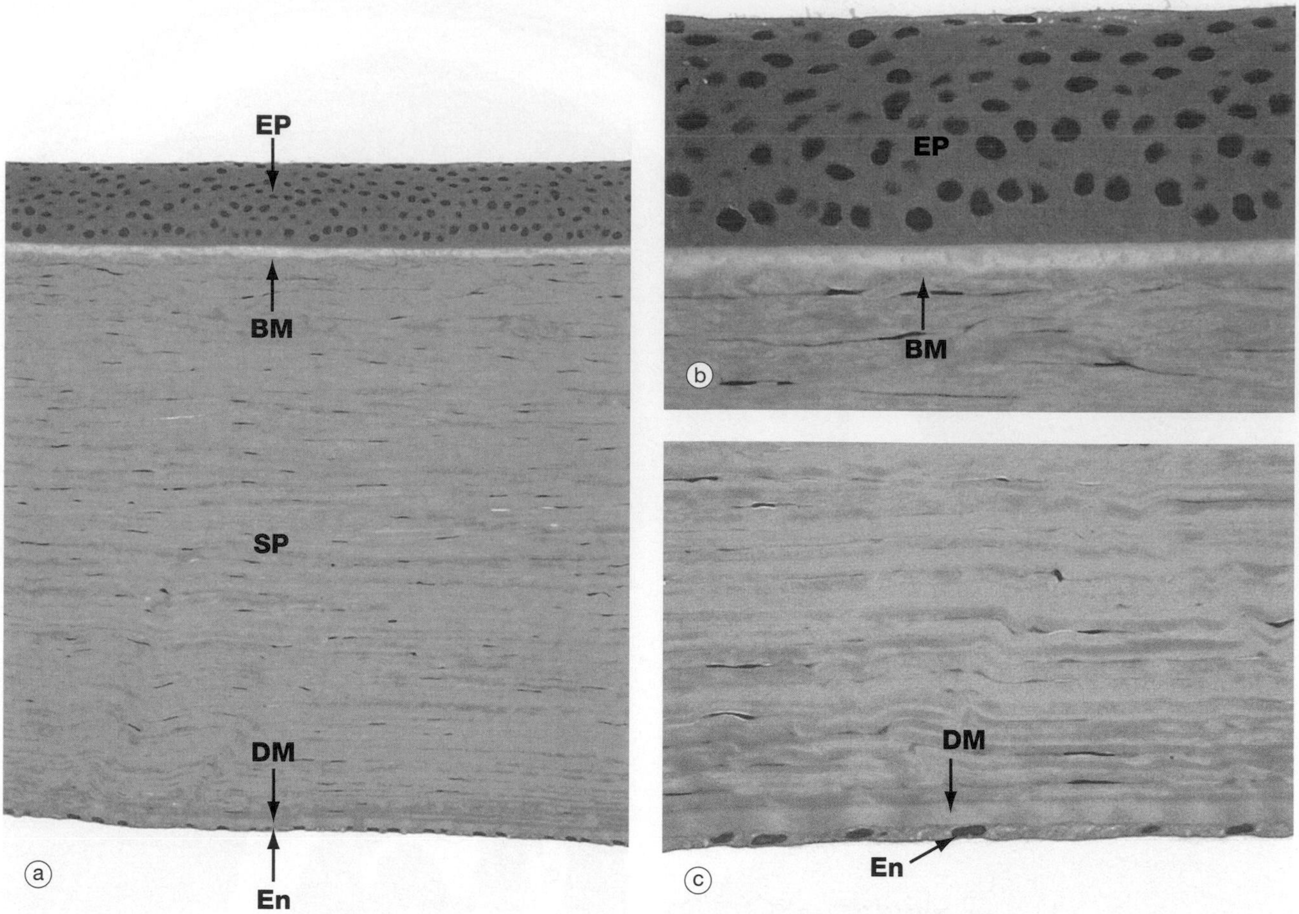

FIG. 21.15 Cornea
(a) H&E (MP) (b) H&E (HP) (c) H&E (HP)

The cornea is the thick transparent portion of the corneo-scleral layer enclosing the anterior one-sixth of the eye. The fixed convexity of the external surface provides the principal mechanism for focusing images upon the retina. Fig. 21.15a shows the full thickness of the cornea, while Figs 21.15b and c show the superficial and deep aspects at higher magnification.

The cornea is an avascular structure consisting of five layers. The outer surface is lined by stratified non-keratinised squamous epithelium **EP** about six cells thick. This epithelium rests on a thin basal lamina, supported by a thick specialised layer of corneal stroma known as ***Bowman's membrane*** **BM**, which is particularly prominent in humans. The bulk of the cornea, the ***substantia propria*** or ***stroma*** **SP**, consists of a highly regular form of dense collagenous tissue forming thin lamellae. Fibroblasts with elongated nuclei and barely visible cytoplasm termed ***keratocytes*** are scattered in the ground substance between the lamellae. The inner surface of the cornea is lined by a layer of flattened endothelial cells **En** which are supported by a very thick basement membrane known as ***Descemet's membrane*** **DM**. The corneal endothelium is highly active in pumping fluid from the substantia propria, preventing excessive hydration which would result in the cornea becoming opaque.

The cornea is sustained by diffusion of metabolites from the aqueous humor and the blood vessels of the limbus; some oxygen is derived directly from the external environment.

There is a rich innervation by free nerve endings, making the cornea very pain sensitive.

Corneal disease

The cornea plays a vital role in refracting light into the eye.

Although the endothelial cell layer looks inconspicuous, it is highly active in pumping fluid out of the corneal stroma. If the endothelial cell layer is damaged or cell numbers are reduced as happens with disease or age, then this fluid pumping function is impaired. Clinically, there is blurring of vision as the corneal stroma becomes waterlogged. The corneal epithelium develops areas of separation from Bowman's membrane, forming small bullae which are very painful and can lead to ulceration of the surface epithelium.

Diseases which cause inflammation of the cornea (e.g. viral infection by herpes zoster) can lead to loss of Bowman's membrane and replacement of the normal highly ordered collagen of the corneal stroma by haphazardly arranged collagenous scar tissue. Corneal scars are not transparent and produce an opacity that interferes with light transmission, so causing poor visual acuity.

If the curvature of the cornea becomes abnormal, there may be loss of visual acuity because light is not focused correctly. An unusual condition called ***keratoconus*** can develop where the cornea develops a conical profile due to remodeling of the corneal collagen.

A damaged cornea may be replaced by a transplant.

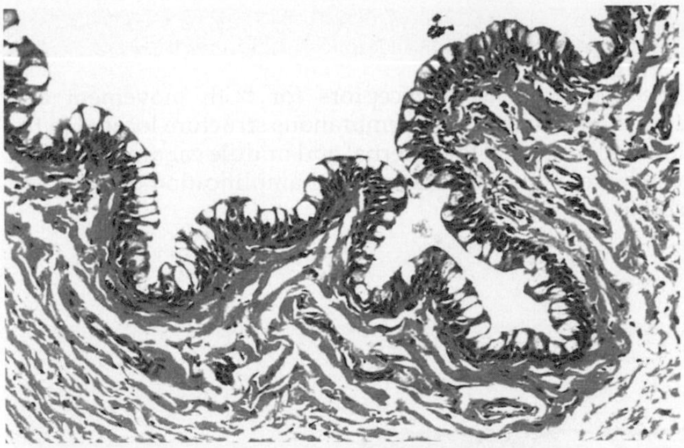

FIG. 21.16 Conjunctiva
H&E (MP)

The ***conjunctiva*** is the epithelium which covers the exposed part of the sclera and inner surface of the eyelids (Fig. 21.16). It is stratified columnar in form and, for a stratified epithelium, is unusual in that it contains goblet cells in the surface layers. Melanocytes are found in the basal layer. The conjunctival mucous secretions contribute to the protective layer on the exposed surface of the eye and allow the eyelids to move freely over the eye.

Beneath the conjunctival epithelium is loose vascular supporting tissue.

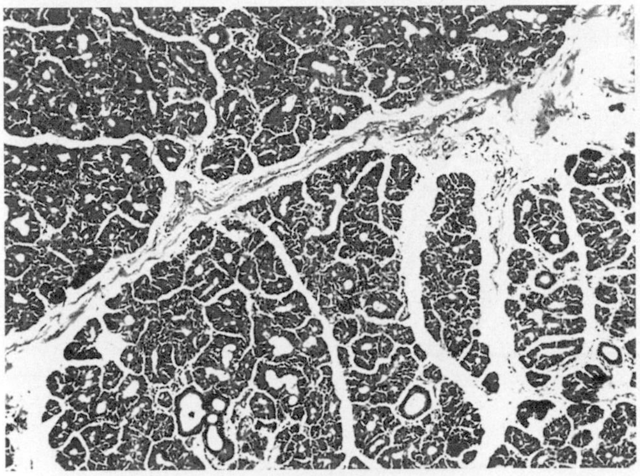

FIG. 21.17 Lacrimal gland
H&E (MP)

The lacrimal gland is responsible for the secretion of tears, a watery fluid containing the antibacterial enzyme lysozyme and electrolytes of similar concentration to plasma.

Histologically, the lacrimal glands are similar to the salivary glands in the lobular structure and compound tubulo-acinar form of the secretory units (Fig. 21.17). The secretory cells have the typical appearance of serous (protein-secreting) cells, with basally located nuclei and strongly stained granular cytoplasm.

Each gland drains via a dozen or more small ducts into the superior fornix. Tears drain to the inner aspect of the eye and then into the nasal cavity via the nasolacrimal duct.

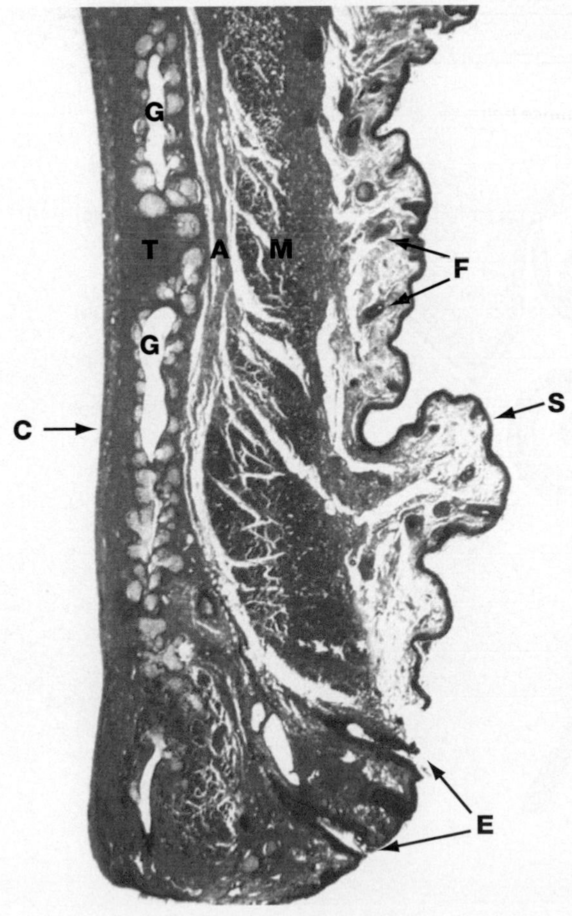

FIG. 21.18 Eyelid
H&E (LP)

Each eyelid (Fig. 21.18) consists of a dense fibroelastic plate, the ***tarsus*** or ***tarsal plate*** **T**, covered externally by thin highly folded skin **S** and, on the internal aspect, by smooth conjunctiva **C**. The skin contains scattered fine hair follicles **F**, and the underlying supporting tissue is extremely loose and devoid of fat.

Skeletal muscle **M** of the ***orbicularis oculi*** (and ***levator palpebrae*** in the upper eyelid) lies immediately superficial to the tarsal plate and is separated from it by a layer of supporting tissue **A** which, in the upper lid, represents a forward continuation of the sub-aponeurotic layer of the scalp. The clinical importance of this is that blood or inflammatory exudates collecting above the scalp aponeurosis may track forward into the superficial planes of the eyelid; being extremely lax, this area may become markedly swollen. This supporting tissue layer also contains the sensory nerves of the eyelid.

Within the tarsal plate lie some 12 to 30 ***tarsal*** (***Meibomian***) ***glands*** **G**, oriented vertically and opening at the free margin of the eyelid via minute foramina. These glands are modified sebaceous glands, each consisting of a long central duct into which open numerous sebaceous acini. Associated with the eyelashes **E** are sebaceous glands known as the ***glands of Zeis*** and modified apocrine sweat glands known as the ***glands of Moll***. Together, the glands of the eyelid produce an oily layer which is thought to cover the tear layer, thereby preventing evaporation of the tears.

A supporting tissue **BM** Bowman's membrane **C** conjunctiva **DM** Descemet's membrane **E** eyelash
En corneal endothelium **EP** corneal epithelium **F** hair follicle **G** Meibomian gland **M** muscle **S** skin
SP substantia propria of cornea **T** tarsal plate

THE EAR

The ear or vestibulo-cochlear apparatus has the dual sensory function of maintenance of equilibrium and hearing (stato-acoustic system).

Structurally, the system may be divided into three parts, the ***external ear***, the ***middle ear*** and the ***internal ear***. The specific sensory receptors for both movement and sound are situated in a membranous structure located in the internal ear, while the external and middle ear are concerned with reception, transmission and amplification of incoming sound waves.

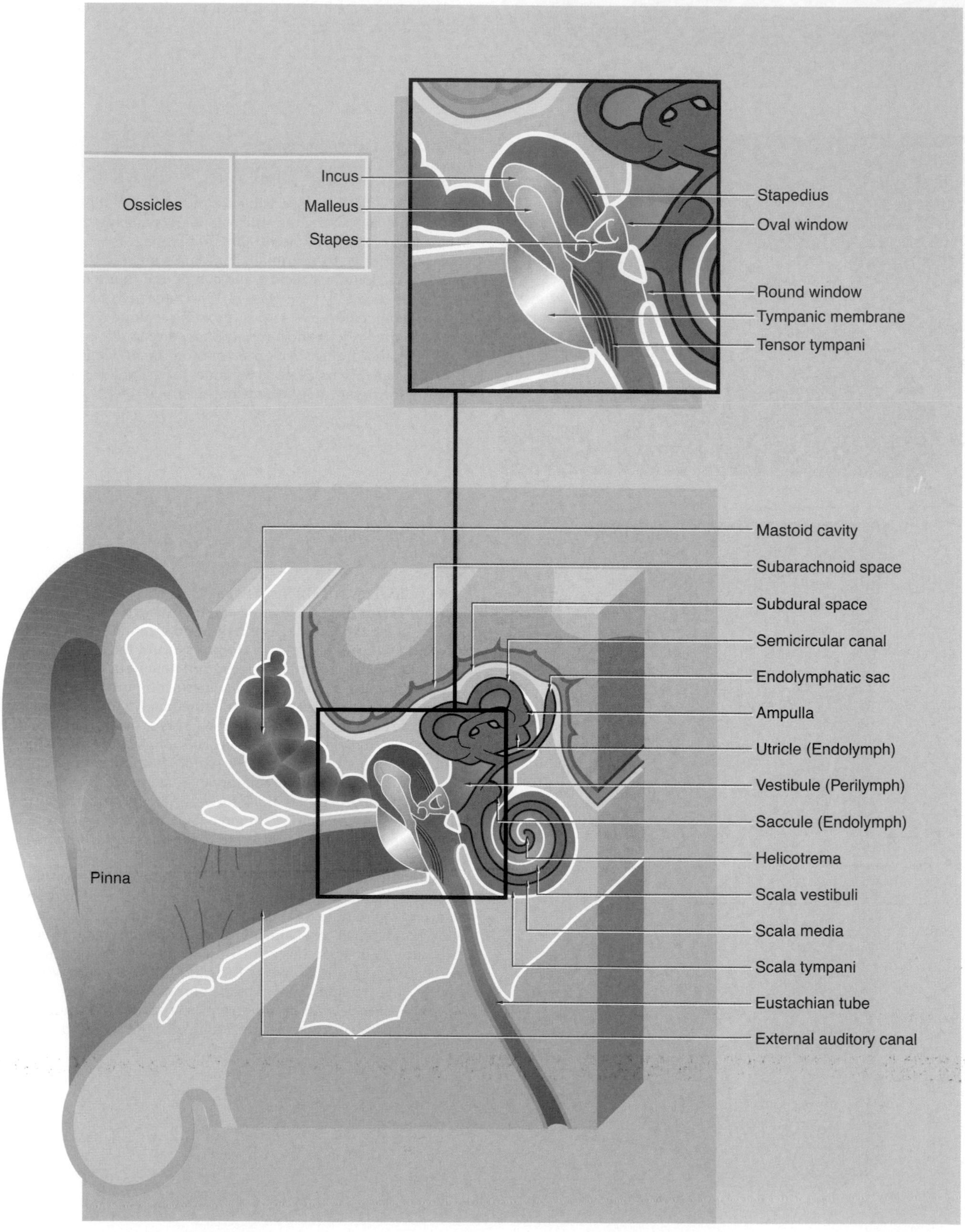

FIG. 21.19 The ear *(caption opposite)*

FIG. 21.19 The ear *(illustration opposite)*

The main structural elements of the vestibulocochlear apparatus are illustrated in this diagram.

External ear

The external ear is responsible for reception of sound waves which are funnelled onto the ear drum (*tympanic membrane*). It consists of the ***auricle*** (***pinna***), a modified cone-shaped structure composed of elastic cartilage covered by skin, which converges onto the ***external auditory meatus*** (***canal***). Elastic cartilage also forms the wall of the outer third of the canal, while the inner two-thirds of the canal lie in the petrous part of the temporal bone. The canal is lined by hairy skin containing sebaceous glands and modified apocrine glands which secrete a waxy material called *cerumen*.

Middle ear

The middle ear is an air-filled cavity, the ***tympanic cavity***, located in the petrous temporal bone and separated from the external auditory canal by the tympanic membrane. Sound waves impinging on the tympanic membrane are converted into mechanical vibrations which are then amplified by a system of levers made up of three small bones called ***ossicles*** (***malleus***, ***incus*** and ***stapes***) and transmitted to the fluid-filled inner ear cavity. The ossicles articulate with one another via synovial joints and the malleus and incus pivot on tiny ligaments which are attached to the wall of the middle ear cavity. Small slips of muscle, the ***tensor tympani*** and ***stapedius***, pass to the midpoint of the tympanic membrane and stapes bone, respectively, and damp down excessive vibrations which might otherwise damage the delicate auditory apparatus. The middle ear cavity communicates anteriorly with the nasopharynx via the ***auditory*** (***Eustachian***) ***tube***, which permits equalisation of pressure changes with the external environment. Posteriorly, the middle ear cavity communicates with numerous interconnected air spaces which lighten the mass of the mastoid part of the temporal bone. The whole of the middle ear and mastoid cavities are lined by simple squamous or cuboidal epithelium.

Internal ear

The internal ear consists of an interconnected fluid-filled ***membranous labyrinth*** lying within a labyrinth of spaces of complementary shape in the temporal bone (the ***osseous labyrinth***). The membranous labyrinth is bound down to the walls of the osseous labyrinth in various places but, in the main, is separated from the bony walls by a fluid-filled space. The fluid within the membranous labyrinth is known as ***endolymph*** and the fluid in the surrounding perimembranous space is known as ***perilymph***. The perimembranous space is directly connected with the subarachnoid space and, like the latter, is crossed by delicate fibrous strands and lined by squamous epithelium; the perilymphatic fluid is thus similar in composition to cerebrospinal fluid. In contrast, the membranous labyrinth is a closed system with a sac, the ***endolymphatic sac***, lying in the subdural space of the underlying brain. The membranous labyrinth is lined by a simple epithelium except in the endolymphatic sac, where the cells are columnar with morphological features suggesting that this is the site of endolymph absorption.

The osseous labyrinth may be divided into three main areas:

- **The vestibule**. The central space of the osseous labyrinth is called the ***vestibule***; it gives rise to three ***semicircular canals*** and to the ***cochlea*** anteriorly. The vestibule contains two components of the membranous labyrinth, the ***utricle*** and the ***saccule***, which are connected by a short Y-shaped duct from which arises the ***endolymphatic duct***. The walls of the utricle and saccule each contain a specialised area of sensory receptor cells known as a ***macula*** (see Fig. 21.27) from which axons pass into the ***vestibular nerve*** as part of sensory inputs to maintain equilibrium.
  Laterally, the vestibule is separated from the middle ear cavity by a thin bony plate containing two fenestrations or windows. The ***oval window*** is occluded by the base of the stapes bone and its surrounding ***annular ligament*** whereby vibrations are transmitted to the perilymph from the tympanic membrane via the ossicle chain. The ***round window*** is closed by a membrane similar to the tympanic membrane and is thus sometimes described as the ***secondary tympanic membrane***. This membrane permits vibrations, which have passed the sensory receptors for sound, to be dissipated.
- **The semicircular canals**. Three semicircular canals arise from the posterior aspect of the vestibule, two being disposed in vertical planes at right angles to one another and the other in a near-horizontal plane. Within each semicircular canal is a semicircular membranous duct filled with endolymph and continuous at both ends with the utricle; near one end of each semicircular membranous duct is a dilated area called the ***ampulla***. In each ampulla, there is a ridge called the ***crista ampullaris*** (see Fig. 21.28) containing sensory receptors with axons converging on the vestibular nerve. Together with the receptors of the maculae of the utricle and saccule, these receptors help maintain balance and equilibrium.
- **The cochlea**. The cochlea occupies a conical spiral-shaped space in the temporal bone, extending from the anterior aspect of the vestibule. The membranous component of the cochlea arises from the saccule and spirals upwards, with its blind end attached at the apex of the osseous space. The membranous canal is triangular in cross-section and attached to the bony walls of the cochlea in such a manner as to divide the osseous space into three spiral compartments (see Fig. 21.24). The middle compartment, the ***scala media***, contains endolymph and the upper and lower compartments contain perilymph. At the base of the cochlea, the upper perilymph compartment is directly continuous with the perilymph of the vestibule and via this space, called the ***scala vestibuli***, vibrations pass through the perilymph towards the apex of the cochlea. At the apex, the scala vestibuli becomes continuous with the lower perilymphatic space of the cochlear spiral via a minute hole called the ***helicotrema***. This lower space terminates at the secondary tympanic membrane covering the round window and 'spent' vibrations are thus dissipated; the lower perilymphatic space is therefore known as the ***scala tympani***. The sensory receptors for sound are located in a spiral-shaped structure known as the ***organ of Corti***, shown in detail in Fig. 21.25.

Cholesteatoma

In this condition, stratified squamous epithelium forms a cyst-like accumulation in the middle ear (see e-Fig. 21.1). It can be congenital, where squamous epithelium remains in the temporal bone during embryogenesis. Secondary causes include repeated infections leading to injury to the tympanic membrane. Cholesteatoma may lead to progressive bony destruction due to ongoing inflammation.

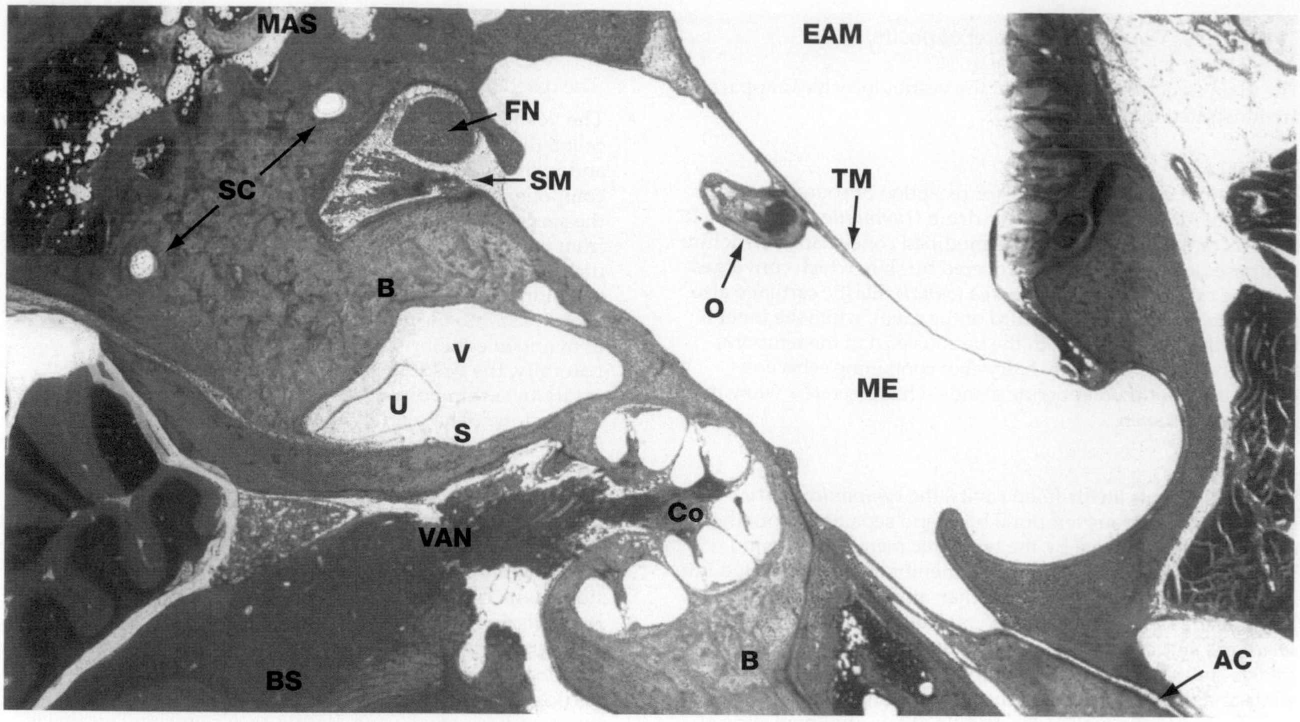

FIG. 21.20 The ear
H&E (LP)

Fig. 21.20 shows a horizontal section through the vestibulo-cochlear apparatus which lies within the temporal bone **B**. The tympanic membrane **TM** can be seen, stretched between the tympanic plate of the temporal bone anteriorly and the lateral part of the petrous temporal bone posteriorly, dividing the external auditory meatus **EAM** from the cavity of the middle ear **ME**. Part of one of the ossicles **O**, the handle of the malleus, can be seen attached to the inner aspect of the tympanic membrane. From the anterior aspect of the middle ear chamber, the auditory canal (Eustachian tube) **AC** passes forwards towards the nasopharynx; in the mastoid part of the temporal bone, there are numerous irregular mastoid air spaces **MAS**.

Near the centre of the field is the vestibule of the inner ear **V**, containing two delicate membranous structures, the utricle **U** and saccule **S**, more anteriorly. Two of the semicircular canals **SC** can be identified deep in the posterior part of the petrous temporal bone. Immediately posterior to the middle ear cavity, the facial nerve **FN** is seen in transverse section as it passes inferiorly; just medial to it lies the stapedius muscle **SM**.

Anterior to the vestibule, the conical spiral of the cochlea **Co** has been cut in longitudinal section through its central bony axis. From the base of the cochlea, the vestibulo-auditory (vestibulo-cochlear) nerve **VAN** passes towards the brainstem **BS**, behind which the cerebellum is easily recognisable.

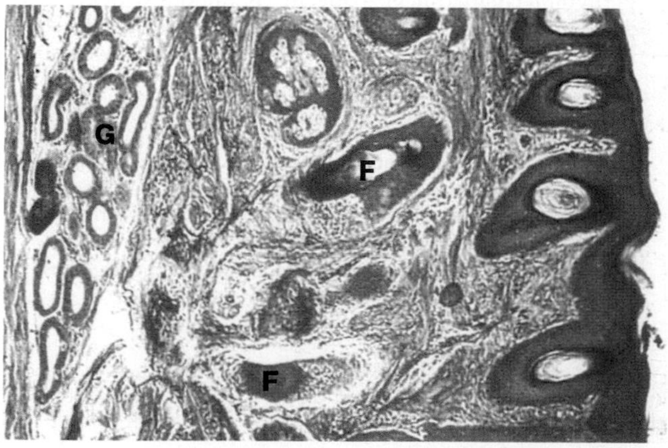

FIG. 21.21 External auditory meatus
H&E (MP)

The external auditory meatus is the canal leading from the auricle to the tympanic membrane. The wall of the outer third is formed by elastic cartilage, whereas the inner two-thirds is formed by the temporal bone. The canal is lined by skin which is devoid of the usual dermal papillae and closely bound down to the underlying cartilage or bone by a dense collagenous dermis. The skin of the outer third (Fig. 21.21) has fine hairs and the dermis contains numerous coiled tubular ***ceruminous glands*** **G** which secrete wax (cerumen) and which represent specialised apocrine glands. The ceruminous glands open directly onto the skin surface or into the sebaceous glands associated with hair follicles **F**. The meatal hairs provide protection from foreign bodies while the cerumen protects the skin of the external meatus from moisture and infection.

AC auditory canal **B** temporal bone **BS** brainstem **C** cuticular layer **Ca** cartilage **CB** compact bone **Co** cochlea **EAM** external auditory meatus **F** hair follicle **Fi** fibrous layer **FN** facial nerve **G** ceruminous gland **M** mucous layer **MAS** mastoid air spaces **ME** middle ear **Mu** tensor tympani muscle **O** ossicle **S** saccule **SC** semicircular canal **SM** stapedius muscle **TM** tympanic membrane **U** utricle **V** vestibule **VAN** vestibulo-auditory nerve

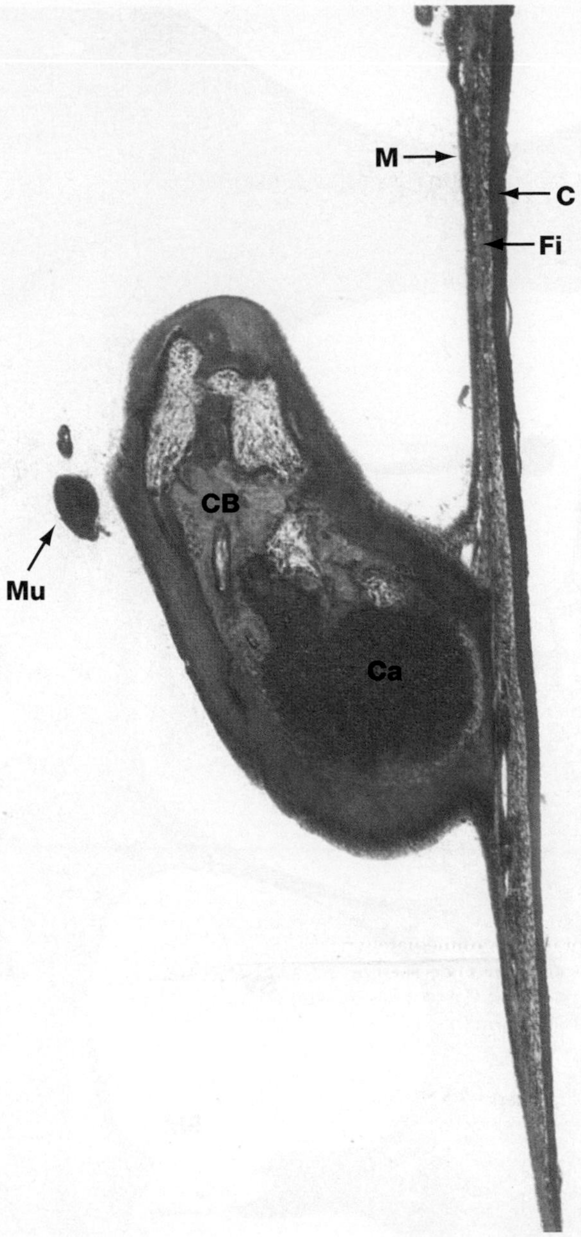

FIG. 21.22 Tympanic membrane and ossicle H&E (LP)

The tympanic membrane (ear drum) is a thin fibrous membrane separating the external auditory canal from the cavity of the middle ear (Fig. 21.22). With the exception of a small triangular area superiorly, the ***pars flaccida***, the membrane is tense (***pars tensa***), being firmly attached to the surrounding bone by a fibrocartilaginous ring. The handle of the malleus is attached to the centre of the membrane, the chain of ossicles pulling the membrane slightly inwards.

The tympanic membrane is made up of three layers: an external ***cuticular layer***, an intermediate ***fibrous layer*** and an inner ***mucous layer***. The cuticular layer **C** consists of thin hairless skin, the epidermis being only about 10 cells thick and the basal layer being flat and devoid of the usual epidermal ridges. The thin dermis contains plump fibroblasts and a fine vascular network.

The intermediate fibrous layer **Fi** consists of an outer layer of fibres radiating from the centre of the membrane towards the circumference and an inner layer of fibres disposed circumferentially at the periphery. These fibres contain a large amount of type II and type III collagen and a small amount of type I collagen, representing a distinct composition especially adapted for the function of the tympanic membrane.

The inner mucous layer **M** represents a continuation of the modified respiratory-type mucous membrane lining the middle ear cavity, but in this situation it is merely a single layer of cuboidal cells devoid of cilia and goblet cells. The underlying lamina propria is thin with a blood supply separate from that of the dermis of the cuticular layer. A similar modified respiratory-type mucosa invests the ossicles, small muscles and nerves exposed to the middle ear cavity.

The ossicles consist of compact bone **CB** formed by endochondral ossification, which accounts for the cartilage **Ca** seen in this specimen from a kitten. Note also the tensor tympani muscle **Mu**.

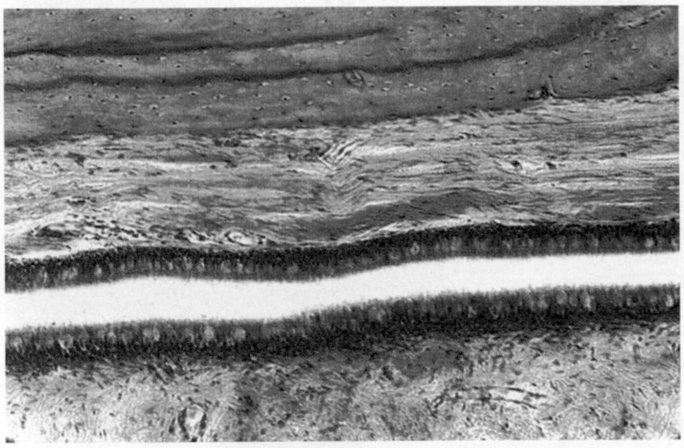

FIG. 21.23 Auditory (Eustachian) canal H&E (HP)

The auditory canal (Fig. 21.23) connects the cavity of the middle ear with the nasopharynx and allows for equalisation of air pressure between the middle ear and the external environment. From the middle ear, the tube first passes through bone, but towards the pharynx, the wall is supported on two sides by cartilage and on the remaining two sides by fibrous tissue.

The tube is lined by typical pseudostratified respiratory epithelium with numerous goblet cells, particularly towards the pharyngeal end. The ***salpingo-pharyngeus***, ***tensor palati*** and ***levator veli palati*** muscles are connected to the fibrocartilaginous part of the tube, causing it to dilate during swallowing.

Conductive deafness

Conductive deafness is caused by disorders that interfere with the conduction of sound through the outer and middle ear, affecting hearing before the sound reaches the cochlea.

- *Accumulated* wax in the external canal is a common cause of impaired hearing.
- Inflammation affecting the middle ear can result in secretions building up within the middle ear cavity (***otitis media***) which usually resolves with appropriate therapy.
- ***Otosclerosis*** is an inherited disease where the ossicles fuse together, preventing conduction of sound. Surgery can re-establish conduction and restore hearing.

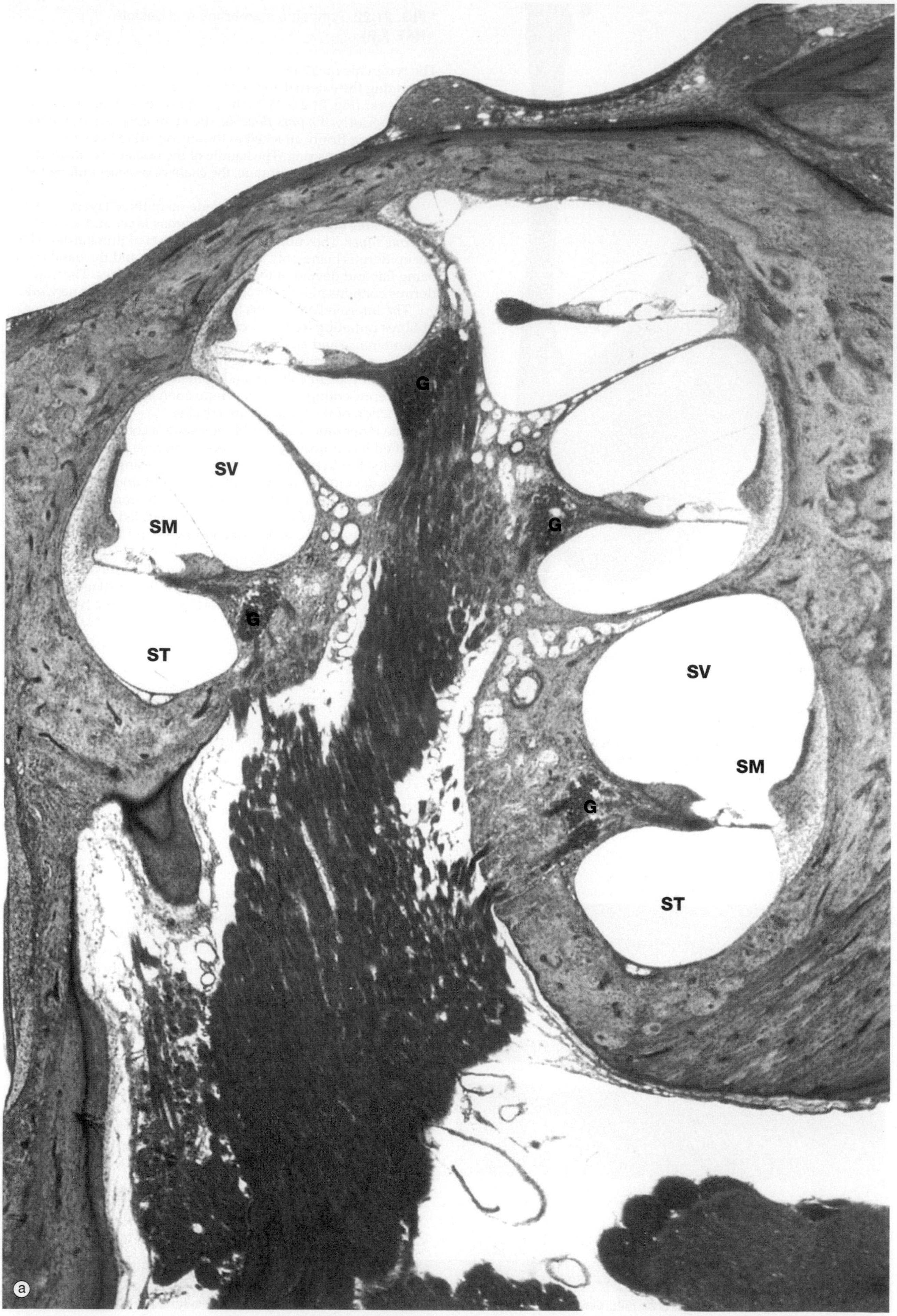

FIG. 21.24 Cochlea *(caption and illustration (b) opposite)*
(a) H&E (LP) (b) H&E (LP)

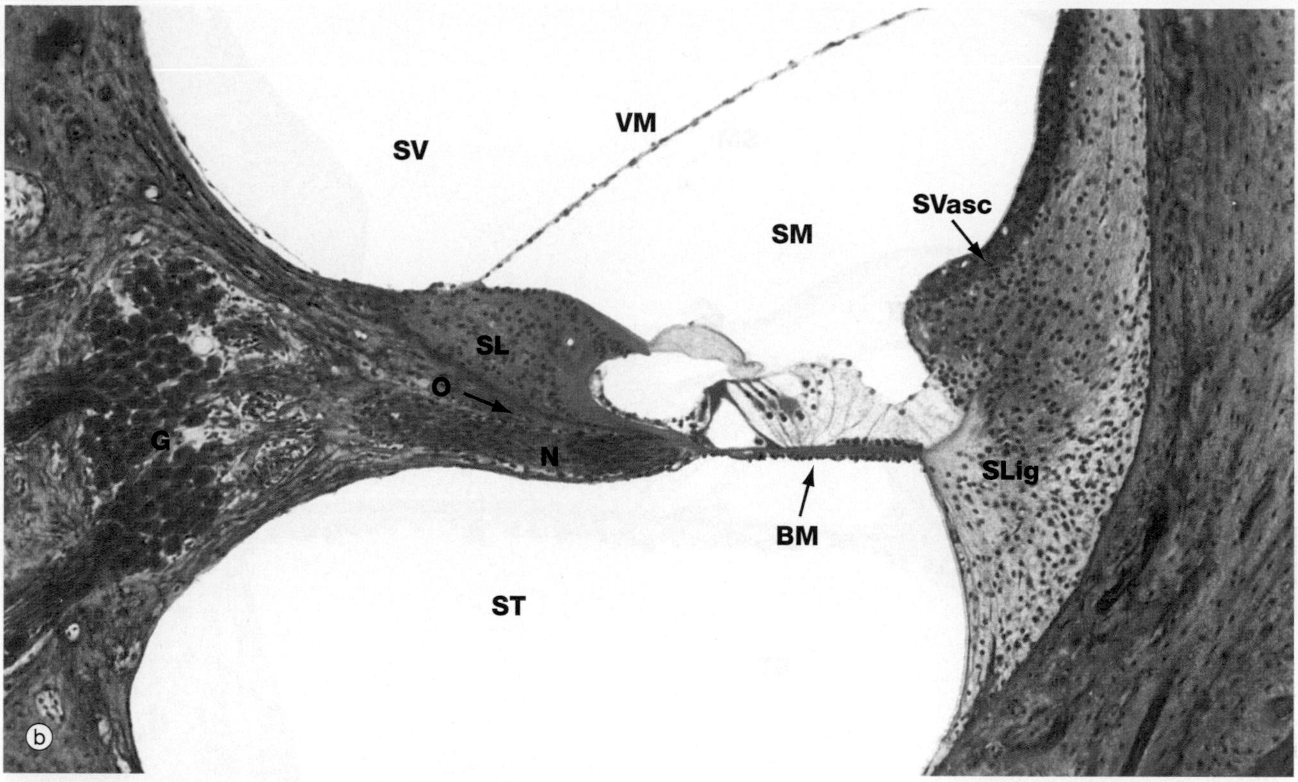

FIG. 21.24 Cochlea *(illustration (a) opposite)*
(a) H&E (LP) (b) H&E (LP)

The cochlea is the component of the internal ear which contains the auditory sense organ. The conical spiral-shaped form of the cochlea can be visualised in Fig. 21.24a which shows a cochlea cut in a plane of section which includes its long bony axis. Note that the cavity in the petrous temporal bone is reminiscent of the space inside a conical snail shell. The cochlea has two-and-a-half full turns; in this section, five separate cross-sections of the cochlea can be seen, each turn of the spiral being separated from the next by a thin plate of bone. A corkscrew-like bony structure, the ***modiolus***, forms the central axis of the cochlea.

Each turn of the cochlear canal can be seen to be divided into three compartments, shown at higher magnification in Fig. 21.24b. The central compartment, the ***scala media* SM**, is roughly triangular in cross-section, with the apex attached to a spicule of bone spiralling outwards from the modiolus and known as the ***osseous spiral lamina* O**. Above the free edge of the osseous spiral lamina is a thickened mass of tissue known as the ***spiral limbus* SL**. The base of the scala media is thickened and attached to the outer wall of the cochlea. The membrane making up the walls of the scala media represents that part of the membranous labyrinth extending up into the cochlea from the saccule and the scala media is thus filled with endolymph.

Above the scala media is the ***scala vestibuli* SV**, originating in the vestibule near the oval window and the base of the stapes; vibrations are conducted towards the apex of the cochlea in the perilymph of the scala vestibuli. Below the scala media is the perilymphatic space which spirals down from the apex to the secondary tympanic membrane, the ***scala tympani* ST**.

The membrane separating the scala media and the scala tympani, known as the ***basilar membrane* BM**, supports the ***organ of Corti*** which contains the auditory receptor cells; the organ of Corti is described in detail in Fig. 21.25. The cells of the organ of Corti are derived from the simple epithelium lining the membranous labyrinth which, embryologically, is of ectodermal origin. The basilar membrane is composed of fibrous tissue. Axially, it is attached to the osseous spiral lamina and laterally to the ***spiral ligament* SLig**, which consists of a marked thickening of the endosteum of the lateral wall of the cochlear canal. The thickened outer wall of the scala media is highly vascular and lined by a stratified epithelium; this area, known as the ***stria vascularis* SVasc**, is responsible for maintaining the correct ionic composition of endolymph.

The membrane between the scala media and scala vestibuli, the ***vestibular* (*Reissner's*) *membrane* VM**, is composed of extremely delicate fibrous tissue lined by simple squamous epithelium on both sides. The scala vestibuli and scala tympani are lined by a simple unspecialised squamous epithelium of mesodermal origin.

In Fig. 21.24b, bundles of afferent nerve fibres **N** can be seen arising from the base of the organ of Corti and converging towards the spiral ganglion **G** in the modiolus at the base of the spiral lamina. These ganglion cells represent the cell bodies of bipolar sensory neurones and their proximal axons form the auditory component of the eighth cranial nerve (see Fig. 21.26).

Sensorineural deafness

Sensorineural deafness is caused by damage to the sensory receptors of the inner ear (hair cells, organ of Corti) or the auditory nerve leading to the brain.

- Children may be born with sensorineural deafness due to intrauterine infection or poor oxygen supply near birth. Cochlear implants can restore hearing.
- Exposure to noise can cause loss of hearing due to damage to sensory elements in the organ of Corti.
- Age-related loss of high-frequency hearing has been called ***presbycusis***.

BM basilar membrane **G** spiral ganglion **O** osseous spiral lamina **N** nerve fibres **SL** spiral limbus **SLig** spiral ligament **SM** scala media **ST** scala tympani **SV** scala vestibuli **SVasc** stria vascularis **VM** vestibular membrane

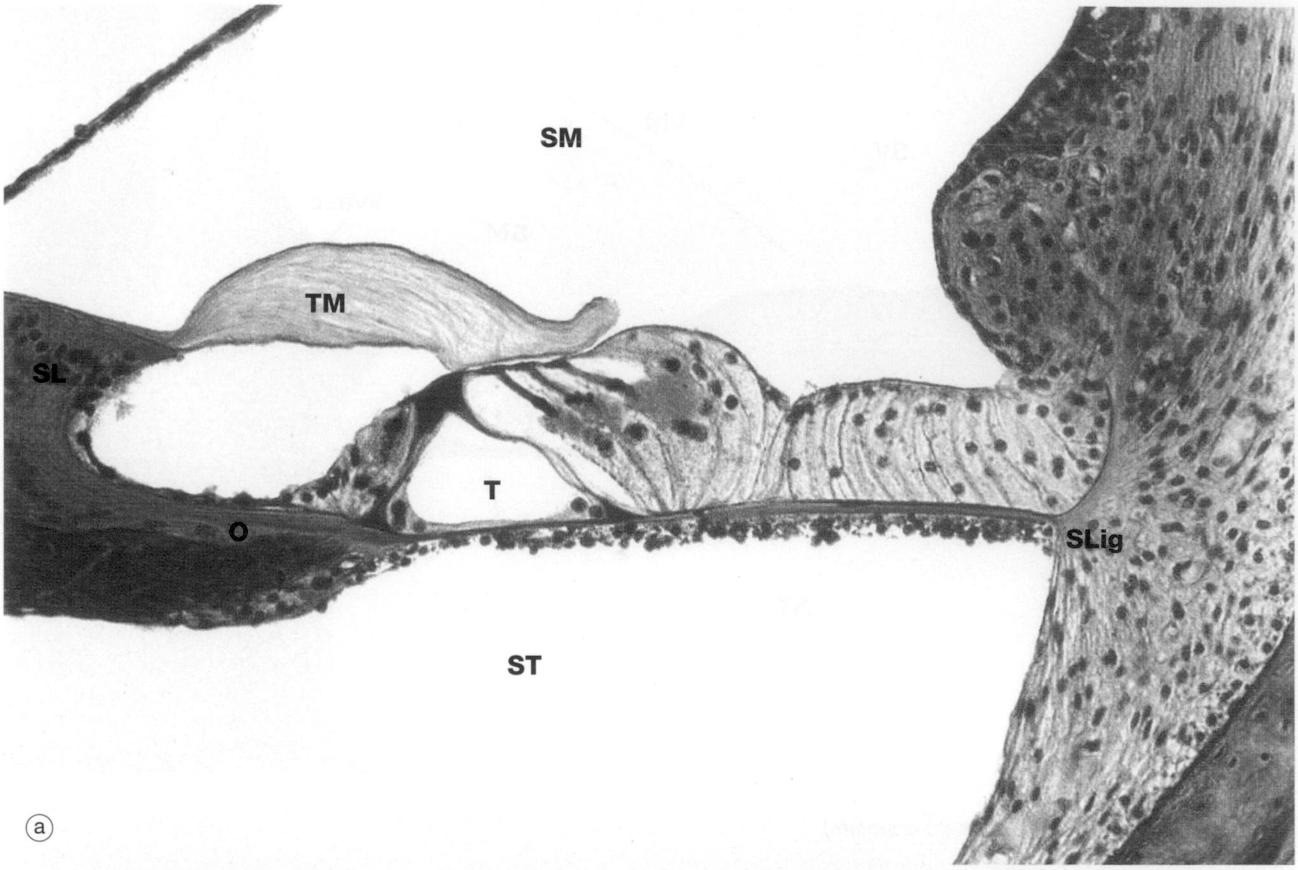

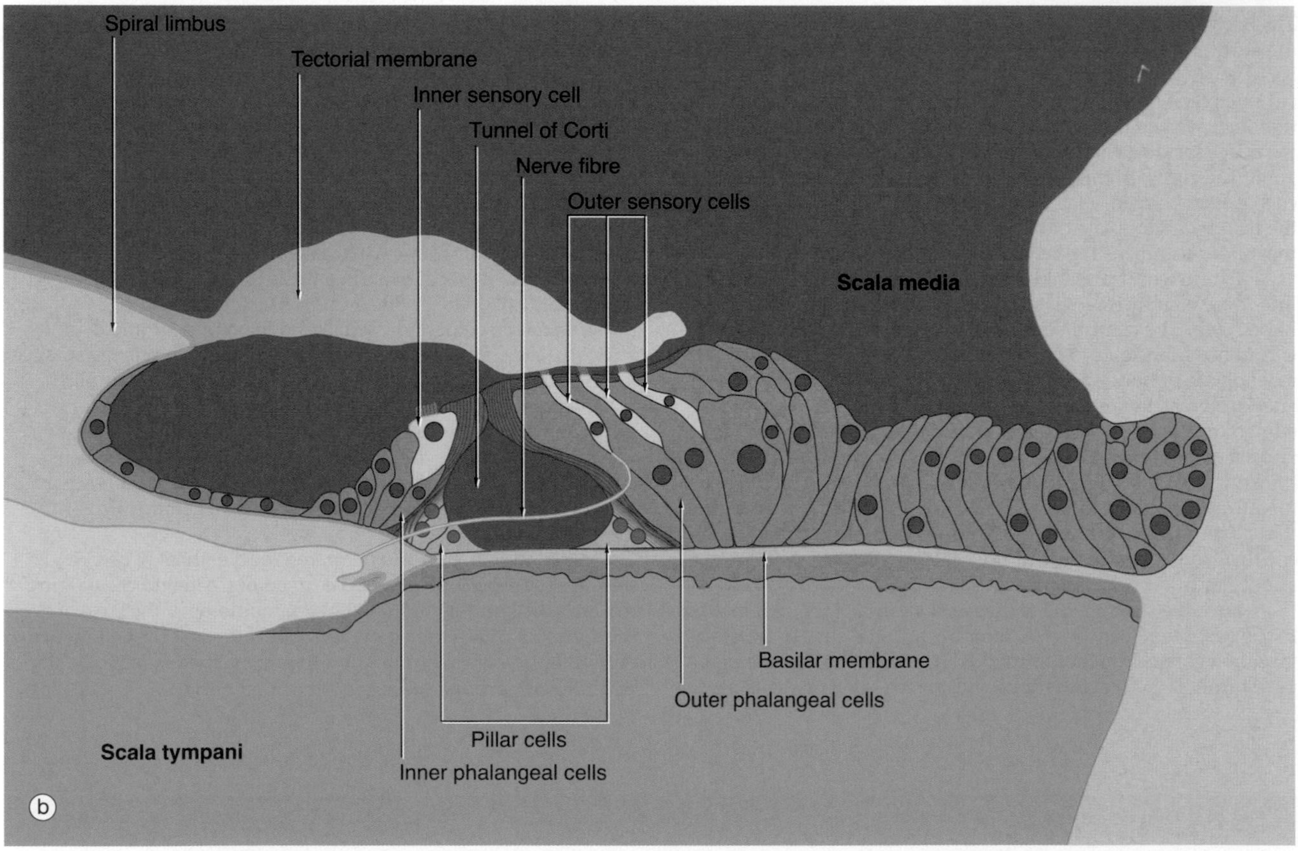

FIG. 21.25 Organ of Corti *(caption opposite)*
(a) H&E (HP) (b) Schematic diagram

O osseous spiral lamina **SL** spiral limbus **SLig** spiral ligament **SM** scala media **ST** scala tympani **T** tunnel of Corti **TM** tectorial membrane

FIG. 21.25 Organ of Corti *(illustrations opposite)*
(a) H&E (HP) (b) Schematic diagram

The ***organ of Corti*** is a highly specialised epithelial structure containing receptor cells which convert (transduce) mechanical energy in the form of vibrations into electrochemical energy, resulting in excitation of auditory sensory receptors (Fig. 21.25a).

The organ of Corti lies in the scala media **SM**, supported on the basilar membrane. The basilar membrane consists of a thin sheet of fibrous tissue stretched between the ***osseous spiral lamina*** **O** of the modiolus and the ***spiral ligament*** **SLig** laterally; its undersurface, exposed to the ***scala tympani*** **ST**, is lined by a simple epithelium. The basilar membrane is thinnest at the base of the cochlea and becomes progressively thicker as it spirals towards the apex.

The organ of Corti consists of two basic types of cells, ***sensory*** (***hair***) ***cells*** and ***support cells*** of several different types, including the ***inner*** and ***outer pillar cells*** and ***inner*** and ***outer phalangeal cells***. At the centre of the organ is a triangular-shaped canal, the inner tunnel or ***tunnel of Corti*** **T**, bounded on each side by a single row of tall columnar cells called ***pillar cells***. Each pillar cell contains a dense bundle (pillar) of microtubules and the pillars on either side of the tunnel of Corti converge at the surface and then curve laterally to form a thin, hood-like structure containing small fenestrations.

The cell bodies of the pillar cells lie in the acute angles formed by the pillars, and the basilar membrane at the floor of the tunnel.

On the inner aspect of the inner row of pillar cells is a single row of flask-shaped cells, the inner phalangeal cells, which support a single row of ***inner sensory*** (***hair***) ***cells***. The phalangeal cells contain microtubules, some of which support the base of the hair cells while others extend to the free surface around the hair cells. Beyond the outer row of pillar cells there are three to five rows of outer phalangeal cells which support the same number of rows of ***outer sensory*** (***hair***) ***cells***.

Cytoplasmic extensions of the phalangeal cells extend to the surface between and around the hair cells and their microtubules support the fenestrated hood-like structure formed by the pillar cells. Through the fenestrations project the free ends of the sensory cells. A variety of other specialised epithelial cells provides the remaining support for the organ of Corti.

The sensory cells are known as hair cells because numerous stereocilia, i.e. very long microvilli (see Fig. 5.15), project from their free ends. The stereocilia are embedded in the surface of the ***tectorial membrane***. As previously described, the spiral ganglion of the cochlea contains bipolar cell bodies of first order sensory neurones. From here, axons pass towards the base of the rows of hair cells, those going to the outer hair cells traversing the tunnel of Corti as shown in Fig. 21.25b. The end of each fibre ramifies into a number of dendrites which make synaptic contact with several hair cells; each sensory cell may synapse with dendrites of several different sensory neurones. In addition, inhibitory neurones arising in the brainstem send fibres which also synapse with the sensory cells and exert a suppressive effect.

From the layer of ***border cells*** which cover the ***spiral limbus*** **SL**, there extends a flap-like mass of glycosaminoglycans called the ***tectorial membrane*** **TM** overlying the sensory cells and within which the tips of the stereocilia are embedded.

Function of the organ of Corti

Only an outline of the mechanism of hearing is presented here; molecular details are being discovered at a rapid pace. Sound waves are funnelled into the external auditory meatus and impinge on the tympanic membrane, which vibrates at the appropriate frequency. These vibrations are transmitted to the stapes bone via the malleus and incus and, in the process, their amplitude is enhanced about 10-fold. The base of the stapes, which lies in the oval window, conducts the vibrations into the perilymph of the vestibule of the inner ear and pressure waves pass from here into the scala vestibuli of the cochlea. These pressure waves are probably conducted directly to the endolymph of the scala media across the delicate vestibular membrane, from which vibrations are induced in the basilar membrane upon which rests the organ of Corti. From here, spent vibrations are transmitted into the perilymph of the scala tympani and dissipated at the secondary tympanic membrane over the round window.

The basilar membrane is thinnest at the base of the cochlea and thickest at the apex. It appears that at every point on the spiral, the membrane is 'tuned' to vibrate to a particular frequency of sound waves reaching the ear; the overall range of frequencies encompassed is of the order of 11 octaves, with the highest frequencies (pitch) being sensed towards the base of the cochlea and progressively lower frequencies being sensed along the spiral towards the apex. For any given sound frequency, only one specific point of the basilar membrane and organ of Corti is thought to vibrate and thereby activate the appropriate hair cells to initiate afferent sensory impulses which then pass to the auditory cortex of the brain. Deformation of the stereocilia of the hair cells results in either depolarisation or hypopolarisation of the cell membrane which, in turn, excites the sensory nerves which synapse with them.

The sensory input from the cochlea is integrated in the brainstem and auditory cortex, from which efferent suppressor pathways can modulate receptor activity to enhance auditory acuity.

Inherited deafness syndromes

Approximately 50% of childhood deafness is caused by mutations in specific genes. Many of these genes have been found to code for proteins that affect function of the specialised sensory elements found in the inner ear. Approximately 70% of genetic hearing loss cases are nonsyndromic, meaning deafness is the only symptom, and 30% are syndromic, where deafness is part of a larger set of medical symptoms.

Mutations in genes coding for connexin proteins involved in formation of gap junctions (see Fig. 5.12) account for a large proportion of cases.

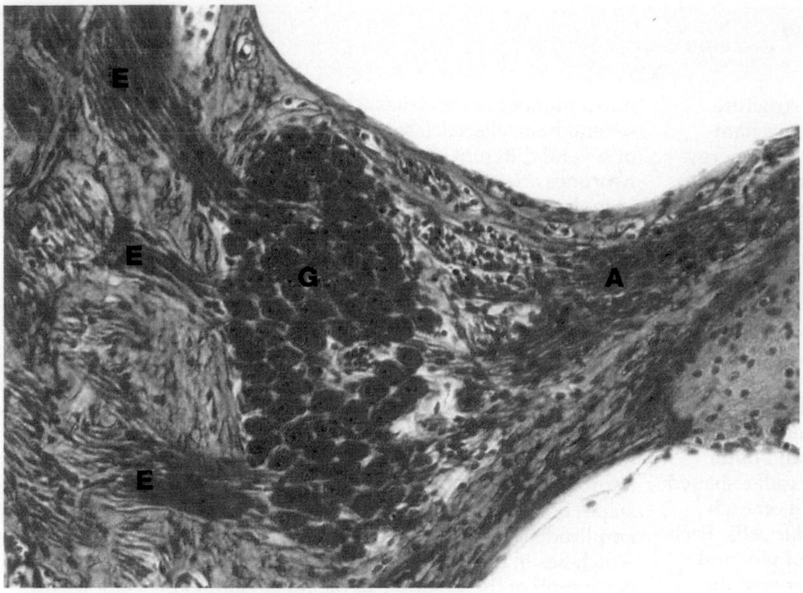

FIG. 21.26 Spiral ganglion
H&E (HP)

The spiral ganglion is a spiral-shaped mass of nerve cell bodies lying in a canal at the extremity of the osseous spiral lamina of the modiolus.

As seen in Fig. 21.26, the ganglion cells **G** have the typical appearance of somatic ganglion cells (see Fig. 7.20) and represent the cell bodies of bipolar sensory neurones, relaying information from the receptors of the organ of Corti to the brain.

Note the afferent fibres **A** entering the ganglion from the organ of Corti and numerous bundles of efferent fibres **E** which pass to the centre of the modiolus to form the cochlear nerve, the auditory component of the eighth cranial nerve; the cochlear nerve is readily seen in Fig. 21.24.

FIG. 21.27 Receptor organs of the saccule and utricle *(illustrations opposite)*
(a) H&E (HP) (b) H&E (HP) (c) SEM ×5000 (d) Schematic diagram

The ***saccule*** and ***utricle*** are two dilated regions of the ***membranous labyrinth***, lying within the vestibule of the inner ear and are filled with ***endolymph***. The walls of each are composed of a fibrous membrane which is bound down in places to the periosteum of the vestibule and, in other areas, is attached to the periosteum by fibrous strands, the intervening space being filled with ***perilymph***. Internally, the saccule and utricle are lined by simple cuboidal epithelium but, in each, there is a small region of highly specialised epithelium called the ***macula***, shown in Fig. 21.27a and b, containing receptor cells which contribute part of the sensory input to that part of the brain responsible for maintaining balance and equilibrium. The macula of the utricle is oriented at right angles to that of the saccule.

The maculae are made up of two basic cell types, ***sensory hair cells*** and ***support cells***. The support cells are tall and columnar with basally located nuclei and microvilli at their free surface. The hair cells lie between the support cells, with their larger nuclei placed more centrally. Each hair cell has a single eccentrically located cilium of typical conformation, often called the ***kinocilium*** (see Fig. 5.13), and many stereocilia (long microvilli; see Fig. 5.15) projecting from its surface, hence the name hair cells. The 'hairs' are embedded in a thick, gelatinous plaque of glycoprotein, probably secreted by the supporting cells; this is lost during histological preparation. At the surface of the glycoprotein layer is a mass of crystals mainly composed of calcium carbonate and known as ***otoliths***. These are shown in Fig. 21.27c.

There are two different forms of hair cells. ***Type I hair cells*** (***goblet cells***) are bulbous in shape and stain poorly, their nuclei tending to lie at a lower level than those of ***type II hair* cells** (***columnar cells***) which are more slender in shape. The type I hair cells are invested by a meshwork of dendritic processes of afferent sensory neurones, whereas the type II hair cells have only small dendritic processes at their bases. The hair cells also have synaptic connections with modulatory (inhibitory) neurones from the central nervous system.

Function of the maculae

The function of the maculae relates mainly to the maintenance of balance by providing sensory information about the static position of the head in space. This is of particular importance when the eyes are closed or in the dark or under water, and the maculae are consequently more developed in animals other than humans.

When the head is moved from a position of equilibrium, the otolithic membrane tends to move with respect to the receptor cells, causing bending of their stereocilia. When the stereocilia are bent in the direction of the cilium, the receptor cell undergoes excitation and, when the relative movement is in the opposite direction, excitation is inhibited. The orientation of the hair cells in different directions in the maculae causes different hair cells to be stimulated with different positions of the head. The pattern of hair cell stimulation allows the central nervous system to determine the position of the head very accurately with respect to gravity.

The neural pathways of the balance and equilibrium mechanism are complex, and the sensory input from the maculae is integrated with that of other proprioceptors, such as muscle spindles, to elicit reflex responses directed towards the maintenance of postural equilibrium.

A afferent nerve fibres **E** efferent nerve fibres **G** ganglion cells

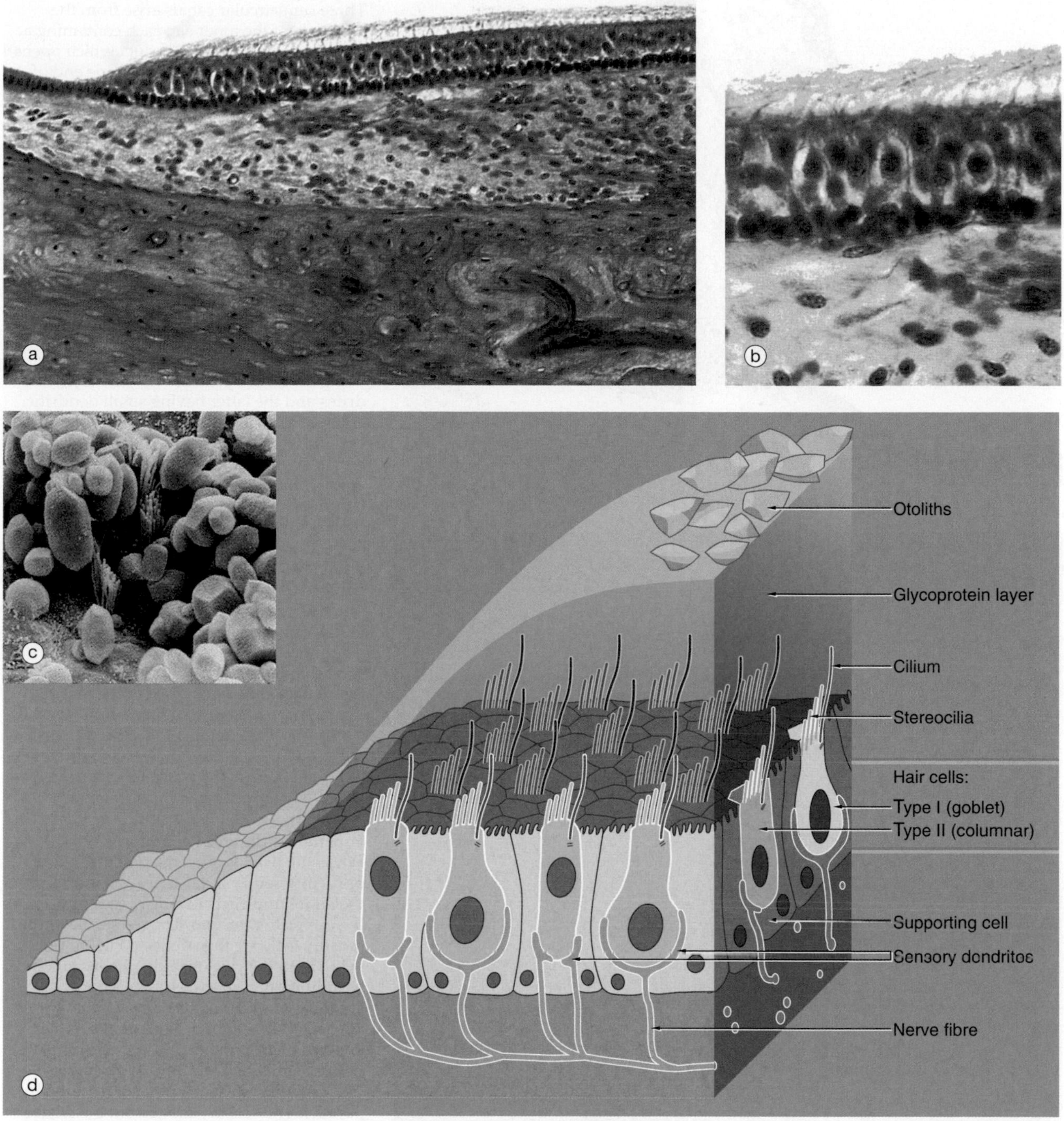

FIG. 21.27 Receptor organs of the saccule and utricle *(caption opposite)*
(a) H&E (HP) (b) H&E (HP) (c) SEM ×5000 (d) Schematic diagram

Diseases of the membranous labyrinth system

Ménière's disease is an abnormality of the inner ear. Clinically, affected patients experience dizziness, disturbance of balance (***vertigo***), a high-pitched rushing or roaring sound in the ears (***tinnitus***) and fluctuating hearing loss.

The symptoms of Ménière's disease are associated with an increase in endolymph volume within the membranous labyrinth system, which is believed to cause the membranous labyrinth to swell (endolymphatic hydrops), leading to development of abnormal signalling from receptors. The cause of this increase in endolymph remains uncertain. One possibility is rupture of the membranous labyrinth which allows the endolymph to mix with perilymph.

For patients with mild disease, treatment with symptomatic medication can be effective. For patients with debilitating disease, surgical ablation of parts of the labyrinthine system are effective but may involve permanent hearing loss.

Infusion of drugs known to be toxic to the sensory-neural apparatus (e.g. gentamicin) in the middle ear is also used for treatment.

Transient dysfunction of the labyrinthine system can be caused by viral infection (viral labyrinthitis). Patients develop severe dizziness, vertigo, nausea and vomiting which reaches a peak after about 24 hours and subsequently resolves within a week.

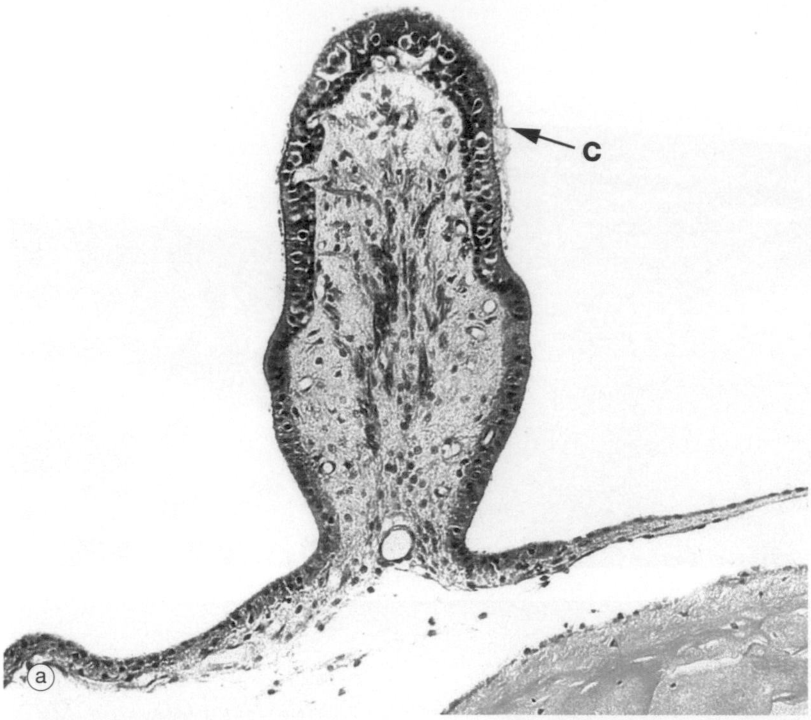

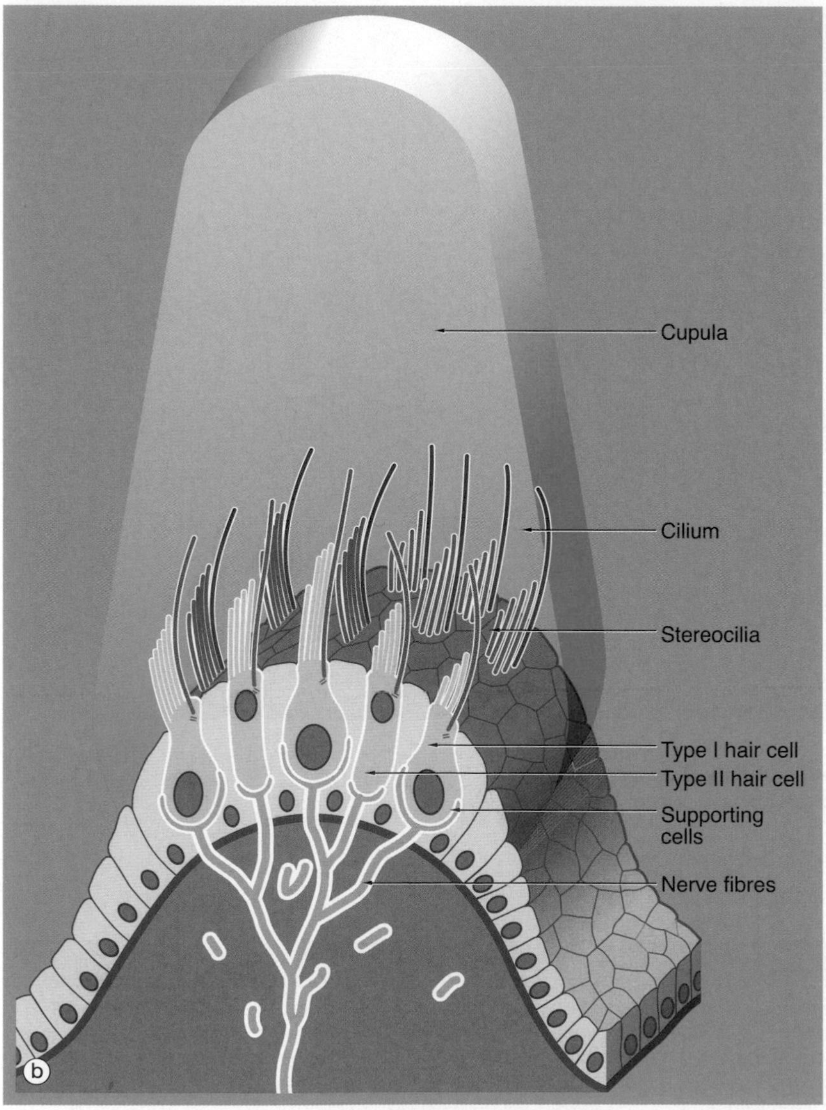

FIG. 21.28 Receptor organs of the semicircular canals
(a) Masson trichrome (MP) (b) Diagram

Three semicircular canals arise from the vestibule of the inner ear, each containing a membranous semicircular duct which opens at both ends into the utricle. At one end of each duct is a dilated portion, the ampulla, which contains a receptor organ called the ***crista ampullaris***, shown in Fig. 21.28a.

Each crista ampullaris is an elongated epithelial structure situated on a ridge of supporting tissue, arising from the membranous wall of the ampulla and oriented at right angles to the direction of flow of the endolymph in the semicircular canal (Fig. 21.28b). Structurally, the cristae ampullares bear many similarities to the maculae of the utricle and saccule (see Fig. 21.27). The hair cells are of the same two morphological forms, ***type I*** and ***type II cells***, the former being invested by a basket of sensory dendrites and the latter having small dendritic endings at the base only. The hair cells are supported by a single layer of columnar cells which is continuous with the simple cuboidal epithelium lining the rest of the membranous labyrinth.

Like those of the maculae, the hair cells of the cristae have numerous ***stereocilia*** and a single ***kinocilium***, the kinocilium being situated at the margin of the cell nearest to the utricle. The stereocilia and the kinocilia of the hair cells are embedded in a ridge of gelatinous glycoprotein which is tall and cone shaped in cross-section, giving rise to the term ***cupula***. In contrast to the macula, the cupula does not contain otolithic crystals.

Traces of the cupula **C** can be seen on the surface of the crista ampullaris in Fig. 21.28a, although most of it has been lost during histological preparation of the specimen.

Function of the crista ampullaris

When the head is moved in the plane of a particular semicircular canal, the inertia of the endolymph acts to deflect the cupula in the opposite direction. The stereocilia of the sensory cells are then deflected towards or away from the cilia, resulting in excitation or inhibition, respectively. In each ear, there are three semicircular canals, two at right angles to each other in vertical planes and one in a near-horizontal plane. Each is paired with a semicircular canal in the other ear, the members of each pair being oriented in parallel. The sensory input from the cristae ampullares mainly concerns changes in the direction and rate of movement of the head. Afferent impulses pass via bipolar sensory neurones with cell bodies in the vestibular ganglion which lies at the base of the internal auditory meatus. Afferent fibres pass via the vestibular part of the eighth cranial nerve to the brainstem, cerebellum and cerebral cortex, where sensory information from various other sources is integrated for the maintenance of balance, position sense and equilibrium.

C cupula

REVIEW

TABLE 21.1 Review of special sense organs

Major structures	Main components or cells	Brief description/ functional attributes	Figure
Taste buds	Chemoreceptors located in the tongue	Mainly located in the circumvallate papilla Taste – bitter, sweet, salty, sour	21.1
Olfactory receptors	Olfactory epithelium in roof of nasal cavity formed of chemoreceptor neurones which connect to olfactory bulbs; outgrowths of the brain but called cranial nerve I	Smell	21.2
Eyes			
Retina	Rods	Light intensity photoreceptors concentrated peripherally	21.6, 21.7
	Cones	Light colour photoreceptors concentrated centrally	
	Fovea	Retinal area in central axis, all colour receptors (cones)	21.9
	Macula lutea	Retina near to fovea; near-maximum vision; mostly cones, some rods	
	Optic disc	Site of exit of optic nerve; no photoreceptors	21.10
Cornea	Epithelium	Transparent stratified squamous epithelium which allows light into the eye	21.15
	Stroma	Densely arrayed specialised collagenous fibres and support cells; no blood vessels; transparent	21.15
Sclera	Fibrous layer forming the eye globe	Supports the globe; continuous with corneal stroma	21.4
Uvea	Choroid	Intermediate layer between sclera and retina; contains blood vessels; supplies retina by diffusion Deeply pigmented to prevent light reflection in globe	
	Ciliary body	Secretes aqueous humor (fluid) into posterior chamber; maintains pressure in globe & globe shape Supports lens; smooth muscle exerts tension on lens via zonule; varies focal length via tension on lens	21.11
	Iris	Soft tissue with smooth muscle and pigment, forming variable-sized diaphragm, the pupil Smooth muscle controls diameter of pupil, varying light entry	21.12
	Canal of Schlemm	Removes fluid from anterior chamber following its circulation from posterior chamber; controls globe pressure	21.13
Lens	Elongated cells containing special proteins which lose their nuclei and form a lens	Attached to ciliary body; tension on lens varies focus	21.14
Ear (hearing)			
External	Pinna and canal	Reception of sound; hair and wax glands protect canal	21.19, 21.20
Middle	Middle ear space and Eustachian tube	An air-filled space Eustachian tube equilibrates air pressure	21.23
	Tympanic membrane	Thin fibrous membrane, separates external and middle ear Vibrates with sound waves	21.22
	Ossicles	Chain of bones, malleus, incus and stapes, with synovial joints and muscle. Incus covers oval window. Transfer sound vibrations to oval window, vibrating perilymph	21.22
Inner	Labyrinth (three parts: vestibule, semi-circular canals and cochlea)	Endolymph fluid in a membrane-bound space, often surrounded by fluid (perilymph) and located in bone Round window dissipates pressure fluctuations	21.20
	Cochlea	Conical spiral-shaped structure containing organ of Corti Converts perilymph vibration to neural signals (i.e. hearing)	21.24
Ear (balance)			
	Semi-circular canals	Sensory ridges in canals detect fluid flow caused by head movements Part of sense of balance for movement	21.28
	Vestibule	Utricle and saccule are perilymph spaces containing sensory areas, maculae with overlying otoliths. Part of sense of balance/ equilibrium for static position	21.27

PART

IV

APPENDICES

APPENDIX

1 Introduction to microscopy

PREPARATION OF A GLASS SLIDE

Histology is about looking at structure, and in this introductory section we aim to provide some guidelines to assist the absolute beginner in examining and interpreting the images in this book. Examination of any biological tissue under a microscope requires a number of preparation steps. These complex techniques are performed by highly skilled professionals known as biomedical scientists who are key members of diagnostic pathology and medical research laboratories. Details of these techniques are outwith the scope of this text, however a brief overview is given below.

Further information is also provided in Chapter 1 of *Wheater's Pathology* (6th edition). Once any fresh tissue (human or animal) is removed, it will generally require the following steps to produce a glass slide for examination under a light microscope. This is vital to ensure the tissue is preserved and remains firm enough for processing, cutting and staining, and also to preserve the slide so that it can be stored and viewed as and when required. Some of these steps are illustrated below and are described in greater detail at the end of this appendix.

1) FIXATION and TRIMMING

Fixation of fresh tissues is essential to prevent autolysis (breaking down) of the tissues. Formalin solutions are normally used for this purpose and help to preserve the tissues for processing and cutting (see below).
Once fixed, the area of interest in the tissue can be trimmed (dissected) so that it will fit onto a glass slide. Smaller samples do not require this step.

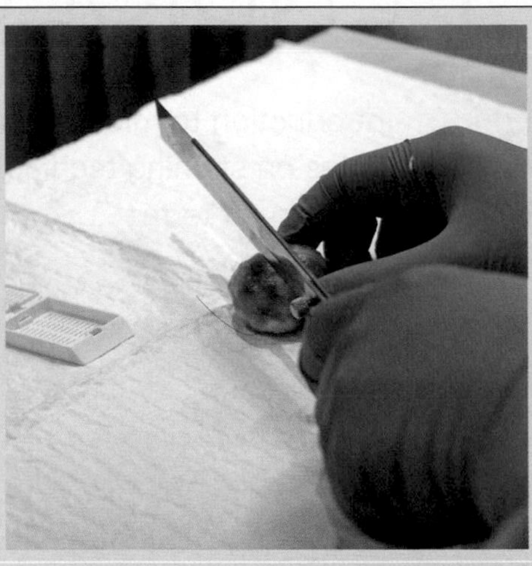

2) PROCESSING and EMBEDDING

Processing includes the steps involved between fixing the tissues and impregnating the tissues with paraffin wax. These steps can be carried out by hand but are most commonly performed using a processor machine. The tissue is dehydrated in graded alcohol solutions.
Embedding is when the processed tissue is infiltrated by hot liquid paraffin wax and placed in a mould. When cool, this solidifies into a block which provides a firm cutting surface for the next step.

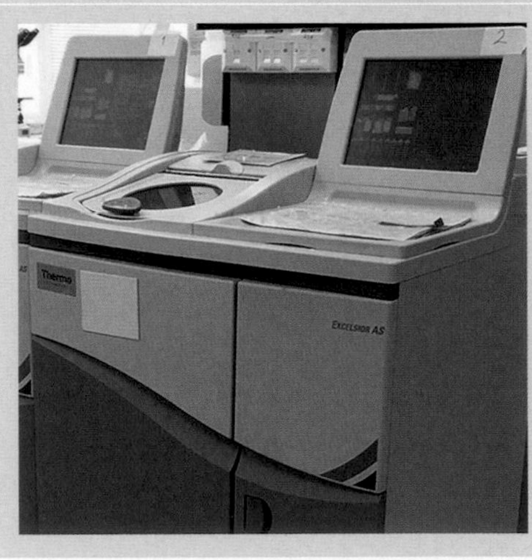

3) MICROTOMY

Very thin slices of tissue (3–5 μm) can be cut from this solid wax block using a special knife called a microtome. These thin tissue sections are floated on a water bath and then mounted on a glass slide.

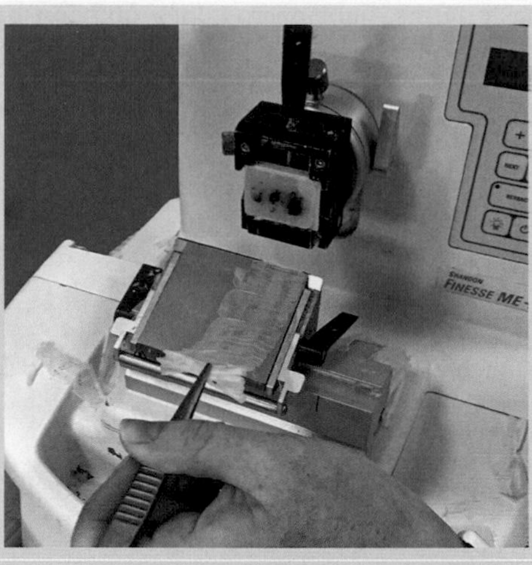

4) STAINING AND COVER SLIPPING

The tissue section is colourless at this point as illustrated and requires staining with special tissue dyes or antibodies in order to view the tissues under a microscope. These stains are further discussed in Appendix 2.
A protective glass cover (cover slip) is applied to protect the underlying tissue.

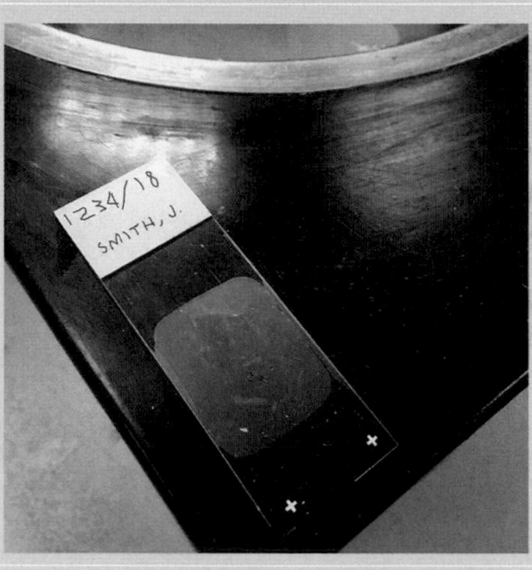

5) FINAL PRODUCT

This is a skin sample which has been stained with haematoxylin and eosin, commonly referred to as 'H&E'. Three tissue sections have been provided on the same slide, allowing easy examination under the microscope.

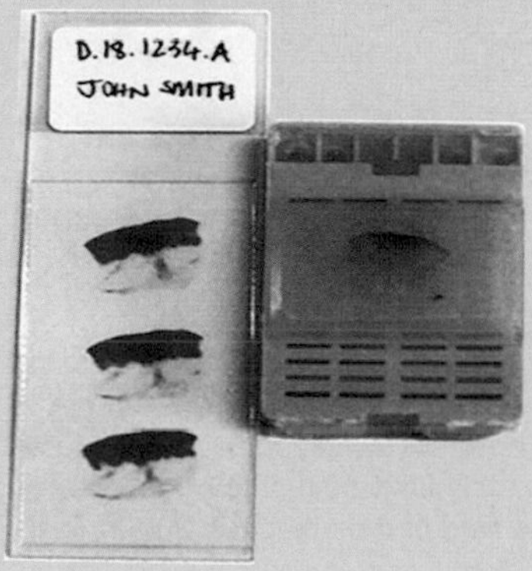

MICROSCOPY

Light microscopy

Light microscopes are an essential tool for most histologists, scientists and pathologists around the world. For histology in particular, light microscopy (LM) has revolutionised our ability to study the structure and function of cells and tissues at high resolution. Many of the images illustrated in this book have been derived from light microscopes. The function of LM is based on the principles of the refractile quality of light when passed through a lens or series of lenses. There are many different types of light microscope, including brightfield, phase contrast and confocal, which allow examination of fixed tissues (see above), organisms or even live cells such as those in cell culture.

In basic terms, light microscopes function by using a beam of light which, when focused through a specimen, produces an image that is then magnified using a lens or objective. With a compound microscope, there are two or more lenses which can further magnify the image. Finally, the image can be viewed by eye using an eyepiece. The component parts of a compound light microscope and the basic steps in setting up a microscope are illustrated below.

SETTING UP A LIGHT MICROSCOPE

A) SET EYEPIECES

1) Turn on the illumination switch, taking care not to set the light too high.
2) Ensure objective lens (×4 or ×10) is in place.
3) Adjust the interpupillary distance between the eyepieces by hand so that the light circles seen through the eyepieces with each eye merge to form one circle.
4) Place a slide on the stage, coverslip upwards
5) Focus using the coarse (large) and then the fine (smaller) focus by closing one eye so that the image appears sharp.
6) Accommodate the other eye by turning the diopter ring on the eyepiece.
7) Repeat the focussing process using the high power ×40 lens.

B) SET CONDENSER

1) Close the diaphragm aperture so that the light field is small.
2) Focus the field diaphragm using the condenser focus.
3) Centre the field diaphragm using the centre adjustment dials on the condenser (see image below).

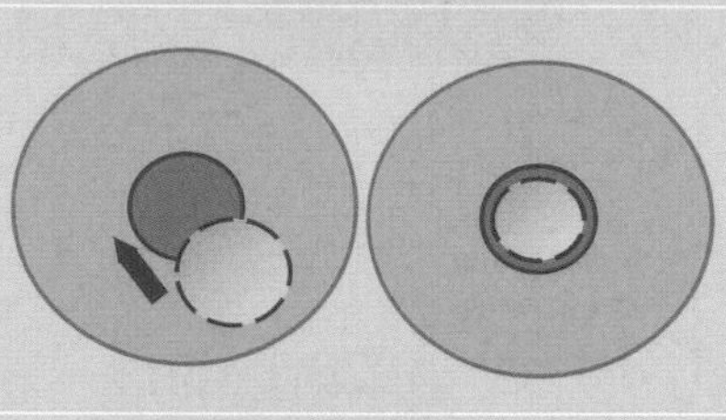

4) Repeat for each objective to check the field diaphragm is centred in each.

C) SET CONTRAST

1) Remove one eyepiece and look down the tubing.
2) Turn the aperture switch up full then reduce by approximately 25% so that aperture diaphragm is just inside the field of the objective.

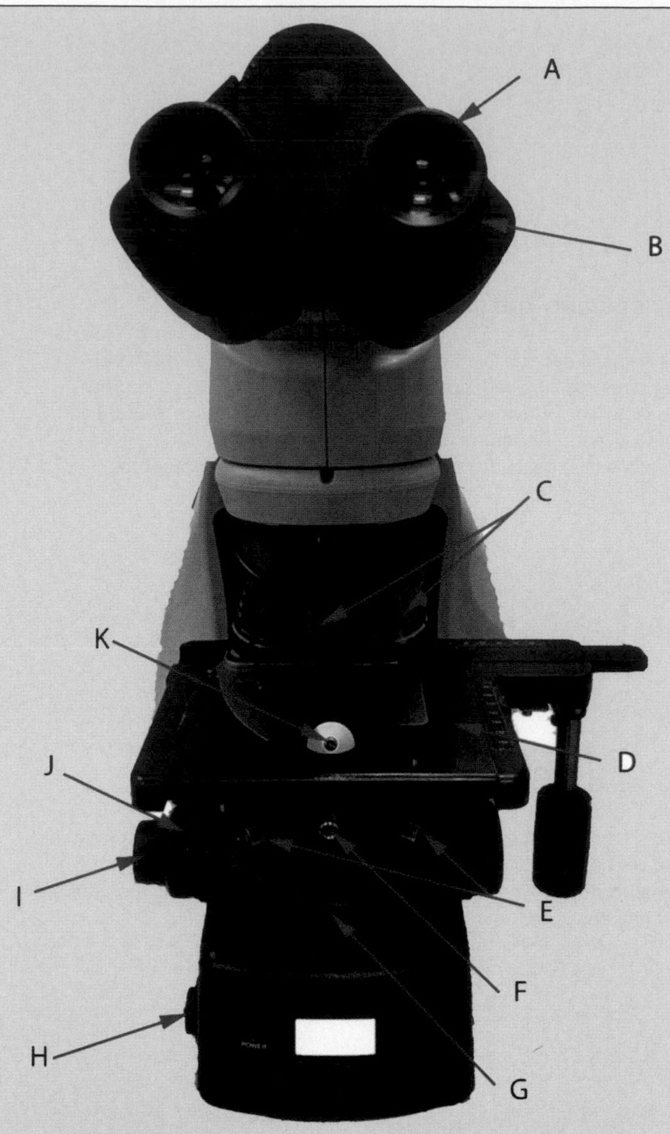

Key:
A – ocular lens (eyepiece)
B – diopter adjustment
C – objective lenses
D – stage
E – centre adjustment dials
F – condenser iris adjustment
G – field diaphragm adjustment
H – light switch
I – fine focus adjustment
J – coarse focus adjustment
K – condenser

Digital microscopy

It is now possible to digitally scan and view histology slides on a high resolution computer screen rather than using a traditional light microscope. These platforms are particularly useful for educational purposes, especially where online learning is required. Many pathology laboratories now use digital pathology instead of microscopes as the primary method for reviewing slides. The technology also facilitates image analysis and is especially valuable in research settings.

Light microscopy versus electron microscopy

This book mainly uses photomicrographs taken with the ***light microscope*** (***LM***) (colour images) and the ***electron microscope*** (***EM***) (black and white images). Simply put, the LM and EM differ in ***optical resolution*** and ***available magnification***. In practical terms, 'resolution' refers to the capacity of an optical system to reveal detail in a specimen. The resolution available from a conventional LM is only about 0.2 μm. Thus, at distances of less than 0.2 μm, objects that are actually separate from one another will appear to merge. In contrast, EM resolution for biological specimens is as little as 1 nm, so that the resolving power is about 200-fold better than LM. In addition, maximum 'available magnification' is limited to about ×1000 in most student LMs, whereas an EM readily achieves 100-fold greater magnification, or about ×100 000. EM images are therefore said to display cell and tissue ***ultrastructure***.

EM images may be two-dimensional or three dimensional

There are two types of electron microscope: ***scanning EM*** and ***transmission EM***. Scanning EM produces three-dimensional (3D) images, but these are restricted to the surface of the object, with the internal structure concealed from view. Transmission EM is so named because the electron beam must pass through the specimen to form an image. To achieve this, ultrathin sections (50–100 nm) must be cut. Transmission of the electron beam through the tissue results in a two-dimensional (2D) image of the plane of the section. In practice, transmission EM is more informative of biological ultrastructure, and these images predominate in this book. We have supplemented these with scanning EM images where it helps with 3D conceptualisation (see Fig. 16.13). As a matter of convention, the abbreviation EM can be assumed to be a transmission EM, while we have identified scanning EMs as SEM.

Light and electron microscopy are complementary

The strengths of LM and EM differ yet complement one another very effectively. With LM, one can observe large areas of a specimen (usually several cm^2). A wide range of staining methods, some empirical, some specific, are available for LM, permitting identification of cell and tissue features; many of these stains are polychromatic, i.e. they produce multiple colours in the specimen which, besides looking pretty, help to identify different components. For certain specimens, sections slightly thicker than usual may be used to demonstrate 3D features. Thus from LM, students can expect to gain an understanding of overall cell and tissue architecture.

The superior resolution and magnification of EM permit visualisation of many features which simply cannot be seen by LM. Yet in some respects, EM is less flexible than LM. For example, the available area in EM specimens is generally less than 1 mm^2 and this may make it difficult to obtain representative fields. Few staining methods are available for EM and these produce only monochromatic (black and white) images. EM is also costly and time-consuming and usually not available to the average student.

Hints and tips for interpreting EM images

Interpretation of EMs can be quite challenging due to the wide range of magnifications available (×500–190 000 in this book). In other words an EM image is not necessarily of very high magnification. In fact, there is an overlap in the magnification ranges of EM and LM. It is a good idea to consciously note the magnification and/or scale bar on each image in the book. The terms ***electron-dense*** and ***electron-lucent*** are used to describe the relative darkness and lightness, respectively, as they appear in transmission EM images. Sections examined by EM are almost featureless unless stained with heavy metals (e.g. uranium and lead salts) that bind to cell and tissue components to varying degrees. Significant binding of metal stain to a particular structure will impede transmission of the electron beam through the specimen at that point; the structure will appear dark grey or black and is said to be electron-dense (really too dense to allow passage of electrons). Other structures with little or no affinity for the stain will appear lighter grey or white and are termed electron-lucent because they permit greater transmission of the electron beam.

A useful starting point in interpreting EMs is to select several commonly found structures that you can confidently identify and memorise their dimensions. These can then be used as 'internal rulers' to gauge the dimensions of numerous other features in the field. For example, plasma membrane and organelle membranes will be visible at medium magnifications as thin electron-dense lines that measure about 10 nm wide. Thus, structures such as intermediate filaments (10 nm in diameter and solid) and microtubules (20–25 nm in diameter but hollow) can be identified. Similarly, individual ribosomes and glycogen particles are 20 to 30 nm in diameter. Being alert to major size differences between organelle types will instill further confidence. For example, nuclear diameter (5–10 μm in most cells) is up to 10 times greater than the diameter of lysosomes and mitochondria (0.2–1.0 μm) and up to 100 times greater than individual Golgi transport vesicles (50–100 nm). The next step is to actively look for the unique set of features that characterises and distinguishes each organelle and inclusion. For example, only mitochondria and the nucleus possess a double membrane, and in mitochondria the inner of these two membranes is thrown into highly characteristic folds.

High-magnification electron micrographs are often required to demonstrate particular features but usually display only a tiny region of the cell. Therefore, do not be surprised if many of the common organelles are not seen in the field. A reliable indicator of high magnification is if an individual membrane appears trilaminar rather than as a single electron-dense line. At low magnification, EM interpretation can actually be more difficult because membranes and the smallest organelles are no longer clearly visible. Get orientated by looking first for the biggest objects, i.e. nuclei and boundaries of the cells themselves and next for the mid-sized organelles such as mitochondria. Regions of interface between cells and extracellular tissue can give clues about tissue heterogeneity. Micrographs of a neutrophil using both LM (left) and EM (right) are illustrated below.

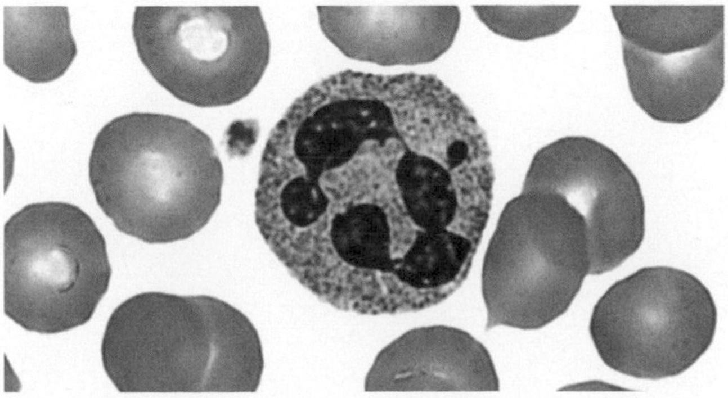

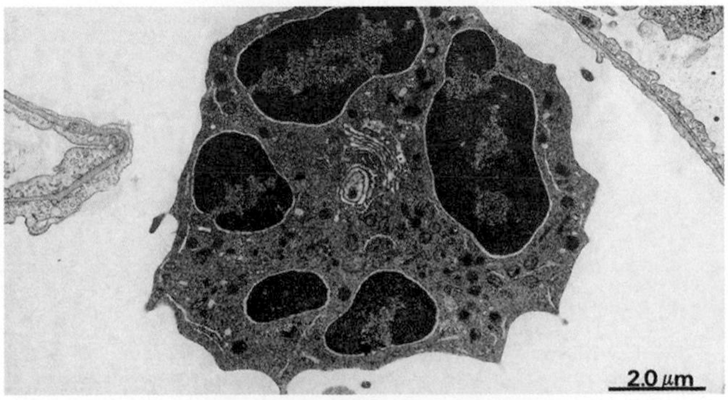

Specific localisation methods for LM and EM

The traditional staining techniques of histology, developed in the last two centuries from dyes used in the textile industry, remain valuable and widely used as empirical methods for LM. Subsequently, a range of specific methods was developed, enabling LM visualisation of defined intracellular and extracellular constituents. More recently, technical refinements have allowed conceptually similar specific localisations to be achieved at EM level.

One major group of specific methods known as ***histochemical techniques*** employs reagents known to react with defined cellular constituents (e.g. lipids, glycogen and DNA), thereby producing selective colouration recognisable by LM. In a subset known as ***enzyme histochemistry*** the activity of enzymes can similarly be demonstrated by staining for their specific substrates or end products; these methods are often applicable for both EM and LM. A further subset termed ***immunohistochemistry*** is very widely used in modern diagnostic pathology. Immunologically based, this newer method offers high specificity and sensitivity of localisation. In essence, antibodies are raised against specific cellular components (in this context, the antigen) and then conjugated with a visual marker appropriate for LM or EM (e.g. dyes, enzymes, tiny particles of colloidal gold). When the antibody is then applied to the tissue under study, it binds to the antigen. Hence, the site of antibody–antigen binding becomes flagged by the chosen visual marker (see Fig. 1.15; Appendix 2, 'Notes on staining techniques').

Constraints in LM and EM – aspects of tissue preparation

A problem common both to light and electron microscopy is the need to prevent autolytic degeneration and to preserve cellular ultrastructure. Fixatives such as ***formaldehyde*** and ***glutaraldehyde*** are used for this purpose. ***Fixation*** causes cross-linking of macromolecules, which reduces and often arrests biological activity, at the same time rendering the cells more amenable to staining. Most tissues are too thick to be examined directly in the microscope and must therefore be cut into very thin slices (***sections***). To facilitate the cutting of thin sections, the tissue is usually ***embedded*** in a hard medium such as paraffin wax (LM) or a plastic resin (EM); fixed tissues generally require dehydration with organic solvents before the embedding step. Each stage in the fixation, dehydration, embedding, sectioning and final staining sequence may induce ***artefacts*** (distortions in cell and tissue architecture, e.g. shrinkage). In situations where preservation of biological activity of cell constituents (e.g. enzymes) is the major objective, thin sections for histochemistry can be obtained from minimally fixed or unfixed frozen tissue; such ***frozen sections*** have their own particular artefactual distortions. As noted above, unstained sections are quite lacking in contrast when viewed by conventional LM or EM. However, special types of LM (***phase contrast***, ***interference contrast***, ***confocal microscopy***) have been developed to address this limitation and are frequently used, for example, to monitor living tissue cultures.

APPENDIX

2 Notes on staining techniques

HISTOCHEMICAL STAINING TECHNIQUES

Most histological stains are dyes which, when applied to tissues, form a chemical bond with proteins within the tissues. Staining tissue sections is essential to differentiate between the different cells and tissues on the slide, permitting examination by light microscopy. Many histological and pathological features can be identified using routine histological stains and by far the most commonly used is haematoxylin and eosin or 'H&E'. This is regarded as the 'bread and butter' stain of both histology and pathology. Additional stains, as detailed below, can help to illustrate particular features within tissues such as collagen or mucin production and to identify infective organisms. If these routine stains do not provide an answer, there are further ancillary stains which can be applied such as immunohistochemistry and immunofluorescence. Further details are provided in the boxes below.

Haematoxylin and eosin (H&E)

This is the most commonly used stain in histology and pathology. Haematoxylin is a basic dye which stains acidic structures a purplish-blue. In contrast, eosin is an acidic dye which stains basic structures pinkish-red. In the mammalian cell, most of the acidic structures reside in the nucleus due to the presence of nuclear DNA, whereas most of the cytoplasmic structures are basic. Thus, nuclei stain purplish-blue and the cytoplasm a pinkish-red. If a cell's cytoplasm contains abundant RNA, then the cytoplasm may have a purplish tint. In the first micrograph, the serous cells of the parotid gland show dense granular purple cytoplasm which is full of zymogen granules.

The intensity of the staining by H&E depends upon many factors including tissue processing and fixation, the thickness of the tissue section and the formulation of the stain. The thickness of the section has the most impact upon the staining intensity as can be seen in some thicker, low-power images throughout this text.

The second micrograph shows early secretory endometrium with subnuclear vacuolation in the glands which are easily demarcated from the background endometrial stroma.

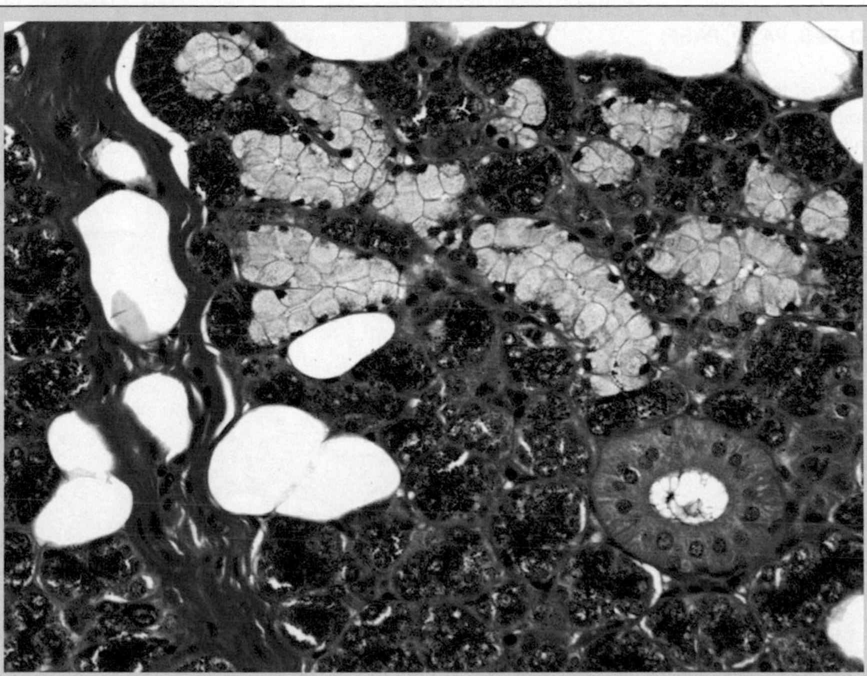

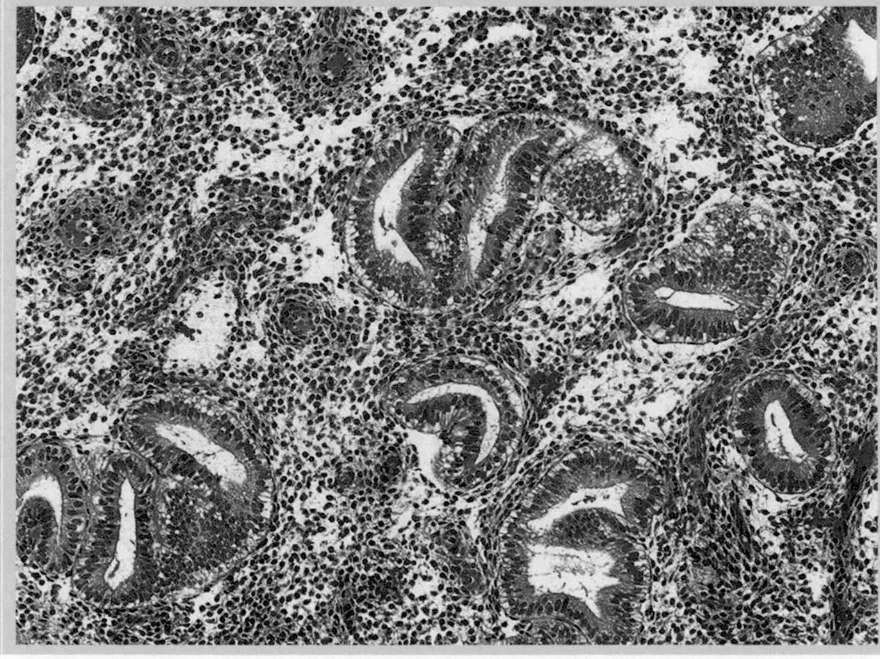

Periodic acid–Schiff (PAS)

The periodic acid–Schiff (PAS) reaction demonstrates the presence of complex carbohydrates by staining them a deep magenta colour. This is referred to as ***'PAS positive'***. PAS will stain pure complex carbohydrates, such as glycogen in hepatocytes and muscle cells, but will also stain carbohydrates when they are bound to lipids and proteins. Basement membranes and the brush borders of kidney tubules and the small and large intestines are PAS positive, as is cartilage and some collagen.

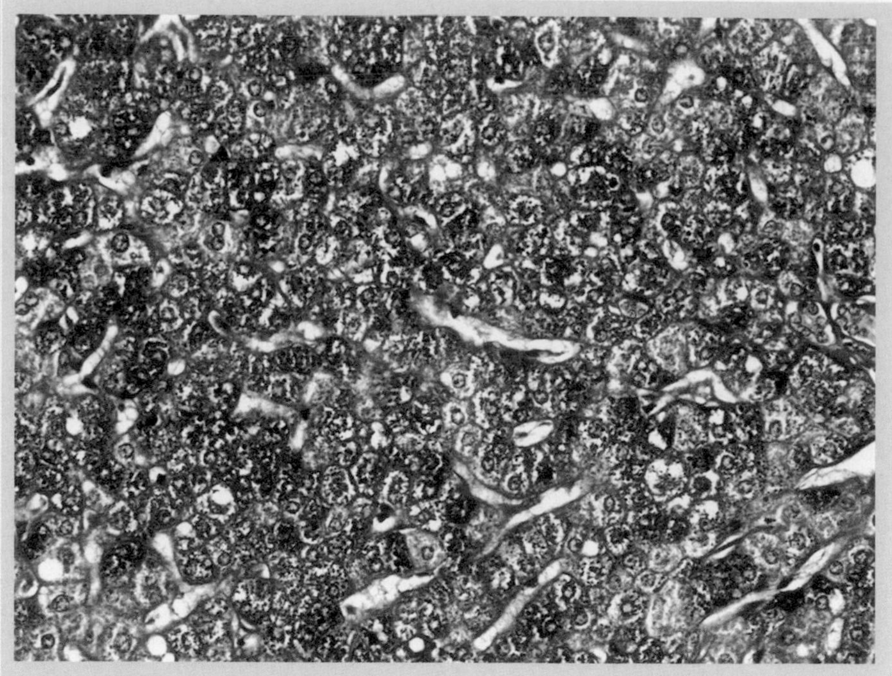

Diastase periodic acid–Schiff (D-PAS, PASD, PASF)

Many of these complex carbohydrate–lipid or protein compounds are present in basement membranes, fungal cell walls and some neutral mucin. In order to differentiate between pure glycogen and these other compounds, glycogen can be eradicated in the tissue section by pre-treatment with the enzyme diastase (amylase) prior to the PAS reaction.

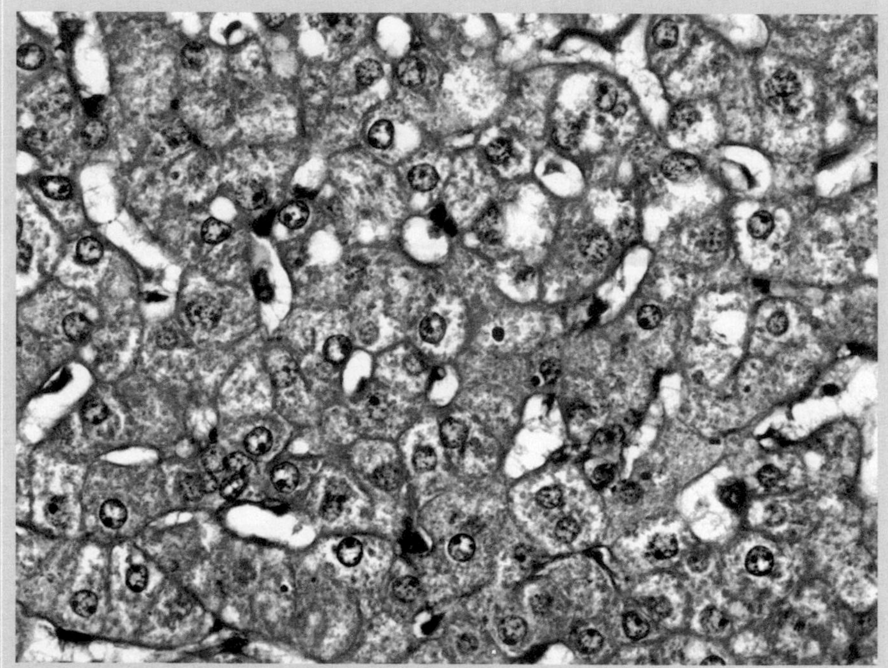

Alcian blue (acid mucin)

Epithelial mucins secreted by epithelial cells are either acidic or neutral. Acidic mucins are present in goblet cells and oesophageal submucosal glands. Most invasive adenocarcinomas also produce acidic mucin. Alcian blue stains acidic mucin a vivid blue colour. In contrast, neutral mucins, e.g. those present in gastric foveolar cells and prostate glands, are PAS positive. Alcian blue can also be used in combination with other stains such as H&E or van Gieson.

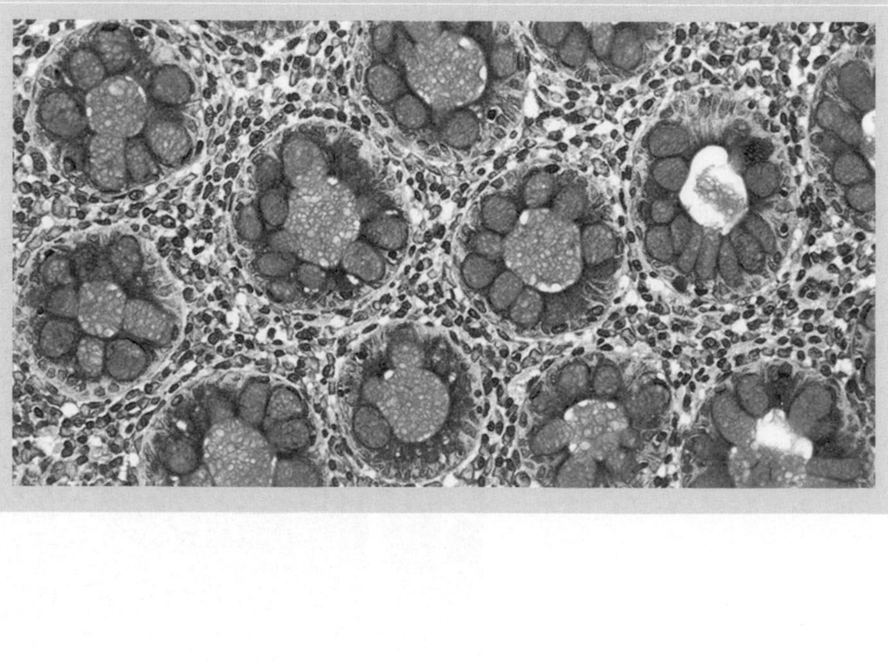

Masson trichrome

Masson trichrome is a connective tissue stain as it is used to demonstrate supporting tissue elements such as collagen. As the name implies, this staining method produces three colours in tissue sections. Nuclei and other basophilic structures are stained black, collagen is stained green or blue depending on which variant of the staining protocol is used, and muscle, erythrocytes and keratin are stained bright red. In pathology, it is used routinely in liver and kidney biopsies.

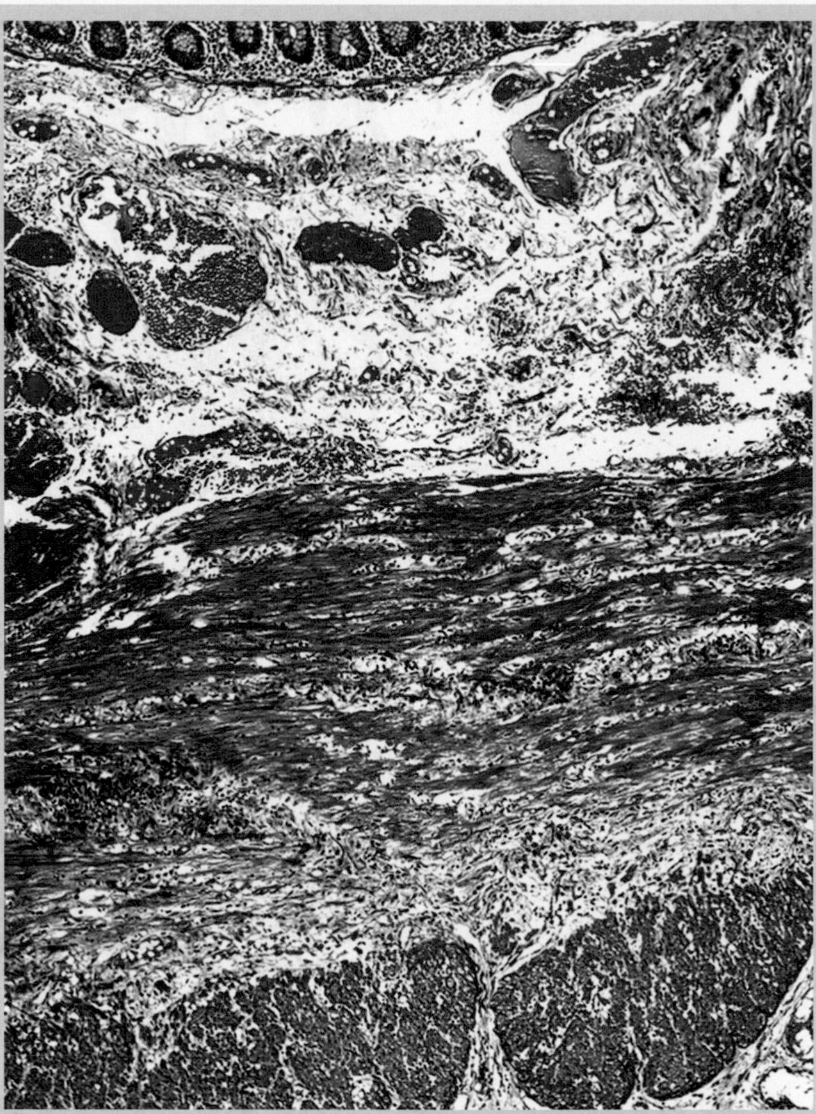

Martius Scarlet Blue (MSB)

MSB is another connective tissue stain. This three-colour staining method stains fibrin red, erythrocytes yellow and collagen blue. It is also useful for the examination of thrombi in histological sections, particularly in the autopsy setting.

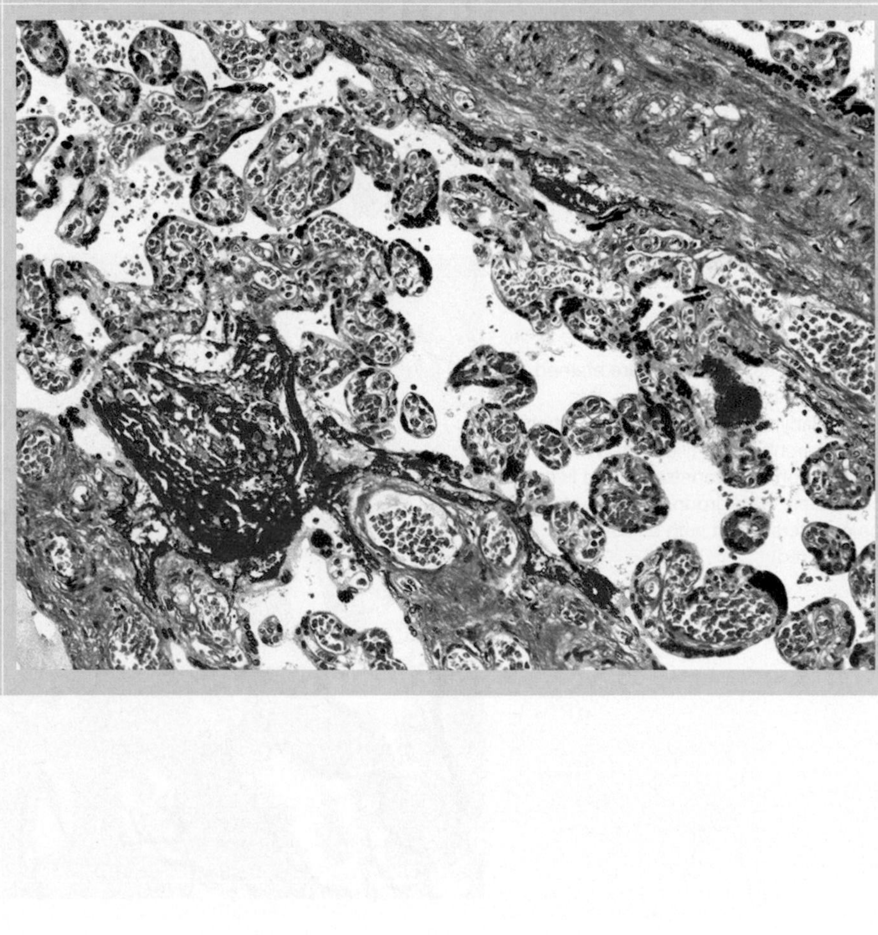

Miller's elastic van Gieson (EVG)

This stains collagen red and elastic fibres black. It is particularly useful in staining the elastic laminae of arteries (black), the smooth muscle of the media and erythrocytes (yellow) and collagenous tissue (red).

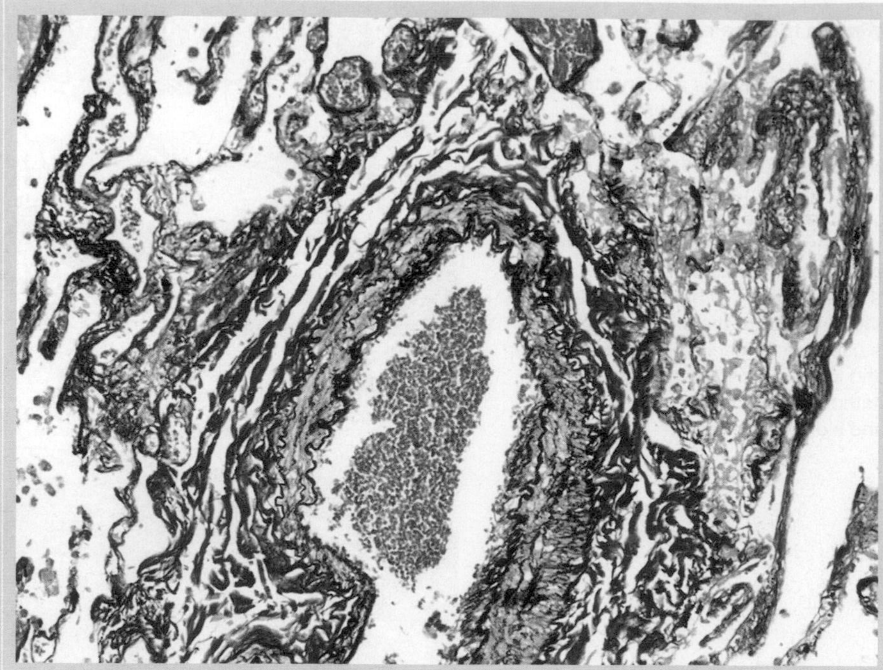

Phosphotungstic acid haematoxylin

This stain demonstrates muscle cross-striations such as in the myocytes of the heart. It may also be used to demonstrate the presence of mitochondria in particular types of tumours.

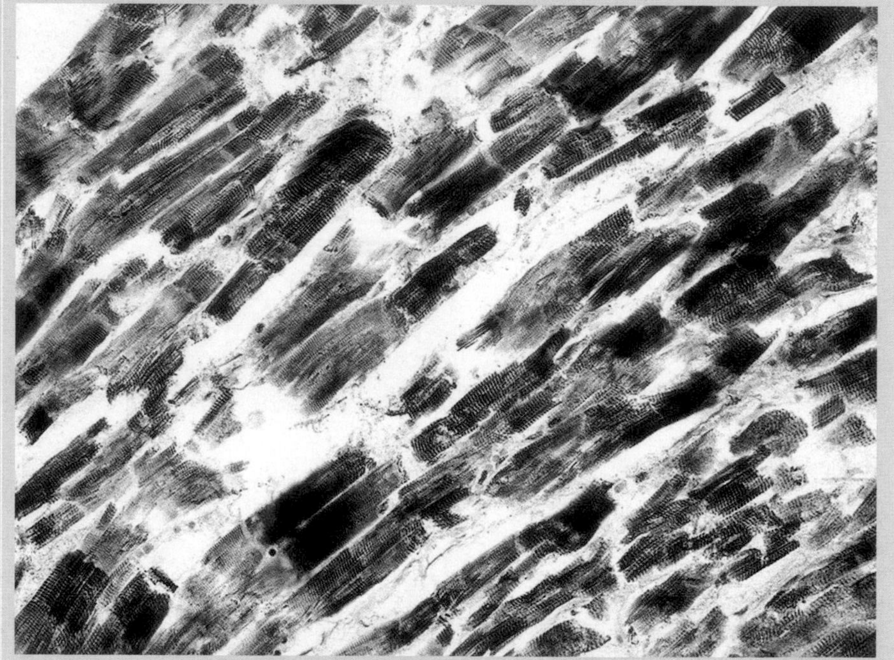

Gordon & Sweet's reticulin

This is a silver-based stain that demonstrates reticulin fibres of supporting tissues which are stained blue/black by this technique. It is particularly useful in the interpretation of liver architecture (illustrated in the micrograph), demonstrating the liver cell plates. Background tissues may be counterstained with a red dye (neutral red).

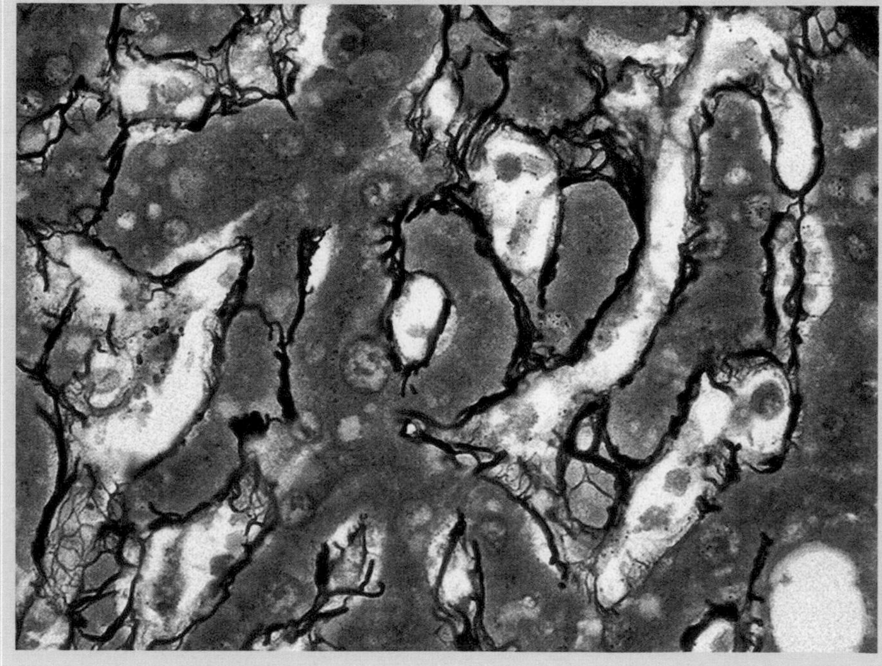

Sirius red

This stain is most commonly used to detect amyloid deposits. These are acidophilic (eosinophilic) deposits of abnormal protein which can occur in many different tissue sites. Amyloid is characterised by beta pleated sheets on electron microscopy. Congo red is a similar stain to Sirius red. Both stain amyloid red and display apple-green birefringence under polarised light.

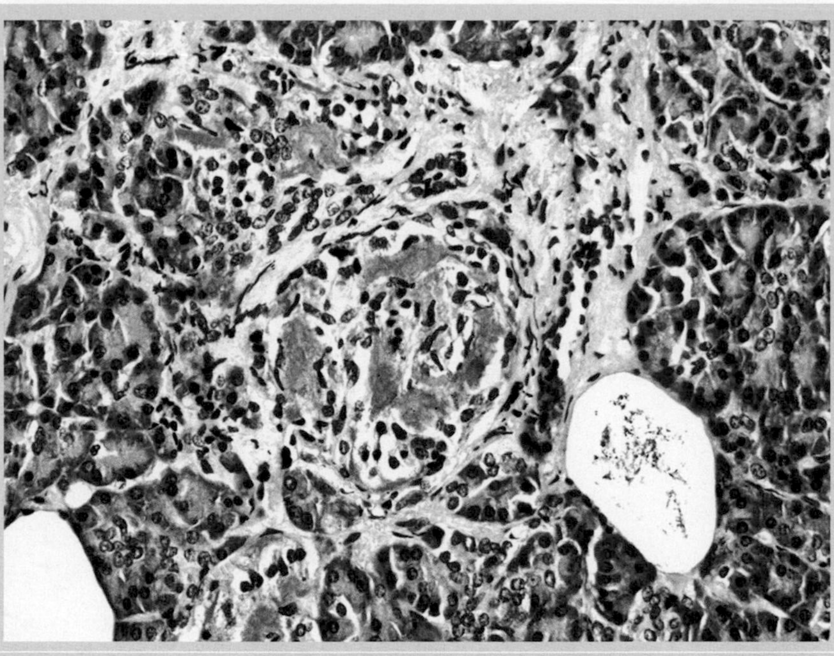

Giemsa stain

This stain is mainly used to stain smears of blood cells and other cells e.g. in bone marrow and in neuropathology. It can also be used to demonstrate some microorganisms. Nuclei are stained dark blue to violet, background cytoplasm pale blue and erythrocytes pale pink.

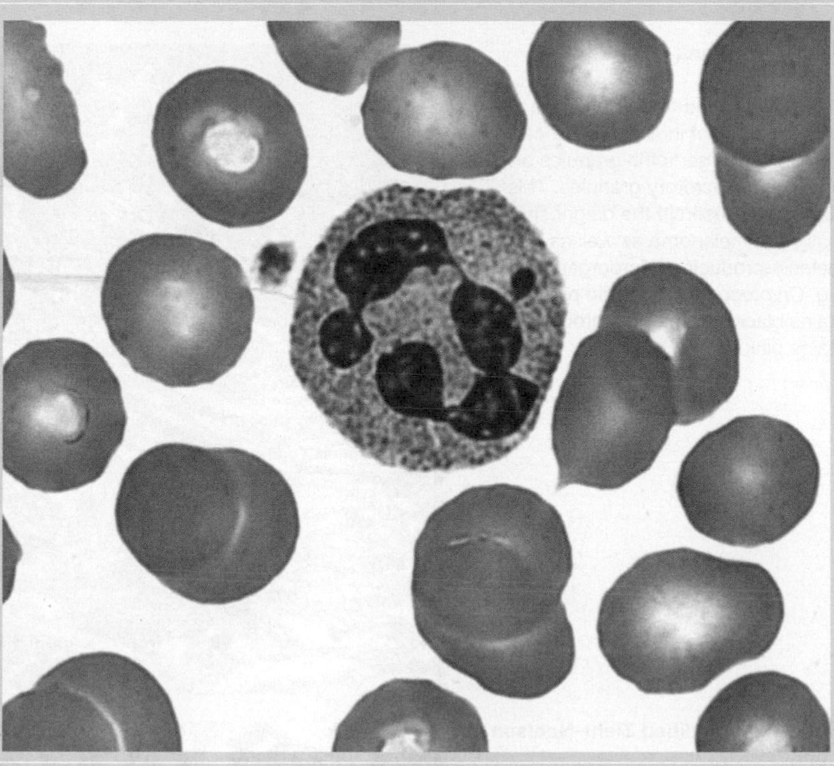

Gram stain

This method is mainly used in smears of bacteria in diagnostic microbiology, but can also be used in histological sections to show whether any bacteria are present and, if so, whether they are Gram-positive or Gram-negative. Gram-positive bacteria stain dark blue as illustrated in the micrograph opposite.

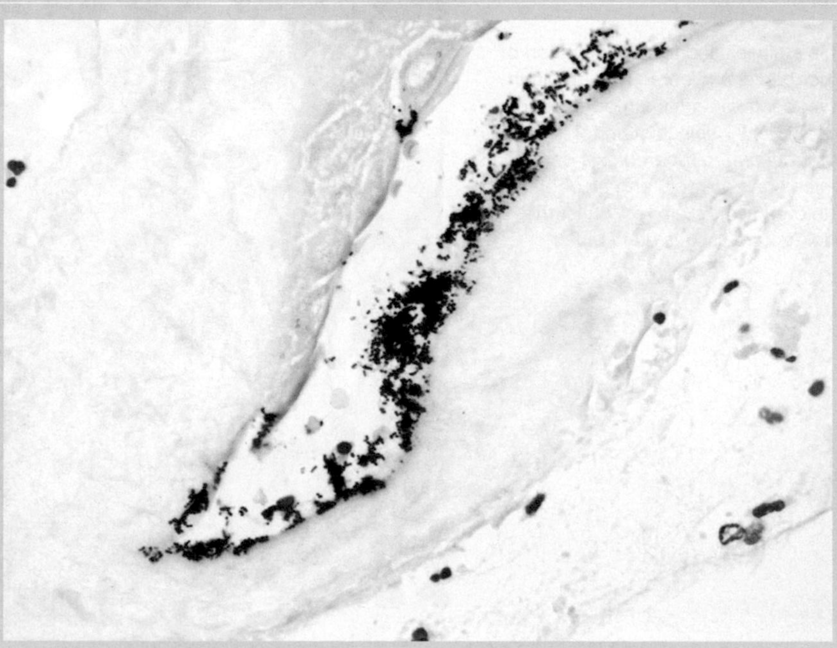

Perls' stain

This stain is used to demonstrate the presence of ferric iron in tissues, usually at the site of old bleeding where the iron-containing pigment, haemosiderin (derived from local haemoglobin breakdown), accumulates. It can also be used to demonstrate accumulation of iron in various tissues in the primary iron storage disease haemochromatosis and can be used for the identification of ferruginous asbestos bodies in lung tissue sections.

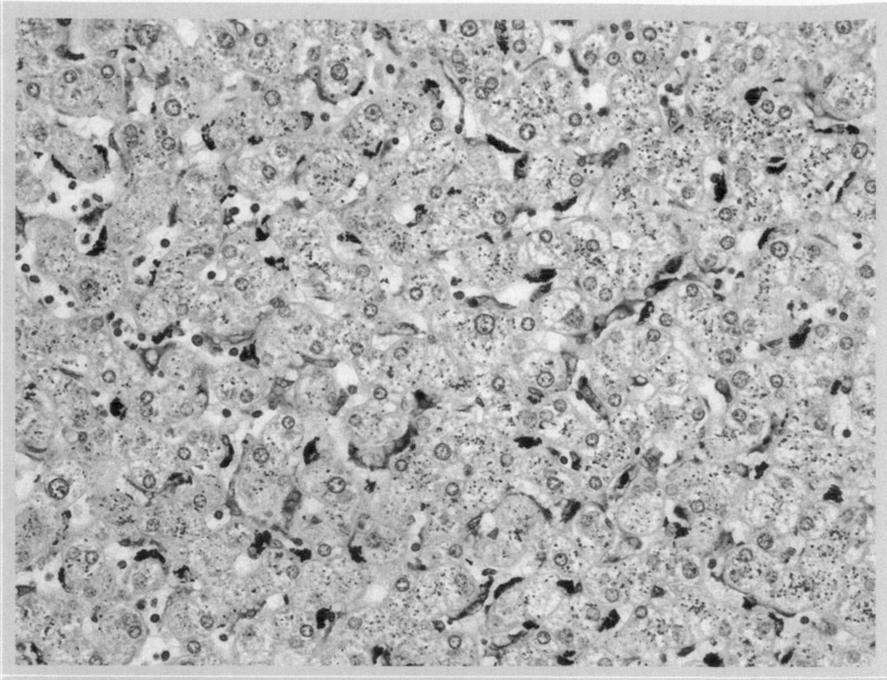

Masson-Fontana

This stain is used to demonstrate melanin pigment in tiss ues but can also identify argentaffin granules and some neurosecretory granules. This stain can be used in the diagnosis of malignant melanoma as well as some melanin-producing microorganisms, e.g. *Cryptococcus*. Melanin pigment stains black and the background tissue stains pink.

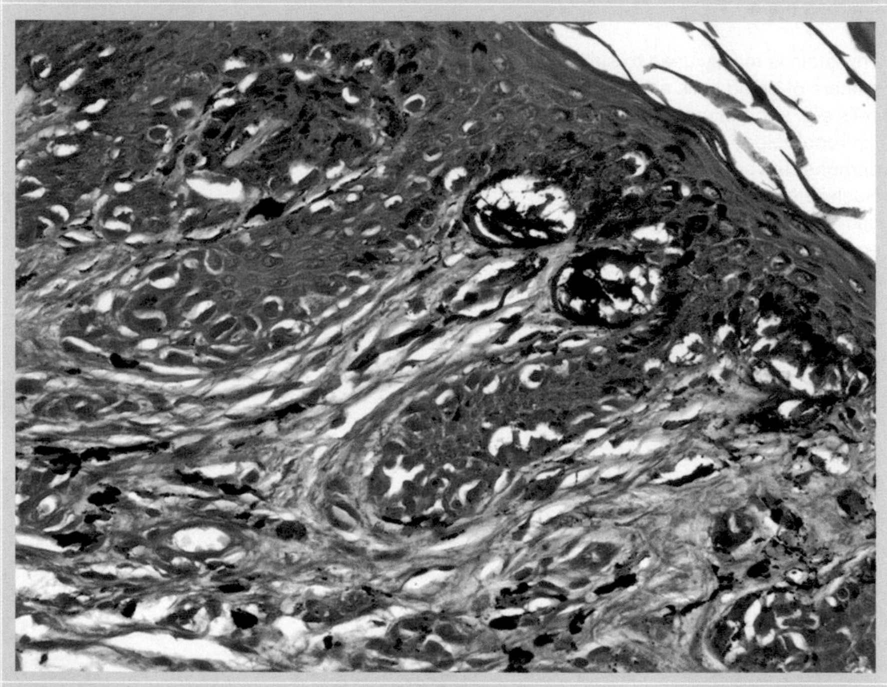

Wade–Fite (modified Ziehl–Neelsen stain)

This stain is used for identification of *Mycobacterium leprae* and atypical *Mycobacteria* and is a modification of the Ziehl–Neelsen stain for *Mycobacterium tuberculosis* organisms which are more acid and alcohol fast. The organisms stain red whilst the background tissues stain blue.

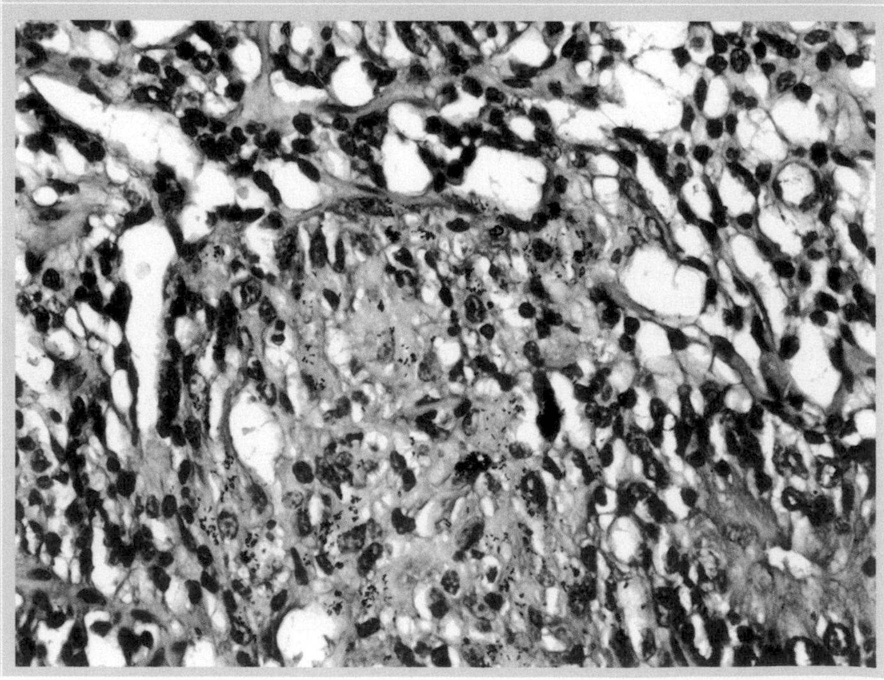

Ziehl–Neelsen

This stain can be used to demonstrate *Mycobacterium tuberculosis*. This bacterium possesses a protective capsule containing lipids that affects the rate at which dyes move into and out of the organism during staining. Two dyes are used, basic fuchsin mixed with phenol and methylene blue. The first dye (which is red) is forced into all the tissues in the section (including any *Mycobacteria*) by heating. The section is then exposed to acid and alcohol which wash the red dye out of everything except the *Mycobacteria*, which hold on to it because of the lipid capsule. All the other tissues are free to take up the contrasting blue dye, but the *Mycobacteria* remain red against a blue background.

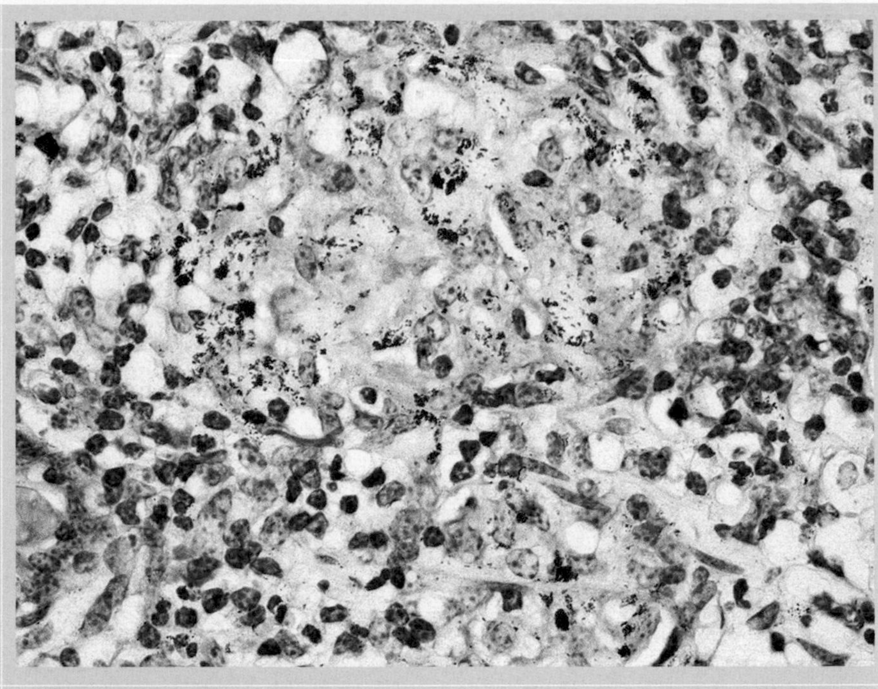

Goldner's trichrome stain

This method is applied to acrylic resin sections of undecalcified bone to distinguish between mineralised bone and unmineralised osteoid. It has a haematoxylin component which also stains the nuclei of osteoblasts, osteocytes, osteoclasts and marrow cells.

The von Kossa silver method stains calcium deposits black. It can be used in a variety of scenarios, including distinguishing between mineralised bone and osteoid and in identifying dystrophic calcium in tissues and in conditions such as pseudogout and malakoplakia.

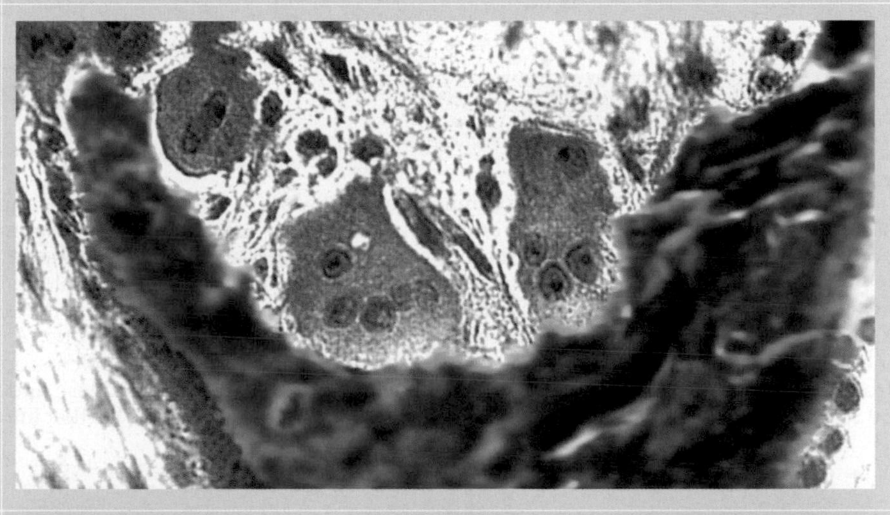

Cresyl fast violet

This is a basic dye commonly used in staining tissues of the brain and spinal cord. The neuropil stains purplish/blue and the Nissl substance of neurones stains dark blue due to the abundance of RNA. A modified version of this stain is also used to stain *Helicobacter pylori* organisms in gastric biopsies as illustrated in the micrograph.

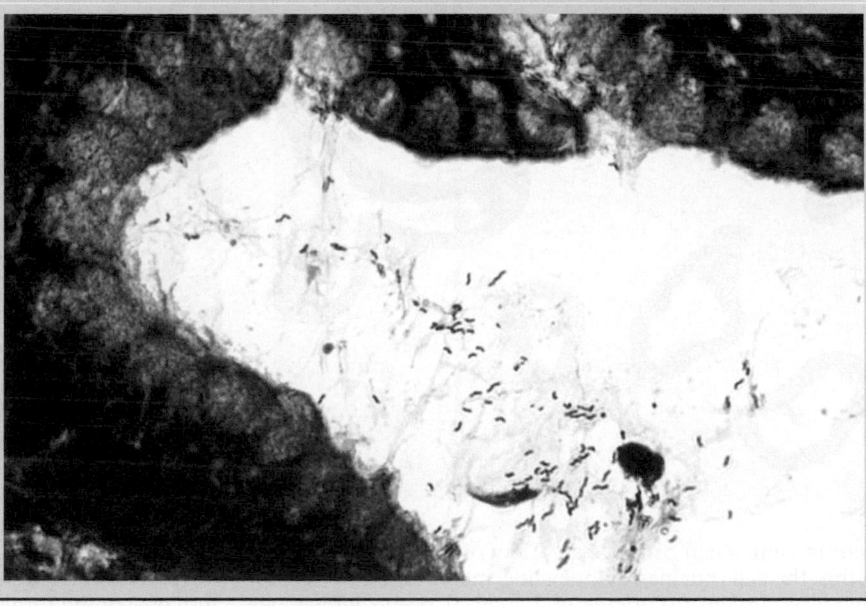

IMMUNOLOGICAL TECHNIQUES

A variety of immunohistochemical techniques are vital for diagnostic purposes in pathology as well as for research. The basis of the technique and some examples are given below. Further examples are also illustrated throughout this book to highlight specific histological features.

Immunohistochemistry (IHC; also known as immunocytochemistry) is a staining method based on the antigen–antibody reaction. IHC markers are antibodies that are produced commercially and target particular antigens (e.g. nuclear proteins, cytoplasmic proteins, cell adhesion proteins) in cells and tissues. There are hundreds of commercially available IHC markers which may highlight different components of tissues, e.g. smooth muscle markers (SMA, desmin and H-caldesmon) stain normal smooth muscle and smooth muscle tumours. IHC can provide useful information in normal histology to identify particular cells or identify the function of a cell/tissue and therefore this technique is often utilised in research laboratories. IHC is also extensively used by diagnostic pathologists for a variety of purposes such as identifying the site of origin of primary tumours, as prognostic and predictive markers in cancer and to screen for genetic diseases. Interpretation of IHC staining is complex and outwith the scope of this book, however some basic points are discussed below and throughout the organ system chapters. There is also more detailed information in Chapter 1 of *Wheater's Pathology* (6th edition).

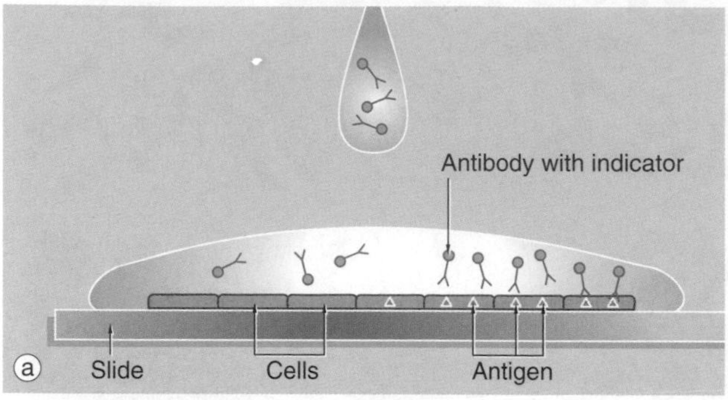

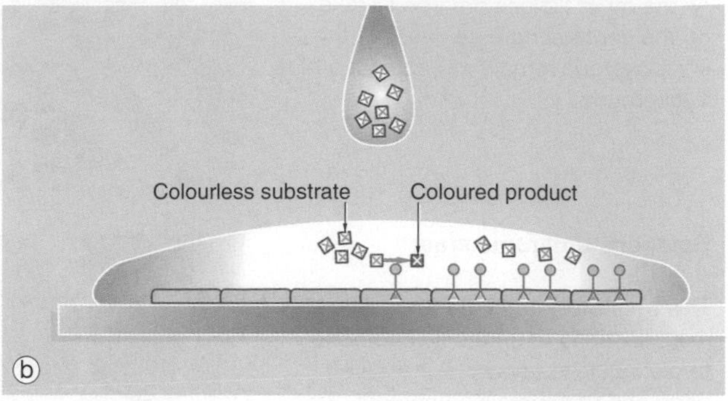

The basic technique of immunostaining is as follows: a section is placed on a glass slide (a) and a solution of antibody is laid over the issue. The antibody binds to the antigen of interest in the tissue and excess antibody is washed away so that only cells with the particular antigen have antibody bound to them. The antibody is pre-linked to an indicator substance (b). This is transformed by an enzyme from a colourless substrate to a coloured product which can be viewed by light microscopy. An enzyme commonly used for this purpose is horseradish peroxidase and the technique is known as the immunoperoxidase reaction. The substrate may also be a fluorescent substance such as fluorescein, in which the technique is known as ***immunofluorescence***, and the position of the antibody can be viewed by a fluorescence microscope. A further modification of this principle for electron microscopy uses antibodies linked to gold which is electron dense and can be detected by EM (immunogold labelling). Further information on EM is given in Appendix 1.

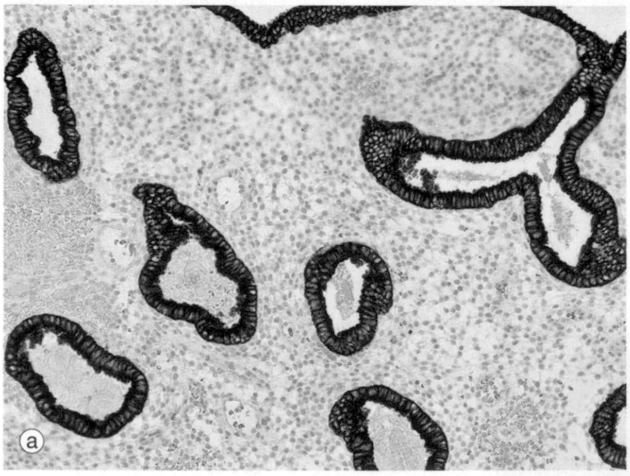

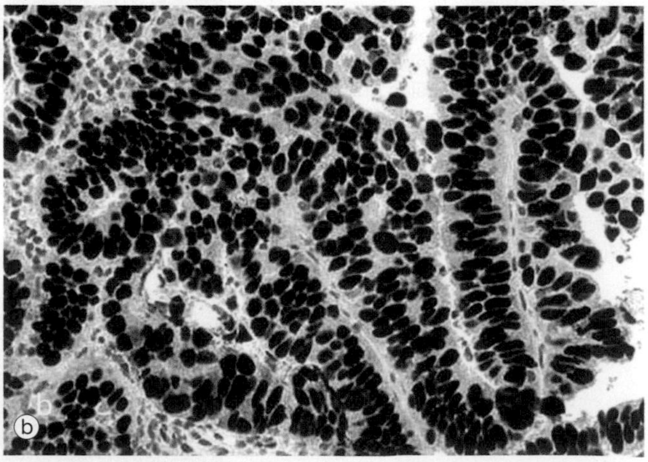

Immunostains can produce a variety of patterns of staining within the cell (nuclear, cytoplasmic, membranous or a combination). Image (a) shows endometrial tissue which has been stained with an epithelial marker (cytokeratin). The positive cytoplasmic brown staining of the glands contrasts to the lack of staining in the endometrial stroma where only the blue counterstain is seen. Image (b) shows a nuclear pattern of staining for the biomarker oestrogen receptor (ER) in a breast carcinoma.

APPENDIX

3 Glossary of terms

Architecture – the organisation and arrangement of cells within a tissue.

ATP – adenosine triphosphate is the small molecule used in cells as the primary source of readily available energy.

Basophilic or haematoxophilic – structures that stain with the basic dye haematoxylin, one of the components of the standard haematoxylin and eosin (H&E) method (see Appendix 2). Acidic molecules such as DNA and RNA take up this dye, thus acquiring a blue colour.

Biomedical scientist – trained scientist who usually works in a variety of laboratory environments carrying out tests and analysing samples for diagnosis and treatment of diseases.

Complement cascade – a group of enzymes found in inactive form in the blood. Binding of immune complexes or certain bacterial products activates the first enzyme, which is then able to activate larger amounts of the second that in turn switches on larger amounts of the third and so on. This cascade can very quickly produce large quantities of effector molecules that fight infection and promote inflammation.

Coronal planes – imaginary vertical planes at right angles to the median/sagittal plane (see below).

Cytokines – proteins or peptides released by cells that convey signals to nearby cells.

Cytology – the study of cells.

Desmosome – a specialised form of intercellular junction, particularly numerous in stratified squamous epithelium and giving rise to the histological appearance of 'prickles' between the cells (also known as **macula adherens**).

Differentiation – the process by which a cell becomes more specialised. Often used in tumour pathology to describe the extent to which a tumour resembles normal tissue.

Distal – anatomical term meaning further from the centre or the root of a limb (e.g. the ankle is distal to the knee).

DNA – deoxyribonucleic acid is the chemical structure that holds the genetic code, which contains the blueprint for every protein produced by an individual. DNA is found in the nucleus where it forms the chromosomes (see Ch. 2).

Ectopic – in the wrong place.

Electron-dense – tissue stained for electron microscopy with heavy metals impedes the passage of electrons to a greater or lesser degree depending on the amount of heavy metal bound. Structures that take up large amounts of heavy metal stains are called electron-dense and appear dark grey to black.

Electron-lucent – tissue stained for electron microscopy with heavy metals impedes the passage of electrons to a greater or lesser degree depending on the amount of heavy metal bound. Those structures that bind little heavy metal and allow the passage of the electron beam are said to be electron-lucent and appear white to pale grey.

EM – two-dimensional electron micrograph views of objects, acquired by passing the electron beam through a thin section of the specimen (see Appendix 1). Almost all of the electron micrographs in this book are transmission electron micrographs and are referred to as 'EMs'. Other authors sometimes use the abbreviation TEM, although by convention the abbreviation EM is assumed to be a transmission EM.

SEM – scanning electron micrographs are three-dimensional views of the surface of objects. SEMs in this book are identified in figure captions as 'SEM' (see Appendix 1 for further details).

Eosinophilic or **acidophilic** – structures that stain with the acidic dye eosin, the other component of the standard haematoxylin and eosin (H&E) method. Most cytoplasmic structures are basic and therefore acidophilic to some extent, so that in most tissues the cell cytoplasm stains with eosin and appears pinkish-red.

ER – endoplasmic reticulum is a membrane-bound cytoplasmic compartment where certain chemical reactions take place sequestered from the rest of the cytoplasm. There are two types – rough and smooth.

- **rER** – rough endoplasmic reticulum is studded with ribosomes and is the site of synthesis and processing of proteins for export.
- **sER** – smooth endoplasmic reticulum is a major site of lipid synthesis.

FISH – fluorescence in situ hydridisation (see Appendix 2).

Haematopoiesis – formation of blood cells.

H&E – haematoxylin and eosin, a standard histological staining method that stains cytoplasm pink and nuclei blue–purple.

Immunohistochemistry – technique which uses specific monoclonal antibodies to identify and stain tissue components (also known as immunocytochemistry and immunoperoxidase staining, see Appendix 2).

In vitro – an experiment taking place outside of a living body (e.g. in a tissue culture dish).

In vivo – occurring in a living body, used in experimental situations to describe events taking place in real life.

Lamellar bone – mature bone with collagen fibres arranged in parallel bands; stronger and more resilient than **woven bone**.

Limiting plate – the layer of hepatocytes around the edge of the portal tracts in the liver.

MALT – mucosa-associated lymphoid tissue.

Microtomy – process of cutting very thin sections from tissues prior to mounting onto a glass slide.

Organelle – a specialised intracellular structure, e.g. Golgi apparatus, mitochondrion, etc.

Osteoid – uncalcified bone matrix produced by osteoblasts.

Pedicel – the foot process of a podocyte, a specialised epithelial cell in the renal glomerulus.

Podocyte – specialised epithelial cell with foot processes, surrounding the glomerular capillaries and forming part of the filtration barrier.

Protein superfamilies – proteins can be grouped into superfamilies by similarities in structure and function. An example is the immunoglobulin superfamily that has a range of functions in antigen recognition and cell–cell interactions.

Proximal – closer to the centre or the root of a limb (e.g. the elbow is proximal to the wrist).

Pseudostratified – a type of epithelium which appears to be multilayered but in which all of the cells sit upon the basement membrane (e.g. respiratory epithelium).

Red pulp – component of the spleen composed of splenic cords and sinuses.

RNA – ribonucleic acid is a chemical structure that exists in three forms: messenger RNA, transfer RNA and ribosomal RNA (see below).

mRNA – messenger RNA is a chemical copy of the sequence of bases in DNA and acts as a template for the synthesis of proteins (see Ch. 1).

rRNA – ribosomal RNA is the type of RNA that makes up the physical structure of the ribosome, the site of protein synthesis. Ribosomal RNA controls the docking of tRNA in the correct order as defined by mRNA to produce the correct sequence of amino acids in a particular polypeptide chain.

tRNA – transfer RNA interacts with mRNA during protein synthesis to assemble the amino acids in the correct order to create a particular protein.

Sagittal or **median plane** – an imaginary vertical plane through the body, dividing it into right and left halves. Additional paramedian or parasagittal planes are parallel to the sagittal plane.

Section or **tissue section** – a very thin slice of tissue that is prepared in one of a number of ways for staining and microscopic examination:

Frozen section – this type of section is used for urgent diagnosis intraoperatively. The tissue is snap frozen, sections cut and stained and a diagnosis given within a short space of time (15–30 minutes). The disadvantage of this method is that tissue preservation is not nearly so good as with routine paraffin sections, and so diagnosis is more difficult. Frozen sections are also used for immunofluorescence microscopy, certain stains to detect lipids in tissue and for enzyme histochemistry.

Paraffin sections – most of the photomicrographs in this book are of paraffin sections. The fixed tissues are dehydrated and infiltrated by hot liquid paraffin wax and cooled until the wax is solid (at room temperature). The wax provides support for the tissue and allows sections as thin as 1–2 μm to be cut. The wax is dissolved away by an organic solvent, and the tissue slice is rehydrated before stains are applied. This procedure requires hours to carry out, and most routine tissue sections are processed overnight (see Appendix 1).

Resin sections – in some circumstances, paraffin wax offers inadequate support for tissue sectioning, and resins are used as the embedding medium. Two main types are used. Acrylic resins are harder than paraffin wax and offer greater support when cutting hard tissues such as fingernail and undecalcified bone. A wide range of stains can be applied. Epoxy resins are even harder and are particularly used in electron microscopy. Using special glass 'knives', very thin sections can be cut and stained with toluidine blue (see Appendix 2) for very high-resolution light microscopy, and even thinner sections (ultrathin sections) stained for transmission electron microscopy.

Starling forces – osmotic and hydrostatic pressures that govern movement of fluid within the microcirculation.

Tight junction – a specialised type of junction between epithelial cells which controls paracellular diffusion (also known as a **zonula occludens**).

Tissue processing – preparation of tissue, including dehydration and impregnation with wax, rendering it firm enough to allow thin sections to be cut for mounting onto a glass slide (see Appendix 1).

Urinary space – the space between the glomerular capillaries and Bowman's capsule.

Vacuole – a membrane bound space within a cell.

White pulp – the lymphoid tissue of the spleen.

Woven bone – immature, non-lamellar bone, with randomly orientated collagen fibres in the osteoid.

Zonula adherens – type of intercellular junction linking the cytoskeletons of adjacent cells to form strong, cohesive epithelia (also known as **adhering belt**).

INDEX

Page numbers followed by "*f*" indicate figures, "*t*" indicate tables, "*b*" indicate boxes, and "*e*" indicate online content.

B

G

M

T